GASTROENTEROLOGY
CLINICAL SCIENCE
AND PRACTICE

GASTROENTEROLOGY
CLINICAL SCIENCE
AND PRACTICE

Ian A. D. Bouchier

CBE, MD, FRCP, FRCP(Edin), HonFCP(SA), FFPHM, FRSA, FIBiol, FRS(Edin),
Professor of Medicine, Department of Medicine (RIE), University of Edinburgh,
The Royal Infirmary, Edinburgh, UK

Robert N. Allan

MD, PhD, FRCP
Consultant Physician, Queen Elizabeth Hospital,
Edgbaston, Birmingham, UK

Humphrey J. F. Hodgson

DM, FRCP
Professor of Gastroenterology, Royal Postgraduate Medical School;
Consultant Physician, Hammersmith Hospital,
London, UK

Michael R. B. Keighley

Barling Professor and Head, Department of Surgery, Queen Elizabeth Hospital,
Edgbaston, Birmingham, UK

SECOND EDITION
VOLUME ONE

W.B. SAUNDERS COMPANY LTD

LONDON   PHILADELPHIA   TORONTO   SYDNEY   TOKYO

This book is printed on acid free paper

W.B. Saunders Company Ltd

24–28 Oval Road
London NW1 7DX

The Curtis Center
Independence Square West
Philadelphia, PA 19106–3399

55 Horner Avenue
Toronto, Ontario M8Z 4X6, Canada

Harcourt Brace & Company (Australia) Pty Ltd
30–52 Smidmore St
Marrickville, NSW 2204, Australia

Harcourt Brace (Japan) Inc.
Ichibancho Central Building, 22-1 Ichibancho
Chiyoda-ku, Tokyo 102, Japan

First published 1984
Second edition 1993

A catalogue record for this book is available from the British Library.

Volume 1 ISBN 0-7020-1803-1
Volume 2 ISBN 0-7020-1804-X
        Set ISBN 0-7020-1500-8

Typeset by Paston Press Ltd., Loddon, Norfolk
Printed and bound in Great Britain by The Bath Press

PREFACE

We are enthusiastic about the preparation of a second edition of our textbook because we have been encouraged by the reviews and by the many requests from our colleagues for a new edition.

The production of this second edition has provided an opportunity to make significant improvements. Many of the contributors have changed. New contributors have joined the team for the first time because of new material which we have introduced while others are no longer active in clinical practice. New issues in the Gastroenterological scene have been included, whereas some topics have been omitted because they no longer seem relevant. The oesophageal chapter has been completely reorganized while the contribution on gastrointestinal bleeding has been combined with gut ischaemia. Systemic disease which may also affect the gastrointestinal tract, and skin diseases relevant to the gut have been combined into a single chapter. An enlarged section concerned with functional disorders incorporates many topics previously included in the nutritional section. We have retained the major chapters on diseases of the gallbladder and bile ducts, which is at the interface between Gastroenterology and Hepatobiliary Disease.

Inevitably the book has grown, but not to a size that is too intimidating. The title now more accurately reflects what we wish to achieve; *Gastroenterology: Clinical Science and Practice*. The original purpose of writing the book remains unchanged. It is an attempt to synthesize theory with practice integrating disease concepts as closely as possible with clinical, diagnostic and therapeutic approaches.

We are grateful to our many contributors who have provided us with texts of high quality. It is a pleasure to acknowledge the continued support and encouragement of our publisher, and in particular we wish to express our thanks to Steven Handley, Richard Cook and Seán Duggan.

IAN A. D. BOUCHIER
ROBERT N. ALLAN

HUMPHREY J. F. HODGSON
MICHAEL R. B. KEIGHLEY

CONTENTS

CONTRIBUTORS

David W. K. Acheson, BSc, MB, BS, MD, MRCP
Division of Geographic Medicine and Infectious Diseases, New England Medical Center, Box 41, 750 Washington Street, Boston, MA 02111, USA.
Shigellosis

John I. Alexander, MB, BS, FCAnaes.
Consultant in Anaesthesia and Pain Relief, Bristol Royal Infirmary, Department of Medicine, Bristol, B52 8HW, UK.
Chronic Functional Abdominal Pain

Arthur Allan, MD, FRCS
Good Hope General Hospital, Rectory Road, Sutton Coldfield, West Midlands, B75 7RR, UK.
Anal and Perirectal Problems

Robert N. Allan, MD, PhD, FRCP
Consultant Physician, Queen Elizabeth Hospital, Queen Elizabeth Medical Centre, Edgbaston, Birmingham, B15 2TH, UK.
Endometriosis; Crohn's Disease: Clinical Presentation, Diagnosis, Medical Treatment

N. S. Ambrose, MB, BS, FRCS, MS
Consultant Surgeon, St James's University Hospital, Leeds, LS9 7TF, UK.
Peritonitis and Perforation; Abdominal Abscesses

Kerry Atkinson, MB, BS, MD, MRCP, FRACP
Senior Staff Specialist, St Vincent's Hospital, Sydney, Australia; Associate Professor, School of Medicine, University of New South Wales, Sydney, Australia.
Graft-Versus-Host Disease

A. T. R. Axon, MD, FRCP
Consultant Physician and Gastroenterologist, Leeds General Infirmary, Great George Street, Leeds, LS1 3EX, UK.
Evaluation of Pancreatic Disease

David J. Ballard, MD, PhD, FACP
Associate Professor, Epidemiology and Medicine, University of Virginia School of Medicine, Charlottesville, Virginia 22908; Director, Thomas Jefferson Health Policy Institute, 400 Peter Jefferson Place, Suite 201, Charlottesville, Virginia 22901, USA.
Aortic Aneurysms

J. E. Banatvala, MA, MD, MRCP, FRCPath
Professor of Clinical Virology, United Medical and Dental Schools of Guy's and St Thomas's Hospitals, St Thomas's Campus, Lambeth Palace Road, London, SE1 7EH; Honorary Consultant Virologist, St Thomas's Hospital, Lambeth Palace Road, London, SE1 7EH, UK.
Virus Infections

J. G. Banwell, MD
Professor, Division of Medicine, Lakeside Hospital, Case Western Reserve, Cleveland, Ohio 44106, USA.
Worm Infestations

R. E. Barry, BSc, MD, FRCP
Consultant Senior Lecturer in Medicine, Clinical Dean, Honorary Consultant Physician with United Bristol Hospitals Trust, Bristol Royal Infirmary, Department of Medicine, Bristol, B52 8HW, UK.
Surgical Causes of Malabsorption: Jejunoileal Bypass

David C. C. Bartolo, MS, FRCS
Consultant, Royal Infirmary of Edinburgh, Lauriston Place, Edinburgh, EH3 9YW, UK.
Physiology of Defaecation and Sphincter Control

Irving S. Benjamin, BSc, MD, FRCS(Glas), FRCS(Engl)

Professor of Surgery and Director, Department of Surgery, King's College School of Medicine and Dentistry, Denmark Hill, London, SE5 9RS, UK.

Gallbladder and Biliary Tract: Anatomy and Embryology, Tumours

Robert W. Beart Jr, MD

Professor of Surgery, Department of Surgery, University of Southern California School of Medicine, USC Consultation Center, 1510 San Pablo Street, Suite 514, Los Angeles, California 90033–4612, USA.

Anal Tumours: Anal Malignancy

John R. Bennett, MD, FRCS

Consultant Gastroenterologist, Hull Royal Infirmary, Anlary Road, Hull, HU3 2JZ, UK.

Pharynx and Oesophagus: Gastro-oesophageal Reflux Disease

S. R. Bloom, MA, MD, DSc, FRCP

Professor of Endocrinology, Endocrinology Unit, Royal Postgraduate Medical School, Hammersmith Hospital, Du Cane Road, London, W12 0NN, UK.

Tumours of the Endocrine Pancreas

I. A. D. Bouchier, CBE, MD, FRCP, FRCP(Edin), Hon FCP(SA), FFPHM, FRSA, FIBiol, FRS(Edin)

Professor of Medicine, University of Edinburgh, Department of Medicine (RIE), Royal Infirmary Edinburgh, EH3 9YW, UK

Pharynx and Oesophagus: Diaphragmatic Hernias; Functional Disorders of the Gut: Flatulence; Gallbladder and Biliary Tract: Clinical Features and Non-surgical Treatment of Gallstones, Cholecystitis and Choledocholithiasis, Other Disorders; The Peritoneum: Ascites

Athos Bousvaros, MD

Instructor in Medicine, Harvard Medical School, Boston Children's Hospital, 300 Longwood Avenue, Boston, MA 02115, USA.

Immunological Disorders Affecting the Small Intestine: Basic Gastrointestinal Immunology

Cedric G. Bremner, MD

Professor of Clinical Surgery, Director of Clinical Research, Department of Surgery, USC Healthcare Consultation Center, 1510 San Pablo Street, #514, Los Angeles, CA 90033–4612, USA.

Pharynx and Oesophagus: Other Conditions

Martin J. Brodie, MD, FRCP

Director, Epilepsy Research Unit, University Department of Medicine and Therapeutics, Gardiner Institute, Western Infirmary, Glasgow, G11 6NT, UK.

Drug Absorption and Bioavailability

Colin Mark Brown, MB, MRCP

Wellcome Trust Clinical Research Fellow, Department of Gastroenterology, Hope Hospital, University of Manchester, School of Medicine, Eccles Old Road, Salford, M6 8HD, UK.

Gastroduodenal Secretion in Health and Disease; Gastroduodenal Motility in Health and Disease

John Calam, BSc, MD, FRCP

Senior Lecturer and Honorary Consultant, Department of Medicine, Royal Postgraduate Medical School, Hammersmith Hospital, Du Cane Road, London, W12 0NN, UK.

Chronic Peptic Ulcer: Epidemiology and Aetiology; Chronic Duodenal Ulcer: Clinical Features, Investigations, Treatment: medical

Michael Camilleri, MD, MPhil(Lond), FRCP(Lond), FRCP(Edin), FACP

Professor of Medicine, Consultant in Gastroenterology and Physiology, Mayo Clinic and Mayo Medical School, Rochester, MN 55905, USA.

Motility Disorders of the Intestine

David C. A. Candy, MB, BS, MSc, MD, FRCP

Professor of Child Health, Department of Child Health, Kings College School of Medicine and Dentistry, London, UK.

Paediatric Gastroenteritis

Martin C. Carey, AM, MD, DSc, LLD, FRCPI
Professor of Medicine, Harvard Medical School; Senior Physician, Brigham and Women's Hospital, Department of Medicine, Division of Gastroenterology, 75 Francis Street, Boston, MA 02115, USA.
Formation of Cholesterol Gallstones; Formation of Pigment Gallstones

Vinton S. Chadwick, BA, Nat Sci Tripos, MA, MB, BChir, MSc, MD, FRCP, FRACP
Professor of Experimental Medicine and Director of Wellcome Medical Research Institute, University of Otago Medical School, PO Box 913, Dunedin, New Zealand; Honorary Consultant Physician, Otago Area Health Board, Dunedin Hospital, Dunedin, New Zealand.
Mechanisms of Malabsorption and Diarrhoea; Clinical Investigation of Patients with Malabsorption and Diarrhoea

Ian L. Chrystie, TD, PhD
Lecturer, Department of Virology, United Medical and Dental Schools of Guy's and St Thomas's, St Thomas's Campus, London, SE1 7EH, UK.
Virus Infections

Paul J. Ciclitira, MD, PhD, FRCP
Senior Lecturer, Clinical and Molecular Medicine, UMBS; Honorary Consultant Physician, St Thomas' and Guy's Hospitals, London, UK.
Coeliac Disease and Related Disorders: Coeliac Disease, Malignant Complications of Coeliac Disease

John G. F. Cleland, MD, MRCP
Senior Lecturer in Medicine and Honorary Consultant Cardiologist, Department of Medicine (Clinical Cardiology), Royal Postgraduate Medical School, Hammersmith Hospital, Du Cane Road, London, W12 0HS, UK
Cardiac Disease

G. C. Cook, DSc, MD, FRCP, FRACP, FLS
Consultant Physician, Hospital for Tropical Diseases, University College Hospital, St Luke's Hospital for the Clergy, London, UK.
Postinfective Malabsorption (Including Tropical Sprue)

B. T. Cooper, BSc, MD, FRCP
Consultant Gastroenterologist, Dudley Road Hospital, Birmingham, B15 3NW; Senior Clinical Lecturer in Medicine, University of Birmingham, Birmingham, UK.
Ménétrièr's Disease; Other Gastroduodenal Disorders; Systemic Endocrine Disorders: Diabetes Mellitus

Peter F. Crookes, FRCS
Assistant Unit Chief, Foregut Service, Department of Surgery, LAC/USC Medical Center, 1200 N. State Street, Los Angeles, CA 90033, USA.
Pharynx and Oesophagus: Indications for, and Outcome of, Surgery for Benign Oesophageal Disease

W. David Cubitt, PhD
Top Grade Virologist, Department of Microbiology, Hospital for Sick Children, Great Ormond Street, London, UK.
Virus Infections

Sidney Cywes, MMed(Surg), FACS(Ped), FRCS(Eng), (Edin), (Glas)
Professor and Head, Department of Paediatric Surgery, University of Cape Town Medical School; Chief of Paediatric Surgery, Red Cross War Memorial Children's Hospital, Rondebosch, Cape Town 7700, Republic of South Africa.
Gall Bladder and Biliary Tract: Congenital Abnormalities

J. S. Davison, PhD
Professor of Physiology, Department of Medical Physiology, University of Calgary Health Science Center, 3330 Hospital Drive NW, Calgary, Alberta, Canada T2N 4NS.
Physiology of Extrahepatic Bile Transport

Deborah M. DeMarco, MD
Assistant Professor of Medicine, Temple University Hospital, Temple University School of Medicine, 3400 N. Broad Street, Philadelphia, PA 19140, USA.
Vasculitic and Connective Tissue Disorders

T. DeMeester, MD
USC Healthcare Consultation Center, 1510 San Pablo Street, Suite 514, Los Angeles, California 90033, USA.
Pharynx and Oesophagus: Indications for, and Outcome of, Surgery for Benign Oesophageal Disease

Anthony V. Dilley, MB, BS
Surgical Research Fellow, Department of Surgery, The St George Hospital, Kogarah, Sydney, NSW 2217, Australia.
Acute Bleeding Peptic Ulcer: Surgery

Caroline M. Doig, ChM, FRCSE, FRCS
Senior Lecturer in Paediatric Surgery, University of Manchester, Booth Hall Children's Hospital, Charlestown Road, Blackley, Manchester, M9 2AA, UK.
Stomach and Duodenum: Embryology and Anatomy, Congenital Abnormalities; Small Intestine: Anatomy, Congenital Abnormalities; Necrotising Enterocolitis; Meconium Ileus

Joanne M. Donovan, MD, PhD
Instructor in Medicine, Harvard Medical School; Associate in Medicine, Brigham and Women's Hospital; Staff Physician, West Roxbury/Brockton VA Medical Center, Division of Gastroenterology, 1400 VFW Parkway, West Roxbury, MA 02132, USA.
Formation of Cholesterol Gallstones: Formation of Pigment Gallstones

Neil J. Douglas, MD, FRCPE
Reader in Medicine, University of Edinburgh; Honorary Consultant Physician, City Hospital, Greenbank Drive, Edinburgh, EH10 5SB, UK.
Pulmonary Associations of Gastrointestinal Disease

S. Dover, MB, MRCP
Medical Registrar, Gastroenterology Unit, Gartnavel General Hospital, Glasgow, G12 0YN, UK.
Systemic Endocrine Disorders: Acute Porphyrias

Graeme S. Duthie, FRCS Ed.
Registrar, Royal Infirmary of Edinburgh, Lauriston Place, Edinburgh, EH3 9YW, UK.
Physiology of Defaecation and Sphincter Control

Olle Ekberg, MD, PhD
Docent, Head, Gastrointestinal Section, Department of Radiology, University of Lund, Malmö General Hospital, S–214 01 Malmö, Sweden.
Pharynx and Oesophagus: Cricopharyngeal Disorders

S. Erlinger, MD
Professor and Chairman, Department of Hepatology, Hôpital Beaujon, 92118 Clichy Cedex, France.
Physiology of Bile Secretion

R. Farouk, FRCS (Glasg.), FRCS Ed.
Research Fellow, Royal Infirmary of Edinburgh, Lauriston Place, Edinburgh, EH3 9YW, UK.
Physiology of Defaecation and Sphincter Control

Michael J. G. Farthing, BSc, MD, FRCP
Professor of Gastroenterology, St Bartholomew's Hospital, West Smithfield, London, EC1A 7BE, UK.
Cholera; Shigellosis; Giardiasis; Campylobacter Infections

Victor W. Fazio, MB, BS, FRACS, FACS
Chairman, Department of Colorectal Surgery, The Cleveland Clinic Foundation, 9500 Evclid Avenue, Cleveland, Ohio 44195, USA.
Perianal Crohn's Disease

J. W. L. Fielding, MD, FRCS
Consultant Surgeon, Queen Elizabeth Hospital, Edgbaston, Birmingham, B15 2TH, UK.
Gastric Carcinoma: Clinical Features, diagnosis and treatment

Carlos Fernández-del Castillo, MD
Instructor in Surgery, Massachusetts General Hospital, Harvard Medical School, 15 Parkman Street, Acc 1464, Boston, MA 02114, USA.
Chronic Pancreatitis

Gordon G. Forstner, MD, FRCP(C)
Professor, Department of Paediatrics, University of Toronto, Division of Gastroenterology, Hospital for Sick Children, 555 University Avenue, Toronto, Ontario, Canada.
Cystic Fibrosis

Christopher P. L. Freeman, MBChB, MPhil, FRCPsych
Consultant Psychotherapist, Royal Edinburgh Hospital, Morningside Terrace, Edinburgh, EH10, UK.
Anorexia Nervosa and Other Psychological Disorders of the Gastrointestinal Tract

Neill V. Freeman, MB, BCh, FRCS(Eng), FRCS(Ed)
Associate Professor, Sultan Qaboos University, Oman; Head of Paediatric Surgery, Royal Hospital, Oman, Department of Paediatric Surgery, CPO Box 2331, SEEB, Sultanate of Oman.
Pharynx and Oesophagus: Congenital Abnormalities

Robert B. Galland, MD, FRCS
Consultant Surgeon, Royal Berkshire Hospital, London Road, Reading, RG1 5AN, UK.
Tumours: Radiation damage

B. G. Gazzard, MA, MD, FRCP
AIDS Coordinator, Chelsea and Westminster Hospital, 369 Fulham Road, London, SW10 9NH, UK.
Sexually Transmitted Diseases Relevant to Gastroenterology; Endoscopic and Surgical Intervention in HIV-positive Individuals

P. Ghosh, MRCP
Section of Digestive Diseases, University of Nebraska Medical Center, 600 South 42nd Street, Omaha, NE 68198–2000, UK.
Bacteriology of the Small Gut and Bacterial Overgrowth

Stephen E. Goldfinger, MD
Massachusetts General Hospital, Fruit Street, Boston, Massachusetts 02114, USA.
Familial Mediterranean Fever (Recurrent Polyserositis)

Sylvia Nancy Gyde, MA, BM, BCh(Oxon), MFCM
Director of Public Health Medicine, North Birmingham Health Authority District Offices, Good Hope Hospital, Sutton Coldfield, West Midlands, UK.
Cancer in Ulcerative Colitis; Cancer in Crohn's Disease

A. Habr-Gama, MD
Associate Professor of Surgery, Faculty of Medicine, University of So Paulo, So Paulo, Brazil.
Chagas' Disease

U. Haglund, MD, PhD
Professor of Surgery, Department of Surgery, University of Uppsala, Akademisk Sjukhuset, Uppsala S–751 85, Sweden.
The Splanchnic Circulation in Shock

John W. Hallett, Jr, MD, FACS
Associate Professor of Surgery, Director of Vascular Surgery Fellowship Program, Mayo Clinic, Rochester, MN 55905, USA.
Aortic Aneurysms

Ian Hamilton, MD, BSc, MRCP, FRACP
Consultant Physician, Royal Infirmary, New Durham Road, Sunderland, Tyne and Wear, SR2 7JE, UK.
Collagenous Colitis

P. J. Hammond, MA, MB, BCh, MRCP
MCRC Training Fellow, Endocrinology Unit, Royal Postgraduate Medical School, Hammersmith Hospital, Du Cane Road, London, W12 0HS, UK.
Tumours of the Endocrine Pancreas

Philip S. E. G. Harland, MB, BCh, FRCP, LRCS, BA (Cantab)
Consultant Paediatrician, West Lane Hospital, Acklam Road, Middlesbrough, TS5 4EE, UK.
Malnutrition in Developing Countries

Peter Hayes, MD, FRCPE
Senior Lecturer, University of Edinburgh and Honorary Consultant Physician, Lothian Health Board, UK.
Haemochromatosis

K. W. Heaton, MA, MD, FRCP
Reader in Medicine, University of Bristol; Honorary Consultant Physician, United Bristol Healthcare Trust, Bristol Royal Infirmary, Bristol, BS2 8HW, UK.
Chronic Functional Abdominal Pain; Irritable Bowel Syndrome

Michael M. Henry, MB, FRCS
Consultant Surgeon, Central Middlesex Hospital, Acton Lane, London, NW6; Senior Lecturer, Academic Surgical Unit, St Mary's Hospital, Praed Street, London W2; Honorary Consultant Surgeon, St Mark's Hospital, City Road, London, EC1V 2PS, UK.
Pelvic Floor Disorders

Graham L. Hill, MD, ChM, FRACS, FRCS, FACS
Professor of Surgery, University Department of Surgery, Auckland Hospital, Aukland 3, New Zealand.
Therapeutic Nutrition

T. Hirayama, MD
Institute of Preventative Oncology, HI Building, 1–2 Sadohara-cho, Ichigaya, Shinjuku-ku, Tokyo 162, Japan.
Gastric Carcinoma: Epidemiology, Screening

Humphrey J. Hodgson, MA, BSc, DM, FRCP
Professor of Gastroenterology, Royal Postgraduate Medical School, Du Cane Road, London, W12 0HS; Consultant Physician, Hammersmith Hospital, Du Cane Road, London, W12 0NN, UK.
Small Intestine: Consequences of Malabsorption; Whipple's Disease; Immunological Disorders Affecting the Small Intestine: Immunodeficiency and the Gut, Amyloidosis, Tumours of the Small Intestine: Carcinoid Tumours and the Carcinoid Syndrome, Other Tumours of the Small Intestine; Vasculitic and Connective Tissue Disorders: Henoch-Schönlein Purpura, Miscellaneous Vasculitic and Other Conditions

Shirley Hodgson, DM, FRCP
Senior Lecturer in Clinical Genetics, Department of Medical and Molecular Genetics, UMDS, Guys Hospital; Honorary Consultant, St Mark's Hospital, City Road, London, EC1V 2PS, UK.
HH Link; Tumours: Hereditary neoplastic diseases of the intestine

A. Victor Hoffbrand, MA, DM, FRCP, FRCPath, FRCP(Ed), DSc
Professor of Haematology, Royal Free School of Medicine; Honorary Consultant Haematologist, Royal Free Hospital, Pond Street, London, NW3 2QG, UK.
Digestion and Malabsorption of Nutrients: Haematinics (Including Gastrointestinal Features of Pernicious Anaemia)

David Hopwood, BSc, MB, ChB, MD, PhD, FRCPath
Reader, Department of Pathology; Honorary Consultant Pathologist, Ninewells Hospital and Medical School, Dundee, DD1 9SY, UK.
Pharynx and Oesophagus: Embryology and Anatomy

Matthew D. A'C. Horton, MB, BS
Surgical Research Fellow, Department of Surgery, The St George Hospital, Kogarah, Sydney, NSW 2217, Australia.
Gastric Tumours: Benign Tumours (Including Gastric Polyps)

Colin W. Howden, MD, FRCP(Glasg), FACG, FCP
Professor, Division of Digestive Diseases and Nutrition, Department of Internal Medicine, University of South Carolina School of Medicine, Columbia, SC 29208, USA.
Drug Absorption and Bioavailability

N. Hyman, MD
Medical Center, Hospital of Vermont, Department of Surgery, Colchester Avenue, Burlington, Vermont 05401, USA.
Perianal Crohn's Disease

C. W. Imrie, BSc, MD, FRCS
Consultant Surgeon, Royal Infirmary, Glasgow, G4 0SF, UK.
Acute Pancreatitis

John R. Jamieson, MD
General Surgeon, Kenridge Hospital, Johannesburgh, South Africa.
Pharynx and Oesophagus: Indications for, and Outcome of, Surgery for Benign Oesophageal Disease

J. Janssens, MD
University Hospital Gasthuisberg, Herestraat 49, Leuven B–3000, Belgium.
Pharynx and Oesophagus: Physiology, Motility Disorders

D. P. Jewell, MA, DPhil, FRCP
Consultant Physician, John Radcliffe Hospital, Oxford, OX3 9DU; Lecturer in Medicine, University of Oxford, Oxford, UK.
Ulcerative Colitis: Pathology, Clinical Presentation, Complications, Treatment: medical

D. Johnston, ChM, FRCS
Professor of Surgery, University Department of Surgery, Leeds General Infirmary, Great George Street, Leeds, LS1 3EX, UK.
Chronic Duodenal Ulcer: Treatment: surgical

Roland T. Jung, MA, MD(Cantab), FRCP(Lond), FRCP(Edin)
Consultant Endocrinologist, Honorary Reader and Clinical Director of Directorate of General Medicine, Ninewells Hospital and Medical School, Dundee, DD1 9SY, UK.
Appetite and Satiety; Obesity

Michael A. Kamm, MD, MRCP, FRACP
Senior Lecturer, Honorary Consultant Physician, Director, Medical Physiology Unit, St Mark's Hospital, City Road, London, EC1V 2PS, UK.
Constipation, Faecal Impaction and Laxative Abuse

Peter Katelaris, MB, BS, FRACP
Research Fellow and Honorary Lecturer, Department of Gastroenterology, St Bartholomew's Hospital, London, EC1A 7BE, UK.
Campylobacter Infections

M. R. B. Keighley, MS, FRCS
Barling Professor and Head of the Department of Surgery, University of Birmingham, Birmingham, UK.
Crohn's Disease: Surgical Treatment; Haemorrhoids; Anal Fissure; Anorectal Sepsis

G. T. Keusch, MD
Division of Geographic Medicine and Infectious Diseases, New England Medical Center, Box 41, 750 Washington Street, Boston, MA 02111, USA.
Shigellosis

Mark Killingback, FRACS, FRCS, FRCS. Ed.
Hornsby Kuringai Hospital, Sydney, New South Wales, Australia.
Diverticular Disease

Barbara S. Kirschner, BA, MD
Professor of Paediatrics and Medicine, Pritzker School of Medicine, Wyler Children's Hospital, University of Chicago, 5841 S. Maryland Avenue, Chicago, Illinois 60637, USA.
Inflammatory Bowel Disease in Childhood

G. J. Krejs, MD
Professor and Chairman, Karl-Franzens Universität, Medizinische Klinik, Auenbruggerplatz 15, Graz A–8036, Austria.
Surgical Causes of Malabsorption: Short Gut Syndrome

D. Kumar, PhD, FRCS
Senior Lecturer in Surgery, University Department of Surgery, Queen Elizabeth Hospital, Edgbaston, Birmingham, B15 2TH, UK.
Obstruction of Small and Large Bowel and Ileus

Parveen J. Kumar, BSc, MD, FRCP
Gastroenterology Department, St Bartholomew's Hospital, London, EC1 7BE, UK.
Food Allergy and Food Intolerance

M. J. S. Langman, MD, FRCP

Professor of Medicine, University of Birmingham Medical School, Queen Elizabeth Hospital, Birmingham, B15 2TH, UK.
Acute Bleeding Peptic Ulcer: Aetiology, Diagnosis, Treatment; Inflammatory Bowel Disease: Incidence, Epidemiology, Genetics

Nicholas F. LaRusso, MD

Professor of Medicine, Mayo Clinic and Mayo Graduate School of Medicine, 200 First Street SW, Rochester, MN 55905, USA.
Primary Sclerosing Cholangitis

J. O. N. Lawson, FRCS

Consultant Paediatric Surgeon, 149 Harley Street, London, W1N 1HG.
Colon: Hirschsprung's Disease, Congital Megacolon, Anorectal Malformations

David John Leaper, MD, ChM, FRCS, FRCSEd

Consultant and Senior Lecturer, University Department of Surgery, Southmead Hospital, Bristol, BS10 5NB, UK.
Acute Appendicitis

John R. Lee, MB, ChB, FRCS, FRCR, DMRD

Consultant Radiologist, The General Hospital, Steelhouse Lane, Birmingham, B4 6NH, UK.
Crohn's Disease: Radiology and Endoscopy

J. E. Lennard-Jones, MD, FRCP

Honorary Consultant in Gastroenterology, St. Mark's Hospital, City Road, London, EC1V 2PS, UK.
Crohn's Disease: Medical Treatment

Robert C. F. Leonard, BSc, MB, BS, MD, FRCPE

Senior Lecturer, Department of Clinical Oncology, University of Edinburgh; Honorary Consultant Physician, Western General Hospital, Edinburgh, UK.
Internal Paraneoplastic Syndromes Associated with Cancer

Paul D. Lewis, DSc, MD, FRCP, FRCPath

Consultant Neuropathologist, Charing Cross Hospital, Fulham Palace Road, London W6 8RF; Emeritus Reader in Histopathology, Royal Postgraduate Medical School; Honorary Consultant, Hammersmith Hospital, Du Cane Road, London, W12 0HS, UK.
Coeliac Disease and Related Disorders: The Neurological Complications of Coeliac Disease

Richard G. Long, MD, FRCP

Clinical Teacher, Nottingham University Medical School; Consultant Physician and Gastroenterologist, City Hospital, Nottingham, NG5 1PB and University Hospital Nottingham, UK.
Systemic Endocrine Disorders

Peter James Lunniss, BSc, MB, BS, FRCS

Clinical Lecturer in Surgery, St Bartholomew's Medical College, West Smithfield, London, EC1A 7BE; Research Registrar, St Mark's Hospital, City Road, London, EC1V 2PS, UK.
Fistula-in-Ano

Michael H. Lyall, MB, ChB, ChM, FRCS(Ed)

Consultant Surgeon, Ninewells Hospital and Medical School, Dundee, DD1 9SY, UK; Honorary Senior Lecturer, University of Dundee, UK.
Colon: Embryology and Anatomy; Congenital Abnormalities of the Anterior Abdominal Wall, Peritoneum and Mesentery

J. R. Malagelada, MD

Professor, Hospital General Vall d'Hebron, Digestive System Research Unit, Barcelona 08035, Spain.
Gut Response to a Meal and its Hormonal Control

Bibhat K. Mandal, FRCP(Ed), FRCP(Glasg)

Director, Regional Department of Infectious Diseases and Tropical Medicine, University of Manchester, Monsall Hospital, Manchester, M10 8WR, UK.
Salmonella Infection

Aylwyn Mannell, MBBS, BSc(Med), FRACS, FRCS(Eng), MS(Syd)
Associate Professor of Surgery, Department of Surgery, University of the Witwatersrand, Medical School, York Road, Parktown, Johannesburg 2193, Republic of South Africa; Visiting Consultant Surgeon, Baragwanath Hospital, Johannesburg; Specialist Surgeon, Rosebank Clinic, Johannesburg, Republic of South Africa.
Pharynx and Oesophagus: Tumours

J. R. Marsden, BSc, BM, MRCP
Consultant Dermatologist, Birmingham General Hospital, Steelhouse Lane, Birmingham, B4 6NH, UK.
Skin Disease in Gastroenterology

I. Martin, MBChB, FRCS
Lecturer in Surgery, Academic Unit of Surgery, Leeds General Infirmary, Great George Street, Leeds, LS1 3EX, UK.
Chronic Duodenal Ulcer: Treatment: surgical

George Masterton, BSc, MD, MRCPsych
Honorary Senior Lecturer, Department of Psychiatry, Edinburgh University; Consultant Liaison Psychiatrist, Royal Infirmary of Edinburgh, 4 Lauriston Place, Edinburgh, EH3 9YW, UK.
Anorexia Nervosa and Other Disorders of the Gastrointestinal Tract

Kenneth E. L. McColl, MD, FRCP
Reader in Gastroenterology, University Department of Medicine and Therapeutics, Western Infirmary, Glasgow, G11 6NT, UK.
Systemic Endocrine Disorders: Acute Porphyrias

Alastair Millar, FRCS(Eng)(Ed), FRACS, DCH
Associate Professor, Department of Paediatric Surgery, University of Cape Town Medical School; Consultant Surgeon, Department of Paediatric Surgery, Red Cross War Memorial Children's Hospital, Rondebosch 7700, Cape Town, Republic of South Africa.
Gall Bladder and Biliary Tract: Congenital Abnormalities

Charles J. Mitchell, MBChB, FRCP, FRCP(Edin), FRCP(Lond)
Consultant Physician, Scarborough Hospital, Scarborough, North Yorkshire, UK.
Evaluation of Pancreatic Disease

Robert Modigliani, MD
Professor of Gastroenterology, Hôpital Saint-Louis, 1 avenue Claude Vellefaux, 75010 Paris, France.
Chronic Non-specific Ulcerative Enteritis

M. R. Moore, PhD, DSc
Reader, Western Infirmary, Department of Medicine and Therapeutics, Gardiner Institute, Glasgow, G11 6NT, UK.
Systemic Endocrine Disorders: Acute Porphyrias

Colm O'Moráin, MD, MSc, FRCPI
Professor, Department of Gastroenterology; Academic Head of Department of Medicine, Meath Adelaide Hospitals, Trinity College, Dublin, Ireland.
Extraintestinal Manifestations of Inflammatory Bowel Disease

A. Gwyn Morgan, MD, FRCP
Consultant Gastroenterologist, Airedale General Hospital, Steeton, Keighley, W. Yorks, BD20 6TD, UK.
Chronic Gastric Ulcer: Clinical Features, Investigations: Treatment: medical

Leon Morgenstern, MD, FACS
Emeritus Director of Surgery, Cedars-Sinai Medical Center, 444 S. San Vicente Blvd, Los Angeles, CA 90048; Emeritus Professor of Surgery, UCLA School of Medicine, Los Angeles, CA, USA.
Radiation Enteropathy

David L. Morris, MB, ChB, FRCS, MD, PhD, FRACS
Presiding Member, Discipline of Surgery, Faculty of Medicine, University of New South Wales; Professor of Surgery, The St George Hospital, Kogarah, Sydney, NSW 2217, Australia.
Acute Bleeding Peptic Ulcer: Surgery; Gastric Tumours: Benign Tumours (Including Gastric Polyps)

Steven F. Moss, BSc, MRCP
Wellcome Research Fellow and Honorary Registrar, Department of Medicine, Royal Postgraduate Medical School, Hammersmith Hospital, Du Cane Road, London, W12 0NN, UK.
Chronic Peptic Ulcer: Epidemiology and Aetiology, Chronic Duodenal Ulcer: Clinical features, Investigations; Treatment: medical

Allen R. Myers, MD
Professor of Medicine and Dean, Temple University School of Medicine, Philadelphia, Pennsylvania 19140, USA.
Vasculitic and Connective Tissue Disorders

G. Neale, FRCP, BSc, MB, CHB
Consultant Physician, Department of Gastroenterology, Addenbrooke's Hospital, Hills Road, Cambridge, CB2 2QQ, UK.
Bacteriology of the Small Gut and Bacterial Overgrowth

John P. Neoptolemos, MA, MB, BChir (Cantab), MD (Leics), FRCS (Eng)
Reader in Surgery, University of Birmingham; Honorary Consultant Surgeon, Dudley Road Hospital, Birmingham, UK.
Clinical Features and Non-surgical Treatment of Gallstones; Cholecystitis and Choledocholithiasis

Mary Ninkovic, MRCP
Registrar, Gastroenterology Unit, Royal Postgraduate Medical School, Hammersmith Hospital, Du Cane Road, London, W12 0NN, UK.
Behçet's Syndrome

T. C. Northfield, MA, MD, FRCP
Consultant Physician, St George's Hospital Medical School, London, UK.
Nutrients: Digestion and Malabsorption of Fat

John M. A. Northover, MS, FRCS
Consultant Surgeon, St Mark's Hospital; Honorary Director, ICRF Colorectal Unit, St Mark's Hospital, City Road, London EC1V 2PS, UK.
Tumours: Hereditary neoplastic diseases of the intestine

Barbara M. Obermayer-Pietsch, MD
Department of Endocrinology and Nuclear Medicine, Department of Gastroenterology, Karl-Franzens-University, 8036 Graz, Auenbruggerplatz 15, Austria.
Surgical Causes of Malabsorption: Short Gut Syndrome

Leslie W. Ottinger, MD
Visiting Surgeon, Massachusetts General Hospital; Associate Professor of Surgery, Harvard Medical School, MGH ACC, 15 Parkman Street, Level 4, Suite 465, Boston, Massachusetts 02114, USA.
Acute and Chronic Ischaemia of the Gut

John H. Pemberton, MD
Associate Professor of Surgery, Mayo Clinic, 200 First Street SW, Rochester, MN 55905, USA.
Ulcerative Colitis: Treatment: surgical

Ole Holger Petersen, MD
Professor of Physiology, University of Liverpool, PO Box 147, Liverpool, L69 3BX, UK.
The Pancreas: Physiology

W. G. Phillips, MA, DCH, MRCGP, MRCP
Wellcome Clinical Research Fellow, Honorary Senior Registrar, St John's Institute of Dermatology, St Thomas's Hospital, Lambeth Palace Road, London, SE1 7EH, UK.
Skin Disease in Gastroenterology

A. B. Price, MA, BM, BCH (Oxford), FRCPath
Consultant Histopathologist, Northwick Park Hospital, Watford Road, Harrow, Middlesex, HA1 3UJ, UK.
Tumours: Benign Tumours – Polyps and Polyposis

John A. Procaccino, MD
Fellow, Department of Colorectal Surgery, The Cleveland Clinic Foundation, 9500 Euclid Avenue, Cleveland, Ohio 44195–5044, USA.
Perianal Crohn's Disease

J.-C. Rambaud, MD
Professor, Hôpital Saint-Lazare, Service de Gastro-Enterologie, 107 rue du Faubourg Saint Denis, Paris 75475 Cedex 10,
France.
Tumours of the Small Intestine: Small Intestinal Lymphomas

A. E. Read, MD, MRCP
Professor of Medicine and Head, University Department of Medicine, Bristol Royal Infirmary, Bristol, BS2 8HW, UK.
Retroperitoneal Fibrosis (Ormond's Disease)

N. W. Read, MA, MD, FRCP
Professor of Human Nutrition, University of Sheffield, Consultant Gastroenterologist, Northern General Hospital,
Sheffield, UK.
Intestinal Transport of Fluid and Electrolytes

William Davis Wynne Rees, MD, FRCP
Consultant Gastroenterologist and Honorary Reader in Medicine, Department of Gastroenterology, Hope Hospital,
University of Manchester School of Medicine, Eccles Old Road, Salford, M6 8HD, UK.
Gastroduodenal Secretion in Health and Disease; Gastroduodenal Motility in Health and Disease

Jonathan M. Rhodes, MA, MD, FRCP
Reader in Medicine and Consultant Gastroenterologist, Department of Medicine, Liverpool University, PO Box 147,
Liverpool, L69 3BX, UK.
Inflammatory Bowel Disease: Aetiology and Pathogenesis – Immunological Aspects

J. M. Richter, MD
Associate Physician, Massachusetts General Hospital, Boston, Massachusetts 02114, USA.
Chronic Pancreatitis

A. Ruskoné-Formestraux, MD
Hôpital Saint-Lazare, Service de Gastro-enterologie, 107 rue du Faubourg Saint Denis, Paris 75475 Cedex 10, France.
Tumours of the Small Intestine: Small Intestinal Lymphomas

R. C. G. Russell, MS, FRCS
Consultant Surgeon, The Middlesex Hospital, Gower Street, London, W1, UK.
The Pancreas: Clinical Anatomy and Congenital Abnormalities

Thomas R. Russell, MD
Chairman, Department of Surgery, California Pacific Medical Center; Clinical Professor of Surgery, University College of
San Francisco, California, USA.
Pruritus Ani; Proctalgia Fugax

G. I. Sandle, BSc, MD, PhD, MRCP
Senior Lecturer in Medicine, University of Manchester and Honorary Consultant Physician, Hope Hospital, Salford, M6
8HD, UK.
Manifestations of Chronic Renal Failure

Christopher T. M. Speakman, MB, FRCS(Edin)
Sir Alan Parks Research Fellow, St Mark's Hospital, City Road, London, EC1V 2PS, UK.
Constipation, Faecal Impaction and Laxative Abuse

John Spencer, MS, FRCS
Reader in Surgery, Royal Postgraduate Medical School, Du Cane Road, London, W12 0NN; Consultant Surgeon,
Hammersmith Hospital, Du Cane Road, London, W12 0HS, UK.
**Pharynx and Oesophagus: Diaphragmatic Hernias; Acute Colonic and Other Lower Gastrointestinal Bleeding; Chronic and
Obscure Gastrointestinal Bleeding**

Robin C. Spiller, MB, BChir, MRCP, MD
Consultant Physician, Department of Therapeutics, University Hospital Medical School, Nottingham, UK.
Digestion and Malabsorption of Nutrients: Carbohydrate, Protein, Minerals, Vitamins

Christopher J. F. Spry, MA, MB, BChir, DPhil, FRCP, FRCPath, FESC
BHF Professor and Honorary Consultant, Department of Cellular and Molecular Sciences and Cardiology, St George's Hospital Medical School, Cranmer Terrace, Tooting, London, SW17 0RE, UK.
Eosinophilic Gastroenteritis

Adrian Steger, MS, FRCS
Senior Registrar in Surgery, Brook Hospital, Shooters Hill Road, London, SE18, UK.
Acute Upper Gastrointestinal Bleeding

J. Stewart, MD, FRCS
Senior Registrar, Leeds General Infirmary, Great George Street, Leeds, LS1 3EX, UK.
Peritonitis and Perforation; Abdominal Abscesses; Blunt Abdominal Trauma

W. Strober, MD
Head, Mucosal Immunity Section, National Institutes of Health, Bethesda, Maryland 20892, USA.
Protein-losing Enteropathy

Rakesh K. Tandon, MD, PhD
Professor and Head, Department of Gastroenterology and Human Nutrition Unit, All India Institute of Medical Sciences, New Delhi 110029, India.
Abdominal Tuberculosis

T. V. Taylor, MD, ChM, FRCS
Consultant Surgeon, Manchester Royal Infirmary, Oxford Road, Manchester, M13 9WL, UK.
Chronic Duodenal Ulcer: The Future of Peptic Ulcer Surgery

J. Temple, ChM, FRCS
Consultant Surgeon, Queen Elizabeth Hospital, Edgbaston, Birmingham, B15 2TH, UK.
Other Causes of Acute Abdomen: Foreign Bodies

John Terblanche, ChM, FRCS(Eng), FCS(SA)
Professor and Head, Department of Surgery, University of Cape Town Medical School, Observatory 7925, Cape Town; Co-director, Medical Research Council Liver Research Centre, University of Cape Town, Republic of South Africa.
Gall Bladder and Biliary Tract: Congenital Abnormalities

Gilbert R. Thompson, MD, FRCP
Honorary Consultant Physician and Honorary Senior Lecturer, MRC Lipoprotein Team, Hammersmith Hospital, Du Cane Road, London, W12 0HS, UK.
Lipid Abnormalities

Henry Thompson, MD, FRCPath
Reader in Pathology, General Hospital and University of Birmingham, Birmingham, UK. Honorary Consultant Pathologist, South Birmingham Health District, Birmingham, UK.
Crohn's Disease: Pathology

J. P. S. Thomson, DM, MS, FRCS
Consultant Surgeon, St Mark's Hospital, City Road, London, EC1V 2PS, UK.
Fistula-in-Ano Anorectal Sepsis; Haemorrhoids; Anal Fissure

James Toouli, MB, FRACS, PhD
Professor of Surgery, Flinders University of South Australia, Bedford Park, SA. Australia 5042; Head, Gastrointestinal Surgery and Liver Transplant Unit, Flinders Medical Centre, Bedford Park, SA. Australia 5042.
Biliary Motor Disorders

S. P. L. Travis, MB, DPhil, MRCP
Senior Registrar in Gastroenterology, John Radcliffe Hospital, Oxford, OX3 9DU, UK.
Ulcerative Colitis: Pathology, Clinical Presentation, Complications, Treatment: medical

Her Hsin Tsai, MB, MRCP
Research Fellow, Department of Medicine, University of Liverpool, PO Box 147, Liverpool, L69 3BX, UK.
Inflammatory Bowel Disease: Aetiology and Pathogenesis – Immunological Aspects

G. N. J. Tytgat, MD
Professor of Medicine Gastroenterology and Chief, Department of Gastroenterology and Hepatology, Academic Medical Center, Meibergdreef 9, 1105 AZ, Amsterdam, The Netherlands.
Gastritis; Duodenitis

G. R. Vantrappen, MD
Professor, University Hospital Gasthuisberg, Herestraat 49, Leuven 8–3000, Belgium.
Pharynx and Oesophagus: Physiology, Motility Disorders

E. P. Variyam, MD
Chief of Gastroenterology, The Wade Park Medical Center, Veterans Administration Medical Center, East Boulevard, Cleveland, Ohio 44106, USA.
Worm Infestations

Christopher W. Venables, MS(Lon), FRCS(Eng), MB, BS
Consultant in Surgical Gastroenterology, Honorary Lecturer, Newcastle University, Freeman Hospital, High Heaton, Newcastle-upon-Tyne, NE7 7DN, UK.
Chronic Gastric Ulcer: Treatment: surgical

W. A. Walker, MD
Professor of Paediatrics, Massachusetts General Hospital, Children's Hospital, 300 Longwood Avenue, Boston, Massachusetts 02115, USA.
Immunological Disorders Affecting the Small Intestine: Basic Gastrointestinal Immunology

J. A. Walker-Smith, MD(Sydney), FRCP(London), FRCP(Edin), FRACP
Professor of Paediatric Gastroenterology, Academic Department of Paediatric Gastroenterology, Queen Elizabeth Hospital for Children and Medical College of St Bartholomew's Hospital, London, UK.
Chronic Diseases of the Small Intestine in Childhood: Coeliac Disease, Other Food-related Disorders, Post-enteritis Syndrome, Toddler's Diarrhoea

Robert P. Walt, MD, FRCP
Senior Lecturer and Honorary Consultant Physician, University of Birmingham, Queen Elizabeth Hospital, Edgbaston, Birmingham, B15 2TH, UK.
Acute Bleeding Peptic Ulcer: Aetiology, Diagnosis, Treatment

Julian R. F. Walters, MA, MB, BChir
Senior Lecturer, Gastroenterology Unit, Royal Postgraduate Medical School, Hammersmith Hospital, Du Cane Road, London, W12 0NN, UK.
Absorption and Malabsorption of Calcium and Vitamin D

Andrew L. Warshaw, MD
Associate Chief of Surgery, Massachusetts General Hospital, Wang Ambulatory Care Center, #336, 15 Parkman Street, Boston, Massachusetts 02113, USA.
Chronic Pancreatitis

P. Watanapa, PhD, FRCS
Staff Surgeon, Department of Surgery, Siriraj Hospital, Bangkok 10700, Thailand.
Cancer of the Exocrine Pancreas

W. C. Watson, MD, PhD, FRCP, FRCP(C), FRCP(G), FACP
Professor of Medicine, University of W. Ontario, Victoria Hospital, 375 South Street, London, Ontario, Canada, N6A 4G5.
Coeliac Axis Compression Syndrome

Gerald Webbe, DSc, MSc(Hon), MD, FIBiol
Professor of Applied Parasitology, Department of Medical Parasitology, London School of Hygiene and Tropical Medicine, Keppel Street, London, WC1E 7HT, UK.
Schistosomiasis

Jane M. Webberley, MB, ChB, MRCPath
Consultant Medical Microbiologist, Worcester Royal Infirmary, Castle Street, Worcester, WR1 3AS; Honorary Senior Clinical Lecturer, University of Birmingham Medical School, Edgbaston, Birmingham, B15 2TT, UK.
Pseudomembranous Colitis and Antibiotic-Associated Colitis; Travellers' Diarrhoea; Yersinia Infections

Russell H. Wiesner, MD
Professor of Medicine, Mayo Clinic and Mayo Graduate School of Medicine, 200 First Street SW, Rochester, MN 55905, USA.
Primary Sclerosing Cholangitis

Christopher B. Williams, BM, FRCP
St Mark's Hospital for Diseases of the Rectum and Colon, St Bartholomew's Hospital, EC1A 7BE, London, UK.
Tumours: Benign Tumours – Polyps and Polyposis

Norman S. Williams, MS, FRCS
Professor of Surgery, The Royal London Hospital, Whitechapel, London, E1 1BB, UK.
Tumours: Malignant tumours

Robin C. N. Williamson, MA(Camb), MD, MChir, FRCS, HonFRCS(Thailand)
Professor and Director of Surgery, Department of Surgery, Hammersmith Hospital, Royal Postgraduate Medical School, Du Cane Road, London, W12 0NN, UK.
Cancer of the Exocrine Pancreas

C. P. Willoughby, MA, DM, FRCP
Consultant Gastroenterologist, Basildon Hospital, Essex, UK.
Inflammatory Bowel Disease and Pregnancy

David Wray, MD, BDS, MBChB, FDS RCS(Ed), FDS RCPS
Professor of Oral Medicine, Department of Oral Surgery and Oral Medicine, Glasgow Dental Hospital and School, 378 Sauchie Hall Street, Glasgow, G2 3JZ; Honorary Consultant, Greater Glasgow Health Board, Glasgow, UK.
Mouth

A. P. Wyatt, MB, BS, FRCS
Consultant Surgeon, Department of Surgery, Brook General Hospital, Shooter's Hill Road, London, SE18 4LW, UK.
Pneumatosis Coli (Pneumatosis Cystoides Intestinalis)

D. Wynick, BSc, MRCP, MD
MRC Clinical Scientist, Endocrinology Unit, Royal Postgraduate Medical School, Hammersmith Hospital, Du Cane Road, London, W12 0NN, UK.
Tumours of the Endocrine Pancreas

I. Zaidman, MD
Head, Department of Gastroenterology, Hospital Pradre Machado, Unidad Clinica Esmeralda IB, Av. Los Proceres, San Bernar, Caracas, Venezuela.
Intestinal Amoebiasis

P. L. Zentler-Munro, MA, MD, FRCP(Edin)
Consultant Physician, Raigmore Hospital, Inverness, IV1 3UJ, UK; Honorary Senior Lecturer in Medicine, University of Aberdeen Medical School, Aberdeen, UK.
Digestion and Malabsorption of Nutrients: Fat

CHAPTER 1

MOUTH, PHARYNX AND OESOPHAGUS

THE MOUTH

ANATOMY AND PHYSIOLOGY

D. Wray

The embryonic oral cavity arises from the primitive stomatodaeum and the oral mucous membranes are derived from both ectodermal and endodermal origins. The mouth is thus susceptible to a range of dermatological disorders in addition to the many diseases that classically involve only the gastrointestinal tract. As a result the mouth displays many symptoms and signs which may not merely reflect local disease but may be a manifestation of systemic disease – in some cases this may be unsuspected before presentation of the oral complaint.

STRUCTURE OF THE ORAL MUCOUS MEMBRANES

The oral cavity is lined by stratified squamous epithelium which is largely non-keratinized or lightly parakeratinized in nature. The palate and gingivae, however, are comprised of mucoperiosteum which is keratinized and immovable whilst the dorsum of the tongue has taste buds scattered throughout its keratinized surface. Clinically, the mucous membranes appear uniformly moist and pink. Variations in texture – 'cobblestoning', atrophy, hyperkeratosis and ulceration – all indicate disease and are discussed later. Dryness (xerostomia) may be transient, due to dehydration or anxiety, or chronic – this may be drug-induced or from an autoimmune disease (Sjögren's disease). Redness of the mucous membranes implies atrophy, inflammation or infection whilst pallor occurs only in significant anaemia (haemoglobin of less than 10 g/dl). Fifty per cent of patients have ectopic sebaceous glands called Fordyce's spots in their mucous membranes, particularly involving the cheeks and lips, which clinically resemble grains of salt and may be quite florid. These are harmless and the patient should be reassured.

SALIVARY CONTROL AND COMPOSITION

Saliva is derived from the parotid (serous) gland, the submandibular and sublingual glands (mixed serous and mucous glands) and numerous minor glands (mucous) sited principally on the inner aspects of the lips and the soft palate.[80] Salivary secretion is under nervous control. Secretion is principally via parasympathetic stimulation whilst the sympathetic nervous system controls composition.[23] Saliva contains urea and electrolytes in addition to a range of organic compounds, including amylase, lysozyme, lactoferrin, hormones and immunoglobulins.[50] Salivary composition is flow dependent; nevertheless its analysis is increasingly used as a non-invasive procedure in clinical investigation, especially in children where many disease states are reflected in alterations in both the inorganic and the organic components of saliva.[18]

ORAL IMMUNITY

The oral cavity is the portal of entry of nutrients into the gastrointestinal tract and so plays an important role in mucosal immunity. It is not physiologically an important absorptive area. Moreover, in contrast to the intestine where antigen stimulates an immunoglobulin A (IgA) response, the nature of the expected oral mucosal immune response is not clear. The oral cavity is bathed with saliva containing secretory IgA. Absence of this immunoglobulin, however, does not usually result in clinical disease. IgA affords little protection to enamel surfaces of

teeth because caries, which results from bacterial acid formation, is endemic. Moreover, human caries vaccines have not been successfully developed and non-immunological protection (e.g. systemic or topical fluoride) is far more important. IgA is produced against food stuffs and its most important role is probably to prevent systemic immune responses to nutritional antigen.

The periodontium which provides ligamentary support for the teeth is in direct communication with the oral cavity via the gingival crevice. Both the periodontium and the crevice are within the domain of the systemic immune response. Thus commensal bacteria around the gingival margins stimulate the IgG response. This may allow the systemic immune system to maintain a response to harmful gut bacteria and prevent their unchallenged absorption. The absence of a clear understanding of oral immunity makes interpretation of immunological profiles difficult in disease states.

MUCOSAL ALLERGY

The oral mucous membranes provide an excellent surface for the absorption of a wide variety of substances. This may be beneficial in the case of nutrients and drugs, e.g. sublingual glyceryl trinitrate, or harmful as in the case of allergy or sensitivity to antigenic substances.[85] Although allergic cheilitis is quite common, allergic reactions within the mouth, even in the presence of a positive skin-patch test, are surprisingly uncommon and there is little evidence for the existence of an oral equivalent to contact dermatitis. Acute swelling and erythema occur occasionally although the exact cause is not invariably identified. Common causes include drugs such as toothpastes usually containing cinnamon derivatives, and some foods. Such IgE-mediated reactions respond to antihistamines or in acute cases to parenteral corticosteroids. Food allergy may manifest itself in the form of oral ulceration (see 'Recurrent oral ulceration', page 6).

Non-IgE-mediated intraoral reactions are more common particularly to drugs and metals. Many systemically administered drugs produce lichenoid drug eruptions especially non-steroidal anti-inflammatory drugs.[65] These reactions may be slow to resolve even on withdrawal of the drug. Clinically, these lesions resemble erosive lichen planus and histologically may mimic lupus erythematosus. Erythema multiforme, often called the Stevens–Johnson syndrome when there is oral involvement, is frequently caused by drugs such as non-steroidal anti-inflammatory preparations.[16]

Allergic reactions are often misdiagnosed when a patient has an adverse reaction to injections of local anaesthetic or dental procedures. The cause is usually emotional and IgE-mediated allergy to local anaesthetic has only rarely been reported. Intradermal challenge, when indicated, should always be performed where adequate resuscitation facilities are available. Perceived acrylic allergy is common when the patient displays a painful erythematous mucosa in contact with the fitting surface of dentures. This is usually chronic erythematous candidiasis (see page 5) and not allergy which is extremely rare. Free acrylic monomer, present in new or incompletely cured dentures, may cause mucosal irritation. In cases of chronic erythematous candidiasis, marked improvement follows appropriate antifungal therapy and proper denture hygiene. Where acrylic allergy is suspected, patch testing is confirmatory either with fresh acrylic or scrapings of acrylic material from the patient's existing denture.

Mercury allergy or toxicity associated with amalgam fillings has been implicated in many diseases including multiple sclerosis and myalgic encephalomyelitis. Mercury allergy is relatively common and may cause lichen planus or lichenoid drug eruptions,[17] but there is no convincing evidence for a role for mercury or amalgam in systemic diseases such as multiple sclerosis or myalgic encephalomyelitis.

ORAL DISEASE

D. Wray

The teeth and their supporting periodontium may become diseased either as a local phenomenon or as a manifestation of a wider disease process. For example, dentinogenesis imperfecta may be seen in association with osteogenesis imperfecta and severe periodontitis occurs in association with the Chediak–Higashi syndrome.[30,81] Similarly oral mucosal disease may occur as an isolated incident, e.g. a fibro-epithelial polyp or the mucosal disease may be a manifestation of an identifiable systemic disease – particularly gastrointestinal disease. Close oral inspection should therefore be an integral part of every patient examination.

DENTAL DISEASE

DENTAL CARIES

Detailed consideration of the aetiology and treatment of dental caries is outside the scope of this text and the interested reader should consult the wide dental literature available on the subject. Caries results from the destruction of the calcified tooth substance by acid derived from bacterial fermentation of dietary sugars. Patients with fructose intolerance are characteristically caries free due to their restricted intake of such dietary sugars. It should be pointed out that there is no evidence to support the notion of focal sepsis arising from the teeth, and significant halitosis even in the absence of adequate oral hygiene is rare. Furthermore, toothache inevitably progresses to abscess formation in the absence of intervention by a dentist. Such alveolar abscess formation improves with antibiotics in the short term but proper surgical drainage, e.g. extraction, is always necessary eventually. Most dental infections are streptococcal in origin and the majority are penicillin sensitive.

TOOTH STAINING

Extrinsic staining of the teeth usually arises from poor oral hygiene, as a result of using chlorhexidine antiseptic mouthwashes, in association with tobacco or food pigments, and can be removed by polishing.[16] Intrinsic stains arise during tooth formation (up to 14 years of age) and may be due to tetracycline ingestion[16] or in association with porphyria erythropoietica (erythrodontia)[89] or blood pigments arising from trauma.

GINGIVITIS AND PERIODONTAL DISEASE

Gingivitis affecting the margins of the gums around the teeth is minimally present in everyone and is an inflammatory response to ubiquitous bacterial plaque. Poor oral hygiene and the resulting plaque accumulation aggravates the condition and leads to bleeding on tooth brushing. More extensive and wider gingival inflammation may result from oral involvement with a dermatosis such as lichen planus or pemphigoid[93] (see later).

Periodontal disease generally arises from the presence of dental plaque in association with altered host defences. This results in the destruction of the periodontium and supporting alveolar bone. The process progresses asymptomatically without obvious clinical signs until loosening of the teeth results. Periodontal disease appears in about 20% of the population and is usually insidious in its progression. Aggressive forms of periodontal disease exist and are usually seen in connection with systemic diseases such as neutrophil abnormalities. Both gingivitis and periodontitis in severe forms are seen in human immunodeficiency virus (HIV) infection which should be suspected in aggressive periodontitis of recent onset.

ORAL SOFT TISSUE DISEASE

The oral mucosa responds in a limited number of ways to disease processes. Thus oral soft tissue disease may present with thickening of the epithelium causing white patches (leukoplakia), epithelial atrophy or ulceration, pigmentation and tumours. Most diseases present in one of these ways including infections: even in acute viral infections the vesicles rapidly break down to form ulcers. Patients with bullous dermatoses also present with oral ulceration due to breakdown of the mucosa overlying the bullae. The differential diagnosis of signs such as ulceration or leukoplakia is therefore broad and is discussed later.

ORAL INFECTIONS

The mouth is the portal of entry of many pathogens which may progress without local destruction to systemic disease. This section, however, deals only with the infections which present as oral disease[48] and are grouped into viral, bacterial and fungal diseases. HIV infection which has many oral manifestations is dealt with later.

Viral infections

Herpes virus infections are the most common cause of acute stomatitis and the most common of these is herpes simplex virus infection. Indeed over 70% of the adult population show serological evidence of previous infection.[48]

Initial infection with herpes simplex virus is either subclinical (particularly in children) or causes primary herpetic gingivostomatitis. The early vesiculation breaks down rapidly to form an ulcerative stomatitis which is associated with fever, malaise and cervical lymphadenopathy. Clinically, primary herpes can be distinguished from common non-viral forms of oral ulceration because viral stomatitis affects the keratinized mucosal surfaces including the palate and gum margins which are spared in

recurrent oral ulceration. Convalescent serology confirms the diagnosis. Clinical recovery takes place spontaneously within 10–14 days. Local symptomatic therapy in the form of analgesics and antiseptic mouthwashes is helpful. Acyclovir is only indicated within 72 hours of onset and may shorten the clinical course. Recurrent herpes labialis (cold sore) results from reactivation of herpes within the trigeminal nerve roots in patients previously infected with the virus. Clinical lesions arise particularly in response to stress, ultraviolet damage or immunosuppression, and can be controlled with the use of topical 5% acyclovir cream.

Herpes zoster is similarly reactivated in previously infected individuals and may cause an intraoral stomatitis with no extraoral manifestations. The clinical diagnosis is suggested by the unilateral nature of the ulceration. Convalescent serology confirms the diagnosis.

Stomatitis may also arise from Coxsackie A virus (herpangina or hand, foot and mouth disease) or Epstein–Barr virus (infectious mononucleosis) infection. The definitive diagnosis of any viral stomatitis relies on direct demonstration of virus or examination of convalescent serology. The self-limiting nature of these infections usually makes such investigations unnecessary.

Bacterial infection

With the exception of the main dental diseases (caries and periodontal disease) oral bacterial infections have now become uncommon. It should be remembered that actinomycetes are often commensal in the mouth and intransigent cervicofacial abscess formation may be the presenting feature of actinomycosis. Microbiological sampling is necessary to confirm such a diagnosis. Sexually transmitted diseases are becoming increasingly prevalent as intraoral infections. Syphilis and gonorrhoea remain uncommon to the extent that they are now only diagnosed when clinical suspicion indicates laboratory investigation.

Fungal infections

With the exception of candidiasis fungal infections of the mouth are rare. Oral fungal infections, such as blastomycosis and coccidiodomycosis, have no pathognomonic clinical features and diagnosis relies on mycological investigation.

Candida species are commensals in the mouth in up to 50% of the population, the most predominant species being *Candida albicans*. Other species may be identified mycologically but are clinically indis-

Table 1.1 Classification of oral candidiasis

	Type	Clinical features
Group 1	Chronic mucocutaneous	Associated immune deficiency syndromes, e.g. Swiss-type agammaglobulinaemia, DiGeorge syndrome
Group 2		
A	Familial chronic mucocutaneous candidiasis	Mouth mainly affected, also skin and nails
B	Diffuse chronic mucocutaneous candidiasis	Extensive involvement of skin
C	Candidal endocrinopathy syndrome	Associated multiple endocrine diseases
D	Chronic hyperplastic candidiasis	Intraoral leukoplakia
Group 3		
A	Pseudomembranous	Medically compromised, e.g. extremes of age, HIV-seropositive individuals
B	Erythematous candidiasis	Antibiotic stomatitis, median rhomboid glossitis, denture stomatitis
C	Angular cheilitis	Sores at angles of mouth

tinguishable and may be managed indentically. As candidal carriage is endemic, mycological culture is unhelpful in diagnosis which relies on the clinical features and direct demonstration of mycelial forms on Gram- or periodic acid–Schiff-stained smears. Oral candidiasis can be separated into three distinct groups[77] (*Table 1.1*): group 1 is very rare and consists of patients with superficial mucocutaneous candidiasis who concurrently have a profound hereditary immune deficiency such as Swiss-type agammaglobulinaemia or DiGeorge syndrome. The immune defect present is usually incompatible with prolonged survival. Group 2 is also rare and comprises four subgroups, three of which are early onset, i.e. familial chronic mucocutaneous candidiasis in which superficial oral candidiasis dominates the clinical picture, diffuse chronic mucocutaneous candidiasis in which skin involvement is usually more extensive and the candidal endocrinopathy syndrome in which chronic superficial candidiasis is associated with multiple endrocrine disorders, especially hypoparathyroidism, thyroiditis and Addison's disease. Chronic hyperplastic candidiasis occurs as a speckled leukoplakia most commonly on the commissure of the buccal mucosa, although it may also occur on the tongue and palate particularly in smokers. Histological demonstration of candidal hyphae in the superficial layers of the epithelium using periodic acid–Schiff stain is required to confirm the diagnosis. Group 3 infections are far more common and are regularly encountered in clinical practice. Pseudomembranous candidiasis (thrush) is usually acute. It classically affects individuals in the extremes of life and is only generally seen in adults who are immunocompromised (*Figure 1.1*). Clinically, the mucosa is erythematous and partially covered with white plaques consisting of candidal

hyphae and squames which can be readily peeled off to leave a raw, bleeding surface. Pseudomembranous candidiasis occurring in an otherwise apparently healthy individual nowadays strongly suggests an underlying HIV seropositivity. Indeed, pseudomembranous candidiasis is a common presenting symptom of such infection.

Erythematous candidiasis may be an acute response to antibiotic therapy (antibiotic stomatitis), when mucosal sensitivity and dryness are common presenting complaints, or chronic in median rhomboid glossitis which is characterized by a smooth, red patch in the centre of the tongue towards the back. Previously this lesion was often diagnosed as a lingual thyroid or persistent tuberculum impar, but it is now recognized to be erythematous candidiasis and should be treated non-surgically. Erythematous candidiasis in both forms is prevalent in HIV-seropositive individuals.

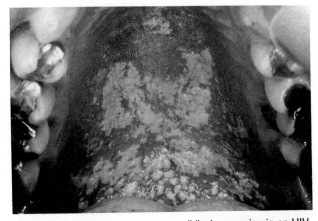

Figure 1.1 Pseudomembranous candidiasis occurring in an HIV-seropositive male homosexual. The palatal mucosa is erythematous and partially covered with white plaques which can be easily scraped off to leave a raw, bleeding surface.

Chronic erythematous candidiasis or denture stomatitis is a common, palatal infection in denture wearers. The condition is usually asymptomatic, although it may be associated with a sense of dryness or a bad taste in the mouth. The erythema is confirmed to the denture-bearing area of the palate and is often misconstrued as an acrylic or cobalt chrome allergy. Removal of the denture at night and appropriate anti fungal therapy results in clinical improvement.

Patients with denture stomatitis often have a concurrent angular cheilitis. This is a common condition and is usually due to candidal superinfection. In dentate individuals staphylococcal or streptococcal infection is more likely. Miconazole cream, which is effective against all three agents, is a suitable topical remedy. Angular cheilitis may also be a manifestation of a nutritional deficiency, especially of folic acid or iron (see later) and is also a feature of oral Crohn's disease.

All types of oral candidiasis are superficial and progression to fungaemia occurs only in immunocompromised patients. Candidal infections are extremely common in association with HIV infection, although fungaemia is rare in these individuals who have elevated serum levels of anticandidal antibodies.[90] Treatment of milder forms of candidiasis may be effected using amphotericin and nystatin lozenges and appropriate denture hygiene. Chronic or mucocutaneous infections respond best to systemic anti-fungals such as fluconazole which may need to be continued to prevent relapse.

ORAL ULCERATION

Oral ulceration is the most common oral mucosal symptom. The causes of oral ulcers are numerous. The main causes include the following:

Traumatic ulcers
Recurrent ulcers (aphthous ulceration including Behçet's syndrome)
Viral stomatitis
Malignant disease (including carcinoma, leukaemia)
Bullous disorders
Gastrointestinal disease
Lichen planus including drug reactions
Bacterial ulcers (including tuberculosis, syphilis).

Those not considered elsewhere in the chapter will be discussed here.

Traumatic ulceration

Simple traumatic ulceration may arise from burns due to hot food, chemicals (aspirin burn), sharp or ragged teeth and ill-fitting dentures. The aetiology is usually obvious and removal of the cause is attended by prompt resolution. Ulceration persisting for more than 2 weeks should be biopsied to exclude malignancy. Recurrent traumatic ulceration often implies that the patient suffers from traumatically induced recurrent aphthae (see below) and should be treated accordingly.

Recurrent oral ulceration (recurrent aphthous stomatitis, recurrent aphthae)

Recurrent aphthous stomatitis is the most common oral soft tissue disease. It has an incidence of 20% and a prevalence of 2% in the general population. Women are affected more than men. The onset is usually within the first two decades and spontaneous remission is common.

Recurrent aphthae occur in three distinct forms: minor, major and herpetiform. Behçet's syndrome, a multisystem disorder, has recurrent aphthae as a major clinical manifestation and will be discussed later.

Pathogenesis

The pathogenesis of recurrent aphthae remains obscure. Immune alterations especially of lymphocytes[63] are thought to be of central importance. No convincing evidence of a role for viruses or bacteria has been forthcoming.[86] There are, however, a number of host and environmental factors which have been shown to be important[87] (*Table 1.2*).

Host factors appear to be important in determining susceptibility whilst environmental causes initiate individual ulcers. The various aetiological factors are not mutually exclusive and may concurrently contribute to the clinical picture. Genetic factors play a small role, as evidenced by an increased incidence of 50% among first-degree relatives of patients and a mild HLA (histocompatibility locus antigen) association with A2 and B12 (relative risk 3.0). Deficiencies of iron, folic acid or vitamin B_{12} occur in 20% of patients either singly or in combination.[91] The majority of deficiencies are

Table 1.2 Aetiological factors in recurrent aphthous stomatitis

Host	*Environmental*
Genetic	Trauma
Haematinics	Allergy
Systemic disease	(Smoking)
Hormones	

latent and hence assay of individual haematinics is essential to identify abnormalities. Replacement therapy is usually attended by clinical remission especially with folic acid and vitamin B_{12}. Nutritional deficiencies are not associated with any particular clinical features and ideally all patients should be haematologically screened. In practice, investigation is restricted to those with severe ulceration or patients with a recent or abrupt onset of ulcers. Once the deficiency has been identified, systemic investigation is mandatory to identify the cause and often severe occult disease is diagnosed, particularly malabsorption.

Hormonal considerations are also important because women are more commonly affected and indeed 5% of women patients experience exclusively premenstrual aphthae.[19] Progestogen therapy is effective in such cases although in practice seldom recommended. Pregnancy is attended by temporary clinical remission in 80% of women.

Environmental factors include trauma and allergy, both of which may mediate their effect by the release of inflammatory mediators causing local immune alteration. Thus, mild trauma, e.g. sharp food or toothbrush trauma, may cause inappropriately severe ulceration[92] and food can be demonstrated to initiate ulcers in one-third of cases,[94,95] especially cheese, chocolate, nuts, tomatoes and citrus fruits. Smoking is negatively associated with ulcers and often patients present first with significant ulceration on cessation of their smoking habit. Interestingly, oral aphthae and carcinoma have never been reported simultaneously in the same patient.

Minor aphthae

These are the most common form and affect 85% of aphthae sufferers. Minor aphthae are 1–10 mm in diameter, round or ovoid with a yellow or grey base and erythematous border, and affect exclusively the non-keratinizing mucosal surfaces (the gingivae and hard palate are spared). The ulcers arise singly or in crops of up to 10 ulcers which last for 3–14 days before healing spontaneously without scarring.

Major aphthae

These are also known as periadenitis mucosa necrotica recurrens and are rarer, affecting only 5–10% of recurrent oral ulcer patients. The ulcers are usually single but are often greater than 10 mm in diameter and persist for weeks or months before healing with significant scarring. Again they affect only non-keratinizing surfaces.

Herpetiform ulcers

These are the least common and affect less than 10% of aphthae sufferers. Recurring crops of up to 100 ulcers of 2–3 mm diameter affect the non-keratinizing surfaces for 2–3 weeks before healing spontaneously without scars. These ulcers are called herpetiform on the basis of their appearance rather than their aetiology, because they are non-infectious and can be distinguished from primary herpetic gingivo-stomatitis due to their mucosal distribution (see above).

Diagnosis

The diagnosis of recurrent aphthous stomatitis is based entirely on a typical history and confirmatory clinical features. Recurrent self-healing oral ulceration confined to the movable (non-keratinized) surfaces is inevitably recurrent aphthous stomatitis.

Treatment

The management of recurrent aphthous stomatitis relies first on the identification and elimination of nutritional or systemic causes in association with dietary manipulation. However, the majority of patients must rely on symptomatic therapy in the form of tetracycline mouthwash, which is effective in 50% of cases, or corticosteroids in the form of triamcinalone in dental paste or beclomethazone sprays. Systemic steroids should be reserved for extreme cases. Thalidomide may be effective in refractory cases occurring in a non-child-bearing population.

Behçet's syndrome

Behçet's syndrome is a multisystem disorder which manifests usually with orogenital ulceration and either skin, ocular, arthritic or neurological complications depending on the HLA status of the patient (*Table 1.3*).[43] Other manifestations include gastrointestinal and emotional disorders. The gastrointestinal manifestations are considered on page 1247. Management is usually with systemic steroids although colchicine 0.5 mg three times daily is effective in controlling symptoms because increased polymorph chemotaxis is a feature of Behçet's syndrome. Immunostimulants have also been tried with limited success.

Table 1.3 Immunogenetic basis for Behçet's syndrome

Clinical type	HLA type
Mucocutaneous	B12
Ocular	B5 (BW51)
Arthritic	B27
Neurological	None

ORAL KERATOSIS

Increased keratinization of the oral mucosa leads to the development of whiteness which may be an effect of several disease processes.

Several forms of oral keratosis can be distinguished; these can usually be diagnosed on the basis of the history and characteristic histology and causes include:

Hereditary
Smoking/friction
Idiopathic leukoplakia
Lichen planus
Lupus erythematosus
Candidal leukoplakia
Hairy leukoplakia.

Leukoplakia

Leukoplakia is defined by the WHO as a white patch of the oral mucosa which cannot be scraped off (thus excluding pseudomembranous candidiasis) and cannot be attributed to any other cause. This definition has been extended to include smoking and frictional keratosis. In practice it is often difficult to quantify the contributions of different aetiological factors and, although removal of the friction or tobacco may be attended by clinical improvement, these white patches should be regarded as leukoplakia until resolution occurs. Also, as in the cases of candidal leukoplakia and hairy leukoplakia, infectious agents are implicated but the term 'leukoplakia' is appropriately used. Leukoplakia as defined above does exclude other diagnosable conditions such as lichen planus and lupus erythematosus.

Leukoplakia is important because it is pre-malignant, some 2–5% of cases progressing to carcinoma. The majority of oral carcinomas arise spontaneously, especially on the lateral borders of the tongue and floor of mouth, but pre-malignant lesions identify some at-risk individuals and allow them to be followed closely. Suspect leukoplakia lesions, especially those with speckled or erythematous areas (erythroplakia) should be biopsied. Lesions show a variable degree of epithelial dysplasia, although in contrast to cervical neoplasia there is no evidence of regular progression through severe dysplasia to frank carcinoma and, in further contrast, there is no evidence to support the notion of a viral aetiology for oral carcinoma.[42] The site of leukoplakia is important and 40% of sublingual keratoses may progress to carcinoma. Management of leukoplakia is usually conservative although excision, thermal surgery and topical cytotoxics have been advocated.

Lichen planus

Lichen planus has been variously associated with abnormal glucose metabolism, liver dysfunction and renal calculi although there is no evidence of a causal relationship.[65] Lichenoid eruptions which can only be subjectively distinguished from lichen planus clinically and histologically may occur in response to metal restorations, especially amalgam containing mercury, and may respond to removal of such fillings in patch test-positive individuals.[17] Also lichen planus occurs in association with ingestion of some drugs, particularly non-steroidal anti-inflammatory drugs, and may respond promptly to withdrawal of the offending medication.[65]

Lichen planus is the most common intraoral keratosis and usually presents with a reticular or papular appearance on the buccal mucosa (*Figure 1.2*), particularly buccal to the last standing lower molars. Plaque or atrophic forms also occur which are difficult to distinguish clinically from leukoplakia or erythroplakia, and the histology may be unhelpful due to the demanding histopathological criteria required for the diagnosis of lichen planus. The distinction is often irrelevant in such patients because the atrophic and erosive forms of lichen planus progress to malignancy in 1–2% of cases and require careful follow-up. Concurrent cutaneous lesions are diagnostic pointers but, in contrast to cutaneous lichen planus which usually resolves in 18 months, oral lichen planus is usually intransigent. Reticular lichen planus can be controlled with a chlorhexidine mouthwash but ulcerated lesions which may be extensive require corticosteroids, often systemically, to resolve the ulceration and discomfort.

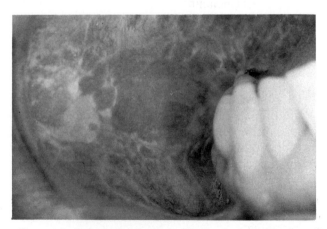

Figure 1.2 Reticular lichen planus affecting the buccal mucosa of a 56-year-old woman. White striae are interspersed with areas of erythematous atrophic mucosa.

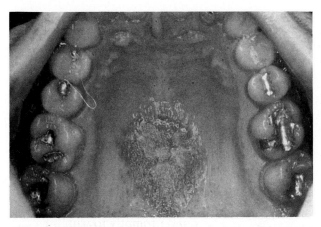

Figure 1.3 Discoid lupus erythematosus occurring as an annular white patch on the hard palate of a 36-year-old woman.

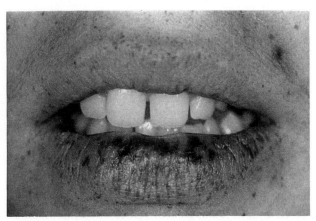

Figure 1.4 Perioral pigmentation occurring in association with intestinal polyposis in a 26-year-old woman with the Peutz–Jeghers syndrome.

Lupus erythematosus

Lupus erythematosus characteristically occurs on the oral mucosa as an annular lesion similar to lichen planus on the palate or buccal mucosa (Figure 1.3).

Histology suggests the diagnosis of lupus erythematosus which is usually discoid rather than systemic. A positive antinuclear factor may not be significant because 50% of patients with oral keratosis in any form have a detectable antinuclear factor.[59]

ORAL PIGMENTATION

Intraoral pigmentation is usually an incidental finding and is harmless but must be distinguished from sinister causes.[37] The main causes of intraoral pigmentation include the following:

Exogenous
    amalgam tattoo
Endogenous (melanin)
    racial
    familial
    congenital
    systemic (e.g. Peutz–Jeghers syndrome and polyostotic fibrous dysplasia)
    Drug-induced
        anti-malarials
        oral contraceptives
        phenothiazines
    trauma (chronic)
    hormonal (e.g. Addison's disease)
    local (naevi)
    malignant melanoma
    idiopathic.

Racial or familial pigmentation is usually diffuse and patchy, and generally involves the labial gingivae. A similar clinical picture may result from drug ingestion, however, or it may be hormonal; Addison's disease always causes other detectable symptoms suggesting the diagnosis, although ACTH-producing bronchogenic carcinomas may present with oral pigmentation. Localized 'pigmented lesions' are often amalgam tattoos due to implantation of metal from fillings often following extractions. These must be distinguished from naevi and malignant melanomas. If clinical doubt exists biopsy is indicated. Chronic irritation causing keratosis may also be associated with increased melanin deposition. The perioral pigmentation associated with Peutz–Jeghers syndrome is characteristic (*Figure 1.4*).

ORAL TUMOURS

Benign tumours

Benign epithelial and connective tissue tumours of the oral mucosa are rare although the incidence of squamous cell papillomas may be increasing.[14] Hyperplastic lesions of the oral mucosa are common and present as a mucosal polyp, denture irritation hyperplasia or gingival epulis. Epulides may be vascular (often associated with pregnancy) or fibrous in nature, or less commonly peripheral giant cell granulomata. These lesions are all reactive and simple excision provides a cure.

Malignant tumours

Squamous-cell carcinoma is the most common intraoral malignancy, although jaw metastases are also common particularly from tumours of the breast, lung, prostate, kidney and stomach. Oral carcinomas may be exophytic but most present as persistent ulcers. Any ulcer which fails to heal within 2 weeks should be biopsied to exclude malignancy. Salivary gland tumours may arise within the minor glands in the oral mucosa and these are discussed below.

SALIVARY GLAND DISEASE

Sialadenitis

Viral sialadenitis (mumps) is suggested by bilateral involvement of the glands. Acute bacterial sialadenitis usually occurs in dehydrated patients postoperatively but is rare nowadays. Chronic sialadenitis arises from recurrent infection causing structural damage to the gland, usually the submandibular. Bacterial sialadenitis persisting despite repeated courses of antibiotics often results in irrevocable structural damage requiring surgical removal of the gland. Obstructive sialadenitis may arise due to stricture of the duct or blockage from a calculus or mucous plug. Unfortunately, the majority of obstructions are due to stricture or mucus and require sialography rather than plain radiography to confirm the diagnosis. Sialography in itself may be therapeutic in relieving the blockage and will, in addition, demonstrate any structural damage present. Significant architectural damage to the gland may predispose to chronic sialadenitis thus necessitating subsequent removal as discussed above. Damage to minor salivary gland ducts, especially in the lower lip, leads to mucocele formation due to extravasation of mucus. Retention mucoceles due to duct obstruction are unusual. The swellings arise quickly and appear as fluid-filled swellings which transilluminate. Excision is required to prevent recurrence. Sublingual swellings can arise in the same way from the sublingual gland giving rise to a ranula. However, ranulae may be caused by tumours and surgical exploration is mandatory.

Xerostomia

Transient dry mouth is most commonly due to simple dehydration or anxiety. However, persistent xerostomia most commonly arises from drug therapy, particularly from tricyclic antidepressants. Salivary gland damage, as discussed above, can also cause xerostomia as can irradiation. Sjögren's syndrome is a significant cause of xerostomia (see later under 'Sjögren's syndrome'). Xerostomia is also an increasingly reported manifestation of HIV infection. Sialosis is painless salivary gland swelling and may be a feature of Sjögren's syndrome, diabetes

mellitus, acromegaly, malnutrition or sarcoidosis. Its pathogenesis remains obscure although its course is benign.

Salivary gland tumours

Salivary gland tumours are uncommon and account for only about 3% of all tumours. The major glands are the most common site but minor intraoral glands can be affected leading to an intraoral presentation of a salivary tumour. Adenomas are the most common salivary gland tumours and the majority are pleomorphic. Pleomorphic salivary adenomas are benign but are locally recurrent. Wide excision rather than radiotherapy is the appropriate treatment. Other rarer tumours occur including the mucoepidermoid and acinic cell carcinoma which can metastasize and behave unpredictably. Several types of carcinoma also occur in the salivary glands including adenoid cystic carcinoma, adenocarcinoma, epidermoid carcinoma and carcinoma arising from pleomorphic salivary adenoma. The most common is the adenoid cystic carcinoma which has a propensity to spread along nerve bundles making excision problematic. The interested reader should consult the specialized texts for more detailed classification and histology.[45]

TONGUE DISEASES

Atrophic glossitis

Atrophic glossitis is characterized by loss of the filiform papillae leaving a smooth red tongue. This is classically associated with iron-deficiency anaemia, although the lingual mucosal atrophy occurs in response to the deficiency of iron rather than the anaemia per se and indeed glossitis may precede changes in the peripheral blood.[89] Papillary atrophy may be quite subtle and patients presenting with a painful or sensitive tongue should be screened for deficiencies of folate and vitamin B_{12} in addition to iron as these haematinics may also be implicated in atrophic glossitis.

Black hairy tongue

Black hairy tongue is characterized by hypertrophy of the filiform papillae which then become discoloured due to superinfection with chromogenic organisms.[69] The condition is not significant but it is difficult to eradicate. Brushing or scraping the surface usually effects an improvement until resolution occurs.

Geographic tongue (benign migratory glossitis)

Geographic tongue is a condition of unknown aetiology which affects both sexes of all ages. Characteristically areas of redness appear due to loss of filiform papillae. These areas are surrounded by an incomplete whitish ring of acanthotic epithelium (*Figure 1.5*). The areas migrate across the surface of the tongue and remit spontaneously at irregular intervals. Symptomatically, the condition is associated with sensitivity to hot or spicy foods; frank discomfort usually indicates superimposed glossitis or glossopyrosis (see later). Intraoral psoriasis occurs rarely and may closely resemble geographic tongue.[56] The presence of cutaneous lesions and a characteristic histology suggest the diagnosis. Significant fissuring and some swelling of the tongue may be an associated feature in patients with geographic tongue. Management consists of reassurance.

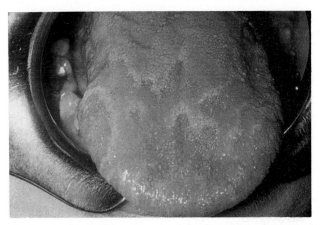

Figure 1.5 Geographic tongue occurring in a 56-year-old man. Marked alteration of the distribution of the lesions occurred within 24 hours.

Median rhomboid glossitis

As mentioned previously, median rhomboid glossitis is now regarded as a form of erythematous candidiasis[78] and is seen most commonly in patients using steroid inhalers and in HIV-seropositive individuals.

Hairy leukoplakia

Hairy leukoplakia occurs almost exclusively in HIV-seropositive patients but has been reported in seronegative immunocompromised patients.[6,27,73] It is due to Epstein–Barr virus infection of the lingual mucosa. Hairy leukoplakia will be discussed later under AIDS and the gastrointestinal tract.

ORAL MANIFESTATIONS OF GASTROINTESTINAL DISEASE

D. Wray

UPPER GASTROINTESTINAL TRACT DISEASE

Oral manifestations seen in association with stomach or oesophageal disease are rare. Acid reflux particularly in patients with bulimia causes erosion of the teeth characteristically on the palatal aspects, but does not cause significant mucositis. There are no oral problems associated with peptic ulceration. Oral disease seen in association with achlorhydria is discussed under pernicious anaemia or below under 'The Kelly–Paterson syndrome'.

THE KELLY–PATERSON SYNDROME (THE PLUMMER–VINSON SYNDROME)

The classic description by Kelly 1919[39] was of iron deficiency, dysphagia and postcricoid oesophageal stricture. The syndrome is also commonly associated with glossitis, angular cheilitis and gastric achlorhydria. The oral manifestations are most probably tissue signs of iron deficiency and should respond to iron replacement. The neoplastic potential[11,38] of the Kelly–Paterson syndrome is between 4% and 16%.[53,66] The majority of carcinomas are postcricoid but they may also occur in the oesophagus and stomach. Carcinoma arising in the associated oral leukoplakia has not been reported. The mechanism whereby iron deficiency causes these changes remains obscure.

LIVER AND PANCREAS

LIVER

Oral complications in liver disease are rare. Sialosis is an occasional complication of alcoholic cirrhosis.

However, Sjögren's syndrome quite often complicates chronic active hepatitis. Bleeding tendencies secondary to hepatic disease may manifest in the mouth. In hepatic porphyria accumulation of unexcreted porphyrin occurs in the tissues and photosensitization results. Dental manipulation may cause mucosal bullae to form which histologically resemble skin lesions.[24] Erythrodontia caused by deposition of porphyrin during formation of the teeth occurs in congenital erythropoietic porphyria but not in hepatic porphyria.[89]

PANCREAS

Cystic fibrosis causes several changes in the mouth: dental manifestations include the delayed eruption of the teeth which are often hypoplastic. In addition repeated courses of tetracycline during childhood often results in intrinsic staining of the teeth. Submandibular salivary gland enlargement occurs but the parotid glands are spared. Significant alterations occur in the composition of the saliva : total protein, and enzyme contents are increased as are concentrations of calcium and phosphorus. However, sodium and potassium levels remain normal[80].

Diabetes mellitus is also occasionally associated with salivary gland swelling (sialosis) and xerostomia is quite common. Reduced salivary flow and increased salivary glucose are thought to contribute to the increased incidence of oral candidiasis among diabetics.[41] Gingival inflammation is also more common in diabetics and severe periodontal disease appears to be more prevalent in some groups of patients perhaps as a result of defective neutrophil chemotaxis.[40]

INTESTINAL DISEASE

COELIAC DISEASE

Recurrent aphthae, glossitis and angular cheilitis are oral aspects of gluten sensitivity. Oral aphthae are the most common manifestation and may occur as a direct result of gluten sensitivity on the oral mucosa or arise in response to malabsorption of haematinics.[91] Patients in the former group develop oral ulceration promptly after ingestion of gluten-containing foods, whilst those with aphthae secondary to nutritional deficiencies only develop ulcers when nutrient levels fall. Four per cent of unselected aphthae patients have coeliac disease which may be asymptomatic.[21] All aphthae patients with folate deficiency should undergo jejunal biopsy. Patients who suffer oral aphthae may have gluten sensitivity without enteropathy and have a clinical response to gluten withdrawal.[85] Sugar absorption tests and secretory antigliadin antibodies in jejunal aspirates may be useful in identifying these patients.[52]

Dental manifestations of coeliac disease include hypoplasia of the teeth and severe osteomalacia may lead to premature tooth loss.

Patients with dermatitis herpetiformis with or without jejunal atrophy also display oral lesions in the majority of cases which show characteristic immunofluorescence staining with IgA (see later).

CROHN'S DISEASE

The original description of the clinical entity by Crohn et al.[13] was of regional ileitis, although it is now apparent that any part of the gut can be affected from the mouth to the anus. The first description of oral Crohn's disease was in 1969[15] and several series have subsequently been published.[4,7,12] The incidence may be increasing. Orofacial granulomatosis may occur in the absence of intestinal involvement and this term has been favoured by some.[75,82]

The term 'orofacial granulomatosis' extends to include, in addition to oral Crohn's disease, sarcoidosis, granulomatous cheilitis and the Melkersson–Rosenthal syndrome. Sarcoidosis is an uncommon cause and accounts for only 3.5% of patients.[82] Granulomatous cheilitis is a descriptive term characterized especially by swelling and granulomatous lesions. The Melkersson–Rosenthal syndrome is a triad of orofacial granulomatosis, fissured tongue and facial nerve palsy which presumably arises due to granulomatous involvement of the seventh nerve. This syndrome affects some 13% of orofacial granulomatosis patients.[82] Ileal or colonic Crohn's disease affects between 10% and 34% of patients but may be asymptomatic.[64,82]

Patients with orofacial granulomatosis have been reported to have a significant incidence of atopy (60%)[35] but this has not been confirmed by other series.[61,83] In addition, food-related allergic reactions have been claimed to be aetiologically important, particularly cinnamon aldehyde, cocoa, carvone and food colourings, and dietary elimination is reputed to cause clinical improvement.[54,71] Other studies have failed to confirm this.[83]

The clinical features of Crohn's disease (orofacial granulomatosis) include the following:

Swelling of lips
Angular cheilitis
Cobblestone appearance

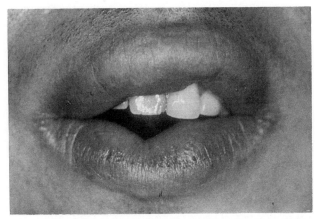

Figure 1.6 Chronic lip swelling and mild angular cheilitis occurring in a 26-year-old man with long-standing intestinal Crohn's disease.

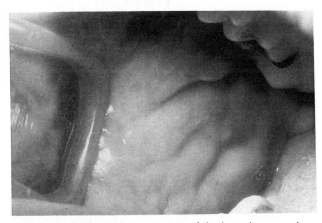

Figure 1.7 Cobblestone appearance of the buccal mucosa in a 35-year-old man with orofacial granulomatosis without evidence of intestinal Crohn's disease.

Linear ulcers
Mucosal tags
Hyperplastic gingivitis
Localized swellings
Recurrent aphthous stomatitis.

Lip swelling (*Figure 1.6*), a 'cobblestone' appearance (*Figure 1.7*) and linear ulcers (*Figure 1.8*) are the most common features. The lip swelling may fluctuate rapidly but seldom regresses significantly. The lip swelling can affect either the upper or the lower lip. Facial infection and angioedema should be included in the differential diagnosis. Cosmetic problems are complicated by soreness of the lips. Cobblestoning and mucosal tags may cause difficulty in eating and speaking. The linear ulcers are painful and intransigent and display the same deep, penetrating tendencies as gut lesions (*Figure 1.9*). Recurrent aphthous stomatitis occurs as an additional form of oral ulceration and occurs in approximately 10–20% of patients.[4,12,25] In contrast to the other oral manifestations, however, which progress independently of the intestinal lesions, recurrent aphthae arise in response to active ileal or colonic Crohn's disease.[4] Pyostomatitis vegetans (see under 'ulcerative colitis') has also been reported in association with Crohn's disease[8] as has an acquired form of epidermolysis bullosa[10].

Investigation

The clinical features of orofacial granulomatosis are often characteristic but biopsy is required to confirm the diagnosis. Biopsy down to muscle is required as granulomata are often deep-seated. Histology is similar to intestinal Crohn's disease and prominent features include non-caseating granulomata and

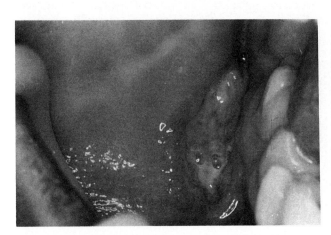

Figure 1.8 Ulceration affecting the buccal sulcus of a 13-year-old girl with oral Crohn's disease without intestinal involvement. The ulcer had been present for 18 months.

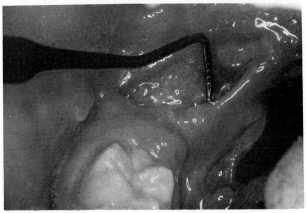

Figure 1.9 Deep penetrating ulceration of the retromolar fossa in the same patient as in Figure 1.8, showing fistula formation with the lateral pharyngeal wall. Note mucosal tags are also present on the buccal mucosa.

perivascular cuffing of lymphocytes in association with intercellular oedema. Healing of biopsy sites is uneventful.

Treatment

Management of orofacial granulomatosis is unsatisfactory. Treatment of lip swelling with intralesional triamcinalone has limited success and surgical reduction of the lips provides only temporary improvement. Approximately one-quarter of patients improve spontaneously but patients with painful ulceration or gross lip swelling warrant early therapy with systemic corticosteroids. Topical steroids are of limited help. Sulphasalazine appears to be of no benefit in reducing oral signs or symptoms.[83]

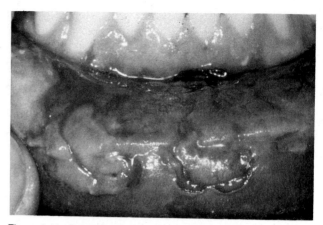

Figure 1.11 Pyostomatitis vegetans affecting a 52-year-old man with an 8-month history of oral bullae and fissuring. Gastrointestinal investigation was completely normal.

ULCERATIVE COLITIS

The oral manifestations of ulcerative colitis include pyostomatitis vegetans, pyoderma gangrenosum and recurrent aphthous stomatitis.

Pyostomatitis vegetans was originally described by McCarthy in 1949 and is a rare manifestation of ulcerative colitis.[46] Clinically, the condition may present as small miliary abscesses (*Figure 1.10*) or as a verrucous stomatitis (*Figure 1.11*). The condition may occur in isolation or secondary to ulcerative colitis or Crohn's disease when oral disease reflects intestinal disease activity.[5] There is a distinctive foetor oris.[88] Histological investigation demonstrates intermucosal abscess formation in a suprabasal distribution with pseudoepithiliomatous hyperplasia and acanthosis (*Figure 1.12*). Immuno-fluorescence staining shows intercellular staining of the prickle-cell layer with IgG similar to pemphigus vulgaris.[88] Treatment comprises topical or systemic corticosteroids combined with sulphasalazine which is of additional therapeutic benefit.[88] Although pyoderma gangrenosum is classically a cutaneous manifestation of ulcerative colitis it has also been reported in the mouth.[3] Chronic ragged ulcers occur (*Figure 1.13*) which are resistant to topical therapy. Sulphasalazine may cause resolution of the oral ulcers.

Recurrent aphthous stomatitis occurs in up to 20% of patients with ulcerative colitis and is usually a result of a secondary nutritional deficiency. Treatment consists of control of the ulcerative colitis and conventional therapy for recurrent aphthous stomatitis (see above).

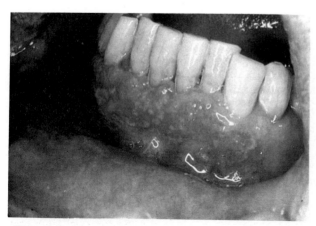

Figure 1.10 Intramucosal abscess formation affecting a 58-year-old man with pyostomatitis vegetans. A colectomy had been performed 1 year previously for caecal carcinoma.

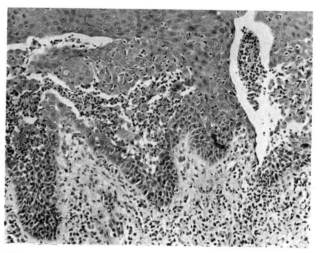

Figure 1.12 Histology of pyostomatitis vegetans showing suprabasal clefting with abundant polymorphonuclear neutrophils.

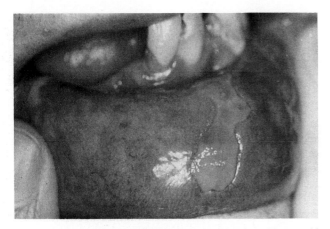

Figure 1.13 Pyoderma gangrenosum occurring in a 36-year-old male with long-standing ulcerative colitis who had been withdrawn from sulphasalazine therapy temporarily due to aspermia. Reintroduction of sulphasalazine caused prompt resolution of the ragged oral ulcers.

FAMILIAL POLYPOSIS COLI

This autosomal dominant syndrome includes a variant which is characterized by soft and hard tissue tumours in addition to the rectal and colonic adenomatous polyps.[37] Soft tissue lesions include dermoid tumours, subcutaneous fibromas and sebaceous cysts. Facial osteomas are characteristic. Hard tissue swellings and dental abnormalities include odontomes and impacted or supernumerary teeth. The extraintestinal manifestations often precede the intestinal manifestations and subsequent neoplastic change by many years. Gastrointestinal tract investigation is mandatory when there is a clinical suspicion.

ORAL MANIFESTATIONS OF SYSTEMIC DISEASE

D. Wray

CONGENITAL ABNORMALITIES

Congenital syndromes affecting the head and neck are innumerable and outside the scope of this text. The interested reader is referred to the authoritative literature on the subject.[26,70] Congenital head and neck syndromes with gastrointestinal manifestations are shown in *Table 1.4*.

IMMUNOLOGICAL DISORDERS

Primary immunodeficiencies are usually inherited and are uncommon. They constitute a large heterogeneous group which has not been fully characterized. The main types seen are shown in *Table 1.5* along with the more common oral manifestations. Although oral ulceration is seen in association with

Table 1.4 Congenital head and neck syndromes with gastrointestinal manifestations

Syndrome	Oral lesions	Gastrointestinal lesions
Acanthosis nigricans	Papillomatosis of oral mucosa	Adenocarcinoma of the stomach
Acrodermatitis enteropathica	Papillomas, erosions, candidiasis	Intermittent diarrhoea
Cowden's syndrome (multiple hamartomatous syndrome)	Papillomatosis of oral mucosa	Colonic polyposis and carcinoma
Familial polyposis coli (Gardner's syndrome)	Osteomas, fibromas, epidermoid cysts, odontomes, supernumerary teeth	Intestinal polyposis
Odontoma–dysphagia syndrome	Odontomas	Dysphagia, cirrhosis
Peutz–Jeghers syndrome	Perioral pigmentation	Intestinal polyposis
Pseudoxanthoma elasticum	Mucosal nodules	Severe gastrointestinal bleeding
White spongy naevus	Hyperkeratosis	Anal keratosis

Table 1.5 Oral manifestations of primary immunodeficiency

Immunodeficiency	*Oral disease*
Cell mediated, e.g. diGeorge syndrome, severe combined immunodeficiency, ataxia telangiectasia and the Wiskott–Aldrich syndrome	Infections (especially candidiasis and herpes) ulceration and gingivitis
Humoral, e.g. agammaglobulinaemia	Oral ulceration
Phagocytic, e.g. chronic granulomatous disease, the Chediak–Higashi syndrome, Job's syndrome, myeloperoxidase deficiency	Periodontal disease Lymphadenopathy
Complement deficiency	Lupus erythematosus, Sjögren's syndrome

agammaglobulinaemias, selective IgA deficiency is usually without oral manifestations.

Secondary immunodeficiency may arise as a result of systemic infection, autoimmunity, neoplasia, drugs, poor nutrition or old age. Most often cellular immunity is depressed and hence viral and fungal infections are the predominant oral disorders. The incidence of oral neoplasia is also increased. The oral manifestations of HIV infection have been extensively documented[28] and are listed in *Table 1.6*. These are discussed in detail later under AIDS and the gastrointestinal tract.

BLOOD DISORDERS

ANAEMIA

The single oral effect of anaemia as such is pallor which is only a valuable indicator when the haemoglobin drops below 10 g/dl. The other tissue changes seen are due to the presence of coexisting deficiency (*Table 1.7*) and respond to replacement therapy.[89] These are discussed individually elsewhere.

Table 1.6 Oral manifestations of HIV infection

Fungal infections	*Viral infections*	*Neurological disturbances*	*Bacterial infections*	*Neoplasms*	*Unknown aetiology*
Candidiasis	Herpetic stomatitis	Trigeminal neuropathy	HIV – necrotizing gingivitis	Kaposi's sarcoma	Recurrent aphthous ulceration
Pseudomembranous	Hairy leukoplakia	Facial palsy	HIV – gingivitis	Squamous-cell carcinoma	Progressive necrotizing ulceration
Erythematous	Herpes zoster		HIV –periodontitis	Non-Hodgkin's lymphoma	Toxic epidermolysis
Hyperplastic	Varicella				
Angular cheilitis	Cytomegalovirus		*Mycobacterium avium intracellulare*	Epitheloid haemangioma	Delayed wound healing
Histoplasmosis	Papilloma virus lesions				
					Idiopathic thrombocytopenia
Cryptococcus neoformans	Verruca vulgaris		*Klebsiella pneumoniae*		Salivary gland enlargement
Geotrichosis	Condyloma acuminatum		*Enterobacterium cloacae*		Xerostomia
	Focal epithelial hyperplasia		Actinomycosis		
			Eschericia coli		HIV – embryopathy
					Submandibular lymphadenopathy
			Sinusitis		Hyperpigmentation
			Exacerbation of apical periodontitis		
			Submandibular cellulitis		

From Pindborg.[55]

Table 1.7 Tissue signs of haematinic deficiency

Condition	Iron	Folate	Vitamin B_{12}
Glossitis	+	+	+
Recurrent aphthous stomatitis	+	+	+
Angular cheilitis	+	±	±
Candidiasis	+	±	±
Leukoplakia	+	−	−
Kelly–Paterson syndrome	+	−	−
Koilonychia	+	−	−

Haemolytic anaemias produce additional oral changes: expansion of the marrow cavity, especially in the haemoglobinopathies and thalassaemias, causes premaxillary remodelling leading to splayed upper anterior teeth and an anterior open bite;[9,51] sickling crisis in sickle-cell disease results in bony infarcts especially in the mandible[31] which are painful and may be radiologically indistinguishable from osteomyelitis.[62]

MYELOPROLIFERATIVE DISEASES

The oral problems arising in myeloproliferative diseases are not specific and occur as a result of defects in the different cell lines. In polycythaemia tissue iron deficiency is common following mobilization of iron stores to sustain the expanded red cell population,[79] leading to oral signs of iron deficiency (*Table 1.7*).

Oral manifestations in the leukaemias are particularly severe in acute leukaemia and may be the presenting complaint. Over two-thirds of patients have oral signs at the time of diagnosis.[68] These signs include adenopathy, gingival hypertrophy, petechiae, oral ulceration and frank haemorrhage.[89] Mucosal infection is also common and arises from immunosuppression caused by the disease or the chemotherapeutic agents used in treatment.[89]

LYMPHORETICULAR MALIGNANCY

In both Hodgkin's and non-Hodgkin's lymphoma cervical lymphadenopathy is common and tonsillar enlargement may occur. Intraoral involvement with lymphomas also occurs. Other effects arise secondary to immunodeficiency.[89]

PLASMA CELL TUMOURS

Plasma cell tumours may arise around the mouth and in addition lead to gingival bleeding and deep, painful ulceration. Oral manifestations of immunodeficiency may arise because normal immunoglobulin production is depressed. Amyloidosis is a common complication of myelomatosis and occurs in a primary amyloidosis distribution with the result that macroglossia may occur.[89]

VASCULAR DISORDERS

PROLIFERATIVE VASCULAR DISORDERS

Proliferative vascular conditions occurring in the mouth may be reactive, hamartomatous or neoplastic in nature. Reactive hyperplasias are relatively common especially in pregnancy and present usually as an epulis in response to local irritation from the teeth or accumulated calculus. Local excision is usually indicated although pregnancy epulides undergo significant regression *post partum*.[20] Oral haemangiomas are quite common as isolated lesions and are usually hamartomatous. The vascular hamartomata include the Sturge–Weber and the Klippel–Trenauney–Weber syndromes in which facial dermal capillary malformation is the dominant clinical feature.[36] Gastrointestinal involvement is not reported, although previously asymptomatic unilateral naevoid telangiectasia may become clinically manifest in cirrhosis.[1]

Osler–Weber–Rendu syndrome[33] is clinically characterized by thin-walled, vascular channels on the mucous membranes and visceral involvement may be extensive. In the similar CRST syndrome (*c*alcinosis, *R*aynaud's phenomenon, *s*clerodactyly and *t*elangiectasia), melaena and haematuria are less common. It should be noted that von Willebrand's disease may not only be associated with vascular malformations of the gastrointestinal tract but associated abnormalities have also been reported in the mouth.[84] The spider naevi which occur in association with cirrhosis also occur on the oral mucous membrane. Malignant vascular neoplasms rarely arise in the mouth except for Kaposi's sarcoma which is now seen in the head and neck region and is associated with AIDS.

ARTERIAL DISEASE

Coronary arterial disease may manifest in the oral cavity with anginal pain. Giant cell arteritis is also occasionally characterized by classic claudication. Vascular disorders such as migraine may present as facial pain. Wegener's granulomatosis and the more sinister midline granuloma may involve the mouth.

Apart from oral ulceration the oral features of the vasculitides are non-specific.

MUSCULOSKELETAL DISORDERS

Musculoskeletal pathology often affects the head and neck region although the oral features are usually non-specific.[47] Some disorders may also be complicated by gastrointestinal manifestations and these are listed below.

OSTEOGENESIS IMPERFECTA

Osteogenesis imperfecta is a rare, usually autosomal dominant, disorder characterized by a defect in type I collagen. In addition to skeletal fragility, dentinogenesis imperfecta is sometimes present resulting in brownish-purple, often translucent, teeth. Joint laxity and hernias occur in addition to the formation of blue sclerae.

OSTEOPETROSIS

Osteopetrosis is characterized by delayed eruption of teeth in addition to skull deformity. Cranial nerve neuropathies complicate the oral features and extramedullary erythropoiesis causes hepatosplenomegaly. Osteomyelitis of the jaws may follow the extraction of teeth.

EHLERS–DANLOS SYNDROME

Ehlers–Danlos syndrome has many oral features: purpura and gingival bleeding are dominant clinical features but early-onset periodontal disease is also extensive and severe (see page 3). Arterial rupture may cause abdominal emergencies.

PSEUDOXANTHOMA ELASTICUM

This is a rare, hereditary disorder of connective tissue in which, as with Ehlers–Danlos syndrome, the skin is hyperextensible and there is joint laxity (see above). The condition is characterized by recurrent, severe gastrointestinal haemorrhage. The oral lesions comprise yellowish intra mucosal nodules in addition to exaggerated perioral skin creases.

ARTHRITIS

Osteoarthritic changes in the temporomandibular joint are common postmortem findings although symptoms related to arthritic changes in the joint are less common. Similarly, although rheumatoid arthritis often affects the temporomandibular joint, pain in this area is rarely the predominant symptom. Patients suffering from rheumatoid arthritis or some other collagen disorder may have Sjögren's syndrome as discussed below.

SJÖGREN'S SYNDROME

Sjögren's syndrome may be divided into primary Sjögren's syndrome (kerato conjunctivitis sicca) which is characterized by xerophthalmia and xerostomia, and secondary Sjögren's syndrome which in addition includes a connective tissue disorder – most commonly rheumatoid arthritis but also systemic lupus erythematosus or systemic sclerosis. In addition to this triad other extraglandular manifestations include primary biliary cirrhosis and chronic atrophic gastritis.[74]

The syndrome is immunologically mediated and the immune abnormalities manifest themselves as infiltration of the affected glands usually with T lymphocytes. In addition B-cell hyperreactivity leads to polyclonal hypergammaglobulinaemia and autoantibody formation: serological tests usually reveal the presence of rheumatoid factor, a positive antinuclear factor, antibodies against nuclear antigens, SS-A (Ro) and SS-B (La) in addition to antigen-specific autoantibodies such as salivary duct antibodies.

The clinical effects of Sjögren's syndrome are dominated by dryness which leads to mucosal cobblestoning, particularly of the tongue and increased susceptibility to candidiasis and increased dental caries.

The histological changes in the salivary glands include focal lymphocytic sialadenitis and significant fibrosis with acinar atrophy. This results in sialectasis, salivary gland enlargement and reduced salivary flow rates. Malignant transformation may ensue usually in the form of a malignant B-cell lymphoma.[97]

Diagnosis relies on the clinical features (xerostomia may be severe) as well as serological and histological features. Histological diagnosis is most easily obtained from the labial salivary glands which reflect major gland involvement and can be obtained with minimal surgery.[29]

Management involves the use of sialogogues and salivary substitutes which may be mucin or methylcellulose based, in addition to antifungals and prophylaxis with topical fluorides. Topical fluoride mouthwashes can arrest the progress of the caries and advanced dental restorative work can maintain the remaining dentition which is important because the ability to wear dentures is compromised by the lack of saliva.

DERMATOLOGICAL DISORDERS

Lichen planus is the most common dermatological disorder to be seen in the mouth. This has been previously considered under 'Lichen planus'. The bullous dermatoses constitute an important group of diseases affecting the oral cavity. The most important diseases with oral manifestations include the following:

Pemphigus vulgaris
Pemphigus vegetans
Benign mucous membrane pemphigoid
Bullous pemphigoid
Linear IgA disease
Dermatitis herpetiformis
Angina bullosa haemorrhagica
Erythema multiforme
Epidermolysis bullosa.

Pemphigus vulgaris is a rare disorder which should be easily distinguishable from common forms of oral ulceration. Intraepithelial splitting causes only transient bullae formation and the patients present with ragged erosions (*Figure 1.14*). Nearly all patients have oral involvement[57] which is the presenting complaint in the majority.[96] Routine biopsy of the erosions is unhelpful as diagnosis relies on immunofluorescent demonstration of immunoglobulin within the epithelium. Nikolsky's sign is positive in the mouth where the mucosa can be peeled away, but this phenomenon occurs in other dermatoses and is not pathognomonic. Treatment is with systemic corticosteroids with or without cytotoxic agents. Pemphigus vegetans is a milder form of disease but oral signs are still present in the majority of cases.[44]

The mouth is involved in both bullous pemphigoid and benign mucous membrane pemphigoid, but mucosal involvement dominates the clinical picture in the latter. The bullae may be blood filled and may persist longer than in pemphigus before rupture. Demonstration of basement membrane zone immunofluorescence usually with IgG is diagnostic. A similar clinical picture arises in association with IgA deposition along the basement membrane zone and this condition is termed 'linear IgA disease' to distinguish it from dermatitis herpetiformis where the distribution of the basement membrane zone immunofluorescence with IgA is granular.[58]

Dermatitis herpetiformis involves the oral cavity in up to 70% of patients. Oral manifestations may be classified as:[22] erythematous lesions which pale on pressure; pseudovesicular lesions which are similar to the above but which are pale in the centre; purpuric lesions; erosions. Dermatitis herpetiformis classically responds to gluten withdrawal and dapsone or sulphamethoxypyridazine.[49] Although gluten withdrawal has no place in the other bullous dermatoses, dapsone or sulphamethoxypyridazine may be useful in their management particularly for pemphigoid, linear IgA disease and erythema multiforme (see earlier). Angina bullosa haemorrhagica is characterized by transient blood-filled bullae which may be large and occur usually on the soft palate. The blisters burst rapidly and heal uneventfully. Immunofluorescence is negative.

Oral mucosal involvement occurs in all cases of epidermolysis bullosa letalis, in 20% of patients with dystrophic epidermolysis bullosa but in only 2% of those with the simplex form. Oral manifestations may be present in the form of bullae, scarring, lingual depapillation, milia and dental hypoplasia. Mucosal fragility may occasionally improve with phenytoin therapy.

DESQUAMATIVE GINGIVITIS

Desquamative gingivitis is a clinical entity characterized by loss of epithelium over the full width of the attached gingivae and occurs in association with bullous dermatoses or secondary to lichen planus when extensive liquefactive degeneration allows desquamation. Allergy and psoriasis are other rare causes of the condition. Maintenance of oral hygiene is important and treatment with topical corticosteroids is helpful. This can be applied on a gingival veneer which also protects the affected mucosa from trauma.[93]

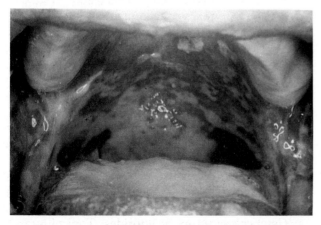

Figure 1.14 Widespread de-epithelialization in the mouth of a 68-year-old woman with pemphigus vulgaris. The remaining patches of epithelium seen on the soft palate and fauces could be easily scraped off with a spatula.

PSORIASIS

Oral involvement in psoriasis is rare but when present usually occurs as geographic tongue (benign migratory glossitis) with fissuring.[2] Small white spots which can be scraped off also occur[56] and diffuse mucosal erythema may parallel cutaneous exacerbations.

RENAL DISEASE

Oral problems in renal failure have become less prevalent with the advent of dialysis.[36] Several oral manifestations still present, however. These include psuedomembranous stomatitis,[34] ulcerative stomatitis, oral haemorrhage, hyperkeratosis, reduced taste sensation perhaps due to zinc deficiency, increased resistance to caries and gingivitis due to increased salivary pH, and increased susceptibility to bacterial stomatitis.[76] Viral warts are also increased in renal transplant patients and hairy leukoplakia, which is due to Epstein–Barr virus and occurs almost exclusively in association with HIV infection, has been described in immunosuppressed renal transplant patients.[27]

PAIN AND NEUROLOGICAL DISORDERS

A comprehensive account of neurological disorders affecting the oral region is outside the scope of this chapter. The most common pain disorders, however, are trigeminal neuralgia and functional pain syndromes.

TRIGEMINAL NEURALGIA

Trigeminal neuralgia is a common disorder which occasionally has trigger zones exclusively within the mouth. Denture trauma may mimic trigeminal neuralgia affecting the dental nerve. A therapeutic response to carbamazepine is, however, diagnostic. Anticonvulsive therapy is the mainstay of treatment which should be life-long in patients over the age of 50 years due to the risk of recurrence. Phenytoin is a useful adjunct to therapy when toxicity from carbamazepine is a problem.[72] In patients who fail to obtain relief with medical therapy, cryosurgery or alcohol block to the affected nerve causes remission. When more than one branch of the trigeminal nerve is affected, coagulation of the gasserian ganglion is required although this is associated with significant morbidity due to the extensive anaesthesia which

results.[67] Trigeminal neuralgia may be a presenting symptom of multiple sclerosis particularly when sensory impairment is also present.[60]

FUNCTIONAL PAIN DISORDERS

The face and mouth are particular targets for functional pain syndromes.[32] These include myofascial pain dysfunction (temporomandibular joint pain dysfunction syndrome), atypical facial pain and oral dysaesthesia, particularly glossopyrosis (burning tongue). These disorders characteristically affect mainly women. Myofascial pain dysfunction and atypical facial pain affect younger women whilst oral dysaesthesia usually affects perimenopausal or postmenopausal women. The symptoms are of chronic discomfort often lasting for years with no locally detectable cause. Symptoms show a diurnal variation and are unresponsive to analgesics. Most patients improve with tricyclic antidepressants or occasionally major tranquillizers after organic causes for their pain have been excluded.

REFERENCES

1. Anderton, R.L. and Smith, J.G. (1975) Unilateral nevoid telangiectasia with gastric involvement. *Archives of Dermatology*, **111**, 617–621.
2. Archard, H.O. (1971) Common stomatologic disorders and stomatologic manifestations of internal and integumental disorders. In *Dermatology in General Medicine* (Eds) Fitzpatrick, T.B., Arndt, K.A., Clark, W.H., Eisen, A.Z., Van Scott, E.J. and Vaughan, J.H. pp. 795–950. New York: McGraw Hill.
3. Basu, M.K. and Asquith, P. (1980) Oral manifestations of inflammatory bowel disease. *Clinics in Gastroenterology*, **9**, 307–321.
4. Basu, M.K., Asquith, P., Thompson, R.A. and Cooke, W.T. (1975) Oral manifestations of Crohn's disease. *Gut*, **16**, 249–254.
5. Basu, M.K. and Chesner, I.M. (1990) Diseases of the gastro-intestinal tract. In *Oral Manifestations Of Systemic Disease*, 2nd edn (Eds.) Jones, J.H. and Mason, D.K. pp. 783–799. London: Baillière Tindall.
6. Birek, C., Patterson, B., Maximiw, W.C. amd Minden, M.D. (1989) EBV and HSV infections in a patient who had undergone bone marrow transplantation: oral manifestations and diagnosis by in situ nucleic acid hybridisation. *Oral Surgery, Oral Medicine, Oral Pathology*, **68**, 612–617.
7. Bishop, R.P., Brewster, A.C. and Antonioli, D.A. (1972) Crohn's disease of the mouth. *Gastroenterology*, **62**, 302–306.
8. Cataldo, E., Covino, M.C. and Tesone, P.E. (1981) Pyostomatitis vegetans. *Oral Surgery, Oral Medicine, Oral Pathology*, **52**, 172–177.

9. Catena, D.L. (1975) Oral manifestations of the haemoglobinopathies. *Dental Clinics of North America*, **19**, 77–85.

10. Cheesborough, M.J. and Kinmont, P.D.C. (1978) Epidermolysis bullosa acquisita and Crohn's disease. *British Journal of Dermatology*, **99**, 53–54.

11. Chisholm, M., Ardrang, M., Callender, S.T. and Wright, R. (1971) Iron deficiency and autoimmunity in post-cricoid webs. *Quarterly Journal of Medicine*, **40**, 421–433.

12. Croft, C.B. and Wilkinson, A.R. (1972) Ulceration of the mouth, pharynx and larynx in Crohn's disease of the intestine. *British Journal of Surgery*, **59**, 249–252.

13. Crohn, D.B., Ginzburg, L. and Openheimer, G.D. (1932) Regional ileitis: a pathologic and clinical entity. *Journal of the American Medical Association*, **9a**, 1323–1328.

14. Cross, D. and Southam, J.C. (1990) Oral squamous cell papillomas – a histological assessment. *Journal of Dental Research*, **69**, 963.

15. Dudeney, T.P. and Todd, I.P. (1969) Crohn's disease of the mouth. *Proceedings of the Royal Society of Medicine*, **62**, 1237–1238.

16. Duxbury, A.J. (1990) Systemic pharmacotherapy. In *Oral Manifestations of Systemic Disease*, 2nd edn (Eds) Jones, J.H. and Mason, D.K. pp. 411–479. London: Baillière Tindall.

17. Eversole, L.K. and Ringer, M. (1984) The role of dental restorative metal in the pathogenesis of oral lichen planus. *Oral Surgery, Oral Medicine, Oral Pathology*, **57**, 383.

18. Ferguson, D.B. (1987) Current diagnostic uses of saliva. *Journal of Dental Research*, **66**, 420–424.

19. Ferguson, M.M., Hart, D.McK., Lindsay, R. and Stephen, K.W. (1978) Progeston therapy in menstrually related aphthae. *International Journal of Oral Surgery*, **7**, 463–470.

20. Ferguson, M.M. and Silverman, S. (1990) Endocrine disorders. In *Oral Manifestations of Systemic Disease*, 2nd edn (Eds) Jones, J.H. and Mason, D.K. pp 593–615. London: Baillière Tindall.

21. Ferguson, M.M., Wray, D., Carmichael, H.A., Russell, R.I. and Lee, F.D. (1980) Coeliac disease associated with recurrent aphthae. *Gut*, **21**, 223–226.

22. Fraser, N.G., Care, N.W. and Donald, D. (1973) Oral lesions in dermatitis herpetiformis. *British Journal of Dermatology*, **89**, 439–450.

23. Garrett, J.R. (1987) The proper role of nerves in salivary secretion: a review. *Journal of Dental Research*, **66**, 420–424.

24. Gilhuus-Moe, O. and Koppang, H.S. (1972) Oral manifestations of porphyria. *Oral Surgery, Oral Medicine, Oral Pathology*, **33**, 926–933.

25. Gocenstein, A.J., Janowitz, H.D. and Sachar, D.B. (1976) The extra-intestinal complications of Crohn's disease and ulcerative colitis: a study of 700 patients. *Medicine*, **55**, 401–412.

26. Gorlin, R.J., Cohen, M.M. and Levin, L.S. (1990) *Syndromes of the Head and Neck*. Oxford: Oxford University Press.

27. Greenspan, D., Greenspan, J.S., de-Souza, Y., Levi, J.A. and Ungar, A.M. (1989) Oral hairy leukoplakia in an HIV-negative renal transplant recipient. *Journal of Oral Pathology and Oral Medicine*, **18**, 32–34.

28. Greenspan, D., Greenspan, J.S., Schiodt, M. and Pindborg, J.J. (1990) *AIDS and the mouth*, Copenhagen: Munksgaard.

29. Greenspan, J.S. and Daniels, T.E. (1990) Connective tissue and granulomatous diseases of doubtful origin. In *Oral Manifestations Of Systemic Disease*, 2nd edn (Eds) Jones, J.H. and Mason, D.K. pp. 271–299. London: Baillière Tindall.

30. Hamilton, R.E. and Giasanti, J.S. (1974) The Chediak–Higashi syndrome. *Oral Surgery, Oral Medicine, Oral Pathology*, **37**, 754–761.

31. Hammersley, N. (1984) Mandibular infarction occurring during a sickle cell crisis. *British Journal of Oral and Maxillofacial Surgery*, **22**, 103–114.

32. Harris, M. and Feinmann, C. (1990) Psychosomatic disorders. In *Oral Manifestations Of Systemic Disease*, 2nd edn (Eds) Jones, J.H. and Mason, D.K. pp. 30–60. London: Baillière Tindall.

33. Harrison, D.F.N. (1964) Familial haemorrhagic telangiectasia. *Quarterly Journal of Medicine*, **33**, 25–38.

34. Hempstead, B.E. and Hench, P.S. (1930) Uremic stomatitis. *Transactions of the American Laryngological, Rhinological and Otological Society*, **36**, 510–522.

35. James, J., Patton, D.W., Lewis C.J., Kirkwood, E.M. and Ferguson M.M. (1986) Orofacial granulomatosis and clinical atopy. *Journal of Oral Medicine*, **41**, 29–30.

36. Jones, J.H. (1990) Cardiovascular and renal diseases. In *Oral Manifestations of Systemic Disease*, 2nd edn (Eds) Jones, J.H. and Mason, D.K. pp. 747–764. London: Baillière Tindall.

37. Jones, J.H. and Sloan, P. (1990) Internal malignancy. In *Oral Manifestations Of Systemic Disease*, 2nd edn (Eds) Jones, J.H. and Mason, D.K. pp. 387–410. London: Baillière Tindall.

38. Jones, R.F. (1961) The Paterson–Brown–Kelly syndrome, its relationship to iron deficiency and post-cricoid carcinoma. *Journal of Laryngology*, **75**, Part I, 529–543: Part II, 544–561.

39. Kelly, A.B. (1919) Spasm at entrance to the oesophagus. *Journal of Laryngology*, **34**, 285–289.

40. Kinane, D.F. and Davis, R.M. (1990) Periodontal manifestations of systemic disease. In *Oral Manifestations of Systemic Disease*, 2nd ed (Eds) Jones, J.H. and Mason, D.K. pp. 512–536. London: Baillière Tindall.

41. Knight, L. and Fletcher, J. (1971) Growth of *Candida albicans* in saliva: stimulation associated with antibiotics, corticosteroids, and diabetes mellitus. *Journal of Infectious Diseases*, **123**, 371–377.

42. Kramer, I.R.H., El-Labban, N. and Lee, K.W.

(1978) The clinical features and risk of malignant transformation in sublingual keratosis. *British Dental Journal*, **144**, 178–80.

43. Lehner, T., Batchelor, J.R., Challacombe, S.J. and Kennedy, L. (1979) An immunogenetic basis for tissue involvement in Behçet's syndrome. *Immunology*, **37**, 895–900.

44. Lever, W.F. 1965) *Pemphigus and Pemphigoid*. Springfield, IL. C.C. Thomas.

45. Lucas, R.B. (1984) *Pathology of Tumours of the Oral Tissues*. Edinburgh: Churchill Livingstone.

46. McCarthy, F.P. (1949) Pyostomatitis vegetans: report of three cases. *Archives of Dermatology and Syphilology*, **40**, 750–764.

47. MacDonald, D.G. and Boyle, I.T. (1990) Skeletal diseases. In *Oral Manifestations Of Systemic Disease*, 2nd edn (Eds) Jones, J.H. and Mason, D.K. pp. 616–659. London: Baillière Tindall.

48. MacFarlane, T.W. and Samaranayake, L.P. (1990) Systemic infections. In *Oral Manifestations Of Systemic Disease*, 2nd edn (Eds) Jones, J.H. and Mason, D.K. pp. 339–386. London: Baillière Tindall.

49. Maddin, S. (1982) *Current Dermatologic Therapy*. Philadelphia: W.B. Saunders.

50. Mason, D.K. and Chisholm, D.M. (1975) *Salivary Glands In Health and Disease*. Philadelphia: W.B. Saunders.

51. Novak, A.J. (1944) The oral manifestations of erythroblastic anaemia. *American Journal of Orthodontics*, **30**, 542.

52. O'Mahony, S., Vestey, J.P. and Ferguson, A. (1990) Similarities in intestinal humoral immunity in dermatitis herpetiformis without enteropathy and in coeliac disease. *The Lancet*, **335**, 1487–1490.

53. Owen, R.D. (1950) The problem of hypopharyngeal carcinoma. *Proceedings of the Royal Society of Medicine*, **43**, 157–170.

54. Patton, D.W., Ferguson, M.M., Forsyth, A. and James, J. (1985) Orofacial granulomatosis: a possible allergic basis. *British Journal of Oral & Maxillofacial Surgery*, **43**, 235–242.

55. Pindborg, J.J. (1989) Classification of oral lesions associated with HIV infection. *Oral Surgery, Oral Medicine, Oral Pathology*, **67**, 292–295.

56. Pindborg, J.J. (1990) Diseases of the skin. In *Oral Manifestations of Systemic Disease*, 2nd edn (Eds) Jones, J.H. and Mason, D.K. pp. 537–592. London: Baillière Tindall.

57. Pisanti, S., Sharav, Y., Kaufman, E. and Posner, L.N. (1974) Pemphigus vulgaris: incidence in Jews of different ethnic groups acording to age, sex, and initial lesion. *Oral Surgery, Oral Medicine, Oral Pathology*, **38**, 382–387.

58. Porter, S.R., Scully, C., Midda, C. and Eveson, J.W. (1990) Adult linear IgA disease manifesting as desquamative gingivitis. *Oral Surgery, Oral Medicine, Oral Pathology*, **70**, 450–453.

59. Robertson, W.D. (1991) Oral keratosis: a clinical, pathological and immunological study. PhD Thesis, University of Edinburgh.

60. Rushton, J.G., Stevens, J.C. and Miller, R.H. (1981) Glossopharyngeal (vagoglossopharyngeal) neuralgia. A study of 217 cases. *Archives of Neurology*, **38**, 201–205.

61. Sainsbury, C.P.Q., Dodge, J.A., Walker, D.M. and Aldred, M.J. (1987) Orofacial granulomatosis in childhood. *British Dental Journal*, **163**, 154–157.

62. Sanner, J.R. and Ramin, J.E. (1977) Osteoporotic haematopoetic mandibular marrow defect: an osseus manifestation of sickle cell anaemia. *Journal of Oral Surgery*, **35**, 986–988.

63. Savage, N.W., Seymour, G.J. and Kruger, B.T. (1985) T-lymphocyte subset changes in recurrent aphthous stomatitis. *Oral Surgery, Oral Medicine, Oral Pathology*, **60**, 175–181.

64. Scully, C., Cochran, K.M., Russell, R.I. *et al.* (1982) Crohn's disease of the mouth: an indication of intestinal involvement. *Gut*, **23**, 198–201.

65. Scully, C. and El-Kom, M. (1985) Lichen planus: review and update on pathogenesis. *Journal of Oral Pathology*, **14**, 431–438.

66. Shamma-a, M.H. and Benedict, E.B. (1958) Oesophageal webs. A report of 58 cases and an attempt at classification. *New England Journal of Medicine*, **259**, 378–384.

67. Sharr, M.M. and Garfield, J.S. (1977) The place of ganglion or root alcohol injection in trigeminal neuralgia. *Journal of Neurology, Neurosurgery and Psychiatry*, **40**, 286–290.

68. Ship, I.I. and Lynch, M.A. (1967) Initial oral manifestations of leukaemia. *Journal of the American Dental Association*, **75**, 932–940.

69. Shklar, G. and McCarthy, P.L. (1976) *The Oral Manifestations Of Systemic Disease*. London: Butterworths.

70. Sofaer, J.A. (1990) Single gene disorders. In *Oral Manifestations Of Systemic Disease*, 2nd edn (Eds) Jones, J.H. and Mason, D.K. pp. 61–111. London: Baillière Tindall.

71. Sweatman, M.C., Tasker, R., Warner, J.O., Ferguson, M.M. and Mitchell, D.N. (1986) Orofacial granulomatosis: response to elemental diet and provocation by food additives. *Clinical Allergy*, **16**, 331–338.

72. Sweet, W.H. (1986) The treatment of trigeminal neuralgia (tic douloureux). *New England Journal of Medicine*, **315**, 174–177.

73. Syrjanen, S., Laine, P., Niemela, M. and Happonen, R.P. (1989) Oral hairy leukoplakia is not a specific sign of HIV-infection but related to immunosuppression in general. *Journal of Oral Pathology and Oral Medicine*, **18**, 28–31.

74. Trevino, H., Tsianose, B. and Schenker, S. (1987) Gastro-intestinal and hepatobiliary features in Sjögren's syndrome. In *Sjögren's Syndrome: Clinical And Immunological Aspects* (Eds) Talal, N., Moutsopoulous, M. and Kassan, S.S. pp. 89–95. Berlin: Springer-Verlag.

75. Tyldesley, W.R. (1979) Oral Crohn's and related conditions. *British Journal of Oral Surgery*, **17**, 1–9.

76. Tyldesley, W.R., Rotter, E. and Sells, R.A. (1977)

Bacterial thrush-like lesions of the mouth in renal transplant patients. *The Lancet*, **1**, 485–486.

77. Walker, D.M. (1975) Candidal infection of the oral mucosa. In *Oral Mucosa in Health and Disease* (Ed.) Dolby, A.E. pp. 467–505. Oxford: Blackwell Scientific.

78. Walker, D.M. (1984) Infectious diseases with oral manifestations. In *Immunological Aspects of Oral Diseases* (Ed.) Ivanyi, L. pp. 101–123. Lancaster: MTP Press.

79. Wassermann, L.R. (1955) Panels in therapy iii. The treatment of polycythaemia vera. *Blood*, **10**, 655–661.

80. Waterhouse, J.P., Beeley, J.A. and Mason, D.K. (1990) Introduction and biological basis. In *Oral Manifestations Of Systemic Disease*, 2nd edn (Eds) Jones, J.H. and Mason, D.K. pp. 1–29. London: Baillière Tindall.

81. Weary, P.E. and Bender, A.S. (1967) The Chediak–Higashi syndrome with severe cutaneous involvement. *Archives of Internal Medicine*, **110**, 381–386.

82. Wiesenfeld, D., Ferguson, M.M., Mitchell, D.N. *et al.* (1985) Orofacial granulomatosis, a clinical and pathological analysis. *Quarterly Journal of Medicine, New Series*, **54**, 101–113.

83. Williams, A.J.K., Wray, D. and Ferguson, A. (1991) The clinical entity of orofacial Crohn's disease. *Quarterly Journal of Medicine, New Series*, **79**, 451–458.

84. Wood, G.M. and Losowsky, M.S. (1982) Angiodysplasia of the tongue with acquired von Willebrand's disease. *Postgraduate Medical Journal*, **58**, 37–38.

85. Wray, D. (1981) Gluten sensitive recurrent aphthous stomatitis. *Journal of Digestive Diseases and Sciences*, **86**, 737–740.

86. Wray, D. (1982) Recurrent aphthous stomatitis and Behçet's syndrome. In *Viruses in Oral Medicine* (Eds) Hooks, J.J. and Jordan, G.W. pp. 279–289. New York: Elsevier North-Holland.

87. Wray, D. (1984) Recurrent aphthous stomatitis. *Journal of the Royal Society of Medicine*, **77**, 1–3.

88. Wray, D. (1984) Pyostomatitis vegetans. *British Dental Journal*, **157**, 316–317.

89. Wray, D. and Dagg, J.H. (1990) Oral manifestations of diseases of the blood and blood forming organs. In *Oral Manifestations of Systemic Disease*, 2nd edn (Eds) Jones, J.H. and Mason, D.K. pp. 663–713. London: Baillière Tindall.

90. Wray, D., Felix D.H. and Cumming, C.G. (1990) Alteration of humoral responses to candida in HIV infection. *British Dental Journal*, **168**, 326–329.

91. Wray, D., Ferguson, M.M., Mason, D.K., Hutcheon, A.W. and Dagg, J.H. (1975) Recurrent aphthae: treatment with vitamin B_{12}, folic acid and iron. *British Medical Journal*, **2**, 490–493.

92. Wray, D., Graykowski, E.A. and Notkins, A.L. (1981) Role of mucosal injury in initiating recurrent aphthous stomatitis. *British Medical Journal*, **2**, 1569–1570.

93. Wray, D. and McCord, J.F. (1987) Labial veneers in the management of desquamative gingivitis. *Oral Surgery, Oral Medicine, Oral Pathology*, **64**, 41–42.

94. Wray, D., Vlagopoulos, T. and Siraganian, R. (1982) The role of food allergens and basophil histamine release in recurrent aphthous stomatitis. *Oral Surgery, Oral Medicine, Oral Pathology*, **54**, 388–395.

95. Wright, A., Ryan, F.P., Willingham, S.E. *et al.* (1986) Food allergy or intolerance in severe recurrent aphthous ulceration of the mouth. *British Medical Journal*, **292**, 1237–1238.

96. Zegarelli, D.J. and Zegarelli, E.V. (1977) Intra-oral pemphigus vulgaris. *Oral Surgery, Oral Medicine, Oral Pathology*, **44**, 384–393.

97. Zulman, J., Jaffe, R. and Talal, N. (1978) Evidence that the malignant lymphoma of Sjögren's syndrome is a monoclonal B-cell neoplasm. *New England Journal of Medicine*, **299**, 1215–1220.

PHARYNX AND OESOPHAGUS

EMBRYOLOGY AND ANATOMY

D. Hopwood

EMBRYOLOGY

Initially the oesophagus is a short tube stretching from the respiratory diverticulum to the fusiform dilatation, which becomes the stomach in the developing part of the foregut. The endodermal lining is at first columnar. With the growth of the embryo and descent of the heart and lungs, the oesophagus lengthens rapidly with a temporary obliteration of the lumen. When this reappears it is lined by stratified squamous epithelium. The visceral mesoderm which surrounds the oesophagus develops into connective and muscular tissue. The upper two-thirds of the muscular tissue becomes mainly striated, whilst the lower one-third, as with the rest of the gut, is mainly non-striated.

ANATOMY

The oesophagus is a muscular tube 25 cm long connecting the pharynx, opposite the sixth vertebra, to the cardia slightly to the left of the eleventh thoracic vertebra and some 40 cm from the incisor teeth. It has three parts: cervical, thoracic and abdominal, each segment has important relationships.

The outermost layer of the oesophagus is a condensation of fascia of the posterior mediastinum. The lower end is fixed by the phreno-oesophageal ligament and posteriorly to the preaortic fascia. The muscular coat has two layers: the outer longitudinal layer and the inner circular layer. In the upper portion both layers are striated with type I fibres predominant (81%). The fibres (30 μm diameter) are significantly smaller than skeletal muscle. There is a fall-out of muscle fibres with age, with an increased variability in fibre diameter.[11] In the lower third both are smooth and continuous with the muscle layers of the stomach. Recently, a muscular lower oesophageal sphincter has been documented in detail.[12] Previously none was thought to be present.[10] Between the muscle layers is the myenteric plexus, but there is no submucosal plexus. Most neurons of the myenteric plexus are cholinesterase positive and probably motor in function; the others

(20–40%) are argyrophilic and thought to be concerned with the coordination of swallowing. The vagi and glossopharyngeal nerves carry motor fibres to the striped muscle (*Figure 1.15*), the vagi supplying parasympathetic fibres. The sympathetic innervation is derived from several sources – the fourth to sixth thoracic segments and the greater splanchnic nerves. There are more autonomic nerves reaching the lower oesophagus than any other segment of the alimentary tract.[15]

The submucosa contains nerve fibres, large blood vessels, lymphatics and oesophageal mucous glands, and scattered lymphocytes and macrophages. The mucosa is formed by a stratified squamous non-keratinized epithelium and is arranged in a series of longitudinal folds. The epithelium changes abruptly to cardiac mucosa[8] 1–2 cm superior to the lower end of the anatomical oesophagus, but merges with that of the mouth proximally. The muscularis mucosae, which is split in the upper part of the oesophagus, fuses in the middle and lower parts and is continuous with the equivalent smooth muscle of the stomach.

The arterial supply is segmental and derived from the inferior thyroid, bronchial, left phrenic and left gastric arteries, and a series of small twigs from the aorta (*Figure 15.1*). There is a well-developed submucous venous plexus which drains into the thyroid, azygos, hemiazygos and left gastric veins. This constitutes an important anastomosis between the systemic and portal venous systems.

The lymphatic drainage from the upper third of the oesophagus is due to the deep cervical, retropharyngeal and para-tracheal nodes. In the middle third the drainage is to the paraoesophageal and tracheobronchial nodes and directly into the thoracic duct. The lower third drains towards the abdomen into the left gastric and pericardial nodes. Papillae (dermal pegs) with capillaries project from the lamina propria up to 33% of the distance towards the luminal surface.

HISTOLOGY AND CELL BIOLOGY

The oesophagus is lined by stratified squamous non-keratinizing epithelium. There are three layers of epithelial cells: basal, prickle and functional.[5]

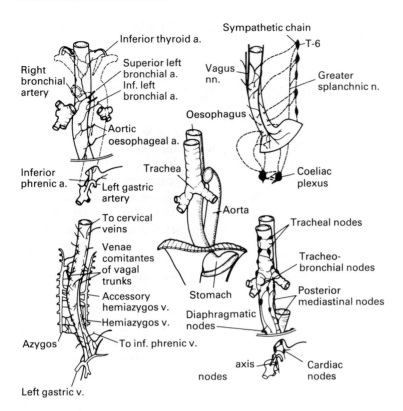

Figure 1.15 Anatomy of the human oesophagus: arterial supply (upper left), venous drainage (lower left), innervation (upper right) and lymphatic system (lower right). (Reproduced from Ellis, F.H. (1981) The oesophagus. In *Davis–Christopher Textbook of Surgery* (Ed.) Sabiston, D.C. p. 794, with kind permission of the author, the editor and the publisher, W.B. Saunders.)

The deepest is the basal cell compartment which is normally one or two cells deep and is the site of mitosis. These cells contain keratin.[9] The basal cell compartment may form up the 15% of the normal epithelial thickness,[8] but in oesophagitis there is an increase in the volume density. There is also a significant increase in labelling of epithelial cells in this compartment in response to cells shed using tritiated thymidine, Ki67 and AgNORS.[3,9] Increased papillary length helps increase the volume of the basal layer by increasing the surface area of the basement membrane and the metabolic exchange with the epithelium. The papillary vessels contain epidermal growth factor.

Above the basal layer, the cells differentiate in the prickle cell layer. Numerous desmosomes on cell processes give the layer its name and, together with abundant tonofilaments, its mechanical strength. The keratins in these and the functional cells are 4, 6 and 13.[3] These suprabasal cells also contain glycogen and membrane-coating granules. The latter also occur in skin and in vaginal and buccal mucosa.[13] In the oral mucosa their volume density rises to about 0.25%. They contain lysosomal enzymes, mucosubstances including carcinoembryonic antigen and Lewis blood group antigens, and a small amount of lipid.[7,14] There are secreted into the intercellular space where the mucosubstances form a partial barrier. A stimulus for their secretion is low pH. The process of exocytosis inserts new undamaged membrane into the cell surface; this can replace damaged plasmalemma which may subsequently be retrieved. Prickle cells and basal cells carry epidermal growth factor receptors[9] (*Figure 1.16*).

Finally, there is the functional layer abutting onto the lumen which consists of largely effete cells capable of withstanding mechanical, chemical and physical trauma from the passing boli of food and regurgitated gastric contents. The lowest 5 cm of the oesophagus is frequently subject to peptic reflux in normal individuals and may show damage which may be produced by various proteases, lipases and the detergent bile acids.[2,4]

Immune mechanisms in the epithelium are represented by Langerhans' cells and cytotoxic T cells (CDT8 positive).[3] Melanocytes are reported among the epithelial cells.[3] Neutral mucosubstances including glycosyl and mannosyl residues are also present in the glycocalyx as well as neuraminidase-sensitive sialyl groups. Sugar residues in the glycocalyx can be seen to increase in amount and become more complex as the cells differentiate towards the luminal surface. Incubation of biopsies with cationized ferritin which labels the plasmalemma, or with horseradish peroxidase demonstrates the fluidity of the prickle-cell membranes and their retrieval.[4] Fine droplets of triacylglycerols (triglycerides) are found in the functional and upper prickle cell layers reflecting the relative hypoxia of these cells.[5]

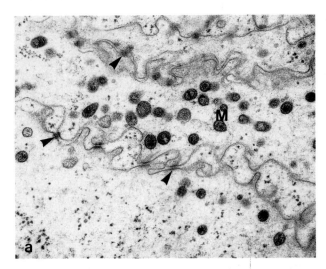 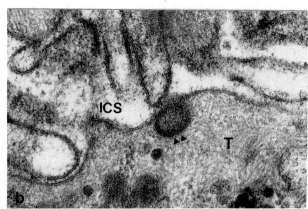

Figure 1.16 (a) Several oesophageal epithelial cells from the functional layer from a patient with a mild oesophagitis. There are moderate numbers of membrane-coating granules (M), showing variation in form but mostly with granular cores. In the intercellular spaces there are glycogen rosettes. The cells are held together by desmosomes (arrowheads). × 22 000. (b) Membrane-coating granule (arrowheads) fusing with cell membrane in exocytosis. The intercellular space is marked ICS. There are abundant tonofilaments (T) in the cytoplasm. × 83 600. (Reproduced from Hopwood, D., Logan, K. and Bouchier, I.A.D. (1978) The electron microscopy of normal human oesophageal epithelium. *Virchows Archiv [B]*, **26**, 345–358, with kind permission of the authors and editors.)

HETEROTOPIAS

Gastric heterotopia is described in about 4% of patients, but probably bears no relation to the metaplastic Barrett's epithelium. Heterotopic pancreas and sebaceous glands have been documented in the oesophagus.[3]

SUBMUCOSAL GLANDS

The submucosal glands, 700–800 in the adult, are similar to the mucus-secreting minor salivary glands with myoepithelial cells and occasional oncocytes as well as the principal and subsidiary mucous cells of the acini.[1] No APUD cells are present (APUD = amine precursor uptake and decarboxylation). Secretion is probably continuous.[3]

FUNCTION

These morphological features reflect defence mechanisms against mechanical trauma, and gastrointestinal secretions which rapidly produce marked damage to the oesophageal epithelium. An excessive loss of cells from the functional layer induces mitosis and extension of the basal compartments.

Refluxing of hydrogen ions induces the exocytosis of membrane-coating granules. Their mucosubstances may act as a partial intercellular barrier to the refluxing materials and also as adhesive molecules, holding the effete functional layer cells together. Parakeratinization may be induced by excess reflux. Acid in the oesophagus also induces peristalsis with clearance of the refluxed material.

REFERENCES

1. Al Yasin, T.M. and Toner, P.G. (1977) Fine structure of squamous epithelium and submucosal glands of human oesophagus. *Journal of Anatomy*, **123**, 703–721.
2. Bateson, M.C., Hopwood, D., Milne, G. and Bouchier, I.A.D. (1981) Oesophageal epithelium ultrastructure after incubation with gastrointestinal fluids and their components. *Journal of Pathology*, **133**, 33–51.
3. Hopwood, D. (1989) The oesophageal lining. In *Gastrointestinal and Oesophageal Pathology*, pp. 3–12. Ed R. Whitehead. Edinburgh: Churchill Livingstone.
4. Hopwood, D., Bateson, M.C., Milne, G. and Bouchier, I.A.D. (1981) The effects of bile acids and hydrogen ion on the fine structure of oesophageal epithelium. *Gut*, **22**, 306–311.
5. Hopwood, D., Jankowski, J., Milne, G. and Wormsley, K. G. (1992) Flow cytometry of oesophageal mucosal biopsies: epidermal growth factor receptor and CD15. *Journal of Pathology* **167**, 321–326.

6. Hopwood, D., Logan, K.R. and Bouchier, I.A.D. (1978) The electron microscopy of normal human oesophageal epithelium. *Virchows Archiv [B]*, **26**, 345–358.
7. Hopwood, D., Ross, P.E. and Bouchier I.A.D. (1981) Reflux oesophagitis. *Clinics in Gastroenterology*, **10**, 505–520.
8. Hopwood, D., Ross, P.E., Logan, K.R., Nicholson, G. and Bouchier, I.A.D. (1979) Changes in enzyme activity in normal and histologically inflamed oesophageal epithelium. *Gut* **20**, 769–774.
9. Jankowski, J. and Treghshis, B., Goghill, G., Grant, H., Hopwood, D. and Wormsley, K.G. (1992) Nucleolar organizer regions in oesophageal cytology and histology. *Gullet*, **2**, 85–90.
10. Lendrum, F.C. (1937) Anatomic features of the cardiac orifice of the stomach. *Archives of Internal Medicine*, **59**, 474.
11. Leese, G. Hopwood, D. (1986) Muscle fibre typing in the human pharyneal constrictors and oesophagus: the effect of ageing. *Acta Anatomica*, **127**, 77–80.
12. Liebermann-Meffert, D., Allgower, M., Schmid, P. and Blum, A.L. (1979) Muscular equivalent of the lower oesophageal sphincter. *Gastroenterology*, **76**, 31–38.
13. Odland, G.F. and Holbrook, K. (1981) The lamellar granules of epidermis. *Current Problems in Dermatology*, **9**, 29–49.
14. Sanders, D.S.A., Kerr, M.A., Hopwood, D., Coghill, G. and Milne, G. (1988) Expression of the 3-fucosyl *N*-acetyllactosamine (CD 15) antigen in normal, metaplastic, dysplastic and neoplastic squamous epithelia. *Journal of Pathology*, **154**, 255–262.
15. Smith, B. (1972) *The Neuropathology of the Alimentary Tract*, London: Arnold.

CONGENITAL ABNORMALITIES

N.V. Freeman

PHARYNX

PHARYNGO-OESOPHAGEAL INCOORDINATION

Cricopharyngeal disorders are seen in the neonate but it is difficult to be certain that they are primary rather than secondary (*Figure 1.17*). Cricopharyngeal achalasia or incoordination is diagnosed and sometimes inappropriately treated with myotomy or dilatation. With careful study of the lower oesophagus, and newer techniques such as manofluorography (which allows simultaneous analysis of manometry and video-fluoroscopy), most cases will be found to be secondary to gastro-oesophageal reflux.[30] The spasm of the cricopharyngeal muscle may even be protective to the larynx.[48]

Iatrogenic perforation of the oesophagus is becoming increasingly common in pre-term and newborn babies. These babies may present with oesophageal atresia or pneumothorax. Treatment is conservative without surgery.[37]

Less common is spontaneous rupture of the lower oesophagus in the neonate – 'neonatal Boerhaave's syndrome'.[23]

Various tumours of the pharynx are seen in the newborn such as epignathus, teratomas, hamartoma, choriostoma,[20] dermoids, heterotopic brain tissue,[68] papilloma, thyroglossal remnants or lingual thyroid, first branchial cleft remnants,[60] branchial fistula (second branchial cleft anomalies), lymphangiomas and haemangiomas.

LARYNGOTRACHEAL CLEFTS

These anomalies are very rare, but important to recognize. The incidence of anomalies of the larynx is approximately 1 in 2000 live births; 0.3% of these are laryngeal or laryngeal tracheo-oesophageal clefts and 20% of clefts are associated with oesophageal atresia or tracheo-oesophageal fistula.[13] Four grades of cleft are recognized (*Figure 1.18a*):

Type I – up to the superior portion of the cricoid plate
Type II – extending to inferior margin of the cricoid plate
Type III – extending into the cervical trachea
Type IV – a cleft into the thoracic trachea and up to the carina.

Symptoms vary according to the length of the defect. The lesser degrees present as a hoarse, weak or absent cry, stridor, cyanosis, recurrent aspiration, pneumonitis and choking on feeding. All except type I require urgent airway management and tracheotomy. Repair is possible via a lateral approach through the cricopharyngeal muscle and lateral pharyngeal wall, or via an anterior laryngofissure. Type IV lesions require a combined cervical and thoracotomy approach. The use of a special bifurcated endotracheal tube as described by Donahoe and Gee[12] facilitates anaesthesia and repair.

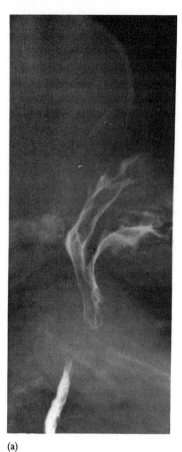

Figure 1.17 (a) Barium study in a baby unable to swallow. Diagnosed as cricopharyngeal achalasia. (b) Repeat contrast study 2 months later still showing spasm of the cricopharyngeal sphincter and spillage into the trachea (bronchogram). (c) This shows a bolus of barium refluxing from the stomach and being stopped at the cricopharyngeal muscle by spasm. (d) This shows a contrast study 2 months after a Nissen fundoplication repair. There is still some nasal regurgitation and hold-up at the cricopharyngeal muscle, but no reflux. The child has considerably improved at this stage.

(a)

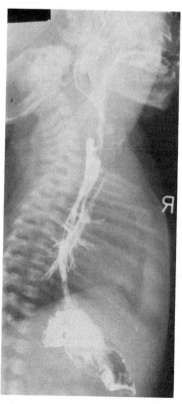

(b)

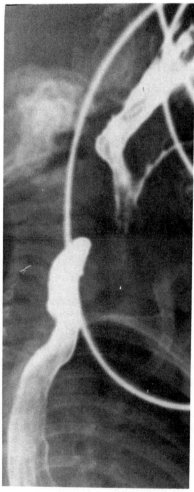

(c)

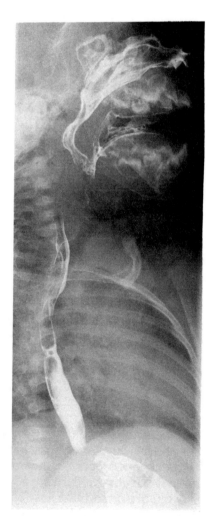

(d)

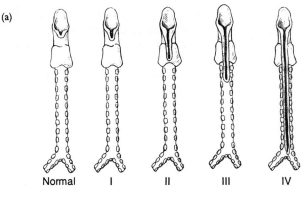

(a)

Normal I II III IV

Figure 1.18 (a) Showing the various types of laryngeal and laryngotracheo-oesophageal clefts. (Reproduced from DuBois, J.J., Pokorny, W.J., Harberg, F.J. and Smith, R.J.H. (1990) Current management of laryngo-tracheo-oesophageal clefts. *Journal of Pediatric Surgery*, **25**, 956, with permission from the editors and publisher.) (b) Diagram showing the various types of oesophageal atresia and the relative incidence.

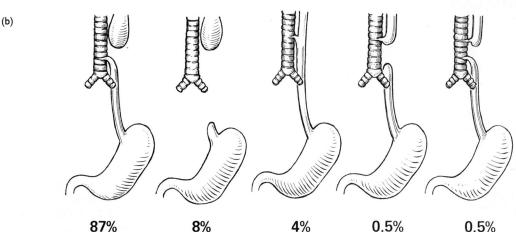

(b)

87%   8%   4%   0.5%   0.5%

OESOPHAGEAL ATRESIA AND TRACHEO-OESOPHAGEAL FISTULA

Although the first survivor of a tracheo-oesophageal fistula following a primary anastomosis was recorded in 1941[22] the outlook today, in at least half of the babies, is excellent. The prognosis depends on early diagnosis, absence of other congenital anomalies, pneumonia or prematurity.

The incidence of oesophageal atresia is between 1 in 3000–4000 live births. Oesophageal atresia without a fistula is uncommon (8%), most being associated with a fistula of the lower oesophagus to the trachea (*Figure 1.18b*).

AETIOLOGY

The aetiology is unknown and the genetic implications unclear. The complete lesion has been found in embryos of 5 weeks' gestation. There are reports of siblings with oesophageal atresia and a report of oesophageal atresia in two generations.[11] Oesophageal atresia has been reported in a father and daughter, and father and son.[36,41] Either one or both

monozygotic twins may be affected; in fact the incidence of twinning in oesophageal atresia is higher then normal.[46]

CLINICAL FEATURES

These babies do not vomit but produce copious salivary secretions which drool from the mouth and require frequent removal by suction. A change in position may precipitate a choking or cyanotic attack, as pooled saliva spills into the trachea.

INVESTIGATIONS

The diagnosis may be suspected antenatally on ultrasound examination of the mother. The presence of hydramnios and an absent fluid-filled stomach are suggestive. Unfortunately this is a diagnosis by exclusion, because only 8% of babies have isolated oesophageal atresia. It is not unusual to fail to identify a fluid-filled stomach, on a single ultrasound examination, in the first 20 weeks of gestation.

Once the diagnosis is suspected a stiff French gauge 10 tube should be passed via the nose. At about 10–12 cm an elastic resistance is felt, which will yield a further 1–2 cm on continued pressure. This feel of stretching the upper pouch is characteristic and almost pathognomonic of oesophageal atresia. An anteroposterior radiograph of the chest and an abdominal radiograph should be taken. This will show the tube held up just above the carina, at about the T4 level. The upper pouch may be outlined by swallowed air or more air can be injected. Contrast media should not be used to delineate the anatomy, except on rare occasions of serious doubt regarding the diagnosis. If contrast is used, not more than 1 ml Micropaque (micronized barium sulphate suspended in methyl cellulose) should be injected, preferably under fluoroscopic control. Lipiodol (iodized oil, viscous injection), Gastrografin (10% sodium diatrizoate and 66% meglumine diatrizoate), Hypaque (sodium diatrizoate) or barium sulphate should not be used, because all have potential dangers. The abdominal radiograph is necessary to observe gas in the stomach, denoting the presence of a fistula, and to exclude associated anomalies of the gut such as duodenal atresia.

Prematurity is common. Fifty per cent of these babies suffer from one or more affiliated anomalies. The acronym VATER (expanded to VACTERL) is a useful reminder of the systems likely to be involved, the anomalies encountered being non-random associations rather than a specific syndrome: V = vertebral anomalies (10% have hemivertebrae or 13 pairs of ribs); A = anal (10% have an anorectal anomaly); C = cardiac (37% have cardiac anomalies, ventricular septal defect, patent ductus anteriosus and tetralogy of Fallot being the most common); TE = tracheo-oesophageal: R = renal (the whole spectrum of renal anomalies has been seen in approximately 18%); and L = limb (skeletal anomalies account for 10%, with thumb deformities and radial dysplasia being the most common). Duplication cysts and bronchopulmonary malformation including pulmonary agenesis, pulmonary hypoplasia, sequestrated lobes, cystic adenomatoid malformation, tracheomalacia and non-ciliated epithelium in the respiratory tree may occur as associated anomalies which influence the prognosis in these babies. Careful examination of the above systems should therefore be undertaken and, if three or more anomalies are present, the VATER or VACTERL association is diagnosed.

TREATMENT

Pre- and perioperative

All personnel dealing with newborn infants should be aware of the symptoms of oesophageal atresia, so that an early diagnosis can be made, before feeding is started. Coughing and spluttering on feeding, excess salivation, excessive bubbly frothing or cyanotic attacks should halt any attempts at feeding until oesophageal atresia has been excluded. Spillage of milk into the lungs is a cause of pneumonitis, but more serious is regurgitation of acid contents, via the fistula, into the lower trachea and the lungs, causing a chemical pneumonitis, which may not be visible on the initial plain radiograph.

Most babies are born away from a specialist centre and need to be transported to the centre for treatment. Adequate precautions are therefore necessary for safe transport. Clear instructions should be issued to the referring hospital. A sample of blood from the mother for cross-matching and operative consent, in case either parent is unable to accompany the baby, are essential. A trained nurse or doctor, who can suck the pharynx frequently with a syringe or portable suction machine, should accompany the baby.

Prior to surgery continuous suction, especially with high negative pressure, may damage the mucosa. High negative suction pressure in the pharanyx may also cause cyanosis by preventing effective inspiration.[52] Therefore a French gauge 10 double-lumen tube (Replogle), should be passed via the nostril into the upper pouch. Intermittent flushing of the side tube keeps the lumen free of saliva. The optimal position in which to nurse the baby is controversial. Head-up (to allow pooling of saliva in the upper pouch and therefore better suction), head-down (to allow free exit of saliva out of the mouth) and flat have all been recommended. Nursing the baby flat, on either side, or supine is satisfactory.

Antibiotics should be started immediately, because it is not possible to predict, or prevent, the vomiting of acid gastric contents into the lungs. The baby must be kept warm, in an incubator if possible, and an intravenous line should be inserted.

Previously oesophageal atresia was treated as an emergency, operation being carried out as soon as the baby was thought to be adequately prepared for the operation. This is now no longer the case with the one exception: if the baby cries a lot, the glottis closes, thereby allowing air to escape via the fistula into the stomach which may cause major distension of the stomach and compromise the breathing by diaphragmatic splinting. In this circumstance emergency operation would be necessary; otherwise, elective surgery, at the next convenient opportunity, is preferable. Babies diagnosed late and suffering from aspiration and pneumonia may benefit from several days of preoperative antibiotic therapy and ventilation. Ventilation, however, can be dangerous because there is a risk of gastric perforation and pneumoperitoneum, until the fistula is ligated or a gastrostomy performed.[35]

Table 1.8 Classification of oesophageal atresia

Group	Description
A	Babies over 2.5 kg and well
B₁	Babies of 1.8–2.5 kg and well
B₂	Babies over 2.5 kg with moderate pneumonia or congenital anomaly
C₁	Babies of birth weight under 1.8 kg
C₂	Babies of any weight and severe pneumonia and severe congenital anomaly

Operative techniques

Babies once diagnosed as suffering from oesophageal atresia must be referred to a specialist centre for treatment if they are to have a reasonable chance of survival, as experience is limited, even in large regional units. In the UK it will take the lifetime of one paediatric surgeon to accumulate the personal experience of 100 cases of oesophageal atresia. A classification, originally described by Waterston,[67] has evolved based on the weight of the baby, the presence of pneumonia or associated congenital anomalies (*Table 1.8*).

Unfortunately this classification does not take into account gestational age in relation to weight. Group A babies should all survive in a specialized unit, whereas 50% of group C₂ are likely to die, mainly from associated anomalies.

Controversies in the surgical management of oesophageal atresia and tracheo-oesophageal fistula

Many differences of opinion regarding the optimal management of these babies still remain.

Emergency or elective surgery
Twenty years ago all presenting infants were regarded as dire emergencies requiring immediate operation at any time of day or night! This attitude has slowly changed over the years and more are now treated as elective procedures. The main theoretical risks of waiting are unseen or undetected acid regurgitation into the lungs, cyanotic attacks from saliva spillage into the lungs or massive gastric distension from an air leak via a large fistula.

Staged procedures
It is recommended, that for ill, low-birth-weight babies with pneumonia (group C₂), the operative procedure should be staged, consisting of an initial gastrostomy and ligation of the fistula, followed by a delayed primary anastomosis in order to increase survival.[31] The efficacy of this technique remains controversial.[64]

Surgical approach
In order to locate the side of the aortic arch, a penetrated plain radiograph, to show the indentation on the tracheal shadow by the aortic arch, should be carefully studied. Supplementary echocardiography may be necessary. A right-sided arch can make the operation very difficult or impossible via the right chest and necessitates a left thoracotomy.

Which incision
The thoracotomy incision can be lateral, posterolateral or vertical (axillary). If a lateral or posterolateral incision is used, it must be low enough not to divide the nerves to latissimus dorsi and serratus anterior, in order to prevent subsequent shoulder girdle deformity.[16]

Extrapleural or transpleural approach
A survey of the American Academy of Pediatrics suggested that there is a better survival with the extrapleural approach.[28] Recent series suggest equal results with the transpleural approach.[2] Once the technique of pleural reflection is mastered there is no increase in operative time – one of the criticisms of the extrapleural approach. If the initial stripping of the pleura is started as far posterior as possible, the pleura is less likely to be torn. Non-collapse of the lung during surgery, and confining any postoperative anastomic leak extrapleurally, are major advantages of this route.

Gastrostomy or transanastomic tube
Over the decades opinion has varied on this issue. Access into the stomach is required for decompression of the stomach and for early feeding. This can be achieved by either a nasogastric tube or a gastrostomy. Gastrostomy alone carries a definite morbidity and mortality. Fixation of the stomach to the abdominal wall leads to increased tension on the anastomosis during coughing and hiccuping. The incidence of gastro-oesophageal reflux is higher following gastrostomy (24%), compared to using a nasogastric tube (12%).[62]

Anastomotic technique
The original two-layered anastomosis described by Haight is not essential.[21] A single-layer anastomosis, using only six to eight sutures, with knots on the inside for the posterior layer and outside for the anterior layer, is safe and adequate. Black silk 4/0 or polyglycolic acid sutures appear to have equal healing properties on experimental evidence.[6,38]

Long-gap oesophageal atresia

Controversy exists in determining which cases are to be considered as 'long-gap', and therefore not suitable for a primary anastomosis. Primary anastomosis should be possible in 75% of all cases. A 'long-gap' may be anticipated and planned for by preoperative bronchoscopy. The finding of a fistula at the carina signals a 'long-gap' atresia.[47] A gap of 2.0–2.5 cm between the oesophageal ends, prior to division of the fistula, should be amenable to a primary anastomosis without undue tension. If the deficit is larger than 2.5 cm, various operative techiques are available to bridge the defect. A circular or spiral myotomy can be performed on the upper pouch to secure extra length.[44] The upper pouch may need to be brought out of the neck temporarily, via a separate cervical incision, for satisfactory exposure.[27] A U-shaped flap cut from the anterior wall of the hypertrophied upper pouch can be tubulated and swung down to bridge the gap.[19] Delayed primary anastomosis may be achieved after 6 or 8 weeks by stretching. Bougienage of the upper and lower pouch is started,[29] but may not be necessary, because natural elongation may take place, aided by gastro-oesophageal reflux. If any of these methods fail, cervical oesophagostomy, on the left or right side, and a gastrostomy overcome the acute situation. The side of the cervical oesophagostomy influences the operative technique of the second procedure. The resultant 'long gap' can be bridged by the use of either a gastric transposition, colon interposition or gastric tube. Gastric transposition and colon interposition can be carried out in the neonatal period.[15] A gastric tube requires a large stomach and has to be delayed to about 1 year of age. Several other ingenious methods of joining the upper and lower ends have been tried, by creating a fistula[4,56] and by electromagnetic bougienage.[26]

Postoperative ventilation

Elective postoperative ventilation has a place in the management of the baby with a tense anastomosis,[62] but need not be used routinely or indiscriminately in group A babies.

Complications

An anastomotic disruption is the major anxiety. Small leaks may go unnoticed and be detected only on subsequent barium studies. Even large extrapleural leaks may be remarkably silent. Intrathoracic leaks can cause a tension pneumo- or pyopneumo-thorax. The disruption can be partial or complete, and a contrast study may be misleading in this respect. Early reoperation and resuture is the procedure of choice when the original anastomosis was not under undue tension. Conservative management, especially in the extrapleural leaks, is effective. Other complications include the following:

- Strictures requiring dilatation may occur early (3–4 weeks) or later (10–12 months) after surgery in 25% of cases.
- Gastro-oesophageal reflux is seen in up to two-thirds of patients 6 years after repair of oesophageal atresia.[34]
- A recurrent fistula develops in 5–15% of patients. It is easily overlooked and difficult to demonstrate. Right upper lobe consolidation, repeated pneumonic episodes and failure to thrive are clues. The recurrent fistula may be overlooked on a single endoscopy and repeated endoscopy may be needed. The fistula may be closed by reoperation or fulguration via a bronchoscope.[55]
- Oesophageal motility following anastomosis is often abnormal.
- Myenteric abnormalities in the oesophagus and stomach have been shown.[51]

'H'-TYPE FISTULA

This variety of oesophageal atresia consists of a normal oesophagus with an isolated tracheo-oesophageal fistula joining the trachea to the oesophagus, at about the seventh cervical to the second thoracic vertebral level. As the direction of the fistula is downwards from the trachea to the oesophagus, feeds do not readily enter the trachea. This anomaly is uncommon, accounting for only 4% of congenital oesophageal atresia anomalies, and is rarely seen in the neonatal period. The diagnosis should be suspected in a baby who appears to feed normally, but suffers from recurrent attacks of pneumonitis, right upper lobe collapse, bouts of coughing and choking during feeds, or a distended tympanitic abdomen on crying. Symptoms are dramatically relieved by gavage feeding. Confirmation of the diagnosis can be difficult. A nasogastric tube can be passed, the open end placed under water and the catheter slowly withdrawn. Air bubbles can be seen or heard. Metrizamide contrast studies using a similar technique with the baby prone can demonstrate the fistula.

Bronchoscopy and oesophagoscopy are mandatory in the management. Once identified most fistulae can be repaired via a right-sided cervical incision.

OESOPHAGEAL OBSTRUCTION

CONGENITAL STENOSIS

Congenital stenosis due to a web or abnormal ectopic tissue in the wall of the oesophagus is extremely rare, and must be distinguished from narrowing in the lower third of the oesophagus, which is caused by gastro-oesophageal reflux and secondary inflammation. Another form of stenosis is associated with oesophageal atresia. Here a diverticulum is formed, as the lower oesophagus joins the upper oesophagus asymmetrically, instead of opening into the trachea.[33] Symptoms develop later when solid food is introduced. Diagnosis is confirmed by barium swallow or oesophagoscopy. The diaphragm or web can be treated by dilatation, repeated if necessary. Excision of a segment of oesophagus is required for ectopic rests of tissue within the wall.

DUPLICATIONS

Duplications may be spherical or tubular structures. They should be firmly attached to one point of the alimentary tract, have smooth muscle in the wall, and a lining of recognizable intestinal epithelium. They may appear anywhere in the alimentary tract from the mouth to the anus. In the chest, the cyst is always situated in the posterior mediastinum and two-thirds will have a spinal deformity involving the cervical or upper thoracic vertebrae. Eighty per cent of the enteric duplications present in the neonatal period;[42] respiratory distress is one of the main features of thoracic duplications. The cysts tend to increase in size because they are lined with mucus-secreting cells. If the lining is gastric in type, autodigestion and ulceration of the oesophagus and bronchus may occur, with haematemesis and haemoptysis. Thoracotomy and excision of the cyst should be carried out as soon as possible. A search for a thoracoabdominal connection must be made and, if found, will require an additional laparotomy. Bronchopulmonary foregut malformations are rare cases of pulmonary sequestrations which communicate with the upper intestinal tract, and may be associated with oesophageal atresia.[14]

INFANTILE GASTRO-OESOPHAGEAL REFLUX AND HIATUS HERNIA

Incompetence of the gastro-oesophageal sphincter is almost universal in newborn babies for the first 4–6 weeks of life. An effective antireflux barrier has developed by 6–7 weeks as shown on manometry.[3] The incidence is uncertain because many cases of vomiting are not investigated. In Liverpool, 114 patients, with 41 proven cases of hiatus hernia, were seen in the neonatal unit, over a period of 30 years.[43] The ratio of male to female was equal. Vomiting, often projectile, is the presenting feature: 25% vomited bile-stained fluid and 10% had haematemesis. In three-quarters of the infants, the vomiting started before the eighth day of life, in contradistinction to babies suffering from pyloric stenosis. In Waterston's study of 602 children with hiatus hernia, 25% were found to have central nervous system disorders such as mental handicap, hydrocephalus and spina bifida.[32] Fifty-two patients were studied adequately, of which 19% were found to have pyloric spasm.

The investigation and classification of gastro-oesophageal reflux and hiatus hernia are similar to those of adults. In 74 children undergoing Nissen fundoplication for persistent gastro-oesophageal reflux, 54% were found to have an associated malrotation.[39]

Treatment is conservative in the first instance, with thickened feeds, upright nursing, antacids and H_2-receptor antagonists. Most cases respond to conservative measures and do not require surgery. There appear to be geographical differences with many more babies apparently requiring surgery in Europe and the USA.

CONGENITAL DIAPHRAGMATIC HERNIA

During the fourth to sixth weeks of embryonic life the diaphragm is formed from a complex process involving the septum transversum (*Figure 1.19*), the pleuroperitoneal membranes and a later contribution from the body wall. The septum transversum forms an incomplete ventral division between the pericardium and the peritoneal cavity. Four main types of hernias are recognized: (1) posterolateral (Bochdalek); (2) unilateral agenesis of the diaphragm; (3) parasternal (Morgagni); (4) ventral (septum transversum) defect (*Figure 1.20*).

Of posterolateral hernias 85–90% are left-sided; 20% have a sac and may be very difficult to distinguish from an eventration (*Figure 1.21*). Parasternal defects account for less than 2% of diaphragmatic defects; 15–30% are bilateral. The ventral defects, probably due to a failure of the development of the septum transversum, are typically associated with a pericardial defect, or combined with a lower sternal defect, upper abdominal

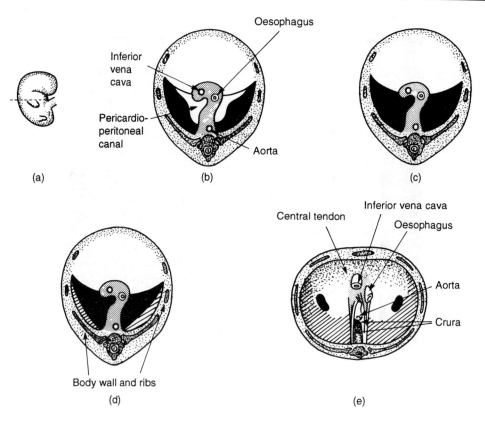

Figure 1.19 This shows the diaphragm viewed from below: (a) sketch of a lateral view of an embryo at the end of the fifth week (actual size) indicating the level of the section; (b) transverse section showing unfused pleuroperitoneal membranes; (c) similar section at the end of the sixth week after fusion of the pleuroperitoneal membranes with the other two diaphragmatic components; (d) transverse section through a 12-week embryo after ingrowth of the fourth diaphragmatic component of the body wall; (e) view of the diaphragm of a newborn infant, indicating the probable embryological origin of its components. □ Septum transversum; ▦ mesentery of the oesophagus; ■ pleuroperitoneal membranes; ▨ body wall. (Reproduced from Moore, K.L. (1988) *The Developing Human: Clinically Orientated Embryology*, 4th edn, by courtesy of the publishers, W.B. Saunders, Philadelphia.)

wall deficiency and intracardiac anomalies to form Cantrell's pentalogy (*Figure 1.22*).

The true incidence of congenital diaphragmatic hernia is difficult to estimate, occurring in approximately 1 in 4500 of live and still births. The outcome in 100 babies born with congenital diaphragmatic hernia is as shown in *Figure 1.23*.

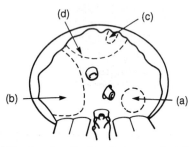

Figure 1.20 Diagram showing the diaphragmatic defects through which hernias occur in the neonate: (a) posterolateral (Bochdalek's); (b) unilateral agenesis of the diaphragm; (c) Morgagni's (parasternal) defect; (d) ventral (septum transversum) defect.

The overall mortality in most large units is around 50%, and almost 80–100% in those diagnosed antenatally, especially if an associated cardiac lesion is present.

CLINICAL FEATURES

Prenatal maternal ultrasonography may show polyhydramnios, mediastinal displacement with herniated organs in the fetal chest, and an absent intra-abdominal stomach bubble. The fetal heart should be examined by fetal echocardiography to exclude serious cardiac malformations.[9] Respiratory distress, tachypnoea, cyanosis and dyspnoea warrant an immediate chest radiograph. The time of onset of symptoms after birth has prognostic significance. Babies presenting with signs and symptoms more than 2 hours after birth should have a good prognosis. Physical examination reveals dextrocardia, a scaphoid abdomen, asymmetry of the chest, absence of breath sounds or the presence of bowel sounds in

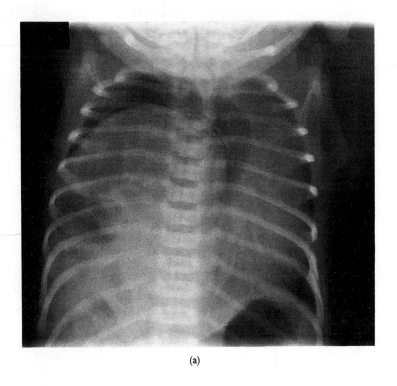

(a)

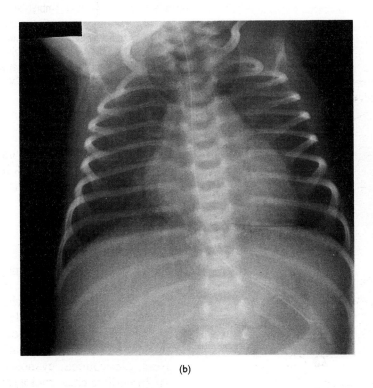

(b)

Figure 1.21 (a) Radiograph of a baby presenting with a right-sided congenital diaphragmatic hernia, and minimal respiratory distress. It is not possible to distinguish this easily from an eventration. (b) Radiograph following repair and plication of the right diaphragm.

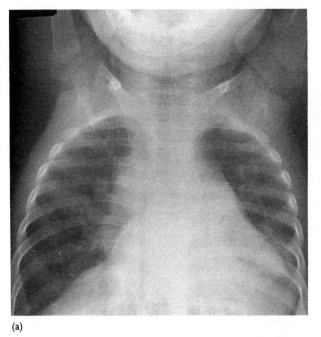

(a)

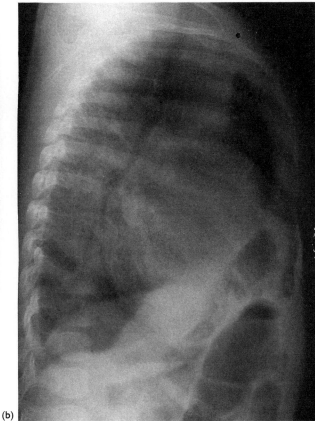

(b)

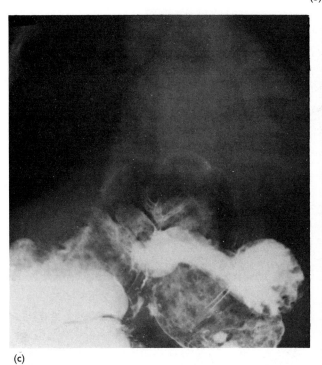

(c)

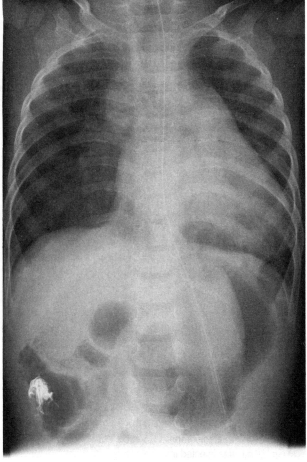

(d)

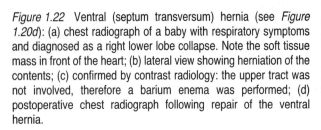

Figure 1.22 Ventral (septum transversum) hernia (see *Figure 1.20d*): (a) chest radiograph of a baby with respiratory symptoms and diagnosed as a right lower lobe collapse. Note the soft tissue mass in front of the heart; (b) lateral view showing herniation of the contents; (c) confirmed by contrast radiology: the upper tract was not involved, therefore a barium enema was performed; (d) postoperative chest radiograph following repair of the ventral hernia.

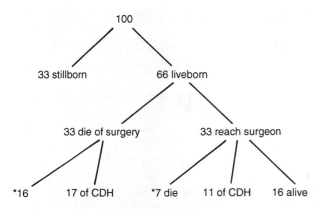

Figure 1.23 Outcome of congenital diaphragmatic hernia (CDH). *Major associated anomalies: anencephaly, hydrocephalus, congenital heart disease and exomphthalos.

injection of a small amount of air may help (*Figure 1.24b*). The position of the stomach should be noted because this has prognostic significance, associated with a 6.2% mortality in the intra-abdominal position, compared to a 58% mortality when found to be in the chest.[18] Other congenital anomalies, apart from those normally associated with viscera in the chest, are present in 40%. This group has a higher mortality.[1]

The condition most likely to be mistaken is cystic adenomatoid malformation of the lung. In these babies the diaphragm is well seen and the abdomen is not scaphoid. Staphylococcal cysts and a localized pneumothorax may give rise to confusion. Agenesis or hypoplasia of the lung with an elevated diaphragm need to be considered.

the chest. Infants with congenital diaphragmatic hernia have a significantly increased chest circumference which may contribute to the postoperative morbidity.[61] A plain radiograph of the chest including the abdomen is all that is necessary for the diagnosis. The radiograph may be difficult to interpret, especially when no air is seen in the chest. The position of the nasogastric tube or the additional

FACTORS CONTRIBUTING TO AN INCREASED MORTALITY

Hypoplasia of the lung, persistent fetal circulation (PFC) and pulmonary hypertension are the three major factors influencing survival.

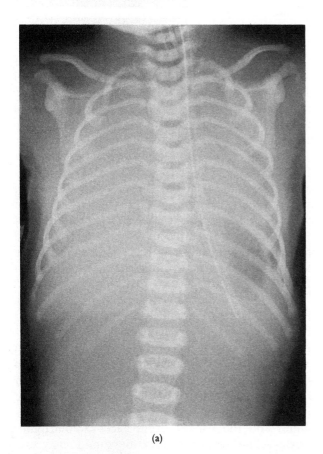

(a)

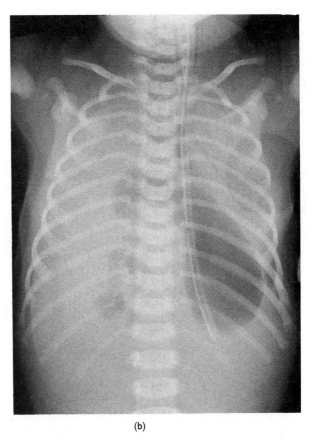

(b)

Figure 1.24 (a) Radiographs of a baby who presented with severe respiratory distress and cyanosis at delivery. Note the airless lungs. (b) Air, 20 ml, was injected into the nasogastric tube to outline the stomach. The baby did not respond to any resuscitative measures and died without surgery being offered.

The development of the lung begins during the fourth week by successive branching, varying between 18 and 25 generations, of the bronchi and pulmonary arteries, and is completed by the sixteenth week.[5] Alveolar development, however, continues to the age of 8 years, but is dependent on the original number of bronchial branches present. Compression of the lung during development will result in a permanent reduction of the number of bronchial divisions. Experimental work on fetal lambs showed that the compressed fetal lung could continue to grow if the obstruction was relieved *in utero*.[24] The compression affects not only the airways but the vasculature and results in a reduction in the total cross-sectional area of the pulmonary bed. The development of the ventricles may also be impaired by compression.

The pulmonary blood flow, pulmonary artery pressure and pulmonary vasculature are exquisitely sensitive to hypoxia and acidosis.[57] Babies dying of diaphragmatic hernia and pulmonary hypertension were found to have an increased muscle mass in the media of the pulmonary arterioles which extended beyond the usual termination of the respiratory bronchiole.[49] It is suggested that the excess muscle enhances the tendency of the arterioles to contrict in response to hypoxia and acidosis.[7]

Prostaglandins must play a role in the pulmonary hypertension, but the pathophysiological function is confusing. Prostaglandins of the E series (PGE_1) and (PGE_2) and prostacyclin (PGI_2) have vasodilator effects on the pulmonary arterioles, whereas the F series are vasoconstrictors.[54] Drugs such as nitroprusside, glyceryl trinitrate, phenoxybenzamine and tolazoline have been used in an attempt to decrease the pulmonary artery pressures.[8]

Score systems have been devized to predict the outcome based on preoperative arterial pH, Pao_2 (arterial oxygen tension), $Paco_2$ (arterial carbon dioxide tension), $A-aDo_2$ (arterial–alveolar oxygen gradient or difference), oxygen gradient, MAP (mean airway pressure).[65]

Survival is unlikely if the initial blood gas analysis shows a pH less than 7.1, a Po_2 less than 50 mmHg, and a Pco_2 greater than 65 mmHg. Postductal Pao_2 of less than 100 has been used as a predictor of hypoplasia. The size of the pulmonary arteries, size of the lungs and perivascular disease was measured on pulmonary arteriograms.[53] Surgery was delayed, or not performed at all, until a Pco_2 of less than 40 mmHg was maintained. High frequency oscillation was used in some of these patients. The group treated by delayed surgery was compared with those who had emergency surgery in the preceding 2 years (1983–85). The mortality was 50% and 58% respectively, which was not statistically significant.[40]

PREOPERATIVE TREATMENT

All, or some, of the following measures may be needed in the management of babies with congenital diaphragmatic hernia.

A nasogastric tube with continuous suction is effective in decompressing the gut in the chest[65] (*Figure 1.25*). An umbilical artery catheter for post-ductal blood gases, and an arterial line in the right radial artery for preductal gases and to calculate the right-to-left shunting, should be inserted. Intubation (not bagging with a face mask which may aggravate the situation), the use of 100% oxygen and hyperventilation, in combination with a bicarbonate drip of 1–2 mmol/kg per h, may enhance the alkalosis and help reduce the pulmonary hypertension. Vasodilators such as tolazoline (a bolus of 1–2 mg/kg per h given over 15 minutes) and treatment of any ipsi- or contralateral pneumothorax may all be necessary. Fluid balance needs to be carefully monitored because two-thirds of babies with congenital diaphragmatic hernia respond inappropriately to postoperative fluid intake by retaining fluid and serious fluid overload may occur.[58] Those who show no response in their oxygenation, pH or carbon dioxide will not respond to surgery and will die (see *Figure 1.24*). Where available extracorporeal membrane oxygenation (ECMO) should be considered because this may salvage some babies.[25]

Surgery is no longer an emergency and patients should be stabilized preoperatively. Reduction of the hernia may actual cause a deterioration in lung compliance.[59] Repair is best via an abdominal approach using a subcostal or oblique incision, along the line of the tenth intercostal nerve.

In the small posterolateral hernias the muscular defect can be closed with sutures. The larger deficiencies (unilateral agenesis) may require the use of muscular flaps, or non-porous Silastic sheeting to close the defect. The use of postoperative chest drain is controversial: recent clinical experience and animal experiments show less barotrauma and a better survival rate without the use of a chest drain.[10]

The group of babies which are the most vexing includes those who demonstrate enough lung tissue for survival and then suddenly deteriorate postoperatively, after the so-called 'honeymoon period'.[8] In this situation ECMO has been used with success in some specialized centres. The deterioration is due to a reversal to a persistent fetal circulation. In these patients ventilation, paralysis, sedation with morphine, and the use of drugs such as tolazoline, prostacycline, dopamine and dobutamine may succeed in reversing the shunting.[45] The rationale of vasodilator therapy in neonates is questioned, be-

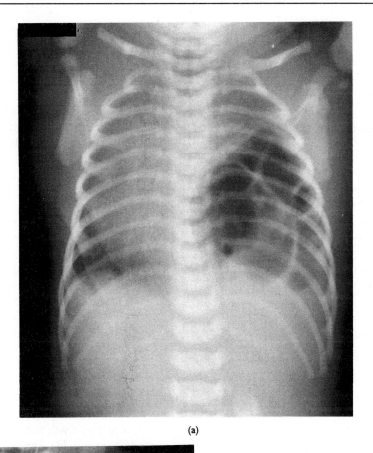

(a)

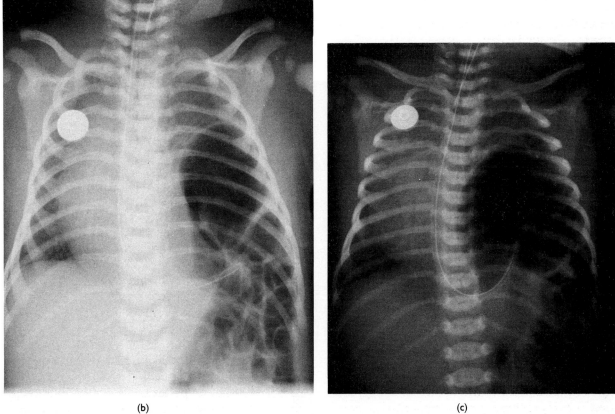

(b)   (c)

Figure 1.25 Three radiographs taken over a period of 24 hours in a baby with little respiratory distress, showing poor management of the nasogastric tube allowing the visceral contents in the chest to distend. It should be possible totally to decompress the viscera with continuous suction.

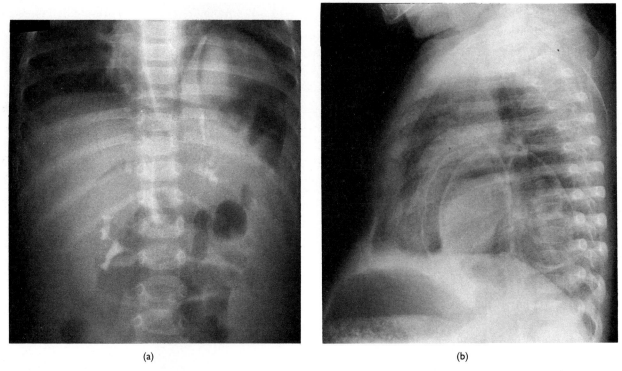

(a)   (b)

Figure 1.26   (a) Anteroposterior and (b) lateral radiographs showing an eventration of the left diaphragm. Note the displacement of the left kidney into the defect.

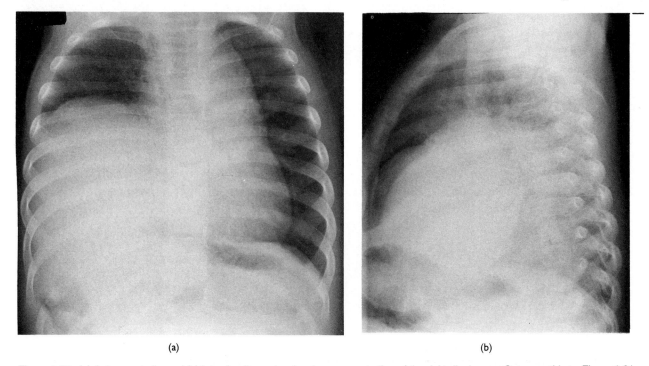

(a)   (b)

Figure 1.27   (a) Anteroposterior and (b) lateral radiographs showing an eventration of the right diaphragm. Compare this to *Figure 1.21* which shows a neonate in acute respiratory distress, with a right-sided congenital diaphragmatic hernia.

cause expansion of the vascular capacitance necessitates additional intravenous fluid; higher inflation pressures are then required, with a consequent reduced cardiac output and the risk of pneumothorax.[66]

ECMO has been used with success in the USA in centres which have the facilities, but is unlikely to become a standard method of treatment. High-frequency ventilation at rates of 2400 cycles per minute has been tried with success. The tidal volumes delivered are less than the dead space and gas exchange appears to take place by diffusion.[17] Experimentally, in fetal lambs, it has been shown that surgery is feasible and beneficial to the developing lung. Surgery on the human fetus raises many ethical issues and should only be contemplated with great caution at present.[50]

Foramen of Morgagni or parasternal hernia

These are rare, accounting for less than 2% of diaphragmatic hernias; they are associated with a sac that protrudes into the chest between the costal and sternal attachments of the diaphragm. They are rare in the neonate, occurring in older children or adults. They are often asymptomatic and are found incidentally on a chest radiograph, as a mass or air–fluid level. They are easily repaired via the abdomen.

Eventration of the diaphragm

Eventration may be congenital or acquired, secondary to phrenic nerve paralysis. The area of affected diaphragm shows hypoplastic muscle fibres. In severe cases the diaphragm is reduced to a thin sac with no muscle fibres. As 20% of congenital diaphragmatic hernias are associated with a sac, it may be impossible to distinguish these from eventration. The small defects, often an anteromedial hump on the diaphragm, may cause no symptoms (*Figure 1.26*) Paradoxical breathing is found in the large defects and is an indication for surgery (*Figure 1.27*). Plication is best achieved via a thoracotomy.[63]

REFERENCES

1. Benjamin, D.R., Juul, S. and Siebert, J.R. (1988) Congenital posterolateral hernia: associated malformations. *Journal of Pediatric Surgery*, **23**, 899–903.
2. Bishop, P.J., Klein, M.D., Philippart, A.I. *et al.* (1985) Transpleural repair of oesophageal atresia without a preliminary gastrostomy: 240 patients treated between 1951 and 1983. *Journal of Pediatric Surgery*, **200**, 823–828.
3. Boix-Ochoa, J. and Canals, J. (1976) Maturation of the lower oesophageal sphincter. *Journal of Pediatric Surgery*, **11**, 749–756.
4. Booss, D., Hollwarth, M. and Sauer, H. (1982) Endoscopic oesophageal anastromosis. *Journal of Pediatric Surgery*, **8**, 9–13.
5. Bucher, U. and Reid, L. (1961) Development of the intrasegmental tree; the pattern of branching and development of cartilage at various stages of intra uterine life. *Thorax*, **16**, 207–218.
6. Carachi, R., Stokes, K.B. and Brown, T.C.K. (1984) Oesophageal anastomosis – an experimental model to study the oesophageal lumen and influence of a transanastomtic tube. *Journal of Pediatric Surgery*, **19**, 9–93.
7. Cloutier R.R., Fournier, L. and Levasseur, L. (1983) Reversion to fetal circulation in congenital diaphragmatic hernia: A preventable postoperative complication. *Journal of Pediatric Surgery*, **18**, 551–555.
8. Collins, D.I., Pomerance, J.J., Travis, K.W. *et al.* (1977) A new approach to congenital posterolateral hernia. *Journal of Pediatric Surgery*, **12**, 149–151.
9. Crawford, D.C., Wright, V.M., Drake, D.P. and Allan, L.D. (1989) Fetal diaphragmatic hernia: the value of fetal echocardiography in the prediction of outcome. *British Journal of Obstetrics and Gynaecology*, **96**, 705–710.
10. de-Luca U., Cloutier, R., Laberge, J.M. *et al.* (1987) Pulmonary barotrauma in congenital diaphragmatic hernia: an experimental study in lambs. *Journal of Pediatric Surgery*, **22**, 311–316.
11. Dennis, N.R., Nicholas, J.L. and Kovar, I. (1973) Oesophageal atresia: 3 cases in 2 generations. *Archives of Diseases of Childhood*, **48**, 980–982.
12. Donahoe, P.K. and Gee, P.E. (1984) Complete laryngotracheoesophageal cleft: Management and repair. *Journal of Pediatric Surgery*, **19**, 143–148.
13. DuBois, J.J., Pokorny, W.J., Harberg, F.J. and Smith, R.J.H. (1990) Current management of laryngeal and laryngotracheoesophageal clefts. *Journal of Pediatric Surgery*, **25**, 855–860.
14. Fowler, C.L., Pokorny, W.J., Wagner, M.L. and Kessler, M.S. (1988) Review of bronchopulmonary foregut malformations. *Journal of Pediatric Surgery*, **23**, 793–797.
15. Freeman, N.V. (1986) Colon interposition. In *Progress in Pediatric Surgery*, Vol. 19 (Ed.) Wurnig, P. pp. 73–87: Berlin: Springer-Verlag.
16. Freeman, N.V. and Walkden, J. (1969) Previously unreported shoulder deformity following right lateral thoracotomy for esophageal atresia. *Journal of Pediatric Surgery*, **4**, 627–636.
17. Fujino, Y., Takezawa, J., Nishimura, M., Imanaka, H., Taenaka, N. and Yoshiya, I. (1989) High frequency oscillation for persistent fetal circulation after repair of congenital diaphragmatic hernia. *Critical Care Medicine*, **17**, 376–377.
18. Goodfellow, T., Hyde, I., Burge, D.M. and Freeman, N.V. (1987) Congenital diaphragmatic

hernia: the prognostic significance of the site of the stomach. *British Journal of Radiology*, **60**, 993–995.

19. Gough, M.H. (1970) Oesophageal atresia: Use of an anterior flap in the difficult case. *Journal of Pediatric Surgery*, **15**, 310–312.

20. Grant, J.W. and Freeman, N.V. (1987) Choriostoma of the soft palate. *Journal of Pediatric Surgery*, **22**, 365–366.

21. Haight, C. (1948) Congenital tracheo-esophageal atresia with esophageal atresia. *Journal of Thoracic Surgery*, **17**, 600–612.

22. Haight, C. and Towsley, H.A. (1943) Congenital atresia of the esophagus with tracheo-esophageal fistula: extrapleural ligation of the fistula and end to end anastomosis of the esophageal segments. *Surgery, Gynecology and Obstetrics*, **76**, 672–688.

23. Harrel G.S., Friedland, G.W., Daily, W.J. *et al.* (1970) Neonatal Boerharave's syndrome. *Radiology*, **95**, 665–668.

24. Harrison, M.R., Bressack, M.A., Churg, A.M. and De Lorimer, A.A. (1980) Correction of congenital diaphragmatic hernia in utero. II. Simulated correction permits fetal lung growth with survival at birth. *Surgery*, **88**, 260–268.

25. Heiss, K., Manning, P., Oldham, K.T. *et al.* (1989) Reversal of mortality for congenital diaphragmatic hernia with ECMO. *Annals of Surgery*, **209**, 225–230.

26. Hendren, W.H. and Hale, J.R. (1975) Electromagnetic bougienage to lengthen esophageal segments in congenital esophageal atresia. *New England Journal of Medicine*, **293**, 428–433.

27. Hoffman, D.G. and Moazan, F. (1984) Transcervical myotomy for wide gap esophageal atresia. *Journal of Pediatric Surgery*, **19**, 680–682.

28. Holder, T.M., Cloud, D.J., Lewis, E. and Pilling, G.P. (1964) Esophageal atresia and tracheo-esophageal fistula. A survey of its members by the Surgical Section of the American Academy of Pediatrics. *Pediatrics*, **34**, 542–549.

29. Howard, R. and Myers, W.A. (1965) Esophageal atresia. A technique for elongation of the upper pouch. *Surgery*, **58**, 725–727.

30. Hunt, P.S., Connel, A.M. and Smiley, T.B. (1970) The cricopharyngeal sphincter in gastro reflux. *Gut*, **11**, 303–306.

31. Ito, T., Sugito, T. and Nagaya, M. (1984) Delayed primary anastomosis in poor risk patients with esophageal atresia associated with tracheoesophageal fistula. *Journal of Pediatric Surgery*, **19**, 243–247.

32. Jewett, T.C. and Waterston, D.J. (1975) Surgical management of hiatus hernia in children. *Journal of Pediatric Surgery*, **10**, 757–761.

33. Jewsbury, P. (1971) An unusal case of oesophageal stricture. *British Journal of Surgery*, **58**, 475.

34. Jolley, S.G., Johnson, D.G., Roberts, C.C. *et al.* (1981) Patterns of gastro-esophageal reflux in children following repair of esophageal and distal tracheoesophageal fistula. *Journal of Pediatric Surgery*, **16**, 857–862.

35. Jones T.B., Kirchner, S.G. and Lee, F.A. (1980) Stomach rupture associated with esophageal atresia, tracheoesophageal fistula, and ventillatory assistance. *American Journal of Roentgenology*, **134**, 675–677.

36. Kashuk, J.L. and Lilly, J.R. (1988) Esophageal atresia in father and son. *Journal of Pediatric Surgery*, **18**, 621–628.

37. Krasna, I.H., Rosenfeld, D., Benjamin, B.G., Klein, G., Hiatt, M. and Hegyi, T. (1987) Esophageal perforation in the neonate: an emerging problem in the new born nursery. *Journal of Pediatric Surgery*, **22**, 784–790.

38. Kullendorf, F., Okmian, L. and Jonsson, N. (1981) Technical considerations of experimental esophageal anastomosis. *Journal of Pediatric Surgery*, **16**, 979–982.

39. Kumar, D., Brereton, R.J., Spitz, L. and Hall, C.M. (1988) Gastro-oesophageal reflux and malrotation in children. *British Journal of Surgery*, **75**, 533–555.

40. Langer, J.C., Filler, R.M., Bohn, D.J. *et al.* (1988) Timing of surgery for congenital diaphragmatic hernia: is emergency surgery necessary? *Journal of Pediatric Surgery*, **23**, 731–734.

41. Lipson, A.H. and Berry, A.B. (1984) Oesophageal atresia in father and daughter. *Australian Paediatric Journal*, **20**, 329.

42. Lister, J. (1990) Duplications of the alimentary tract. *In Neonatal Surgery*, 3rd edn (Eds) Lister, J. and Irving, I. pp. 474–484. London: Butterworths.

43. Lister, J. (1990) Gastro-oesophageal reflux and hiatus hernia. In *Neonatal Surgery*, 3rd edn (Eds) Lister, J. and Irving, I. p. 224. London: Butterworths.

44. Livaditis, A. (1975) Long gap between oesophageal segments. *Zeitschrift für Kinderchirurgie*, Suppl. 17, 54–59.

45. Long, W.A. and Rubin, L.J. (1987) Prostacylin and PGEI treatment in pulmonary hypertension. *American Review of Respiratory Diseases*, **136**, 773–776.

46. McConnell, R.B. (1966) *The Genetics of Gastro-intestinal Disorders*, London: Oxford University Press.

47. McKinnon, L.J. and Kosloske, A.M. (1990) Prediction of the anastomotic complications of esophageal atresia and tracheoesophageal fistula. *Journal of Pediatric Surgery*, **25**, 778–781.

48. Mendelsohn, M.S. and McConnel, F.M. (1987) Function of the pharyngo-oesophageal segment. *The Laryngoscope*, **97**, 483–489.

49. Murphy, J.D., Rabinovich, M., Goldstein, J. *et al.* (1981) The structural basis of persistent pulmonary hypertension in the newborn infant. *Journal of Pediatrics*, **98**, 962–965.

50. Nakayama, D.K., Harrison, M.R., Serron-Ferre, M. *et al.* (1984) Fetal surgery in the primate. II. Uterine electromyographic response to operative procedures and pharmacological agents. *Journal of Pediatric Surgery*, **19**, 333–337.

51. Nakazato, Y., Landing, B.H. and Wells, T.R. (1986) Abnormal Auerbach plexus in the oesophagus and stomach of a patient with esophageal atresia and tracheo-esophageal atresia. *Journal of Pediatric Surgery,* **21**, 831–837.

52. Noblett, H.R. and Wright, V.E.M. (1978) A complication of continuous upper pouch suction in esophageal atresia. *Journal of Pediatric Surgery,* **13**, 369–370.

53. O'Rourke, P.P., Vacanti, J.P., Crone, R.K., Fellows, K., Lellehei, C. and Hougen, T.J. (1988) The use of post ductal PaO$_2$ as a predictor of pulmonary vascular hyplasia in infants with congenital diaphragmatic hernia. *Journal of Pediatric Surgery,* **23**, 904–907.

54. Philips, J.B. and Lyrene, R.K. (1984) Prostaglandins, related compounds and perinatal pulmonary circulation. *Clinical Pathology,* **11**, 565–570.

55. Rangecroft, L., Bush, G.H. and Irving, I.M. (1984) Endoscopic diathermy of recurrent tracheo-esophageal fistula. *Journal of Pediatric Surgery,* **19**, 41–43.

56. Rehbein, F. (1971) Reconstruction of the oesophagus without colon transplant in cases of atresia. *Journal of Pediatric Surgery,* **6**, 746–752.

57. Rowe, M.I. and Uribe, F.L. (1971) Diaphragmatic hernia in the newborn infant: Blood gas and pH considerations. *Surgery,* **70**, 758–761.

58. Rowe, M.I., Smith, S.D. and Cheu, H. (1988) Inappropriate fluid response in congenital diaphragmatic hernia: first report of a frequent occurrence. *Journal of Pediatric Surgery,* **23**, 1147–1153.

59. Sakai, H., Tamura, M., Hosokawa, Y., Bryan, A.C., Barker, G.A. and Bohn, D.J. (1987) Effect of surgical repair on respiratory mechanics in congenital diaphragmatic hernia. *Journal of Pediatrics,* **111**, 432–438.

60. Schuring, A.G. (1964) Accessory auricle in the nasopharynx. *The Laryngoscope,* **74**, 111–113.

61. Siebert, J.R. and Benjamin, D.R. (1987) Chest size and symmetry in congenital diaphragmatic hernia. *Journal of Pediatric Surgery,* **22**, 394–396.

62. Spitz, L., Kelly, E. and Bereton, R.J. (1987) Esophageal atresia: five year experience with 148 cases. *Journal of Pediatric Surgery,* **22**, 103–108.

63. Stauffer, U.G. and Rickham, P.P. (1972) Acquired eventration of the diaphragm in the newborn. *Journal of Pediatric Surgery,* **7**, 635–643.

64. Templeton, J.M., Templeton, J.J. and Schnaufner, L. (1985) Management of esophageal atresia in the neonate with severe respiratory distress syndrome. *Journal of Pediatric Surgery,* **20**, 394–397.

65. Tibboel, D., Bos, A.P., Pattenier, J.W., Hazebroek, F.W., Madern, G.C. and Molenaar, J.C. (1989) Preoperative stabilisation with delayed repair in congenital diaphragmatic hernia. *Zeitschrift für Kinderchirurgie,* **44**, 139–143.

66. Vacanti, J.P., Crone, R.K., Murphy, J.D. *et al.* (1984) The pulmonary haemo-dynamic response to peri-operative anaesthesia in the treatment of high-risk infants with congenital diaphragmatic hernia. *Journal of Pediatric Surgery,* **19**, 672–679.

67. Waterson, D.J., Bonham-Carter, R.E. and Aberdeen, E. (1962) Oesophageal atresia. Tracheo-oesophageal fistula. *The Lancet,* 1, 819–822.

68. Zarem, H.A., Gray, G.F. Morehead, D. *et al.* (1967) Heterotopic brain tissue in the nasopharynx and soft palate: Report of two cases. *Surgery,* **61**, 483–485.

CRICOPHARYNGEAL DISORDERS

O. Ekberg

The transition between the relatively wide pharynx and the relatively narrow cervical oesophagus is clinically important because of the prevalent dysfunctions in the cricopharyngeal muscle. However, the cricopharyngeal muscle is only one part of the pharyngo-oesophageal segment. The cricopharyngeal muscle acts in concert with the anatomically related and functionally integrated adjacent segments of the pharyngo-oesophageal segment thereby constituting the upper-oesophageal sphincter. The interrelationship between the cricopharyngeal muscle and the oral and pharyngeal function superiorly, as well as the oesophageal function inferiorly, is important in patients with dysphagia. This chapter will therefore focus on disorders of the cricopharyngeal muscle in a setting of the dysphagic patient who suffers from abnormal function. Structural abnormalities in the pharyngo-oesophageal segment, such as diverticulum, web, stenosis and neoplasm, are covered elsewhere.

ANATOMY

The transverse portion of the cricopharyngeal muscle is attached symmetrically to each side of the inferior two-thirds of the cricoid cartilage (*Figure 1.28*). A minor superior portion extends obliquely superiorly and mingles with the inferior pharyngeal

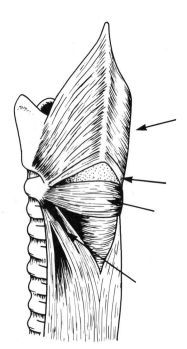

Figure 1.28 Drawing of the pharyngo-oesophageal junction, showing the three portions of the cricopharyngeal muscle as seen from the left and behind: pars obliqua (curved arrow), pars transversa (thin arrow) and pars longitudinalis (thick arrow). The inferior pharyngeal constrictor (open arrow) is also shown. (From Ekberg, O. and Nylander, G. (1982) Dysfunction of the cricopharyngeal muscle. *Radiology*, **143**, 481–486, with permission.)

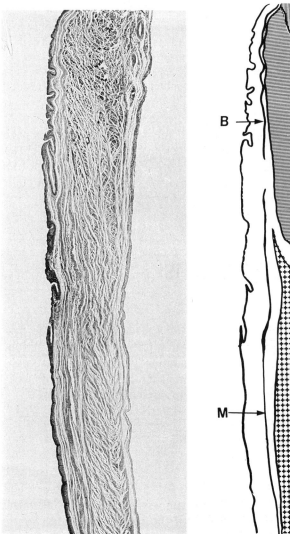

(a)   (b)

Figure 1.29 (a) Histological specimen and (b) diagram of the pharynx and cervical oesophagus corresponding to the pharyngo-oesophageal segment. Haematoxylin and eosin. B = buccopharyngeal aponeurosis; T = thyropharyngeal muscle; CR = cricopharyngeal muscle; E = circular musculature of the cervical oesophagus; M = muscularis mucosae of the oesophagus. (From Ekberg, O. and Lindström, C. (1987) The upper oesophageal sphincter area. *Acta Radiologia*, **28**, 173–176, with permission.)

constrictor (the thyropharyngeal muscle). There is a potentially weak area between these two muscles and it is in this area that a Zenker's diverticulum may protrude. There is also a small longitudinal portion of the cricopharyngeal muscle which extends inferiorly on both sides of the oesophagus and acts as part of the elevators of the oesophagus. However, the bulk of the cricopharyngeal muscle extends in a transverse direction to join the contralateral muscle. The muscle has a height of about 1 cm. In further descriptions this transverse portion will be referred to as the cricopharyngeal muscle. In contrast to the pharyngeal constrictors the cricopharyngeal muscle has no midline connective tissue raphe posteriorly.

No macroscopic well-defined space exists between the oblique and transverse portions of the cricopharyngeal muscle, or between the cricopharyngeal muscle and the musculature of the cervical oesophagus inferiorly (*Figure 1.29*). However, on microscopic examination a variable amount of connective tissue, blood vessels, nerves and ganglion cells was found in a recent study.[32] Moreover, the cricopharyngeal muscle has about the same thickness as the thyropharyngeal muscle above and the musculature of the cervical oesophagus below. The cricopharyngeal muscle also overlaps muscle bundles in the thyropharyngeal muscle and the cervical oesophagus, the muscle fibres of the former being coarser and containing less connective tissue. There is no muscularis mucosa in the pharynx but this starts 2–3 cm below the cricopharyngeal muscle. There is, however, a distinct submucosal layer called the pharyngeal aponeurosis. This is attached to the basicranium and also to peri- and endomysium as well as to the submucosal connective tissue.

HISTOLOGY

Histological and chemical examination of the cricopharyngeal muscle in human beings shows that this muscle is similar to the quadriceps. However, muscle fibres are generally much smaller and more variable in size. The endomysial connective tissue is markedly increased in the cricopharyngeal muscle and muscle spindles are not present. Certain features normally considered to be pathological are also noted in the normal cricopharyngeal muscle. Many of the muscle fibres are histochemically of a high oxidative type and are slow-twitch. This finding is consistent with a proposed function of the muscle as a sphincter.[7,8]

NEUROANATOMY AND NEUROPHYSIOLOGY

The cricopharyngeal muscle is a striated muscle innervated from the nucleus ambiguus which is the somatic efferent nucleus in the brain stem of the vagus nerve. Neurotransmission seems to be the classic nicotinic, cholinergic transmission. Contrary to prior belief there is no sympathetic or parasympathetic innervation.[49,59] This is in contrast to the pharynx proper in which the majority of the contraction is due to non-cholinergic, non-adrenergic transmission.[59]

There is an abundance of neuropeptides in the pharyngo-oesophageal segment most of which are located in the submucosa and around the blood vessels.[77] However, calcitonin gene-related peptide (CGRP) is found on motor end plates in the cricopharyngeal muscle and may have modulating or trophic effects on the end plates.[62]

FUNCTION

The cricopharyngeal muscle is the main portion of the upper oesophageal sphincter and therefore acts to separate the oesophagus from the pharynx between swallows. Functionally integrated are the inferior portion of the thyropharyngeal muscle (above) and the cervical oesophagus (below). Thereby the upper oesophageal sphincter comprises three segments each of which has a length of about 1 cm. The pharyngo-oesophageal segment has three functions: (1) to act as a sphincter of the upper oesophagus between swallows; (2) to open up during swallowing, rumination, belching and vomiting; and (3) to function as an integrated part with the constrictors during the peristaltic transportation of the tail of the bolus into the oesophagus.

The pharyngo-oesophageal segment should open synchronously and symmetrically at the initiation of pharyngeal swallow. This starts at the elevation of the larynx and pharynx which in turn is synchronous with elevation of the hyoid bone and contraction of the thyrohyoid muscle. Opening of this segment is due first to relaxation of the tonic contraction, and second to elevation and anterior movement of the segment which results from activation of the myelohyoid, genohyoid, stylohyoid, thyrohyoid, stylopharyngeal and salpingopharyngeal muscles. The laryngeal movement is an early event in swallowing; indeed myelohyoid activity is the first activity to appear in response to swallowing.[21] Finally, the intraluminal pressure created by the bolus also acts to open the pharyngo-oesophageal segment. The cricopharyngeal muscle participates in the constricting wave which traverses with a speed of about 10 cm/s in the distal direction. Eventually there is a short time lapse at the lower extreme of the cricopharyngeal muscle before the constricting wave reaches into the oesophagus.

RADIOLOGY

Radiologically, the pharyngo-oesophageal segment is identified as that particular segment of the transition between the pharynx and the oesophagus that is collapsed (i.e. not air filled) on lateral radiographs obtained during quiet breathing between swallows (*Figure 1.30*).

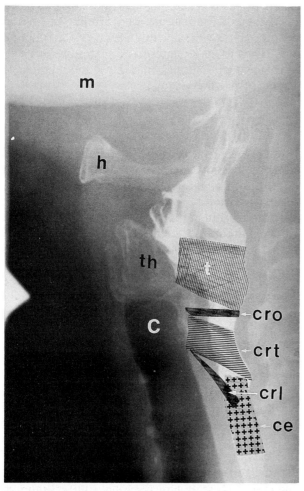

Figure 1.30 Lateral pharyngogram with schematic representation of pertinent muscles of the pharyngo-oesophageal segment. m = mandible; h = hyoid bone; th = lamina of thyroid cartilage; c = cricoid cartilage; t = thyropharyngeal muscle; cro = oblique portion of the cricopharyngeal muscle; crt = transverse portion of the cricopharyngeal muscle; crl = longitudinal portion of the cricopharyngeal muscle; ce = circular and longitudinal musculature of the cervical oesophagus. (From Ekberg, O. and Lindström, C. (1987) The upper esophageal sphincter area. *Acta Radiologica*, **28**, 173–176, with permission.)

The best way to examine the cricopharyngeal muscle radiologically is by video or cineradiographic technique. The patient is examined in an erect position in lateral projection during swallowing of high density liquid barium (250% w/v $BaSO_4$).

MANOMETRY

Manofluorography has shown an intriguing pattern of response in the pharyngo-oesophageal segment during normal swallow. For optimal monitoring, a low-compliance infusion catheter system or a solid state system, as well as a 3-cm sleeve, have proved necessary.[66] The transfer system ought to be capable of recording a flat frequency response of up to 2000 Hz to reduce the distortion of the high-frequency signals generated in the segment.

The closure pressure in the pharyngo-oesophageal segment between swallows varies somewhat with the experimental circumstances in which measurements are made. The pressure profile of the segment shows marked radial and axial asymmetry,[2,45,82] the pressures being much higher when the catheter tip faces either the anterior or posterior walls than when it is oriented laterally. Welch and colleagues have constructed a three-dimensional profile.[82] The pressure increases with inspiration at the high pressure zone (cricopharyngeal muscle) but decreases above and below.[39] The anterior and posterior pressures during suspended respiration are between 100 and 130 mmHg but laterally only one-third of this. The upper oesophageal sphincter pressure is about 35 mmHg with a non-oriented intraluminal strain gauge system or high-fidelity perfused recording system. There is usually a short period of slight increase in the upper oesophageal sphincter tone preceding the deglutitive relaxation. The pressure in the cervical oesophagus may reach subatmospheric levels and it is thought that the bolus is to some extent sucked into the oesophagus.[58]

ELECTROMYOGRAPHY

Electromyographically, there is a continuous spike activity in the cricopharyngeal muscle between swallows. This increases shortly before swallow; thereafter, an inhibition is seen which is followed by a spike corresponding to the peristalsis lasting about 1 second.[64]

ENDOSCOPY

During endoscopy the level of the cricopharyngeal muscle is recognized as a confluence of several folds to a central point and usually located 15–18 cm from the incisor teeth. The muscle, as well as adjacent structures, is covered by a pale mucosa of squamous type. The cricopharyngeal muscle and its closed central opening are regularly found just to the left of the centre.

DEFECTIVE OPENING OF CRICOPHARYNGEAL MUSCLE

EPIDEMIOLOGY

The frequency of this dysfunction varies considerably between reported series most of which have relied solely on radiological techniques. Crichlow, who was probably the first to develop the technique, claimed that the normal cricopharyngeal muscle was never seen, and when seen as a posterior bar this was always abnormal.[13] The frequency of dysfunction was very high with such a wide criterion. Using stricter criteria for abnormality the frequency was found to be 22% and there was a marked increase in patients with non-specified neurological disease and dysphagia, particularly in elderly females.[33]

In a study of 101 dysphagic patients over 80 years, 33% had defective opening of the pharyngo-oesophageal segment. These patients usually showed other motor dysfunctions in the segment.[9]

AETIOLOGY AND PATHOGENESIS

Defective opening of the cricopharyngeal muscle may be due either to an intrinsic abnormality of the muscle such as fibrosis, hypertrophy or hyperplasia or to abnormal relaxation.[76] Delayed but complete opening of the pharyngo-oesophageal segment represents spasm whilst incomplete relaxation may indicate either spasm, hypertrophy, hyperplasia or fibrosis or other deposits. There might even be infiltration of inflammatory cells as in oculopharyngeal muscular dystrophy and polymyositis or dermatomyositis.[18,67,81] A patient with Crohn's disease of the cricopharyngeal muscle has been reported who presented with complete dysphagia and was successfully treated by balloon dilatation.[69]

Oculopharyngeal muscular dystrophy is an autosomal dominant myopathy that exhibits the symptoms of progressive dysphagia with ptosis usually occurring after the age of 40 years. There is a high incidence of the disease in the French Canadian population, as well as in other ethnic groups. Radiological studies show a cricopharyngeal bar and aspiration. Results of electron-microscopic examinations of muscle biopsy specimens from the vastus lateralis and cricopharyngeal muscles confirm the presence of a chronic, active, severe, myopathic process which is more pronounced in the cricopharyngeal muscle.[18,81]

Hannah and Henderson used electron microscopy of the cricopharyngeal muscle in 7 patients and found non-specific degeneration, they concluded that the disorder is a local muscular dysfunction.[40]

Shaw *et al.* reported that in an aged population the upper oesophageal sphincter compliance diminished which was recognized as a decrease in the opening area of the sphincter during swallowing.[71] Another study concluded that degeneration, regeneration, and interstitial fibrosis of the cricopharyngeal muscle was secondary to dysfunction in the pharyngo-oesophageal segment and not a primary lesion.[15] No evidence of underlying vascular or neurological disease was found, but there was a marked increase with advancing years.[28,33] Therefore, altered swallowing in the elderly may be a natural consequence of ageing.

Defective opening of the cricopharyngeal muscle may also be due to involvement of the suprahyoid muscles causing defective upward movement of the pharyngo-oesophageal segment during deglutition.

In the majority of patients with a posterior indentation at the level of the cricopharyngeal muscle, the gullet above and below is wider than in those without such an indentation. This suggests that in the majority of patients the posterior indentation from the cricopharyngeal muscle dysfunction does not cause a substantial mechanical obstacle for swallowing, but the dysphagia is due to paresis of the muscle segments above and below,[23] indeed there is widespread dysfunction or incoordination of the pharyngo-oesophageal segments in patients with such a posterior bar. Therefore, a cricopharyngeal indentation is just one aspect (but a conspicuous one) of segment incoordination.

The elevation of the pharynx is more pronounced in patients with defective opening of the cricopharyngeal muscle compared to controls. The defective opening of the muscle during swallowing has no relationship to defective pharyngolaryngeal elevation,[24] a narrowing immediately below the muscle being regularly seen. However, when the width in an anteroposterior (AP) projection is less than three-quarters of the width in the lateral projection, an abnormally narrow cervical oesophagus is suggested and is an indication for endoscopic evaluation. Treatment is by myectomy.[25]

Jones and colleagues studied the interrelationship between the pharynx and oesophagus extensively and suggested that, neurological disease having been excluded, isolated cricopharyngeal prominence during radiological examination is often an indication of associated oesophageal disease. Detection of a prominent cricopharyngeal muscle during dynamic radiological study of the pharynx should lead to a careful search for oesophageal disease such as gastro-oesophageal reflux, oesophagitis and neoplasm.[44] A comparison of pharyngeal function and gastro-oesophageal reflux revealed that 12% of patients without gastro-oesophageal reflux had defective opening of the pharyngo-oesophageal segment seen as a posterior indentation of the cricopharyngeal muscle. In patients with gastro-oesophageal reflux, 40% had such indentations. No other types of pharyngeal dysfunction showed a correlation with gastro-oesophageal reflux.[29]

It has been suggested that the cricopharyngeal muscle dysfunction, such as delayed or defective relaxation, is secondary to acid reflux. The hyperactive cricopharyngeal muscle is believed to hinder regurgitation of refluxed material into the pharynx, eventually preventing aspiration pneumonia.[5,6,41–43,52] However, no significant difference was demonstrated in a manometric study in sphincter pressure compared to normals.[72,73] It has even been suggested that pharyngo-oesophageal dysphagia resulting from cricopharyngeal muscle spasm may be relieved by treatment of the gastro-oesophageal reflux either medically or surgically.[41,84] However, regurgitation occurs between swallows and assessment of the cricopharyngeal muscle in the above two studies was confined to the behaviour of the muscle only during swallowing.

Experimental observations may help to account for the cricopharyngeal muscle impression in the lumen of patients with gastro-oesophageal reflux. Increased pressure in the oseophageal sphincter has been registered manometrically as a response to distension of the oesophagus by either a foreign body, liquids, or an intraluminal balloon.[36,37,68] The causal relationship between gastro-oesophageal reflux and cricopharyngeal muscle dysfunction/incoordination is not clear. Both segments develop from the foregut and there may be a common defect in neuromuscular control resulting in abnormal function.

Cooke et al. found that the globus sensation, i.e. the feeling of a lump in the throat between swallows, was elicited by distension of a balloon in the proximal and mid-oesophagus in patients with dysphagia but infrequently in asymptomatic patients.[12] The upper oesophageal sphincter pressure increased during insufflation but there was a poor correlation between the upper oesophageal sphincter pressure and the presence of dysphagia. Acid infusion into the oesophagus neither altered basal upper oesophageal sphincter pressure significantly nor elicited

dysphagia. In another study, the upper oesophageal pressure in response to stress did not differ between patients with globus symptoms and asymptomatic volunteers. Even if the upper oesophageal sphincter tone did not correlate with acute mental stress (dichotic listening task), it is possible that those upper oesophageal sphincters that show hyper-responsiveness to other stimuli or subjective intolerance to changes in pharyngo-oesophageal segment pressure might account for symptoms of globus sensation.[11] In a study by Vakil et al,[78] using pH monitoring and manometry of the pharyngo-oesophageal segment, basal segment pressure was similar in normal volunteers and in patients with oesophagitis. Episodes of spontaneous gastro-oesophageal reflux were not associated with any change in segment pressure and oesophageal perfusion with hydrochloric acid did not alter the segment pressure. Vakil et al. concluded that the upper oesophageal sphincter exhibits normal basal pressure in patients with oesophagitis and that oesophageal acid exposure, either spontaneous or experimental, does not affect pharyngo-oesophageal segment either in normal volunteers or in patients with oesophagitis.

Watson and Sullivan[80] reported high resting upper oesophageal sphincter pressures in patients with globus sensation in the neck, with sphincter pressures of 140–220 mmHg (mean 176 mmHg) in patients as compared to pressures of 70–140 mmHg (mean 96 mmHg) in controls. The authors suggest that cricopharyngeal hypertension between swallows may be caused by globus sensation. Interestingly, these patients did not show any radiological abnormalities in the cricopharyngeal muscle during swallowing.[80]

The relationship between globus sensation in the neck, which is not felt during swallows, and defective opening (whether delayed opening or too early closure) is controversial. Whilst it is the belief of many that such a relationship exists, scientific evidence is missing.

CLINICAL FEATURES

Symptoms are usually those of dysphagia with the feeling that something 'gets stuck in the neck' after swallowing. Dysphagia may be severe and there may be complete functional obstruction at the level of the cricopharyngeal muscle. No barium may pass into the oesophagus but in these patients the elevation of the pharyngo-oesophageal segment is usually completely absent.

Lindgren and Ekberg[54] reported that cricopharyngeal muscle incoordination is significantly associated with obstructed symptoms during eating. Defective opening of the cricopharyngeal muscle may be asymptomatic for many years. More commonly, and especially with progression of narrowing, the symptoms of obstruction are likely to develop and the patient experiences a feeling that the bolus or part of the bolus has become lodged in the neck during swallowing. The patient is also likely to choke which may be due to misdirected swallowing with part of the bolus reaching the airways. However, it is more likely that the feeling of choking is from reflexive laryngeal spasm when the bolus lodges in the pharyngo-oesophageal segment. These symptoms lead to restriction or change in the selection of food and the patient will prefer softer food that is easy to chew and/or fragment. Meal-times may become longer and longer and the patient cuts the food into smaller and smaller pieces.

Individuals with defective opening of the cricopharyngeal muscle are likely to experience impaction of foreign bodies at this level, but the majority also have other oral and pharyngeal dysfunctions. The clinical presentation may therefore be dominated by these latter features which present as difficulties initiating swallow and coughing during eating. Therefore, any swallowing symptoms require a thorough clinical evaluation and additionally a video or cine recording of barium swallow.

Spasm in the cricopharyngeal muscle is believed to be a major cause of failed speech rehabilitation following laryngectomy. The poor distension of the pharyngo-oesophageal segment hinders the airflow and thereby restricts the vibratory property of the new pharynx. Voluntary control of pharyngo-oesophageal opening in these patients is impaired. The cause of the spasm in these patients is likely to be the surgical procedure that divides the levators of the hyoid, larynx and pharynx which effectively removes the function of the main contributor to opening.

INVESTIGATIONS

Radiology

There is regularly an early closure in patients with defective opening of the cricopharyngeal muscle which is due to delayed peristalsis in the segment above the muscle. Retention follows dysfunction/incoordination and retention in the segment above is always minimal[26] (Figure 1.31) However, a pseduo-Zenker's diverticulum may be seen indicating the incoordination. Major retention is always due to weak peristalsis in the inferior pharyngeal constrictor (Figure 1.32).

The interrelationship between defective opening of the cricopharyngeal muscle and other oral and pharyngeal dysfunctions is often conspicuous during the barium swallow (Figure 1.31). Defective opening of the muscle is also present, together with a cervical oesophageal web in one-third of patients with neurological disease. This is twice as common as the frequency of webs in dysphagic patients without defective opening of the cricopharyngeal muscle.

Manometry

There is poor correlation between the radiological observations of the posterior cricopharyngeal muscle and increased sphincter pressure monitored during manometry. It is important to realize that the radiological study does not provide any information about the tonicity in the sphincter between swallows: between swallows, it reveals only the length of collapsed segment. In the same way manometry reveals nothing about the pressure circumstances in the cricopharyngeal muscle except between swallows, when the wall is in direct contact with the manometric device. When the lumen opens up, even minimally, and there is air or fluid surrounding the orifice or sensor, the pharynx above and the oesophagus below is open and the pressure which is registered is always the pressure in the fluid between the sensor and the surrounding structure. The pressure is the mean of the pressure over a long segment.

The inconsistency between manometric and radiological observations of the cricopharyngeal muscle can be explained as follows. The incomplete nature of the defective relaxation may cause partial opening of the lumen which may be wider than the diameter of the manometric device so that normal relaxation is missed by the manometric catheter. Secondly, in these patients the cricopharyngeal muscle may relax normally but the lumen is not fully open due to the weakness of the adjoining muscles which should generate pressure to bolus.

COMPLICATIONS

Perforation may occur during oesophagoscopy if the pharyngo-oesophageal segment does not open up normally. This occurs above the cricopharyngeal muscle, usually through the left piriform sinus.[61] The oesophageal inlet is located close to the cricoid lamina and this is anterior to the oesophageal axis at

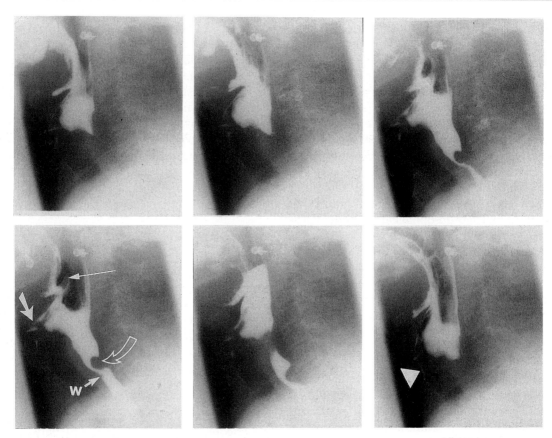

Figure 1.31 Defective opening of the pharyngo-oesophageal segment: sequence of a cineradiographic study during barium swallow. There is a constant posterior inbulging by the cricopharyngeal muscle (bent open arrow). Barium reaches into the laryngeal vestibule (arrow) and further down into the trachea (arrow head). The epiglottis is immobile (thin arrow). There is a tiny web in the anterior wall of the PES (w). Only the most inferior portion of the pharyngeal constrictor musculature is acting normally. (From Ekberg, O. and Wahlgren, L. (1985) Dysfunction of pharyngeal swallowing. A cineradiographic investigation in 854 dysphagial patients. *Acta Radiologica Diagnostica* **26**, 389–395, with permission.)

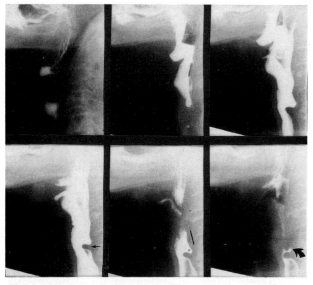

Figure 1.32 Incoordination of the pharyngo-oesophageal segment: there is a posterior inbulging due to the cricopharyngeal muscle (small arrow). The contractility in the most inferior portion of the inferior pharyngeal constrictor is weak (bar). This leads to retention (bent arrow). (From Ekberg, O. (1986) The cricopharyngeus revisited. *British Journal of Radiology*, **59**, 875–879, with permission.)

which the endoscope is introduced. Furthermore the wall of the pharynx is thin. Prompt cervical mediastinotomy is usually advocated to provide drainage for the prevertebral space.

There is a consistent disagreement over the relationship between the cricopharyngeal muscle and Zenker's diverticulum. It has been claimed that premature closure of the cricopharyngeal muscle during swallow is important for the development of Zenker's diverticulum,[34,48,70] this assumption being based on radiological observations of the posterior bar.[1,5,14,19,57,60,75,83] Others have observed that the cricopharyngeal muscle does not obstruct the bolus but that it closed too soon which resulted in pouch formation.[61,70] Such minor retention above the muscle does not progress to a full-blown diverticulum, and in these patients with a so-called pseudo-Zenker's diverticulum, the outpouching is absent because the barium does not extend beyond the level of the distended pharynx. Manometric studies in patients with Zenker's diverticulum have regularly failed to show a consistent pattern of increased pressure.[34,50,51,79]

TREATMENT

No pharmacological therapy for the defective opening of the cricopharyngeal muscle is available and treatment focuses on either compensatory strategies such as change in food consistencies or postural changes. Patients with defective opening of this muscle often voluntarily and subconsciously change their diets. Dieticians are largely involved in treatment planning. They offer advice and determine what food consistency the patient can handle with safety. The patient might even have to change to thin liquids when the opening of the pharyngo-oesophageal segment is small.

A change in posture may be recommended in addition to the dietary regimen. If elevation of the pharyngo-oesophageal segment is defective, the Mendelsohn manoeuvre can be effective in which the patient elevates the hyoid bone with the hand until it reaches in under the mandible. This can prove very helpful when undertaken before and during swallowing. However, to be effective, at least some thyrohyoid apposition is necessary as well as the preservation of reasonable tongue thrusts. Turning the head steeply to one side is also thought to decrease tonus in the cricopharyngeal muscle and thereby facilitate opening.

Cold stimulation of the anterior faucial folds has also been utilized in rehabilitation of patients with neurological swallowing disorders.[56] This is assumed to facilitate the pharyngeal swallow including the crucial elevation of the pharyngo-oesophageal segment. The mechanism has been ascribed to recruitment leading to return of swallowing function,[17] but this assumption was not substantiated in a recent manofluorographic study.[49]

Myotomy

Division of the cricopharyngeal muscle was described in 1951 by Kaplan for treatment of dysphagia in patients with bulbar poliomyelitis.[27] Later Sutherland performed cricopharyngeal myotomy in patients with Zenker's diverticulum because he assumed a relationship between the muscle and the diverticulum.[75] If the myotomy is performed under local anaesthesia the surgeon is able to check the effect of the procedure by demonstrating improved distension when the patient swallows. Should myotomy be performed under general anaesthesia, a nasogastric tube is passed via the rigid hypopharyngoscope into the stomach and the tube is used as a guide. The myotomy includes the inferior 1 cm of the thyopharyngeal muscle and 2–3 cm of the upper cervical oesophagus. Care is taken not to open the musoca because this leads to more frequent leakage

and even to a pharyngocutaneous fistula.[27] Both complications are rare and are treated simply by prolonged nasogastric feeding.[27]

Myectomy is preferred in patients with a cervical oesophageal web and a narrowing of the pharyngo-oesophageal segment. This implies the removing of a 1-cm strip of the cricopharyngeal muscle and adjacent oesophagus together with submucous fibrotic tissue. This provides a more effective mode of distension.[53,55] In patients with cervical oesophageal web there is frequently additional circular narrowing of the pharyngo-oesophageal segment which is due to submucosal fibrosis or fibrosis in the cricopharyngeal muscle. Such fibrosis may be important for the development of the ring.

Myotomy has proven effective in relieving dysphagia in patients with neuromuscular disease.[16,55] Retention of bolus in the pharynx from cricopharyngeal muscle dysfunction is rare and always due to poor oral pharyngeal propulsion – in other words the tongue thrust and compliance of pharyngeal constrictors. Aspiration in such patients may cause or trigger symptoms of chronic obstructive pulmonary disease such as wheezing and severe dyspnoea. These symptoms may be relieved by myotomy in selected patients.[74] Protection of the airways, as judged by tilting down of the epiglottis and closure of the laryngeal vestibule, may improve after myotomy. Such improvement adds to the decrease in bolus retention after the myotomy.[30]

Patients with poor pharyngeal function do not benefit from myotomy[35] because they lack the ability to initiate sufficient elevation of the pharynx and oropharyngeal propulsion in order to overcome the pressure surrounding the pharyngo-oesophageal segment. Instead of improving function, a myotomy in patients with severe swallowing impairment may induce further deterioration of function and should be avoided. The barium swallow can select appropriate patients in this category for myotomy.

Regardless of the aetiological relationship between Zenker's diverticulum and the cricopharyngeal muscle, and even if the tonicity of the muscle may be decreased in these patients, myotomy with or without diverticulum suspension or diverticulectomy was reported to be effective in several series.[5,10,22,35,55,79] Current opinion is that the myotomy should be combined with diverticulectomy for better results.[34]

Myotomy has proved to be effective in relieving dysphagia in patients thought to have gastro-oesophageal reflux-induced cricopharyngeal muscle dysfunction.[24] The myotomy is unlikely to cause regurgitation of refluxed material into the pharynx, a circumstance which potentially could lead to aspiration; however, severe symtomatic regurgitation has been reported in such a patient with reflux undergoing myotomy.[84]

Placement of a stent has been advocated in patients with stenosis of the proximal cervical oesophagus close the cricopharyngeal muscle.[38]

Those patients who received a tracheo-oesophageal fenestration after total laryngectomy to create more fluent speech may experience failure due to defective opening of the cricopharyngeal muscle; an extended myectomy including the inferior pharyngeal constrictor and distal half of the middle constrictor has been performed in these patients with satisfying results.[4]

The passive dilatation of the pharyngo-oesophageal segment with a dilator immediately before a meal has gained limited popularity because the defective opening is usually due to incoordinated motor function, but it is only in those with fibrosis or other structural abnormalities that the dilatation is likely to be effective.

DEFECTIVE TONICITY (CHALASIA)

Defective tonicity of the cricopharyngeal muscle between swallows is a relatively uncommon phenomenon which is usually iatrogenic. There are no reports of any histological or microscopic changes in the cricopharyngeal muscle that could lead to defective tonicity.

PATHOPHYSIOLOGY

The tonic closure of the cricopharyngeal muscle is due to myoneural activity and therefore disorders in such activities may lead to hypotension. The causes of cricopharyngeal muscle hypotension are diseases that involve the lower motor neurons, e.g. myasthenia gravis and myotonic dystrophy. Chalasia has been described as a pathognomonic feature of myotonic dystrophy,[20,63,65] and dysphagia can be an early and prominent symptom in this disease. The mechanism by which myotonic dystrophy causes the chalasia is not known but is probably part of the same degenerative process that affects skeletal musculature in other parts of the body. There is a correlation between chalasia and ageing because this is observed with increasing frequency in otherwise asymptomatic elderly patients in whom no other causes can be found.

Another study reported that several patients with chalasia gave a history of radiotherapy to the neck, often several years before the onset of symptoms.[31] It is unclear why radiation should have a more profound effect on tonicity than on either relaxation or peristalsis in the cricopharyngeal muscle and it is also unclear to what extent the radical neck dissection might have added to the dysfunction. Defective tonicity of the cricopharyngeal muscle has also been reported after myotomy.[27,31,47] However, it is surprising that an adequately performed myotomy does not lead more frequently to lack of tonicity.

Defective tonicity of the upper oesophageal sphincter has been described in patients with Parkinson disease during 'off' periods on L-dopa therapy. These patients suffer from episodic belching and the symptoms subside when apomorphine is given subcutaneously. As the patients were on domperidone it is likely that the effect of the dopamine agonist was central because domperidone causes peripheral dopamine receptor blockage.[47]

CLINICAL FEATURES

Defective tonicity of the cricopharyngeal muscle is often asymptomatic. Impairment of other oral and pharyngeal functions, often present, is much more likely to be the cause of the patients complaining of difficulty during swallowing, including coughing during or after swallow and feeling the sensation of 'sticking' in the neck during or after swallow. As during normal conditions the cricopharyngeal muscle acts as a barrier to air reaching the oesophagus during inspiration, chalasia may lead to aerophagy: during inspiration part of the inhaled air reaches the oesophagus. If persistent, the oesophagus may dilate. The air will be expelled into the pharynx when the intrathoracic pressure increases during expiration or when the oesophagus contracts, i.e. secondary contractions. This is then experienced as belching which can be profuse and may severely inhibit the patient's enjoyment of social activities.[47] Refluxed material may reach the pharynx if gastro-oesophageal reflux is present and even reach the mouth. Such retching, when it incorporates acid or previously swallowed food, is uncomfortable. Cricopharyngeal muscle myotomy should not therefore be performed in those patients with gastro-oesophageal reflux, and tests for such reflux should always be performed in the assessment of patients for myotomy.[31]

INVESTIGATIONS

Radiology

Defective closure of the cricopharyngeal muscle is seen as air in the pharyngo-oesophageal segment between swallows (*Figure 1.33*). It is important to appreciate that most diseases that produce crico-

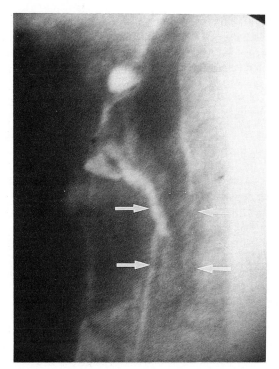

Figure 1.33 Chalasia of the pharyngo-oesophageal segment including the cricopharyngeal muscle. Lateral radiograph after barium swallow. Between swallowing the pharyngo-oesophageal segment is open (arrows). (From Ekberg, O., Lindgren, S. and Nylander, G. (1986) Chalasia of the upper esophageal sphincter. *Acta Radiologica Diagnostica*, **26**, 557–561, with permission.)

pharyngeal muscle hypotension also produce weakness of the pharynx. The oesophagus is often distended if air enters the oesophagus during inspiration.

Manometry

Manometrically defective tonicity of the cricopharyngeal muscle is present when the pressure is below 10 mmHg.

TREATMENT

Symptomatic gastro-oesophageal reflux has to be treated. The patient should be given enforced instructions if regurgitation into the pharynx and mouth occurs. Because the chalasia cannot be treated a fundoplication or some other antireflux procedure should be considered.

DEFECTIVE PERISTALSIS

Defective peristalsis of the cricopharyngeal muscle is extremely uncommon. However, such motor dys-

function is frequent in both the segment above (thyropharyngeal muscle) and that below (cervical oesophagus).

AETIOLOGY

The cause of defective peristalsis in the cricopharyngeal muscle is not fully understood but defective peristalsis is regularly seen in patients with cerebrovascular disease and in those who have other features of a brain-stem lesion. It is therefore likely that any disease to that may cause oral and pharyngeal dysfunction is also able to cause defective peristalsis in the cricopharyngeal muscle.

CLINICAL FEATURES

Patients with defective peristalsis in the cricopharyngeal muscle always have concomitant dysfunction which is likely to obscure any specific symptomatology. The dysfunction in the short cricopharyngeal muscle is often conspicuous but not necessarily symptomatic. Concomitant dissociation between oral and pharyngeal swallow, abnormal closure of the laryngeal vestibule and pharyngeal constrictor paresis is much more likely to be experienced by the patient. Therefore, impaired transport of bolus material over the 10-mm cricopharyngeal muscle is overshadowed by such dysfunction.

INVESTIGATION

Radiology

Defective peristalsis in the cricopharyngeal muscle is an infrequent, isolated finding and the adjacent dysfunctions may overshadow poor peristalsis in the muscle. Normally, the peristaltic wave traverses from the level of the superior pharyngeal constrictor inferiorly through the cricopharyngeal muscle. The short interruption at this level marks the beginning of the oesophageal stage of peristalsis.

Manometry

Manometrically defective peristalsis is seen as an uncoordinated or even absent increase in pressure in relation to the pharynx proper superiorly and the cervical oesophagus inferiorly. The main technical problem is lack of definition of the position of the pressure probe in relation to the cricopharyngeal muscle.

TREATMENT

Defective peristalsis as described above is not an isolated phenomenon but often occurs in association with a multitude of other dysfunctions. Treatment should focus on the initiation of a pharyngeal swallow, oropharyngeal propulsion and closure of the airways. Alteration of food texture, viscosity and head posture is necessary to compensate for these abnormalities. Radiology plays an important role in documenting how such regimens improve swallowing.

REFERENCES

1. Adran, G.M. and Kemp, F.H. (1961) The radiography of the lower lateral food channels. *Journal of Laryngology and Otology*, **75**, 358–370.
2. Asoh, R. and Goyal, R.K. (1978) Manometry and electromyography of the upper esophageal sphincter in the opposum. *Gastroenterology*, **74**, 514–520.
3. Bain, W.M., Harrington, J.W., Thomas, L.E. and Schaefer, S.D. (1983) Head and neck manifestations of gastroesophageal reflux. *The Laryngoscope*, **93**, 93–175.
4. Baugh, R.F., Baker, F.S.R. and Lewin, J.S. (1988) Surgical treatment of pharyngoesophageal spasm. *The Laryngoscope*, **98**, 1124–1126.
5. Belsey, R. (1966) Functional disease of the esophagus. *Journal of Thoracic and Cardiovascular Surgery*, **52**, 164–188.
6. Blakely, W.R., Garety, E.J. and Smith D.E. (1968) Section of the cricopharyngeus muscle for dysphagia. *Archives of Surgery*, **96**, 745.
7. Bonington, A., Mahon, M. and Whitmore, I. (1988) A histological and histochemical study of the cricopharyngeus muscle in man. *Journal of Anatomy*, **156**, 27–37.
8. Bonington, A., Whitmore, I. and Mahon, M. (1987) A histological and histochemical study of the cricopharyngeus muscle in the guinea-pig. *Journal of Anatomy*, **153**, 151–161.
9. Borgström, P.S. and Ekberg, O. (1988) Pharyngeal dysfunction in the elderly. *Journal of Medical Imaging*, **2**, 74–81.
10. Clagett, O.T. and Payne, W.S. (1960) Surgical treatment for propulsion diverticula of the hypopharynx: one stage resection in 478 cases. *Diseases of the Chest*, **37**, 257–261.
11. Cook, J.J., Dent, J. and Collins, S.M. (1989) Upper esophageal sphincter tone and reactivity to stress in patients with a history of globus sensation. *Digestive Diseases and Sciences*, **34**, 672–676.
12. Cook, I.J., Deut, J., Shannon, S. and Collins, S.M. (1987) Measurement of upper esophageal sphincter pressure effect of acute emotional stress. *Gastroenterology*, **93**, 526–532.
13. Cricklow, T.V.L. (1956) The cricopharyngeus in radiography and cineradiography. *British Journal of Radiology*, **29**, 546–556.
14. Cross, F.S. (1968) Esophageal diverticula: related neuromuscular problems. *Annals of Otology, Rhinology and Laryngology*, **77**, 358–370.
15. Cruse, J.P., Edwards, D.A.W., Smith, J.F. and Wyllie, J.H. (1979) The pathology of cricopharyngeal dysphagia. *Histopathology*, **3**, 223–232.
16. David, V.C. (1985) Relief of dysphagia in motor neuron disease with cricopharyngeal myotomy. *Annals of the Royal College of Surgeons of England*, **67**, 229–231.
17. de Lama, G., Lazzara, G. and Logemann, J.H. (1986) Impact of thermal stimulation in the triggering of the swallowing reflux. *Dysphagia*, **1**, 73–77.
18. Dobrowski, H.M., Zajtchuk, J.T., LaPiana, F.G. and Hensley, S.D. Jr (1986) Oculopharyngeal muscular dystrophy: clinical and histopathologic correlations. *Otolaryngology and Head and Neck Surgery*, **95**, 131–142.
19. Dohlman, G. and Mattsson, O. (1959) The role of the cricopharyngeal muscle in cases of hypopharyngeal diverticula: a cineroentgenographic study. *American Journal of Roentgenology*, **81**, 561–569.
20. Donner, M.W. and Siegel, C.I. (1965) The evaluation of pharyngeal neuromuscular disorders by cinefluorography. *American Journal of Roentgenology*, **94**, 299–307.
21. Doty, R.M. and Bosma, J.F. (1956) An electromyographic analysis of reflux deglutition. *Journal of Neurophysiology*, **19**, 44–60.
22. Duranceau, A., Rheault, M.J. and Jamieson, G.G. (1983) Physiologic response to cricopharyngeal myotomy and diverticulum suspension. *Surgery* **94**, 655–662.
23. Ekberg, O. (1986) Dimension of the pharyngoesophageal segment in dysfunction of the cricopharyngeal muscle. *Acta Radiologica Diagnostica*, **27**, 539–541.
24. Ekberg, O. (1986) Elevation of the pharynx and the width of the pharyngo-esophageal segment during swallow. *Acta Radiologica Diagnostica*, **27**, 290–295.
25. Ekberg, O. (1986) The width of the pharyngo-oesophageal junction area. *Acta Radiologica Diagnostica*, **27**, 205–208.
26. Ekberg, O. (1986) The cricopharyngeus revisited. *British Journal of Radiology*, **59**, 875–879.
27. Ekberg, O., Besjakov, J. and Lindgren, S. (1987) Radiographic findings after cricopharyngeal myotomy. *Acta Radiologica*, **28**, 555–558.
28. Ekberg, O. and Feinberg, M. (1992) Altered swallowing function in elderly patients without dysphagia: Radiologic findings in 56 cases. *American Journal of Roentgenology*, in press.
29. Ekberg, O. and Lindgren, S. (1986) Gastroesophageal reflux and pharyngeal swallow. *Acta Radiologica Diagnostica*, **27**, 421–423.

30. Ekberg, O. and Lindgren, S. (1987) Effect of cricopharyngeal myotomy on pharyngoesophageal function: pre- and postoperative cineradiographic findings. *Gastrointestinal Radiology,* **12**, 1–6.

31. Ekberg, O., Lindgren, S. and Nylander, G. (1985) Chalasia of the upper esophageal sphincter. *Acta Radiologica Diagnostica,* **26**, 557–561.

32. Ekberg, O. and Lindström, C. (1987) The upper esophageal sphincter area. *Acta Radiologica,* **28**, 173–176.

33. Ekberg, O. and Wahlgren, L. (1985) Dysfunction of pharyngeal swallowing: a cineradiographic investigation of 854 dysphageal patients. *Acta Radiologica Diagnostica,* **26**, 389–395.

34. Ellis, F.J. Jr, Schlegel, J.F., Lynch, V.P. and Payne, W.S. (1969) Cricopharyngeal myotomy for pharyngoesophageal diverticulum. *Annals of Surgery,* **170**, 340–349.

35. Ellis, F.H. and Crozier, R.E. (1981) Cervical esophageal dysphagia. Indications for and results of cricopharyngeal myotomy. *Annals of Surgery,* **194**, 279–289.

36. Enzmann, D.R., Hareil, G.S. and Zboralske, F.F. (1977) Upper esophageal responses to intraluminal distension in man. *Gastroenterology,* **72**, 1292.

37. Gerhardt, D.C., Schuck, B.S. Bordeaux, R.A. and Winship, D.H. (1978) Human upper esophageal sphincter. Response to volume, osmotic and acid stimuli. *Gastroenterology,* **75**, 268.

38. Goldschmid, S., Boyce, H.W. Jr, Nord, H.J. and Brady, P.G. (1988) Treatment of pharyngo-esophageal stenosis by polyvinyl prosthesis. *American Journal of Gastroenterology,* **83**, 513–518.

39. Goyal, R.K., Sangree, M.H. and Hersh, T. (1970) Pressure inversion point at the upper high pressure zone and its genesis. *Gastroenterology,* **59**, 754–759.

40. Hanna, W. and Henderson, R.D. (1980) Nemaline rods in cricopharyngeal dysphagia. *American Journal of Clinical Pathology,* **74**, 186–191.

41. Henderson, R.D. and Marrayait, G. (1977) Cricopharyngeal myotomy as a method of treating cricopharyngeal dysphagia secondary to gastroesophageal reflux. *Journal of Thoracic and Cardiovascular Surgery,* **74**, 721.

42. Hutcheon, D.F. and Hendrix, T.R. (1977) Esophageal reflux diagnosis and therapy. *Postgraduate Medicine,* **61**, 131–137.

43. Jacob, P., Kahrilas, P.J., Logemann, J.A., Shah, V. and Ha, T. (1989) Upper esophageal sphincter opening and modulation during swallowing. *Gastroenterology,* **97**, 1469–1478.

44. Jones, B., Ravich, W.J., Donner, M.W., Kramer, S.S. and Hendrix, T.R. (1985) Pharyngoesophageal interrelationship: Observations and working concepts. *Gastrointestinal Radiology,* **10**, 225–230.

45. Kahrilas, P.J., Dodds, W.J., Deut, J., Logemann, J.A. and Shaker, R. (1988) Upper esophageal sphincter function during deglutition. *Gastroenterology,* **95**, 52–62.

46. Kaplan, S. (1951) Paralysis of deglutition. *Annals of Surgery,* **133**, 527–573.

47. Kempster, P.A., Lees, A.J., Crichton, P., Frankel, J.P. and Shorvour, P. (1989) Off-period belching due to a reversible disturbance of esophageal motility in Parkinson's disease and its treatment with apomorphine. *Motility Disorders,* **4**, 47–52.

48. Killian, G. (1907) The mouth of the esophagus. *The Laryngoscope,* **17**, 421–428.

49. Knauer, C.M., Castell, J.A., Dalton, C.B., Novak, L. and Castell, D.O. (1990) Pharyngeal/upper esophageal sphincter pressure dynamics in humans. Effects of pharmacologic agents and thermal stimulation. *Digestive Diseases and Sciences,* **35**, 774–780.

50. Knuff, T.E., Benjamin, S.B. and Castell, D.O. (1982) Pharyngoesophageal (Zenker's) diverticulum: a reappraisal. *Gastroenterology,* **82**, 734–736.

51. Kodicek, J. and Creamer, B. (1961) A study of pharyngeal pouches. *Journal of Laryngology,* **75**, 406–414.

52. Larrain, A., Lira, E., Otero, M. and Pope, C.E. II. (1981) Posterior laryngitis. A useful marker of esophageal reflux. (Abstract). *Gastroenterology,* **80**, 1204.

53. Lindgren, S. (1992) Endoscopic dilatation and myectomy of symtomatic cervical esophageal web. *Dysphagia,* in press.

54. Lindgren, S. and Ekberg, O. (1988) Swallowing complaints and cineradiographic abnormalities of the pharynx. *Dysphagia,* **3**, 97–110.

55. Lindgren, S. and Ekberg, O. (1990) Cricopharyngeal myotomy in the treatment of dysphagia. *Clinical Otolaryngology,* **15**, 221–227.

56. Logemann, J.A. (1983) *Elevation and Treatment of Swallowing Disorders.* San Diego, CA, College-Hill Press. CA

57. Lund, W.S. (1968) The cricopharyngeal sphincter: its relationship to the relief of pharyngeal paralysis and the surgical treatment of the early pharyngeal pouch. *Journal of Laryngology and Otology,* **82**, 353–367.

58. McConnel, F.M.S. (1988) Analysis of pressure generation and bolus transit during pharyngeal swallowing. *The Laryngoscope,* **98**, 71–78.

59. Malmberg, L., Ekberg, O. and Ekström, J. (1992) Effects of drugs and electrical field stimulation on isolated muscle strips from rabbit pharyngo-esophageal segment. *Dysphagia,* in press.

60. Negus, V.E. (1957) The etiology of pharyngeal diverticula. *Bulletin of the Johns Hopkins Hospital,* **101**, 209–223.

61. Norman, E.A. and Sosis, M. (1986) Iatrogenic oesphageal perforation due to tracheal or nasogastric intubation. *Canadian Anaesthetists Society Journal,* **33**, 222–226.

62. Ohhaski, T. and Jacobowitz, D.M. (1988) Effects of calcitonin gene-related peptide on neuromuscular transmission in the isolated diaphragma. *Peptides,* **9**, 613–617.

63. Palmer, E.D. (1976) Disorders of the

cricopharyngeal muscle. A review. *Gastroenterology,* **71**, 510–519.

64. Palmer, J.B. (1989) Electromyography of the muscles of oropharyngeal swallow: basic concepts. *Dysphagia,* **3**, 192–198.

65. Pierre, J.W., Craemer, B. and MacDermot, V. (1965) Pharynx and esophagus in dystrophia myotonia. *Gut,* **6**, 392–395.

66. Richter, J.E. and Castell, J.A. (1989) Esophageal manometry. In *Dysphagia – Diagnosis and Management* (Eds) Gelfand D.W., Richter, J.E. pp. 83–114. New York: Igaku-Shoin

67. Romans, B. and Cohen, S. (1988) A rheumatologist's view of polymyositis/ dermatomyositis: extracutaneous and extramuscular involvement and overlap syndromes. *Clinical Dermatology,* **6**, 15–22.

68. Rosenberg, S.J. and Harris, L.D. (1971) A single physiologic mechanism for changing strength of both esophageal sphincters (Abstract). *Gastroenterology,* **60**, 798.

69. Rowe, P.H., Taylor, P.R., Sladen, G.E. and Owen, W.J. (1987) Cricopharyngeal Crohn's disease. *Postgraduate Medical Journal,* **63**, 1101–1102.

70. Seaman, W.B. (1973) Roentgenology of pharyngeal disorders. In *Alimentary Tract Roentgenology,* pp. 305–336. Margulis, A.R. and Burhenne, H.J. (Eds), St Louis: C.V. Mosby.

71. Shaw, D.W., Coole, I.J., Dent, J. *et al.* (1989) Age influences oropharyngeal and upper esophageal sphincter function during swallowing. *Gastroenterology,* **98**, A390.

72. Sokol, E.M., Heitmen, P., Wolfe, B.S. and Cohen, B.R. (1966) Simultaneous cineradiographic and manometric study of the pharynx, hypopharynx and cervical esophagus. *Gastroenterology,* **51**, 960–974.

73. Stanciu, C. and Bennett, J.R. (1974) Upper esophageal sphincter yield pressure in normal subjects and in patients with gastroesophageal reflux. *Thorax,* **29**, 259–262.

74. Stein, M., Williams, A.J., Grossman, F.,

Weinberg, A.S. and Zuckerbraun, L. (1990) Cricopharyngeal dysfunction in chronic obstructive pulmonary disease. *Chest,* **97**, 347–352.

75. Sutherland, H.D. (1962) Cricopharyngeal achalasia. *Journal of Thoracic and Cardiovascular Surgery,* **43**, 110–126.

76. Torres, W.E., Clements, J.L., Austin, G.E. and Knight, K. (1984) Cricopharyngeal muscle hypertrophy: radiology–anatomic correlation. *American Journal of Roentgenology,* **141**, 927–930.

77. Uddman, R., Ekberg, O., Malmberg, L. *et al.* (1990) Neuropeptide-containing nerve fibres in the pharynx in the rabbit. *Dysphagia,* **4**, 220–226.

78. Vakil, N.B., Kahrilas, P.J., Dodds, W.J. and Vanaguas, A. (1989) Absence of an upper esophageal sphincter response to acid reflux. *American Journal of Gastroenterology,* **89**, 606–610.

79. van Overbeck, J.J.M. and Behlem, H.C. (1979) Cricopharyngeal myotomy in pharyngeal paralysis, cineradiographic and manometric indications. *Annals of Otology, Rhinology and Laryngology,* **88**, 596–602.

80. Watson, W.C. and Sullivan, S.N. (1974) Hypertonicity of cricopharyngeal sphincter: cause of globus sensation. *The Lancet,* **2**, 1417–1418.

81. Watters, M.R. and Herbers, J.E. (1985) Premortem examination of the cricopharyngeus muscle in oculopharyngeal muscular dystrophy: inflammatory cells and tubular aggregates – case report. *Military Medicines,* **150**, 686–688.

82. Welch, R.N., Lucmann, K., Ricks, P.M., Drake, S.T. and Gates, G.A. (1979) Manometry of the upper esophageal sphincter and its alteration in laryngectomy. *Journal of Clinical Investigations,* **63**, 1036–1041.

83. Wilson, C.P. (1962) Pharyngeal diverticula: their cause and treatment. *Journal of Laryngology and Otology,* **76**, 151–180.

84. Woolfe, C. and Marryait, G. (1976) Pharyngoesophageal dysphagia and gastroesophageal reflux. *The Laryngoscope,* **86**, 1531.

PHYSIOLOGY

G.R. Vantrappen and J. Janssens

INTRODUCTION

Swallowing induces a contraction wave which starts high up in the pharynx, progresses down the oesophagus, and pushes food and drink ahead of it. In between swallows both ends of the normal oesophagus are closed most of the time by sphincteric mechanisms. The upper oesophageal sphincter prevents air from entering the oesophagus during inspiration. The lower oesophageal sphincter is of primary importance in the prevention of gastro-oesophageal reflux. Both sphincters relax temporarily after deglutition to allow passage of the swallowed bolus.

THE NEUROMUSCULAR SUBSTRATE OF OESOPHAGEAL MOTOR FUNCTION

THE MUSCULAR WALL

The muscular wall of the human oesophagus, about 20 cm in length, consists of an outer longitudinal and an inner circular layer of equal thickness. The upper oesophageal sphincter and the proximal 2–6 cm of the oesophageal body are composed of striated muscle fibres. The distal half of the oesophagus contains only smooth muscle fibres. The transition from striated to smooth muscle is gradual, beginning at a distance 2–6 cm below the upper oesophageal sphincter. Striated muscle fibres extend more distally in the longitudinal than in the circular layer.

In the transitional zone, striated and smooth muscle cells can be seen running together in the same fascicle. Junctional structures between these two types of muscle cells, such as a nexus or close contact, are not observed in the human oesophagus.[82]

The smooth muscle fibres of the human oesophagus resemble those of gastrointestinal smooth muscle elsewhere. Cell-to-cell contact is common, particularly in the circular muscle layer. Electron microscopic studies of the lower oesophageal sphincter muscle show that the muscle cells of the sphincter have extensive evaginations, which are not seen in the circular muscle of the oesophageal body and may be related to the tonic contraction of the sphincter muscle.[77] Ultrastructural studies in the opossum oesophagus indicate that interstitial cells of Cajal make numerous gap junctions with smooth muscle cells and also have contacts with nerve ending. These observations suggest that the interstitial cells of Cajal may function to transmit nerve impulses to the muscle cells.[17]

DEGLUTITION CENTRE

Once it has been initiated, the act of deglutition and all its complex associated activities follow a stereotyped pattern, regardless of the provocative stimulus.[31,47] Physiological evidence indicates that coordination of the various muscle contractions involved in the pharyngeal phase of swallowing is achieved by a well-organized central nervous mechanism, the deglutition centre, rather than by sequential linkages between motor neurons. Although the structure and precise localization of this swallowing centre have not yet been determined, it is known that it is located in the reticular formation of the rhombencephalon and consists of two half centres.[7,32,58] Bilateral coordination of deglutition is brought about by connections between the two half centres, rather than via projections from one centre towards bilateral motor centres. The rhombencephalic deglutition centre receives afferent information from the sensory nucleus of the tractus solitarius, which in turn receives sensory stimuli from the periphery and from the cortical deglutition centre (*Table 1.9*).

MOTOR INNERVATION

The motor nerves of the upper oesophageal sphincter and the oesophagus originate in the motor nuclei of the vagus.[30] The motor neurons of the striated muscle cells lie mainly in the nucleus ambiguus. The nerve fibres are of the somatic type and terminate on motor end plates in the striated muscle fibres, without synapsing with ganglion cells in the muscular wall. Innervation of the upper oesophageal sphincter is predominantly through the vagus nerve, although there are contributions from the glossopharyngeal and the spinal accessory nerves. Nerve fibres arrive in the sphincter via the superior pharyngeal, the laryngeal and the recurrent laryngeal nerves. The motor neurons of the smooth muscle cells of the oesophagus lie in the dorsal motor nucleus of the vagus.[87] Oesophageal branches of the vagi form a network on the surface of the oesophagus. The oesophageal branches from this plexus are autonomic nerve fibres which make contacts with ganglion cells in the oesophagus wall. Some of these nerve fibres run for considerable distances within the oesophageal wall before entering nerve ganglia.

SENSORY INNERVATION

Sensory information from the periphery converges into the solitary tract, the afferent reception portion of the deglutition centre. This sensory information can serve to initiate deglutition and its associated swallowing sequence. It may also alter previously initiated activity, thereby modifying ongoing motor activity. Finally, it may function within reflexes affecting the oesophageal body and its sphincters independently of swallowing. Sensory information from the entire oesophagus, including the sphincters, is carried in the vagus.

The vagal sensory nerves of the oesophagus arise from cell bodies of the nodose ganglion, the principal sensory ganglion of the vagus. Vagal afferent nerve fibres from the pharynx reach the central

Table 1.9 Central organization of deglutition

Level	Afferent impulses	Integration	Efferent impulses
Cortical	Deglutition centre II		
Rhombencephalon	N. tractus solitarius II, X	II, X → Reticular formation (organization in rhombencephalic deglutition centre) Heterolateral centre	II, X, a → Motor neurons of: Trigeminal nerve (II) Facial nerve (II) Hypoglossal nerve (II) Nucleus ambiguus (II X) Dorsal nerve (II X)
Peripheral:	Glossopharyngeal nerve Trigeminal nerve Superior laryngeal nerve Recurrent laryngeal nerve Vagus (rami oesophagei)		Trigeminal nerve Facial nerve Hypoglossal nerve Vagus nerve

→, stimulation; ↔, inhibition; II, homolateral connection; X, heterolateral connection; a, crossed for inferior (and middle) constrictor pharyngis in case of deglutition, not in case of respiration or inhibition.

nervous system via the glossopharyngeal nerve; those from the upper part of the cervical oesophagus pass through the superior laryngeal nerve, whereas those from the lower part of the cervical and the upper part of the thoracic oesophagus run in the recurrent laryngeal nerve. The afferent fibres from the lower part of the oesophagus traverse the oesophageal branches of the vagus.[8] Oesophageal sensation also uses sympathetic pathways that pass through dorsal roots T3–T12.[46]

SENSORY RECEPTORS

Both mechanoreceptor and thermoreceptor mechanisms have been described in the oesophagus of several animal species.[8] The vagal mechanoreceptors are concentrated at both ends of the oesophagus. They are located not only in the muscular wall and the mucosa, but also in the serosa. The sympathetic mechanoreceptors are found mainly among the muscles whilst some lie in the serosa. The mechanoreceptors of the striated muscle layer probably correspond to the richly innervated muscle spindles observed in the canine oesophagus.[3] The mechanoreceptors in smooth oesophageal muscles have not yet been clearly identified, but the intraganglionic

laminar endings (IGLEs) of Rodrigo et al.[69,70] are the most suitable candidates.

The subepithelial plexus, consisting of nonmyelinated varicose fibres just beneath the epithelial layer, contains laminae that lie in apposition to the cells of the basal epithelial layer.[71] Whether these laminar structures constitute the mucosal mechanoreceptor mechanism described by Clerc and Mei[14] remains an open question. Three types of vagal thermoreceptors have been described.[33] Warm receptors respond to temperatures between 39°C and 50°C and cold receptors to temperatures between 10°C and 35°C. Mixed receptors discharge at temperatures in both ranges. It was found that stimulation of warm receptors depresses and stimulation of cold receptors enhances proximal oesophageal contractions. The structures carrying out these sensory mechanisms have not yet been identified. It is possible that they correspond to intraepithelial nerve endings that extend from the subepithelial plexus, pass among the dendritic cells of Langerhans and terminate at various levels between the epithelial cells.[71]

Rodrigo et al.[72] described yet another type of receptor-like structure in the submucosa of the mid-oesophagus of cats and monkeys. Non-varicose nerve fibres formed a series of laminar structures on the surface of blood vessels. The function of these putative arterial receptors is unknown.

THE INTRAMURAL NERVE PLEXUS

The intramural nerve plexus has been studied intensively in silver-stained stretch preparations of the opossum oesophagus.[13] The main plexus is the myenteric plexus located between the longitudinal and circular muscle layers. The submucosal plexus is very sparse. Geboes and Mebis[34,61] studied histochemically stained stretch preparations of the human oesophagus. The submucosal plexus was limited to the deeper layers of the submucosa. Nerve endings were absent in the epithelium. In the subepithelial region, along the muscularis mucosae, enzyme histochemistry was practically negative, suggesting that Meisner's plexus is absent or very sparse in the human oesophagus. The nerve bundles in the plexus of Henle were sparse and formed a polygonal network that was less irregular than that of the myenteric plexus. Ganglia were rare and were usually small, containing only three to four cells.

The myenteric plexus of the human oesophagus showed the same irregularities in the nerve bundle network as the opossum oesophagus, and contained few ganglia. The ganglion density in the striated muscle part increased from about $1/cm^2$ in the uppermost segment to about $10/cm^2$ in the zone of transition from striated to smooth muscle cells. In the smooth muscle part of the oesophagus the density amounted to about 25 ganglia/cm^2. In the lower oesophageal sphincter it decreased to about 15 ganglia/cm^2. The ganglia in the striated muscle part of the oesophagus are bigger (but less compact) and contain more cells than those of the smooth muscle part. Parafascicular ganglia, similar to those described in the opossum oesophagus, occur in the human oesophagus. The plexus of the striated muscle portion of the oesophagus probably serves mainly a sensory role. It is generally believed that the postganglionic fibres pass directly to innervate the striated muscle fibres through cholinergic, nicotinic receptors. Two important effector neurons are operating in the smooth muscle segment of the oesophagus. One mediates cholinergic excitation of both longitudinal and circular muscle layer; the other mediates non-adrenergic, non-cholinergic inhibition, mainly of the circular layer.[9,15,24,25,37,38,75] The neurotransmitter released by the non-adrenergic, non-cholinergic neurons is unknown. Purine nucleotides, peptide hormones, such as vasoactive intestinal polypeptide (VIP), and nitrogen oxide have all been proposed.[9,43,44] Cholinergic excitation of the excitatory neuron is nicotinic whilst that of the non-adrenergic, non-cholinergic can be muscarinic (M1 receptor). Both types of neurons innervate the smooth muscle of body and lower oesophageal sphincter.

Sympathetic nerves of the myenteric plexus probably modulate the activity of other neurons and their neurotransmitter release, and hence can modify the amplitude and velocity of oesophageal contraction and the tone of the lower oesophageal sphincter.[40,59] β-Adrenergic effect is inhibitory and α-adrenergic effect is excitatory.

CONTROL OF PERISTALSIS

The swallowing centre controls the peristaltic progression in the striated muscle portion of the oesophagus by sequential activation of motor neurons, resulting in activation of progressively more distal oesophageal muscle segments.[73] A similar sequencing mechanism may conceivably be responsible for peristalsis on the smooth muscle part of the oesophagus. In several animal species with intrinsic nerves intact, continuity of the intramural mechanism is not necessary for primary or secondary peristalsis to cross a level of transection, regardless of whether the ends are reanastomosed, or are separated with deviation of the bolus.[53–56]

However, a central mechanism is not essential for peristalsis to occur because (1) peristaltic contractions can be elicited in vitro in the smooth muscle oesophagus by balloon distension[62] and other stimuli,[12,41] and (2) in vivo electrical stimulation of the distal cut end of the vagus may result in a peristaltic contraction, in spite of the apparently simultaneous activation of the entire gullet.[25,85] These observations do not exclude the possibility of a central sequencing mechanism resulting in sequential activation of oesophageal smooth muscles.

Two theories for the control of peristalsis have been proposed. According to the first theory the control programme directs the cholinergic excitatory neurons as the final common pathway, with the intramural mechanism normally serving to modulate activity and to provide a local mechanism for distal inhibition. Sequential activation of vagal preganglionic fibres causing sequential activation of postganglionic cholinergic excitatory neurons, has been reported in baboons.[76] Direct recording of swallowing-evoked action potentials in single vagal preganglionic fibres indicate that two types of vagal fibres innervate the thoracic oesophagus of the opossum.[36] The short-latency fibres discharge within 1 second of myelohyoid activation. The long-latency fibres show a range of latencies (1–5 s) which is similar to the latencies of peristaltic contractions. The short-latency fibres could mediate the fast-moving wave of deglutitive inhibition that precedes the peristaltic contraction in oesophagus and lower oesophageal sphincter, whereas the long-latency fibres would be responsible for sequential activation of cholinergic excitatory neurons, as described by Roman and Gonella.[74] The best candidate for this sequential cholinergic activation would seem to be the longitudinal muscle layer. Indeed, longitudinal muscle contraction of the opossum oesophagus has been shown to occur in an aboral sequence after swallowing but simultaneously upon vagal efferent stimulation. In contrast, the circular muscle contraction is sequential for both swallowing and vagal stimulation.[79] This observation indicates that the sequential activation of longitudinal muscle during peristalsis is centrally mediated. Whether the central sequencing mechanism has a role in modulating the sequential contraction of the circular muscle layer remains to be determined.

Studies on the influence of vagal efferent stimulation on peristalsis in the opossum oesophagus[35] showed that the speed of propagation of the contraction could be changed and that simultaneous, or even anti-peristaltic, contractions could be induced by changing the stimulus parameters. Antiperistalsis or simultaneous responses occurred near threshold stimulus parameters, whereas higher stimuli produced peristaltic contractions. These observations suggest that the central nervous system may modulate the occurrence, polarity and speed of propagation of oesophageal contractions by modifying the intensity and frequency of vagal activation.

A second theory attributes the peristaltic contraction of the smooth muscle oesophagus to an aborally increasing latency gradient in oesophageal smooth muscle contraction, an entirely peripheral intramural mechanism.[10,12,18,19,88] According to this theory, the swallowing centre activates an inhibitory pathway in which preganglionic fibres excite secondary nerve cells in the myenteric plexus which then inhibit circular muscle. This inhibition occurs almost simultaneously over the entire length of the smooth muscle oesophagus and results in hyperpolarization of the muscle due to accumulation of potassium in the cell. At the end of the inhibition, potassium escapes from the cell which leads to the entrance of sodium and a rebound contraction. The mechanism of the latency gradient of the rebound contraction remains unexplained.

Two intramural neural mechanisms have been proposed for control of peristalsis in the opossum and the cat.[25,29,37] The 'on-contraction', a peristaltic contraction starting near the onset of vagal stimulation or balloon distension, has a propagation ve-locity comparable to that of swallow-induced peristalsis. This response is atropine sensitive and is induced by low frequency stimulation. The 'off-contraction' has a much more rapid propagation, similar to the delays in 'off-response' observed in vitro in serial muscle strips. This contraction is atropine resistant and occurs at higher stimulation frequencies. The former mechanism is attributed to activation of excitatory cholinergic neurons; the latter would be mediated through the non-adrenergic, non-cholinergic inhibitory neuron, causing hyperpolarization of the smooth muscles and a rebound contraction developing with an aborally increasing latency gradient.

Peristaltic oesophageal contractions are modulated by afferent information emanating from the oesophageal wall during passage of a bolus. Receptors in the mucosa, muscularis and serosa of the oesophagus elicit afferent impulses in vagal afferent fibres. These reach the swallowing centre in the rhombencephalon via the nucleus of the solitary fasciculi[6] and influence the motor neurons of the nucleus ambiguus and the dorsal nerve. Roman studied the vagal output destined to the oesophagus of sheep by connecting the vagus nerve to the accessory nerve and recording the electrical activity of the trapezius muscle.[73] He clearly demonstrated that the pattern of discharge in various efferent units was strongly affected by afferent feedback. Manometric studies in human beings[28,51] also indicate that liquid boluses are associated with a greater amplitude and duration and a slower speed of progression of the peristaltic pressure complexes, and with a longer duration of lower oesophageal sphincter relaxation than a dry swallow is.

The presence of an intraluminal bolus not only changes quantitative variables of oesophageal peristaltic contraction, but it may also change the deglutitive response qualitatively.[53–56] Experiments with oesophageal transection and bolus deviation in dogs indicate that the presence of an intraluminal bolus is a prerequisite for the primary peristaltic contraction to occur in the cervical oesophagus, whereas in the thoracic part of the gullet a bolus, although not necessary, greatly improves the peristaltic performance of the oesophagus. In monkeys with transection and bolus deviation at the level of the smooth muscle segment of the oesophagus, the peristaltic progression of the deglutitive contraction is better when the deglutition is induced by a solid bolus than when a liquid bolus is swallowed. In humans also, liquid boluses of 2 ml elicit a higher incidence of normal peristaltic sequences than do dry swallows. Increasing the volume of the bolus does not yield better results.[28,51] A possible scheme for the control of oesophageal peristalsis is presented in *Figure 1.34*.

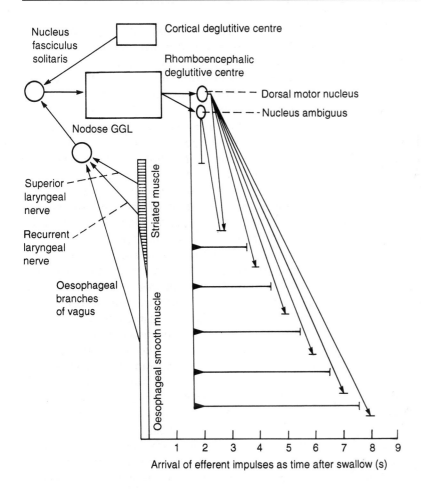

Figure 1.34 Scheme of control mechanisms of oesophageal peristalsis. Peristalsis of the striated muscle part of the oesophagus is controlled by the deglutition centre, acting as a central sequencing mechanism. Control of oesophageal smooth muscle peristalsis is complex. The swallowing centre activates inhibitory neurons over the entire gullet almost simultaneously to produce hyperpolarization of circular muscle. Sequencing results from a latency gradient in the rebound contraction of circular muscles. The longitudinal muscle is activated sequentially by the central sequencing mechanism. The mechanism of coordination between striated and smooth muscles and between both smooth muscle coats is unknown. The deglutition centre may have a role in this coordination because it can modulate the progression characteristics of circular muscle contraction by changing inhibitory stimulus parameters.

CONTROL OF LOWER OESOPHAGEAL SPHINCTER FUNCTION

The basal tone of the lower oesophageal sphincter is an important factor in the prevention of gastro-oesophageal reflux, and is due to a tonic contraction of circular muscle. This active tone is not, at least in the opossum lower oesophageal sphincter, produced by continuous excitatory nerve activity, because tetrodotoxin (which blocks sodium-dependent conduction of action potentials in nerves) does not change the lower oesophageal sphincter pressure when administered intravascularly in large doses[42] and does not reduce the tone of transverse strips of the opossum sphincter.[11] The role of cholinergic excitatory input in the genesis of (part of) the basal lower oesophageal sphincter tone in cats, dogs and humans remains controversial.[26,39,66,92]

The basal lower sphincter tone seems to be mainly of myogenic origin. Careful in vivo studies indicate that the opossum lower sphincter shows continuous spike activity at rest[4] and that sphincter relaxation is associated with disappearance of this spike activity. The resting membrane potential of cat lower sphincter smooth muscle (-40 mV) is lower than that recorded in oesophageal body smooth muscle, which ranged from -53 mV to -43 mV.[91] this lower transmembrane potential difference may allow a constant inward leak of calcium ions leading to tonic contraction. However, a considerable part of basal lower oesophageal sphincter pressure persists in the absence of any spike activity. The genesis of the major (spike-independent) component of the sphincter tone may be related to intrinsic characteristics of the sphincter smooth muscles.

The basal lower oesophageal sphincter tone is modulated by neural influences and by circulating or local hormones. Increases in intra-abdominal pressure[63] and oesophageal body acidification[67] increase the sphincter pressure, whereas ingestion of fat and alcohol, and smoking, reduce sphincter pressure.

Reflex relaxation of the lower oesophageal sphincter is an active inhibitory phenomenon, which occurs in association with swallowing oesophageal distension. The role of the central nervous system in producing deglutitive lower sphincter relaxation is confirmed by studies in cats, showing that electrical stimulation of the dorsal motor nucleus of the vagus, the nucleus ambiguus and adjacent area evokes relaxation, and that this relaxation is abolished by bilateral cervical vagotomy.[5]

Lower oesophageal sphincter relaxation may be induced by oesophageal distension via intramural nerve pathways. The central nervous system may modulate this reflux, because the threshold for inducing sphincter relaxation is increased after vagal blockage by cooling.[66] Lower oesophageal sphincter relaxation may also occur as a consequence of an increase in gastric pressure as in the belching reflux,[60] and it is brought about by activation of postganglionic inhibitory neurons that are neither cholinergic nor adrenergic.[45,65]

CLINICAL PHYSIOLOGY

OESOPHAGEAL TRANSIT

Primary peristaltic contraction, induced by swallowing, is the main mechanism of active propulsion of swallowed material. The wave of inhibition that precedes the peristaltic contraction results in relaxation of the upper and lower oesophageal sphincters and inhibits contractile activity going on in the oesophageal body, thereby assuring that passage of the bolus is not hampered by any functional obstruction. Gravity only has a role for liquids swallowed in the upright position.

Transport can also be achieved by 'secondary' peristalsis. This is a progressive contraction in the oesophageal body that is not induced by a swallow, but rather by stimulation of sensory receptors in the oesophageal body. Secondary peristalsis is usually caused by distension with refluxed gastric content, or following incomplete clearing of the oesophageal content by a primary peristaltic contraction. Secondary peristalsis is mediated by the swallowing centre.

When swallows are taken in rapid succession, two phenomena may interfere with the stereotyped deglutitive response, i.e. deglutitive inhibition and the refractory period following peristalsis. The deglutitive inhibition accompanying the second of two consecutive swallows may inhibit the first deglutitive response. Conversely, the second deglutitive response may be affected by the refractory period following the first contraction sequence.

Based upon manometric, electromyographic and radiocinematographic observations, the following picture of deglutitive inhibition in humans can be constructed.[49,53] If a second swallow occurs when the peristaltic contraction elicited by the first deglutition is still in the striated muscle part of the oesophagus (i.e. after an interval of less than 2–3 s), this contraction stops immediately. If the first deglutitive contraction had already reached the smooth muscle part of the oesophagus at the time of the second deglutition (i.e. if the interval is more than 4 or 5 s), the ongoing contraction is not wiped out but the distal progression of the contraction is inhibited (*Figure 1.35*).

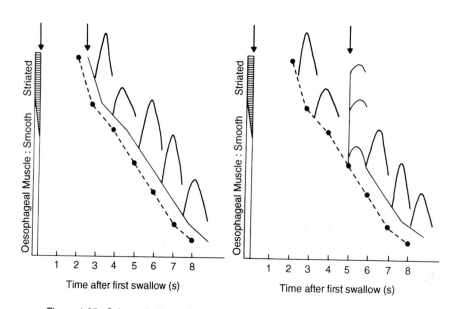

Figure 1.35 Schematic illustration of deglutitive inhibition in the human oesophagus.

The contraction which follows the second deglutition is often abnormal itself. When swallows are taken with an interval of less than 3 s, the first deglutitive contraction is wiped out by the deglutitive inhibition and replaced by a contraction wave with an earlier onset, but which is otherwise normal. However, when the interval between the two deglutitions is 4 s or more, the first deglutitive contraction wave will have already passed down the upper 5 or 6 cm of the oesophagus; the second deglutition then produces simultaneous pressure peaks in the upper part of the gullet or a peristaltic wave with a high progression velocity. It is as though the second contraction catches up with the first. When the two contractions join, the first is inhibited and the second proceeds in a normal peristaltic way. Even if the interval between two deglutitions is as long as 10–12 s, the pressure complex of the second contraction may be of low amplitude and occur simultaneously at different levels. An interval of 20–30 s is required for consecutive swallows to produce normal deglutitive responses.[81]

CLOSING MECHANISM OF THE CARDIA

Several mechanisms have been proposed to have a role in the closing mechanism of the cardia. They include the lower oesophageal sphincter tone, the normal anatomical position of the lower oesophageal sphincter across the diaphragmatic hiatus, the diaphragmatic crura, the acute angle at the gastro-oesophageal junction (the angle of His) and a mucosal plug (the cardiac 'rosette'). Methods to evaluate the importance of many of these factors are not yet available. Only the lower oesophageal sphincter function has been studied in sufficient detail to allow valid conclusions.

Incompetence of the lower oesophageal sphincter, caused by a defective basal sphincter tone, has long been considered the main mechanism of gastro-oesophageal reflux. As many patients with reflux disease have normal basal lower oesophageal sphincter pressures, another mechanism must be involved as well. Recent studies indicate that transient relaxation of the lower oesophageal sphincter is an important contributory mechanism to spontaneous episodes of gastro-oesophageal reflux in normal subjects as well as in patients with reflux oesophagitis.[21,27] In normal subjects gastro-oesophageal reflux occurs exclusively as a result of transient lower sphincter relaxation. A prerequisite for the occurrence of gastro-oesophageal reflux is a fall of lower sphincter pressure to a minimal value of 3 mmHg or less. Even during intervals of increased intra-abdominal pressure, gastro-oesophageal reflux[22] does not occur unless the sphincter pressure is less than 4 mmHg. A low sphincter pressure is often an intermittent phenomenon, presenting as transient relaxations of long duration (15–30 seconds).

The mechanism of transient lower oesophageal sphincter relaxation has not been fully elucidated. There is evidence, that 'transient lower oesophageal sphincter relaxation' can be evoked from below by distension of the gastric fundus,[60] whereas 'isolated lower oesophageal sphincter relaxation' can be evoked from above, by incomplete expression of the deglutitive reflex or the peripheral reflex mediating secondary peristalsis. Whether the transient sphincter relaxation of Dent et al.[21] and the isolated sphincter relaxations of Paterson et al.[64] represent the same phenomenon is not known.

CLINICAL INVESTIGATION OF OESOPHAGEAL MOTILITY

The main method of studying oesophageal motility in humans is manometry, although video-recording of a radio-opaque bolus and radionuclide scintigraphy are also used for oesophageal transit studies. Electromyography is still in the experimental stage.[48,50]

Manometric techniques have been widely used to examine the motor function of the oesophagus and its sphincters. For clinical purposes a bundle of tubes having lateral openings at different levels is used in connection with external strain gauges and a continuous low compliance perfusion technique.[2] Details of the manometric methods have been published in many recent publications.[2,83] Intraluminal pressure measurements yield information on tension developed in circular muscles, but not on changes in longitudinal muscle tension. This technique is particularly useful in studying motor events in the LOS and the oesophageal body; its frequency response, however, is at the very limit for an adequate recording of the fast motor events occurring in the pharynx and the upper oesophageal sphincter. Intraluminal solid state transducers have a much higher frequency response and prevent the need for perfusion, but they are more expensive and vulnerable. Solid-state transducers are used in ambulatory recording systems that monitor oesophageal pressures (and pH) for prolonged periods of time in patients with angina-like chest pain of non-cardiac origin.[57,86]

THE OESOPHAGUS AT REST: INTERDEGLUTITIVE ACTIVITY

Based upon conventional studies it is generally believed that the oesophageal body is flaccid at rest, in the interdeglutitive phase, whereas upper and lower oesophageal sphincters are closed. Prolonged pressure recordings, however, indicate that resting lower oesophageal sphincter pressures vary a great deal in relation to meals and the various phases of the migrating motor complex.[23,78] Both short- and long-lasting inappropriate relaxations also occur. In the oesophageal body, bursts of 'spontaneous' activity (not induced by swallowing or gastro-oesophageal reflux) occur in most normal subjects. They consist of simultaneous repetitive pressure peaks of rather low amplitude in the distal 10–15 cm of the oesophagus, often accompanying the gastric phase III of the migrating motor complex[1] (*Figure 1.36*).

The resting pressure in the upper oesophageal sphincter shows marked radial and axial asymmetry, laterally.[46,90] Its normal maximal value in the resting state is fairly high, up to 100–130 mmHg above atmospheric pressure.

The lower oesophageal sphincter also shows radial asymmetry with maximal pressure left laterally, primarily due to the crus sinistrum of the diaphragm and the angled aspect of the lower oesophagus.[89] Because of this asymmetry, lower oesophageal sphincter resting pressures should be evaluated manometrically using three or four tubes, with the lateral openings facing in different directions 120° or 90° apart. The lower sphincter pressure

can also be evaluated by means of a rapid or a step-wise pull-through. The latter usually measures a slightly higher sphincter pressure than the step-wise pull-through.[89] The best way to monitor continuously maximal sphincter pressure over a prolonged period of time is performed with the Dent sleeve.[20] Normal values of lower oesophageal sphincter pressure vary from +10 to +40 mmHg above gastric fundic pressure.

The competence of the lower oesophageal sphincter is best evaluated by 24-hour intraoesophageal pH measurements. A few reflux episodes (less than 50 peaks/24 h) or a pH below 4 for less than 4.2% of time are normal and represent the so-called physiological reflux.

THE OESOPHAGUS IN ACTION: DEGLUTITIVE ACTIVITY

The upper oesophageal sphincter relaxes after deglutition to allow easy passage of the swallowed bolus. The relaxation may even reach subatmospheric pressures. It starts upon swallowing, lasts for about 0.5–1.0 s and is followed by a contraction which is the start of a primary peristaltic contraction in the oesophageal body. The deglutitive pressure complex comprises several components. An initial short negative pressure peak is elicited by a short inspiration just prior to the swallowing movement (*Schluckatmung*).[84] The main pressure component of the normal deglutition complex is a large positive pressure wave which represents the peristaltic con-

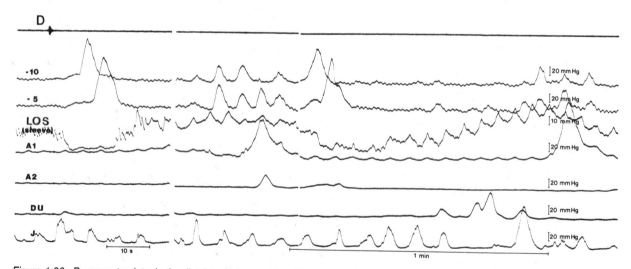

Figure 1.36 Pressure tracings in the distal oesophagus 10 and 5 cm above the lower oesophageal sphincter (−10 and −5), in the lower sphincter, at two levels in the distal antrum (A1,A2), in the duodenum (Du) and in the upper jejunum (J). At the left hand side, the deglutition produces a normal deglutitive response in the oesophagus and the lower oesophageal sphincter. At the right-hand side there is spontaneous activity in the distal oesophagus and in the lower oesophageal sphincter, coinciding with a phase 3 of the MMC.

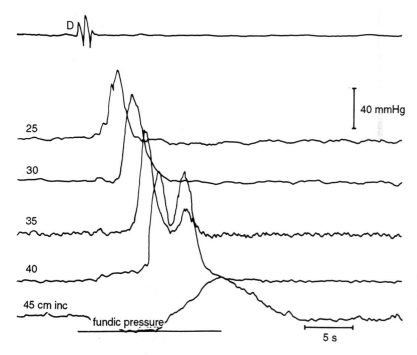

Figure 1.37 Intraluminal pressure recording with a catheter assembly consisting of five perfused catheters with side openings 5 cm apart. The post-deglutitive (D) peristaltic contraction shows an M-shaped pressure wave at level of 41 cm from the incisors.

traction. In most instances it is a single-peaked wave but double-peaked waves (M-waves) are seen in healthy volunteers after about 11% of wet swallows (*Figure 1.37*).[68] The amplitude of the peristaltic contraction varies considerably from one individual to another and, in the same individual, from one segment of the oesophageal body to another. Measured with intraluminal solid state transducers the mean amplitude was found to be 69.5 ± 12.1 mmHg in the lower oesophagus, 53.4 ± 9.0 mmHg in the upper gullet and 35.0 ± 6.4 mmHg in the mid-oesophageal segment which corresponds to the transition zone between striated and smooth oesophageal muscle.[52] The speed of progression of the peristaltic wave increases from 3 cm/s in the upper segment to 5 cm/s in the lower oesophagus, but slows down to 2.5 cm/s just above the lower oesophageal sphincter. The peristaltic contraction reaches to the sphincter 5–6 s after swallowing. The duration of a single peaked peristaltic wave varies from 2 to 4 s but never exceeds 6.5 s.[84]

Deglutitive pressure peaks have to reach values of more than 140 mmHg[80] or over 180 mmHg[16] in order to be considered abnormally high.

REFERENCES

1. Annese, V., Janssens, J., Vantrappen, G. and Coremans, G. (1990) In man not only the LES but also the smooth muscle portion of the esophageal body takes part in phase 3 of the MMC (Abstract). *Gastroenterology,* **98**, A322.

2. Arndorfer, R.C., Stef, J.J., Dodds, W.J., Linehan, J.H. and Hogan, W.J. (1977) Improved infusion system for intraluminal esophageal manometry. *Gastroenterology,* **73**, 23–27.

3. Asaad, K., Abd-El Rahman, S., Nawar, N.N.Y. and Mikhail, Y. (1983) Intrinsic innervation of the oesophagus in dogs with special reference to the presence of muscle spindles. *Acta Anatomica,* **115**, 91–96.

4. Asoh, R. and Goyal, R.K. (1978) Electrical activity of the opossum lower esophageal sphincter in vivo. *Gastroenterology,* **74**, 835–840.

5. Barone, F.C., Lombardi, D.M. and Ormsbee, H.S. III (1984) Effect of hindbrain stimulation of lower esophageal sphincter pressure in the cat. *American Journal of Physiology,* **247**, G70–G78.

6. Car, A. and Jean, A. (1971) Potentials in the rhombencephalon of sheep evoked by stimulation of the superior laryngeal nerve. Contribution to the study of the localization of the deglutitory center. *Journal of Physiology (Paris),* **63**, 715–730.

7. Car, A. and Roman, C. (1970) Deglutitions and oesophageal reflex contractions induced by electrical stimulation of the medulla oblongata. *Experimental Brain Research,* **11**, 75–92.

8. Christensen, J. (1984) Origin of sensation in the esophagus. *American Journal of Physiology (Gastrointestinal Liver Physiology 9),* **246**, G221–G225.

9. Christensen, J. (1986) Motor functions of the pharynx and esophagus. In *Physiology of the Gastrointestinal Tract* 2nd edn, pp. 595–612. (Ed), Johnson, L.R. New York: Raven Press.

10. Christensen, J., Arthur, C. and Conkin, J.L. (1979) Some determinants of latency of off-response to

electrical field stimulation in circular layer of smooth muscle of opossum esophagus. *Gastroenterology,* **77**, 677–681.

11. Christensen, J., Freeman, B.W. and Miller, J.K. (1973) Some physiological characteristics of the esophagogastric junction in the opossum *Gastroenterology,* **64**, 1119–1125.

12. Christensen, J. and Lund, G.F. (1969) Esophageal responses to distension and electrical stimulation. *Journal of Clinical Investigation,* **48**, 408–419.

13. Christensen, J. and Robison, B.A. (1982) Anatomy of the myenteric plexus of the opossum esophagus. *Gastroenterology,* **83**, 1033–1042.

14. Clerc, N. and Mei, N. (1983) Vagal mechanoreceptors located in the lower oesophageal sphincter of the cat. *Journal of Physiology (London),* **336**, 487–498.

15. Crist, J., Gidda, J.S. and Goyal, R.K. (1984) Intramural mechanism of esophageal peristalsis: roles of cholinergic and noncholinergic nerves. *Proceedings of the National Academy of Science of the United States of America,* **81**, 3595–3599.

16. Dalton, C.B., Castell, D.O. and Richter, J.E. (1988) The changing faces of the nutcracker esophagus. *American Journal of Gastroenterology,* **83**, 623–628.

17. Daniel, E.E. and Posey-Daniel, V. (1984) Neuromuscular structures in opossum esophagus: role of interstitial cells of Cajal. *American Journal of Physiology,* **246**, G305–G315.

18. De Carle, D.J., Christensen, J., Szabo, A.C., Templeman, D.C. and MacKinley, D.R. (1977a) Calcium dependence of neuromuscular events in esophageal smooth muscle of the opossum. *American Journal of Physiology,* **232**, E547–E552.

19. De Carle, D.J., Szabo, A.C. and Christensen, J. (1977b) Temperature dependence of responses of esophageal smooth muscle to electrical field stimulation. *American Journal of Physiology,* **232**, E432–E436.

20. Dent, J. (1976) A new technique for continuous sphincter pressure measurement. *Gastroenterology,* **71**, 263–267.

21. Dent, J., Dodds, W.J., Friedman, R.H. *et al.* (1980) Mechanism of gastroesophageal reflux in recumbent asymptomatic human subjects. *Journal of Clinical Investigation,* **65**, 256–267.

22. Dent, J., Dodds, W.J., Hogan, W.J. and Toouli, J. (1988) Factors that influence induction of gastroesophageal reflux in normal human subjects. *Digestive Diseases and Sciences,* **33**, 270–275.

23. Dent, J., Dodds, W.J., Sekiguchi, T., Hogan, W.J. and Arndorfer, R.C. (1983) Interdigestive phasic contractions of the human lower esophageal sphincter. *Gastroenterology,* **84**, 453–460.

24. Diamant, N.E. (1987) Physiology of the esophagus. In *Physiology, Diagnosis and therapy in Gastrointestinal Motility Disorders* (Eds) Champion, M.C. and McCallum, R.W., pp. 1–14. Canada: The Medicine Publishing Foundation.

25. Dodds, W.J., Christensen, J., Dent, J., Wood, J.D. and Arndorfer, R.C. (1978) Esophageal contractions induced by vagal stimulation in the opossum. *American Journal of Physiology,* **235**, E392–E401.

26. Dodds, W.J., Dent, J., Hogan, W.J. and Arndorfer, R.C. (1978) The effect of atropine on esophageal motor function in man. *Gastroenterology,* **74**, 1028.

27. Dodds, W.J., Dent, J., Hogan, W.J. *et al.* (1982) Mechanisms of gastroesophageal reflux in patients with reflux esophagitis. *New England Journal of Medicine,* **307**, 1547–1552.

28. Dodds, W.J., Hogan, W.J., Reid, D.P., Stewart, E.T. and Arndorfer, R.C. (1973) A comparison between primary esophageal peristalsis following wet and dry swallows. *Journal of Applied Physiology,* **35**, 851–857.

29. Dodds, W.J., Steff, J.J., Stewart, E.T., Hogan, W.T., Arndorfer, R.C. and Cohen, E.B. (1978) Responses of feline esophagus to cervical vagal stimulation. *American Journal of Physiology,* **235**, E63–E73.

30. Doty, R.W. (1968) Neural organisation of deglutition. In *Handbook of Physiology.* Section 6, Vol. 4, pp. 1861–1902 (Ed.) Code, C.F. Washington DC: American Physiological Society.

31. Doty, R.W. and Bosma, J.F. (1956) Electromyographic analysis of reflex deglutition. *Journal of Neurophysiology,* **19**, 44–60.

32. Doty, R.W., Richmond, W.H. and Storey, A.T. (1967) Effect of medullary lesions on coordination of deglutition. *Experimental Neurology,* **17**, 91–106.

33. El-Ouazzani, T. and Mei, N. (1982) Electrophysiologic properties and role of the vagal thermoreceptors of the lower esophagus and stomach of cat. *Gastroenterology,* **83**, 995–10001.

34. Geboes, K., Mebis, J. and Desmet, V. (1988) The oesophagus: normal ultrastructure and pathological patterns. In *Ultrastructure of the Digestive Tract* (Eds) Motta, P.M. and Fujita, H., pp. 17–34. Boston: Martinus-Nijhoff.

35. Gidda, J.S., Cobb, B.W. and Goyal, R.K. (1981) Modulation of esophageal peristalsis by vagal efferent stimulation in opossum. *Journal of Clinical Investigation,* **68**, 1411–1419.

36. Gidda, J.S. and Goyal, R.K. (1984) Swallow-evoked action potentials in vagal preganglionic efferents. *Journal of Neurophysiology,* **52**, 1169–1180.

37. Gilbert, R.J. and Dodds, W.J. (1986) Effect of selective muscarinic antagonists on peristaltic contractions in opossum smooth muscle. *American Journal of Physiology,* **250**, G50–G59.

38. Gilbert, R., Rattan, S. and Goyal, R.K. (1984) Pharmacologic identification, activation and antagonism of two muscarinic receptor subtypes on the lower esophageal sphincter. *Journal of Pharmacology and Experimental Therapeutics,* **230**, 284–291.

39. Gonella, J., Niel, J.P. and Roman, C. (1977) Vagal control of lower oesophageal sphincter motility in

the cat. *Journal of Physiology (London)*, **273**, 647–664.

40. Gonella, J., Niel, J.P. and Roman, C. (1979) Sympathetic control of lower esophageal sphincter motility in the cat. *Journal of Physiology (London)*, **287**, 177–190.

41. Goyal, R.K. and Cobb, B.W. (1981) Motility of the pharynx, esophagus, and esophageal sphincter. In *Physiology of the Gastrointestinal Tract*, pp. 359–391. (Ed.) Johnson, L.R. New York: Raven Press.

42. Goyal, R.K. and Rattan, S. (1976) Genesis of basal sphincter pressure: effect of tetrodotoxin on lower esophageal sphincter pressure in opossum in vivo. *Gastroenterology*, **71**, 62–67.

43. Goyal, R.K. and Rattan, S. (1978) Neurohumoral, hormonal, and drug receptors for the lower esophageal sphincter. *Gastroenterology*, **74**, 598–619.

44. Goyal, R.K., Rattan, S. and Said, S. (1980) VIP as a possible neurotransmitter of non-cholinergic non-adrenergic inhibitory neurones. *Nature*, **288**, 378.

45. Goyal, R.K., Said, S. and Rattan, S. (1979) Influence of VIP antiserum on lower esophageal sphincter relaxation: possible evidence for VIP as the inhibitory neurotransmitter. *Gastroenterology*, **76**, 1142.

46. Hazarika, N.H., Coote, J. and Downmann, C.B.B. (1964) Gastrointestinal dorsal root viscerotomes in the cat. *Journal of Neurophysiology*, **27**, 107–116.

47. Hellemans, J., Pelemans, W. and Vantrappen, G. (1981) Pharyngoesophageal swallowing disorders and the pharyngoesophageal sphincter. *Medical Clinics of North America*, **65**, 1149–1171.

48. Hellemans, J. and Vantrappen, G. (1967) Electromyographic studies on canine esophageal motility. *American Journal of Digestive Diseases*, **12**, 1240–1255.

49. Hellemans, J. and Vantrappen, G. (1974) Electromyography of the Esophagus. In *Diseases of the Esophagus* pp. 40–102 (Eds) Vantrappen, G. and Hellemans, J. New York: Springer Verlag.

50. Hellemans, J., Vantrappen, G., Valembois, P., Janssens, J. and Vandenbroucke, J. (1968) Electrical activity of striated and smooth muscle of the esophagus. *American Journal of Digestive Diseases*, **13**, 320–339.

51. Hollis, J.B. and Castell, D.O. (1975) Effect of dry swallows and wet swallows of different volumes on esophageal peristalsis. *Journal of Applied Physiology*, **38**, 1161–1164.

52. Humphries, T.J. and Castell, D.O. (1977) Pressure profile of esophageal peristalsis in normal humans as measured by direct intraesophageal transducers. *American Journal of Digestive Diseases*, **22**, 641–645.

53. Janssens, J. (1978) *The Peristaltic Mechanism of the Esophagus*. Leuven: Acco.

54. Janssens, J., De Wever, I., Vantrappen, G. and Hellemans, J. (1976) Peristalsis in smooth muscle esophagus after transection and bolus deviation. *Gastroenterology*, **71**, 1004–1009.

55. Janssens, J., Valembois, P., Hellemans, J., Vantrappen, G. and Pelemans, W. (1974) Studies on the necessity of a bolus for the progression of secondary peristalsis in the canine esophagus. *Gastroenterology*, **67**, 245–251.

56. Janssens, J., Valembois, P., Vantrappen, G., Hellemans, J. and Pelemans, W. (1973) Is the primary peristaltic contraction of the canine esophagus bolus-dependent? *Gastroenterology*, **65**, 750–756.

57. Janssens, J., Vantrappen, G. and Ghillebert, G. (1986) 24-hour recording of esophageal pressure and pH in patients with noncardiac chest pain. *Gastroenterology*, **90**, 1978–1984.

58. Jean, A. (1972) Localization and activity of medullary swallowing neurones. *Journal of Physiology (Paris)*, **64**, 227–268.

59. Lyrenas, E. and Abrahamsson, H. (1986) Beta adrenergic influence on oesophageal peristalsis in man. *Gut*, **27**, 260–266.

60. Martin, C.J., Patrikios, J. and Dent, J. (1986) Abolition of gas reflux and transient lower esophageal sphincter relaxation by vagal blockade in the dog. *Gastroenterology*, **91**, 890–896.

61. Mebis, J., Geboes, K., Janssens, J., Vantrappen, G., Moerman, P. and Desmet, V. (1989) Immunohistochemistry of efferent and afferent pathways in components neural plexuses of the human pharyngo oesophagus. In *Nerves and the Gastrointestinal Tract*, pp. 562–566 (Eds) Singer, H.V. and Goebell, H. Lancaster: MTP Press.

62. Netter, F.H. (1959) In *Ciba Collection of Medical Illustrations*, Vol. 3(1), pp. 34–46. Ciba Pharmaceutical Products.

63. Ogilvie, A.L. and Atkinson, M. (1984) Influence of the vagus nerve upon the reflex control of the lower oesophageal sphincter. *Gut*, **25**, 253–258.

64. Paterson, W.G., Rattan, S. and Goyal, R.K. (1986) Experimental induction of isolated lower esophageal sphincter relaxation in anesthetized opossum. *Journal of Clinical Investigation*, **77**, 1187–1193.

65. Rattan, S., Said, S.I. and Goyal, R.K. (1977) Effect of vasoactive intestinal polypeptide. *Proceedings of the Society for Experimental Biology and Medicine*, **155**, 40–43.

66. Reynolds, R.P.E., El-Sharkawy, T.Y. and Diamant, N.E. (1984) Lower esophageal sphincter function in the cat: role of central innervation assessed by transient vagal blockage. *American Journal of Physiology*, **246**, G666–G674.

67. Reynolds, J.C., Ouyang, A. and Cohen, C. (1984) A lower esophageal sphincter reflex involving substance P. *American Journal of Physiology*, **246**, G346–G354.

68. Richter, J.E., Wu, W.C., Johns, D.N., Blackwell, J.N., Nelson, J.L., Castell, J.A. and Castell, D.O. (1987) Esophageal manometry in 95 healthy adult volunteers: variability of pressure with age and frequency of 'abnormal' contractions. *Digestive Diseases and Sciences*, **32**, 583–92.

69. Rodrigo, J., De Filipe, J., Robles-Chillida, E.M., Perez Anton, J.A., Mayo, I. and Gomez, A. (1982) Sensory vagal nature and anatomical access paths to esophagus laminar nerve endings in myenteric ganglia. Determination by surgical degeneration methods. *Acta Anatomica*, **112**, 45–57.

70. Rodrigo, J., Hernandez, C.V., Vidal, M.A. and Pedrosa, J.A. (1975) Vegetative innervation of the esophagus. II. Intraganglionic laminar endings. *Acta Anatomica*, **92**, 79–100.

71. Rodrigo, J., Hernandez, C.J., Vidal, M.A. and Pedrosa, J.A. (1975) Vegetative innervation of the esophagus. III. Intraepithelial endings. *Acta Anatomica*, **92**, 242–258.

72. Rodrigo, J., Nava, B.E. and Pedrosa, J. (1970) Study of vegetative innervation in the oesophagus. I. Perivascular endings. *Trabajos des Instituto Cajal de Investigaciones Biologicas*, **62**, 39–65.

73. Roman, C. (1966) Nervous control of esophageal peristalsis. *Journal of Physiology*, **58**, 79–108.

74. Roman, C. and Gonella, J. (1981). Extrinsic control of digestive tract motility. In *Physiology of the Gastrointestinal Tract*, pp. 289–333 (Ed.) Johnson, L.R. New York: Raven Press.

75. Roman, C. and Gonella, J. (1986) Extrinsic control of digestive tract motility. In *Physiology of the Gastrointestinal Tract*, 2nd edn, pp. 507–554 (Ed.) Johnson, L.R. New York: Raven Press.

76. Roman, C. and Tiefenbach, L. (1972) Recording the unit activity of vagal motor fibres innervating the baboon esophagus. *Journal of Physiology (Paris)*, **64**, 479–506.

77. Seelig, L.L. Jr and Goyal, R.K. (1978) Morphological evaluation of opossum lower esophageal sphincter. *Gastroenterology*, **75**, 51–58.

78. Smout, A.J.P.M., Bogaard, J.W., Grade, A.C., Ten Thye, O.J., Akkermans, L.M.A. and Wittebol, P. (1985) Effects of Cisapride, a new gastrointestinal prokinetic substance, on interdigestive and postprandial motor activity of the distal oesophagus in man. *Gut*, **26**, 246–251.

79. Sugarbaker, D.J., Rattan, S. and Goyal, R.K. (1984) Swallowing induces sequential activation of esophageal longitudinal smooth muscle. *American Journal of Physiology (Gastrointestinal Liver Physiology* 10), **247**, G515–G519.

80. Traube, M., Abbili, R. and McCallum, R.W. (1983) High-amplitude peristaltic esophageal contractions associated with chest pain. *Journal of the American Medical Association*, **250**, 2655–2659.

81. Vantrappen, G.(1971) Measurements in the electrical activity. In *Postgraduate Course 'The Esophagus'*, pp. 26. Florida: American Gastroenterological Association.

82. Vantrappen, G. (1987) Esophageal transit and motility. In *Cellular Physiology and Clinical Studies of Gastrointestinal Smooth Muscle*, pp. 287–309 (Ed.) Szurszewski, J.H. Amsterdam: Elsevier Science.

83. Vantrappen, G., Clouse, R., Corazziari, E., Janssens, J. and Wienbeck, M. (1989) Standardization of oesophageal manometry: An outline of required measurements and technical standards. *Gastroenterology International*, **2**, 150–154.

84. Vantrappen, G. and Hellemans, J. (1967) Studies on the normal deglutition complex. *American Journal of Digestive Diseases*, **12**, 255–260.

85. Vantrappen, G. and Hellemans, J. (1970) Esophageal motility. *Rendiconti Romani di Gastroenterologia*, **2**, 7–19.

86. Vantrappen, G., Servaes, J., Janssens, J. and Peeters, T. (1982). Twenty-four-hour esophageal pH- and pressure recording in outpatients. In *Motility of the Digestive Tract*, pp. 293–297 (Ed.) Wienbeck, M. New York: Raven Press.

87. Weisbrodt, N.W. (1974). In *Gastrointestinal Physiology*, pp. 139–183 (Eds) Jacobson, E.D. and Shanbour, L.L. Baltimore, MD: University Park Press.

88. Weisbrodt, N.W. and Christensen, J. (1972) Gradients of contractions in the opossum esophagus. *Gastroenterology*, **62**, 1159–1166.

89. Welch, R.W. and Drake, S.T. (1980) Normal lower esophageal sphincter pressure: a comparison of rapid vs slow pull through techniques. *Gastroenterology*, **78**, 1446–1451.

90. Welch, R.W., Luckmann, K., Ricks, P.M., Drake, S.T. and Gates, G.A. (1979) Manometry of the normal esophageal sphincter and its alteration in laryngectomy. *Journal of Clinical Investigation*, **63**, 1036–1041.

91. Zelcer, E. and Weisbrodt, N.W. (1984) Electrical and mechanical activity in the lower esophageal sphincter of the cat. *American Journal of Physiology*, **246**, G243–G247.

92. Zwick, R., Bowes, K.L., Daniel, E.E. and Sarna, S.K. (1976) Mechanism of action of pentagastrin on the lower esophageal sphincter. *Journal of Clinical Investigation*, **57**, 1644–1651.

MOTILITY DISORDERS

G. R. Vantrappen and J. Janssens

Primary oesophageal motility disorders constitute a spectrum including achalasia, diffuse oesophageal spasm and intermediate conditions.[91] In addition, non-specific oesophageal motility disorders have been described, which include conditions such as hypertensive lower oesophageal sphincter and the nutcracker oesophagus.[6,35] The latter two conditions have been identified on the basis of high resting or contractile pressures not accompanied by abnormalities of peristalsis or sphincteric relaxation. The relationship between these manometric findings and clinical symptoms remains controversial. The irritable oesophagus denotes a condition in which the gullet appears hypersensitive to various stimuli, such as acid or motility disorders.[85]

Secondary oesophageal motility disorders include secondary forms of achalasia (due to malignancy, Chagas' disease or pseudo-obstruction), postsurgical conditions, amyloidosis, sarcoidosis, etc. Severe gastro-oesophageal reflux may induce oesophageal motility disturbances mimicking the manometric picture of diffuse oesophageal spasm. Diabetic and alcoholic neuropathy, and striated and smooth muscle diseases, may also produce secondary motility disturbances.

PRIMARY OESOPHAGEAL MOTILITY DISORDERS

ACHALASIA (ACHALASIA OF THE CARDIA)

Typical achalasia is a disease of unknown aetiology characterized by aperistalsis in the body of the oesophagus and defective relaxation of the lower oesophageal sphincter, which is often hypertonic. Loss of propulsive peristaltic contractions, together with defective sphincter relaxations, cause stasis of food in a progressively dilating gullet. The oesophageal stasis is the common factor in most of the symptoms and complications of achalasia.

Incidence

The incidence of achalasia is in the range of 1 per 100 000 population per year. The disease can occur at any age, but only 5% of the patients have onset of symptoms before the age of 14 years.

Pathology and pathophysiology

The pathology of achalasia is still incompletely understood. Lesions have been demonstrated in the dorsal vagal nucleus,[13] in the vagal nerve fibres,[14] in Auerbach's plexus and in the oesophageal muscle.[82] There is pharmacological evidence of denervation.[51] Direct cholinergic stimulation by methacholine (Mecholyl) results in a strong contractile reaction in both the oesophageal body and the lower oesophageal sphincter. The denervation, however, cannot be complete because a cholinesterase inhibitor (edrophonium) will increase the pressure in the LOS.[20] There is also pharmacological evidence that the non-adrenergic, non-cholinergic, inhibitory, postganglionic nervous system is impaired in achalasia patients. This system mediates sphincter relaxation in the opossum and may also have a role in the peristaltic progression of oesophageal contractions.[29,41]

Clinical features

Dysphagia, regurgitation, weight loss and pain are the most important symptoms.[86] Characteristically, the patient has dysphagia for liquids as well as solids from the onset of the disease. This 'functional dysphagia' differs from organic dysphagia, which is initially for solids, and only later for both solids and liquids. The degree of swallowing difficulty varies considerably from day to day, but tends to get worse with time. Prandial or postprandial regurgitation is often mistaken for vomiting. Retention of large quantities of food in a dilated gullet may lead to regurgitation when the patient is in the recumbent position or to aspiration in the airways and bronchopulmonary complications. The degree of weight loss is related to the severity of the dysphagia. Retrosternal pain occurs more often in the younger age groups and in the initial stages of the disease. The frequency of these various symptoms is summarized in *Figure 1.38*.

Investigations

The diagnosis can be made in most instances by radiological examination. However, manometry allows a better appreciation and a quantitative evaluation of the diagnostically important motor disorders.

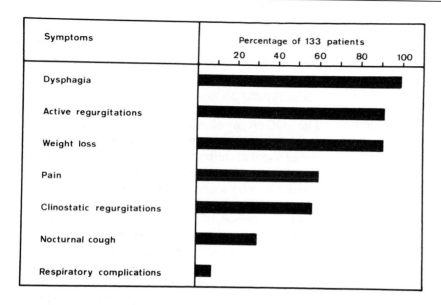

Symptoms	Percentage of 133 patients

Dysphagia

Active regurgitations

Weight loss

Pain

Clinostatic regurgitations

Nocturnal cough

Respiratory complications

Figure 1.38 Frequency of symptoms of achalasia.

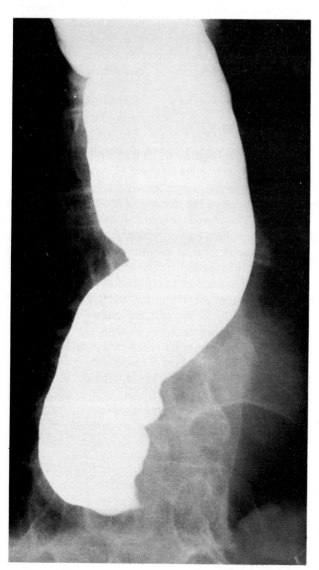

Figure 1.39 Barium swallow showing classic achalasia.

Radiology

Cineradiography may visualize the absence of peristaltic contraction waves and the disorganized and non-propulsive nature of the contractions. Because the lower oesophageal sphincter fails to open normally following deglutition, the head of the barium column takes a smoothly tapered 'bird's beak' appearance (*Figure 1.39*). The oesophageal body gradually becomes dilated, and eventually elongated and tortuous: the gastric air bubble disappears.

Manometry

On manometric examination the deglutitive pressure peaks develop shortly after swallowing and occur simultaneously throughout the oesophageal body (*Figure 1.40*). In some patients progressive contractions still occur in the upper few centimetres of the gullet, corresponding to the striated muscle portion. After treatment the oesophageal diameter decreases in nearly one-third of the patients and peristaltic contractions may reappear.[91]

The amplitude of the pressure waves decreases when the oesophagus becomes dilated and they assume a typical broad-based shape. When the amplitude of the contraction waves is high, the pressure waves are repetitive, and spontaneous contractions occur, the condition is called 'vigorous achalasia'.[72] The hyperactive deglutitive motility response of the oesophageal body and some clinical features of vigorous achalasia resemble the pattern of symptomatic diffuse oesophageal spasm. As in achalasia, however, peristaltic waves are not seen, and the sphincteric relaxations are defective.

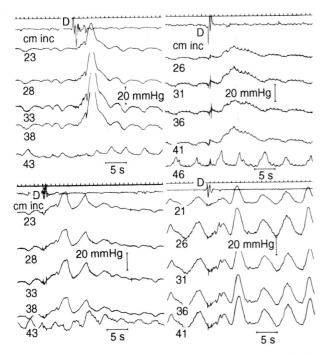

Figure 1.40 Manometric patterns in achalasia (D = deglutition): simultaneous waves of normal amplitude (upper left); simultaneous waves in dilated oesophagus (upper right); simultaneous repetitive waves (lower left); vigorous achalasia (lower right).

The resting pressure of the lower oesophageal sphincter is increased in achalasia.[21] Pressures above 30 mmHg have been measured in from 40%[8] to 90%[21] of patients. Furthermore, sphincter relaxation upon swallowing is incomplete (about 30% relaxation), in contrast to the normal sphincter, which relaxes completely. The residual sphincter pressure seems responsible for the obstruction to the passage from the oesophagus into the stomach.

Differential diagnosis

A mega-oesophagus with a smooth distal narrowing has been found in children with familial dysautonomia (Riley–Day syndrome), but in these patients oesophageal peristalsis is preserved.[47] Amyloidosis may cause a mega-oesophagus which resembles achalasia on both radiological and manometric examination. Bulbar paralysis and intestinal pseudo-obstruction can also cause an atonic oesophagus. In these instances extra-oesophageal manifestations will point to the diagnosis. In scleroderma the skeletal muscle portion of the oesophagus is usually not involved, some degree of peristalsis may be preserved in the smooth muscle portion, the oesophageal contractions are weak and the tone of the lower oesophageal sphincter is decreased. Barium is readily evacuated in the upright position but not in the recumbent position.

Carcinoma of the cardia may pose a difficult diagnostic problem. Oesophagoscopy with biopsy may be necessary to rule out carcinomatous involvement of the distal oesophagus. Endoscopy is also the best way to recognize carcinomatous change (usually in the body of the oesophagus), which may complicate long-standing achalasia.

Pancreatic, bronchial and gastric cancer, and lymphoma of the distal oesophagus, may produce an achalasia-like picture.[48,83] The manometric features are identical to those in idiopathic achalasia, but the clinical history is slighly different. Patients are usually more than 50 years old, have a short duration of dysphagia (less than 1 year) and weight loss is prominent. The mechanism of this type of secondary achalasia is unknown.

Treatment

Current treatment of achalasia is palliative and aims at improving oesophageal emptying by reducing the resistance at the cardia to a sufficiently low level to allow aboral flow but not sufficiently to allow gastro-oesophageal reflux.

Drug treatment

Early trials with anticholinergics and β-adrenergic agonists did not demonstrate any substantial benefit. More recently the effect of nitrates and calcium channel blockers has been evaluated because these agents have been shown to decrease lower oesophageal sphincter pressure.

Prolonged treatment with nifedipine, a calcium channel blocker, significantly reduced symptoms of dysphagia, but only slightly reduced lower oesophageal sphincter pressure (28% reduction) and had no effect on oesophageal emptying as measured by scintigraphy.[11,79] Side effects were common. The effect of diltiazem, another calcium channel blocker, on lower oesophageal sphincter pressure and on symptoms was marginal.[73]

A randomized cross-over study compared the effect of a 2-week treatment with isosorbide dinitrate, the long-acting form of glyceryl trinitrate (nitroglycerin), with that nifedipine in 15 achalasia patients. Isosorbide dinitrate resulted in better subjective improvement, but also had a higher incidence of side effects.

With the current drug therapy available it seems

hard to justify its life-long use when other treatment modalities, e.g. pneumatic dilatation or surgery, result in excellent or good long-term results in 80% of patients. It seems reasonable to restrict drug therapy to the following indications:

1. As a temporary measure until more definitive treatment is performed.
2. As adjuvant therapy for patients in whom dilatation or surgery was only partially successful.
3. As palliative therapy in patients with an unacceptably high risk for more invasive therapy.

In these circumstances nifedipine 10–20 mg or isosorbide dinitrate 5 mg sublingually before each meal is recommended.

Dilatation

Most authors report excellent to good results in about 67% of the patients after a single dilatation with a hydrostatic or pneumatic bag of fixed diameter, whilst about 18% are not improved (*Table 1.10*). Treatment by repeated dilatations with bags of progressively larger diameter yields excellent to good results in 77% of the patients, whereas 7% are not improved.[88] The technique of progressive pneumatic dilatation consists of a series of two to four dilatations with bags of diameters of 3–4.5 cm. Disappearance of dysphagia, ease in emptying the oesophagus on fluoroscopy and, particularly, a substantial reduction of the lower oesophageal sphincter pressure are used as a guide to the required number of dilatations.[89] Contraindications to pneumatic dilatation are (1) poor patient cooperation because of young age or psychiatric illness, (2) inability to exclude an organic stenosis, (3) the presence of lesions of the cardia or the stomach which make surgery mandatory, such as carcinoma, and (4) the occurrence of an epiphrenic diverticulum, which increases the risk of perforation.

The major immediate complication of progressive forcible dilatation is perforation at the lower end of the oesophagus. In the experience of the authors this occurred in 13 of 570 patients (2.3%).[88] Conservative treatment with antibiotics and total parenteral feeding produced complete healing in 10 of the 13 patients. Two other patients were treated by surgical drainage, and one patient died. The late results were excellent or good in 80% of this subgroup of patients.

Myotomy

The modified Heller procedure yields excellent to good results in 65–88% of the patients (*Table 1.11*).[2,5,10,55,88] The incidence of reflux and reflux oesophagitis (3–52%) has been sufficiently high for many surgeons to combine the Heller myotomy with an antireflux procedure.[10,62] Excellent to good results are reported in 54–100% of patients treated in this way. Because the follow-up period of this type of surgery has not been sufficiently long and the number of patients so treated not sufficiently large, it is too early to draw firm conclusions on its value. As good prospective trials are lacking, a reasonable choice between forceful dilatation and surgery must be based on retrospective studies.[90] The only prospective study published thus far yielded excellent or good long-term results in 95% of the patients after myotomy as compared to 65% after dilatation, which, however, is an unusually low figure for outcome following a forceful dilatation.[23] The two retrospective studies which are reasonably comparable in various aspects are the Mayo Clinic myotomy study and the Leuven dilatation study.[88,90] *Table 1.12* compares the results of these two studies. The number of excellent or good results is higher in the Mayo Clinic study (85% vs 77%) whereas early morbidity and mortality are similar. Late strictures occurred in only 0.7% of the Leuven patients as compared to 3% in the Mayo Clinic series (which

Table 1.10 Late results of forcible dilatation in achalasia

	Number of patients	Duration of follow-up (years)	Symptomatic results (%)			
			Excellent	Good	Fair	Poor
Single hydrostatic dilatation						
Olsen *et al.*[56]	452	4–16	68.2		30.2	
Sanderson *et al.*[71]	313	2.5	28.2	37	16	19
Progressive pneumatic dilatation						
Vantrappen and Hellemans[88]	403	7.8	37.5	39.5	8.7	14.4

Table 1.11 Late results of surgery in achalasia

	Number followed up	Follow-up (years)	Symptomatic results (%)			
			Excellent	Good	Fair	Poor
Myotomy						
Okike et al.[55]	456	6, 6.5	50	35	9	6
Akuamoa[2]	84	6	53.6	17.8	16.7	11.9
Black et al.[10]	53	4	67.9	15.1		17
Barker and Franklin[5]	30	1	93.3	3.3		3.3
	14	10–20	35.7	28.6	35.7	
Myotomy + antireflux procedure						
Black et al.[10]						
+ anterior suture	44	4	54.5	38.7		6.8
+ formal repair	11	4	100	0	0	0
Ribet et al.[62]	45	2–10	38	41	21	

Table 1.12 Comparison of myotomy and forcible dilatation

	Myotomy (Mayo Clinic)	Progressive dilatation (Leuven)
Number of patients with follow-up	427	403
Duration of follow-up (years)	6; 6.5	7.8
Results:		
excellent or good (%)	85	77
fair (%)	9	8.7
poor (%)	6	14.4
improved (%)	94	93
Early morbidity (%)		
(surgical oesophageal leak; perforation)	1	2.6
Mortality (%)	0.21	0.17
Late stricture (%)	3	0.7

has an unusually low incidence of severe peptic complications after myotomy). Therefore, it seems reasonable to perform forceful dilatations as the initial treatment and to reserve cardiomyotomy for those patients who fail to benefit from dilatations.

DIFFUSE OESOPHAGEAL SPASM

Symptomatic diffuse oesophageal spasm is characterized by clinical symptoms of intermittent chest pain, dysphagia or both in the absence of a demonstrable organic lesion, and by abnormal, non-peristaltic contractions on manometry or radiological examination.[30,34,40]

Incidence

Typical diffuse spasm is a rare disorder, being less than one-fifth as frequent as achalasia. It can occur in either sex and at any age, but is more common in individuals over 50 years of age.

Pathology

The pathology of diffuse oesophageal spasm is not well known. Oesophageal wall thickening has been ascribed to both hyperplasia and hypertrophy of smooth muscle cells.[13,36] The nervous tissue changes are less pronounced than in achalasia but show the same pattern, i.e. decreased number of ganglion cells,[1] degenerative nerve endings[13] and inflammation.[74]

Pathophysiology

The oesophageal motility disorders of patients with diffuse oesophageal spasm are less severe than those of achalasia patients. The oesophagus has not completely lost the capacity to produce normal peristaltic contractions and normal lower oesophageal sphincter relaxation. In the typical patient peristalsis progresses in a normal way from the pharynx along the oesophagus over a length of several centimetres. Once in the middle third of the gullet the peristaltic contraction is replaced by 'tertiary contractions' which develop simultaneously over the entire length of the remaining distal oesophagus. The tertiary contractions of diffuse oesophageal spasm often produce pressure waves of high amplitude and longer duration. Not infrequently deglutition results in repetitive contractions (several waves in reponse to a single swallow).[22] Sometimes the peristaltic progression seems to be interrupted in a segment of several centimetres and reappears in the more distal part of the oesophagus. The propulsion of the swallowed bolus may be hindered by 'spastic' tertiary contractions which obliterate the lumen prior to the passage of the bolus. This is one mechanism for dysphagia, another being defective relaxation of the lower oesophageal sphincter. Pain is probably produced by strong contractions following deglutition or occurring 'spontaneously'.

Described in 1960[17,92] when oesophageal manometry was still performed with an unperfused catheter system, the 'hypertensive lower oesophageal sphincter' syndrome remains a controversial issue. The mean resting sphincter pressure in this syndrome was 45.9 mmHg as compared to 18 mmHg in a control series. A hypertensive sphincter may occur as an isolated finding, or it may be accompanied by distal oesophageal body contraction abnormalities which may range from the nutcracker oesophagus (abnormally increased distal oesophageal body contraction amplitude)[21,80] to diffuse oesophageal spasm.[21,37,61,87] Most[35,59,80] but not all[93] manometric studies in patients with the hypertensive lower oesophageal sphincter syndrome have shown that the percentage relaxation of the sphincter after swallowing does not differ significantly from that of controls. Consequently, the residual pressure after swallowing is higher than in controls, which may contribute to the development of dysphagia.

The symptoms that have been ascribed to a hypertensive lower oesophageal sphincter include chest pain and dysphagia. As for the nutcracker oesophagus it is unclear whether the hypertensive lower oesophageal sphincter is merely an abnormal manometric finding or constitutes a clinically important abnormality. It is possible that a hypertensive lower oesophageal sphincter is an epiphenomenon from an exaggerated response to various stimuli such as chest pain or environmental stress.[3]

Clinical features

Most patients have both pain and dysphagia; these occur intermittently and vary from being mild and occasional to severe and daily. The pain is precipitated by a meal in approximately 50% of patients, is often associated with dysphagia, and may worsen during periods of emotional stress. However, the pain may be unrelated to meals, occur at night and mimic pain of myocardial origin. Both types of pain are relieved by glyceryl trinitrate. The dysphagia is of variable severity and lacks the persistence seen in achalasia or organic stenosis.

Investigations

The diagnosis of diffuse oesophageal spasm is based on a combination of clinical symptoms and a poorly defined complex of manometric abnormalities (*Figure 1.41*) in a gullet which has not completely lost its capability of producing peristaltic contractions and lower oesophageal sphincter relaxations.

One of the main problems is the relationship between symptomatic diffuse oesophageal spasm and acid sensitivity. Both conditions may coexist. Pressure monitoring and 24-hour pH may prove to be useful for the recognition of pain of oesophageal origin and for the identification of gastro-oesophageal reflux or spasm as the cause of pain.

Manometry

There are no uniform, generally accepted criteria for the manometric diagnosis of diffuse oesophageal spasm. The following criteria have been proposed.

1. According to Richter and Castell[65] more than 10% of wet swallows should produce simultaneous pressure peaks. For others[30,53] 30% of the deglutitive reponses should consist of simultaneous waves of high amplitude and long duration. A duration of more than 6 seconds has been proposed as the definition of prolonged contractions, because this value is greater than the mean + 2 standard deviations in normal subjects.[6,53,64] The concept of high amplitude has not yet been well defined. However, with intraluminal transducers or a low compliance perfu-

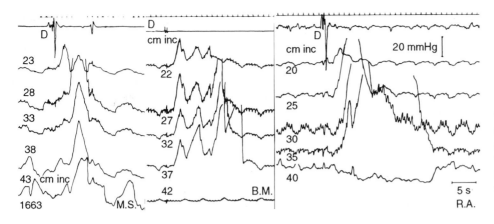

Figure 1.41 Manometric patterns in diffuse oesophageal spasm (D = deglutition): peristaltic waves becoming simultaneous in the distal oesophagus (left); repetitive waves (centre); peristaltic 'giant' waves (right).

sion system and wet swallows, pressure peaks in the distal oesophagus of 190 mmHg or more are generally considered to be of high amplitude.

2. Repetitive waves (several pressure peaks in response to a single swallow) are seen in the majority (56–95%) of patients,[40,69] and spontaneous contractions (not induced by swallows) occur in more than half of these patients.[92]

3. Incomplete (<75%) lower oesophageal sphincter relaxations and high (>50 mmHg) sphincter pressure may also be seen.

Radiology

The radiological appearance of symptomatic diffuse oesophageal spasm (*Figure 1.42*) is described as curling, segmental spasm, ladder spasm, rosary bead oesophagus, spastic pseudodiverticulosis, corkscrew oesophagus, etc. These terms refer to segmental, non-peristaltic contractions, which may trap the barium and push it back and forth. This is best demonstrated when the patient is in the recumbent position. A second, but less common, picture is a tight contraction of the oesophagus over a length of several centimetres or a slight diffuse narrowing of the lower half of the oesophagus with a slightly dilated upper segment.[87] Marked dilatation of the oesophagus and prolonged stasis of food and fluids are rare in diffuse spasm.

The extent and severity of the radiological abnormalities may vary widely from patient to patient and from one time to another in the same patient.[7] The severity of the radiological changes correlates poorly with the clinical, manometric or pathological findings. Patients with diffuse oesophageal spasm may appear normal on routine radiological examination and typical radiological pictures may occur in asymptomatic patients (mainly the elderly) or in patients with diffuse spasm at a symptom-free moment.

Diagnostic tests

The lack of strict diagnostic criteria and the need to distinguish diffuse spasm from achalasia on the one hand and from non-specific or asymptomatic motor disorders on the other, make provocation tests highly desirable. The oesophagus of many patients with symptomatic diffuse oesophageal spasm is

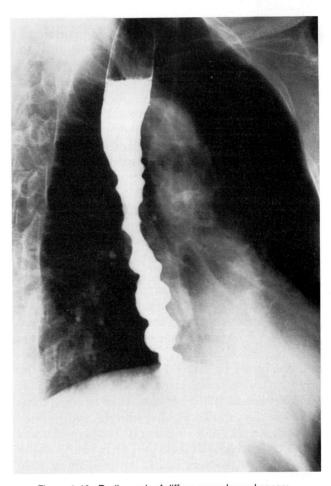

Figure 1.42 Radiograph of diffuse oesophageal spasm.

hypersensitive to cholinergics such as methacholine (Mecholyl)[49] and bethanechol[53] and is also hypertensive to the cholinesterase inhibitor edrophonium chloride.[53] However the methacholine test is also positive in patients with primary achalasia, those with Chagas' disease and in some patients with carcinomatous infiltration of Auerbach's plexus.[44] The test can be useful to distinguish diffuse spasm from asymptomatic similar motor disorders[50] and from reflux-related spasm.[53] The oesophagus of patients with diffuse spasm has been reported to be supersensitive to pentagastrin or gastrin administration.[33,52] The pentagastrin test has proved to be disappointing because it is often negative in patients with symptomatic diffuse oesophageal spasm and positive in patients with achalasia[58] and in some elderly patients.[42]

Ergometrine maleate (Ergonovine), an α-adrenergic agonist, has been used as a provocative test for coronary artery spasm[45] and for oesophageal spasm.[26] However, serious side effects may occur and the test should not be used routinely.

Treatment

A variety of medical treatments has been offered to these patients but few have proved to be efficient. Anticholinergic drugs are not indicated because they worsen the peristaltic performance of the oesophagus and favour gastro-oesophageal reflux, which in itself may trigger motor abnormalities. Long-term symptomatic and manometric improvement has been reported with the use of long-acting nitrates, but the tolerated dose is usually low owing to the side effects, especially headache, they produce.[57,76]

Calcium channel blockers have been suggested as potentially beneficial. Nifedipine is able to reduce the amplitude and also the frequency of non-peristaltic contractions in patients with diffuse spasm, but the results of long-term trials have been controversial. No significant effect on symptom relief has been obtained in double-blind studies prolonged for more than 1 month.[27,28,54]

Symptomatic diffuse oesophageal spasm should only be treated by pneumatic dilatations if the lower oesophageal sphincter is functioning poorly and dysphagia is the main symptom. The same technique as for achalasia patients will be used but the results are less favourable. In the authors' own limited experience only 45% of patients treated in this way reported excellent or good long-term results.[88] Relief of dysphagia was clearly better than relief of pain. The same holds true for cardiomyotomy – long

oesophageal myotomy for pain is only indicated exceptionally.

PRIMARY OESOPHAGEAL MOTILITY DISORDERS OF THE INTERMEDIATE TYPE

Although achalasia and symptomatic diffuse oesophageal spasm have distinctive properties, a number of patients do not fit into this simple classification. Some patients who would otherwise fit the criteria have occasional peristaltic waves or sphincter relaxations. Up to 24% of those with motility disorders severe enough to justify treatment with dilatation did not fit well into the two classic categories.[91] Furthermore, after dilatation as many as 45% of the patients fell into the intermediate category. These patients presented with either complete absence of peristalsis and the presence of (at least some) normal lower oesophageal sphincter relaxations, or with some degree of peristalsis and complete absence of normal lower oesophageal sphincter relaxation. These observations suggest that the primary oesophageal motility disorders constitute a spectrum of motor disorders composed of achalasia, diffuse spasm and intermediate types (*Figure 1.43*).[91] Moreover, transition from symptomatic diffuse oesophageal spasm to achalasia has been documented,[50,91] although most patients with diffuse spasm remain unchanged over long periods of time. Radiological examination shows an oesophagus that resembles achalasia rather than diffuse spasm.

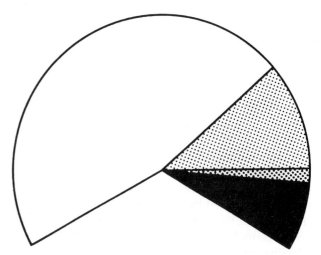

Figure 1.43 Spectrum of primary oesophageal motility disorders. □ Achalasia: no peristalsis, no normal relaxations; ■ diffuse oesophageal spasm: some peristalsis, some normal relaxations; □ intermediate type: no peristalsis, some normal relaxations; ▦ intermediate type: some peristalsis, no normal relaxations.

Treatment with pneumatic dilatation results in a success rate comparable to that of achalasia.

NUTCRACKER OESOPHAGUS (SYMPTOMATIC OESOPHAGEAL PERISTALSIS)

The development of measurement systems able to pick up rapid pressure rises has led to the description of a syndrome characterized clinically by angina-like chest pain and/or dysphagia and manometrically by oesophageal peristaltic contractions of markedly increased amplitude and/or duration.

Originally identified by Brand et al.,[12] this condition has been studied intensively in recent years and is usually termed 'nutcracker oesophagus'.[6,24,77,78] The manometric criteria proposed for the diagnosis of nutcracker oesophagus are a mean amplitude of deglutitive pressure peaks above 180 mmHg in the lower one-third of the oesophagus after swallowing 5-ml liquid boluses.[24,68] The most common symptom is angina-like chest pain. High-amplitude, distal oesophageal body contractions have been reported in 27–48% of patients with non-cardiac chest pain. Others have doubted the relationship between the amplitude of the contraction peaks and symptoms in patients with nutcracker oesophagus,[18] because calcium channel blockers may decrease the amplitude without improving the symptoms.[66] Because the amplitude of oesophageal contractions increases during psychological stress, particularly in patients with the nutcracker oesophagus, high amplitude contractions may simply be an epiphenomenon from an exaggerated reponse to various stimuli such as chest pain or environmental stress.

IRRITABLE OESOPHAGUS

The irritable oesophagus concept was derived from the observation that some patients with non-cardiac chest pain, when studied by 24-hour pH and pressure measurements, sometimes developed pain associated with reflux alone (without motor disorders), and on other occasions during the same study experienced the same pain together with motility disorders alone (without) acid reflux.[85] The oesophagus of these patients appears to be hypersensitive to a variety of stimuli. The diagnosis of irritable oesophagus, is therefore, based on the demonstration that the patient's familiar chest pain can be elicited by both mechanical and chemical stimuli. To demonstrate the association of pain with endogenous stimuli (acid reflux, motor disorders),

24-hour pH and pressure measurements are used. Provocation tests can also be used as exogenous stimuli. These include the acid perfusion test of Bernstein,[9] the edrophonium test,[67] the balloon distension test[63] and the vasopressin test.[39] A positive acid perfusion test indicates that the oesophagus is acid sensitive, but does not prove that the spontaneous pain attacks are induced by acid reflux.[46] Likewise, a positive edrophonium test or a positive balloon distension test indicates that the oesophagus is mechanosensitive, but does not prove that motor disorders are the cause of the spontaneous chest pain episodes. At present the best way to determine the cause of spontaneous pain attacks of non-cardiac chest pain is by 24-hour intraoesophageal pH and pressure recordings.[39]

It is obviously important to identify the specific abnormality that causes the chest pain because this will determine the type of treatment. Patients with chest pain due to acid reflux will be treated primarily by measures that reduce or eliminate acid exposure of the oesophageal mucosa. Hyperactive motility disturbances will be treated by muscle relaxants such as nitrates or calcium channel blockers. Patients with an irritable oesophagus constitute a difficult management problem. These patients may need drugs that reduce pain perception rather than drugs that combat gastro-oesophageal reflux or motor disturbances. Clouse et al.[16] have successfully used the non-tricyclic antidepressant trazodone in patients with chest pain.

SECONDARY OESOPHAGEAL MOTOR DISORDERS

Various generalized diseases may cause motor disorders of the oesophagus (Table 1.13), but only some of these will be discussed here.

Systemic sclerosis and other collagen diseases

The oesophagus is abnormal in 50–80% of patients with scleroderma;[43] the degree of oesophageal involvement bears no relation to the degree of involvement of other organs. Sometimes the skin lesions improve while the oesophageal involvement progresses. Histological studies of the oesophagus show that the smooth muscle layers are atrophied with some fibrous replacement whilst the striated muscle fibres are remarkably well preserved.[4,25,32,81] Inflammatory and fibrous changes also occur in the mucosa and submucosa. At least some of the mucosal lesions are due to gastro-oesophageal reflux. Intraluminal pressure measure-

Table 1.13   Diseases causing oesophageal motility disorder

Collagen diseases
    Systemic sclerosis
    Systemic lupus erythematosus
    Polymyositis–dermatomyositis
 	
Muscle diseases
    Myotonic dystrophy
    Ocular and oculopharyngeal myopathy
    Myasthenia gravis
	Central nervous system diseases
	    Brain-stem lesions
	    Poliomyelitis
	    Motor neuron disease
	    Extrapyramidal disturbances
	    Stiff-man (Moersch–Woltmann) syndrome
	    Dysautonomia
	    Intestinal pseudo-obstruction
	
	Peripheral neuropathies
	    Diabetic neuropathy
	    Alcoholic neuropathy

ments indicate that peristalsis usually remains normal in the upper, striated portion of the gullet, whereas in the smooth muscle portion the contractions are often non-peristaltic, weak and may eventually disappear completely (*Figure 1.44*).[11,38,84] The lower oesophageal sphincter pressure is frequently lower than normal, which may lead to gastro-oesophageal reflux and oesophagitis. The loss of coordinated peristalsis in the distal oesophagus is fairly well correlated with the development of Raynaud's phenomenon.[75]

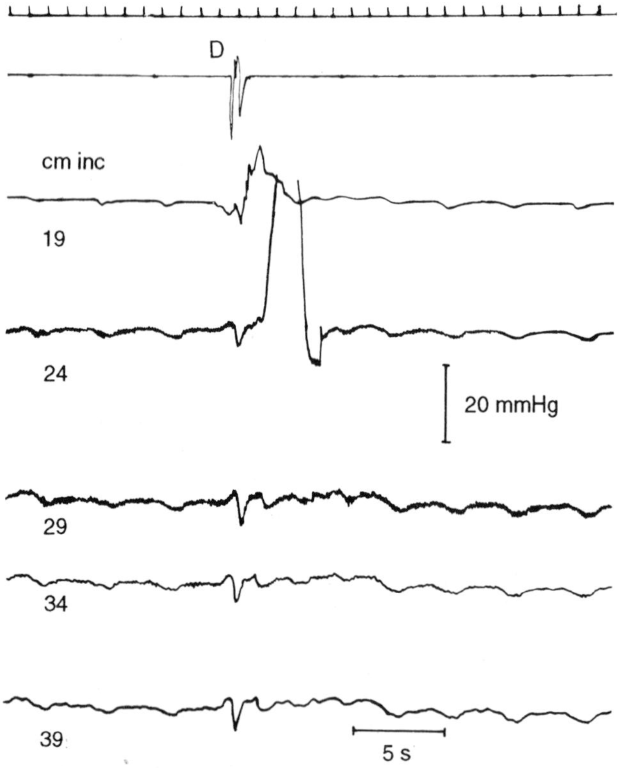

Oesophageal motility disorders may be present in early scleroderma, in the presence of normal oesophageal smooth muscle at autopsy.[81] Moreover, some patients with scleroderma have a preserved response to muscle stimulants but not to agents requiring intact cholinergic innervation.[19] Although these observations suggest that smooth muscle atrophy is a secondary phenomenon, ultrastructural and light microscopic studies have failed to give morphological supporting evidence.[37,70]

The oesophagus is involved in 10–25% of patients with systemic lupus erythematosus. The motility disorders resemble those of systemic sclerosis but are less pronounced.[75]

More than 60% of patients with dermatomyositis or polymyositis complain of high dysphagia.[15,31,60] The degree of dysphagia parallels the course and severity of the muscle involvement. Initially the motility disturbances are most prominent in the pharynx and upper oesophagus; later, smooth muscles are involved as well. Weakness of oesophageal contractions often leads to tracheal aspiration and nasal reflux. Radiological examination reveals an atonic upper oesophageal sphincter, and pooling of barium in the valleculae and pyriform sinuses. When the lower oesophagus is involved the contractions become weak and non-peristaltic and the lower oesophageal sphincter pressure decreases, which may lead to reflux oesophagitis.

Figure 1.44 Manometric pattern of oesophageal motility in scleroderma. Normal peristaltic contractions in the upper part; absence of deglutitive response in the lower part.

REFERENCES

1. Adams, C.W.M., Brain, R.H.F. and Trounce, J.R. (1976) Ganglion cells in achalasia of the cardia. *Virchows Archiv [A]*, **327**, 75–79.
2. Akuamoa, G. (1971) Achalasia oesophagi. *Acta Chirurgica Scandinavica*, **137**, 782–788.
3. Anderson, K.O., Dalton, C.B., Bradley, L.A. and Richter, J.E. (1989) Stress induces alteration of esophageal pressures in healthy volunteers and noncardiac chest pain patients. *Digestive Diseases and Sciences*, **34**, 83–91.

4. Atkinson, M. and Summerling, M.D. (1966) Oesophageal changes in systemic sclerosis. *Gut,* **7,** 402–408.

5. Barker, J.R. and Franklin, R.H. (1971) Heller's operation for achalasia of the cardia. A study of the early and late results. *British Journal of Surgery,* **58,** 466–468.

6. Benjamin, S.B., Gerhardt, D.C. and Castell, D.O. (1979) High amplitude peristaltic esophageal contractions associated with chest pain and/or dysphagia. *Gastroenterology,* **77,** 478–483.

7. Bennett, J.R. and Hendrix, T.R. (1970) Diffuse esophageal spasm: a disorder with more than one cause. *Gastroenterology,* **59,** 273–279.

8. Berger, K. and McCullum, R.W. (1981) The hypertensive lower esophageal sphincter: a clinical and manometric study. *Gastroenterology,* **80,** 1109.

9. Bernstein, L.M. and Baker, L.A. (1958) A clinical test for esophagitis. *Gastroenterology,* **34,** 760–781.

10. Black, J., Vorbach, A.N. and Collis, J.L. (1976) Results of Heller's operation for achalasia of the esophagus. The importance of hiatal repair. *British Journal of Surgery,* **63,** 949–953.

11. Bortolotti, M. and Labo, G. (1981) Clinical and manometric effects of nifedipine in patients with esophageal achalasia. *Gastroenterology,* **80,** 39–44.

12. Brand, D.L., Martin, D. and Pope, C.E. (1977) Esophageal manometries in patients with angina-like chest pain. *American Journal of Digestive Diseases,* **22,** 300–304.

13. Cassella, R.R., Brown, A.L. Jr, Sayre, G.P. and Ellis, F.H. Jr (1964) Achalasia of the esophagus: pathologic and etiologic considerations. *Annals of Surgery,* **160,** 474–486.

14. Cassella, R.R., Ellis, F.H. Jr and Brown, A.L. (1965) Fine-structure changes in achalasia of the esophagus. I. Vagus nerves. *American Journal of Pathology,* **46,** 279–288.

15. Christianson, H.B., Brunsting, L.A. and Perry, H.L. (1956) Dermatomyositis: unusual features, complications, and treatment. *Archives of Dermatology (Chicago),* **74,** 581–589.

16. Clouse, R.E., Lustman, P.J., Eckert, T.C., Ferney, D.M. and Griffith, L.S. (1987) Low dose trasodone for symptomatic patients with esophageal contraction abnormalities. *Gastroenterology,* **92,** 1027–1036.

17. Code, C.F., Schlegel, J.F., Kelly, M.L., Olsen, A.M. and Ellis, J.H. (1960) Hypertensive gastroesophageal sphincter. *Proceedings of the Mayo Clinic,* **35,** 391–399.

18. Cohen, S. (1987) Esophageal motility disorders: the sphinx revisited. *Gastroenterology,* **93,** 201–203.

19. Cohen, S., Fisher, R., Lipshutz, W., Turner, R., Myers, A. and Schumachter, R. (1972) The pathogenesis of esophageal dysfunction in scleroderma and Raynaud's disease. *Journal of Clinical Investigation,* **51,** 2663–2668.

20. Cohen, S., Fisher, R. and Tuch, A. (1972) The site of denervation in achalasia. *Gut,* **13,** 556–558.

21. Cohen, S. and Lipschutz, W. (1971) Lower esophageal sphincter dysfunction in achalasia. *Gastroenterology,* **61,** 814–820.

22. Creamer, B., Donoghue, F.E. and Code, C.F. (1958) Pattern of esophageal motility in diffuse spasm. *Gastroenterology,* **34,** 782–796.

23. Csendes, A., Velasco, N., Braghetto, I. and Henriquez, A. (1981) A prospective randomized study comparing forceful dilatation and esophagomyotomy in patients with achalasia of the esophagus. *Gastroenterology,* **80,** 789–795.

24. Dalton, C.B., Castell, D.O. and Richter, J.E. (1988) The changing faces of the nutcracker esophagus. *American Journal of Gastroenterology,* **83,** 623–628.

25. d'Angelo, W.A., Fries, J.F., Masi, A.T. and Schulman, L.E. (1969) Pathologic observations in systemic sclerosis (scleroderma). *American Journal of Medicine,* **46,** 428–440.

26. Dart, A.M., Alban Davies, H., Lowndes, R.H., Dalal, J., Ruttley, M. and Henderson, A.H. (1980) Oesophageal spasm and 'angina': diagnostic value of ergometrine provocation. *European Heart Journal,* **1,** 91–95.

27. Davies H.A., Lewis, M., Rhodes, J. and Henderson, A. (1982) Nifedipine for relief of esophageal chest pain? *New England Journal of Medicine,* **307,** 1274.

28. Davies, H.A., Lewis, M.J., Rhodes, J. and Henderson, A.H. (1987) Trial of nifedipine for prevention of oesophageal spasm. *Digestion,* **36,** 81–83.

29. Diamant, N.E. and El-Sharkawy, T.Y. (1977) Neural control of esophageal peristalsis. A conceptual analysis. *Gastroenterology,* **72,** 546–556.

30. DiMarino, A.J. Jr and Cohen, S. (1974) Characteristics of lower esophageal sphincter function in symptomatic diffuse esophageal spasm. *Gastroenterology,* **66,** 1–6.

31. Donoghue, F., Winkelmann, R. and Moersch H. (1960) Esophageal defects in dermatomyositis. *Annals of Otology,* **69,** 1139–1145.

32. Dornhorst, A.C., Pierce, J.W. and Whimsler, I.W. (1954) The esophageal lesion in scleroderma. *The Lancet,* **1,** 698–699.

33. Eckhardt, V.F., Krüger, J., Holtermüller, K.H. and Ewe, K. (1975) Alteration of esophageal peristalsis by pentagastrin in patients with diffuse esophageal spasm. *Scandinavian Journal of Gastroenterology,* **10,** 475–479.

34. Fleshler, B. (1967) Diffuse esophageal spasm. *Gastroenterology,* **52,** 559–564.

35. Freidin, N., Traube, M., Mittal, R.K. and McCallum, R.W. (1989) The hypertensive lower esophageal sphincter. Manometric and clinical aspects. *Digestive Diseases and Sciences,* **34,** 1063–1067.

36. Friesen, D.L., Henderson, R.D. and Hanna, W. (1983) Ultrastructure of the esophageal muscle in achalasia and diffuse esophageal spasm. *American Journal of Clinical Pathology,* **79,** 319–325.

37. Garrett, J.M. and Goodwin, D.H. (1969) Gastroesophageal hypercontracting sphincter. *Journal of American Medical Association,* **208**, 992–998.

38. Garrett, J.M., Winkelmann, R.K., Schlegel, J.F. and Code, C.F. (1971) Esophageal deterioration in scleroderma. *Mayo Clinic Proceedings,* **46**, 92–96.

39. Ghillebert, G., Janssens, J., Vantrappen, G., Nevens, F. and Piessens J. (1990) Ambulatory 24 hour intraoesophageal pH and pressure recordings vs provocation tests in the diagnosis of chest pain of oesophageal origin. *Gut,* **31**, 738–744.

40. Gillies, M., Nicks, R. and Skyring, A. (1967) Clinical, manometric and pathological studies in diffuse oesophageal spasm. *British Medical Journal,* **2**, 527–530.

41. Goyal, R.K. and Rattan, S. (1978) Neurohumoral, hormonal and drug receptors for the lower esophageal sphincter. *Gastroenterology,* **84**, 589–619.

42. Guelrud, M., Simon, C., Gomez, G. and Villalta, B. (1981) Pentagastrin supersensitivity of the lower esophageal sphincter (LES) in the elderly. *Gastroenterology,* **80**, 1165.

43. Hellemans, J. and Vantrappen, G. (1974) Motor disorders due to collagen diseases. In *Diseases of the Esophagus,* pp. 383–393 (Eds) Vantrappen, G. and Hellemans, J. Berlin: Heidelberg; New York: Springer-Verlag.

44. Herrera, A.F., Colon, J., Valdes-Dapena, A. and Roth, J.L.A. (1970) Achalasia or carcinoma? The significance of the mecholyl test. *American Journal of Digestive Diseases,* **15**, 1073–1081.

45. Heupler, F.A. Jr, Proudfit, W.L., Razavi, M., Shirley, E.K., Greenstreet, R. and Sheldon, W.C. (1978) Ergonovine maleate provocative test for coronary arterial spasm. *American Journal of Cardiology,* **41**, 631–640.

46. Janssens, J., Vantrappen, G. and Ghillebert, G. (1984) 24-hour recording of esophageal pressure and pH in patients with noncardiac chest pain. *Gastroenterology,* **90**, 1978–1984.

47. Joseph, R. and Job, J.C. (1963) Dysautonomie familiale et mégaoesophage. *Archives Françaises de Pédiatrie,* **20**, 25–33.

48. Kolodny, M., Schrader, Z.R., Rubin, W., Hochman, R. and Sleisenger, M.H. (1968) Esophageal achalasia probably due to gastric carcinoma. *Annals of Internal Medicine,* **69**, 569–573.

49. Kramer, P., Fleshler, B., McNally, E. and Harris, L.D. (1967) Oesophageal sensitivity to mecholyl in symptomatic diffuse spasm. *Gut,* **8**, 120–127.

50. Kramer, P., Harris, L.D. and Donaldson, R.M. Jr (1967) Transition from symptomatic diffuse spasm to cardiospasm. *Gut,* **8**, 115–119.

51. Kramer, P. and Ingelfinger, F.J. (1951) Esophageal sensitivity to mecholyl in cardiospasm. *Gastroenterology,* **19**, 242–253.

52. Lane, W.H., Ippoliti, A.F. and McCallum, R.W. (1979) Effect of gastrin heptadecapeptide (G17) on oesophageal contractions in patients with diffuse oesophageal spasm. *Gut,* **20**, 756–759.

53. Mellow, M. (1977) Symptomatic diffuse esophageal spasm, Manometric follow-up and response to cholinergic stimulation and cholinesterase inhibition. *Gastroenterology,* **73**, 237–240.

54. Nasrallah, S.M., Tommaso, C.T., Singleton, R.T. and Backhaus, E.A. (1985) Primary esophageal motor disorders: clinical responses to nifedipine. *Southern Medical Journal,* **8**, 312–315.

55. Okike, N., Payne, W.S., Neufeld, D.M., Bernatz, P.E., Pairolero, P.C. and Sanderson, D.R. (1979) Esophagotomy versus forceful dilators for achalasia of the esophagus: results in 899 patients. *Annals of Thoracic Surgery,* **28**, 119–125.

56. Olsen, A.M., Harrington, S.W., Moersch, H.J. and Anderson, H.A. (1951) The treatment of cardiospasm analysis of a twelve-year experience. *Journal of Thoracic Cardiovascular Surgery,* **22**, 164–167.

57. Orlando, R.C. and Bozymski, E. (1973) Clinical and manometric effect of nitroglycerin in diffuse esophageal spasm. *New England Journal of Medicine,* **289**, 23–25.

58. Orlando, R.C. and Bozymski, E. (1979) The effects of pentagastrin in achalasia and diffuse esophageal spasm. *Gastroenterology,* **77**, 472–477.

59. Orr, W.C. and Robinson, M.G. (1982) Hypertensive peristalsis in the pathogenesis of chest pain: further exploration of the 'nutcracker' esophagus. *American Journal of Gastroenterology,* **77**, 604–607.

60. Pearson, C.M. (1969) Polymyositis and related disorders. In *Disorders of Voluntary Muscle,* 2nd edn, pp. 501–539. (Ed.) Walton, J.N. London: Churchill.

61. Pederson, S.A. and Alstrup, P. (1972) The hypertensive gastroesophageal sphincter. A manometric and clinical study. *Scandinavian Journal of Gastroenterology,* **7**, 531–534.

62. Ribet, M., Callafi, R. and Hamon, Y. (1975) Mégaoesophage idiopathique. Résultats et séquelles do son traitement chirurgical. *Archives Françaises des Maladies de l'Appareil Digestif,* **64**, 629–637.

63. Richter, J.E., Barish, C.F. and Castell, D.O. (1968) Abnormal sensory perception in patients with esophageal chest pain. *Gastroenterology,* **91**, 845–852.

64. Richter, J.E., Bradley, L.A. and Castell, D.O. (1989) Esophageal chest pain: current controversies in pathogenesis, diagnosis and therapy. *Annals of Internal Medicine,* **110**, 66–78.

65. Richter, J.E. and Castell, D.O. (1984) Diffuse esophageal spasm: a reappraisal. *Annals of Internal Medicine,* **100**, 242–245.

66. Richter, J.E., Dalton, C.B., Bradley, L.A. and Castell, D.O. (1987) Oral nifedipine in the treatment of non-cardiac chest pain in patients with the nutcracker esophagus. *Gastroenterology,* **93**, 21–28.

67. Richter, J.E., Hackshaw, B.T., Wu, W.C. and Castell, D.O. (1985) Edrophonium: a useful provocative test for esophageal chest pain. *Annals of Internal Medicine,* **103**, 14–21.

68. Richter, J.E., Wu, W.C., Johns, D.N. *et al.* (1987) Esophageal manometry in 95 healthy adult volunteers. *Digestive Diseases and Sciences,* **34**, 583–592.

69. Roth, H.P. and Fleshler, B. (1964) Diffuse esophageal spasm. *Annals of Internal Medicine,* **61**, 914–923.

70. Russel, M.L., Friezen, D., Henderson, R.D. and Hanna, W.M. (1982) Ultrastructure of the esophagus in scleroderma. *Arthritis and Rheumatology,* **25**, 1117–1123.

71. Sanderson, D.R., Ellis, F.H. Jr and Olsen A.M. (1970) Achalasia of the esophagus results of therapy by dilatation, 1950–1967. *Chest,* **58**, 116–121.

72. Sanderson, D.R., Ellis, F.H. Jr, Schlegel, J.F. and Olsen, A.M. (1967) Syndrome of vigorous achalasia: clinical and physiologic observations. *Diseases of the Chest,* **52**, 508–517.

73. Silverstein, B.D., Kramer, C.M. and Pope, C.E. (1982) Treatment of esophageal motor disorders with a calcium-blocker, diltiazem. *Gastroenterology,* **82**, 1181.

74. Sloper, J.C. (1954) Idiopathic diffuse muscular hypertrophy of the lower oesophagus. *Thorax,* **9**, 136–146.

75. Stevens, M.B., Hookman, P., Siegel, C.I., Esterly, J.R., Shelman, L.E. and Hendrix, T.R. (1964) Aperistalsis of the esophagus in patients with connective-tissue disorders and Raynauds's phenomenon. *New England Journal of Medicine,* **270**, 1218–1222.

76. Swamy, N. (1977) Esophageal spasm: clinical and manometric responses to nitroglycerine and long acting nitrites. *Gastroenterology,* **72**, 23–27.

77. Traube, M., Aaronson, R.M. and McCallum, R.W. (1987) Transition from nutcracker esophagus to diffuse esophagus spasm. *Archives of Internal Medicine,* **146**, 1844–1847.

78. Traube, M., Abibi, R. and McCallum, R.W. (1983) High amplitude peristaltic contractions associated with chest pain. *Journal of American Medical Association,* **250**, 2655–2659.

79. Traube, M., Dubovik, R., Lange, R.C. and McCallum, R.W. (1989) The role of nifedipine therapy in achalasia: results of a randomized, double-blind placebo-controlled study. *American Journal of Gastroenterology,* **84**, 1259–1262.

80. Traube, M. and McCallum, R.W. (1987) Comparison of esophageal manometric characteristics in asymptomatic subjects and symptomatic patients with high-amplitude esophageal peristaltic contractions. *American Journal of Gastroenterology,* **82**, 831–835.

81. Treacy, W.L., Baggenstoss, A.H., Slocumb, C.H. and Code, C.F. (1963) Scleroderma of the esophagus. A correlation of histologic and physiologic findings. *Annals of Internal Medicine,* **59**, 351–356.

82. Trounce, J.R., Deucher, D.C., Kauntze, R. and Thomas, G.A. (1957) Studies in achalasia of the cardia. *Quarterly Journal of Medicine,* **28**, 433–443.

83. Tucker, H.J. Snape, W.J. Jr and Cohen, S. (1978) Achalasia secondary to carcinoma: manometric and clinical features. *Annals of Internal Medicine,* **89**, 315–318.

84. Turner, R., Lipshutz, W., Miller, W., Rittenberg, G., Schumacher, H.R. and Cohen, S. (1973) Esophageal dysfunction in collagen disease. *American Journal of Medical Sciences,* **265**, 191–199.

85. Vantrappen, G., Janssens, J. and Ghillebert, G. (1987) The irritable esophagus – a frequent cause of angina-like pain. *The Lancet,* **1**, 1232–1234.

86. Vantrappen, G. and Hellemans, J. (1974) Achalasia. In *Diseases of the Esophagus* (Ed.) Vantrappen, G. & Hellemans, J. pp. 287–354. Berlin, Heidelberg, New York: Springer-Verlag.

87. Vantrappen, G. and Hellemans, J. (1976) Diffuse muscle spasm of the oesophagus and hypertensive oesophageal sphincter. *Clinics in Gastroenterology,* **5**, 59–72.

88. Vantrappen, G. and Hellemans, J. (1980) Treatment of achalasia and related motor disorders. *Gastroenterology,* **79**, 144–154.

89. Vantrappen, G. and Hellemans, J. (1981) Achalasia. In *Therapeutic Endoscopy and Radiology of the Gut,* pp. 73–86 (Ed.) Bennett, J.R. London: Chapman & Hall.

90. Vantrappen, G. and Janssens, J. (1983) To dilate or to operate? That is the question. *Gut,* **24**, 1013–1019.

91. Vantrappen, G., Janssens, J., Hellemans, J. and Coremans, G. (1979) Achalasia, diffuse esophageal spasm, and related motility disorders. *Gastroenterology,* **76**, 450–457.

92. Vantrappen, G., Van Derstappen, G.V. and Vandenbroucke, J. (1960) The syndrome of hypertonic gastroesophageal sphincter. In *Proceedings of the International Congress of Gastroenterology,* pp. 377–384. Leiden, Amsterdam: Excerpta Medica.

93. Waterman, D.C., Dalton, C.B., Ott, D.J. *et al.* (1989) Hypertensive lower esophageal sphincter: What does it mean? *Journal of Clinical Gastroenterology,* **11**, 139–146.

GASTRO-OESOPHAGEAL REFLUX DISEASE

J.R. Bennett

REFLUX OESOPHAGITIS

DEFINITION

If digestive juices frequently reflux from the stomach to the lower oesophagus their irritant effect may give rise to symptoms such as pain and dysphagia, or even complications such as haemorrhage or stricture. This is known as gastro-oesophageal reflux disease, a term preferred to reflux oesophagitis because at least 30% of patients with such symptoms have no detectable inflammatory change in the oesophagus.

AETIOLOGY

Reflux of gastric juice into the oesophagus is normally prevented by barrier mechanisms, which include the anatomical arrangements at the diaphragmatic oesophageal hiatus, and the lower oesophageal sphincter (gastro-oesophageal sphincter). The barrier mechanism is necessarily incomplete because it at least has to allow belching and vomiting. Reflux of gastric contents across the barrier into the lower oesophagus occurs in everyone several times a day due to transient relaxations of the gastro-oesophageal sphincter, the errant juices being quickly returned to the stomach by gravity, primary peristalsis induced by swallowing or secondary peristalsis triggered by oesophageal distension. To produce symptoms or oesophagitis (or both) other factors must be involved. Compared with normal subjects, patients with gastro-oesophageal reflux disease may have:

1. More frequent episodes of reflux
2. Abnormalities of gastric function
3. Slower oesophageal emptying ('reduced clearance')
4. More irritant juice
5. Diminished mucosal resistance.[12,44]

The importance of each factor varies from patient to patient and may alter in any individual patient from time to time. An element of self-perpetuation may be present, because the presence of reflux oesophagitis may itself promote poorer clearing and diminish mucosal resistance, and reversibly weaken the gastro-oesophageal sphincter. Each causative factor is influenced by changes in a number of physiological control mechanisms.

FREQUENCY OF REFLUX

It is impossible to determine the contribution of each factor but, in some patients, deficiency of one or more may be a major contribution to reflux.

The gastro-oesophageal sphincter is a band of specialized muscle squeezing the oesophageal lumen. Innumerable influences, especially hormones, have been shown to affect sphincter tone, though uncertainty continues as to which of these are true physiological effects. Those that may contribute causatively to reflux oesophagitis include the following:

Myogenic
– oesophagitis[18]
– systemic sclerosis[29]
– after achalasia therapy[13,110]
Neural
– oesophagitis[47,48]
– early systemic sclerosis[29]
– smoking[39,100]
– alcohol[60,66]
Hormonal
– menstruation[109]
– pregnancy[108]
– fat/chocolate ingestion[6,44,82,120]
– coffee[40]

The strength of the sphincter is not high – normally 1.5–25 kPa (15–25 cm H_2O) – but this is sufficient to keep the sphincter segment narrow and resist opening force from below, following the general principles of La Place's law which shows that the force required to distend a pliable tube is inversely proportional to the tube's diameter.[87]

It was believed that the refluxed material forced its way through a weakened sphincter at rest but it has now been shown that the sphincter frequently relaxes transiently and not in response to a swallow.[42] Although the mechanism of these transient relaxations is not known, they seem to account for the episodes of diurnal reflux seen in normal subjects, and for much of the reflux in patients with symptomatic reflux disease both in adults[42,79] and infants.[77] Reflux may also occur when the sphincter relaxes after swallowing,[33] especially in infants who regurgitate.[75]

Hiatus hernia

Early descriptions of gastro-oesophageal reflux stressed its relationship with herniation of the stomach through the oesophageal hiatus of the diaphragm, and much more effort was expended in trying to demonstrate such hiatus hernias radiologically. A hiatus hernia may be produced transiently in most normal individuals, and such herniation is part of the normal vomiting mechanism, so it is not a useful diagnostic finding. A fixed hiatus hernia may play a part in the pathogenesis of reflux disease (perhaps by delaying oesophageal clearance[78]), but it is not the most important causative factor and its radiological demonstration is neither a sensitive nor a specific way to confirm a diagnosis of reflux disease. Moreover, patients often become unnecessarily perturbed when they are told that they 'have a hiatus hernia', believing it likely to be subjected to the same hazards and complications as an inguinal or femoral hernia, and that it will necessarily require surgical treatment.

It would be desirable if the term 'hiatus hernia' ceased to be used as a diagnostic label in patients with reflux symptoms.

GASTRIC FACTORS

Potentially, three abnormalities of gastric function could contribute to gastro-oesophageal reflux disease:

1. Gastric secretion
2. Gastric emptying
3. Duodenogastric reflux.

Gastric secretion in reflux oesophagitis has been the subject of many studies with discrepant findings. It is usually similar to that in normal subjects, although subtle differences have been detected (see page 198).

Gastric emptying may be slower, especially for solids, in some patients with gastro-oesophageal reflux.[73,74] Duodenogastric reflux may occur more commonly in patients with reflux oesophagitis.[67]

OESOPHAGEAL CLEARANCE

The oesophagus deals with refluxed, acidic juice in two ways. Most is returned to the stomach by peristalsis[58] which may be primary (induced by a swallow)[85] or secondary (induced by oesophageal stimulation of the refluxed material).[69] In normal people 90% of swallows induce an effective, propagated peristaltic sequence. In conditions such as systemic sclerosis, in which peristalsis is lost, the oesophagus loses this mechanical clearing action and becomes especially vulnerable to reflux and the development of oesophagitis. With increasing degrees of oesophagitis the proportion of ineffective or non-propagated peristaltic waves increases.[65] Whether this is the result of oesophagitis, or whether oesophagitis has developed in an oesophagus in which peristalsis has failed, is uncertain; nevertheless, it is clear that this phenomenon is one element in the tendency of reflux disease to be self-perpetuating.

The second, and auxiliary, method of disposing of acid is neutralization by swallowed alkaline saliva.[58] Salivary secretion increases during heartburn and stimulated saliva has a greater neutralizing capacity.[57]

COMPOSITION OF REFLUXED JUICE

The constituents of refluxed juice which are mainly responsible for the epithelial damage are acid, pepsin and perhaps bile; the contribution of pancreatic enzymes is uncertain. Under experimental conditions each of these elements may cause oesophagitis but how they interact to induce reflux oesophagitis remains speculative. Oesophagitis may occur in achlorhydric subjects, or even after total gastrectomy when it is speculated that bile may be the cause, but in most patients acid and pepsin are the important factors.

Although major differences in gastric acid secretion have not been clearly shown in reflux subjects there is a linear correlation between the dose of histamine H_2-receptor antagonist necessary to induce remission of reflux disease and the basal acid secretion; thus subtle increases in acid concentration may determine the severity of reflux disease.[30]

Studies of bile salt concentrations in oesophageal fluid have yielded conflicting results. If present the quantities are certainly small, although even small amounts could have a deleterious effect on mucosal permeability (see below).[80,93]

MUCOSAL SENSITIVITY (TISSUE RESISTANCE)

Oesophageal mucosal defences may be considered as pre-epithelial, epithelial and post-epithelial.[84]

Pre-epithelial defences

These include the unstirred layer of mucus, mainly derived from swallowed saliva but partly from submucous glands. There is also a thin glycocalyx over the stratum corneum.[72]

Epithelial defences

The intercellular junctions of the stratum granulosum resist acid attack until a late stage in the inflammatory process. Beneath this, the prickle cell layer contains Na^+/K^+ ATPase which maintains cellular integrity. At a late stage of H^+ ion penetration the activity of this enzyme is reduced and causes cell swelling and rupture.

Post-epithelial defences

These depend on blood flow, dispersing penetrating H^+ ions and delivering HCO_3^- ions.

SUMMARY

Gastro-oesophageal reflux of greater than normal frequency results usually from altered gastro-oesophageal sphincter function. The oesophagus, nevertheless, has a series of defences against refluxed material, and reflux disease will occur only if the refluxed material is unusually corrosive, if normal peristalsis is defective, if salivation is impaired or if the mucosal defence mechanisms are breached. A downward spiral of worsening oesophageal function and increasing mucosal damage may then ensue.

CLINICAL FEATURES

Infants

Regurgitation often occurs in infants. In a few it causes frequent vomiting which may impair nutrition and lead to aspiration pulmonary complications. In 60% it resolves spontaneously by 18 months;[24] the symptoms will respond to thickening of the feeds and keeping the infant prone with the head raised by 30°. However, in 10% it causes pain, and there may be severe oesophagitis with haemorrhage or stricture formation.[35] More vigorous treatment with alginates, histamine H_2-receptor antagonists and pro-kinetic drugs are necessary in these infants and, if the response is inadequate, surgical intervention may be required.[77]

Adults

Gastro-oesophageal reflux may exist for years without symptoms; indeed, the severity of symptoms is a poor guide to the degree of reflux. The initial presentation of many patients is with a stricture, an oesophageal ulcer or a columnar lined oesophagus (all considered to be complications of chronic reflux) in the absence of any preceding reflux symptoms.

Heartburn (pyrosis)

This is the most common symptom of gastro-oesophageal reflux and is due to direct mucosal irritation by refluxed juice. Discomfort or pain, usually burning in character, is felt behind the sternum, often appearing to rise from the epigastrium and move towards or into the throat, and sometimes radiating into the back. Occasionally the sensation may be experienced entirely in the throat or in the epigastrium.

This is an intermittent symptom, occurring particularly within 30 minutes of meals, on exercise, after bending or on lying down; it may waken patients from sleep. A large meal, especially if it contains fat, chocolate, coffee or alcohol, is particularly likely to precipitate heartburn. The discomfort often disappears quickly on drinking water or milk, or after taking an antacid. If heartburn occurs frequently it can interfere with the patient's way of life, particularly work or pleasure involving lying or bending, including gardening and sexual intercourse.

About 50% of people in Britain have experienced heartburn at some time. Of the 40% of the population who experience dyspepsia in a 6-month period, more than half have heartburn.[63] However, only when heartburn becomes more frequent, or sufficiently easily precipitated to interfere with normal life, need it be considered pathological. Only a quarter of British patients with dyspepsia consult their general practitioner.[63] Heartburn is not synonymous with gastro-oesophageal reflux;[68] it may be a symptom of some other disease process such as peptic ulceration or of non-organic disease such as functional dyspepsia.

Heartburn occurs in about two-thirds of all pregnant women especially in the second and third trimesters.[108]

Other oesophageal pain

The disordered oesophagus may present with pain other than heartburn. This can be of any character but often is described as 'gripping' or 'knife-like'. The pain is usually central sternal in origin but may radiate widely to abdomen, back, neck and arms, and can be severe. The character, radiation and severity may cause diagnostic difficulty, simulating cardiac, biliary or duodenal pain. As many as one-third of patients admitted to hospital with a provisional diagnosis of cardiac pain may prove to have only oesophageal disease.[14]

Oesophageal pain may be experienced entirely in the epigastrium, when it may mimic peptic ulceration.

Odynophagia

This term describes a transitory discomfort, usually of burning character, felt behind the sternum when food or fluid (usually a hot or an alcoholic drink or citrus juice) is swallowed. It is characteristic and diagnostic of oesophagitis, occurring both in reflux disease and infective oesophagitis.

Regurgitation and vomiting

Fluid may enter the mouth when the patient lies down, bends or strains, and may even wake him or her at night. Acid regurgitation and heartburn are the two most specific symptoms of reflux disease.[68] The fluid may taste bitter (bile) or sour (acid). There may be vomiting and, in some patients with gastro-oesophageal reflux, the predominant symptom is of frequent, effortless vomiting.

Dysphagia

A sensation of delay at the lower end of the sternum as food is swallowed may be experienced in reflux oesophagitis.[105] If it is more than mild and occasional it suggests that a stricture is present or that there is an associated motor abnormality. The degree of dysphagia correlates as closely with the severity of oesophagitis as it does with the degree of stricture formation.

Haemorrhage

Overt bleeding from reflux oesophagitis accounts for about 4% of all gastrointestinal haemorrhage. Occult bleeding is also uncommon. Identification of the oesophagus as the sole site of haemorrhage can be achieved only by gastrointestinal endoscopy. An ulcer in the oesophagus or in the intrathoracic portion of a herniated stomach bleeds more often than uncomplicated oesophagitis. 'Hiatus hernia', diagnosed radiologically and previously accepted as a satisfactory explanation for alimentary haemorrhage or occult bleeding, can no longer be regarded as adequate; in such patients, endoscopic confirmation of the bleeding site is essential, and if there is no visible abnormality the remaining gastrointestinal tract must be investigated.

Respiratory symptoms

Large volume regurgitation may cause recurrent aspiration pneumonia or segmental pulmonary collapse.

The link between gastro-oesophageal reflux and asthma is less well understood.[53] There is an increased incidence of gastro-oesophageal reflux in asthmatic patients compared with the 'normal population', the figures varying between 30% and 89% with the consensus being around 50%. All ages are affected and the association is well recognized in children who have a shorter lower oesophageal sphincter and are liable to more frequent reflux. In infants it is particularly important to diagnose pulmonary aspiration which may be amenable to surgical treatment. In adults aspiration is uncommon and the respiratory symptoms must be explained by other mechanisms. The theory of 'microaspiration' of gastric contents into the airways is supported by some animal experiments.[106] The oesophagus and the bronchial tree share embryological origins in the foregut, and acid reflux may initiate bronchoconstriction by a vagally mediated reflex through their shared autonomic innervation.[76]

Asthma may be the *cause* of gastro-oesophageal reflux in some patients. Increased transdiaphragmatic pressure during airflow obstruction could pump gastric contents into the oesophagus, and a low flat diaphragm interferes with lower oesophageal sphincter function. Drugs used in asthma such as the theophyllines and β_2-agonists might also have a detrimental effect on the antireflux barrier and promote gastro-oesophageal reflux. However, maximum inspiratory efforts in normal subjects can produce transdiaphragmatic pressures of 300 cmH_2O without causing gastro-oesophageal reflux. Histamine-induced bronchoconstriction has been shown to have little effect in asthmatic patients taking theophylline.

A rational approach to treatment of patients with gastro-oesophageal reflux and asthma would first select those with reflux-associated respiratory symptoms. Treatment of their gastro-oesophageal reflux should be along standard lines (see below). Treatment of the asthma should include inhaled corticosteroids with β_2-adrenergic agonists for symptomatic relief. Withdrawing theophyllines may improve oesophageal and possibly respiratory symptoms. Patients who are refractory to this regimen may benefit from cisapride or omeprazole. Surgical intervention is indicated only in cases of severe and intractable oesophagitis or documented recurrent pulmonary aspiration.

INVESTIGATIONS (*Figure 1.45*)

In many patients the diagnosis is easy. The patient complains of heartburn with the characteristic postural and dietary associations, and without dysphagia, vomiting or weight loss. Investigations are unnecessary in these individuals, although follow-up is desirable to ensure that appropriate therapy has given relief, and that no new symptom has arisen.

Upper gastrointestinal endoscopy is desirable if the symptoms arise unexpectedly, are less typical, or are associated with epigastric pain or dysphagia, or if typical symptoms fail to respond to treatment; this is not only to confirm reflux oesophagitis but also particularly to discover a peptic ulcer or carcinoma of cardia or pylorus which may cause reflux symptoms.

If chest pain is less typically oesophageal, especially if it resembles cardiac pain, more careful assessment is needed, particularly using tests to provoke oesophageal pain.

Investigations must be categorized according to what abnormalities they might demonstrate because reflux symptoms may be present without oesophagitis, reflux oesophagitis may not cause symptoms, and pathological reflux may exist without oesophagitis or symptoms.

Tests for reflux

Barium radiology is an insensitive and unreliable test for gastro-oesophageal reflux[89] despite attempts to improve its discriminatory value by modification of technique[28] or methods of interpretation.[119] Scintiscanning, in which the oesophagus is scanned by a gamma camera after swallowing a technetium-labelled liquid meal and applying abdominal pressure by a binder, provides a semi-quantitative measure of reflux[49] but, because it is cumbersome, uncomfortable and involves radioactivity, it has not become popular. Detection of reflux by real-time ultrasound scanning is practicable but operator-dependent and not yet adequately standardized.

Intraluminal pH measurement

Although acid is not the sole cause of reflux disease, acid frequently refluxes abnormally in the great majority of patients with this disorder, except in those few patients with achlorhydria – e.g. after gastric surgery. Thus, measuring the frequency with which acid enters the lower oesophagus using a small pH electrode is a relatively simple way of quantifying at least the frequency of reflux. This has been achieved in various ways. The best known short test (sometimes known as the standard acid reflux test – SART) is to have the subject perform a series of provocative movements such as coughing or the Valsalva manoeuvre in different positions; in normal subjects there will be three or four spurts of acid in twelve manoeuvres. This test is specific but insensitive.[10]

Oesophageal pH can be monitored continuously over 12–24 hours using a solid state recorder with subsequent computerized play-back and analysis. Measurements, such as the frequency of acid spurts, their mean duration or the proportion of recording time under pH 4 or 5 may be automatically computed and compared with results in normal subjects. Although currently regarded as the best test for gastro-oesophageal reflux, it is beset by practical difficulties, and careful attention to detail, for example the positioning of the electrode, is essential if the results are to be useful and reliable.[15,26] Complicated 'scores' are probably unnecessary for interpretation; the percentage time that the pH in the lower oesophagus is less than 4 is the single best criterion for reflux. However, the 'normal' is age-related and in people over 45 years up to 12% of 'normal' subjects may have a low pH.[95]

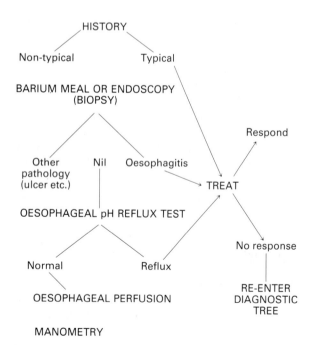

Figure 1.45 Diagnosis of gastro-oesophageal reflux.

Tests for oesophagitis

These tests are also performed to exclude other pathology.

Barium swallow and meal

The presence of oesophagitis is suggested by irregularity of the mucosa in profile, thickening of oesophageal folds or granularity of the mucosa,[104] but these subtle signs are present only when oesophagitis is marked and radiology is an insensitive and poorly specific method to diagnose mucosal inflammation.

A barium meal is effective in detecting or excluding alternative pathology, such as peptic ulceration or malignancy, and will usually detect motility abnormalities of the oesophagus.

Fibreoptic upper gastrointestinal endoscopy

Endoscopy provides more information about oesophageal disease than does radiology even though it is more uncomfortable and slightly more hazardous to the patient, and unsatisfactory for detecting motility abnormalities. It will detect ulcers and carcinoma at least as well as radiology but also enables an accurate assessment of oesophagitis to be made, and permits mucosal biopsies.

The mildest mucosal changes of oesophagitis are one or two red spots just above the gastro-oesophageal junction, especially posteriorly. Diffuse reddening of the lower oesophageal mucosa is not a reliable sign. Exudate on the surface of the spots increases their importance. More advanced damage is shown by elongation of these erosions to longitudinal streaks, usually on the crests of mucosal folds, and their extension around the circumference so that advanced degrees show confluence of erosions around the whole circumference of the cardia, extending several centimetres up the lumen of the oesophagus.

Observer error is frequent and written descriptions of changes should be provided. A number of classifications of endoscopic oesophagitis have been proposed, none being entirely satisfactory.[2] Until there is universal agreement, a description (and perhaps a diagram) in the hospital record is the most reliable method of communication.

About one-third of patients with gastro-esophageal reflux will have no detectable oesophagitis. The severity of oesophagitis correlates with the degree of reflux, but symptoms are not proportional to mucosal change and severe symptoms can occur in patients with no oesophagitis, whilst advanced mucosal disease is sometimes discovered in individuals with few symptoms.

Oesophageal biopsy

Up to 30% of patients with undoubted reflux symptoms do not have endoscopically visible oesophagitis but some will have histological abnormalities in mucosal biopsies. Conventional histological changes of inflammation are not always present, but hyperplasia of the basal cell layers of the squamous mucosa with elongation of papillae towards the surface are characteristic.[62] A biopsy should be taken 5 cm above the gastro-oesophageal mucosal junction if reflux is suspected and the oesophageal mucosa looks normal through the endoscope. although the small biopsies usually taken through fibreoptic endoscopes pose interpretative problems.[64]

Tests for oesophageal pain

Oesophageal perfusion

The discomfort can be precipitated or reproduced in almost all patients with pain from reflux oesophagitis by dripping 0.1 M hydrochloric acid into the oesophagus[17] in a 'single-blind' manner, using saline as a control. The patient compares any induced discomfort with his or her spontaneous pain. The pain of reflux oesophagitis is usually precipitated by acid but not saline, although in a few 'hyperreactors' saline also causes pain. Some patients have retrosternal burning generated by the acid perfusion which is different from their spontaneous pain; this is termed a 'positive unrelated response' and indicates that the spontaneous pain is probably not oesophageal in origin. This test is sometimes useful in differentiating oesophageal and cardiac pain.[16,37]

The irritable oesophagus

A relationship exists between pain and abnormal oesophageal motility in some patients with oesophageal pain, particularly if it is severe and cardiac-like. This spasm may be triggered spontaneously by injected provocative agents such as ergometrine or edrophonium, by balloon distension in the oesophagus or by episodes of acid gastro-oesophageal reflux. This has been termed 'the irritable oesophagus'.[51,86,111] Its practical relevance is that in any patient with oesophageal pain reflux should be searched for by a sensitive test such as intraluminal pH monitoring because reflux is the most treatable cause of such pain.[51]

Other tests

Oesophageal manometry

Pressure recording in the oesophagus permits measurement of lower oesophageal sphincter tone, and assessment of oesophageal peristalsis. However, it is of little value in the *diagnosis* of gastro-oesophageal reflux[25] because, although gastro-oesophageal sphincter tone tends to be lower in reflux subjects, there is considerable overlap with the normal population and the test has poor discrimination. Manometry is helpful as a preliminary to surgery in patients who respond poorly to medical treatment to assess oesophageal peristalsis and sphincter tone, and it will also detect aperistalsis as in systemic sclerosis in which reflux oesophagitis is common. Motor abnormalities, such as diffuse oesophageal spasm, may be detected which may themselves cause oesophageal pain in the absence of gastro-oesophageal reflux, or spasm associated with reflux; however, these spasm disorders are often intermittent and may not be apparent during a single, short-term recording.

Differential diagnosis of reflux oesophagitis

Peptic ulcer

Gastro-oesophageal reflux often complicates or coexists with peptic ulceration,[50,112,113] probably due to changes in gastric motility, gastro-oesophageal sphincter dysfunction, and the high acid content of the gastric juice. An ulcer may be suggested in a patient with reflux symptoms by unusually rapid progress of the symptoms, epigastric pain as well as heartburn or periodicity (of the duodenal ulcer type). A peptic ulcer should be sought radiologically or endoscopically in most patients with reflux oesophagitis as an ulcer modifies the management approach.

Cardiac pain

Characteristic heartburn with postural and postcibal aggravation is unlikely to be confused with cardiac pain. However, some patients with gastro-oesophageal reflux experience more severe pain which may simulate cardiac pain, sometimes even radiating into the arms or jaws, and occurring particularly during or after exercise. Conversely, cardiac pain is occasionally of burning character and sometimes predominantly postcibal or nocturnal. Careful elicitation of all details of the pain leads to accurate diagnosis in most patients, but standardized exercise electrocardiograms and tests for reflux oesophagitis may be necessary. Acid perfusion of the oesophagus is helpful. It must be emphasized that ischaemic heart disease and reflux oesophagitis are both common conditions in the middle-aged, and some patients will have pain from both causes, which can give rise to problems with therapy if the patient has difficulty in differentiating between the two pains.[14]

Functional dyspepsia

The syndrome of functional dyspepsia embraces a number of symptoms including upper abdominal fullness, nausea, early satiety, anorexia, morning vomiting, belching and also heartburn. Although its causation is not fully understood, in some patients it may be due to disordered gastric fundal accommodation or to disordered antral and duodenal motility with delayed gastric emptying and perhaps duodenogastric reflux. The heartburn may partly respond to antireflux measures but the other symptoms will not. Antireflux surgery should be avoided in such patients because they respond poorly. Prokinetic agents, such as metoclopramide or cisapride, may be more helpful.

Flatulent dyspepsia occurs in patients with gallstones. However, an equal number of people with flatulent dyspepsia have normal cholecystograms because they do not have gallstones, and removal of the gallbladder relieves the symptoms in fewer than half the patients. There is, therefore, no point in performing a 'routine' search for gallbladder disease in patients with gastro-oesophageal reflux disease; however, if a patient with gallstones has significant reflux oesophagitis, consideration may be given to performing an antireflux procedure at the same time as cholecystectomy.

TREATMENT

Most sufferers from intermittent heartburn find quick relief from any antacid preparation. Others require more treatment and, although the various available therapies may be tried empirically, it is helpful to consider their modes of action. As reflux oesophagitis is usually caused by a number of interacting abnormalities (see page 82), treatment may be directed at one or other of these factors.[11,12]

Frequency of reflux

Certain foods reduce lower oesophageal sphincter tone and should be avoided – particularly fat, chocolate, coffee, alcohol and spices. Cigarette smoking weakens the sphincter and allows reflux and should be stopped.

The lower oesophageal sphincter may be strengthened (i.e. its resting tone increased) by prokinetic drugs, of which cisapride is currently the most effective. However, reflux is frequently not due to weakness of the resting sphincter, but rather to its inappropriate relaxation (especially during sleep), or from spurts of reflux when the sphincter relaxes in response to a swallow, and at present this is not susceptible to pharmacological control.

Compounds containing sodium alginate and antacid interact with gastric acid to produce a floating, viscous foam which diminishes the frequency and duration of acid reflux.

Surgical antireflux operations markedly diminish reflux (see page 107).

Gastric factors

The volume of gastric contents should be kept small by avoiding large meals. Gastric emptying may be accelerated by a prokinetic agent such as metoclopramide or cisapride. Gastric secretory volume is lowered by anti-secretory drugs such as histamine H_2-receptor antagonists or proton pump inhibitors.

Oesophageal clearing

Any refluxed juices should be cleared from the oesophagus as quickly as possible to shorten contact with the mucosa. Swallowing induces primary peristalsis and is encouraged by antacids given as chewable tablets, which also stimulate secretion of alkaline saliva. At night, propping the bed-head up 20 cm reduces acid contact time and improves symptoms and oesophagitis.

Constituents of refluxed juice

The acid content can be neutralized by antacids, or reduced by histamine H_2-receptor antagonists or proton-pump inhibitors. At present no effective agent is available to lower concentrations of pepsin or bile salts, although the amount of duodeno-gastric reflux of bile may be lessened by prokinetic agents.

Mucosal sensitivity

Drugs such as corticosteroids or non-steroidal anti-inflammatory agents may be particularly irritant to the oesophagus and should be discontinued if possible, or at least reduced to the minimum practicable dose. Local anaesthetic agents do not diminish mucosal pain sensitivity. Cigarette smoke diminishes mucosal resistance to H^+ ion penetration and patients are advised to stop smoking; drugs including antibiotics and non-steroidal anti-inflammatory drugs may have a similar effect. Carbenoxolone increases mucosal repair mechanisms but has not been widely used, partly because of its aldosterone-like side effects. Sucralfate enhances resistance of the mucosa to acid, pepsin and bile, although its performance in clinical trials has not been uniformly good.

Vicious circles

The inflamed oesophagus is more sensitive and has an increased permeability to H^+ ions. Improving the oesophagitis, by whatever means, may itself be helpful in controlling gastro-oesophageal reflux. Experimental studies have shown that oesophagitis weakens the lower oesophageal sphincter but that this is reversible.[7,48] Oesophagitis diminishes oesophageal acid clearing which improves after medical treatment. Thus, if a period of intensive treatment can improve the condition, relapse is not inevitable when treatment is partially or wholly withdrawn.

A PRACTICAL APPROACH TO TREATMENT[11]

'Lifestyle modification'

Obese patients are advised to lose weight which can be a most effective therapeutic step although the mechanism is uncertain. Smoking should be discontinued and the patient advised not to eat fatty foods and chocolate. Alcohol and coffee are discouraged. meals must be of small volume and not taken late at night. Drugs which may aggravate the condition such as the non-steroidal anti-inflammatory, anticholinergic and calcium-channel blocking agents, and the theophylline compounds, should be stopped or at least reduced if possible.

Initial medication

An antacid–alginate compound is prescribed after meals and at bedtime supplemented by antacid tablets sucked frequently, every 1–2 hours between meals.

Further medication

If symptoms are more severe or persist a histamine H_2-receptor blocking drug may be given. The standard dose (as for peptic ulcers) may suffice but often higher and more frequent doses, e.g. cimetidine 400 mg four times daily, ranitidine 300 mg twice daily or famotidine 40 mg twice daily are needed.

The bed-head should be elevated on 20 cm blocks if the response remains inadequate or a prokinetic agent such as cisapride 5–20 mg before meals and at bedtime should be added. The proton-pump inhibitor omeprazole (20–40 mg with breakfast) provides a high rate of symptom reduction and healing of oesophagitis.

Most patients will respond to this regimen which should be maintained for about 12 weeks. Thereafter one measure at a time is withdrawn whilst any recurrence of symptoms indicates its restitution. In this way the minimum maintenance treatment may be determined.

Surgery is considered if improvement is inadequate or can only be maintained at the cost of continuous irksome measures, but it is necessary to be certain that the symptoms are due exclusively to gastro-oesophageal reflux (see page 87). Acid-reducing operations alone are inadequate, although they may be combined with an antireflux procedure if there is evidence of hypersecretion or associated peptic ulceration. The most widely used effective antireflux procedure is the Nissen fundoplication or one of its variants (see page 109). A silicone ring tied round the lower oesophagus below the diaphragm[1] has produced some good results but complications (such as dysphagia) are too frequent for its recommendation. Bile diversion, using a Roux-en-Y anastomosis may relieve heartburn dramatically, especially when oesophagitis has followed gastric surgery or a cardiomyotomy for achalasia, or if the cardia is inaccessible for technical reasons.

OESOPHAGEAL ULCER

An ulcer may complicate reflux oesophagitis. Ulcers usually occur at the junction between oesophageal squamous mucosa and the distal mucosa. Other ulcers occur within Barrett's epithelium (Barrett's ulcer – see below) at the junction of the two epithelia (Wolf–Marshak–Som ulcer) or within the squamous mucosa proximal to the junction (Savary ulcer). The symptoms of reflux oesophagitis do not necessarily change when an ulcer occurs but many patients report pain in the lower sternal region which is more persistent, penetrating and severe than before. Dysphagia is usually present even if there is no demonstrable stricture.

An oesophageal ulcer is an occasional cause of haematemesis; spontaneous perforation rarely occurs.

Oesophageal erosions or ulcers may be caused by corrosives and particularly by tablets. The patient notices the rapid or sudden onset of retrosternal pain and dysphagia which may prevent any food or solids being swallowed. The ulcer may be seen endoscopically.

The majority heal readily with a standard antireflux medication whilst those that are resistant require a proton-pump inhibitor.[70] Ulcers heal quickly if the offending medication is stopped.

BARRETT'S SYNDROME (COLUMNAR-LINED OESOPHAGUS)

Barrett described[8,9] an oesophagus in which the lower part was lined not by stratified squamous epithelium but with columnar epithelium similar to that found in the stomach. This phenomenon has been observed frequently although the reason for ulcerated squamous epithelium being replaced by columnar remains obscure.

DEFINITION

An extension of columnar epithelium of more than 3 cm, either as a cylinder or as 'tongues', above the cardia is considered to constitute the columnar-lined oesophagus.[32,92,118] There is the possibility of readily confusing a tubular hiatus hernia with columnar-lined oesophagus but in practice the decision is not difficult for the experienced endoscopist. The tubular columnar-lined oesophagus lacks the folds usually seen in a herniated stomach. A more common error is for an endoscopist to fail to recognize that the squamocolumnar junction lies high in the oesophagus, thereby overlooking the diagnosis.

AETIOLOGY

Although it is agreed that patients with columnar-lined oesophagus have gastro-oesophageal reflux[61] and often a weak gastro-oesophageal sphincter,[61,116] the factors which cause substitution of the squamous lining by columnar epithelium remain obscure. Credence was attached to the idea that recurrent ulceration of the squamous lining healed by metaplastic columnar epithelium, a process which slowly crept up the oesophagus.[55] The number of instances in which this has been observed are few and the degree of 'creep' is small and hardly explains the extent of columnar-lined oesophagus which may be 15–20 cm. In one carefully documented series when patients were endoscoped regularly there was no evidence of extension of columnar-lined oesophagus; moreover older patients did not have a greater extent than younger patients, favouring the view that the development of columnar-lined oesophagus may be a sudden event, perhaps consequent upon severe and extensive loss of mucosa.[22] A defect created in the squamous mucosa of dogs, and separated from the gastric mucosa by a strip of normal squamous epithelium, heals by columnar epithelium derived from cells lining oesophageal gland ducts when there is free reflux of acid.[52]

The incidence of columnar-lined oesophagus is reported to be from 0.6% to 4% of all endoscopies[21,38,59,83] and from 10% to 20% of all patients with endoscopic oesophagitis.[32,83,90,102,118]

CLINICAL FEATURES

Most patients with columnar-lined oesophagus have symptoms indistinguishable from uncomplicated gastro-oesophageal reflux. Dysphagia, even without a stricture, is relatively common; consequently, 40% of patients reported by Cooper and Barbezat[32] had this symptom, probably because of the frequently defective peristalsis. Oesophageal ulcers in association with columnar-lined oesophagus may give particularly severe pain or even lead to haemorrhage (see page 85). Strictures often occur and may be the cause of the presenting symptom; one report found dysphagia in 44% of columnar-lined oesophagus in patients with chronic oesophageal strictures.[99] Strictures are usually at or immediately above the squamo-columnar junction although a few occur within the columnar-lined oesophagus, probably at the site of a healed Barrett's ulcer. Ulcers and strictures probably occur only in patients with circumferential columnar-lined oesophagus, and lesser degree of substitution may not be at risk of these complications.[59]

MALIGNANT POTENTIAL

The propensity of columnar-lined oesophagus to develop adenocarcinoma is the chief cause of concern and a main reason for interest in this condition. The exact risk is uncertain; *prevalence* studies have reported figures from zero to 46.5%.[5,97] More importantly retrospective studies of *incidence* show figures from 1 adenocarcinoma per 46 'patient-years' of follow-up to 1 per 441 patient-years; however, such studies are fraught with statistical difficulties, not least because the duration of the columnar-lined oesophagus before surveillance began is unknown. Three large studies [23,98,107] found incidences of 1/175, 1/441 and 1/170 patient-years, an estimated risk 30–40 times greater than the 'general population', although Atkinson[5] comments that 'general population' incidence figures are unreliable because some of these growths will be gastric in origin and others will have arisen in unrecognized columnar-lined oesophagus.

Unfortunately, established adenocarcinomas tend to be advanced by the time of diagnosis;[54,92,94,97] therefore the possibilities of detecting pre-malignant change have aroused considerable interest. Dysplasia can be recognized and is often found to be associated with established adenocarcinoma in columnar-lined oesophagus.[54,92,94,97] There is a strong likelihood of invasive carcinoma being present where there is high-grade dysplasia if the oesophagus is removed,[71,88] but the significance and importance of milder degrees of dysplasia is less clear.

The cost-effectiveness of endoscopic screening of patients with columnar-lined oesophagus has not been established. A practical approach may be to undertake annual endoscopic examination of patients with columnar-lined oesophagus of more than 8 cm in extent, provided the patients are suitable candidates for oesophagectomy should severe dysplasia be reliably detected.[5]

OESOPHAGEAL STRICTURES

DEFINITION

An oesophageal stricture is a narrowing of the lumen caused by an abnormality of the oesophageal wall. Strictures, other than those caused by carcinoma, are due to inflammation, usually with mucosal ulceration and fibrous scarring. The oesophagus behaves as other parts of the alimentary tract which may also respond to mucosal damage by cicatricial narrowing. Strictures are rigid and inelastic.

Narrowing of the oesophagus may, however, be transient and may disappear after being stretched or after removal of an irritant agent. The stricture may be visible radiologically and yet cause no obstruction to the passage of food or an endoscope. Such abnormalities are rarely removed surgically or explored at autopsy and their nature remains in doubt. They are sometimes called 'elastic strictures' with the implication that circular muscle fibre spasm is responsible, although this can rarely be demonstrated by pressure measurements, or due to 'webs' or 'rings'. Their relation, if any, to fibrous strictures is unclear.

AETIOLOGY

Corrosive strictures

Diffuse

Strong alkali or strong acid if the concentration, volume and duration of contact are sufficient can lead to necrosis, which may be deep and extend over a considerable area, sometimes leading to perforation. Within 3 weeks fibrous scarring develops and readily leads to stricture formation graded as:

Grade I: Shelf strictures, involving a short segment but not circumferential

Grade II: Annular strictures, less than 1 cm in length

Grade III: Dense annular strictures, less than 1 cm long extended through all layers

Grade IV: Tubular strictures with peri-oesophageal adhesions

Local corrosion

Various tablets cause oesophagitis locally if they adhere to the mucosa. Those implicated include non-steroidal anti-inflammatory drugs, potassium chloride, tetracycline and related antibiotics.[31] Swallowed tablets often remain in the oesophagus for longer than 5 minutes and may produce a small area of oesophagitis or an ulcer with accompanying pain or dysphagia. This sometimes progresses to stricture formation by fibrous scarring.

Infections (Candida sp.)

Severe or prolonged candidiasis can lead to a stricture.

Gastro-oesophageal reflux

Fibrous oesophageal strictures result from reflux but the pathogenesis is uncertain. Severe, prolonged oesophagitis, with mucosal and penetrating ulceration, is likely to lead eventually to a stricture but strictures are found in patients who acknowledge few previous symptoms of reflux, and particularly occur in the elderly (*Figure 1.46*). Sometimes the strictures appear quickly, e.g. after a period of recumbency or the prolonged placement of a nasogastric tube. It is hard to understand how a fibrous cicatrix can evolve so quickly if the usual explanation of recurrent ulceration and associated fibrous reaction is accepted, unless there has been pre-existing painless oesophagitis, and the intubation or recumbency has simply caused a major exacerbation.

In Britain almost all oesophageal strictures are due to reflux oesophagitis as corrosive swallowing is rare. An association with the ingestion of non-steroidal anti-inflammatory drugs has been observed.[56,118]

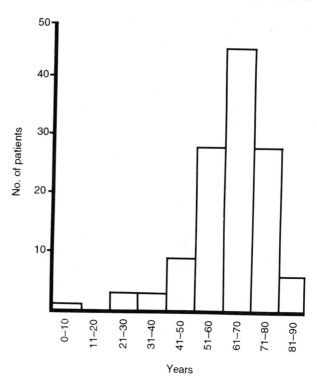

Figure 1.46 Age distribution of patients with oesophageal strictures seen at Hull Royal Infirmary 1980–1990.

Webs and rings

Schatzki–Kramer ring

Ring-like narrow constrictions of the lower oesophagus may be evanescent, are often invisible to the endoscopist (though mucosal diaphragms have been seen and biopsied), and dysphagia is often absent or occurs only occasionally at widely spread intervals. Some probably represent the early stage of a stricture following gastro-oesophageal reflux, whilst others are a motor phenomenon, either a strongly contracting gastro-oesophageal sphincter, a longitudinal muscle contraction throwing up a pleat of mucosa, or an area of circular muscle 'spasm'.

Sideropenic web (Patterson–Brown–Kelley syndrome)

A web is sometimes seen at the level of the cricopharyngeal sphincter in patients who are iron deficient. The webs are slender and usually detected radiologically on the anterior aspect of the pharynx. They may cause intermittent, high dysphagia.

CLINICAL FEATURES

The main symptom of an oesophageal stricture is dysphagia, the complaint being a feeling of food 'sticking' or being delayed in its passage through the oesophagus. Corrosive strictures, especially if long, often lead to severe dysphagia affecting even liquids, and the lumen may be completely obliterated. Benign 'peptic' strictures usually have a slow onset with dysphagia developing gradually over several years. Even when the lumen is severely narrow, dysphagia only affects solids, and it is rare for a benign stricture to cause difficulty in drinking liquids, unless a solid bolus becomes impacted. The degree of dysphagia is related to the diameter of the residual lumen but this is not the only factor. The severity of associated oesophagitis is an equally important determinant of dysphagia and failure of motility is a further contributory factor. There may also be pain on drinking hot liquids or strong alcohol due to the associated mucosal changes. A past history of heartburn or reflux for some years may be present but is denied by up to half the patients.

A malignant stricture must be considered if the dysphagia progresses rapidly or leads to complete dysphagia for fluids as well as solids, or if a solid bolus impacts with pain due to strong secondary peristalsis.

INVESTIGATIONS

Radiology

Radiological screening of swallowed radio-opaque medium is the desirable first step in the investigation of any patient with dysphagia, although if a stricture is suspected, endoscopy by an experienced operator without preceding radiology is permissible. Barium is usually used unless a perforation is suspected. The purpose of radiology is to demonstrate if there is a stricture, its site, its length and its nature.

A stricture is best demonstrated if the oesophagus is well distended by a large volume of swallowed barium with the patient prone (*Figure 1.47a*). Barium should be allowed to pass through the stricture into the stomach and, by tipping the patient head-down, the oesophagus may be filled from below, demonstrating the lower extent of the stricture and hence its length. It is not always easy to decide whether the stricture is benign or malignant. Distension and complete filling aid differentiation by demonstrating the abrupt transition to normal,

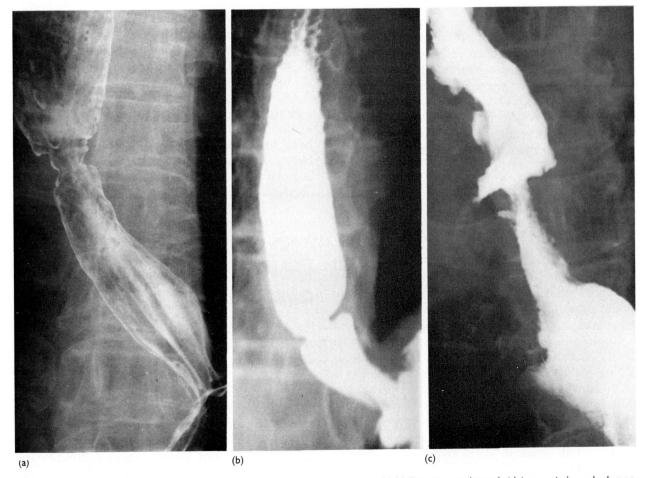

(a) (b) (c)

Figure 1.47 (a) Benign 'peptic' stricture of oesophagus: note smooth tapering. (b) Malignant oesophageal stricture: note irregular lumen and abrupt transition between normal and abnormal ('shouldering'). (c) Oesophageal web: note the thin web with a wide lumen.

distensible oesophagus ('shouldering'), and the irregularity of the channel through a carcinoma (*Figure 1.47b*), whereas a benign stricture shows a smooth tapering.

The diameter of the stricture may be measured by comparing the width of the barium stream using a radio-opaque ruler placed behind the patient, or by asking the patient to swallow a series of radio-opaque balls, of increasing size, until one impacts. Such balls can be made of wax which melt at body temperature.[46]

Endoscopy

Any patient with dysphagia requires endoscopy whether or not a lesion has been shown radiologically. If a stricture is visible on a radiograph its nature requires elucidation by inspection and biopsy; if no abnormality is seen radiologically a stricture may still be detectable by the endoscope.

The purpose of endoscopy is to confirm the presence of a stricture, to assess its nature, to obtain biopsies and cytology specimens, and (sometimes) dilatation by bougienage.

Presence of the stricture
Usually the narrowing of the oesophageal lumen will be apparent as the endoscope proceeds down the oesophagus. Often oesophagitis will be seen at the narrowest point or extending a few centimetres above. Occasionally no clear narrowing is observed which may be because the stricture lumen is greater than the diameter of the endoscope or that the stricture seen radiologically is predominantly a motor phenomenon ('spasm').

Assessment of its nature
It is essential to determine whether the stricture is benign or malignant. Characteristically a benign stricture is smooth, not very narrow, and there may be associated oesophagitis or mucosal peptic ulceration. A malignant stricture is usually irregular with polypoid projections, friable and haemorrhagic with some necrotic areas, and it may be very narrow. However, appearances can be misleading. Severe oesophagitis near a benign stricture may render the wall oedematous, haemorrhagic and friable, simulating the appearances of malignancy, whereas a malignant stricture may be relatively smooth and non-friable. A particular problem is the gastric fundal carcinoma which infiltrates the cardia submucosally. This may cause narrowing that is symmetrical and smooth because it is covered by normal epithelium.

Webs and rings may be invisible to the endoscopist, either because they are stretched by the rapid passage of the instrument, or because inadequate distension of the lumen with air fails to demonstrate these slender structures whose bore is usually wide (*Figure 1.47c*). If seen and displayed by distension with air, the appearance is of a thin, featureless ring of normal mucosa. Biopsies show normal histological features but the mucosa immediately below a lower oesophageal ring is usually columnar in type.

An uncommon but important differentiation is between achalasia and a stricture, particularly in a patient known to have had achalasia treated in the past, whether by surgery or dilatation. In this difficult setting manometry and the endoscopic appearances are the only ways of achieving the diagnosis. In achalasia the endoscope will usually pass with slight pressure through the high-pressure, pliable sphincter. A stricture will be appreciated as a firm obstruction which will either not yield, or will do so abruptly as the fibrous tissue is stretched. Oesophagitis is often not visible although these strictures are due to reflux.

Biopsies and cytology specimens
Tissue specimens for histology and cytology should always be taken except in the case of a known corrosive stricture, or an obvious mucosal ring or web. Cytology specimens are obtained by brushing the lumen of the stricture. Ideally, biopsies of the narrowest part of the stricture are taken from each quadrant, plus two further specimens after passing the forceps through the stricture. Further specimens distal to the stricture can be obtained at repeat endoscopy after dilatation. The tangential approach of the forceps to the lumen may make specimens hard to obtain but crocodile-toothed or spiked biopsy forceps are helpful. The combination of cytology and biopsies should lead to a correct distinction between benign and malignant strictures in over 95% of cases.

TREATMENT

Corrosive stricture

Local strictures following corrosive tablet ingestion are usually short and not dense. They are easily dilated and may require only one course of bougienage.

Strictures caused by liquid corrosives may be more difficult to manage and are dealt with according to their grade. Grades I, II and most of III can be treated by intermittent bougienage, beginning 3 weeks after the burn. Bougienage carried out earlier has a high incidence of perforation. Weekly dilatations are performed initially with lengthening intervals according to response. If the intervals between dilatations cannot be lengthened to a convenient period, the patient may be taught self-bougienage using Maloney mercury bougies.

Those strictures of grade III which are tough, and most of the long grade IV strictures, may be difficult and hazardous to dilate. However, this is hard to predict and a trial of bougienage is always justified. Surgery should be recommended if dilatation by bougies is impossible or if it is required too frequently and the patient is fit enough. Short strictures can be excised with reanastomosis but long ones require excision and replacement by colon or jejunum.

Reflux (peptic) strictures

The choices of therapy are either medical alone or medical plus stricture dilatation, or surgery. If standard antireflux medical therapy is provided, up to one-third of patients will require no other treatment, presumably because of the reduction of spasm. However, the propensity for reflux continues even if the stricture resolves or is alleviated. It is therefore necessary to maintain the patient on a permanent medical regimen if it is to be effective and lasting, and if the effects of dilatation by bougies are to be maximized.

Stricture dilatation

Dilatation of strictures using unguided bougies through an open rigid oesophagoscope cannot be recommended for routine use because of the risk of perforation. Current choice for dilatation lies between bougies passed over a guide wire, or balloons or mercury-weighted rubber bougies.

Bougies over guide wire

The original Eder–Puestow dilators, the efficacy and safety of which has transformed the modern management of benign strictures, have been superseded by new designs which are faster, more comfortable and safer. The best available are shown in Table 1.14 which records their sizes and calculated 'angle of incidence' because a narrow angle makes for easier and smoother dilatation. All are passed over a guide wire introduced through the channel of the endoscope which is then removed. Benzodiazepine sedation is usually the only required medication but occasionally pethidine may be added.

Balloons[36]

Polyethylene balloons, derived from Grunzig angioplasty balloons, have been used for stricture dilatation. They are inelastic and when fully inflated retain their fixed size; increasing pressure renders the balloon harder but not larger. They may be passed over a guide wire under radiological direction, or under direct vision passed down the endoscope channel. The balloons may be convenient under some circumstances but they are expensive and there is no evidence that they are safer and, indeed, they may be less effective than bougies.[34]

Mercury-weighted bougies

The mercury-weighted flexible rubber bougies designed by Maloney are generally safe and can be passed with the patient sitting without sedation. The patient may learn to pass his or her own. They will not dilate a narrow stricture and are unsafe if the lumen is eccentric or irregular, so their real value is in maintaining an adequate lumen after dilatation by some other technique.

Table 1.14 Bougies over guide wire

Dilator	Wire needed?	Radiograph needed?	Min. diameter (tip) (mm)	Max. diameter (body) mm	Fr	Tip to max. diameter* (cm)	Angle of incidence (°)†	Number of passages‡
Balloon (Rigiflex)	Yes	Yes	2.8	20	60	8	–	1
Balloon (Rigiflex TTS)	Yes	No	1.8	20	60	8	–	1
Celestin	Yes	No	3.7	18	54	16	6	2
Eder–Puestow	Yes	No	3.7	19.3	58	2.1	49	Multiple
Hurst	No	No	4.0	19.5	59	14	8	3
KAD	Yes	No	3.0	17.3	52	8.2	12	3 or less
Maloney	No	No	4.4	16	48	11.5	8	Multiple
Pilling	No	No	4.4	19.8	60	14	8	Multiple
Savary	Yes	No	5.0	20	60	17.7	6	Multiple
Tridil	Yes	No	3.7	18	54	2.1	46	3 or less

Reproduced with permission from *Therapeutic Endoscopy and Radiology of the Gut* (eds) J.R. Bennett and R.H. Hunt, Chapman & Hall, London, 1990.

Dilatation of the stricture is usually necessary at least once, whether medical or surgical treatment is employed, but in many patients recurrent dilatation is needed. A second dilatation may be performed in association with a medical regimen 1–2 weeks after the first dilatation but, unless the stricture is clearly narrowing rapidly, the intervals between dilatation can soon be lengthened. After the first 6 months few patients should need more than two or three dilatations a year and many will find them unnecessary.[115]

It is desirable that cytology and biopsy specimens should be taken from the stricture annually at the time of dilatation because of the possibility of malignant transformation.

SURGERY (see page 109)

Many patients may retain relatively trouble-free swallowing by medical treatment plus bougienage but the need for more than occasional dilatation is irksome and not without hazard. Treatment by surgery should be recommended for younger fit patients if control of dysphagia by bougienage is imperfect. Unless oesophagitis and perioesophagitis have so damaged the oesophagus that its replacement by a segment of intestine is desirable, an operation to prevent gastro-oesophageal reflux, or to modify the nature of the refluxed material, is usually combined with preoperative dilatation of the stricture, and if necessary postoperative bougienage.[114] Such surgery is difficult and carries a definite morbidity and mortality even in the young. It should not be considered as the first choice for treating a condition which predominantly affects the middle-aged and elderly, intermittent bougienage offering such patients the best long-term outcome.

REFERENCES

1. Angelchik, J.P. and Cohen, R. (1979) A new surgical procedure for the treatment of gastro-esophageal reflux and hiatal hernia. *Surgery, Gynecology and Obstetrics*, **148**, 246–248.
2. Armstrong, D., Monnier, P.H., Nicolet, M., Blum, A.C. and Savary, M. (1991) Endoscopic assessment of oesophagitis. *Gullet*, **1**, 63–67.
3. Atkinson, M. (1981) Bleeding from the oesophagus. In *Gastrointestinal Haemorrhage*, (Eds) Dykes, P.W. and Keighley, M.R.B., pp. 23–33, London: Wright PSG.
4. Atkinson, M. and Summerling, M.D. (1954) The competence of the cardia after cardiomyotomy. *Gastroenterologia*, **92**, 123–134.
5. Atkinson, M. (1989) Barrett's oesophagus – to screen or not to screen? *Gut*, **30**, 2–5.
6. Babka, J.C. and Castell, D.O. (1973) On the genesis of heartburn; the effects of specific foods on the lower oesophageal sphincter. *American Journal of Digestive Diseases*, **18**, 391–397.
7. Baldi, F., Ferrarini, F. and Longanesi, A. *et al.* (1988) Oesophageal function before, during, and after healing of erosive oesophagitis. *Gut*, **29**, 157–160.
8. Barrett, N.R. (1950) Chronic peptic ulcer of the oesophagus and oesophagitis. *British Journal of Surgery*, **38**, 175–182.
9. Barrett, N.R. (1957) The lower oesophagus lined by columnar epithelium. *Surgery*, **41**, 881–894.
10. Behar, J., Biancini, P. and Sheahan, D.G. (1976) Evaluation of esophageal tests in the diagnosis of reflux esophagitis. *Gastroenterology*, **71**, 9–15.
11. Bennett, J.R. (1988) Medical therapy for gastro-oesophageal reflux. In *Reflux Oesophagitis* (Eds) Hennessy, T.P.J., Cuschieri, A. and Bennett, J.R., pp. 123–141. London: Butterworths.
12. Bennett, J.R. (1978) Medical management of gastro-oesophageal reflux. *Clinics in Gastroenterology*, **5**, 175–185.
13. Bennett, J.R. (1980) Treatment of achalasia, a review. *Journal of the Society of Medicine*, **73**, 649–653.
14. Bennett, J.R. (1983) Chest pain – heart or gullet? *British Medical Journal*.
15. Bennett, J.R. (1987) pH measurement in the oesophagus. *Baillière's Clinical Gastroenterology*, **1**, 747–768.
16. Bennett, J.R. and Atkinson, M. (1966) Oesophageal acid perfusion in the diagnosis of precordial pain. *The Lancet*, **2**, 1150–1152.
17. Bernstein, L., Fruin, R. and Pacini, R. (1962) Differentiation of esophageal pain from angina pectoris. *Medicine*, **41**, 143–162.
18. Biancini, P., Barwick, K., Selling, J. and McCallum, R. (1984) Effects of acute experimental esophagitis on mechanical properties of the lower esophageal sphincter. *Gastroenterology*, **87**, 8–16.
19. Booth, D.J., Kemmerer, M.D. and Skinner, D.B. (1968) Acid clearing from the distal esophagus. *Archives of Surgery*, **76**, 732–734.
20. Branicki, F.J., Evans, D.F., Ogilvie, A.L., Atkinson, M. and Hardcastle, J.D. (1982) Ambulatory monitoring of oesophageal pH in reflux oesophagitis using a portable radiotelemetry system. *Gut*, **23**, 992–998.
21. Burbige, E.S. and Radigan, H. (1978) Characteristics of the columnar-lined oesophagus. *Gastroenterology*, **74**, 1015.
22. Cameron, A.J. (1984) A follow-up study of Barrett's esophagus: does the length of columnar mucosa progress or regress? *Proceedings of Fourth World Congress of the International Society for Diseases of the Esophagus*, Chicago.
23. Cameron, A.J., Ott, B.J. and Payne, W.G. (1985) The incidence of adenocarcinoma in columnar-lined (Barrett's) esophagus. *New England Journal of Medicine*, **313**, 857–859.
24. Carre, I.J. (1959) The natural history of the partial

thoracic stomach (hiatus hernia) in children. *Archives of the Diseases in Childhood*, **34**, 44–53.

25. Castell, D.O. (1982) Clinical application of esophageal manometry. *Digestive Diseases and Sciences*, **27**, 769–771.

26. Castell, D.O. (1990) Ambulatory monitoring in esophageal disease. *Gastroenterology International*, **3**, 40–44.

27. Celestin, L.R. and Campbell, W.B. (1981) A new and safe system for oesophageal dilatation. *The Lancet*, **1**, 74–75.

28. Christiansen, T., Funch-Jensen, P., Jacobsen, N.O. and Thommesen, P. (1987) Radiologic quantitation of gastro-oesophageal reflux. *Acta Radiologica*, **28**, 731–734.

29. Cohen, S., Fisher, R. and Lipschutz, W. (1972) The pathogenesis of esophageal dysfunction in scleroderma and Raynaud's disease. *Journal of Clinical Investigation*, **51**, 2663–2668.

30. Collen, M.J., Lewis, J.H. and Benjamin, S.B. (1990) Gastric acid hypersecretion in refractory gastro-esophageal reflux disease. *Gastroenterology*, **98**, 654–661.

31. Collins, F.J., Matthews, H.R., Baker, S.E. and Strakava, J.M. (1971) Drug-induced oesophageal injury. *British Medical Journal*, **1**, 1673–1676.

32. Cooper, B.J. and Barbezat, G.O. (1987) Barrett's oesophagus: a clinical study of 52 patients. *Quarterly Journal of Medicine*, **62**, 97–100.

33. Corazziari, E., Bontempo, I., Anzini, F. and Torsoli, A. (1982) Motility of the distal esophagus and gastro-esophageal reflux. First European Symposium on Gastro-intestinal Motility. *Gut*, **25**, 7–13.

34. Cox, J.G.C., Winter, R.K., Maslin, S.C. *et al.* (1988) Balloon or bougie for dilatation of benign oesophageal strictures? An interim report of a randomised controlled trial. *Gut*, **29**, 1741–1747.

35. Curci, M. and Dibbins, A. (1982) Gastro-esophageal reflux in children: an under-rated disease. *American Journal of Surgery*, **143**, 413–416.

36. Dakkak, M. and Bennett, J.R. (1991) Balloon technology and its applications in gastrointestinal endoscopy. *Baillière's Clinical Gastroenterology*, **5**, 195–208.

37. Davies, H.A., Jones, D.B. and Rhodes, J. (1982) 'Esophageal angina' as the cause of chest pain. *Journal of the American Medical Association*, **248**, 2274–2278.

38. Dees, J., Van Blankenstein, M. and Frenkel, K. (1978) Adenocarcinoma in Barrett's esophagus: a report of 13 cases. *Gastroenterology*, **74**, 1119.

39. Dennish, G.W. and Castell, D.O. (1971) Inhibitory effect of smoking on the lower esophageal sphincter. *New England Journal of Medicine*, **284**, 1136–1137.

40. Dennish, G.W. and Castell, D.O. (1977) Caffeine and the lower esophageal sphincter. *American Journal of Digestive Diseases*, **17**, 993–996.

41. De Meester, J.R. and Johnson, L.F. (1976) The evaluation of objective measurements of gastro-esophageal reflux and their contributions to patient management. *Surgical Clinics of North America*, **56**, 39–53.

42. Dent, J., Dodds, W.J., Friedman, R.H. *et al.* (1980) Mechanism of gastro-esophageal reflux in recumbent asymptomatic human subjects. *Journal of Clinical Investigation*, **65**, 256–267.

43. Dent, J., Holloway, R.H., Toouli, J. and Dodds, W.J. (1988) Mechanisms of lower oesophageal sphincter incompetence in patients with symptomatic gastro-oesophageal reflux. *Gut*, **29**, 1024–1028.

44. Dodds, W.J., Dent, J., Hogan W.J. *et al.* (1982) Mechanisms of gastro-esophageal reflux in patients with reflux esophagitis. *New England Journal of Medicine*, **307**, 1549–1552.

45. Dodds, W.J., Hogan, W.J., Helm, J.F. and Dent, J. (1981) Pathogenesis of reflux esophagitis. *Gastroenterology*, **81**, 376–394.

46. Dyet, J.F., Bennett, J.R., Buckton, G.K. and Ashworth, D. (1983) The radiological measurement of oesophageal stricture diameter. *Clinical Radiology*, **34**, 647–649.

47. Eastwood, G.L., Beck, G.D., Castell, D.O. *et al.* (1981) Beneficial effects of Indomethacin in acid-induced esophagitis in cats. *Digestive Diseases and Sciences*, **26**, 601–608.

48. Eastwood, G.L., Castell, D.O. and Higgs, R.H. (1975) Experimental esophagitis in cats impairs lower esophageal sphincter pressure. *Gastroenterology*, **69**, 146–163.

49. Fisher, R.S., Malmud, L.S., Roberts, G.S. and Lobis, I.F. (1976) Gastroesophageal scintiscanning to detect acid gastro-esophageal reflux. *Gastroenterology*, **70**, 301–308.

50. Flook, D. and Stoddard, C.J. (1985) Gastro-oesophageal reflux and oesophagitis after vagotomy for duodenal ulcer. *British Journal of Surgery*, **72**, 804–807.

51. Ghillebert, G., Janssens, J., Vantrappen, G., Nevens, F. and Pressens, J. (1990) Ambulatory 24h intra oesophageal pH and pressure recordings v. provocation tests in the diagnosis of chest pain of oesophageal origin. *Gut*, **31**, 738–744.

52. Gillen, P., Keeting, P., Byrne, P.J., West, A.G. and Hennessey, T.P.J. (1988) Experimental columnar metaplasia in the canine oesophagus. *British Journal of Surgery*, **75**, 117–115.

53. Goldman, J.M. and Bennett, J.R. (1990) Gastro-oesophageal reflux and asthma: a common association but of what clinical importance? *Gut*, **31**, 1–3.

54. Harle, I.A., Finlay, R.J., Balsheim *et al.* (1985) Management of adenocarcinoma in columnar-lined esophagus. *American Thoracic Surgery*, **40**, 330–336.

55. Hayward, J. (1961) The treatment of fibrous stricture of the oesophagus associated with hiatal hernia. *Thorax*, **16**, 45–52.

56. Heller, S.R., Fellows, I.W., Ogilvie, A.L. and Atkinson, M. (1982) Non-steroidal anti-inflammatory drugs and benign oesophageal stricture. *British Medical Journal*, **2**, 167–168.

57. Helm, J.F., Dodds, W.J. and Hogan, W.J. (1987) Salivary response to esophageal acid in normal subjects and patients with reflux esophagitis. *Gastroenterology*, **93**, 1393–1397.

58. Helm, J.F., Dodds, W.J., Riedel, D.R. *et al.* (1983) Determinants of esophageal acid disease in normal subjects. *Gastroenterology*, **85**, 607–612.

59. Herlihy K.J., Orlando, R.L. and Bryson, J.L. (1984) Barrett's oesophagus – clinical, endoscopic, histologic, manometric and electrical potential characteristics. *Gastroenterology*, **86**, 436–443.

60. Hogan, W.J., de Andrado, V. and Winship, D.H. (1982) Ethanol-induced esophageal motor dysfunction. *Journal of Applied Physiology*, **32**, 755–760.

61. Iascone, C., de Meester, T.R., Little, A.G. *et al.* (1983) Barrett's esophagus: functional assessment, proposed pathogenesis and surgical management. *Archives of Surgery*, **118**, 543–549.

62. Ismail-Beigi, F., Horton, P.E. and Pope. C.W. II (1970) Histological consequence of gastroesophageal reflux in man. *Gastroenterology*, **58**, 163–169.

63. Jones, R.H., Lydeard, S.E., Hobbs, F.D. *et al.* (1990) Dyspepsia in England and Scotland. *Gut*, **31**, 401–405.

64. Kaboyoshi, S. and Kasugai, T. (1974) Endoscopic and biopsy criteria for the diagnosis of oesophagitis with a fibreoptic esophagoscope. *Digestive Diseases*, **19**, 345–353.

65. Kahrilas, P.J., Dodds, W.J., Hogan, W.J. *et al.* (1986) Esophageal peristaltic dysfunction in peptic esophagitis. *Gastroenterology*, **91**, 897–904.

66. Kaufman, S.E. and Kaye, M.D. (1978) Induction of gastro-oesophageal reflux by alcohol. *Gut*, **19**, 336–338.

67. Kaye, M.D. and Showalter, J.P. (1974) Pyloric incompetence in patients with symptomatic gastroesophageal reflux. *Journal of Laboratory and Clinical Medicine*, **83**, 198–206.

68. Klauser, A.B., Schindlebeck, N.E. and Muller-Lissner, S.A. (1990) Symptoms in gastro-oesophageal reflux disease. *The Lancet*, **1**, 205–208.

69. Kruse-Anderson, S., Wallin, L. and Madsen, T. (1987) Acid gastro-oesophageal reflux and oesophageal pressure activity during post-prandial and nocturnal periods. *Scandinavian Journal of Gastroenterology*, **22**, 926–930.

70. Lee, F.I. and Isaacs, P.E.T. (1989) Peptic ulcer of the esophagus (Barrett ulcer). Healing in response to standard dose ranitidine, high dose ranitidine and omeprazole. *American Journal of Gastroenterology*, **940**, 926.

71. Lee, R.G. (1985) Dysplasia in Barrett's esophagus. *American Journal of Surgical Pathology*, **9**, 845–852.

72. Logan, K.R., Hopwood, D. and Milne, G. (1977) Ultrastructural demonstration of a cell coat on the cell surface of normal oesophageal epithelium. *Histochemistry Journal*, **9**, 495–504.

73. McCallum, R.W., Berkowitz, D.T. and Lerner, E. (1981) Gastric emptying in patients with gastroesophageal reflux. *Gastroenterology*, **80**, 285–291.

74. Maddern, G.J., Chatterton, R.E., Collins, P.T. *et al.* (1985) Solid and liquid gastric emptying in patients with gastro-oesophageal reflux. *British Journal of Surgery*, **72**, 344–347.

75. Mahony, M.J., Migliovacca, M., Spitz, L. and Milla, P.J. (1989) Motor disorders of the esophagus in gastro-oesophageal reflux. *Archives of Diseases in Childhood*, **63**, 333–338.

76. Mansfield, L.E. and Stern, M.R. (1981) Gastro-esophageal reflux and asthma: a possible reflex mechanism. *Annals of Allergy*, **41**, 224–226.

77. Milla, P.J. (1990) Reflux vomiting. *Archives of Diseases in Childhood*, **65**, 996–999.

78. Mittal, R.K., Large, R.C. and McCallum, R.W. (1987) Identification and mechanism of delayed esophageal acid clearance in subjects with hiatus hernia. *Gastroenterology*, **92**, 130–135.

79. Mittal, R.K. and McCallum, R.W. (1988) Characteristics and frequency of transient relaxation of the lower esophageal sphincter in patients with reflux esophagitis. *Gastroenterology*, **95**, 593–599.

80. Mittal, R.K., Reuben, A., Whiting, J.O. and McCallum, R.W. (1987) Do bile acids reflux into the esophagus? A study in normal subjects and patients with gastroesophageal reflux disease. *Gastroenterology*, **192**, 371–375.

81. Mittal, R.K., Rochester, D.F. and McCallum, R.W. (1987) Effect of diaphragmatic contraction in lower oesophageal sphincter pressure in man. *Gut*, **28**, 1564–1568.

82. Nebel, O.T. and Castell, D.O. (1972) Lower esophageal sphincter changes after food ingestion. *Gastroenterology*, **63**, 778–783.

83. Niaf, A.P., Savary, M. and Oziello, L. (1975) Columnar-lined esophagus: an aquired condition with malignant predisposition. *Journal of Thoracic and Cardiovascular Surgery*, **70**, 826–835.

84. Orlando, R.C. (1986) Esophageal epithelial resistance. *Journal of Clinical Gastroenterology*, **8**, 12–16.

85. Orr, W.C., Robinson, M.G. and Johnson, L.F. (1981) Acid clearance during sleep in the pathogenesis of reflux esophagitis. *Digestive Diseases and Sciences*, **26**, 423–427.

86. Peters, L., Maas, L., Petty, D. *et al.* (1988) Spontaneous non-cardiac chest pain. Evaluation by 24 hour ambulatory esophageal motility and pH monitoring. *Gastroenterology*, **94**, 878–886.

87. Petterson, G.B., Bombeck, C.T. and Nyhus, L.M. (1980) The lower esophageal sphincter: mechanism of opening and closure. *Surgery*, **88**, 307–314.

88. Reid, B.J., Lewin, K., van Deventer *et al.* (1986) Barrett's esophagus: high grade dysplasia and intra mucosal carcinoma detected by endoscopic biopsy. *Gastroenterology*, **90**, 1801.

89. Richter, J.E. and Castell, D.O. (1982) Gastro-oesophageal reflux. Pathogenesis, diagnosis and therapy. *Annals of Internal Medicine*, **97**, 93–103.

90. Sarr, M.G., Hamilton, S.R., Marrone, G.L. and Cameron, J.L. (1985) Barrett's esophagus: its prevalence and association with adenocarcinoma in patients with symptoms of gastro-esophageal reflux. *American Journal of Surgery*, **149**, 187–193.

91. Schatzki, R. and Carey, J.R. (1953) Dysphagia due to a diaphragm-like localized narrowing in the lower esophagus. *American Journal of Roentgenology*, **70**, 911.

92. Skinner, D.G., Walthen, R.C. and Riddek, R.H. (1983) Barrett's esophagus: comparison of benign and malignant cases. *American Journal of Surgery*, **198**, 554-565.

93. Smith, M., Buckton, G.K. and Bennett, J.R. (1984) Bile acid levels in stomach and oesophagus in patients with acid gastro-oesophageal reflux. *Gut*, **25**, A556.

94. Smith, R.R.L., Hamilton, S.R., Boitnott, J.K. *et al.* (1984) The spectrum of carcinoma occurring in Barrett's esophagus: a clinicopathological study of 26 patients. *American Journal of Surgical Pathology*, **8**, 563–573.

95. Smout, A.T.P., Breed, J.K.M., Van der Zoun *et al.* (1989) Physiological gastro-esophageal reflux and esophageal motor activity studies with a new system for 24 hour recording. *Digestive Diseases and Sciences*, **34**, 372–376.

96. Sontag, S.J., O'Connell, S., Khandelwal, S. *et al.* (1990) Most asthmatics have gastro-esophageal reflux with or without bronchodilator therapy. *Gastroenterology*, **99**, 613–620.

97. Spechler, G.J. and Goyal, R.K. (1986) Barrett's esophagus. *New England Journal of Medicine*, **315**, 362–371.

98. Spechler, G.J., Robbins, A.H., Rubin. H.B. *et al.* (1984) Adenocarcinoma and Barrett's esophagus: an over-rated risk? *Gastroenterology*, **87**, 927–933.

99. Spechler, S.J., Sperber, N., Doos, W.G. *et al.* (1983) The prevalence of Barrett's esophagus in patients with chronic peptic strictures. *Digestive Diseases and Sciences*, **28**, 769–774.

100. Stanciu, C. and Bennett, J.R. (1972) Smoking and gastro-oesophageal reflux. *British Medical Journal*, **2**, 793–795.

101. Stanciu, C., Hoare, R.C. and Bennett, J.R. (1977) Correlation between manometric and pH tests for gastro-oesopheageal reflux. *Gut*, **18**, 536–540.

102. Starnes, V.A., Adkins, E.S., Ballinger, J.R. and Sawyers, J. L. (1984) Barrett's esophagus: a surgical entity. *Archives of Surgery*, **119**, 563–567.

103. Thomas, F.B., Sterbough, J.T., Frankes, J.J., Mekhjian, H.A. and Caldwell, J.H. (1980) Inhibitory effect of coffee on lower esophageal sphincter pressure. *Gastroenterology*, **79**, 1262–1266.

104. Trenker, S.W. and Laufer, R. (1984) Double contrast examination: oesophagus, stomach and duodenum. *Clinical Gastroenterology*, **13**, 41–43.

105. Triadafilopoulos, G. (1989) Non-obstructive dysphagia in reflux esophagitis. *American Journal of Gastroenterology*, **84**, 614–618.

106. Tuchman, D.N., Boyle, J.T. and Pack, A.I. (1984) Comparison of airway responses following tracheal or oesophageal acidification in the cat. *Gastroenterology*, **87**, 872–881.

107. Van der Veen, A.H., Dees, J., Blankenstein, J.D. and Blankenstein, M.V. (1985) Adenocarcinoma in Barrett's oesophagus: an over-rated risk. *Gut*, **30**, 14–18.

108. Van Thiel, D.H., Gavalar, G.S., Joshe, S.N., Sara, R.T. and Stremple, J.F. (1977) Heartburn of pregnancy. *Gastroenterology*, **72**, 666–668.

109. Van Thiel, D.H., Gavalar, G.S. and Stremple, J.F. (1979) Lower eosphageal sphincter strength during the menstrual cycle. *American Journal of Obstetrics and Gynecology*, **134**, 64–67.

110. Vantrappen, G. and Hellemans, J. (1980) Treatment of achalasia and related disorders. *Gastroenterology*, **79**, 144–154.

111. Vantrappen, G. and Janssens, J. (1988) What is irritable esophagus? *Gastroenterology*, **94**, 1092–1097.

112. Wallin, L. (1980) Gastro-oesophageal function in duodenal ulcer patients. *Scandinavian Journal of Gastroenterology*, **15**, 145–150.

113. Wallin, L. (1980) Acid gastro-oesophageal reflux pattern in duodenal ulcer patients related to dyspeptic symptoms. *Scandinavian Journal of Gastroenterology*, **15**, 151–155.

114. Watson, A. (1987) Reflux stricture of the oesophagus. *British Journal of Surgery*, **74**, 443–448.

115. Wesdorp, K.E., Bartelsman, J.F.W.M, des Hartlog Jeger, P.C.A., Huibregtse, K. and Tytgat, G.N. (1982) Results of conservative treatment of benign oesophageal stricture. *Gastroenterology*, **82**, 487–493.

116. Wesdorp, E., Bartelsman, J.F.W.M., Skipper, M.E. *et al.* (1981) Effect of long term treatment with cimetidine and antacids in Barrett's oesophagus. *Gut*, **22**, 724–727.

117. Wilkins, W.E., Ridley, M.S. and Pozniak, A.L. (1984) Benign stricture of the oesophagus: use of non-steroidal anti-inflammatory drugs. *Gut*, **25**, 479–480.

118. Winters, C., Spurling, T.J. and Chobanson, S.J. (1987) Barrett's esophagus: a prevalent occult complication of gastro-esophageal reflux disease. *Gastroenterology*, **92**, 118–124.

119. Wolf, B.S. (1973) Sliding hiatus hernia: the need for redefinition. *American Journal of Roentgenology*, **117**, 231–247.

120. Wright, L.E. and Castell, D.O. (1975) The adverse effect of chocolate on lower esophageal sphincter pressure. *American Journal of Digestive Diseases*, **20**, 703—707.

DIAPHRAGMATIC HERNIAS

J. Spencer and I.A.D. Bouchier

The common diaphragmatic hernia of adult life is the sliding hernia through the oesophageal hiatus. Rolling (or paraoesophageal) hernias are less common but clinically important. Other hernias of adult life are either associated with traumatic rupture or incision of the diaphragm or, most rarely, due to late presentation of hernias through congenital defects.

Congenital diaphragmatic hernias occur either through the posterolateral space of Bochdalek or anteriorly through the foramen of Morgagni.

SLIDING HIATUS HERNIA

Sliding hernias of the stomach occur through the oesophageal hiatus of the diaphragm, and are 'axial' hernias, i.e. the oesophagus–cardia–stomach axis remains intact but the cardia is elevated above the diaphragm. By contrast, in a paraoesophageal or rolling hernia the cardia remains below the diaphragm and the fundus of the stomach herniates out of the abdomen, carrying with it an anterior sac of peritoneum.

Herniation through the hiatus occurs during vomiting and eructation. It must therefore be considered in its intermittent form as a physiological phenomenon. Extreme manoeuvres sometimes employed by radiologists can produce herniation of the stomach on screening, indicating a mobility of the cardia that is not necessarily of clinical significance. These observations add fuel to the controversy as to what is 'significant' herniation.

Aetiology and natural history

Little is known of the aetiology of herniation. Much of the past literature has discussed ways in which the stomach may be forced up into the chest, but this concept ignores a dominant anatomical feature, namely the longitudinal muscle of the oesophagus. This powerful muscle, attaching the cardia – via the median raphe of the pharynx – to the base of the skull, elevates the cardia when it contracts. Appropriate, and ill-understood, reflexes control elevation of the cardia during eructation and emesis, eliminating the intra-abdominal oesophagus and permitting reflux. Basic research in the 1930s and 1940s indicated that stimulation of intra-abdominal organs such as the gallbladder induced such contraction of the oesophagus. This, and much clinical evidence

assembled by Johnson,[7] suggest that hernias are produced by an excessively frequent or forceful exercise of this reflex, the stomach being actively drawn into the chest. Such a hypothesis explains the association of reflux and heartburn with other upper abdominal disease, and the common association between gallstones and hiatus hernia. Clinical measurement of longitudinal muscle function presents difficulties which have hampered useful investigation of such phenomena.

Significant clinical reflux, with or without herniation, may be a transient phenomenon, particularly in pregnancy. Although it is tempting to attribute this to increased abdominal pressure, such an increase does not occur except as a direct hydrostatic effect on the hiatus in the supine position, and hormonal effects are almost certainly of much greater importance. Obesity contributes to reflux and herniation in a way that is reversible.

Small hernias associated with minimal symptoms may remain unchanged for years. Those with more marked symptoms tend to worsen if not actively treated. Observed hernias tend to enlarge with the passage of time.

A clinical assumption often made is that patients with mild oesophagitis will inevitably progress to severe inflammation and stricture if not treated; in fact, this rarely occurs. The majority of strictures, especially in the elderly, are of sudden onset, often with absent or minimal preceding symptoms.

The association between herniation and reflux is the cause of much debate, amidst which some loose thinking is often in evidence. In a classic paper in 1971 Cohen and Harris demonstrated in large groups of selected subjects that whether or not a hernia was present, symptoms occurred only if an incompetent sphincter barrier could be demonstrated,[5] and these data have been used as an indication that the hernia is irrelevant. Prevention of reflux is normally dependent on two main factors. The first is the existence of an intra-abdominal segment of oesophagus. Surgically creating and maintaining such a segment, or a substitute for it, prevents reflux. The second factor is the lower oesophageal sphincter, the activity of which is determined neurally and hormonally. The effects of hormones on the sphincter are readily demonstrable, but the doses needed tend to be pharmacological rather than physiological. Various drugs increase the tone of the lower oesophageal sphincter and both metoclopramide and cisapride have been claimed to be therapeutically useful.

It is possible that a hiatus hernia may follow a sequence of events initiated by gastro-oesophageal reflux. An initiating factor stimulates longitudinal muscle contraction of the oesophagus so that the intra-abdominal oesophagus is eliminated for varying periods of time. This enables reflux into the oesophagus to occur, causing irritation of the oesophageal mucosa. The irritation provokes further contraction and the intra-abdominal oesophagus is eliminated for longer periods. The cardia eventually becomes elevated above the diaphragm. Depending on the interplay of factors involved, various courses are now possible: herniation may be increased; inflammation may be increased, with stricture formation; or volume and reflux may be increased, causing mechanical reflux symptoms to dominate.

The nature of the refluxed material is probably of crucial significance, particularly the presence of bile: this causes a much more severe oesophagitis than acid reflux alone. The bile salts have been implicated in this: at low pH conjugated bile salts cause oesophagitis, but at neutral pH deconjugated salts are more damaging. In some animal models pancreatic juice causes severe oesophagitis. Salo found that in acid-free conditions deoxycholate and cheno-deoxycholate, together with trypsin, caused severe damage in rabbits.[10] In humans it is known that anastomosis of the oesophagus to small bowel after total gastrectomy in a way that permits biliopancreatic reflux causes severe oesophagitis.

Oesophageal clearance is a factor that helps determine the contact time between refluxed material and the mucosa. It is affected by gravity and salivation as well as by motility. The latter is disordered in oesophagitis and especially in scleroderma.

Clinical features

Most sliding hernias are probably asymptomatic. Many produce mild symptoms that are easily controlled and do not demand extensive investigation. Although many symptoms and sequelae are described, only four are commonly important: heartburn (pyrosis), reflux, respiratory symptoms and dysphagia. Other less frequent complications include anaemia and the possibility of oesophageal carcinoma if oesophagitis persists over a long period. The incidence of the latter progression is low and varies in different reports.

Heartburn

This is the most common symptom associated with reflux. It is characteristically burning and most often associated with bile in the oesophageal aspirates. The sensation appears to arise in the oesophageal mucosa, and can be reproduced by acid perfusion of the gullet as described by Bernstein and Baker.[2] It does, however, occur commonly in patients with gallbladder disease and duodenal or gastric ulcer, possibly implying that reflux occurs in these patients and might be prevented by treating the primary disease. The severity of pyrosis is not related directly to the degree of inflammation in the oesophagus, although histological changes exist that are characteristically associated with the existence of reflux.[6] These consist of a thinning of the epidermis, with a thickened basal cell layer and more deeply penetrating dermal pegs (papillae). Such changes are often wrongly referred to as 'oesophagitis': strictly speaking, they are changes associated with reflux, which appear to precede the appearance of inflammation. It has been suggested that thinning of the epithelium brings sensitive nerve endings nearer to the surface, making painful an acid insult that would not be noticed by a normal individual.

Reflux

This may be the dominant symptom in some patients, who experience the regurgitation of bitter fluid into the throat or mouth, especially on exertion or postural change. The symptom may or may not be associated with pyrosis. Clinical experience suggests that prolonged reflux of low volumes of gastric juice may be sufficient to sensitize the mucosa to produce pyrosis and oesophagitis. Whereas the majority of patients with a sliding hiatus hernia do not have oesophagitis, most patients with moderate or severe oesophagitis have a hiatus hernia. The dominance of reflux itself as a symptom implies a larger volume of refluxed material. This is a symptom complex that is less readily managed medically, except in the obese if weight can be lost and at the end of a pregnancy, and it therefore has logistic implications as regards therapy.

Chest infections

These are a consequence of overspill of refluxed material. In the adult infection seems less frequent in patients with gastro-oesophageal reflux than in those with achalasia, unless stricture formation occurs. In infants, however, evidence is emerging that asthma may well be initiated by gastro-oesophageal reflux, and that in some individuals a life-time of asthma and bronchitis begins with reflux of this kind. Indeed, it is now postulated that surgical correction of reflux in infancy may avert life-long pulmonary problems in many individuals.

Dysphagia

Dysphagia associated with reflex occurs in two forms. Clinical observation reveals that patients with dysphagia, contrary to much previous teaching, are very poor indicators of the true site of obstruction. The major discrepancy is due to the sensation of food sticking in the cricopharyngeal area, whereas the only radiological pathology is the existence of a sliding hiatus hernia with reflux. Manometric evidence is being produced, albeit not all consistent, that there is pharyngocricopharyngeal dyscoordination in these subjects. Most patients once described as having a 'globus hystericus' are now thought to have such a cricopharyngeal syndrome, and in many this is associated with reflux. It is not yet certain whether all patients respond to therapy directed towards the lower end of the oesophagus, although most do.

The more readily recognised dysphagia is that associated with oesophagitis, with or without stricture. As in other parts of the alimentary canal, inflammatory narrowing has three components – spasm, oedema and fibrosis. It is not often appreciated how much the first two components contribute to peptic oesophageal 'strictures'. Such strictures are remarkably reversible if the causative factors are relieved. Dysphagia of any kind is likely to be associated with overspill causing respiratory symptoms.

Rarely, a sliding hiatus hernia is present without reflux, and causes aching discomfort in the epigastrium or left hypochondrium which may be relieved by eructation. This appears to be analogous to the pain occurring in other abdominal hernias, and is relieved by operative repair.

INVESTIGATIONS

In the majority of patients with clinically significant sliding hiatus hernias there is no difficulty in diagnosis. Clinical suspicion leads to a request for a barium 'swallow and meal' during which the diagnosis is confirmed.

The existence of a hernia is confirmed if the radiologist can recognize the gastro-oesophageal junction lying above the diaphragm. The site of the hiatus is usually indicated by its compression on the herniated stomach; surprisingly it may be above or below the projected curve of the diaphragmatic dome. The mucosal pattern usually separates oesophagus and stomach readily, and a sphincter zone can be identified. Sometimes this is ring-like as described by Schatzki; if dilatation of such a ring is limited to a diameter of 12 mm or less then dysphagia is usual. The existence of free reflux without undue provocation is of great clinical significance, and probably more important than the documentation of an anatomical hernia. Double-contrast techniques permit the detection of quite early

changes in oesophagitis. In more severe inflammation ulceration may be seen. Strictures due to peptic digestion are almost always short, but may appear long because the portion below the stricture cannot be distended with contrast medium. One exception is the stricture associated with nasogastric intubation in sick, and especially in comatose, patients; such strictures are long and tapering and occur in the lower third of the oesophagus. High strictures, usually at the level of the aortic arch, are seen associated with Barrett's columnar-lined gullet.

Inflammatory strictures often occur in the elderly, and may present as dysphagia with little in the way of previous symptoms. A significant event must have occurred in these subjects. This may be a change in the nature of previously refluxing gastric juice, perhaps by the addition of *bile*. This is hypothetical at the moment.

Endoscopy

This has an important role in the diagnosis of dysphagia, being mandatory in every patient with this symptom. Fibreoptic examination is a simple outpatient procedure permitting biopsy of the oesophageal mucosa and of strictures. Cytological brushings should be obtained. If repeated biopsies do not exclude malignancy in doubtful cases, rigid endoscopy under anaesthesia permits more accurate and much larger biopsies.

The Bernstein acid-perfusion test

This has been widely used in the diagnosis of reflux oesophagitis. Hydrochloric acid (0.1 mol/l) is infused through an oro-oesophageal tube so that it perfuses the lower third of the oesophagus; the symptomatic effects of this are compared with those of a similar infusion of physiological saline as a control. This is basically a pain-reproduction test. In most patients a good clinical history will tell everything that a Bernstein test can reveal.

The greatest disadvantage of the test, however, is its poor specificity, the test often being positive, for example, in subjects with gallstones (*Table 1.15*). If

Table 1.15 Bernstein oesophageal perfusion test: incidence of positive results in 140 subjects

Diagnosis	n	Positive results
Normal	11	2 (18%)
Peptic ulcer	17	5 (29%)
Gallstones	3	2 (67%)
Dyspepsia	27	10 (37%)
Hiatus hernia	82	40 (49%)

there remains any clinical use for this test, it is in the differentiation of cardiac and oesophageal pain in the occasional difficult patient. Other clinical features help in this differentiation, especially the persistence of pain after exercise has ceased.

Oesophageal pH measurements

These demonstrate both increased frequency of gastro-oesophageal reflux and prolonged acid clearance in patients with hiatus hernia. Ambulatory pH monitoring allows precise and prolonged evaluation for evidence of gastro-oesophageal reflux.

Radionuclide transit

This is a safe test in which liquid boluses, labelled with an isotope such as ^{99m}Tc-sulphur colloid are swallowed on the transit time determined. However, this test is still under evaluation because it is not widely accepted as a reliable screening procedure.

Acid-clearing tests

These are a development in which a pH probe is used to determine the time taken for the oesophageal muscle to clear away an instilled acid bolus. Patients with hiatus hernia and reflux have delayed (impaired) acid clearance. Mittal *et al.*[8] described a biphasic pH response. An initial fall in pH due to acid reflux is followed by a rise, due to acid clearance. Impaired acid clearance is a particular feature of non-reducing hiatus hernias.[1]

Oesophageal manometry

This is a well-established method of assessing motility and sphincter tone. It is perhaps more accurate to refer to sphincter 'squeeze' rather than 'pressure'. Results depend on whether or not the hernia is reducing. Impaired emptying in reducing hernias is due to late retrograde flow of gastric contents during the time that the hernia is emptying; impaired emptying in non-reducing hernias occurs because of early retrograde flow of material from the hernia occurring immediately after gastro-oesophageal relaxation. Patients with non-reducing hernias have reduced competence of the diaphragmatic crura which is conducive to gastro-oesophageal incompetence.

PARAOESOPHAGEAL (ROLLING) HERNIA

A paraoesophageal hiatus hernia is quite different from a sliding hernia. This is herniation of the stomach through the oesophageal hiatus, the cardia remaining in its normal anatomical position below the diaphragm. One school of thought claims that such hernias are variants of the Bochdalek hernia, there sometimes being residual tissue indicating that the hernia did not originally occur through the oesophageal hiatus; in most, this tissue is atrophied, or destroyed unnoticed at operation. The majority opinion is that the herniation is through the true oesophageal hiatus. Most often the gastric fundus herniates first. There may be progressive herniation of the stomach, usually with volvulus, so that the greater curve becomes uppermost, and eventually colon or other organs may be involved. A complete peritoneal sac is present.

These hernias are usually seen late in life, often as a finding on chest radiograph or else on a barium meal examination. Symptoms are often vague, with retrosternal or hypochondrial discomfort, nausea or fullness after meals. Vomiting is not common, and heartburn is not a feature. Dysphagia is not usual.

Mild symptoms may persist for years, but a rolling hernia is dangerous and not amenable to any conservative therapy. The major complications are (1) bleeding from gastritis or gastric ulcer, (2) gastric volvulus and (3) incarceration or strangulation.

Anaemia due to bleeding is common, one series indicating an incidence of 30%. The so-called 'riding ulcer' seen adjacent to the hiatus in these patients may be intractable until herniorrhaphy, implicating mechanical factors in its causation.

An intra-abdominal gastric volvulus may be organo- or mesentero-axial. Organo-axial volvulus is more frequent and is commonly associated with rolling hernia, with much or all of the stomach lying in the chest. Acute presentation of such volvulus is characterized by a triad described by Borchardt in 1904:[3]

1. Severe epigastric pain or distension.
2. Vomiting, followed by retching with inability to vomit.
3. Difficulty in passing a nasogastric tube.

This triad suggests initial blockage of the pylorus followed by cardiac obstruction and gastric dilatation. Acute strangulation may follow.

In a series of 25 patients with acute gastric volvulus[4] 18 were associated with paraoesophageal hernia, 3 with traumatic change to the diaphragm, 2 with eventration of the diaphragm and 1 with a Bochdalek hernia. Only one was not associated with a diaphragmatic defect of some kind.

As a consequence of the high incidence and the severity of complications, all paraoesophageal hernias should ideally be treated surgically; in practice, however, they are seen most often in the extremely aged, often as an incidental finding. In patients who are considered fit for operation, an abdominal approach usually permits reduction of the hernia; anterior approximation of the crura to narrow the hiatus prevents recurrence.

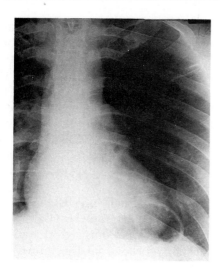

Figure 1.48 Traumatic diaphragmatic hernia after a motor-cycle accident. Stomach is seen in the chest.

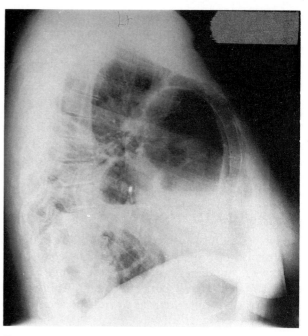

Figure 1.49 Incisional hernia through the diaphragm, occurring through a surgical incision in the left dome. The whole stomach and splenic flexure of the colon lie in the chest.

TRAUMATIC DIAPHRAGMATIC HERNIA

Rupture of the diaphragm may follow either thoracic or abdominal trauma; iatrogenic trauma consists of surgical incisions in the diaphragm (*Figures 1.48* and *1.49*). Herniation may occur through resulting defects soon after the trauma or many years later; to confuse the issue further, early herniation may be symptomless and cause later complications. Presumably because of males' predisposition to trauma there is a 6:1 male:female ratio in incidence of traumatic diaphragmatic hernias.[6] The aetiology in any series is determined largely by social factors. Thus, crushing injuries due to car accidents are a common cause, and penetrating wounds are important where stab wounds are common. Rupture due to crushing requires considerable force, and is associated with a high incidence of other injuries. Lower thoracic stab wounds are commonly associated with diaphragmatic trauma.

Crushing trauma damages the left diaphragm more commonly than the right. This may be mainly because of the presence of the liver on the right side, but cadaver studies have also demonstrated a relative weakness in the posterior part of the left diaphragm. Traumatic herniation must be considered in all patients with lower thoracic or upper abdominal trauma. Pain and dyspnoea occur and may be exacerbated by meals. Bowel sounds heard in the chest are an important sign. Examination of the chest reveals dullness and poor air entry. Chest radiographs may reveal bowel in the chest, elevated or indistinct diaphragm, or effusion. Barium studies may be necessary to confirm the diagnosis.

In both acute and chronic traumatic herniation the treatment is surgical (see page 115). Laparotomy, reduction and repair of the diaphragm are performed. In long-standing hernias thoracotomy may be preferred because the adhesions may bleed on division; a high incidence of empyema has been reported following repair of such hernias from below.

REFERENCES

1. Behar, J., Sheahan, D.G., Biancani, P. *et al.* (1975) Medical and surgical management of reflux esophagitis. *New England Journal of Medicine*, **293**, 263–268.
2. Bernstein, L.M. and Baker, L.A. (1958) A clinical test for esophagitis. *Gastroenterology*, **34**, 760–781.
3. Borchardt, M. (1904) Zur Pathologie and Therapie des Magnevolvulus. *Arhiv für klinische Chirurgie*, **74**, 243.
4. Carter, R., Brewer, L.A. and Hinshaw, D.B. (1980) Acute gastric volvulus. A study of 25 cases. *American Journal of Surgery*, **140**, 99–106.
5. Cohen, S. and Harris, L.D. (1971) Does hiatus hernia affect the competence of the gastroesophageal sphincter? *New England Journal of Medicine*, **284**, 1053–1056.
6. Ismail-Beigi, F., Horton, P.F. and Pope, C.E. (1970) Histological consequences of gastroesophageal reflux in man. *Gastroenterology*, **58**, 163–174.

7. Johnson, H.D. (1968) *The Cardia and Hiatus Hernia*. London: Heinemann.
8. Mittal, R.K., Lange, R.C. and McCallum, R.W. (1987) Identification and mechanism of delayed esophageal acid clearance in subjects with hiatus hernia. *Gastroenterology*, **92**, 130–135.
9. Payne, J.H. and Lellin, A.E. (1982) Traumatic diaphragmatic hernia. *Archives of Surgery*, **117**, 18–24.
10. Salo, J.A. and Kivilaakso, E. (1983) Role of bile salts and trypsin in the pathogenesis of experimental alkaline eosophagitis. *Surgery*, **93**, 525–532.
11. Sloan, S. and Kahriles, P.J. (1991) Impairment of esophageal emptying with hiatal hernia. *Gastroenterology*, **100**, 596–605.

INDICATIONS FOR, AND OUTCOME OF, SURGERY FOR BENIGN OESOPHAGEAL DISEASE

P.F. Crookes, J.R. Jamieson and T. DeMeester

SLIDING HIATUS HERNIA

The clinical significance of sliding hiatus hernia lies in its association with gastro-oesophageal reflux, and only exceptionally does the hernia cause symptoms or require treatment for any other reason. The chief exception is in a small group of patients with dysphagia in whom a pouch of upper stomach may be partially obstructed by the crura of the diaphragm, causing accumulation of swallowed material. This is seen radiologically as 'abnormal hiatal flow'.[27] There may be no reflux, but surgical correction by an antireflux procedure is curative.[44]

This exception aside, the 'surgery of hiatus hernia' is the surgery of gastro-oesophageal reflux, although the relationship between these two entities is not cause and effect; either may exist without the other. Contrary to what was thought in the past, the physical presence of the hernial sac in the chest does not mean that there is no 'abdominal' sphincter. The peritoneal sac transmits the changes of intra-abdominal pressure. What determines whether or not the sphincter is deficient depends on the attachment of the phreno-oesophageal ligament. The dissections of Bombeck *et al.*[8] showed that, regardless of the presence of a hiatus hernia, a high attachment of the phreno-oesophageal ligament above the gastro-oesophageal junction reduced the distraction of the sphincter, allowing it to function normally, whereas when the insertion was displaced inferiorly, the sphincter was held open and oesophagitis was more common (*Figure 1.50*). In the authors' own study of hiatus hernia patients, some with and some without reflux, it was possible to confirm this concept by finding that patients with hiatus hernia and proven reflux had a lower oesophageal sphincter manometrically shorter in abdominal length than patients with hiatus hernia and no reflux (*Figure 1.51*).[18]

There is abundant evidence to show that hiatus hernia is associated with less efficient peristalsis and impaired clearance.[54,66] *Figure 1.51a* shows this phenomenon indirectly by demonstrating that the number of episodes of reflux lasting longer than 5 minutes is greater in refluxing patients who have a hiatus hernia compared with those who do not. This may be due to loss of distal fixation of the oesophagus with consequent alteration of the length/tension relationship in the longitudinal muscle. The effect is independent of sphincter incompetence. Similar results have been found by Mittal *et al.*[54] in a study using a standard acid load and measuring time to clearance above pH 5 (*Figure 1.52*). It is important to note that the patient with hiatus hernia and an incompetent sphincter has a triply compromised mechanism: there is lack of an adequate pressure to protect the oesophagus against acid reflux during changes in intragastric pressure, a lack of adequate abdominal length to protect against rises in intra-abdominal pressure, and a reduced ability to clear acid when the exposure occurs. Gastro-oesophageal reflux, although not caused by the hiatus hernia, is therefore likely to be more severe than when the disease occurs in the absence of a hernia.

Pathogenesis of complications of gastro-oesophageal reflux disease

Once gastro-oesophageal reflux disease has developed, what factors predispose to the development of complications?

The incidence of a mechanically defective sphincter is strongly correlated with the develop-

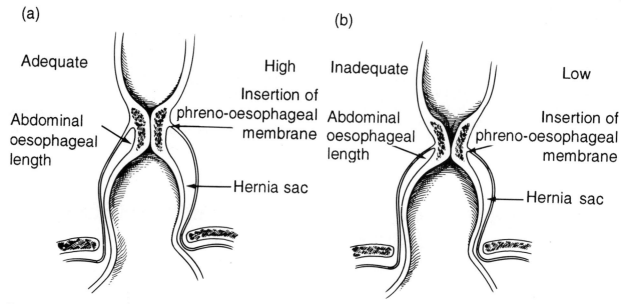

Figure 1.50 (a) The attachment of the phreno-oesophageal ligament (membrane) and its relationship to the abdominal length of the lower oesophageal sphincter. (From DeMeester, T.R., *et al.*, (1981) (b) Relationship of a hiatal hernia to the function of the body of the esophagus and the gastroesophageal junction. (*Journal of Thoracic and Cardiovascular Surgery*, **82**, 547–558, with permission.)

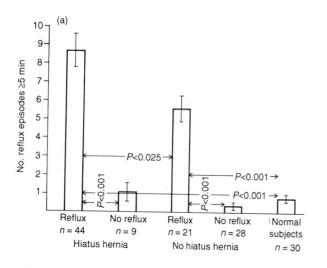

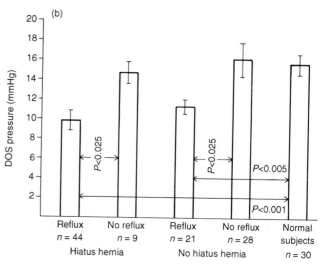

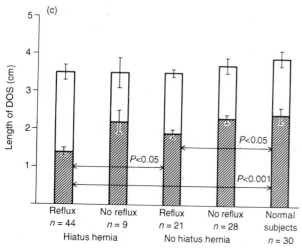

Figure 1.51 The relationship of hiatus hernia to the functional components of the lower oesophageal sphincter. (a) Impaired clearance as shown by increased number of prolonged episodes of reflux; (b) sphincter pressure unrelated to presence of hiatus hernia; (c) abdominal length but not total length reduced in hiatus hernia: □ above rip; ▨ below rip. DOS = distal oesophageal sphincter. (From DeMeester, T.R., *et al.* (1981) Relationship of a hiatal hernia to the function of the body of the esophagus and the gastroesophageal junction. *Journal of Thoracic and Cardiovascular Surgery*, **82**, 547–558, with permission.)

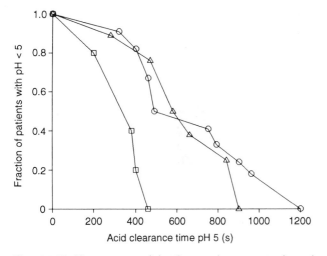

Figure 1.52 Measurement of the time to clear an oesophageal bolus of acid to pH 5 in three groups of subjects. Acid clearance time is significantly faster in group 2 (□) (symptomatic non-hiatus hernia patients) than in group 1 (⊖) (symptomatic hiatus hernia) or group 3 (△) (asymptomatic hiatus hernia). (From Mittal, R.K., Large, R.C. and McCallum, R.W. (1987) Identification and mechanism of delayed esophageal and clearance in subjects with hiatus hernia. *Gastroenterology*, **92**, 130–135, with permission.)

ment of complications, i.e. oesophagitis, stricture and Barrett's oesophagus. *Table 1.16* shows the relationship of a defective sphincter to complications in 150 consecutive patients with gastro-oesophageal reflux.[23] Whereas the incidence of a defective sphincter in uncomplicated gastro-oesophageal reflux disease is 42%, it is 77% when oesophagitis is present and 80–90% when stricture is present. Barrett's oesophagus is almost always associated with a grossly defective sphincter. This suggests that a mechanically defective sphincter is a major factor in the pathogenesis of complications. The commonly advanced argument that sphincter damage is secondary to reflux damage does not explain the fact that a mechanically defective sphincter also occurs in 42% of patients who do not have a complication of increased oesophageal exposure to gastric juice. This observation suggests that the defect in the sphincter is primary and not the result of inflammation or tissue damage.

The composition of the refluxed material also has an effect on the development of complications. The injurious effect of refluxed juice depends on a number of interacting components. Pepsin-induced mucosal damage is likely only in an acid environment, but in the presence of bile salts and a higher pH, trypsin may be more important. In the clinical situation, complications of gastro-oesophageal reflux disease are more common when there is an alkaline component to the refluxate. In Barrett's oesophagus, the development of complications such as stricture and ulceration is strongly associated with increased alkaline exposure.[3]

Any defect of oesophageal clearance which prolongs the contact time between the refluxate and the mucosa is likely to lead to increased tissue injury. When it occurs in combination with either of the above factors, the tissue injury is likely to be severe, as in scleroderma or hiatus hernia.

The place of surgery in uncomplicated gastro-oesophageal reflux disease

Many patients with gastro-oesophageal reflux do not seek medical aid, and of those who do, many respond to simple advice about lifestyle and short-term antacids. Surgery is only considered in those patients whose symptoms require long-term medication for their control, those who do not respond to medical therapy or those who develop complications while on therapy.

Aim of surgery

The aim of surgery is to restore the patient to a life free of symptoms, without the need to take regular medications, and without undue social, dietary or other lifestyle restrictions. The status of a patient whose reflux symptoms are only controlled by taking regular antacids, H_2-receptor blockers and pro-kinetic agents, avoiding late meals and spicy food, eschewing alcohol, tobacco, chocolate and peppermint, wearing only loose clothes and sleeping propped up,[7] perhaps in a double bed, cannot be considered ideal. The social and domestic disruption imposed by such a regimen has not been sufficiently attended to.

Chronic atypical symptoms of reflux, e.g. chest pain, chronic cough, recurrent pneumonias, episodes of nocturnal choking, waking up with gastric

Table 1.16 Complications of gastro-oesophageal reflux disease*

Complication	No.	Normal sphincter (%)	Defective sphincter (%)
None	59	58	42
Oesophagitis	47	23†	77
Stricture	19	11	89
Barrett's oesophagus	25	0	100

*In 150 consecutive cases with documented gastro-oesophageal reflux disease (by 24-hour pH monitoring, endoscopy and motility).

†Grade more severe with defective cardia.

contents in the mouth or soilage of the bed pillow, may also indicate the need for surgical therapy. If 24-hour pH monitoring confirms the presence of increased oesophageal acid exposure and a mechanical defect of the lower oesophageal sphincter and normal oesophageal body motility is found on manometry, an antireflux procedure may be expected to produce a good result.[25] It is not unusual for these patients to have a non-specific motor abnormality of the oesophageal body which tends to propel the refluxed material towards the pharynx. In some of these patients the motor abnormality will disppear following reflux control by a surgical antireflux procedure. In others, the motor disorder will persist and may cause postoperative aspiration of swallowed saliva and food. Consequently, the results of an antireflux procedure in patients with a motor disorder of the oesophageal body are variable.

Medical or surgical therapy

It is surprising that in such a common disease so few randomized trials have compared the relative merits of medical versus surgical treatment. One early report in 31 randomized patients followed up over a 38-month period showed a good symptomatic response in 73% of the surgical group compared with 19% of the medical group.[5] The relevance of this study to modern practice may be criticized because the medically treated group did not receive H_2-receptor blockers, which are a mainstay of current medical therapy. The results of a large multicentre Veterans' Administration study have recently become available: in this study patients were randomized to receive either conventional medical therapy, intensive medical therapy or surgery. A total of 247 patients was randomized, and the 2-year follow-up data show a clear advantage in the surgically treated patients.[69] Although 'intensive medical therapy' did not include omeprazole, the findings are highly relevant to current practice, because the long-term effect of this drug is unknown. Other interesting observations emerged. Many side effects often attributed to surgical intervention, e.g. abdominal swelling and fullness, occurred with equal frequency in the medically treated groups.[68] Secondly, 8% of patients free of stricture on entry to the study developed a stricture while on medical treatment.[45]

As against this, the poor results of ill-conceived or poorly executed surgery have made many physicians wary of recommending surgery for what is regarded as a benign disease. There are two major reasons for poor surgical results: (1) inappropriate patient selection and (2) technical errors in the performance of the operation. These topics will be addressed in turn.

Who benefits from antireflux surgery?

The first requirement for consideration of antireflux surgery is the objective demonstration of the presence of gastro-oesophageal reflux disease. It has been emphasized already that this is best done by prolonged 24-hour pH monitoring. Secondly, the patient must have either symptoms or complications of the disease. Thirdly, the disease should be caused by a defect that is correctable by surgery, such as a mechanically deficient sphincter. The algorithm in *Figure 1.53* summarizes the common situations in which surgery may be recommended.

If 24-hour oesophageal pH monitoring is normal in a patient with unequivocal endoscopic oesophagitis, then possibilities of alkaline, drug-induced or retention oesophagitis should be considered. If the sphincter is manometrically normal in a patient with increased oesophageal exposure to gastric juice, the patient should be evaluated for an oesophageal or gastric cause of increased acid exposure. In this situation, the most common abnormality is gastric hypersecretion.[4] Some patients with increased acid exposure and a mechanically defective sphincter, and who have no complication of the disease, respond well to medical therapy but they require long-term medication for continued relief. These patients should be given the option of surgery as a cost-effective alternative.[30]

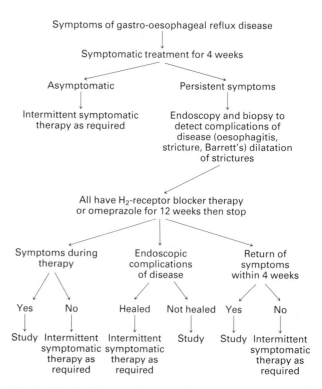

Figure 1.53 Decision tree for treatment of symptomatic gastro-oesophageal reflux disease.

Choice of antireflux surgery

The development of effective antireflux surgery parallels our understanding of the deranged physiology in gastro-oesophageal reflux disease. The earliest attempts at surgery were aimed simply at reducing the hiatus hernia. Radiological and symptomatic recurrence were common after these procedures. Allison is generally regarded as being the first to perform an operation specifically designed to reduce reflux, with somewhat better results, but his long-term results were disappointing – recurrence was reported in 49%.[1] Although a bewildering variety of operations has since been described, only three with adequate long-term follow-up data are commonly employed world wide – those of Hill, Belsey and Nissen. Only one randomized controlled trial comparing these three operations has been published.[17] The results showed that the Nissen procedure was the most effective in preventing reflux and restoring manometric characteristics to normal, but at the expense of a higher incidence of temporary postoperative dysphagia and inability to vomit. The results of subsequent uncontrolled series from many different centres have substantiated these findings and it is now possible to evaluate their relative merits and provide guidelines for the use of each. In brief, the Hill operation carries the risk of iatrogenic damage to the coeliac axis, and despite Hill's insistence has not been widely used outside his own centre.[38] It may be especially valuable in a patient with a previous gastric resection where there is not enough stomach to fashion a normal wrap.

Both the Belsey and the Nissen operations create a fundic wrap round the lower oesophagus. The Belsey operation is a partial fundoplication performed through the chest, which provides excellent relief of symptoms provided that the wrap is not placed under tension.[6] The thoracic approach allows extensive mobilization of the oesophagus up to the aortic arch. Because the wrap is incomplete, it is less prone to cause obstruction than the Nissen operation. This feature makes it more suitable in patients where peristaltic efficiency is impaired. For the same reason, inability to belch or vomit is less than after a Nissen operation. It is more technically exacting to perform than a Nissen operation, and Belsey reported a recurrence rate of 15% when the operation was performed by registrars, compared with 6% when performed by consultants. Postthoracotomy pain is a problem which may be reduced, but not abolished, by making the thoracotomy high (sixth rib), resecting a small segment of rib posteriorly, and avoiding vigorous rib retraction. The early enthusiastic reports of the intraoperative use of cryotherapy to the intercostal nerves[49,50] to reduce post-thoracotomy pain have not been substantiated by more recent controlled studies.[55]

The Nissen operation is the most widely performed procedure for uncomplicated gastro-oesophageal reflux disease, but it has necessitated several modifications to the original description to reduce the incidence of side effects. These have been well documented both by the authors[19] (see below) and by Donahue et al.[26] The dysphagia and tendency to bloating noted in early reports can be minimized by making the wrap shorter and looser, and also by ensuring that only appropriate patients are operated on. Performing fundoplication on patients with a normal sphincter who reflux due to gastric dilatation secondary to aerophagia is another cause of the 'gas bloat syndrome' described by Woodward et al.[82] The Nissen procedure is usually performed transabdominally, but the transthoracic route may be preferred in a very obese patient when exposure is likely to be difficult, or where a fixed hiatus hernia is present, because more extensive mobilization of the oesophagus will be required.

Other factors to consider prior to antireflux surgery

Prior to proceeding with an antireflux operation, the authors would routinely consider several factors that may cause the operative strategy to be modified. First, the propulsive force of the body of the oesophagus should be evaluated in order to determine whether it has sufficient power to propel a bolus of food through a newly reconstructed valve. This can be carried out with standard or 24-hour ambulatory oesophageal manometry.[70] Patients with normal peristaltic contractions do well with a 360° Nissen fundoplication. When peristalsis is absent, severely disordered or of low magnitude (peak amplitude below 20 mm Hg), the Belsey two-thirds partial fundoplication is the procedure of choice. This is usually the case in patients with strictures or Barrett's oesophagus.

Secondly, anatomical shortening of the oesophagus can compromise the ability to carry out adequate repair without tension, and can lead to an increased incidence of breakdown or thoracic displacement of the repair. Oesophageal shortening is identified radiologically by a sliding hiatus hernia which will not reduce in the upright position or which measures more than 5 cm between the diaphragmatic crura and the gastro-oesophageal junction on endoscopy. When present, the motility of the oesophageal body must be carefully evaluated and, if adequate, a Collis-type gastroplasty should be performed to obtain extra length.[59] This may be combined with either a Belsey or a Nissen wrap, and the choice depends on the propulsive power of the oesophageal body. In practice oesophageal body shortening is usually combined with loss of peristaltic efficiency, and consequently the Belsey procedure will be added most often. In patients with absent contractility, more than 50% interrupted or dropped contractions or those who had several failed previous antireflux procedures, oesophageal resection should be considered as an alternative.

Thirdly, the surgeon should specifically query the patient regarding complaints of epigastric pain, nausea, vomiting and loss of appetite. In the past, these symptoms were accepted as part of the reflux syndrome, but it is now realized that they can be due to excessive duodenogastric reflux which occurs in about 11% of patients with gastro-oesophageal reflux disease.[31] This problem is usually seen in patients who have had previous upper gastro-intestinal surgery, although this is not always the case. In such patients, the correction of only the incompetent cardia will result in a disgruntled individual who continues to complain of nausea and epigastric pain on eating. In these patients, 24-hour pH monitoring of the stomach may help to detect and quantify duodenogastric reflux.[32] The diagnosis can also be documented with a ^{99m}Tc-HIDA (hydroxy imino diacetic acid) scan if excessive reflux of bile from the duodenum into the stomach can be demonstrated.[71] If surgery is necessary to control gastro-oesophageal reflux and if severe duodeno-gastric reflux is present, consideration should also be given to performing a bile diversion procedure as well.[20] When diagnosed after an anti-reflux repair, the administration of sucralfate may relieve the persistent complaint of nausea and epigastric pain.

Fourthly, approximately 30% of patients with proven gastro-oesophageal reflux on 24-hour pH monitoring will have hypersecretion on gastric analysis;[4] 2–3% of patients who have an antireflux operation will develop a gastric or duodenal ulcer. These factors may modify the proposed antireflux procedure by the addition of a highly selective vagotomy. The authors' policy is to add a vagotomy only when there is a documented history of, or currently active, duodenal ulcer.

Lastly, delayed gastric emptying is found in approximately 40% of patients with gastro-oesophageal reflux disease and can contribute to postoperative symptoms after antireflux repair. Usually, however, mild degrees of delayed gastric emptying are corrected by the antireflux procedure and only in patients with severe emptying disorders and recognized gastric pathology is there need for an additional gastric procedure at the time of antireflux repair.[39]

Results of the Nissen fundoplication

Modifications to original technique

To evaluate the durability and the long-term side effects of a primary antireflux procedure, the authors assessed the results of 100 consecutive primary Nissen repairs performed for uncomplicated reflux disease over a 13-year period in patients selected as outlined above.[19] *Figure 1.54* shows that the actuarial success rate of the operation to control reflux symptoms over a 10-year period is 91%. From the patients' perspective 90% were satisfied with the results of the operation, and 92% would have the operation if the decision had to be made again.

Three modifications in surgical technique were made as experience was gained with the procedure to minimize the side effects: first, the calibre of the bougie used to size the fundoplication was increased from 36 to 60 F. This reduced the incidence of temporary postoperative swallowing discomfort from 83% to 39%. Secondly, the length of the fundoplication was decreased from 4 cm to 1 cm. This decreased the incidence of persistent dysphagia (i.e. any discomfort with swallowing) from 21% to 3%. To shorten the wrap required reduction in the numbers of sutures and reinforcing them to prevent unravelling. This was accomplished by one permanent 2-0 Prolene (polypropylene) horizontal mattress suture reinforced by Teflon pledgets. Thirdly, the gastric fundus was mobilized prior to construction of the fundoplication. This increased the incidence of complete lower oesophageal sphincter relaxation on swallowing from 31% to 71%.

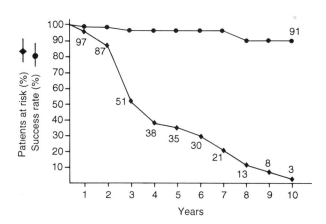

Figure 1.54 Long-term follow-up of 100 patients after Nissen fundoplication for uncomplicated gastro-oesophageal reflux disease. Relief of symptoms expressed as actuarial survival curve. (From DeMeester, T.R., Bonavina, L. and Albertucci, M. (1986) Nissen fundoplication for gastroesophageal reflux disease. *Annals of Surgery*, **204**, 9–20, with permission.)

Effect of operation on physiology

Preoperatively the patients had a lower mean resting pressure of the lower oesophageal sphincter, shorter mean sphincter overall length, shorter mean sphincter abdominal length and lower mean amplitude of contractions in the distal oesophagus as compared to healthy controls (*Figure 1.55*). The Nissen fundoplication corrected the deficiences of the lower oesophageal sphincter as shown by the manometric measurements in 36 patients who volunteered for postoperative studies. The procedure restored the lower oesophageal sphincter pressure, overall length, and abdominal length to normal values (*Figure 1.55 a–c*). The ability of the Nissen fundoplication to re-establish the lower oesophageal sphincter can be appreciated by comparing the pre- and postoperative three dimensional sphincter images. *Figure 1.56* shows how fundoplication restored the sphincter pressure profile to normal in a patient with a defective sphincter. Calculation of the volume of the three dimensional images pre- and postoperatively showed that restoration of the sphincter vector volume to normal correlated with the success of the operation.[72] The Belsey procedure produced a smaller increase in the sphincter vector volume. Adding a fundoplication did not change the amplitude of contractions in the distal oesophagus (*Figure 1.55d*).

On the basis of the authors' experience, in a patient with increased oesophageal exposure to gastric juice due to a mechanically defective lower oesophageal sphincter, the Nissen fundoplication provides effective and durable relief of reflux with minimal side effects. This is accomplished by restor-

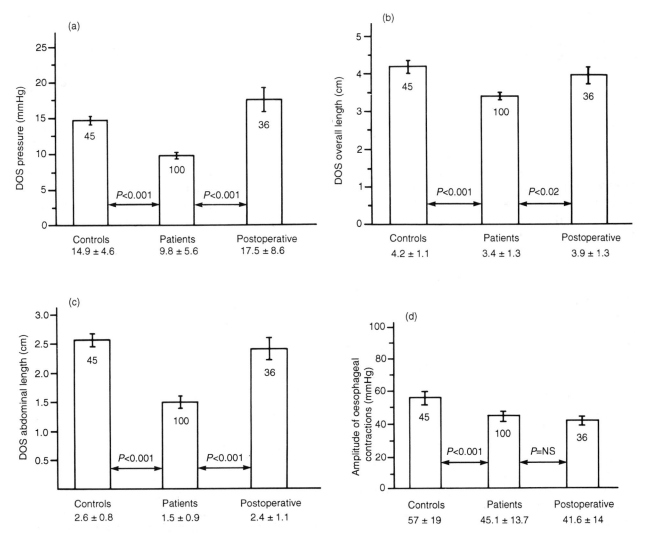

Figure 1.55 Effect of Nissen fundoplication on oesophageal function: (a) sphincter pressure; (b) total length; (c) abdominal length; (d) amplitude of oesophageal contractions. NS = non-significant; DOS = distal oesophageal sphincter. (From DeMeester, T.R., Bonavina, L. and Albertucci, M. (1986) Nissen fundoplication for gastroesophageal reflux disease. *Annals of Surgery*, **204**, 9–20, with permission.)

(a)

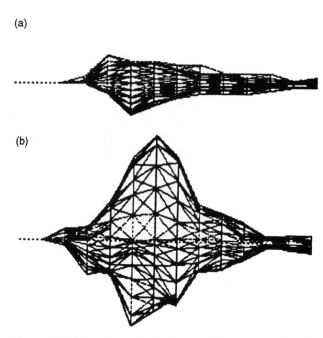

(b)

Figure 1.56 Three-dimensional image of lower oesophageal sphincter in a patient with a mechanically defective sphincter: (a) preoperatively; (b) after Nissen fundoplication.

ing normal mechanical characteristics to a defective lower oesophageal sphincter. These results from the authors' unit are comparable to those reported from other specialist centres.[26,62] Similar long-term results for the Belsey procedure have also been reported from several centres, although there is a slightly higher incidence of long-term failure.[6]

Poor results

There is a steadily increasing volume of literature on the subject of failures of antireflux surgery,[46,48,51,58] from which several important lessons are emerging. The most significant is the importance of attention to technical details during the operation. Common faults in performing the intra-abdominal Nissen procedure include insufficient mobilization of the gastric fundus and the lower oesophagus. The result is that the wrap may be constructed from the body of the stomach rather than the fundus, or that the wrap is placed too low, round the body of the stomach, instead of the lower oesophagus. It is well recognized that if the wrap is too long or too tight, postoperative dysphagia will result. The modifications to the original procedure which the authors have studied have been confirmed by several other workers.

Complications

In all antireflux operations splenic damage is a risk, often reported to be about 10%;[61] it can be mini-

mized by providing good exposure and avoiding excessive traction on the gastrosplenic ligament. Many minor injuries can be repaired and will not require splenectomy.

Local sepsis may result from penetration of the sutures into the lumina of the stomach or oesophagus in creating the wrap. Most of the unusual fistulous complications such as gastropericardial fistula or gastropleural or gastrobronchial fistulas have arisen in this way, with sepsis leading to abscess formation which later ruptures into an adjacent cavity. The necessity of using non-absorbable sutures and reinforcing materials such as Teflon pledgets may add to this risk, but it can be minimized by care in placing sutures at the correct depth.

Other antireflux operations

A number of alternative procedures have been proposed for which good results have been claimed, usually by the originators of the operation. In Europe, the repair of Lorat-Jacob continues to be popular, but has not been as extensively studied in a controlled situation. The same is true of the series of repairs using the ligamentum teres as a sling round the angle of His.[56] More recently Taylor *et al.*[74] have proposed an operation analogous to vertical banded gastroplasty, claiming good short-term results, but there are no indications that will offer any significant advantage over more established techniques.

Recently, there has been a resurgence of interest in the partial fundoplication of Toupet (1963),[10,76] due to the increasing reports of distressing side effects of the Nissen fundoplication. This is recommended by Cuschieri,[15] and a recent randomized controlled trial comparing Nissen fundoplication with the Toupet procedure showed a clear symptomatic advantage for the latter, especially in the low incidence of side effects, in a follow-up period of 5 years. Possible criticisms of this study are the small sample size (only 31 patients), relatively high incidence of slipped Nissen fundoplications in the Nissen group (3 of 12), suggesting that technical problems have still not been solved, and the lack of documentation of the results by 24-hour pH monitoring.[75] The problem with partial fundoplication procedures has always been lack of durability, and only the Belsey operation has stood the test of time in this regard, because the thoracic approach allows extensive mobilization of the oesophagus and construction of the wrap without tension.[65] It is not widely appreciated that a partial fundoplication performed through the abdomen requires a greater length of oesophagus than a short Nissen wrap, and the tension of the partial wrap is the major reason for the higher incidence of disruption. It remains to be seen whether these other partial fundoplications performed without the ability to mobilize the infra-aortic oesophagus will provide adequate long-term control of reflux. In the authors' own view, a properly executed Nissen fundoplication in appropiate patients will avoid most of these problems.

The Angelchik antireflux prosthesis was introduced in 1979 with a view to simplifying antireflux surgery.[2] This device, – a Silastic-filled 'doughnut' – which was simply tied round the gastro-oesophageal junction, was initially associated with a wide range of complications, some of them bizarre, but mostly related to design faults or inappropiate use. Erosion is a problem if the device is used where there is a fresh suture line in the gastrointestinal tract, and migration occurs if the tied tapes come adrift, or the oesophagus is shortened and the prosthesis pulled into the chest. These problems have been reduced to some extent as experience of the complications has been gained, but the value of the device is still not clear. One recent, randomized, controlled trial showed no difference in either reflux control or side effects between Nissen fundoplication and the Angelchik device, though there were non-significant increases in the degrees of oesophagitis in the Angelchik group.[73] Another smaller and non-randomized comparison found a similar proportion of good results in the Angelchik group, but 2 of the 22 patients died postoperatively and 4 of the remaining 20 patients had to have the prosthesis removed.[16] In general, even if the prosthesis is associated with the same frequency of good results, a bad result is more likely to require a second operation to remove it. One alleged advantage of the device is the ease with which it can be inserted. In the authors' view, there is no place for an inexperienced surgeon performing antireflux surgery, and this feature of the Angelchik device is not relevant to modern scientific surgical practice, as it may lead to inappropriate use. In particular, the unpremeditated intraoperative decision to 'repair a hiatus hernia' by a procedure thought to be quick and easy is especially to be deplored.

Until long-term controlled studies using these operations are reported, there seems little prospect of the established procedures being replaced. The future of antireflux surgery is likely to be moulded by the expanding role of laparoscopic techniques, and there are indications that the development of laparoscopic/endoscopic antireflux procedures is already far advanced.

Role of surgical treatment for the complications of gastro-oesophageal reflux

Oesophagitis: prevention of stricture

The presence of endoscopic oesophagitis in symptomatic patients with a mechanically defective lower oesophageal sphincter should encourage surgical therapy because these patients commonly receive little long-term benefit from medical therapy.[47] Even if the patient responds symptomatically to medical therapy but endoscopic oesophagitis persists, there is a strong case for recommending surgery. The reason is that these patients can still progress to develop a stricture or Barrett's oesophagus while on therapy because reflux of alkaline gastric contents continues through a mechanically defective sphincter. In this situation, an antireflux procedure corrects the mechanically defective sphincter, prevents formation of a stricture or Barrett's oesophagus, and heals the oesophagitis. Support for this view comes from the results of a randomized trial by Watson, who found that antireflux surgery significantly reduced the need for dilatation in a small study of 32 patients over a 22-month period.[81] The much larger Veterans' Administration cooperative study found that, of the medically treated group, 8% of the patients without a stricture at entry developed one during the study period.[44]

Established stricture

The development of a stricture in a patient with a mechanically defective sphincter is usually associated with loss of oesophageal contractility.[83] It can not be emphasized too strongly that in most cases the development of a stricture represents a failure of medical therapy, and is an indication for a surgical antireflux procedure. Sometimes a patient presents for the first time with a stricture in the absence of heartburn, but careful history taking usually reveals a history of antacid intake in the past, or the possibility of a drug induced stricture. In the initial assessment, a malignant aetiology of the stricture should be excluded and the stricture progressively dilated up to a 60 F bougie. When fully dilated, the relief of dysphagia is evaluated and oesophageal manometry is performed to determine the adequacy of peristalsis in the distal oesophagus. If dysphagia is relieved and the amplitude of oesophageal contractions is adequate, an antireflux procedure should be performed; if the amplitude of oesophageal contractions is poor, caution should be exercised in performing an antireflux procedure with a complete fundoplication and a partial fundoplication such as a Belsey should be considered, combined with oesophageal lengthening if necessary. If the dysphagia persists and the amplitude of contractions is deficient, an oesophageal resection and colon interposition should be considered.[21] This is because the stricture has caused such extensive transmural injury that the creation of any antireflux mechanism overcomes the propulsive power of the oesophagus, and dysphagia inevitably results. Even in milder strictures, the abnormalities of peristalsis rarely revert to normal after antireflux surgery.[63] In rare situations dysphagia persists after dilatation despite the presence of an adequate amplitude of oesophageal contractions. In this situation the authors recommend prolonged ambulatory monitoring of oesophageal motor activity to search for an unrecognized motor disorder prior to proceeding with an antireflux procedure. If the 24-hour oesophageal pH record in a patient with a stricture is normal, the stricture is probably secondary to drug ingestion and dilatation may be all that is needed. Usually in these patients the lower oesophageal sphincter is normal.[9] Care must be taken to ensure that the tightness of the stricture has not prevented obtaining meaningful pH test results, because there is anecdotal evidence that acid exposure decreases as the stricture narrows.

Barrett's oesophagus

Barrett's columnar-lined oesophagus is almost always associated with a severe mechanical defect of the lower oesophageal sphincter, poor contractility of the oesophageal body, acid hypersecretion, duodenogastric reflux and mucosal insensitivity.[24,41,67] Patients with Barrett's oesophagus are at risk of progression of the mucosal abnormality up the oesophagus, formation of a stricture, haemorrhage from a Barrett's ulcer, and the development of an adenocarcinoma. A surgical antireflux procedure can arrest the progression of the disease, heal ulceration and resolve strictures. Some workers have noted a regression of the Barrett's epithelium after antire-flux surgery, but only in a minority of patients.[11] An antireflux procedure may also reduce the degree of pleomorphism and dysplasia. The risk of adenocarcinoma developing in Barrett's oesophagus is still debated, but even conservative estimates put it at 40–50 times that of the general population.[13,67] Although adenocarcinoma has occasionally been noted in patients following an antireflux procedure, the weight of evidence suggests that antireflux surgery does protect against malignant change. The report on the Barrett's registry study by the American College of Gastroenterology has recently indicated that of the patients who entered the study free of dysplasia or cancer and treated medically, 20% have developed

dysplasia and 1.3% developed carcinoma, but there have been no cancers in the surgically treated group.[52] It concluded that 'antire-flux surgery in the form of fundoplication significantly prevented the development of dysplasia and cancer during long-term follow-up when compared to medical therapy ($p < .025$)'. The situation is more urgent if severe dysplasia is found on mucosal biopsies and confirmed by a second opinion. The authors recommend an oesophageal resection for this situation because it has been reported that 50% of such specimens will show early invasive carcinomas.

PARA-OESOPHAGEAL HERNIA

It is well established that the optimal treatment for para-oesophageal hernia is surgical. In the classic report of Skinner and Belsey,[95] 21 patients with para-oesophageal hernia were followed expectantly, because their symptoms were mild. Six of these presented with acute complications and died and, as a result, the remaining 15 patients had their hernias repaired electively without incident. The presence of a para-oesophageal hernia is sufficient indication for it to be repaired unless the patient is a very poor operative risk. Published reports of the complications of elective surgery show a mortality of less than 1%,[65] 2%[28,60] and many smaller series have been reported with no mortality, despite the advanced age (mean 70 years) of many of the patients.[79,80] By contrast, the mortality in patients presenting acutely with complications is much higher[34,37] ranging from 10% to 50%.

There are two important controversies in this connection: first, the route of approach can be either through the chest or the abdomen. The advantages of laparotomy include speed and more direct access to other abdominal organs, and it is the preferred approach in elective cases. However, when incarcerated it is sometimes necessary to enlarge the hiatus in order to deliver the stomach safely. When the viability of the stomach is in doubt, thoracotomy is preferred. If proximal gangrenous stomach is encountered, no attempt should be made to perform a primary repair. A grossly contaminated mediastinum greatly increases the risk of anastomotic breakdown. In this situation, the necrotic stomach should be excised, the gastric remnant closed, and the whole thoracic oesophagus mobilized and stuffed into the posterosuperior mediastinum. The thoracotomy can then be closed, and the patient placed supine for insertion of a feeding jejunostomy and construction of a cervical oesopohagotomy. Retaining as much length as possible makes subsequent reconstruction easier.

Secondly, not all surgeons perform a concomitant antireflux procedure because symptoms of gastro-oesophageal reflux are not usually prominent, and extensive preoperative testing is not commonly performed. However, in the large series from Adelaide, 75% of patients had heartburn and regurgitation.[77] The only study to perform pH and manometry on patients preoperatively was by Walther et al.[80] which showed abnormal acid exposure in 9 of 15 patients. They also noted that the positive pH tests could not be inferred from the patients' symptoms. The patients had a manometrically short overall length of the lower oesophageal sphincter. For this reason, and because the hiatal attachments are usually disrupted during the mobilization and repair of the hernia, the authors recommend the addition of a Nissen fundoplication to the repair of the crural defect.

INTRATHORACIC STOMACH

A totally intrathoracic stomach can result from sliding or para-oesophageal hiatus hernia. In the latter, it is sometimes called 'upside-down stomach', and is an intrathoracic form of gastric volvulus. Other reported causes include hernias through the foramen of Bochdalek and penetrating diaphragmatic injuries. Gastric volvulus in the abdomen can be confused with intrathoracic stomach if it follows phrenic nerve injury or eventration of the diaphragm. The significance of intrathoracic stomach is that it is likely to cause obstruction, with the rapid development of distension, leading to both mediastinal shift and strangulation of the incarcerated stomach. About one-third of all cases of complete gastric volvulus present in this way. In the series of 25 patients with acute gastric volvulus reported by Carter et al.[14], 7 presented with gangrene of the stomach, and death occurred in 3.

It may be possible to decompress the stomach by passing a nasogastric tube, and endoscopic decompression has been described. This manoeuvre can buy some time to allow adequate preparation for surgery. More commonly, the site of the volvulus has occluded the gastro-oesophageal junction and it is not possible to pass a tube in which circumstance an emergency operation must be performed. The priority is to decompress the distended stomach and resect any gangrenous tissue. In elective cases, the best protection against recurrence is closure of the diaphragmatic defect and a Nissen fundoplication, but various gastropexies have been reported with satisfactory results in the short term.[54]

TRAUMATIC DIAPHRAGMATIC HERNIA

Penetrating or blunt injuries to the diaphragm may allow abdominal contents to pass into the chest. There are two distinct presentations of this event: usually it is detected at the time of the initial assessment of the traumatic episode, and treated simultaneously with concomitant injuries: these patients are unlikely to present to a gastroenterologist. In the second type of presentation the defect is only discovered months or even years later, and such patients may present with symptoms suggestive of upper gastrointestinal disorders.

Acute diaphragmatic rupture

This condition occurs most commonly after blunt trauma to the trunk, usually following road traffic accidents or a fall from a height. In most patients, the clinical picture is dominated by the presence of other injuries; two-thirds have fractures of the ribs, pelvis or long bones, and half have injury to the liver or spleen. Rupture and herniation are much more common on the left side, presumably owing to the protective effect of the liver.[12,35,43,78]

The important step in management is to consider the diagnosis. The chest radiograph shows abnormalities in 50%. Suggestive signs are a raised hemidiaphragm, or the presence of an air-containing viscus in the thorax. Peritoneal lavage may indicate the need for laparotomy, and the presence of lavage fluid coming from the chest drain is pathognomic. The associated injuries requiring surgical correction are usually abdominal. Most diaphragmatic tears on the left are in the dome and extend into the hiatus. They can be easily repaired through the abdomen. The importance of carefully inspecting the domes of the diaphragm during any laparotomy for trauma cannot be over-emphasized. A separate thoracotomy is usually needed to close a defect accurately on the right. This is preferable to extending the incision across the costal margin. Repair must be with stout non-absorbable material, and buttressing with Teflon pledgets is helpful if there is no gross contamination of the peritoneal cavity. The outcome is related to the severity of the associated injuries. The diaphragmatic defect usually heals without incident.

Penetrating trauma from stab or gunshot wounds to the chest or abdomen may traverse the diaphragm and permit herniation. The principles of treatment are the same as for blunt trauma. Associated injuries are more localized but more likely to perforate a hollow viscus. The surgical approach depends on the other probable injuries, but usually the abdominal route will be chosen.

Delayed presentation of diaphragmatic rupture

Occasionally a patient is found to have a hernia through the dome of the diaphragm months or even years after an episode of severe trauma, and it is concluded that the rupture was missed at the time of initial presentation.[33,40,64] It has been observed after an admission where the patient had a laparotomy and the diagnosis was presumably missed.[36] The trauma is usually penetrating (stab or gunshot), but may be iatrogenic in which case it usually follows a procedure necessitating a diaphragmatic incision, such as an Allison repair.[42] As in other types of diaphragmatic hernia, the left hemidiaphragm is almost always affected.[29] These injuries are unlikely to heal spontaneously because of the constant pleuroperitoneal pressure gradient tending to force abdominal contents into the chest. Because the symptoms are often insidious these patients may present to a general physician or gastroenterologist, and one-third do so in this way. However, it is also important to be aware of the possibility of complications of incarceration and strangulation.

Strangulation is a common presentation in these hernias because the diaphragmatic defect is usually small. The authors recommend that all stab wounds to the abdomen and chest be followed up with a radiograph 3 months after discharge. As in para-oesophageal hernia, the mortality of cases operated on as acute emergencies may be up to ten times that of elective operation.[36]

Between 5% and 15% of all traumatic ruptures of diaphragm present in this late manner.[34,64] The diagnosis is often suspected on chest radiograph and confirmed by contrast radiology. Once established, the treatment is surgical. A thoracotomy is often preferred as it allows dissection of the adhesions to the lungs under direct vision. The diaphragmatic defect must be repaired with non-absorbable sutures; if the defect is so large that it cannot be primarily repaired without tension, a prosthetic patch of GoreTex or Marlex mesh can be safely used if there is no sepsis. The early practice of crushing the phrenic nerve is unnecessary and harmful.

REFERENCES

1. Allison, P.R. (1973) Hiatus hernia (A 20-year retrospective survey). *Annals of Surgery*, **178**, 273–276.
2. Angelchik, J.P. and Cohen, R. (1979) A new surgical procedure for the treatment of gastroesophageal reflux and hiatal hernia. *Surgery, Gynecology and Obstetrics*, **148**, 246–248.
3. Attwood, S.E.A., DeMeester, T.R., Bremner, C.G., Barlow, A.P. and Hinder, R.A. (1989) Alkaline gastroesophageal reflux: Implications in the development of complications in Barrett's columnar-lined esophagus. *Surgery*, **106**, 764–770.
4. Barlow, A.P., DeMeester, T.R., Ball, C.S. and Eypasch, E.P. (1989) The significance of the gastric secretory state in gastroesophageal reflux disease. *Archives of Surgery*, **124**, 937–940.
5. Behar, J., Sheahan, D.G., Biancani, P., Spiro, H.M. and Storer, E.H. (1975) Medical and surgical management of reflux esophagitis. A 38-month report on a prospective clinical trial. *New England Journal of Medicine*, **293**, 263–268.
6. Belsey, R. (1977) Mark IV repair of hiatal hernia by the transthoracic approach. *World Journal of Surgery*, **1**, 475–483.
7. Bennett, J.R. (1989) Medical therapy for gastro-oesophageal reflux. In *Reflux Oesophagitis* (Eds) Hennessy, T.P.J., Cuschieri, A. and Bennett, J.R., pp. 123–141. London: Butterworths.
8. Bombeck, C.T., Dillard, D.H. and Nyhus, L.M. (1966) Muscular anatomy of the gastroesophageal junction and role of the Phrenoesophageal Ligament. *Annals of Surgery*, **164**, 643–654.
9. Bonavina, L., DeMeester, T.R., McChesney, L., Schwizer, W., Albertucci, M. and Bailey, R.T. (1987) Drug-induced oesophageal strictures. *Annals of Surgery*, **206**, 173–183.
10. Boutelier, P. and Jonsell, G. (1982) An alternative fundoplicative maneuver for gastroesophageal reflux. *American Journal of Surgery*, **143**, 260–264.
11. Brand, D.L., Ylvsiaker, J.T., Gelfand, M. and Pope, C.E. (1980) Regression of columnar esophageal (Barrett's) epithelium after anti-reflux surgery. *New England Journal of Medicine*, **302**, 844–848.
12. Brown, G.L. and Richardson, J.D. (1985) Traumatic diaphragmatic hernia: A continuing challenge. *Annals of Thoracic Surgery*, **39**, 170–173.
13. Cameron, A.J., Ott, B.J. and Payne, W.S. (1985) The incidence of adenocarcinoma in columnar-lined lower esophagus. *New England Journal of Medicine*, **313**, 857–858.
14. Carter, R., Brewer, L.A. and Hinshaw, D.B. (1980) Acute gastric volvulus – A study of 25 cases. *American Journal of Surgery*, **140**, 99–106.
15. Cuschieri, A. (1989) Surgical treatment of reflux disease. In *Reflux Oesophagitis*, pp. 143–169. (Eds) Hennessy, T.P.J., Cuschieri, A. and Bennett, J.R. London: Butterworths.
16. Deakin, M., Mayer, D. and Temple, J.G. (1989) Surgery for gastro-oesophageal reflux: the Angelchik prosthesis compared to the floppy Nissen fundoplication. Two-year follow-up study and a five-year evaluation of the Angelchik prosthesis. *Annals of the Royal College of Surgeons of England*, **71**, 249–252.

17. DeMeester, T.R., Johnston, L.F. and Kent, A.H. (1974) Evaluation of current operations for the prevention of gastresophageal reflux. *Annals of Surgery*, **180**, 511–525.

18. DeMeester, T.R., LaFontaine, E., Joelsson, B.E. *et al.* (1981) Relationship of a hiatal hernia to the function of the body of the esophagus and the gastresophageal junction. *Journal of Thoracic and Cardiovascular Surgery*, **82**, 547–558.

19. DeMeester, T.R., Bonavina, L. and Albertucci, M. (1986) Nissen fundoplication for gastroesophageal reflux disease. *Annals of Surgery*, **204**, 9–20.

20. DeMeester, T.R., Fuchs, K.F., Ball, C.S., Albertucci, M., Smyrk, T.C. and Marcus, J.N. (1987) Experimental and clinical results with proximal end-to-end duodenojejunostomy for pathologic duodenogastric reflux. *Annals of Surgery*, **216**, 414–426.

21. DeMeester, T.R., Johansson, K-E., Franze, I. *et al.* (1988) Indications, surgical technique, and long-term functional results of colon interposition or bypass. *Annals of Surgery*, **208**, 460–474.

22. DeMeester, T.R. and Bonavina, L. (1989) Paraesophageal hiatal hernia. In *Hernia*, 3rd ed (Eds) Condon, R.E. and Nyhus, L.M., pp. 684–693. Philadelphia: J.B. Lippincott.

23. DeMeester, T.R. and Stein, H.J. (1989) Gastroesophageal reflux disease. In *The Surgical Treatment of Digestive Disease*, 2nd edn, (Eds) Moody, F.G., Carey, L.C., Jones, R.S., Kelly, K.A., Nahrwold, D.L. and Skinner, D.B., pp. 65–108. Chicago: Year Book Medical Publishers.

24. DeMeester, T.R., Attwood, S.E.A., Smyrk, T.C., Therkildsen, D.H. and Hinder, R.A. (1990) Surgical therapy in Barrett's esophagus. *Annals of Surgery*, **212**, 528–542.

25. DeMeester, T.R. Bonavina, L., Iascone, C., Courtney, J.V. and Skinner, D.B. (1990) Chronic respiratory symptoms and occult gastroesophageal reflux. *Annals of Surgery*, **211**, 337–345.

26. Donahue, P.E., Samelson, S., Nyhus, L.M. and Bombeck, C.T. (1985) The floppy Nissen fundoplication. *Archives of Surgery*, **120**, 663–668.

27. Edwards, D.A.W. (1982) Radiological examination and quantitation of reflux in the hiatal hernia-reflux syndrome. In *Pathological Gastroesophageal Reflux*, pp. 47–53 (Eds) Van Heukelem, H.A., Gooszen, H.G., Terpstra, J.B. *et al.* Amsterdam: Zuid Nederlandse Uitgevers Maatschappij BV.

28. Ellis, F.H., Crozier, R.E. and Shea, J.A. (1986) Paraesophageal hiatus hernia. *Archives of Surgery*, **121**, 416–420.

29. Feliciano, D.V., Cruse, P.A., Mattox, K.L. *et al.* (1988) Delayed diagnosis of injuries to the diaphragm after penetrating wounds. *Journal of Trauma*, **28**, 1135–1144.

30. Fuchs, K.H. and DeMeester, T.R. (1987) Cost benefit analysis in the management of gastroesophageal reflux disease. In *Diseases of the Esophagus*, pp. 857–861 (Eds) Siewert, J.R. and Hölscher, A.H. New York: Springer-Verlag.

31. Fuchs, K.H., DeMeester, T.R., Schwizer, W. and Albertucci, M. (1987) Concomitant duodenogastric and gastroesophageal reflux: The role of twenty-four hour gastric pH monitoring. In *Diseases of the Esophagus*, pp. 1073–1076 (Eds) Siewert, J.R. and Hölscher, A.H. New York: Springer-Verlag.

32. Fuchs, K.H., DeMeester, T.R., Hinder, R.A., Stein, H.J., Barlow, A.P. and Gupta, N.C. (1991) Computerized identification of pathologic duodenogastric reflux using 24-hour gastric pH monitoring. *Annals of Surgery*, **213**, 13–19.

33. Griffin, S.M. and Rich, A.J. (1986) Late presentation of traumatic diaphragmatic hernia. *Journal of the Royal Society of Medicine*, **79**, 45.

34. Haas, O., Rat, P., Christophe, M., Friedman, S. and Favre, J.P. (1990) Surgical results of intrathoracic gastric volvulus complicating hiatal hernia. *British Journal of Surgery*, **77**, 1379–1381.

35. Harms, B., Helgerson, R. and Starling, J. (1987) Diaphragmatic injuries following blunt trauma. *The American Surgeon*, **53**, 325–328.

36. Hegarty, M.M., Bryer, J.V., Angorn, K.B. and Baker, L.W. (1978) Delayed presentation of diaphragmatic hernia. *Annals of Surgery*, **188**, 229–233.

37. Hill, L.D. (1973) Incarcerated paraesophageal hernia – A surgical emergency. *Americal Journal of Surgery*, **126**, 286–291.

38. Hill, L.D. (1977) Progress in the surgical management of hiatal hernia. *World Journal of Surgery*, **1**, 425–438.

39. Hinder, R.A., Stein, H.J., Bremner, C.G. and DeMeester, T.R. (1989) Relationship of a satisfactory outcome to normalization of delayed gastric emptying after Nissen fundoplication. *Annals of Surgery*, **210**, 458–464.

40. Holm, A., Belley, P.Q. and Aldrette, J.S. (1988) Diaphragmatic rupture due to blunt trauma. Morbidity and mortality in 42 cases. *Southern Medical Journal*, **81**, 956–962.

41. Iascone, C., DeMeester, T.R., Little, A.G. and Skinner, D.B. (1983) Barrett's esophagus: Functional assessment, proposed pathogenesis, and surgical therapy. *Archives of Surgery*, **118**, 543–549.

42. Johnston, C.D. and Shandall, A. (1987) Incisional hernia of the diaphragm causing large bowel obstruction. *Journal of the Royal College of Surgeons of Edinburgh*, **32**, 51–52.

43. Johnston, C.D. (1988) Blunt injuries of the diaphragm. *British Journal of Surgery*, **75**, 226–230.

44. Kaul, B.K., DeMeester, T.R., Oka, M. *et al.* (1990) The cause of dysphagia in uncomplicated sliding hiatal hernia and its relief by hiatal herniorraphy. *Annals of Surgery*, **211**, 406–410.

45. Lanspa, S.J., Spechler, S.J., DeMeester, T.R., Zetterman, R., Williford, W.O., Krol, W.F. and VA Cooperative Study Group #277 (1991) Incidence of stricture formation in patients with complicated gastroesophageal reflux disease (GERD). *Gastroenterology*, **100**, A107.

46. Leonardi, H.K., Crozier, R.E. and Ellis, F.H.

(1981) Reoperation for the complications of the Nissen fundoplication. *Journal of Thoracic and Cardiovascular Surgery*, **81**, 50–56.

47. Liebermann, D.A. (1987) Medical therapy for chronic reflux esophagitis; long-term follow-up. *Archives of Internal Medicine*, **147**, 1717–1720.

48. Little, A.G., Ferguson, M.K. and Skinner, D.B. (1986) Reoperation for failed fundoplication. *Journal of Thoracic and Cardiovascular Surgery*, **91**, 511–517.

49. Lloyd, J.W., Barnard, J.D.W. and Glynn, C.J. (1976) Cryoanalgesia: a new approach to pain relief. *The Lancet*, **ii**, 932–934.

50. Maiwand, O. and Makey, A.R. (1981) Cryoanalgesia for relief of pain after thoracotomy. *British Medical Journal*, **282**, 1749–1750.

51. Martin, C.J. and Crookes, P.F. (1990) Reoperation for failed antireflux surgery. *Australian and New Zealand Journal of Surgery*, **60**, 773–778.

52. McCallum, R.W., Polepalle, S., Davenport, K., Frierson, H. and Boyd, S. (1991) Role of anti-reflux surgery against dysplasia in Barrett's esophagus. *Gastroenterology*, **100**, A121.

53. Menguy, R. (1988) Surgical management of large paraesophageal hernia with complete intrathoracic stomach. *World Journal of Surgery*, **12**, 415–422.

54. Mittal, R.K., Lange, R.C. and McCallum, R.W. (1987) Identification and mechanism of delayed esophageal acid clearance in subjects with hiatus hernia. *Gastroenterology*, **92**, 130–135.

55. Muller, J. Ch., Salzer, G.M., Ransmayr, G. and Neiss, A. (1989) Intraoperative cryoanalgesia for postthoracotomy pain relief. *Annals of Thoracic Surgery*, **48**, 15–18.

56. Narbona, B. (1989) The sling approach to the treatment of reflux peptic esophagitis in: *Hernia*, 3rd edn, pp. 668–683 (Eds) Nyhus, L.M. and Condon, R.E. Philadelphia: J.B. Lippincott.

57. Nebel, O.T., Fornes, M.F. and Castell, D.O. (1976) Symptomatic gastroesophageal reflux: Incidence and precipitating factors. *Digestive Diseases*, **21**, 953–956.

58. Negre, J.B. (1983) Post-fundoplication syndromes. Do they restrict the success of Nissen fundoplication? *Annals of Surgery*, **198**, 698–700.

59. Pearson, F.G., Cooper, J.D., Patterson, G.A., Ramirez, J. and Todd, T.R. (1987) Gastroplasty and fundoplication for complex reflux problems. *Annals of Surgery*, **296**, 473–480.

60. Pearson, F.G., Copper, J.D., Ilves, R., Todd, T.R.J. and Jamieson, W.R.E. (1983) Massive hiatal hernia with incarceration: A report of 53 cases. *Annals of Thoracic Surgery*, **35**, 45–51.

61. Polk, H.C. (1976) Fundoplication for reflux esophagitis: Misadventures with the operation of choice. *Annals of Surgery*, **183**, 645–652.

62. Rosetti, M. and Hell, K. (1977) Fundoplication for the treatment of gastroesophageal reflux disease. *World Journal of Surgery*, **1**, 439–444.

63. Russell, C.O.H., Pope. C.E., Gannan, R.M. (1981) Does surgery correct esophageal motor dysfunction in gastroesophageal reflux? *Annals of Surgery*, **194**, 290–296.

64. Saber, W.L., Moore, E.E., Hopeman, A.R. and Aragon, W.E. (1986) Delayed presentation of traumatic diaphragmatic hernia. *Journal of Emergency Medicine*, **4**, 1–7.

65. Skinner, D.B. and Belsey, R.H.R. (1967) Surgical management of esophageal reflux and hiatus hernia. *Journal of Thoracic and Cardiovascular Surgery*, **53**, 33–54.

66. Sloan, S and Kahrilas, P.J. (1991) Impairment of esophageal emptying with hiatal hernia. *Gastroenterology*, **100**, 596–605.

67. Spechler, S.J. and Goyal, R.K. (1986) Barrett's esophagus. *New England Journal of Medicine*, **315**, 362–371.

68. Spechler, S.J., Williford, W.O. and the VA Cooperative Study Group #277 (1990) Complications of medical and surgical therapies for gastroesophageal reflux disease (GERD). *Gastroenterology*, **98**, A130.

69. Spechler, S.J. and the VA Gastroesophageal Reflux Disease Group (1992) Comparison of medical and surgical therapy for complicated gastroesophageal reflux disease in Veterans. *New England Journal of Medicine*, **326**, 786–792.

70. Stein, H.J., Eypasch, E.P., DeMeester, T.R., Smyrk, T.C. and Attwood, S.E.A. (1990) Circadian esophageal motor function in patients with gastroesophageal reflux disease. *Surgery*, **108**, 769–778.

71. Stein, H.J., Hinder, R.A., DeMeester, T.R. (1990) Clinical use of 24-hour gastric pH monitoring vs O-diisopropyl Iminodiacetic Acid (DISIDA) scanning in the diagnosis of pathologic duodenogastric reflux. *Archives of Surgery*, **125**, 966–971.

72. Stein, H.J., DeMeester, T.R., Naspetti, R., Jamieson, J. and Perry, R.E. (1991) Three-dimensional imaging of the lower esophageal sphincter in gastroesophageal reflux disease. *Annals of Surgery*, **214**, 374–384.

73. Stuart, R.C., Dawson, K., Keeling, P., Bryne, P.J and Hennessy, T.P.J. (1989) A prospective randomized trial of Angelchik prosthesis versus Nissen fundoplication. *British Journal of Surgery*, **76**, 86–89.

74. Taylor, T.V., Knox, R.A. and Pullan, B.R. (1989) Vertical gastric plication: an operation for gastro-oesophageal reflux. *Annals of the Royal College of Surgeons of England*, **71**, 31–36.

75. Thor, K.B.A. and Silander, T. (1989) A long-term randomized prospective trial of the Nissen procedure versus a Modified Toupet Technique. *Annals of Surgery*, **210**, 719–724.

76. Toupet, A. (1963) Technique d'oesophago-gastroplastie avec phréno-gastropexie appliquée dans la cure radicale des hernies hiatales et comme complément de l'opération de Heller dans les cardiospasmes. *Memoires d'Académie de Chirurgie*, **89**, 394–399.

77. Treacy, P.J. and Jamieson, G.C. (1987) An

approach to the management of paraoesophageal hernias. *Australian and New Zealand Journal of Surgery*, **57**, 813–817.

78. Troop, B., Myers, R.M. and Agarwal, N.N. (1985) Early recognition of diaphragmatic injuries from blunt trauma. *Annals of Emergency Medicine*, **2**, 97–101.

79. Vitelli, C.E., Jaffe, B.M. and Kahng, K.U. (1989) Paraesophageal hernia. *New York State Journal of Medicine*, **89**, 654–657.

80. Walther, B., DeMeester, T.R., LaFontaine, E., Courtney, J.V., Little, A.G. and Skinner, D.B. (1984) Effect of paraesophageal hernia on sphincter function and its implication on surgical therapy. *American Journal of Surgery*, **147**, 111–115.

81. Watson, A. (1985) Randomized study comparing medical and surgical reflux control in peptic oesophageal stricture treated by intermittent dilatation. *Gut*, **26**, A555.

82. Woodward, E.R., Thomas, H.F. and McAlhany, J.C. (1971) Comparison of crural repair and Nissen fundoplication in the treatment of esophageal hiatus hernia with peptic esophagitis. *Annals of Surgery*, **173**, 782–792.

83. Zaninotto, G., DeMeester, T.R., Bremner, C.G., Smyrk, T.C. and Cheng, S-C. (1989) Esophageal function in patients with reflux-induced strictures and its revelance to surgical treatment. *Annals of Thoracic Surgery*, **47**, 362–370.

TUMOURS

A. Mannell

BENIGN TUMOURS OF THE OESOPHAGUS

Benign tumours of the oesophagus are usually small, asymptomatic and frequently incidental findings at autopsy or during radiological investigations for other gastrointestinal conditions. However, the occasional bizarre and life-threatening presentations of these rare tumours continues to fascinate the clinician and the differentiation of a benign lesion from the more common oesophageal malignancies is obviously important to the patient.

Although rare, sufficient data on benign oesophageal tumours have been accumulated to establish the characteristic clinical pictures, to enable the diagnosis to be made when endoscopic biopsy may be contraindicated and to select the appropriate method of treatment.

INCIDENCE

Many benign tumours of the oesophagus are asymptomatic so the true incidence of these lesions is best reflected by autopsy studies. However, the incidence has shown considerable variation between reported series. Moersch and Harrington[15] found 44 benign tumours in 7459 autopsies, Schaffer and Kitles[23] found no reports of benign oesophageal tumours in the records of 6000 autopsies, but Plachta[21] was able to collect 90 cases from 20 000 autopsies performed over a 50-year period at the

New York Medical College, Metropolitan Medical Center.

The variations in incidence may reflect the care with which the oesophagus is examined for very small tumours. Postlethwaite[22] reviewed the results of over 86 000 autopsies to find only 48 cases of oesophageal leiomyomas, the most common benign tumour of the oesophagus. However, in a personal series of 1000 autopsies, he was able to identify 51 oesophageal leiomyomas most of which varied from 1.0 to 4.0 mm in diameter.

CLASSIFICATION

The most widely used system is that proposed by Nemir *et al.*[16] in which benign tumours are classified according to the tissue of origin within the oesophagus:

A. Epithelial tumours
    (1) papilloma
    (2) polyps
    (3) adenoma
    (4) cysts
B. Non-epithelial tumours
    (1) myoma:
        (a) leiomyoma
        (b) fibromyoma
        (c) lipomyoma
        (d) fibroma
    (2) vascular tumours
        (a) haemangioma
        (b) lymphangioma

  (3) mesenchymal and others
   (a) reticuloendothelial tumour
   (b) lipoma
   (c) myxofibroma
   (d) giant cell tumour
   (e) neurofibroma
   (f) osteochondroma
C. Heterotopic tumours
  (1) gastric mucosa
  (2) melanoblastic elements
  (3) sebaceous gland
  (4) granular cell myoblastoma
  (5) pancreatic gland
  (6) thyroid nodule.

It must be noted that the Nemir classification includes lesions that are congenital rather than neoplastic and those that arise from ectopic cell nests. An alternative system has been described by Totten[29] and Schmidt[25] in which benign oesophageal tumours are divided into (1) mucosal (intraluminal) and (2) extramucosal (intramural), depending on their predominant relationship with the oesophageal wall. This is a useful classification because polyps, the most common epithelial tumours, are usually intraluminal in origin whilst most benign oesophageal tumours are intramural leiomyomas. There is, however, some overlap between these two categories: a small number of oesophageal leiomyomas will present as polypoid intraluminal lesions.

LEIOMYOMA

Incidence

Leiomyomas account for 50–70% of benign oesophageal tumours[16,21,22,26] but these tumours are encountered much less frequently in the oesophagus than in stomach and intestine. Oberhelman et al.[17] found that only 6% of gastrointestinal leiomyomas arise in the oesophagus whilst Seremetis et al.,[26] reviewing the results of over 180 000 autopsies in the world literature, noted that the autopsy incidence of oesophageal leiomyomas was 1 in 1120 cases. Unlike oesophageal cancer, the authors found no racial or geographical differences in the incidence of this uncommon tumour. Although it is possible that most single lesions are not reported, they are a very rare cause of oesophageal symptoms: Moersch and Harrington[15] were able to identify only 15 leiomyomas among 11 000 patients investigated for dysphagia. Males are affected twice as commonly as women, most often in the fifth decade (range 12–80 year, mean 44 years). Leiomyomas arise from the smooth muscle cells and therefore are most common in the lower two-thirds of the oesophagus. In the 838

cases collected by Seremetis et al.,[26] 56% occurred in the distal oesophagus and 33% in the midoesophagus with 11% of cases arising from the small amount of smooth muscle in the upper oesophagus.[3]

Ninety-seven per cent oesophageal leiomyomas are intramural tumours, 2% are extraoesophageal or subserosal in origin and 1% are polypoid intraluminal lesions.[17,26] Most are single lesions, 2–5 cm in diameter, but 'giant' leiomyomas of the oesophagus, weighing up to 5000 g, have been reported.[5,9,12] Less than 3% leiomyomas are multiple and must then be differentiated from the very rare condition of diffuse oesophageal leiomyomatosis which may represent hypertrophy of the oesophageal wall in response to diffuse oesophageal spasm.

Pathology

The oesophageal leiomyoma is a firm, round, encapsulated tumour with greyish-white or yellow appearance on cross-section. It is localized to one area of the oesophageal wall in 90% of patients although 10% of symptomatic cases are found to have a leiomyoma partly or completely encircling the oesophageal lumen. Cystic degeneration, characteristic of large leiomyomas at other sites, is not seen in the oesophagus and less than 2% of tumours are calcified.[26]

Histologically the leiomyoma consists of bundles of elongated cells containing intracellular myofibrils. The smooth muscle cell bundles are surrounded by hypovascular connective tissue in which fat or fibroblasts may be prominent, leading to categorization of the tumour as a lipomyoma or fibromyoma.[21] Palisading may be seen and, if present, microscopic interdigitation into adjacent muscle tissue must be distinguished from sarcomatous infiltration. Malignant transformation of oesophageal leiomyomas is, in fact, very rare with only two cases documented in the world literature up to 1970.[7]

Clinical features

These lesions grow very slowly and remain asymptomatic until they are more than 5 cm in size, have encircled the oesophagus or involve the gastro-oesophageal junction. Characteristically, the patient is a middle-aged or elderly man with a long history of intermittent dysphagia associated with a vague sense of retrosternal discomfort or pressure. Occasionally pain is felt in the left chest and, if severe, must be differentiated from angina pectoris. Less common symptoms include weight loss, regurgitation and salivation. Haemorrhage may result from peptic ulceration of the overlying mucosa where a leiomyoma involves the cardio-oesophageal junction.[3] Very large leiomyomas can compress the tracheobronchial tree resulting in episodes of dyspnoea, stridor and repeated pulmonary infection.[16] Pedunculated oesophageal leiomyomas have been regurgitated into the oropharynx, leading to asphyxia from glottic destruction, but this is exceptionally rare. The association of hypertrophic osteoarthropathy with leiomyoma of the oesophagus has been reported.[30]

Investigations

It is usually not difficult to make the diagnosis of oesophageal leiomyoma from the long duration of slight intermittent dysphagia combined with the typical radiographic and endoscopic appearance of the tumour. The barium swallow displays a smooth well-demarcated defect in the contour of the oesophageal lumen (*Figure 1.57*) with no evidence of

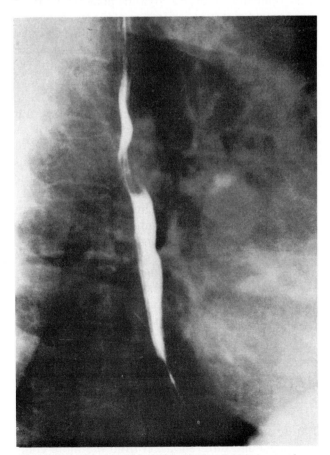

Figure 1.57 The typical radiographic appearance of an oesophageal leiomyoma on barium swallow examination (Courtesy of Mr P.A. Game.) From Game, P.A. (1988) *Survey of the Oesophagus* (Ed.) G.G. Jamieson, Churchill Livingstone, Edinburgh, with permission.)

mucosal ulceration.[24] Although the mucosal folds may be obliterated over the lesion in the postero-anterior view, these are often evident on the opposite wall in the oblique or lateral view (smear effect). Retention of contrast and proximal oesophageal dilatation are very uncommon even with large tumours which have produced considerable distortion in the longitudinal axis of the oesophagus. However, leiomyomas at the gastro-oesophageal junction have been mistaken for achalasia prior to the routine use of computed tomography (CT). The tumour may be evident on a chest radiograph as a soft tissue swelling. This can be identified as a hypovascular tumour by contrast CT scanning and distinguished from mediastinal cysts, pulmonary granulomata and thoracic aortic aneurysms.

At endoscopy, the oesophageal mucosa appears normal and bulges into the lumen, but there is usually no obstruction to the passage of the oesophagoscope. Unless the tumour is the rare polypoid pedunculated variety, the intact mucosa should not be biopsied because this may interfere with subsequent surgical removal.

Treatment

The serendipitous discovery of a small asymptomatic intramural tumour in the older patient is not an indication for treatment. It can be safely observed because the risk of malignant change is so small. Surgical removal is indicated when the tumour is large or pedunculated, associated with either oesophageal or respiratory symptoms and if it involves the gastro-oesophageal junction. Most tumours can be safely removed by enucleation unless the overlying mucosa is inflamed or has been damaged by endoscopic biopsy. The approach, through either the right or left side of the chest, is determined by the site of the lesion; the overlying muscle layer is split and a plane developed between tumour and mucosa without entering the oesophageal lumen. In 10% of cases reported by Seremetis *et al.*,[26] oesophageal resection was required for large and annular tumours, those densely adherent to the mucosa and for tumours crossing the gastro-oesophageal junction. Endoscopic removal is possible only for very small pedunculated tumours.

POLYPS

Long before Roentgen's discovery of X-rays and the invention of the oesophagoscope, the oesophageal polyp was recognized clinically from the bizarre effect of regurgitation into or beyond the mouth.

Postlethwaite[22] found that this rare tumour was first described in 1559 and that death from laryngeal obstruction by oesophageal polyps had been reported by early writers.

Incidence

Polyps are the second most benign tumour of the oesophagus but account for less than 5% of benign oesophageal neoplasms.[21] In collected series, oesophageal polyps predominated in elderly men, and 80% were cervical in origin and usually attached at the level of the cricoid cartilage.[22]

Pathology

The typical polyp is a solitary, cylindrical tumour on a stalk which is progressively lengthened by oesophageal peristalsis. Polyps consist of vascular fibroblastic tissue which varies from loose myxoid to dense collagen fibres covered by mucosa. Polyps may also be composed of fat, eosinophilic granulomatous tissue or glandular, hamartomatous elements and must be distinguished from polypoid malignancies. Malignant change in an oesophageal polyp has been reported.[22]

Clinical features

The most common symptoms are those secondary to oesophageal obstruction and include dysphagia, weight loss, regurgitation and pain. Respiratory symptoms from aspiration or compression of the tracheobronchial tree are much less common.[25] Haemorrhage from ulceration of the overlying mucosa and regurgitation of the polyp with protrusion from the mouth or glottic obstruction are potentially lethal complications.

Investigation

The polyp may be seen on barium swallow as an intraluminal defect with a rounded lower border. Complete oesophageal obstruction is uncommon because the oesophagus dilates as the tumour enlarges, and a polyp extending into the distal oesophagus has been mistaken for a food bolus in the presence of achalasia.[7]

The polyp is soft, mobile, covered with normal mucosa and may be missed during passage of the oesophagoscope if the pedicle is not seen.

Treatment

All polyps must be removed and the method selected will depend on the size and level of attachment. Small polyps with narrow pedicles can be removed by endoscopic snare and electrocautery. Excision is advised where the pedicle is broad and well vascularized but must be preceded by accurate assessment of the level of attachment. This will determine the surgical approach and oesophagotomy should be performed through the opposite, unaffected wall of the oesophagus.

CYSTS

Although cysts account for 3–20% of benign oesophageal tumours in reported series,[21,28,29] these lesions are not true neoplasms and are either congenital in origin or retention cysts of the oesophageal mucous glands.

Congenital or duplication cysts arise from abnormal endodermal remnants of the neural tube, from developmental errors during vacuolization of primitive foregut or during separation of the tracheobronchial bud from the foregut.[6] Duplication cysts may be associated with vertebral abnormalities and intraspinal connections can be present. Therefore spinal radiographs are essential in all children with oesophageal duplication cysts, particularly if these extend into posterior mediastinum. Where vertebral abnormalities are present, careful examination of the spinal cord by CT scanning, magnetic resonance imaging (MRI) or myelography is mandatory. Congenital oesophageal cysts may be lined by ciliated or squamous epithelium and ectopic gastric mucosa: unlike cysts of bronchial origin they do not contain cartilage. Complete reduplication of the oesophagus, another variety of foregut cyst, is rare but can present in adults.[25] However, most congenital cysts present in infancy or childhood with symptoms of respiratory or oesophageal obstruction, but may become symptomatic in adults when complications such as bleeding, infection or secretion of gastric acid cause the cyst to enlarge or perforate.

Retention cysts result from obstruction of the duct of mucous glands in the adult oesophagus.[6] Most are small, varying in size from a few millimetres to 3 cm, and symptoms are due to the associated chronic oesophagitis rather than the cysts themselves.[11] Rarely, a solitary cyst in the adult may present with dysphagia and differentiation from the more common leiomyoma can be difficult unless the cystic nature of the lesion is identified by CT scanning or MRI. The treatment of choice for oesophageal cysts is enucleation with complete removal of the epithelial lining.

HAEMANGIOMAS

The oesophagus is a rare site for vascular tumours of the gastrointestinal tract, haemangiomas accounting for 2–3% of benign oesophageal tumours.[21,22] They arise from submucosal blood vessels, may be capillary, cavernous or mixed lesions and are often encapsulated. Usually asymptomatic, most cases have been incidental discoveries at autopsy.[8,22] The main symptom is haematemesis which is minor and self-limiting, although torrential haemorrhage has been reported.[18]

Investigations

The diagnosis may be made at endoscopy from the finding of a sessile red granular lesion, a dark purplish nodule or a collection of dilated greyish blue submucosal vessels.[6,22] If a vascular lesion is suspected, biopsy is not recommended because this may be followed by haemorrhage. Contrast CT scanning is useful to identify this highly vascular tumour and may show the characteristic multiple calcifications within it.[6]

Treatment

Intervention is recommended for all haemangiomas complicated by bleeding and the method will depend on the size of the tumour. Sclerotherapy or laser coagulation may be considered for small lesions but large haemangiomas should be excised. Where a small asymptomatic haemangioma is an incidental finding during upper gastrointestinal endoscopy, it can be observed safely with periodic endoscopic assessment.[6]

GRANULAR CELL TUMOURS

First described by Abrikossoff in 1926 as 'granular cell myoblastoma',[1] this name is a misnomer because the tumour does not arise from primitive muscle cells or, as was subsequently believed, from fibroblasts.[21] Using electron microscopy and wallerian degeneration studies, Fisher and Weschler[4] identified the cell of origin as the Schwann cell. The oesophagus is a rare site for granular cell tumours which are more common in the tongue, skin, breast, oral cavity and upper respiratory tract.[19,20]

Granular cell tumours account for less than 2% benign oesophageal tumours.[13,27] Johnson and Helwig found that less than one-third of intestinal and perianal granular cell tumours arise from the oesophagus.[10]

Oesophageal granular cell tumours are most common in middle-aged women[6] and more than half have been found in the distal oesophagus, often associated with a granular cell tumour at another site. Less than 5% are malignant with local invasion and, rarely, lymph node metastases.[22]

The tumour varies in size from 0.5 to 4 cm, consisting of sheets of cells with small dark nuclei and granular esinophilic cytoplasm. Symptoms, present in half of the cases reported, include dysphagia, nausea, vomiting and retrosternal discomfort. The diagnosis is usually made from the endoscopic finding of small, well-circumscribed, firm, yellow plaques which Cohle et al.[2] have described as similar to seborrheic keratoses on the skin. Submucosal in origin, the mucosa over the plaque or nodule may be so atrophic that the tumour appears to arise from the mucosa and biopsy is indicated. Endoscopic removal of very small lesions has been reported[2] and surgical excision is only recommended for larger, symptomatic tumours. Cases with infiltrative margins have been described[19] and local excision, rather than enucleation, is advised.

SUMMARY

Compared to oesophageal cancer, benign tumours of the oesophagus are rare. Most are small, asymptomatic and have been incidental autopsy findings. The most common benign tumour is an intramural leiomyoma but oesophagus polyps are well known for the dramatic way in which they may present with regurgitation into the mouth or larynx. Because the malignant potential of these tumours is very small, surgical removal is recommended only for relief of symptoms and for very large tumours. The procedure of choice for the majority of intramural tumours is enucleation.

REFERENCES

1. Abrikossoff, A.I. (1926) Uebermyome, ausghend con der guergest – reiften wivfurlichen muskulatur. *Virchows Archives of Pathology and Anatomy*, **260**, 214–233.
2. Cohle, S.D., McKechnie, J.C., Truong, L. and Jurco, S. (1981) Granular cell tumour of the esophagus. *American Journal of Gastroenterology*, **75**, 431–435.
3. Deverall, P.B. (1968) Smooth-muscle tumours of the oesophagus. *British Journal of Surgery*, **55**, 457–461.
4. Fisher, E.R. and Wechsler, H. (1962) Granular cell myoblastoma – a misnomer. Electron microscopic and histochemical evidence concerning its Schwann

cell derivation and nature (granular cell Schwannoma) *Cancer*, **15**, 936–954.

5. Gallinger, S., Steinhardt, M.I. and Goldberg, M. (1983) Giant leiomyoma of the esophagus. *American Journal of Gastroenterology*, **78**, 708–711.

6. Game, P.A. (1988) Cysts and duplications of the oesophagus. In: *Surgery of the Oesophagus*, pp. 887–892 (Ed.) Jamieson, G.G. New York: Churchill-Livingstone.

7. Game, P.A. and Jamieson, G.G. (1988) Benign tumours of the oesophagus. In: *Surgery of the Oesophagus*, pp. 893–898 (Ed.) Jamieson, G.G. New York: Churchill-Livingstone.

8. Gentry, R.W., Dockerty, M.B. and Clagett, O.T. (1949) Collective review; vascular malformations and vascular tumors of the gastrointestinal tract. *International Abstracts in Surgery*, **88**, 281–323.

9. Haber, K. and Winifield, A.C. (1974) Multiple leiomyomas of the esophagus. *Digestive Diseases*, **19**, 678–680.

10. Johnson, J. and Helwig, E.B. (1981) Granular cell tumours of the gastrointestinal tract and perianal region. *Digestive Disease and Science*, **26**, 807–816.

11. Kahle, M. and Weber, A.E. (1980) Cysts of the esophagus. *Hepato-Gastroenterology*, **27**, 372–376.

12. Kennedy, L.J. (1953) Giant intramural leiomyoma of the esophagus – a care report. *Journal of Thoracic Surgery*, **26**, 93–100.

13. Lack, E.E., Worsham, G.F., Calliham, M.O. *et al.* (1980) Granular cell tumor, a clinicopathologic study of 110 patients. *Journal of Surgical Oncology*, **13**, 301–316.

14. Lortat-Jacob, J.C. (1950) Myomatoses localizé es et myomatoses diffuses de l'oesophage. *Archives des Maladies l'Apparell Digestif et des Maladies de la Nutrition*, **39**, 519–524.

15. Moersch, H.J. and Harrington, S.W. (1944) Benign tumor of the oesophagus. *Annals of Otorhinolaryngology*, **53**, 800–817.

16. Nemir, P., Wallace, H.W. and Fallahnejad, M. (1976) Diagnosis and surgical management of benign disease of the esophagus. *Current Problems in Surgery*, **XIII** (3), 38–45.

17. Oberhelman, H.A., Condon, J.B. and Guzauskas, A.C. (1952) Leiomyoma of the gastrointestinal tract. *Surgical Clinics of North America*, **32**, 111–122.

18. Palchick, B.A., Alpert, M.A., Holmes, R.A., Tully, R.J. and Wilson, R.C. (1983) Esophageal hemangioma: diagnosis with computed tomography and radionucleotide angiography. *Southern Medical Journal*, **76**, 1582–1584.

19. Paskin, D.L., Hull, J.D. and Cookson, P.J. (1972) Granular cell myoblastoma: a comprehensive review of 15 years experience. *Annals of Surgery*, **175**, 501–504.

20. Peterson, P.A., Soule, E.H. and Bernatz, P.E. (1957) Benign granular cell myoblastoma of the bronchus: report of two cases. *Journal of Thoracic Surgery*, **34**, 95–104.

21. Platcha, A. (1962) Benign tumours of the esophagus. Review of the literature and Report of 99 cases. *American Journal of Gastroenterology*, **38**, 639–652.

22. Postlethwaite, R.W. (1979) Benign tumors of the esophagus. In: *Surgery of the Esophagus*, pp. 318–314 (Ed.) Postlethwaite, R.W. New York: Appleton–Century–Crofts.

23. Schaffar, P.W. and Kittle, C.F. (1947) Esophageal leiomyoma, report of successful resection. *Journal of the American Medical Association*, **1933**, 1202–1205.

24. Schatzi, R. and Howes, L.E. (1950) Tumours of the oesophagus below the mucosa and their roentgenological differential diagnosis. *Reviews in Gastroenterology*, **17**, 971–1014.

25. Schmidt, H.W., Clagett, T. and Harrison, E.G. (1961) Benign tumors and cysts of the esophagus. *Journal of Thoracic and Cardiovascular Surgery*, **41**, 717–732.

26. Seremetis, M.G., Lyons, W.S., de Guzman, V.C. and Peabody, J.W. (1976) Leiomyomata of the esophagus. *Cancer*, **38**, 2166–2177.

27. Stout, A.P. (1953) Tumors of the soft tissue. In: *Atlas of Tumor Pathology*, 1st edn, Vol. 5. Washington Armed Forces Institute of Pathology.

28. Tapia, R.H. and White, V.A. (1985) Squamous cell carcinoma arising in a duplication cyst of the esophagus. *American Journal of Gastroenterology*, **80**, 325–329.

29. Totten, R.S., Stout, A.P., Humphreys, G.H. and Moore, R.L. (1953) Benign tumours and cysts of the esophagus. *Journal of Thoracic Surgery*, **25**, 606–622.

30. Ullal, S.R. (1972) Hypertrophic osteoarthropathy and leiomyoma of the esophagus. *American Journal of Surgery*, **123**, 356–358.

MALIGNANT TUMOURS OF THE OESOPHAGUS

SQUAMOUS CELL CARCINOMA

Incidence, epidemiology and pathogenesis

Squamous carcinoma of the oesophagus is one of the 10 most common cancers in the world[19] and no adult, irrespective of age, sex or race, is immune from this lethal disease. However, there are enormous and changing variations in the incidence of oesophageal cancer, not only across international borders but between provinces or even districts within certain countries.

The annual incidence rate in the USA over the 10 years ending 1982 was 2.6 per 100 000 population.[54]

This is similar to the overall European incidence of 2–8 cases per 100 000.[44] But even within Europe there are major differences between countries, e.g. the incidence in France is threefold greater than in Spain,[10,45] and French national averages of 13 rises to 30 per 100 000 populations in the provinces of Burgundy and Normandy.[45]

The incidence rates of oesophageal cancer in the Western World are, however, dwarfed by those of China and Iran. In Linxian County (Henan province) in Northern China, oesophageal cancer is the most common cause of death[31] with an age-adjusted mortality rate of 151 per 100 000 men and 115 per 100 000 women.[30] But an even higher incidence is reported from Mazanderan Province of the Caspian Littoral of Iran: in the districts of Gonbad and Gorgan (Turkoman, Sahara) the incidence of oesophageal cancer is the highest in the world with 195 cases per 100 000 females and 165 per 100 000 males.[12,32]

The risk of oesophageal cancer rises with each increasing decade of life.[54] The mean age at diagnosis in the Black population of South Africa is 51 years,[34] a decade younger than their white counterparts but it is probably that, as the number of Blacks living into the elderly segments of the population increase, so the mean age of those suffering from oesophageal cancer will rise. In low incidence areas there is a male predominance but the male-to-female ratio in high-risk areas approaches 1 and the ratio is reversed in Iran.[32]

Although there has been a decline in the mortality from oesophageal cancer in younger age groups in north China,[31] disturbing trends in the incidence rates of oesophageal cancer been reported from other parts of the world. In contrast to China and Iran, where the disease has been endemic for centuries, a dramatic increase in oesophageal cancer has occurred in South Africa over the last 40 years: virtually unknown in Black peoples before 1950,[15] incidence rates of 28.4 and 17.8 per 100 000 (men and women, respectively) have been documented in the Transkei.[22] Yang[54] also noted a 30% increase of oesophageal cancer in Black men and women in the USA. Another alarming trend is the apparent rise in incidence in young Black people in South Africa. McGlashan found that very few people with oesophageal cancer were less than 40 years of age when death certificate data for 1980–1982 were analysed, but of 1926 new cases of oesophageal cancer collected in South Africa 1986–1988, 8.8% occurred in the third and fourth decade of life.[34,35]

Despite the incidence of oesophageal cancer in South Africa, the incidence rate in Nigeria remains low, ranging from 1 to 2.8 per 100 000 people and it is evident that the disease is not peculiar to a single racial group.[32,53]

Pathogenesis

The cause of the overwhelming majority of human cancers is not known and squamous cell carcinoma of the oesophagus is no exception. But the high incidence of this disease in geographically distinct areas throughout the world has resulted in mass epidemiological studies of environmental factors, specific to those areas, which increase the risk of oesophageal cancer. In certain countries where oesophageal cancer is endemic, large-scale screening programmes have been undertaken to identify the precursor lesions in the oesophagus.

Precursor lesions

Dysplasia

The cancer precursor role of dysplasia in the pathogenesis of oesophageal cancer has received strong support from the mass cytological sampling projects in high-risk areas of northern China. Using an abrasive balloon technique, Yang[56] and Shu[42] showed that severe dysplasia progressed to cancer in 30% of cases followed for 7–10 years. Further evidence for the concept of dysplasia as a premalignant lesion is provided by endoscopic surveys of asymptomatic individuals in Henan Province: Guanrei and Songliong[14] identified dysplasia in 38% of the inhabitants of high-risk areas compared to 5% of those in low-risk areas. Furthermore, endoscopic follow-up for 30–78 months revealed that one-third of cases with dysplasia developed early stage carcinoma. The results of similar studies in Iran[6] and South Africa[23] have also identified cytological abnormalities among high-risk groups.

It is probable that the relationship between dysplasia and the development of oesophageal cancer is a complex one. The observation that patients with minor dysplasia appear to be at equal risk of oesophageal cancer as those with severe dysplasia is unexplained, as is the finding that dysplasia either fails to progress or even disappears in two-thirds of the cases examined. The three-fold discrepancy in the prevalence of early oesophageal cancer diagnosed by cytological screening and the incidence of invasive cancer in the same region of northern China[55,56] could represent regression, or difficulty with interpretation of oesophageal cytology.

Oesophagitis

Chronic oesophagitis is considered to be a precursor of oesophageal cancer by some workers,[17,23] but this is controversial. Guanrei and Songliong[14] found that the prevalence of oesophagitis in endoscopic surveys was similar in high- and low-risk areas of Henan, although there appeared to be a correlation between the severity of oesophagitis and the incidence of dysplasia. Jacob et al.[21] reported difficulties in distinguishing squamous cell dysplasia from inflammation with balloon mesh cutological examination, and concluded that squamous cell dysplasia identified by this technique is seldom a precursor of oesophageal cancer in the high-risk US population. It is possible that chronic inflammation could make the oesophagus more vulnerable to carcinogens,[14] but caution is advised in the interpretation of studies which correlate risk factors with the incidence of dysplasia and oesophagitis.

Risk factors

Geographically based epidemiological research in high-incidence areas has identified factors associated with an increased risk of oesophageal cancer. The most important of these appear to be the following.

Nutritional deficiency

Carcinoma of the oesophagus is a disease of poverty and malnutrition: the factor common to all high-incidence areas is the low socioeconomic status of the population. Research studies in China, Iran and South Africa suggest that exposure to trace element and vitamin deficiencies early in life increases the risk of oesophageal cancer in later years.[4,12,23] But there is no strong correlation between specific micronutrient deficiencies and the incidence of precursor lesions in the oesophagus;[7] randomized, controlled, vitamin intervention studies have failed to demonstrate an effect on oesophagitis or dysplasia.[50] However, animal studies have shown that dietary factors can alter the response to oesophageal carcinogens[37] and vitamin supplements reduce endogenous production of mutagenic nitrosamines. Even in Western countries where cancer of the oesophagus occurs sporadically, poor nutritional status is a major risk factor: the susceptibility of urban Black men in the USA is attributed in part to malnutrition[57] and the intake of vitamin A inversely correlates with risk of oesophageal cancer in Norway and Japan.[28]

Dietary contaminants

Eating mouldy or pickled foods contaminated by Candida and Fusarium species is common in north China and the Transkei, and increase the intake of nitrosamine precursors which are carcinogenic in animal models. Other dietary factors implicated include tannins,[56] mate herbal tea,[47] ingested opium and pipe tobacco residues,[6,48] drinking water contaminated by petrol[17] and pomegranate spice.[11] However, case-controlled studies have failed to demonstrate strong associations between dietary customs and oesophageal cancer.[29,30,47] More research is necessary to distinguish cultural differences from environmental carcinogens.

Alcohol, tobacco and opium

There is compelling epidemiological evidence for the association between alcohol, tobacco and oesophageal cancer in France, South Africa and the USA[15,39,46] where studies have shown that the risk of oesophageal cancer increases with the amount of alcohol consumed and the number of cigarettes smoked. The type of alcohol and the cigarettes used may also contribute to the risk: in France, drinkers of apple brandy, in which benzo[α]pyrene and volatile nitrosamines are present, have a greater risk than the general population. In northern Italy, cigarettes with a heavy tar content have been incriminated. The carcinogenic properties of tobacco lie in the polynuclear aromatic hydrocarbons and nitrosamines released when tar fraction burns, with alcohol acting as a solvent for these. In the Caspian littoral, alcohol and heavy smoking are not risk factors but opium use, identified by urinary morphine metabolites, is much more common in high- than in low-risk area. Experimental studies have identified mutagenic substances with carcinogenic potential in opium and morphine pyrolysates.[13,33]

Infective agents

Human papilloma virus (HPV) has been demonstrated in a small number of squamous cancers at different sites and HPV has been identified in squamous papillomas of the oesophagus.[26,43] In South Africa the presence of HPV antigens was demonstrated by immunohistochemical staining in 10% of oesophageal specimens taken from patients with invasive squamous cell carcinoma.[18] In north China, HPV DNA was detected in cytologically normal, dysplastic and malignant oesophageal epithelium.[3] HPV may simply colonize damaged squamous epithelium but it could be an oesophageal carcinogen acting in concert with chemical and/or nutritional factors. One hypothesis suggests that the effect of persistent HPV infection on mucosal immune surveillance (Langerhans' cells and intraepithelial lymphocytes) could increase the risk of neoplastic transformation[36] and several cases of rapidly progressive oesophageal cancer have been reported in patients infected by the human immunodeficiency virus (HIV). Indirect evidence for the existence of a transmissable agent of low infectivity in the pathogenesis of oesophageal cancer has come from studies of domestic fowls in north China. Chickens in the low-risk areas in Henan Province do not suffer from gullet cancer, but a small number of indigenous chickens raised by immigrants from high-risk areas have developed oesophageal cancer.[16] In Soweto, the largest Black urban community in South Africa, the incidence of oesophageal cancer now exceeds that of rural areas[24] with the majority of cases localized to areas of serious overcrowding, irrespective of income per capita (A. Mannell, 1988, unpublished data).

Genetic factors

Tylosis palmarum et plantarum, in which there is hyperkeratosis of the interphalangeal epithelium and soles of the feet, is an inherited condition, transmitted as an autosomal dominant. Tylosis was first identified in two Liverpool families, later in a south Indian family,[20] and affected individuals have a very high risk of developing squamous oesophageal cancer. Certain families in China and Iran have an inherited tendency to develop oesophageal cancer in the second decade of life.[40,56]

But in the vast majority of cases there is no direct evidence that oesophageal cancer is an inherited disease. However, Li et al.[27] identified an increased risk of oesophageal cancer in north China among those whose parents had oesophageal cancer. The incidence of numerical and structural chromosome aberrations is higher in patients with oesophageal cancer and a positive family history than in sufferers from the disease without a family history.[51] It is possible that subtle and as yet unidentified genetic differences may increase the likelihood of transformation in oncogenes associated with human oesophageal neoplasia when individuals or races are exposed to environmental carcinogens.

Oesophageal diseases

CAUSTIC STRICTURES

The risk of oesophageal cancer in patients with corrosive oesophageal strictures is twenty-two fold more than that of the normal population, the interval between caustic injury and the development of oesophageal cancer varying from 40 to 50 years.[8] It is suggested that stasis secondary to the stricture and prolongation of exposure to oesophageal carcinogens are the causative factors.[9] However, cancers that develop in scarred skin after burns, irradiation and in lupus are well known and it is possible that repetitive cycles of damage to vulnerable epithelium followed by epithelial hyperplasia can be incriminated in the oesophagus.

PLUMMER–VINSON SYNDROME

This is an uncommon condition in which dysphagia combined with iron-deficient anaemia occurs in women and is associated with an increased risk of carcinoma of the hypopharynx or cervical oesophagus. Atrophy of the oropharyngeal mucosa, shrinkage of the opening of the mouth, koilonychia and loss of teeth are common clinical features of the syndrome. Affected women have associated vitamin deficiencies and the development of malignancy has been related both to iron and riboflavine deficiency and to scarring in the atrophic mucous membranes.[1]

ACHALASIA OF THE CARDIA

An association between achalasia and oesophageal cancer has been reported by many authors and is believed to result from retention oesophagitis secondary to oesophageal stasis.[9] It would appear, however, that the treatment of achalasia does not influence the risk of malignant disease.[49,52]

The prevalence of oesophageal cancer in achalasia patients varies in different series. Petri and Imre[38] reported a prevalence of 2%, rising to 29% in autopsy studies. The concept of achalasia as a risk factor for oesophageal cancer has been challenged by Chuong et al.[5] who found no cases in 91 patients with achalasia followed for a mean of 77.6 months. But the diagnosis of achalasia may precede the development of oesophageal cancer by 15–21 years[38] and it is evident that long-term surveillance of patients with achalasia is necessary before the association can be refuted.

REFLUX OESOPHAGITIS

In contrast to the development of adenocarcinoma there is little evidence that oesophageal reflux is associated with an increased risk of squamous cell carcinoma of the oesophagus. A few cases of squamous oesophageal cancers have been reported in patients with evidence of oesophageal reflux[2,25] but the relationship is unproven.

REFERENCES

1. Ahlbom, H.E. (1986) Simple achlorhydria anaemia, Plummers–Vinson syndrome carcinoma of the mouth, pharynx and esophagus in women. *British Medical Journal*, **2**, 331–333.
2. Bremner, C.G. (1982) Benign strictures of the esophagus. *Current Problems in Surgery*, **19**, 444–449.
3. Chang, F. Sheng, Q., Zhuo, J. et al. (1990) Detection of human papilloma virus DNA in cytologic specimens derives from esophageal precancer lesions and cancer. *Scandinavian Journal of Gastroenterology*, **25**, 383–388.

4. Chang-Claude, J.C., Wahrendorf, S., Liang, O.S. *et al*. (1990) An epidemiological study of precursor lesions of esophageal cancer among young persons in a high-risk population in Huixian China. *Cancer Research*, **50**, 2268–2274.

5. Chuong, J.J.H., DuBovik, S. and McCallum, R.W. (1984) Achalasia as a risk factor for esophageal carcinoma. *Digestive Disease Sciences*, **29**, 1105–1108.

6. Crespi, M., Munoz, N., Grassi, A. *et al*. (1979) Oesophageal lesions in Northern Iran: a premalignant condition. *The Lancet*, **2**, 217–220.

7. Crespi, M., Munoz, N., Crassi, A. *et al*. (1984) Precursor lesions of oesophageal cancer in a low-risk population in China: comparison with a high-risk population. *International Journal of Cancer*, **34**, 599–602.

8. Csikos, M., Horvath, O., Petri, A. and Imre, J. (1985) Late malignant transformation of chronic corrosive oesophageal strictures. *Langenbecks Archives of Surgery*, **365**, 231–238.

9. Devitt, P.C., Iyer, P.V. and Rowland, R. (1988) Pathogenesis and clinical features of cancer of the oesophagus. In: *Surgery of the Oesophagus*, pp. 551–558 (Ed.) Jamieson, G.G. New York: Churchill-Livingstone.

10. Faivre, J., Milan, C., Martin, F. *et al*. (1981) Cancer of the esophagus: an incidence study in Cote D'Or (Burgundy). *Oncology*, **38**, 1–3.

11. Ghadirian, P. (1987) Food habits of the people of the Caspian Littoral of Iran in relation to oesophageal cancer. *Nutrition and Cancer*, **9**, 147–157.

12. Ghadirian, P. (1987) Thermal irritation and oesophageal cancer in Northern Iran. *Cancer*, **60**, 1909–1914.

13. Ghadirian, P., Stein, C.F., Gorodetsky, C. *et al*. (1985) Oesophageal cancer studies in the Caspian Littoral of Iran: Some residual results, including opium use as a risk factor. *International Journal of Cancer*, **35**, 593–597.

14. Guanrei, Y. and Songliong, Q. (1987) Endoscopic surveys in high-risk and low-risk populations for oesophageal cancer in China with special reference to precursors of oesophageal cancer. *Endoscopy*, **19**, 91–95.

15. Harrington, J.S. and Bradshaw, E. (1985) The changing pattern of cancer mortality in South Africa 1949–1979. *South African Medical Journal*, **68**, 455–465.

16. Haocai, L. and Yu, S.L. (1983) Esophageal cancers in migrants from high- or low-risk areas in China. *Ecological Diseases*, **214**, 249–253.

17. Hecker, E. (1987) Co-carcinogens of the diterpene esther type as principal risk factors of cancer in Curacao and possible in South China. Identification of second order risk factors of cancer in multifactorial carcinogenesis. In: *Cancer of the Liver, Esophagus and Nasopharynx*, pp. 101–113 (Eds) Wang, G. and Zhang, Y.H. New York: Springer-Verlag.

18. Hille, J.J., Margolius, K.A., Markovitz, S. and Isaacson, C. (1986) Human papillomavirus infection relation to oesophageal carcinoma in black South Africans. A preliminary study. *South African Medical Journal*, **69**, 417–420.

19. Hollstein, M., Bos, J., Galiana, G. *et al*. (1988) Mutation and amplipeation of cellular oncogenes in human esophageal cancer (Meeting abstract). *Proceedings of the Annual Meeting of American Association for Cancer Research*, **29A**, 1034.

20. Howel-Evans, W., McConnell, R.B., Clarke, C.A. and Sheppard, P.M. (1958) Carcinoma of the oesophagus with keratosis palmaris et plantaris (tylosis). *Quarterly Journal of Medicine*, **27**, 413–429.

21. Jacob, P., Kahrilas, P.J., Desai, T. *et al* (1990) Natural history and significance of esophageal squamous cell dysplasia. *Cancer*, **65**, 2731–2739.

22. Jaskiewicz, K., Marasas, W.F. and Van Der Watt, F.E. (1987) Oesophageal and other main cancer patterns in four Districts of the Transkei, 1981–1984. *South African Medical Journal*, **72**, 27–30.

23. Jaskiewicz, K. (1989) Oesophageal carcinoma: cytopathology and nutritional aspects in aetiology. *Anticancer Research*, **9**, 1847–1852.

24. Kneebone, R.L. and Mannell, A. (1985) Cancer of the oesophagus in Soweto 1985. *South African Medical Journal*, **67**, 839–842.

25. Kuylenstierna, R. and Munck-Wikland, E. (1985) Esophagitis and cancer of the esophagus. *Cancer*, **56**, 837–839.

26. Lesec, E., Goguser, J., Fernaud, H., Gorce, D., Lemaitre, J.P. and Verdier, A. (1985) Presence of papilloma group viral antigens in an oesophageal condyloma. *Gastroenterology and Clinical Biology*, **9**, 166–168.

27. Li, J.Y., Ershaw, A.G., Chen, Z.J. *et al*. (1989) A case-control study of cancer of the esophagus and gastric cardia in Linxian. *International Journal of Cancer*, **43**, 755–761.

28. Lohle, L., Scholmerich, J., Kollgen, E., Weisser, H. and Vuilleumier, J.P. (1982) The influence of vitamin A on carcinogenesis in otorhinolaryngology (Meeting abstract). *Blut*, **45**, A193.

29. Lu, S.H., Montesano, R., Zhang, M.S. *et al*. (1986) Relevance of N-nitrosamines in esophageal cancer in China. *Journal of Cellular Physiology* (suppl.) **4**, 51–58.

30. Lu, S.H., Montesano, R., Zhang, M.S. *et al*. (1987) Effect of *N*-nitrosamines on human esophageal epithelium collected from populations from a high-risk area for esophageal cancer in Northern China. In: *Cancer of the Lower Esophagus and Nasopharynx*, pp. 126–131 (Eds) Wagner, G. and Zhang, Y.H. New York: Springer-Verlag.

31. Lu, J.B., Yang, W.X., Lu, J.M., Li, Y.S. and Qin, Y.M. (1985) Trends in morbidity and mortality for oesophageal cancer in Linxian country, 1959–1983. *International Journal of Cancer*, **43**, 755–761.

32. Mahboubi, E. (1977) Epidemiology of oral cavity, pharyngeal and esophageal cancer outside of North

American and Western Europe. *Cancer*, **40**, 1879–1886.

33. Mahboubi, E.O. and Aramesh, B. (1980) Epidemiology of esophageal cancer in Iran, with special reference to nutritional and cultural aspects. *Preventative Medicine*, **9**, 613–624.

34. Mannell, A. and Murray, W. (1989) Esophageal cancer in South Africa. A review of 1926 cases. *Cancer*, **64**, 2604–2608.

35. McClashan, W.D. (1988) Oesophageal cancer in the black peoples of South Africa 1980–1982. *South African Journal of Science*, **84**, 92–99.

36. Morris, H. and Price, S. (1986) Langerhans' cells, papillomaviruses and oesophageal carcinoma. A hypothesis. *South African Medical Journal*, **69**, 413–417.

37. Newberne, P.M. (1985) Dietary factors affecting biological responses to esophageal and colon chemical carcinogenesis. *ACS Symposium Services*, **277**, 163–76.

38. Petri, A. and Imre, J. (1980) Esophageal carcinoma in patients with achalasia. *Orv Hetil*, **121**, 1643–1645.

39. Pottern, L.M., Morris, L.E., Blot, W.J., Ziegler, R.C. and Fraumeni, J.F. (1981) Esophageal cancer among black men in Washington DC. Alcohol, tobacco and other risk factors. *Journal of Neoplastic and Cancer Incidence*, **67**, 777–783.

40. Pour, P. and Ghadirian, P. (1974) Familial cancer of the esophagus in Iran. *Cancer*, **33**, 1649–1652.

41. Silber, W. (1982) Comparative prevalence of GI cancer in the young (Meeting Abstract). The World Congress in Stockholm, Sweden. June 14–19, 1982. *The Sweden Society of Medical Sciences*, p. 558.

42. Shu, Y.J. (1983) Cytopathology of the esophagus. An overview of the esophageal cytopathology in China. *Acta Cytologica (Baltimore)*, **27**, 7–16.

43. Syranjanen, K., Pyrhönen, S., Aukee, S. and Koskela, E. (1982) Squamous cell papilloma of the esophagus: a tumour probably caused by human papilloma virus (HPV). *Diagnostic Histopathology*, **5**, 291–296.

44. Thompson, J. (1982) Esophageal cancer and the premalignant changes of esophageal diseases. In: *Diseases of the Esophagus*, pp. 239–276 (Eds) Cohen, S. and Soloway, R.C. New York: Churchill-Livingstone.

45. Tuyns, A.J. and Masse, G. (1975) Cancer of the oesophagus in Brittany: An incidence study in Illie et Vilaine. *International Journal of Epidemiology*, **4**, 55–59.

46. Tuyns, A.J. and Gricuite, L.L. (1980) Carcinogenic substances in alcoholic beverages. *Excerpta Medical International Congress Services*, **(484)**, 130–135.

47. Victora, C.G., Munoz, N., Day, N.E. *et al.* (1987) Aor beverages and oesophageal cancer in Southern Brazil. A case control study. *International Journal of Cancer*, **39**, 710–716.

48. Warwick, P. and Harrington, G.S. (1973) Some aspects of the epidemiology and etiology of esophageal cancer with particular emphasis on the Transkei, South Africa. *Advances in Cancer Research*, **17**, 81–229.

49. Walters, P.F. and DeMeester, T.R. (1981) Foregut motor disorders and their surgical management. *Medical Clinics of North America*, **65**, 1235–1268.

50. Waldendorf, F., Munoz, N. and Lu, J.B. (1987) Vitamin intervention of precancerous lesions of the esophagus in a high-risk population of China. In: *Cancer of the Liver, Esophagus and Nasopharynx*, pp. 124–125 (Eds) Wagner, C. and Zhang, Y.H. New York: Springer-Verlag.

51. Wu, Y. and Puan, X. (1981) Genetic etiology of esophageal cancer. II Cytogenetic studies on peripheral blood cells of esophageal cancer and epithelial dysplasia patients with positive family history in Linxian County. *Zhonghua Zhongliu Zazhi*, **2**, 12–15.

52. Wychulis, A.R., Woolan, G.L., Anderson, H.A. and Ellis, F.H. (1971) Achalasia and carcinoma of the esophagus. *Journal of American Medical Association*, **215**, 1638–1641.

53. Wynder, E.L. and Mabuchi, K. (1973) Etiology and environmental factors. *Journal of the American Medical Association*, **226**, 1546–1548.

54. Yang, P.C. and Davis, S. (1988) Incidence of cancer of the esophagus in the US by histologic type. *Cancer*, **61**, 612–617.

55. Yang, G., Huang, H., Qui, S. and Chang, Y. (1982) Endoscopic diagnosis of early esophageal carcinoma. *Endoscopy*, **14**, 157–161.

56. Yang, C.S. (1980) Research on esophageal cancer in China: A review. *Cancer Research*, **40**, 2633–2644.

57. Ziegler, R.C. (1986) Epidemiologic studies of vitamins and cancer of the lung, esophagus and cervix. *Advances of Experimental Biology*, **206**, 11–26.

Histopathology

When cases of adenocarcinoma of gastric origin spreading into the distal oesophagus are excluded, 95% of primary oesophageal malignancies are squamous cell cancers with the classification of squamous cell cancers being into the following:

1. Carcinoma in situ
2. Invasive cancer
   (a) well differentiated
   (b) moderately differentiated
   (c) poorly differentiated
3. Variants of squamous cell carcinoma
   (a) spindle-cell carcinoma
   (b) 'pseudosarcoma'
   (c) verrucous carcinoma
   (d) basaloid (basal cell carcinoma)
   (e) epidermoid cancer with glandular features.

Primary adenocarcinomas of the Oesophagus (see under 'Adenocarcinoma of the oesophagus') which include cancer arising from the mucous glands of the oesophagus and from the columnar epithelium in a Barrett's oesophagus, account for 3–4%. The remaining 1–2% of oesophageal malignancies are exceptionally rare tumours of epithelial and non-epithelial origin.

Histology

Carcinoma *in situ*

This carcinoma, described as 'intraepithelial' or 'occult' cancer, is a microscopically early form of oesophageal carcinoma in which dysplastic cells with abnormal chromatic nuclei occupy the full thickness of the epithelium without breaching the basement membrane. Carcinoma in situ has been identified in inhabitants of the high-risk areas of China and affects patients between the ages of 40 and 50 years. It is usually symptomless but its significance lies in the observation that progression to frankly invasive carcinoma has been observed within 3–4 years of diagnosis.[7]

Carcinoma in situ is commonly found in resection specimens lying adjacent to the invasive squamous cell carcinoma. However, distant foci carcinoma in situ may be present and, if found at the proximal line of resection, can lead to anastomotic recurrence.[10]

Invasive squamous cell carcinoma

Only a small number of tumours are well differentiated, with the characteristic features of keratin formation (epithelial pearls), intercellular bridges and minimal pleomorphism. A large group of squamous carcinomas is poorly differentiated with marked nuclear and cellular pleomorphism, absence of intercellular bridges and presence of occasional foci of keratinization. The remaining tumours can be described as moderately differentiated, consisting of obviously malignant cells with evidence of intercellular bridges and keratinization. Sugimachi et al.[14] noted that histological grade did not significantly influence prognosis after curative oesophagectomy and Rosenberg et al.[13] were unable to correlate degree of differentiation with survival or incidence of nodal metastases.

Variants of squamous carcinoma

The spindle-cell carcinoma is a variant of poorly differentiated squamous cell cancer. It consists of spindle-shaped cells resembling fibroblasts which give the appearances of a sarcoma. A 'pseudo-sarcoma' is a polypoid tumour containing nests of malignant squamous cells within a spindle cell stoma

which may have undergone pseudomalignant change.

Verrucous squamous cell carcinoma is well differentiated, has a papillary appearance and pursues a less aggressive course. The rare basaloid type consists of closely packed hyperchromatic cells with peripheral palisading which resemble basal cell cancers of the skin. Those epidermoid cancers which show minor glandular changes are also described as variants of squamous cell carcinoma.

Macroscopic appearance

Early

When carcinoma is limited to the mucosa and submucosal, the endoscopic appearances are subtle and can be missed or mistaken for oesophagitis. Usually involving the midoesophagus these early cancers have been classified by Chinese workers are plaque-like, erosive, occult or papillary.[15]

1. Plaque-like: this type is the most common form of endoscopically identifiable early cancer and appears as a slightly raised, dark-red granular patch of mucosa, with coarse ridging and superficial erosions if large.
2. Erosive: a sharply demarcated area of dark-red mucosa which is slightly depressed or erosive is the second most common form.
3. Occult: in this type of early cancer the only abnormality apparent is an area of mucosa that is darker than normal.
4. Papillary: the least common type, this lesion is less than 3 cm in diameter, darker than adjacent mucosa and slightly polypoid in appearance.

Advanced

SITE

An oesophageal cancer may be considered advanced when the tumour has spread into or beyond the muscle coat of the oesophagus. The site of advanced squamous cell carcinoma varies from series to series and depends to some extent on the system used to describe the oesophageal segments. The Japanese Society for Esophageal Diseases[8] has divided the oesophagus into five segments including the short abdominal oesophagus as a separate segment, and uses adjacent soft tissue structures (tracheal bifurcation, inferior pulmonary vein) to define the upper and middle thoracic segments. The oesophageal segment may be described in terms of endoscopic distances from the incisor teeth but these distances will vary with the height of the patient, the oesophagus being longer in tall subjects, and with the type of endoscope used; the proximal limit of a

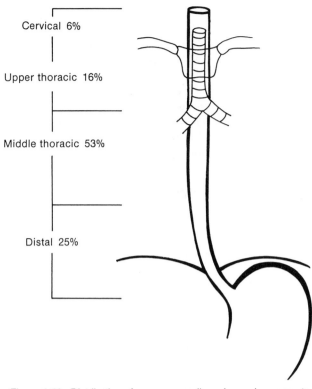

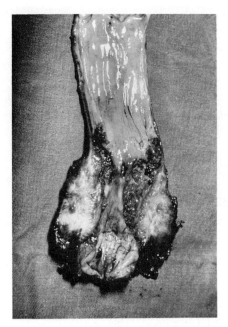

Figure 1.59 A fungating squamous cancer in the distal oesophagus.

Figure 1.58 Distribution of squamous cell carcinoma in segments of the oesophagus.

tumour is detected with the rigid scope at a level 2.4 cm distal to that diagnosed by the fibrescope.[18]

The oesophagus can be conveniently divided into four segments (*Figure 1.58*):

1. Cervical – from the oesophageal opening to the suprasternal notch.
2. Upper thoracic – from the suprasternal notch to a point opposite the lower margin of the fourth thoracic vertebra (radiologically).
3. Middle thoracic – from the lower margin of the fourth thoracic vertebra to a point opposite the lower margin of the eighth thoracic vertebra.
4. Distal – from the lower margin of the eighth thoracic vertebra to the cardio-oesophageal junction which is usually located approximately adjacent to the lower margin of the twelfth thoracic vertebra.

This system has the advantage of using fixed bony points to define the oesophageal segments rather than soft tissue structures, which may be difficult to identify clinically. In addition, these four divisions of the oesophagus are commonly used by clinicians to select the appropriate method of treatment.

In a collected series of 15 000 cases,[3,12] 50% of cancers were located in the mid-thoracic oesophagus, 30% involved the distal oesophagus and 20% in the cervical with upper thoracic segments. In a recent study of 1926 new cases of oesophageal cancer in South Africa, the mid-thoracic oesophagus was involved in 53% of cases, the distal segment in 25%, the upper thoracic in 16% and the cervical oesophagus in 6% of cases.[10] In this study, the length of tumours measured by barium swallow varied from 3 to 15 cm (mean length 6 cm) with cancers involving two or more adjacent segments in 8.3% of patients.

Most symptomatic oesophageal cancers are 5 cm or more in length, almost or completely circumferential, and have penetrated deeply into the oesophageal wall. Three macroscopic types have been recognized, depending on whether the growth is predominantly exophytic, endophytic or intramural; these are fungating, ulcerative and infiltrative (*Figures 1.58–1.61*).

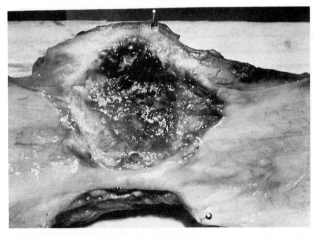

Figure 1.60 An ulcerative squamous cancer in the mid-thoracic oesophagus.

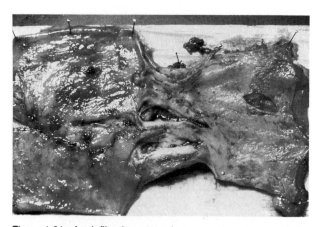

Figure 1.61 An infiltrative stenosing squamous cancer of the oesophagus.

FUNGATING

The fungating tumours grow into the oesophageal lumen as nodular or plaque-like masses, identified on barium swallow examination by single or multiple filling defects. The intraluminal surface which is usually ulcerated may also consist of multiple polypoid excrescences or, in the rare verrucous papillary form, as a finely nodular lesion.

ULCERATIVE

This type appears as a malignant ulcer with irregular everted edges and a shaggy, often haemorrhagic base. Intramural infiltration is associated with a fibrous tissue response which narrows the oesophageal lumen so that the tumour appears as an irregular, ulcerated, stenotic lesion on barium swallow.

INFILTRATIVE

Also known as 'desmoplastic-stenosing' or 'ulcerative type with scar', the infiltrative tumour is characterized by extensive intramural spread. The infiltrating malignant cells excite a marked desmoplastic response producing severe degrees of stricturing. Shallow ulceration is often present but as most of the tumour lies deep to the mucosa this form is difficult to biopsy effectively. The severe stricturing prevents passage of the oesophagus to the site of mucosal involvement. The infiltrative type is easily distinguished from the superficial spreading form in which tumour has infiltrated only the superficial layers of the oesophageal wall. Superficial spreading cancers, well described by the Japanese Society for Esophageal Diseases,[8] are far less common than the other macroscopic types in European and African patients.

MULTIPLE PRIMARY CARCINOMAS

The existence of multiple primary cancers in the oesophagus is well known: in one series,[1] 41 out of 532 patients with oesophageal cancer had synchronous lesions, a phenomenon most probably related to field carcinogenesis.

Synchronous cancers may also arise in other organs, usually in the oral cavity, pharynx and larynx (OPL), on the skin and in the stomach.

With improved methods of treatment the patient with oesophageal cancer may survive long enough to develop metachronous cancer and it appears that the risk of developing a second tumour is twice that of the normal population.[6] Botha *et al.*[3] found that as many as 6% of patients with an oesophageal neoplasm developed a metachronous cancer or had synchronous squamous cancer of the OPL. The importance of patient follow-up with repeated and careful examination of these areas to detect the development of a second primary is obvious.

Spread of oesophageal cancer

Intraoesophageal

An important route for dissemination of malignancy is along the submucosal plane, microscopic spread of tumour being far more extensive than the macroscopic limits. Allowing for shrinkage of the oesophagus in formalin, Miller[11] found evidence of proximal microscopic spread up to 6 cm beyond visible tumour in 22% of cases, at a distance of 9 cm in 11% and as far as 10.5 cm in 3% of cases. These findings were confirmed by Mannell[10] who noted that the proximal lines of excision was involved in 3% of oesophagectomy specimens where a 10-cm margin of macroscopically normal tissue had been excised above the tumour. Microscopic spread below the inferior limit of visible tumour is said to be less extensive,[12] but distal microscopic spread may be similar in extent to proximal spread.[9] These histological findings have important implications for the clinician. Microscopic intraoesophageal spread is the most common cause of inadequate surgical resection leading to anastomotic recurrence. Curative treatment of oesophageal cancer should include virtually all the oesophagus.

Malignant cells may be carried in the submucosal lymphatics to sites 2 cm or more from the main growth, producing 'skip' or satellite nodules and, more rarely so-called 'double' carcinomas separated by radiologically intact epithelium. The prognosis for patients with this variety of intraoesophageal spread is very poor; there is a high incidence of lymph node metastases and almost all patients are dead within a year of diagnosis, irrespective of treatment.[16]

Extraoesophageal

DIRECT

A carcinoma of the oesophagus can penetrate the muscle layer spreading beyond the oesophagus before the lumen is obstructed by the malignant growth and before the patient experiences dysphagia. In a recent series of 1926 African patients, 84% had evidence of extraoesophageal spread at the time of presentation. Once cancer has spread through the muscle coat, invasion of vital structures readily occurs. The cervical, upper thoracic and mid-thoracic segments lie immediately behind the tracheobronchial tree. The thin fibromembranous posterior wall of the airway offers no barrier to malignant invasion. It is not surprising, therefore, that direct spread into the trachea and bronchi has occurred in 22% of patients by the time of diagnosis, with an established oesophageal-airway fistula present in 13% of those admitted to hospital.

In the neck the oesophagus is intimately related to recurrent laryngeal nerves to the thyroid and to the carotid sheath, all of which may be invaded by cervical cancers. In the thorax, oesophageal cancer frequently infiltrates the left recurrent laryngeal nerve, the adventitia of the aorta, the pleura and the lung. Although the muscle coat of the aorta and the fibrous pericardium are relatively resistant to invasion, aorto-oesophageal and oesophagoatrial fistulas are sometimes observed in fatal cases. Thoracic cancers often invade the azygous vein, the thoracic duct and the diaphragm. Cancer at any level in the oesophagus may infiltrate the prevertebral fascia and, rarely, the vertebral bodies. The prognosis for a patient with extraoesophageal spread is grave: the local effects of invasion into the airways are lethal and even microscopic spread beyond the oesophagus reduces the chance of 2-year survival to less than 20%, regardless of radical surgery.[4]

LYMPHATIC

The lymphatic drainage of the oesophagus consists of an extensive interconnecting network of submucosal, muscular and adventitial lymphatics. Lymphatic flow is predominantly longitudinal rather than segmental, and it is this feature more than any other that accounts for the poor response to radical local treatment.

Tumour cells in the oesophageal lymphatics can be carried considerable distances proximal and distal to the cancer, so that nodal metastases are found far from the primary tumour. The abdominal nodes are involved in 30% of upper thoracic and in 38% of mid-thoracic cancers. The cervical nodes are involved in 4% of mid-thoracic cancers and, on occasion, by spread from distal oesophageal cancers. The phenomenon of 'skip' metastases is well known

in carcinoma of the oesophagus: Fekete et al.[5] reported that lymph node metastases distant to regional nodes were present in nearly half of the patients undergoing surgical resection without involvement of the regional nodes. These figures support the concept of non-segmental drainage of lymph and of major intramural longitudinal lymphatic drainage of the oesophagus.

At the time of surgical exploration over half the patients are found to have lymph node metastases. Lymph node involvement is an important determinant of prognosis: 5-year survival rates of over 50% can be expected after curative treatment for node-negative cases, but if the lymph nodes are positive the 5-year survival falls to 10%.[17]

BLOOD

Metastatic spread via the blood stream is not a common finding in the untreated patient with oesophageal cancer and is evident in less than 10% of cases at the time of diagnosis.[10] Pulmonary metastases are more frequent than liver metastases, unless the cancer involves the distal oesophagus which drains into the portal venous system. Visceral metastases are, however, present in more than half of fatal cases: metastatic involvement of ribs, vertebrae and adrenal glands is not an uncommon finding in autopsy series.[19]

Staging of oesophageal cancer

Not all patients with oesophageal cancer are candidates for surgical exploration because of either physical debility or another modality of treatment being selected. Surgical exploration is the most accurate method of determining the extent of involvement and the stage of disease. Because the oesophagus is a deep-seated organ, spread of cancer is difficult to assess by non-invasive modalities and clinical staging is frequently inaccurate. Nevertheless, clinical staging may aid in comparing the effectiveness of various forms of therapy in similar patient populations. The most common method used is the TNM system of staging devised by the American Joint Committee in 1977 (Tables 1.17 and 1.18).[2] In stage I and II disease, there must be no clinical evidence of local extraoesophageal spread of distant metastases. Length of lesions and circumferential involvement in thoracic cancers, and presence of mobile lymph nodes in cervical carcinoma, are used to differentiate between these two stages. Stage III disease includes all cases with evidence of local extraoesophageal invasion (see under 'Extraoesophageal' earlier), extracapsular spread from involved lymph nodes and distant metastases to either viscera, bones or remote lymph nodes.

Table 1.17 TNM staging for oesophageal cancer

A Primary tumour (T)
  T0 No demonstrable tumour
  TIS Carcinoma in situ
  T1 Tumour involves 5 cm or less of oesophageal length with no obstruction or no complete circumferential involvement or no extraoesophageal spread
  T2 Tumour involves more than 5 cm of oesophagus and produces obstruction with circumferential involvement of the oesophagus, but no extraoesophageal spread
  T3 Tumour with extension outside the oesophagus involving mediastinal structures

B Regional lymph nodes (N)
  Cervical oesophagus (cervical and supraclavicular lymph nodes)
  N0 No nodal involvement
  N1 Unilateral involvement (movable)
  N2 Bilateral involvement (movable)
  N3 Fixed nodes
  Thoracic oesophagus (nodes in the thorax, not those of the cervical, supraclavicular or abdominal areas)
  N0 No nodal involvement
  N1 Nodal involvement

C Distant metastases (M)
  M0 No metastases
  M1 Distal metastases; cancer of thoracic oesophagus with cervical, supraclavicular, or abdominal lymph node involvement is classified as M1

Table 1.18 Stage grouping from TNM classification

A Stage I
  1 TIS N0 M0
    Carcinoma in situ
  2 T1 N0 M0
    T1 NX M0
    Tumour in any region of the oesophagus, which involves 5 cm or less of oesophageal length, produces no obstruction, has no extraoesophageal spread, does not involve the entire circumference, and shows no regional lymph node metastases or remote metastases

B Stage II
  1 A tumour of any size with no extraoesophageal spread and with no distant metastasis
  A Cervical oesophagus:
    (1) T1 N1 M0
        T1 N2 M0
        T2 N1 M0
        T2 N2 M0
    Any tumour with palpable, movable, regional nodes
    (2) T2 N0 M0
    A tumour more than 5 cm in length with negative nodes
  B Thoracic oesophagus:
    (1) T2 NX MO
    Lymph nodes cannot be assessed (clinical–diagnostic evaluation)
    (2) T2 N0 M0
    A tumour more than 5 cm in length or a tumour of any size with obstruction or circumferential involvement with no lymph node involvement (postsurgical treatment – pathological evaluation)

C Stage III
  1 Any T3
  2 Any N3 (cervical)
  3 Any N1 (thoracic)
  4 Any M1
  5 Any oesophageal cancer at any level with:
    A Distant metastasis
    B Extraoesophageal spread or
    C Fixed lymph node metastasis
      Any intrathoracic oesophageal carcinoma including either upper and mid-thoracic region or lower thoracic region with any positive findings in regional lymph nodes

Table 1.19   Japanese Society for Esophageal Diseases: Staging for oesophageal cancer

Tumour (T)
  m, sm – confined to mucosa, submucosa
  m_p – confined to muscularis propria
  a_1 – invasion reaching the overlying adventitia
  a_2 – invasion into the adventitia
  a_3 – invasion into neighbouring structures

Lymph node metastases (N)
  n_0 – no metastases
  n_1 – metastases to paraoesophageal nodes of the involved segment
  n_2 – metastases to paraoesophageal nodes of the segments of oesophagus
         adjacent to the tumour and/or metastases to perioesophageal nodes of
         the involved or adjacent oesophageal segments
  n_3 – metastases to paraoesophageal or perioesophageal nodes or distant
         oesophageal segments and/or metastases to lateral oesophageal nodes
  n_4 – metastases to nodes beyond group n_3

Organ metastases (M)
  m_0 – no organ metastases noted
  m_1 – organ metastases positive

Pleural dissemination (P)
  pl_0 – no plural dissemination noted
  pl_1 – pleural dissemination positive

Table 1.20   Japanese Society for Esophageal Diseases: Stage grouping

Histo-logical stage	Tumour	Lymph node meta-stases	Organ meta-stases	Pleural dissem-ination
0	m, sm	n_0	m_0	pl_0
I	mp	n_0	m_0	pl_0
II	a_1	n_1	m_0	pl_0
III	a_2	n_2	m_0	pl_0
IV	a_3	n_3, n_4	m_1	pl_1

The Japanese Society of Esophageal Diseases has described a more detailed system based both on histological examination of the resected oesophagus and lymph nodes and on the presence or absence of visceral metastases and pleural involvement (*Table 1.19*). Tumours submitted to surgical excision are then classified into one of five histological stages (*Table 1.20*).

REFERENCES

1. Akiyama, H. and Tsurumaru, M. (1988) Basic principles of resectional therapy for cancer of the oesophagus. In: *Surgery of the Oesophagus*, pp. 605–610 (Ed.) Jamieson, G.G. New York: Churchill-Livingstone.

2. American Joint Committee (1978) Staging of Cancer of the Esophagus. In: *Manual for Staging of Cancer*, pp. 65–70. Philadelphia: J.B. Lippincott.

3. Botha, J.R.C., Bowen, R.M. and Uys, C.J. (1978) The pathology of carcinoma of the esophagus. In: *Carcinoma of the Oesophagus*, pp. 117–130 (Ed.) Silber, W. Cape Town: A.A. Mulkema.

4. DeMeester, T.R. and Lafontaine, E.R. (1985) Surgical therapy. In: *Cancer of the Esophagus*, pp. 141–197 (Eds) DeMeester, T.R. and Levin, B. Orlando, FL: Grune & Statton.

5. Fekete, F., Gayer, B., Molas, G.J.M. (1988) Prophylactic operative techniques: thoracic esophageal squamous cell cancer surgery, with special references to lymph node removal. In: *Esophageal Cancer. International Trends in General Thoracic Surgery*, Vol. 4, pp. 130–135 (Eds) Delarue, N.C., Wilkins, E.W. and Wong, J.

6. Fitzpatrick, P.J. Tepperman, B.S. and de Boer, G. (1984) Multiple primary squamous cell carcinoma in the upper digestive tract. *International Journal of Radiology, Oncology, Biology and Physics*, **10**, 2273–2279.

7. Guanrei, K., Hettu, H., Sunglian, Q. and Yuming, C. (1982) Endoscopic diagnosis of 115 cases of early esophageal cancer. *Endoscopy*, **14**, 157–161.

8. Japanese Society for Esophageal Diseases (1976) Guidelines of clinical and pathological studies for carcinoma of the esophagus (2). *Japanese Journal of Surgery*, **6**, 69–78, 79–86.

9. Kirk, R.M. (1983) Double indemnity in oesophageal carcinoma? *British Medical Journal*, **286** (6365), 582–583.

10. Mannell, A. and Murray, W. (1989) Oesophageal Cancer in South Africa. A review of 1926 cases. *Cancer*, **64**, 2604–2608.

11. Miller, C. (1962) Carcinoma of thoracic oesophagus and cardia: a review of 405 cases. *British Journal of Surgery*, **49**, 507–522.

12. Postlethwaite, R.W. (1979) *Surgery of the Esophagus*, pp. 341–395, 439–467. New York: Appleton–Century–Crofts.

13. Rosenberg, J.C., Schwane, J.G., Vairkevicius, V.K. (1982) Cancer of the esophagus. In: *Cancer Principles and Practice of Oncology*, pp. 499–533 (Eds) De Vita, V.T., Hellman, S. and Rosenberg, S.A. Philadelphia: J.B. Lippincott.

14. Sugimachi, K., Matsuura, H., Kai, H. *et al.* (1986) Prognostic factors of esophageal carcinoma: univariate and multivariate analyses. *Journal of Surgical Oncology*, **31**, 108–112.

15. Tumour Prevention Treatment and Research Group, Chenchow, Honan (1977) Esophageal Cancer Research Group, Chinese Academy of Medical Sciences Peking and Linhsien County People's Hospital, Honan.

16. Watanabe, H., Iizuka, N. and Hirata, K. (1979) Examination of esophageal cancer with intramural skip or separate satellite nodules. *Geka Shinryo*, **21**, 1096–1100.

17. Watson, A. (1988) Pathologic changes affecting survival in esophageal cancer. In: *Esophageal Cancer International Trends in General Thoracic Surgery*, Vol. 4, pp. 36–44 (Eds) Delarue, N.C., Wilkins, E.W. and Wong, J. St Louis: CV Mosby.

18. Wong, J. and Branicki, F.J. (1988) Esophagoscopy and bronchoscopy. In: *Esophageal Cancer International Trends in General Thoracic Surgery*, Vol. 4, pp. 36–44 (Eds) Delarue, N.C., Wilkins, E.W. and Wong, J. St Louis: CV Mosby.

19. Yamashita, N. (1979) A statistical analysis of the dissemination routes of esophageal cancer based on autopsy records, particularly the role of liver and lung. *Nippon Gan Chiyo Gakkai Shi*, **14**, 1146–1149.

ADENOCARCINOMA OF THE OESOPHAGUS

Incidence, epidemiology and pathogenesis

Primary oesophageal adenocarcinoma is an uncommon tumour, and the true incidence is difficult to determine because cancers arising from the gastric cardia or fundus of the stomach may spread into the lower oesophagus. To differentiate prevalence of oesophageal adenocarcinoma in certain high-risk patient groups from the incidence of this tumour, it is necessary to analyse data from population-based cancer registries. Yang and Davis[35] examined the demographic characteristics related to the occurrence of oesophageal adenocarcinoma in the USA:

from a review of nine population-based cancer registries, the overall annual incidence of adenocarcinoma was 0.4 per 100 000 persons. Although this malignancy is not confined to a single racial group, Whites have a threefold higher rate of adenocarcinoma than Blacks. The male-to-female ratio for adenocarcinoma is seven in Whites and ten in Blacks and there is evidence that the rate of oesophageal adenocarcinoma has increased among White men. This observation is supported by historical comparison of the rate of adenocarcinoma in other tumour-based registries: Bosch *et al.*[4] noted that adenocarcinoma accounted for less than 8% of all cases of oesophageal cancer, whereas Hesketh *et al.*[14] reported that adenocarcinoma accounted for 18% of oesophageal malignancy in the Massachusetts' tumour registries from 1982 to 1984.

Adenocarcinoma of the oesophagus can arise from the oesophageal mucosal glands, the submucosal glands, ectopic islands of gastric mucosa or from metaplastic columnar-lined epithelium (Barrett's metaplasia).

The most accurate way of defining the relative importance of these sources to the occurrence of adenocarcinoma in the oesophagus is by subsite analysis.[9] Using data from tumour registries (*Figure 1.62*), adenocarcinoma represents 1–2% of malignancies arising in the upper one-third of the oesophagus, 3% in the middle one-third and 19% of lower oesophageal malignancies.[9] The oesophageal

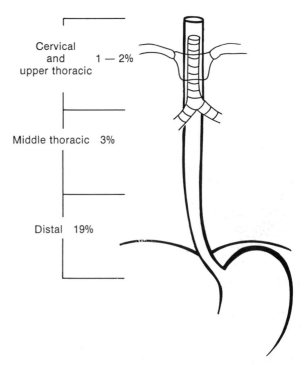

Figure 1.62 Adenocarcinomas as a percentage of oesophageal malignancies in the oesophageal segments.

glands are normally distributed throughout the length of the oesophagus, heterotrophic gastric mucosa is most frequent in the upper thoracic or low cervical oesophagus and metaplastic columnar epithelium predominantly affects the lower oesophagus. Subsite analysis therefore supports the concept that most oesophageal adenocarcinomas arise in metaplastic columnar epithelium,[6] and in one study 86% of cases of adenocarcinomas revealed Barrett's metaplasia in adjacent mucosa.[13] It has also been suggested that all adenocarcinomas involving the lower oesophagus arise from Barrett's metaplasia with, in some cases, the cancer destroying all evidence of benign metaplasia by the time of diagnosis.[28]

In 1950, Barrett drew attention to the condition in which the squamous epithelium of a variable segment of the oesophagus proximal to the lower oesophageal sphincter is replaced by metaplastic columnar epithelium. Originally believed to be congenital in origin, recent studies suggest that most cases are acquired secondary to gastro-oesophageal reflux.[3]

Symptoms suggestive of reflux oesophagitis are present in 60% of patients with Barrett's metaplasia, and it has been estimated that in 10% of patients with reflux oesophagitis the oesophageal mucosa will undergo columnar metaplastic changes.[28] Because patients with Barrett's metaplasia were found, in one study,[30] to have a much higher incidence of colonic tumours, it has been suggested that genetic factors may determine which cases with gastro-oesophageal reflux will undergo metaplasia. However, the true incidence of Barrett's metaplasia is unknown because gastro-oesophageal reflux may be asymptomatic and many patients presenting with an adenocarcinoma of the lower oesophagus and Barrett's metaplasia deny antecedent symptoms of reflux or even dyspepsia (page 90).

It is difficult to estimate the risk of malignancy and Barrett's metaplasia. On one hand, the age- and sex-adjusted survival rate for patients with benign Barrett's metaplasia appears to be identical to those of the general population;[23] on the other hand, the prevalence of malignancy in patients with Barrett's oesophagus (using the Mayo Clinic series) was 15%, with a reported incidence of 227 per 100 000. This is an incidence of 30 times the expected rate.

Varying degrees of dysplasia may occur in the columnar mucosa of Barrett's oesophagus and, in resected specimens containing adenocarcinoma, many writers have identified areas of dysplasia and carcinoma in situ in the adjacent epithelium forming Barrett's metaplasia[13,23] It has been suggested that the risk of developing dysplasia and adenocarcinoma may be related to additional factors such as cigarette smoking and alcohol abuse: Sanfrey et al.[27] found that most patients with adenocarcinoma developing in a Barrett's oesophagus admitted to regular alcohol intake and cigarette smoking. Additional risk factors such as alcohol and tobacco use may also explain why columnar epithelium of the oesophagus does not return to squamous epithelium when reflux has been surgically corrected.[19]

Pathology

Site

Adenocarcinoma of the oesophagus is commonly located in the lower one-third of the oesophagus (*Figure 1.70*), and the gross appearances are similar to those of squamous cell carcinomas. Cancers arising within Barrett's metaplasia may be multiple: Payne et al.[23] reported a 13% incidence of multicentricity in the adenocarcinomas found in resected specimens of Barrett's oesophagus.

Histology

Adenocarcinoma of the oesophagus can be classified histologically as follows:

Adenocarcinoma
  papillary
  poorly differentiated
  signet ring
Variants of adenocarcinoma
  adenocanthoma
  adenosquamous carcinoma
  mucoepidermoid
  adenoid cystic.

The degree of differentiation of adenocarcinoma of the oesophagus varies from the well-differentiated papillary type to a poorly differentiated carcinoma containing small glands or single cells. Oesophageal adenocarcinomas arising in heterotopic gastric mucosa are microscopically similar to the intestinal type of gastric carcinoma, and signet-ring cell carcinomas have been described.[17]

Barrett's metaplasia includes gastric fundus-type epithelium, gastric cardial epithelium and intestinal type epithelium; the multidirectional differentiation seen in the columnar-lined oesophagus is also present in the cells of the tumour arising from this epithelium. Banner et al.[2] identified gastrin and somatostatin in these adenocarcinomas. Focal areas of dysplasia, leading to neoplastic transformation, are found in association with 50% of the adenocarcinomas arising from Barrett's oesophagus.[9] More than half of these adenocarcinomas are poorly differentiated with transmural spread through the muscularis propria.[23]

Adenocanthoma is essentially an adenocarcinoma containing foci of benign squamous epithelium. When both squamous and glandular epithelium are histologically malignant, the tumour is best described as an adenosquamous carcinoma.

Although Ming[21] postulated that mucoepidermoid cancer arose from ectopic islands of gastric mucosa, it is probable that the mucoepidermoid tumours actually arise from the multipotential cells of the excretory ducts of submucosal mucous glands. The mucoepidermoid cancer has microscopic features similar to those of mucoepidermoid tumours of the salivary glands, having mucus-secreting cells, squamous cells and intermediate cells. Ultrastructural studies have identified features of squamous cell cancer (numerous cell functions and tonofibrillar aggregates) and adenocarcinoma (microvillae, basal lamina formation and secretory granules).[24] Further evidence of the origin of mucoepidermoid cancers from the deep oesophageal glands lies in the observation that these tumours may be present as intramural growths, frequently with deep infiltration through the muscle coat of the oesophagus.

Adenoid cystic adenocarcinoma is an uncommon tumour. It resembles the adenoid cystic carcinoma of salivary glands but has a poorer prognosis, usually with widespread metastases by the time of diagnosis. Almost certainly arising from the submucosal mucous glands, this form of adenocarcinoma typically presents as a nodular mass in the middle third of the oesophagus. It is slightly more common in men than in women, the age of the patients ranging from the sixth to the eight decade of life. The adenoid cystic carcinoma has a characteristic microscopic appearance, consisting of irregular masses – trabeculae of small round cells with darkly staining nuclei and scanty cytoplasm. Mucus is present between the epithelial glands which are surrounded and separated by pink hyaline material.[17]

Spread

The spread of adenocarcinomas of the oesophagus is similar to that of squamous cell carcinoma. By the time of diagnosis, there is extensive infiltration of the oesophageal wall and lymphatic metastases. Because adenocarcinomas arise predominantly in the distal oesophagus, the most commonly involved lymph nodes are paraoesophageal, coeliac and splenic groups.

Lymph node metastases are found in 70% of resected specimens of adenocarcinoma of the distal oesophagus,[1] and in 10% of patients having nodal metastases around the common hepatic artery and in the superior mediastinum. Adenocarcinomas tend to be associated with greater degrees of nodal metastases than squamous cell carcinoma.[33]

The pattern of local spread is determined by the location of the tumour and may involve stomach, diaphragm, pleura, pericardium, lung, liver or aorta. Haematogenous spread to the liver and lungs is not uncommon, and autopsy series have shown that almost any organ may contain metastases from an adenocarcinoma of the oesophagus.[17]

Staging

Adenocarcinoma of the distal oesophagus frequently spreads into the stomach and, unless the tumour is confined to the oesophagus,[8] the exact site or origin may be difficult to define. The Japanese Society for Esophageal Diseases has therefore described carcinoma involving the gastro-oesophageal junction as EC where the major portion of the tumour lies within the oesophagus and as E = C where there is an equal length of tumour in the oesophagus and stomach. With this system those cancers that have probably arisen in the fundus of the stomach, and have spread proximally into the oesophagus, are described as cardio-oesophageal or CE.

The TNM system of staging proposed by the American Joint Committee on Cancer is commonly used to stage adenocarcinomas of the oesophagus. In the Mayo Clinic series,[23] 19% of patients undergoing resection of adenocarcinomas arising in a Barrett's oesophagus have stage I disease, 21% presented with stage II cancers and 60% of cases were found to have stage III disease. Patients with visceral metastases were excluded from that particular series.

Unusual malignant disease of the oesophagus

The uncommon malignant disorders involving the oesophagus can be any of the following:

Primary
  epithelial
    oat-cell carcinoma
    carcinosarcoma
    carcinoid
    malignant melanoma
    choriocarcinoma
  non-epithelial
    haemangio-endothelioma
    Kaposi's sarcoma
    leiomyosarcoma
    rhabdomyosarcoma
    fibrosarcoma
    Hodgkin's lymphoma
    reticulum cell sarcoma
    plasmacytoma

Secondary
  metastatic
    breast carcinoma
    melanoma
    hepatocellular cancer.

OAT-CELL CARCINOMA

This is a rare tumour, accounting for less than 1% of oesophageal malignant disease in Western series, although Japanese authors have reported an incidence of up to 9% of malignant oesophageal tumours. Macroscopically, the most frequent type is a fungating polypoid lesion but malignant strictures or ulcers have been described.[17] The oat-cell carcinoma usually involves either the middle or distal oesophagus and consists of masses or sheets of small cells with darkly staining nuclei resembling small-cell anaplastic bronchial carcinoma. Two variants have been described, one with malignant squamous cells and the other containing adenocarcinoma.[9] These admixtures of tumour cells have led to debate concerning the histogenesis of oat-cell carcinomas of the oesophagus. It has been suggested that the cell of origin may lie in squamous mucosa, in the submucosal glands or in embryonic tracheobronchial rests.[9] Argyrophil cells have been demonstrated in the basal epithelium of the normal oesophagus.[32] Following the identification of cytoplasmic argyrophilic and neurosecretary granules in the cells of oat-cell carcinoma, as well as the demonstration of somatostatin, calcitonin and ACTH activity within these tumours, it has been suggested that cells derived from the enterochromaffin system give rise to oat-cell carcinomas of the oesophagus.[25,31]

Oat-cell carcinoma is a very aggressive neoplasm, most patients dying of metastatic disease within 6 months of diagnosis regardless of treatment.

CARCINOSARCOMA

This very rare tumour is composed of a mixture of malignant epithelioid and sarcoma cells; the epithelial element is typically squamous carcinoma whereas the sarcomatous component consists of malignant spindle cells. The histogenesis of this tumour is uncertain: it is possible that the carcinosarcoma has arisen from some malignant epithelial and stromal elements, that it represents a tumour arising from a single stem cell with divergent differentiation, or that it is composed of an oesophageal squamous cancer and a gastric adenocarcinoma with independent origins that have 'collided' at some point.[22]

Most cases have been described in middle-aged or elderly men and they account for approximately 1% of primary oesophageal tumours in China.[34] The most frequent macroscopic type consists of large polypoid masses within a dilated oesophagus, but ulcerative and stenosing varieties have been described. The distal two-thirds of the oesophagus is most often affected and, on biopsy, the lesion has been mistaken for a leiomyosarcoma.[9,17]

Metastases from a carcinosarcoma are usually composed of sarcomatous elements, but may consist of carcinomatous elements or a mixed carcinosarcomatous pattern. The overall prognosis of carcinosarcoma is poor with a 2–6% 5-year survival rate.[15]

MALIGNANT MELANOMA

Primary malignant melanoma is a rare tumour of the oesophagus, accounting for 0.1–0.4% of oesophageal carcinomas in reported series.[9,18] The existence of primary melanomas of the oesophagus was disputed until De La Pava et al.[7] demonstrated that melanocytes are occasionally found in the normal oesophagus. Primary malignant melanoma is a disease of older age, predominantly affecting men in the sixth and seventh decade, with a male-to-female ratio of 2.[26]

The tumour commonly arises in the distal oesophagus, it is almost always a bulky polypoid lesion, frequently pigmented and often associated with melanosis of adjacent oesophageal mucosa.[12] Most tumours are ulcerated, friable and bleed readily on contact. Despite the characteristic appearance the diagnosis is often not made before surgery or is made at autopsy.[26] Endoscopic biopsies may fail to reveal microscopic pigmentation unless special techniques, such as the Masson–Fontana stain, are used to identify melanin.[7]

It has been suggested that melanocytic junctional activity in the juxtapositional epithelium or melanosis of the oesophageal mucosa must be present before the diagnosis of primary oesophageal melanoma can be made.[16] However, in the collected series of 139 cases reviewed by Sabananthan et al.,[26] these changes were present in less than half the cases. An oesophageal tumour can be diagnosed as primary malignant melanoma when the malignant cells contain melanin or show ultrastructural evidence of melanomacytic differentiation in the form of cytoplasmic pre-melanosomes, and the patient has no history of evidence of another mucosal or cutaneous melanoma.[20] The oesophagus is an uncommon site for metastatic melanoma,[8] and symptomatic metastases are even more rare than primary melanoma in the oesophagus with only seven cases reported in the world literature.[26]

The prognosis in primary melanoma is grave; less than 2% of patients survive for 5 years after diagnosis. The tumours are usually advanced by the time of presentation and a survival rate of less than 5% is reported for cases undergoing oesophagectomy.[26]

However, the response to other modalities of treatment for this biologically aggressive tumour is even worse and, provided the resection margins are sufficient to encompass the extensive submucosal spread, surgical excision remains the treatment of choice.

World literature contains isolated case reports of other rare malignant tumours which may arise in the oesophagus (see above). Hodgkin's lymphoma, reticulum cell sarcoma, lymphosarcoma and plasmocytomas usually involve the oesophagus by direct infiltration from mediastinal nodes; but very rarely they may be primary in the oesophagus.[24]

The malignant mesenchymal tumours of muscle origin, leiomyosarcomas and rhabdomyosarcomas are much less common than their benign counterparts. It is difficult to determine the incidence of leiomyosarcomas because many cures were described in the older literature in which the descriptions and diagnostic terms used make interpretation difficult. Ming[21] noted that leiomyosarcomas are grossly polypoid tumours with a broad base which may infiltrate adjacent organs and can metastasize to viscera, the liver being the most common organ affected by secondary spread. Rhabdomyosarcomas are exceptionally rare as are fibrosarcomas and Postlethwaite[24] found only 13 of the former and 10 of the latter reported in world literature up to 1979.

Secondary tumours of the oesophagus may result from invasion from malignant tumours involving adjacent structures, by metastatic spread through mediastinal lymphatics and by blood spread (see above).

Excluding spread from gastric cancer, involvement of the oesophagus by cancer of the larynx, thyroid and bronchus, and by leukaemic infiltrates is most frequently reported. Carcinoma of the breast is thought to involve the oesophagus by spread through the intercostal veins and lymphatics. Bloodstream metastases from malignant melanoma, prostatic carcinoma, testicular tumours, pancreatic adenocarcinomas, chondrosarcomas and hepatomas have been reported.[11,24]

REFERENCES

1. Akiyama, H., Tsurumaru, M., Kawamura, T. and Ono, Y. (1981) Principles of surgical treatment for carcinoma of the esophagus. Analysis of lymph node involvement. *Annals of Surgery*, **194**, 438–445.
2. Banner, B.F., Memoli, V.A., Warren, W.H. and Gould, V.E. (1983) Carcinoma with multidirectional differentiation arising in Barrett's esophagus. *Ultrastructural Pathology*, **4**, 205–217.
3. Barrett, N.R. (1950) Chronic peptic ulcer of the oesophagus and 'oesophagitis'. *British Journal of Surgery*, **38**, 175–182.
4. Bosch, A., Frias, Z. and Caldwell, W.L. (1979) Adenocarcinoma of the esophagus. *Cancer*, **43**, 1557–1561.
5. Cameron, A.J., Ott, B.J. and Payne, W.S. (1985) The incidence of adenocarcinoma in columnar-lined (Barrett's) esophagus. *New England Journal of Medicine*, **313**, 857–859.
6. De Baecque, C., Potet, F., Molas, G. *et al.* (1990) Superficial adenocarcinoma of the oesophagus arising in Barrett's mucosa with dysplasia: a clinico pathological study of 12 patients. *Histopathology*, **16**, 213–220.
7. De La Pava, S., Nigogosyan, E., Pickren, J.N. and Caberra, A. (1963) Melanosis of the esophagus. *Cancer*, **26**, 48–50.
8. Eng, J., Pradhan, G.M., Sabananthan, S. and Mearns, A.J. (1989) Malignant melanoma metastatic to the esophagus. *Annals of Thoracic Surgery*, **4**, 287–288.
9. Faintuch, J., Shephard, K.V. and Levin, B. (1984) Adenocarcinoma and other unusual variants of esophageal cancer. *Seminars in Oncology*, **11**, 196–202.
10. Fujimaki, M., Soga, J., Wada, K. *et al.* (1972) Total gastrectomy for gastric cancer. Clinical considerations on 431 cases. *Cancer*, **30**, 660–664.
11. Gowing, N.F.C. (1961) The pathology of oesophageal tumours. In: *Tumours of the Oesophagus*, pp. 91–135 (Eds) Tanner, N.C. and Smithers, D.W. Edinburgh: E&S Livingstone.
12. Guzman, R.P., Wrightman, R., Ravinsky, E. and Unruh, H.N. (1989) Primary malignant melanoma of the esophagus with diffuse melanocytic atypia and melanoma in situ. *American Journal of Clinical Pathology*, **92**, 802–804.
13. Haggitt, R.C., Tryzelaar, J., Ellis, F.H. and Colcher, H. (1978) Adenocarcinoma complicating columnar epithelium-lined (Barrett's) esophagus. *American Journal of Clinical Pathology*, **70**, 1–5.
14. Hesketh, P.J., Clapp, R.W., Doos, W.G. and Spechler, S.J. (1989) The increasing frequency of adenocarcinoma of the esophagus. *Cancer*, **64**, 526–530.
15. Hinderleider, C.D., Aguam, A.S. and Wilder, J.R. (1979) Carcinosarcoma of the esophagus. A case report and review of the literature. *International Surgery*, **64**, 13–19.
16. Isaacs, J.L. and Quirke, P. (1988) Two cases of primary malignant melanoma of the oesophagus. *Clinical Radiology*, **39**, 455–457.
17. Iyer, P.V. and Rowland, R. (1988) The Pathology of oesophageal cancer. In: *Surgery of the oesophagus*, pp. 559–570 (Ed.) Jamieson, G.G. Edinburgh: Churchill-Livingstone.
18. Kormano, M.J. and Yrjana, J. (1981) Radiology of uncommon esophageal neoplasms. *European Journal of Radiology*, **1**, 51–56.
19. Mangla, J.C. (1980) Barrett's epithelium: regression or no regression? *New England Journal of Medicine*, **303**, 529–530.
20. Mannell, A., Hunter, S.J.S. and Hale, M.J. (1991)

Primary malignant melanoma of the oesophagus: report of a case with flow cytometric DNA analysis. *South African Journal of Surgery*, in Press.

21. Ming, S.C. (1973) Tumors of the esophagus and stomach. *Atlas of Tumor Pathology*, Second Series, Fascicle 7. Armed Forces Institute of Pathology, Washington DC.

22. Morson, B.C. and Dawson, I.M.P. (1979) *Gastrointestinal Pathology*. Oxford: Blackwell.

23. Payne, S.W., McAfee, M., Trastek, V.F., Unni, K.K. and Cameron, A.J. (1988) Adenocarcinoma of the columnar epithelial-lined lower esophagus of Barrett. In: *International Trends in General Thoracic Surgery*, Vol. 4, pp. 256–261 (Eds) Delarue, N.C., Wilkins, E.W. and Wong, J. *Esophageal Cancer*. St Louis: CV Mosby.

24. Postlethwaite, R.W. (1979) *Surgery of the Esophagus*, pp. 415–438, New York: Appleton–Century–Croft.

25. Reid, H.A.S., Richardson, W.W. and Corrin, B. (1980) Oat cell carcinoma of the Esophagus. *Cancer*, **45**, 2342–2347.

26. Sabananthan, S., Eng, J. and Pradhan, G.N. (1989) Primary malignant melanoma of the esophagus. *American Journal of Gastroenterology*, **84**, 1475–1481.

27. Sanfrey, H., Hamilton, S.R., Smith, R.R. and Cameron, J.L. (1985) Carcinoma arising in Barrett's esophagus. *Surgery, Gynecology and Obstetrics*, **161**, 570–574.

28. Sjörgren, R.W. and Johnson, L.T. (1983) Barrett's esophagus. A review. *American Journal of Surgery*, **74**, 313–321.

29. Smith, J.L. (1981) Pathology of adenocarcinoma of the esophagus and gastroesophageal region and 'Barrett's esophagus' as a predisposing factor. In: *Gastrointestinal Cancer*, pp. 125–135 (Eds) Stroehlein, J.R. and Romsdall, M.M. New York: Raven Press.

30. Sontag, S.J., Cheyfer, G., Stanley, M.M. *et al.* (1985) Barrett's oesophagus and colonic tumours. *The Lancet*, **1**, 946–948.

31. Tanone, S., Shimeda, T., Suzuki, M., Ikegani, M., Ishikawa, E. and Sano, T. (1983) Anaplastic carcinoma of the esophagus. *Acta Pathologica (Japan)*, **33**, 831–841.

32. Tateishi, R., Taniguchi, H., Wada, A., Horai, T. and Taniguchi, K. (1974) Argyrophil cells and melanocytes in esophageal mucosa. *Archives of Pathology*, **98**, 87–89.

33. Watson, A. (1988) Pathologic changes affecting survival in oesophageal cancer. In: *International Trends in General Thoracic Surgery*, Vol. 4, (Eds) Delarue, N.C., Wilkins, E.W. and Wong, J. St Louis: C.V. Mosby.

34. Xu, L., Sun, C., Wu, L., Chang, Z. and Liu, T. (1984) Clinical and pathological characteristics of the esophagus: report of four cases. *Annals of Thoracic Surgery*, **37**, 197–203.

35. Yang, P.S. and Davis, S. (1988) Incidence of cancer of the esophagus in the US by histologic type. *Cancer*, **61**, 612–617.

Clinical features

Early

Until mass screening programmes are introduced for all patient populations known to be at increased risk, or whenever oesophageal cancer is endemic, the clinician must be alert to the symptoms of early carcinoma of the oesophagus. These are mild but definite symptoms related to deglutition such as retrosternal discomfort, slight odynophagia or a sense of delayed passage of food, particularly hard solids[4] and can be expanded as follows:

Intermittent dysphagia (minimal)
Mild odynophagia
  'tingling'
  'burning'
Sensations of
  'foreign body in the throat'
  'delayed passage' of hard foods
  postprandial 'fullness' over the distal oesophagus.

These early symptoms only occur on swallowing and are usually intermittent; patients may therefore attach no significance to symptoms until late in the disease when dysphagia is persistent. Studies in high-incidence areas have shown that nearly 90% of patients with early oesophageal carcinoma are symptomatic.[4] Even minor symptoms connected with the oesophagus in populations or individual patients at risk for oesophageal cancer are an indication for cytological and endoscopic investigation.

Advanced

Symptoms of established oesophagus cancer include the following:

Dysphagia
Regurgitation
Weight loss
Pain on swallowing
Chronic cough
Haematemesis.

Symptoms associated with extraoesophageal spread are shown in Table 1.21. Dysphagia is well recog-

Table 1.21 Symptoms associated with extraoesophageal spread

Symptom	Significance
Anorexia	Large tumour load
Constant pain	Mediastinal infiltration
Hoarseness	Recurrent laryngeal nerve invasion
Coughing when swallowing	Oesophageal-airway fistula
Haemoptysis	Tracheobronchial invasion

nized as the definitive and often the first symptom of oesophageal cancer. It is a late symptom of this lethal disease because the cancer must have encircled at least half the oesophageal lumen before obstructive symptoms develop: by this time the cancer has spread outside the oesophagus and lymphatic metastases are present. In a small number of patients, dysphagia is preceded by intermittent retrosternal pain but, once dysphagia occurs, it is unremitting – a feature that differentiates malignant from benign disease – and progresses rapidly. Most patients, whether in Western or less developed countries, only seek medical attention 2–4 months after the onset of dysphagia. By then, 24% cannot swallow liquids.[14] Duration of symptoms cannot be correlated with size or grade of lesion or with its resectability: an occasional patient with a very low-grade malignancy will have suffered dysphagia for 12 months or more before presentation.

Severe dysphagia is invariably associated with *regurgitation* and *marked weight loss*, despite constant hunger. *Anorexia*, however, is a sinister symptom usually indicative of a large tumour load. *Fatigue* and *weight loss* are common complaints largely due to the loss of weight but anaemia, due to either dietary cause or occult bleeding from an ulcerated tumour, can be a contributory factor. Frank *haematemesis* is unusual and associated with fungating friable cancer of the distal oesophagus.

Pain on swallowing is characteristic of an oesophageal lesion, and is felt retrosternally radiating to the neck and interscapular areas or, if the distal oesophagus is affected, to the epigastrium and lower back. Pain may precede the development of dysphagia but is usually not the predominant symptom. However, constant pain, or pain at times other than swallowing, has serious implications; this means that the cancer has spread transmurally, to excite a perioesophageal inflammatory response, and/or invaded the soft tissues of the mediastinum neck or abdomen.[13]

Aspiration is a common complication of oesophageal cancer. Food particles and saliva accumulate above the lesion and are silently aspirated when the patient lies down to sleep. This most probably occurs weeks or months before admission, even before the patient has dysphagia because most patients, including non-smokers, have evidence of chronic pulmonary damage with cough and signs of basal pneumonitis. If pulmonary aspiration is severe, the patient may suffer exertional dyspnoea, pleuritic pain and fever due to an underlying aspiration pneumonia affecting, most often the lower lobe of the right lung.

If coughing is directly related to the act of swallowing, the patient has either a malignant oesophageal-airway fistula or a very high lesion which interferes with the mechanics of digestion. In these cases, a lung abscess may be present. In less developed countries with endemic tuberculosis, reactivation of the pulmonary lesions can occur when the nutritional status of the patients deteriorates. This is one cause of haemoptysis but bleeding from malignant invasion of the airways is the usual reason for this symptom.

Hoarseness is sometimes due to the laryngitis associated with chronic aspiration, but is more often due to invasion of the recurrent laryngeal nerves. Cancer of the midoesophagus will invade the left recurrent laryngeal nerve as it crosses the arch of the aorta. Cancer of the cervical oesophagus can involve the right or left recurrent laryngeal nerve as can extracapsular spread from nodal metastases.

Signs

The oesophagus is a deeply placed organ so that the signs of oesophageal cancer are those resulting from oesophageal obstruction and/or spread of the tumour. On general examination, weight loss is usually obvious and in high-incidence endemic areas the patient may be emaciated with hypoproteinaemic oedema, pellagra and the respiratory complications of aspiration; foetor is due to decomposing food debris in the obstructed oesophagus and, if associated with grossly purulent sputum, is strongly suggestive of a lung abscess. When dysphagia is severe, constant spitting up of saliva is characteristic and dehydration may be evident.

Examination of the chest will reveal evidence of pneumonitis or pneumonia. On auscultation reduced air entry to one lung, with a fixed rhonchus on that side, is a sign of ipsilateral bronchial invasion or compression by tumour.

A careful search must be made for signs of tumour spread. The cervical and supraclavicular lymph nodes may be palpable, and epigastric tenderness in all but the very debilitated is suggestive of involvement of the stomach wall either by extension of a distal tumour or by extracapsular spread from gross coeliac and left gastric nodal metastases. Hepatic secondaries are most common when the distal oesophagus is affected.

Tenderness in the neck or stridor is very suggestive of extraoesophageal spread from cancer of the cervical oesophagus which is infiltrating the soft tissues of the neck and invading the trachea or the recurrent laryngeal nerves.

Metastases to lungs or bones are infrequent but pleural effusion or bone pain would indicate that these have occurred. Other signs of blood-stream spread, such as subcutaneous nodules, are rare and usually only found as a late manifestation after apparently successful treatment of the local lesion.

Investigations

The objectives of investigation in oesophageal cancer, namely confirmation of disease, assessing spread of the cancer and selection of appropriate treatment for the individual patient, are met with combinations of the following.

Barium swallow

In patients with dysphagia, the barium swallow examination will almost certainly demonstrate the oesophageal malignancy. It cannot detect carcinoma in situ but the *double-contrast* technique is effective in detecting superficial and early tumours.[20] The positive radiographic findings in early cases consist of thickening, interruption and/or tortuosity of mucosal folds, localized rigidity of the oesophageal wall and superficial filling defects. With the double-contrast technique, 50% of early cases will have positive radiographic signs of the disease,[4] but detection of these changes require considerable skill on the part of the radiologist.

In advanced oesophageal cancer, the characteristic radiographic picture is that of a long irregular stricture in the oesophagus with a ragged mucosal pattern (*Figure 1.63*). If the cancer is of the infiltrative type, a tight stricture is evident and the oesophagus above the lesion is dilated (*Figure. 1.64*). However, the extreme tortuosity and dilatation present in a late case of achalasia are not seen with carcinoma. Fungating tumours (*Figure 1.65*) appear as multiple filling defects with ulcerated margins in an expanded segment of the oesophagus. The solitary malignant ulcer, with a filling defect in the oesophageal lumen and single ulcers protruding beyond the margin of the oesophagus (*Figure 1.66*) are uncommon.

Certain radiological features on the barium swallow are diagnostic of extraoesophageal invasion and

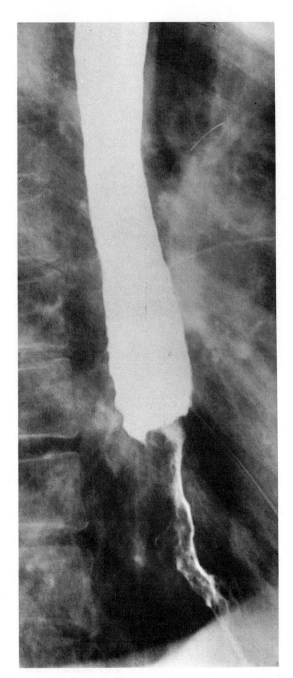

Figure 1.63 Barium swallow showing the typical long irregular stricture of oesophageal cancer.

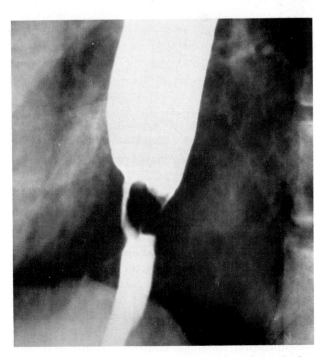

Figure 1.64 Barium swallow appearance of a desmoplastic–stenosing oesophageal cancer.

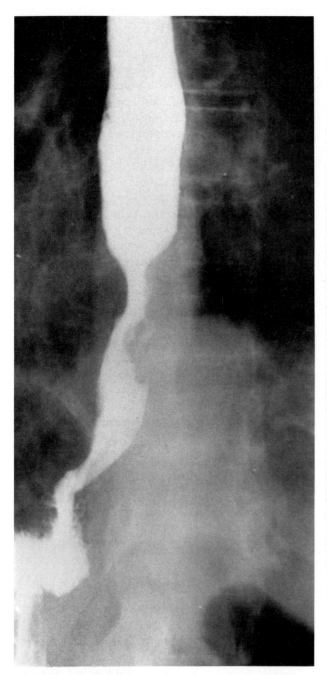

Figure 1.65 A fungating oesophageal cancer with stenosis on barium swallow examination.

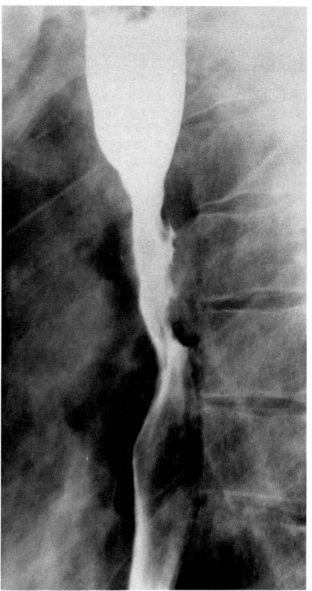

Figure 1.66 Barium swallow appearance of an ulcerative squamous cell carcinoma in the mid-oesophagus.

of the unsuitability of the lesion for radical local treatment. These features include passage of contrast through an oesophageal-airway fistula (*Figure 1.67*), communication between the malignant stricture and pulmonary tissue (*Figure 1.68*), and a sinus into the mediastinum (*Figure 1.69*). The barium swallow can be used to measure the length of the lesion; even with a radio-opaque rule to correct for magnification, the single-contrast examination is not as reliable as the double-contrast technique[3,6] in the determination of the extent of involvement.

Although length of lesion has no direct relationship to depth of invasion, assessment of length is important: tumours greater than 10 cm in length are usually incurable.[12]

With extraoesophageal spread, the cancerous segment of the oesophagus becomes fixed and immobile. Two changes then occur in the longitudinal axis of the oesophagus: proximal dilatation and tortuosity of the oesophagus above the tumour, and angulation or deviation of the oesophageal axis above and below the malignant segment. The longitudinal axis of the oesophagus can be assessed by posteroanterior and lateral views on a single-contrast barium swallow. A normal oesophageal axis in both projections reliably excludes

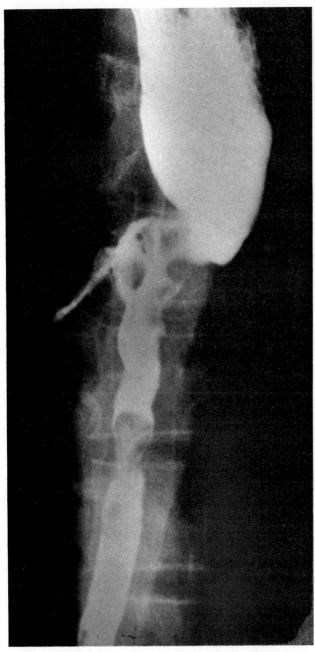

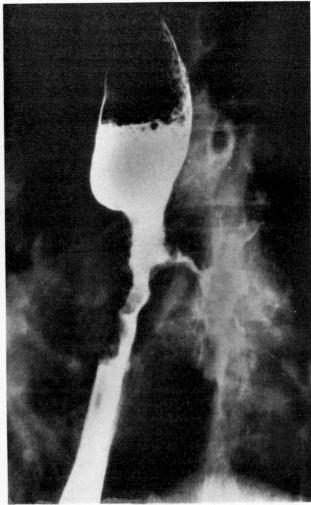

Figure 1.68 Barium examination showing an oesophago-pulmonary fistula.

Chest radiograph

The chest radiograph is an essential part of the work-up of all patients with carcinoma of the oesophagus, and provides invaluable information about the cardiovascular and pulmonary systems.

Over 40% of patients with oesophageal cancer have radiological abnormalities, including air on an air–fluid level in the oesophagus (*Figure 1.71*), distortion of the tracheal air shadow in relation to the tumour (*Figure 1.72*), a widened mediastinum, lymphadenopathy and, infrequently, hilar lymphadenopathy.[9] A normal chest radiograph in patients with oesophageal cancer is of little prognostic significance because it cannot exclude extraoesophageal spread or lymphatic metastases.[10]

Azygos venography

Extraoesophageal spread from cancers of the mid-thoracic and distal oesophagus can result in distortion or obstruction of the azygos vein which lies in

Figure 1.67 Barium study of a malignant oesophageal–airway fistula.

gross malignant invasion,[13] whilst obvious distortion (*Figure 1.70*) of the oesophageal axis at, above or below the malignant segments is associated with extraoesophageal spread in 75–80% of cases. Minor deviation in the oesophageal axis can result from local inflammatory changes with false positives in 10–16% of cases.[1] The oesophageal axis is more accurate than evaluation of tumour length and type in the preoperative assessment of resectability.

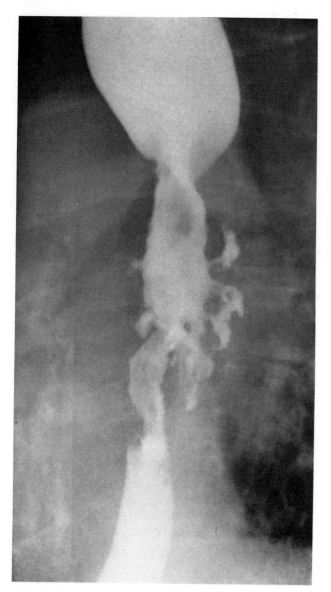

Figure 1.69 Oesophageal cancer with gross mediastinal invasion on barium swallow.

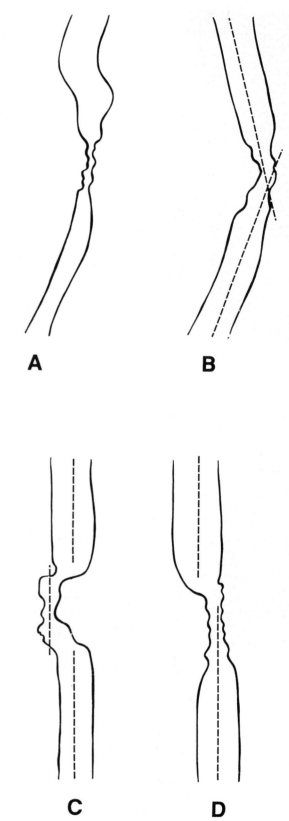

Figure 1.70 Deformities of the oesophageal axis associated with extraoesophageal invasion: (a) proximal dilatation and tortuosity; (b) angulation; (c) deviation of the tumour axis; (d) deviation of the oesophageal axis.

close relationship to these segments. Azygos venography is an invasive procedure that has been used extensively by Japanese workers[1] to assess extent of spread of oesophageal cancer, although there is a false-positive rate of 10% in patients with localized disease. Because computed tomography is an accurate and non-invasive method for definition of the relationship of the azygos vein to an oesophageal cancer, enthusiasm for azygos venography has waned.[20]

Computed tomography (CT) scans

The thoracic and abdominal segments of the oesophagus are easily recognised on a CT scan: the normal oesophagus is seen as a thin-walled structure containing air and easily delineated by far planes

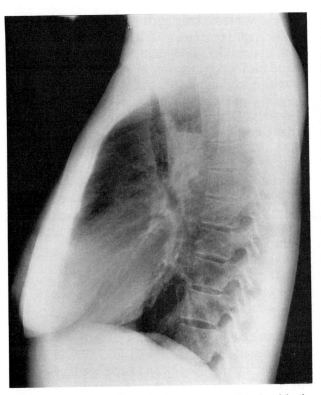

Figure 1.71 Chest radiograph showing an air–fluid level in the obstructed oesophagus.

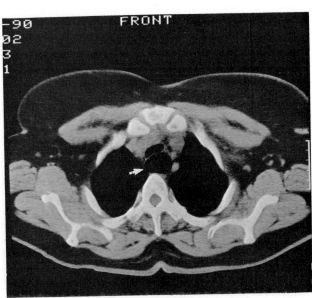

Figure 1.73 A CT scan showing a dilated but otherwise thin-walled thoracic oesophagus (arrow).

from adjacent mediastinal and intra-abdominal structures (*Figure 1.73*). Oesophageal cancer appears as an irregular thickening of the oeso-phageal wall or as a mass lesion of the oesophagus (*Figure 1.74*).

CT scanning has not proved to be as accurate as double-contrast barium examination in defining the length of a lesion, but is more reliable in identifying extramucosal extent.[20] A CT scan which shows gross distortion of mediastinal anatomy (*Figure 1.75*) is reliable evidence of the unresectability of oeso-phageal cancer, and has replaced the invasive, and

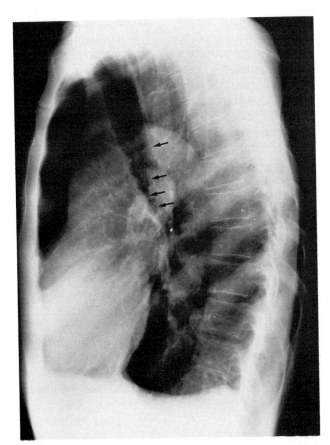

Figure 1.72 Malignant invasion of the trachea (arrows) evident on a chest radiograph.

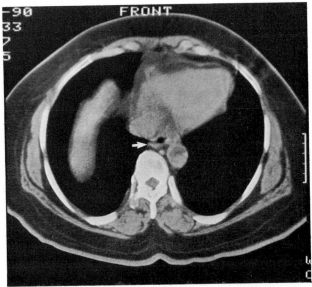

Figure 1.74 A CT scan showing thickening and irregularity of the oesophagus at the site of oesophageal cancer (arrow).

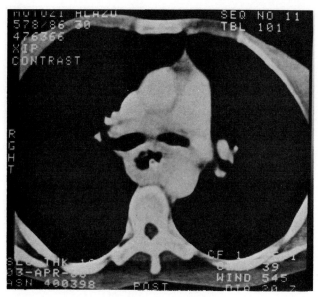

Figure 1.75 Gross distortion of mediastinal anatomy by an advanced unresectable oesophageal cancer.

potentially dangerous, techniques of staging laparotomies or exploratory thoracotomies in these cases.

However, CT scanning has its limitations. In the neck, absence of sufficient paraoesophageal fat makes differentiation of the oesophagus from adjacent soft tissues difficult; density artefacts from cervical vertebrae and bones of the shoulder girdle also detract from the image. Obliteration of the perioesophageal fat planes due to severe weight loss or inflammatory adhesions around the tumour cannot be distinguished easily from extraoesophageal spread.[13] CT scans cannot resolve the thin membranous back wall of the tracheobronchial tree as a distinct layer and careful fibreoptic bronchoscopy is essential to distinguish contiguous compression from direct invasion of the airway.[2] The incidence of a false-positive diagnosis of extraoesophageal spread in the prospective evaluation of 103 patients with oesophageal cancer was 56%[13] and recent studies have reported similar findings.[7,15]

CT scanning is not helping in the diagnosis of mediastinal node metastases: it is not possible to identify micrometastatic disease or to distinguish lymph nodes enlarged by reactive hyperplasia from nodal metastases with a CT scan.[13,20] However, specificity of this diagnostic modality for invasion and node involvement is high (85–95%) and CT scanning is relatively reliable when it predicts a 'negative result' for either extraoesophageal spread or lymphatic metastases.[7] CT scanning is therefore a valuable adjunct to radiological and endoscopic examination in the identification of the patient with oesophageal cancer who is a candidate for radical local treatment.

Magnetic resonance imaging (MRI)

This imaging is capable of detecting tissue characteristics and, unlike radiography, does not depend on radio-opacity for creation of an image. MRI is a promising technique for the non-invasive assessment of oesophageal malignancy and structural relationships can be examined in transaxial, coronal and sagittal planes. Experience with this new modality of imaging is limited. Halvorsen et al.[5] have found sagittal images to be valuable in determining the longitudinal extent of the primary tumour and transaxial images to be superior in the detection of tracheobronchial invasion. MRI has a sensitivity of 88%, specificity of 87% and, when indeterminate results are excluded, an accuracy of 87% in the identification of extraoesophageal spread.[5]

MRI is still under development but MRI staging of oesophageal carcinoma does not appear to be more accurate than CT scans.[17]

Endoscopic ultrasonography (EUS)

The normal oesophageal wall is depicted as five layers by high-frequency endoscopic ultrasonography (EUS) and, provided the echo endoscope can be passed through a malignant stricture, EUS is proving highly accurate in the assessment of transmural invasion of oesophageal cancer. Overall accuracy rates in predicting depth of tumour infiltration of 82–90% have been reported.[19,21] When the instrument cannot be passed through the cancerous segment, CT is superior to EUS in the assessment of extraoesophageal spread.

EUS is also more accurate than CT in the assessment of regional lymph node metastases unless there is severe stenosis.[21] Sugimaki et al.[19] reported a visualization rate for mediastinal lymph nodes of 92–97% when the nodes were more than 10 mm in diameter but the detection of lymph nodes less than 5 mm in diameter is poor. In addition, EUS cannot reliably distinguish reactive hyperplasia or lymphadenitis from micrometastatic lymph node involvement.[21,22] High-frequency EUS, with a limited depth of penetration, is not effective for the evaluation of distant metastases, but it is proving valuable in the diagnosis of locally recurrent oesophageal cancer, identified by nodular hyperechoic thickening at the anastomosis.[11]

CT and EUS provide complementary information in the evaluation patients with oesophageal cancer. Technical improvements such as a smaller diameter echo endoscope may further enhance the diagnostic accuracy and application of EUS.

Electronic endoscopy

The video-endoscope, incorporating a small light-sensitive microprocessor chip, can transmit electronic signals to a video-processor which converts these signals into a visual display on a television screen. This will allow the endoscopist to demonstrate the oesophageal lesions to other gastroenterologists and pathologists, and to store the images for subsequent review. With the incorporation of microcomputers to analyse and store endoscopic data, diagnoses of macroscopic oesophageal lesions may be enhanced by these electronic video-endoscopes.

Radioactive isotopes

The ability of malignant cells to accumulate radioactive isotopes has been used in the detection of oesophageal malignancy. One of the earliest methods described was the use of radioactive phosphorus (^{32}p).[16] However, the necessity for specially designed Geiger counters to be positioned within a few millimetres of the tissue being examined made this investigation cumbersome and impractical.

There was subsequent enthusiasm for oesophageal scintigraphy using gallium-67. Although oesophageal cancers are gallium-avid, the results were disappointing: ^{67}Ga accumulation had a sensitivity of 67% for extraoesophageal spread and a sensitivity of 27% in the detection of lymph node metastases.[8] This limited success rate reduced the use of gallium scintiscanning for oesophageal cancer, although recently Sostre et al.[18] have suggested that these studies should be performed with single photon emission computed tomography (SPECT) imaging to overcome interference from sternum and spine. The imaging characteristics of technetium-99m are superior to those of ^{67}Ga and a new tumour imaging agent, technetium-99m–dimercapto-succinic acid (^{99m}Tc-DMSA) has been used to evaluate squamous carcinoma of the head and neck.[23] The preliminary results of a study of ^{99m}Tc-DMSA with SPECT imaging in patients with oesophageal cancer, investigated at Baragwanath Hospital, Johannesburg, appear promising (Figure 1.76) with a sensitivity approaching 100% in lesion detection in untreated patients (personal communication). Use of this tumour-imaging agent will depend on the results of a prospective study which has been undertaken to determine if the oesophageal uptake of ^{99m}Tc-DMSA can be correlated with extent of the primary lesion, and on its sensitivity in the detection of regional and distant lymphatic metastases.

Oesophagoscopy

Oesophagoscopy is obviously mandatory in any patient with symptoms related to swallowing and is the most reliable procedure for diagnosing oesophageal cancer. The subtle endoscopic changes in the appearance of the mucosa, that are suggestive of early oesophageal cancer have been described earlier and, in patients with minimal symptomatology, diagnostic accuracy can be increased with chromo-oesophagoscopy. In this technique, vital dyes are sprayed onto the oesophageal mucosa, either 2% toluidine blue or 3% iodine (Lugol's) solution. Using toluidine (or methylene) blue, the oesophagus is washed with water and dried by aspiration: carcinomatous tissue appears blue, whilst the normal mucosa remains unstained. Directed endoscopic biopsies are taken for histological identification of the abnormal mucosa because areas of oesophagitis and peptic ulceration also stain blue. After spraying with Lugol's iodine, normal mucosa turns dark brown and the malignant tissue remains unstained.[2]

Advanced oesophageal carcinoma is easy to recognize: as the oesophagoscope passes through the cricopharyngeal muscle, it encounters a characteristic foul-smelling pool of frothy saliva and debris. After aspiration of the oesophageal contents, the cancer is seen as a pinkish-white friable mass in the lumen. In the desmoplastic-stenosing variety, the lumen is severely narrowed by oedematous mucosa and frankly malignant tissue may not be obvious. Less commonly, the carcinoma is evident as an ulcer with raised edges and a haemorrhagic base. It is important to record accurately the upper limit of the lesion and the presence of any satellite nodules of growth in the proximal oesophagus. Gentle handling of the endoscope is essential, regardless of whether this is of rigid or flexible type.

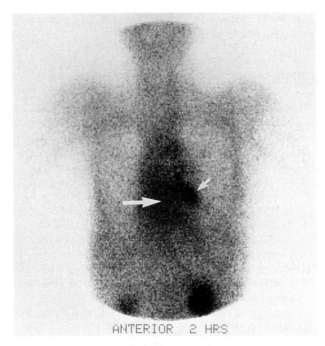

ANTERIOR 2 HRS

Figure 1.76 99 mTc(V)–DMSA scan in oesophageal cancer (large arrow) with malignant lymphadenopathy (small arrow).

When more than 50% of the oesophageal circumference is involved, no attempt should be made to introduce the rigid scope through the tumour: the walls of the oesophagus are weakened by malignant infiltration and such an attempt could rupture the oesophagus. Undoubtedly more traumatic than the flexible fibreoptic gastroscope, the rigid scope does allow the collection of deeper biopsy specimens which is valuable in tumours with extensive submucosal spread. Where surgery is considered for cancers of the upper one-third of the oesophagus, the rigid scope is more accurate than the flexible instrument in defining the distance between the cricopharyngeal muscle and the proximal edge of the tumour.[24]

Oesophagoscopy with the flexible scope can be performed under local anaesthesia and, after dilatation of the malignant stricture, can be passed through the tumour to estimate its length and to identify coexistent gastroduodenal pathology.

Bronchoscopy

The cervical and proximal two-thirds of the thoracic oesophagus lie immediately behind the tracheobronchial tree: bronchoscopic abnormalities ranging from distortion and invasion to malignant fistulas are found in 50–60% of patients with upper third cancers and in 40% of cases with middle third cancer.[24] Abnormal appearances at bronchoscopy are present in 17.5% of patients with cancer of the distal oesophagus. Bronchoscopy is mandatory in the assessment of oesophageal cancers irrespective of the size or location of the tumour.

Fibreoptic bronchoscopy offers the advantages of a local anaesthetic procedure, a more complete examination of the vocal folds, posterior walls of the bronchi and the peripheral bronchi. But many patients with oesophageal cancer have obstructive airway disease and respiratory impairment. Under these circumstances, the rigid bronchoscope should be used with general anaesthesia and intermittent jet (Venturi) ventilation: the flexible bronchoscope, unlike the rigid bronchoscope which is an open tube, acts as a space-occupying lesion in the trachea and could lead to a critical reduction in Po_2. Indirect laryngoscopy should be used to examine the vocal folds in patients undergoing rigid bronchoscopy.

Node biopsy

Fine-needle aspiration cytology is advised to confirm or exclude metastatic spread to palpable scalene and cervical nodes. Mediastinoscopy will provide additional information regarding spread of oesophageal cancer in the upper and mid-thoracic oesophagus to the anterior mediastinal nodes. However, the presence of micrometastatic disease is not considered to be a contraindication to oesophagectomy if the primary tumour can be safely resected.[12]

Mediastinoscopy is an invasive procedure, requiring a general anaesthetic, and is not widely used in the pre-treatment assessment of patients with oesophageal cancer.

Laboratory tests

Laboratory tests form an essential part of the management of carcinoma of the oesophagus and are chiefly directed at assessment of the state of nutrition, hydration, renal function and haematological status of the individual patient. Serial measurement of the blood urea concentration is a useful guide to fluid replacement in the severely dysphagic. Following correction of fluid deficits, anaemia is frequently unmasked and blood transfusion or haematinics may be considered. Many patients with oesophageal cancer have a history of alcohol abuse and liver function studies with a coagulation profile are essential. The serum albumin is a valuable index of nutritional status and is a simple way of assessing the patient's response to nutritional support. Respiratory status must be carefully assessed by means of lung function tests, including the forced expiratory volume in 1 second (FEV_1) and serial blood gas analyses: severe impairment of respiratory function may contraindicate surgery, radical radiotherapy and use of certain cytotoxic drugs. Clinical evaluation and electrocardiography are essential: the gated radionuclide pool scan, a coronary arteriogram and a ventriculogram may be indicated in older patients. Any gross defects in the patient's general condition must be corrected before invasive procedures are planned.

REFERENCES

1. Akiyama, H. (1980) Surgery for carcinoma of the esophagus. *Current Problems in Surgery*, **SVII**, 55–120.
2. Endo, M. (1988) Special techniques in the endoscopic diagnosis of esophageal carcinoma. In: *International Trends in General Thoracic Surgery*, Vol. 4, pp. 45–68 (Eds) Delarue, N.C., Wilkins, E.W. and Wong, J. St Louis: C.V. Mosby.
3. Goldstein, H.M., Zornoza, J. and Hopens, T. (1981) Intrinsic diseases of the adult oesophagus: benign and malignant tumours. *Seminars in Roentgenology*, **XVI**, 183–197.
4. Guojun, H., Lingfang, S., Dawer, Z. *et al.* (1981) Diagnosis and surgical treatment of early esophageal carcinoma. *Chinese Medical Journal*, **94**, 229–232.
5. Halvorsen, R.A. Herfkins, R.T., Wolfe, W.G. and Thompson, W.M. (1987) Comparison of magnetic resonance to computed tomography for staging

esophageal carcinoma (Meeting Abstract) Eighty-seventh Annual Meeting of the American Society, April 26–May 1, 1987, p. 133, Miami Beach, FL.

6. Khan, M.F. and Mannell, A. (1988) A radiographic and tomographic examination of the length and volume of oesophageal cancers (abstract). *South African Journal of Surgery*, **26**, 125.

7. Kirk, S.J., Moorehead, R.J., McIrath, E., Gibbons, J.P. and Spence, R.A. (1990) Does preoperative computed tomography scanning aid assessment of oesophageal carcinoma. *Postgraduate Medical Journal*, **66**, 191–194.

8. Kondo, M., Hashimoro, S., Kubo, A., Kakegawa, T. and Ando, N. (1979) 67-Ga scanning in the evaluation of esophageal cancer. *Radiology*, **131**, 723–726.

9. Levy, J.I. (1978) Some aspects of the radiology of oesophageal cancer in Johannesburg Blacks. In: *Carcinoma of the Oesophagus*, pp. 162–168 (Ed.) Silber, W. Cape Town: A.A. Balkema.

10. Lindell, M.M., Hill, C.A. and Libsritz, H.F. (1979) Esophageal cancer: radiographic chest findings and their prognostic significance. *American Journal of Roentgenology*, **133**, 461–465.

11. Lightdale, C.J., Botet, J.F., Kelsen, D.F., Turnbull, A.D. and Brenan, M.C. (1989) Diagnosis of recurrent gastrointestinal cancer at the surgical anastomosis by endoscopic ultrasound. *Gastrointestinal Endoscopy*, **35**, 407–412.

12. Mannell, A. (1988) Carcinoma of the oesophagus. In: *Modern Surgery in Africa*, pp. 165–187 (Ed.) Pantanowitz, D. Johannesburg: Southern Book Publishers.

13. Mannell, A., Epstein, B., Patel, V., Omar, G.M. and Diamantes, T. (1984) The spread of oesophageal cancer: an evaluation of clinical barium and computed tomography assessments. *Australian and New Zealand Journal of Surgery*, **54**, 119–126.

14. Mannell, A. and Murray, W. (1989) Oesophageal cancer in South Africa: a review of 1926 cases. *Cancer*, **64**, 2604–2608.

15. Markland, C.G., Manhire, A., Davies, P. *et al.* (1989) The role of computed tomography in assessing the operability of oesophageal carcinoma. *European Journal of Cardiothoracic Surgery*, **3**, 33–36.

16. Nakayama, K. (1961) The diagnosis of cancer of the oesophagus with radioactive phosphorus. In: *Tumours of the Oesophagus*, pp. 157–162 (Eds) Tanner, N.C. and Smithers, D.W. Edinburgh: E&S Livingstone.

17. Siewert, J.R. (1989) Esophageal cancer from the German point of view. *Japanese Journal of Surgery*, **19**, 11–20.

18. Sostre, S., Romero, I., Riviera, J.V., Baez, L. and Clinton, E. (1990) Gallium imaging of esophageal carcinoma: increased sensitivity with lateral views of the thorax. *Clinical Nuclear Medicine*, **15**, 163–167.

19. Sugimaki, K., Ohno, S., Fugishima, H. *et al.* (1990) Endoscopic ultrasonographic detection of carcinomatous invasion and of lymph nodes in the thoracic esophagus. *Surgery*, **107**, 366–371.

20. Thompson, W.M. (1983) Esophageal cancer. *International Journal of Radiation Oncology Biology Physics*, **9**, 1533–1565.

21. Tio, T.L., Cohen, P., Coene, P.P. *et al.* (1989) Endosonography and computed tomography of esophageal carcinoma. Preoperative classification compared to the new (1987) TNM Classification. *Gastroenterology*, **96**, 1478–1486.

22. Tio, T.L., Coene, P.P., Schouwink, M.H. and Tygat, G.N. (1989) Esophagogastric carcinoma: preoperative TNM classification with endosonography. *Radiology*, **173**, 411–417.

23. Watkinson, J.C., Allen, S., Lazarus, C.R. *et al.* (1990) Pharmacokinetics biodistribution and dosimetry of 99Tcm(V) DMSA in humans with squamous cell carcinoma. *Nuclear Medicine Communications*, **11**, 343–359.

24. Wong, J. and Branicki, F.J. (1988) Esophagoscopy and bronchoscopy. In: Esophageal carcinoma. *International Trends in General Thoracic Surgery*, vol. 4, pp. 36–44 (Eds) Delarue, N.C., Wilkins, E.W. and Wong, J. St Louis: C.V. Mosby.

TREATMENT

Oesophageal cancer is a distressing and lethal disease. Without treatment, the patient will die of starvation. But before death occurs, he or she may suffer the miseries of pneumonia and lung abscess secondary to aspiration from the obstructed oesophagus, paroxysms of coughing with each swallow if the cancer has fistulated into the airways and constant pain from malignant invasion of extraoesophageal tissues.

The principle aims of treatment, whether curative or palliative, are relief of oesophageal obstruction and to prolong life in comfort. But whatever treatment is selected for the patient with oesophageal cancer, success of the treatment is critically dependent on the general condition of the patient.

Preparation of the patient

The most serious complications of oesophageal obstruction are aspiration and starvation; the effects of these must be at least partly reversed before treatment can begin.

To stop the patient aspirating, oral intake must be restricted to a diet that the patient can swallow at a normal rate. Difficulty with swallowing liquids necessitates passage of a fine-bore Silastic tube for enteral feeding. Dilatation of the malignant stricture may be required to enable the feeding tube to be passed into the stomach. Intravenous alimentation is indicated for patients with impassable strictures and for those with oesophageal-airway fistulas. A tube passing across the oesophagogastric junction leads to incompetence of the inferior sphincter and gastro-oesophageal reflux which may exacerbate pulmonary contamination in patients with malignant fistulas. Feeding gastrostomies or jejunostomies, which can be complicated by leakage, sepsis and bowel obstruction, should be avoided, particularly in patients considered to be candidates for oesophageal surgery. The serum albumin, the patient's weight and gain in strength must be closely monitored in order to ensure that nutritional state has improved and that the negative nitrogen balance is reversed.

Many patients with oesophageal cancer are heavy smokers with chronic obstructive airway disease.[62] Repeated aspiration from the obstructed oesophagus leads to airway damage, destruction of pulmonary tissue and fibrosis.[10] Therefore careful attention must be given to improving respiratory status. The patient must stop smoking; evidence of wheezing is an indication for bronchodilator therapy; chest physiotherapy is essential in order to assist the patient in clearing secretions. Purulent sputum or evidence of pulmonary tuberculosis, common in less developed countries, will require appropriate antibiotic therapy. The improvement in pulmonary function can be monitored by simple spirometric tests such as the forced expiratory volume in 1 second (FEV_1), maximum voluntary ventilation (MVV) and serial blood gas analyses. At the bedside the patient's progress should be assessed by daily examination of the lungs and by watching the patient's efforts with incentive spirometry.[59]

The large number of techniques applied to the treatment of oesophageal cancer indicates that no single treatment is appropriate for all patients with this disease. *Three factors influence the selection of therapy*:

1. The stage of the disease, whether potentially curable or advanced.
2. The general condition, age and decision of the patient.
3. The experience, and field of expertise, of those responsible for the patient's management.

Oesophageal resection

This is a widely accepted method of treatment for oesophageal cancer for two reasons: first, a successful resection with reconstruction of the gastrointestinal tract offers complete and lasting relief from dysphagia; secondly, resection is potentially curative in patients with cancer localized to the oesophagus.

How effectively the goals of safe, successful resec-

tion and cure of oesophageal cancer are achieved by surgery was questioned in the critical review of a collected series of over 80 000 cases published by Earlam and Cunha-Melo.[22] These authors analysed the results of surgical treatment for oesophageal cancer in the 25-year period ending 1978, and found that the average hospital mortality after oesophagectomy was an alarming 33%. However, this review included 36 papers published over 20 years previously, some dating back to the 1950s, with at least 21 authors reporting an experience of less than 30 resections. Hospital mortality has been reduced substantially in the last decade by perioperative nutritional support,[73] by the introduction of prophylactic antibiotics, and by advances in anaesthesia and intensive care medicine. In a more recent report, Muller et al.[74] reviewed 1201 papers on surgical treatment of oesophageal cancer during the period 1980 to 1988 and found the average hospital mortality to be 13%. Thus, hospital mortality rates have more than halved over the last 10 years compared to the figures reported by Earlam and Cunha-Melo in 1980. It appears that oesophagectomy has become a safer method of treatment, with the proviso that it is undertaken by those experienced in the technique: Mathews et al.[68] showed that a negative correlation exists between the number of oesophagectomies performed per annum and hospital mortality, among surgeons. Most surgeons resect and replace the oesophagus using an 'open' or transthoracic approach[74] but an increasing number favour transhiatal resection without thoracotomy – the so-called 'blunt' or blind oesophagectomy – for reduction of the operative risk to the patient.[82] The combination of a thoracotomy wound with an upper abdominal incision produces significant impairment in respiratory function and theoretically avoidance of thoracotomy should reduce the pulmonary complication rate.[29] Respiratory complications are seen less often after transhiatal compared to right transthoracic resection.[74] However, many authors report that hospital mortality, the number of days spent in the intensive care and the duration of hospital stay are not significantly reduced by selection of the transhiatal approach.[32,45,97] It is quite probable that the results of 'blunt' oesophagectomy are adversely affected if high-risk patients are selected for this procedure. However, the results of 'blunt' oesophagectomy will be favourably influenced if the procedure is performed mainly for the distal oesophageal tumours which can be mobilized at least partially under vision and, unlike middle third cancers, are not adherent to the tracheobronchial tree. Prospective, controlled, randomized trials comparing 'blunt' with transthoracic resection for tumours at different levels in the oesophagus are not available to evaluate accurately the role of these surgical approaches.

Complete and lasting relief from dysphagia can only be achieved by oesophageal resection if the anastomosis heals soundly and the margins of resection are sufficient to obviate the risk of anastomotic recurrence. Healing of the anastomosis without leakage or stricture depends less on the technique selected to fashion the anastomosis than on the condition of the patient before and during operation. McManus et al.[71] and Muller et al.[74] found that the incidence of leakage and strictures was not significantly influenced by choice of sutures versus stapling devices. However, the risk of anastomotic leakage and subsequent stricturing is increased in patients in whom cancer hypercatabolism and malnutrition cannot be reversed before surgery; another modality of treatment should be selected for these patients. The dangers of perioperative hypotension leading to anastomotic breakdown has been confirmed by both clinical and experimental studies.[60,87] This observation offers an explanation for the better surgical results in the hands of experienced surgeons who can perform oesophageal resections with the minimum of trauma and blood loss.

The risk of anastomotic recurrence is reduced by resecting 10 cm of macroscopically normal tissue proximal to the cancer. In practice, however, the extent of proximal resection depends on the location of the tumour. It is not always possible to resect 10 cm of normal oesophagus above a cancer in the upper thoracic oesophagus; the surgeon and patient may have to accept the 8% risk of anastomotic recurrence where the proximal resection margin is reduced to less than 10 cm.[104]

Controversy still exists concerning the extent of resection distal to the tumour. Skinner et al.[100] advocate a 10-cm distal margin, but Tam et al.[104] found the incidence of anastomotic recurrence to be solely dependent on the proximal resection margin and Mannell and Becker[61] noted that extending the distal margin of resection from 5 to 10 cm in all cases would benefit less than 1% of patients.

Over the last 10 years, oesophageal resection has not substantially improved the long-term prognosis of patients with oesophageal cancer, despite adoption of such techniques as en-bloc resection[100] and use of adjuvant radiotherapy and/or chemotherapy.[74] In their collected series, Earlam and Cunho-Melo[22] reported a 2-year survival after oesophagectomy of 29%, with 18% of surgical cases surviving 5 years. A decade later, Muller et al.[74] noted that 34% of patients survive 2 years and 20% survive 5 years after oesophageal resection.

Regardless of the surgical approach, operative technique and the type of lymph node dissection, the principal determinants of long-term survival are extent of transmural spread and lymphatic metastases. For those with cancer confined to the oesophagus and no lymph node metastases, the 5-year survival rates range from 22% to 58% for patients undergoing standard techniques of oesophagectomy, extended en-bloc resection or 'blunt' oesophagectomy.[74]

Removal of involved lymph nodes, by whatever method of lymph node dissection, will achieve cure for not more than 10–15% of patients. This supports the observation that the presence of positive lymph nodes is indicative of disseminated disease for the majority of patients.

Adjuvant radiotherapy

Adjuvant radiation therapy, administered preoperatively, offers the theoretical advantages of increasing resectability rate by shrinking bulky tumours, of reducing the risk of tumour inplantation or distant metastases during operation, and of sterilizing the tumour bed. However, the results of studies of preoperative radiotherapy are conflicting. One prospective randomized study from China[44] reported a 46% 5-year survival rate when patients were given preoperative radiotherapy compared to a 25% 5-year survival in those healed by surgery alone. But it is not certain if the two groups in that study were similar with respect to stage of disease. Three other randomized studies[35,46,54] failed to show any benefit from preoperative radiation therapy with respect to resectability rate median or long-term survival. The study by Launois et al.,[54] in which high-dose radiotherapy was administered over 8–12 days increased postoperative mortality. The failure of preoperative radiotherapy to improve survival in these trials is both disappointing and unexpected. However, preoperative radiation therapy has been found to impair cellular immunity significantly in patients with oesophageal cancer.[111,112] It is possible that reduction in the number of total lymphocytes and natural killer (NK) T lymphocytes impairs the host's defence against tumour cells, and this could provide an explanation for the increase in lymphatic invasion and metastases observed by Maeta et al.[58] in irradiated patients.

Muller et al.[74] reviewed the results of five uncontrolled, retrospective studies of postoperative radiation therapy. These showed that radiotherapy significantly improved survival when compared to non-irradiated controls. Kasai et al.[49] observed that postoperative radiotherapy benefited patients with minimal disease, and Mannell and Becker[61] found that survival of patients in whom lateral resection margins were microscopically involved by cancer was significantly improved by radiation therapy to the tumour bed; where all lines of excision were clear of microscopic tumour, radiotherapy had no effect on survival.

Adjuvant chemotherapy

Autopsy studies have shown that 73–85% of patients with squamous cancer of the oesophagus have disease that has disseminated to lymph nodes, liver and lungs.[1,5] These findings have stimulated interest in the use of preoperative chemotherapy to destroy systemic micrometastases. At present nine drugs have been adequately evaluated in the treatment of oesophageal cancer: bleomycin, cisplatin, vindesine, methotrexate, chloroethyl-cycloethyl-nitrosourea (CCNU), mitomycin C, doxorubicin (Adriamycin), 5-fluorouracil, methylglyoxal bisguanylhydrazone (methyl-GAG). Used as single agents, responses to each are similar, occurring in 15–20% of patients and lasting from 1 to 3 months.

Combination of cytotoxic agents will increase the response rate to 40–50% where cisplatin is included in the combination, and prolong the duration of response by several months. Oesophageal cancer can no longer be regarded as resistant to chemotherapy but the response rate is not as favourable as in other solid tumours, such as testicular and ovarian carcinomas. The toxicity of multi-drug therapies can be severe[36] and these are not without risk when given before surgery. Using cisplatin, mitomycin C, bleomycin and prednisone, Kukla et al.[5] reported a postoperative mortality of 45%, with four of the five deaths drug related. In a review of collected series in which chemotherapy was given before surgery, Mannell[62] found no irrefutable evidence that preoperative chemotherapy improved with the resectability or long-term survival rate. Promising results from the combination of cisplatin and methotrexate had been reported by Desai (1985) although the study suffered the disadvantage of using historical controls.[19] Muller et al.[74] reviewed the results of 11 prospective and prospectively randomized trials of preoperative chemotherapy. These authors concluded that preoperative chemotherapy did not increase the resectability rate and that there was no evidence that preoperative chemotherapy substantially improved long-term prognosis.

Preoperative chemoradiation therapy

Response rates using combined preoperative chemotherapy and radiotherapy are much higher than when each modality is used alone, but the collected series reviewed by Mannell et al.[65] and Muller et al.[74] suffer the disadvantage of comparison with historical controls. The substantial morbidity and postoperative mortality rates reported in several studies must be emphasized.[55,63,86] Pulmonary toxicity is a common problem associated with many cytotoxic drugs, and those that sensitize the lungs to the effects of oxygen and infection should be avoided. In their review of 11 prospective and prospectively randomized trials, Muller et al.[74] concluded that resectability was not increased and, in most studies, there was no difference in long-term survival rates and these reported in most studies not using adjuvant therapy.

One hopeful finding has been the absence of residual disease in resected specimens. This is remarkably similar in many of the studies: 27% for methotrexate,[108] 26% for 5-fluorouracil + mitomycin,[33] 33% for 5-fluorouracil + cisplatin.[55] Where a true complete response to preoperative adjuvant therapy is confirmed by pathological examination of resected specimens, the late results are very good: Poplin et al.[92] reported a 45% 3-year survival in the patients who had a complete response to preoperative chemoradiation therapy using cisplatin and 5-fluorouracil.

Although satisfactory long-term control of the primary tumour was achieved in the majority of patients in studies of preoperative chemoradiation therapy, most recurrences develop outside the irradiated volume. This supports the observation that the cytotoxics available for treatment of oesophageal cancer are inadequate and advances in adjuvant therapy awaits the discovery of new and more potent agents.[36] At this time, chemotherapy must be regarded as under evaluation and not a treatment suitable for routine clinical use.

Radiation therapy

Between 40% and 85% of patients with oesophageal cancer present at a late stage of the disease,[25,62] when there is evidence of local spread into the mediastinum, lungs, tracheobronchial tree, recurrent laryngeal nerves and distant metastases. For most surgeons, extraoesophageal spread is a contraindication to surgical resection. Thus, in collected series, the resectability rate has ranged from 25%[24] to 39%.[22] In a review of recent world literature on surgical treatment for oesophageal cancer, Muller et al.[74] found that the average resectability rate was 56%. The percentage of resections in some series increased to over 80% when palliative, incomplete resections were included.[28]

Radiotherapy is generally used in those patients with unresectable tumours and in those who are considered unfit for surgery; there has been no controlled prospective randomized trial of radiotherapy versus surgery for localized oesophageal cancers which are clinically assessed as resectable. However, results published from centres where radiation therapy is the standard treatment for oeso-phageal cancer do indicate what can be achieved by radical therapy given with curative intent. Earlam and Cunha-Melo[23] noted that radical radiotherapy for tumours apparently localized to the oesophagus resulted in a median survival of approximately 12 months and a mean 5-year survival rate of 6%. Slevin and Stout[101] found that the 1-year survival of cases treated by radiation therapy was 40% which is similar to the 48% 1-year survival rate for patients undergoing oesophagectomy.[74]

The response to radiation therapy depends on the site, length, radiological type and histology of the tumour and the results of radiotherapy can be further improved by selecting patients with favour-able lesions. These include those with the following:

1. Cancer of the cervical oesophagus.[89] Newaishy et al.[77] reported a 5-year survival rate of 18.9% for tumours of the cervical oesophagus treated by radiation therapy.
2. Tumours less than 5 cm in length: Beatty et al.[8] found that all T1 lesions (of length less than 5 cm, incomplete circumferential involvement) re-sponded to treatment, and Newaishy et al.[77] reported a 5-year survival rate of 11.9% for patients with tumours less than 5 cm in length.
3. Proliferative or superficial lesions: Morita et al.[72] found that 25% of these tumours were cured by radiotherapy.
4. Well-differentiated squamous carcinomas.[8]

Other factors associated with a good response to treatment include patients aged 70 years or more[8] and female patients.[8,77] Factors associated with a poor response to radiation therapy are tumours longer than 5 cm in men[77] and intrathoracic lesions with radiological evidence of stenosis before treat-ment.[72] However, survival figures do not indicate how effectively complete and lasting relief of dysphagia – the principle goal of treatment – is achieved by radiotherapy.

Beatty et al.[8] found that of 146 patients treated by radical irradiation, the tumour failed to respond to irradiation in one-third of these and, in the other two-thirds, malignant oesophageal obstruction re-curred after the initial response. Gill[36] in reviewing the results of 227 patients treated with radiotherapy at the Royal Adelaide Hospital, noted that only 2% were free of dysphagia in the final phase of their illness.

There is no easy solution to the problem of recur-rent dysphagia after irradiation. 'Salvage' oeso-phagectomy following irradiation is associated with a prohibitive mortality and little hope of cure.[8,90] Earlam[25] has advised repeated oesophageal dila-tations for this problem with insertion of a rigid tube

if dilatation has to be performed too frequently. However, the insertion of an oesophageal tube for postradiation recurrence carries a high mortality with a mean survival of 35 days.[8]

The main attraction of radiotherapy is its safety. The treatment can be stopped when complications occur and, in the hands of expert radiation thera-pists, using doses less then 60 Gy, the incidence of radiation pneumonitis, myocardial damage, peri-cardium and spinal cord injury is very small. How-ever, the final selection of patients for radical radiotherapy must depend on the overall treatment results at the individual institutions.

At centres where both radical radiotherapy and oesophageal resection are treatment options for localized oesophageal cancers, each patient must be assessed with respect to the likelihood that the particular tumour will respond to irradiation, the risks of surgery, and the results of an audit of treatment outcome for these two modalities at the particular centre. If the results of operation in a particular institution compare unfavourably with those obtained by irradiation then, despite its limi-tations, radiotherapy would be the treatment of choice of oesophageal cancer at that institution.

Palliation of oesophageal cancer

At least 50% of patients with oesophageal cancer are obviously incurable by the time they are admit-ted to hospital. These include patients with the symptoms and signs of extraoesophageal spread of tumour and patients who are too ill to safely undergo radical treatment. The modality of treatment selected for patients with advanced disease must satisfy certain criteria: there must be acceptably low mortality and morbidity rates and it must offer prompt relief from dysphagia and pain. The thera-peutic modalities for palliation of advanced oeso-phageal cancer include oesophageal resection, radiation therapy with or without chemotherapy, oesophageal bypass, intubation and fulguration of intraluminal tumour using laser, diathermy or photodynamic therapy.

Oesophageal resection

Successful surgical reconstruction of the oesophagus is the most certain way permanently to restore normal swallowing. This observation, and the knowledge that over 80% of oesophageal cancers are incurable, has led to an aggressive surgical approach to palliation in some centres.

Ellis[27] recorded an overall operability rate of 81.3% in a total of 385 patients with carcinoma of the oesophagus and cardia treatment at the Lahey

Clinic: of the 238 patients undergoing oesophago-gastrectomy, resection was incomplete or palliative in 16.8%. Wong and Siu[110] reviewed the treatment of 311 patients admitted to the Queen Mary Hospital, Hong Kong: 189 patients had an oesophagectomy which was noted to be palliative in 95 patients. In both series the 30-day mortality rates were less than 10% and the quality of palliation was said to be 'good' with most patients able to eat a normal meal. Wong and Siu[110] reported an actuarial 3-year survival of 10% and Ellis[27] a median survival of 7 months for palliative oesophageal resection. Median survival after incomplete tumour excision was similar in the small series reported by Mannell and Becker[61] who also found that survival was not significantly improved by postoperative irradiation of residual tumour.

It is evident that resection can be performed with a low mortality in centres where surgery is the principal modality of treatment, for both cure and palliation. However, the results of palliative surgery from other institutions are less encouraging. Muller et al.,[74] reviewing the results of over 120 000 oesophageal resections, found that the average hospital mortality rate for palliative resection was 19%. The advisability of a treatment that offers the patient almost a one in five chance of dying in hospital with no prospect of cure can be questioned and has led many authors to select non-operative modalities for palliation of oesophageal cancer.

Radiotherapy

The aim of external beam radiotherapy (EBR) is to debulk the luminal content of advanced oesophageal tumours, restoring the ability to swallow. EBR is a widely accepted modality of palliative therapy but a tumour response is not likely to be achieved with doses less than 45 Gy, commonly given from a linear accelerator over a 4- to 5-week period.

However, EBR is contraindicated in patients in poor general health, those too ill to complete the course and those with severe pulmonary disease or a lung abscess which can be exacerbated by 'scatter' into the lungs. Also excluded from EBR are those with malignant invasion of the airways, where radiotherapy may precipitate an oesophageal-airway fistula, and patients with very large tumours or visceral metastases in whom the primary lesion will almost certainly fail to respond to radiation therapy. In the Edinburgh series reported by Pearson[89] only half of the patients with incurable lesions were in fact suitable for radiotherapy and data from the West Midlands Cancer Registry[25] suggest that not more than 20% of patients in Western communities with oesophageal cancer are treated by EBR.

Twenty-one per cent of patients with locally advanced disease undergoing palliative EBR do experience worthwhile improvement in swallowing.[8] This fraction can be increased to 50%[107] with careful selection of patients and supportive care of the patient during treatment. Palliative radiotherapy may be selected as the initial treatment for tumours not longer than 10 cm which are of the fungating or polypoid type (*Figure 1.77*), where the patient has suffered only moderate weight loss and has no serious respiratory impairment. EBR should be considered for all cancers of the cervical oesophagus because a malignant stricture at this site cannot be intubated, an oesophageal resection necessitates laryngectomy plus a tracheostomy for the remaining months of life, and laser fulgarization has a higher risk of complications in the cervical oesophagus.

Nutritional support is essential during treatment: response to radiation therapy is less likely in debilitated cases.[65] If the patient is taking an oral diet the ability to swallow must be assessed repeatedly or a fine-bore Silastic tube passed through the malignant stricture for enteral feeding. Respiratory status should be carefully monitored during EBR: an

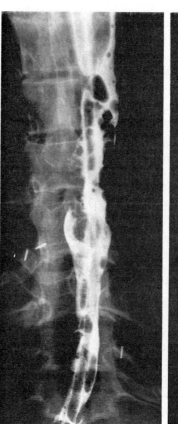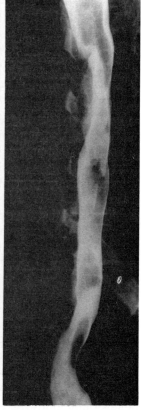

(a) (b)

Figure 1.77 (a) Fungating cancer of the thoracic oesophagus with feeding tube in situ; (b) after palliative radiotherapy.

inflammatory response to radionecrosis can transiently worsen dysphagia with increased risk of aspiration pneumonia and lung abscess. After completion of therapy, swallowing must be re-evaluated: persistent dysphagia will require oesophageal bougienage or insertion of a prosthetic tube.

There is no evidence that the overall results of EBR are influenced by hypoxic cell radiosensitizers, fast neutron teletherapy or helium charged-particle radiotherapy.[3,14,53] However, drug therapy and synchronous or sequential radiotherapy provide a promising avenue of investigation for the palliative management of oesophageal cancer. In experimental models, cisplatin has improved the response rate to radiation therapy.[83] Sequential chemotherapy and radiotherapy regimens using cisplatin or vindesine have extended median and long-term survival in patients with a good performance status.[16,67]

Brachytherapy or intracavitary radiation (ICR) is a recent addition to the modalities of treatment for advanced oesophageal cancer. A radioactive source is inserted into the oesophagus for the administration of a high-dose single fraction. This offers the advantage of a single treatment for rapid palliation. However, administration of ICR requires preliminary oesophageal dilatation, positioning of an applicator under fluoroscopy, a computerized remote afterloading system for the radioactive materials, and special screening rooms to observe the treatment by closed circuit television. Facilities of such a sophisticated nature are not readily available to patients in rural or less developed endemic areas.

Pilot studies have shown that most patients can tolerate the long treatment session of ICR (1–2 hours) and experience an improvement in swallowing,[84] although Bryer *et al.*[11] found that ICR did not influence patient survival. The addition of ICR to EBR is an attractive concept for palliation of oesophageal cancer. The exophytic, hypoxic, necrotic, intraluminal disease is irradiated at higher doses by the intracavitary treatment without affecting adjacent normal tissues, and external irradiation permits a better dose in depth to the peripheral, more oxygenated and hence more sensitive part of the tumour. Hishikawa *et al.*[43] found that the mean survival of patients and ability to swallow were improved by the addition of ICR to EBR, compared to treatment with EBR alone. The results of prospective studies from centres equipped to administer these treatments are awaited in order to evaluate the role of ICR in palliative management of oesophageal cancer.

Hyperthermia, shown in laboratory studies to have a demonstrable anti-tumour effect, has attracted increasing interest as an additional modality for the treatment of oesophageal cancer. Using radiofrequency energies by means of electrodes placed in the oesophagus and on the chest, an anatomical segment of the oesophagus can be made hyperthermic. Sugimachi *et al.*[102] treated 17 tumours with EBR, hyperthermia to 42–43°C for 30 minutes and intravenous bleomycin: 4 patients had a complete response and 10 patients had a partial response. These authors considered that hyperthermo-chemo-radiotherapy has great promise in treating patients with oesophageal cancer.[103] However, prospective randomized trials must be undertaken to allow analysis of the effects of hyperthermia versus chemoradiotherapy before the value of hyperthermia can be assessed.

Bypass surgery

The major disadvantages of radiation or chemoradiation therapy for advanced oesophageal cancer is persistent dysphagia in 50% of patients and recurrence of dysphagia in two-thirds of those in whom the tumour has responded. Recurrence of dysphagia usually occurs 3 months after the therapy.[52]

Palliative resection can permanently restore the ability to swallow but has an unacceptable mortality rate in many centres.[74] Oesophageal bypass surgery is a theoretically attractive alternative to palliative resection: the gastrointestinal tract can be surgically reconstructed without the morbidity and mortality associated with thoracotomy, and a tumour with an intact blood supply is more likely to respond to irradiation than hypoxic residual tumour deposits left in situ after either 'open' or 'blunt' oesophagectomy.

However, the role of bypass surgery in the management of advanced oesophageal cancer is controversial. Some authors in small series[20,96] have reported mortality rates of less than 10% with normal swallowing restored to almost all patients, but large series have reported mortality rates of 28–37%.[80,109] This suggests that results of bypass operations depend more on the selection of patients than on the experience of surgeons, although techniques utilizing stomach are less likely to be complicated than colonic bypass procedures. Mannell *et al.*[66] reviewed the early and late results of bypass surgery and radiotherapy in 124 cases of unresectable oesophageal cancer in an attempt to identify those patients who should be selected for this combined approach and those in whom bypass operations are contraindicated. Hospital mortality rate was an acceptable 7.5% in patients with tumours less than or equal to 10 cm in length and with local extra-oesophageal spread: survival in these patients was significantly improved by the addition of EBR. Bypass surgery offered distinct advantages to those with malignant invasion of the airways who could be made fit for operation: after the oesophagus was bypassed and aspiration prevented, radiation therapy could be safely given. But oesophageal bypass was not safe in those patients with extensive tumours (greater than 10 mm in length and/or fixed nodal metastases), because the hospital mortality rose to 18% and radiation therapy did not improve survival beyond a median of 3 months. For patients in the latter group, in whom no response to EBR can be expected, safer methods of palliation should be selected. Endoscopic intubation, laser fulgurization, photodynamic therapy or ICR may be appropriate for these cases.[66]

Oesophageal intubation

For more than 100 years, attempts have been made to relieve dysphagia by oesophageal bougienage and to maintain the ability to swallow by insertion of a semi-rigid tube through the malignant strictures. These treatments, aimed simply at restoring oesophageal patency, are usually selected for patients with advanced, unresectable disease or who are medically unfit for radical treatment.

Oesophageal bougienage is simple, can be safely performed at endoscopy with fluoroscopic screening[26] and has a low complication rate.[56] However, the method suffers the major disadvantage of rapid recurrence of dysphagia requiring repeated dilatations at monthly intervals (or less). There is little information on the survival of patients managed by dilatation alone. Intubation after initial oesophageal bougienage is a time-honoured method to maintain oesophageal patency. The observation that operative insertion of traction tubes of the Celestin type is associated with mortality rates of 27–30%[20,41,94] led to a search for other techniques of intubation. Pulsion intubation, using a rigid oesophagoscope under general anaesthesia, has a hospital mortality of 16–36% depending on the general status of the patient.[2,93] However, the advent of the flexible fibreoptic oesophagoscope, and the development of tubes suitable for endoscopic placement, have diminished the need for operative and rigid endoscopic intubation. Flexible endoscopic intubation is a safer method, with a technical mortality rate of less than 5% and hospital mortality rates of less than 20% in many series.[34] But the inherent disadvantages of a semi-rigid oesophageal prosthesis remain. Bolus obstruction, dislodgement of the prosthesis and aspiration where the tube crosses the cardio-oesophageal junction are common complications. The quality of palliation is often disappointing: few patients return to a normal diet, about 50% of those intubated are able to swallow soft foods and the remainder are restricted to liquids.[20,34,64]

Oesophageal intubation is usually reserved for patients with advanced malignancy, so short survival after intubation is not unexpected, median survival varying from 2.2 months to 3.2 months.[15,34,93]

Chavy et al.[15] and Oliver et al.[81] found that survival after intubation was not affected by the extent of disease or the administration of radiotherapy. This suggests that in many patients the major factor affecting survival is the presence of the tube; the prosthesis must be incompressible to remain patent and constant pressure on the oesophageal wall will ultimately lead to necrosis and erosion. Delayed perforation from pressure necrosis is one explanation for the short survival following oesophageal intubation.

Nevertheless, endo-oesophageal prostheses continue to have a role in the palliation of oesophageal cancer. They are the method of choice for patients with malignant oesophageal-airway fistulas who cannot reach the level of fitness necessary for bypass surgery, and have been used extensively for large numbers of patients presenting with advanced oesophageal carcinoma in circumstances where resources are severely limited.[17] This method may be selected for frail elderly patients and for those where other methods of palliation have failed.

Endoscopic laser therapy (ELT)

ELT is now recognized world-wide as an acceptable form of palliation for oesophageal cancer. An endoscope is advanced to the oesophageal neoplasm and the laser beam is focused on the tumour tissue. The type of laser usually employed is the neodymium:yttrium–aluminium–garnet (ND:YAG) laser with some variation in technical applications (antegrade versus retrograde, non-contact versus contact, high power versus low power), each of which have their advantages and disadvantages.[30]

Since laser was introduced as a treatment for oesophageal cancer,[31] sufficient experience has accumulated to identify the value and limitations of the method. Destruction of tumour tissue to restore luminal patency can be achieved in 97% of patients in an average of two or three treatment sessions,[69] but up to 30% of patients cannot take an adequate diet after laser treatment.[69,75] Reasons for the discrepancy between luminal patency and functional success include anorexia, a large extraoesophageal tumour mass compressing the oesophagus, treatment complications and poor performance status.[30] However, in this patient group with advanced cancers, any method of palliation is likely to achieve less than ideal results.

A good response to ELT can be expected in exophytic asymmetrical tumours less than 8 cm in length in a straight segment of the mid- or distal oesophagus. The results are not as good and the technical difficulty greatest for tumours of the cervical oesophagus,[30] malignancies resulting in acute angulation of the oesophagogastric junction for tumours with a large submucosal component, especially if these are of the desmoplastic–stenotic variety, and in very long stenotic lesions. ELT is contraindicated in patients with malignant oesophageal-airway fistulas where, unless the fistula is small and the patient can be made fit for bypass surgery, oesophageal intubation is necessary.

ELT is a comparatively safe treatment. Buset et al.[12] compared ELT to intubation; relief from dysphagia was similar for both techniques but morbidity and mortality were higher for oesophageal intubation. The major complication is oesophageal perforation which occurs in 4–5% of patients.[30] However, Murray et al.[75] found that the risks from laser therapy increase with each session of treatment and that complications such as aspiration or perforation are more frequent in older patients with advanced disease. The major disadvantage of ELT is that treatments have to be repeated on average every 4 weeks to maintain luminal patency.[39] Intubation provides more lasting relief of dysphagia.[95] This was confirmed by the results of the prospective randomized trial of ELT versus ELT followed by intubation reported by Barr et al.[7] The complication rate was higher in those treated by intubation than in those receiving ELT alone, but the latter group suffered more frequent recurrence of dysphagia.

To overcome the short-lived effect of ELT, several studies have been undertaken using ELT combined with endoluminal irradiation and with chemoradiation therapy. Using the combination of ELT and endoluminal iridium-192, Bader et al.[6] achieved long-term relief of dysphagia in 80% of patients and observed recurrent stenosis in 20% of cases. Hagenmuller et al.[39] compared ELT alone with ELT and endoluminal radiation but were unable to reproduce the results achieved by Bader et al. Hagenmuller et al. found that restenosis occurred in almost all patients but their dysphagia-free interval could be increased using endoluminal radiation.

Simko and Esseese[98] combined laser with chemoradiation therapy. This is an attractive concept; if swallowing is restored by ELT, the physical and psychological sense of well-being should be improved and the patient better able to tolerate the chemoradiation therapy. They noted that ELT combined with chemoradiation therapy achieved similar survival in patients with advanced disease to those with localized tumours undergoing oesophageal resection. It is evident that prospective trials of ELT combined with other modalities of treatment are necessary to establish the therapeutic choreography of the different treatment options.

Photodynamic therapy

The development of photosensitizing agents in the form of haematoporphyrin derivatives has provided another technique for treating oesophageal cancer with lasers.

Injected intravenously into the patient, haematoporphyrin derivatives are distributed uniformly throughout all tissues of the body but are excreted rapidly from normal tissue and selectively retained in cancer tissue. When these derivatives within the tumour are exposed to laser light of the appropriate wavelength, the haematoporphyrin is activated and converts triplet oxygen to excited singlet oxygen which has a cytotoxic effect. Activation of haematoporphyrin derivatives is possible with both Nd:YAG laser and the argon laser. Because the technique is not dependent on thermal destruction of tissue by high energy levels, it is less likely to be complicated by perforation.[78] However, Thomas and Morstyn[105] found that if the cancer has penetrated the entire oesophageal wall, full-thickness necrosis can occur producing mediastinitis and pleural effusions. Use of haematoporphyrin derivatives results in skin photosensitivity to sunlight for periods of up to 3 months; patients receiving this treatment have to stay out of direct sunlight, wear protective clothing, use sunscreens and assume a nocturnal lifestyle. Good results from photodynamic therapy have been obtained in patients with superficial tumours,[50] but the palliative results in patients with advanced tumours is dependent on the Karnofsky performance status[78] and does not offer greater benefit than conventional ELT.

Electrocoagulation

Johnston et al.[48] developed a large tumour probe which employs bipolar electrocoagulation for its thermal effect. This has been used to palliate oesophageal cancer as a less expensive alternative to laser. Jensen et al.[47] compared the efficacy and safety of low-power YAG laser with the Bipolar Coagulation Probe (BICAP) tumour probe (BTP) for palliation of patients with oesophagogastric cancer. In this non-randomized study, the treatment results and survival were not significantly different in the two groups, although minor complications such as pain and oedema were less frequent in those treated with BTP and strictures developed in 21%

of patients treated with YAG laser. However, laser was safer than BTP for exophytic non-circumferential tumours because it could be focused endoscopically. Both Jensen et al.[47] (1988) and Nava et al.[76] found that relief of dysphagia after electro-coagulation was similar to that achieved by ELT. The average number of treatments required to re-store luminal patency (two) was similar in the two groups of patients and both treatments had to be repeated at an average of every 4 weeks. BTP had the advantage of a lower cost, being readily avail-able in all operating rooms without installation of special equipment and is likely to replace YAG laser for the palliation of circumferential malignant tumours. Prospective randomized trials to compare the two methods should now be undertaken.

Other treatments

Payne-James et al.[88] have used endoscopic injection of ethanol to induce tumour necrosis in a small series of patients with inoperable, unresectable or recur-rent oesophagogastric cancer. The results appear to be similar to those of ELT and BTP. Patients required an average of two treatments to restore luminal patency and the treatment had to be re-peated monthly. There were no complications associated with ethanol-induced tumour necrosis and the method may have potential for palliation of malignant dysphagia.

Management of adenocarcinoma

Adenocarcinomas of the distal oesophagus and car-dia form a specific subgroup of oesophageal malig-nancies. Although the spread of these cancers is similar to that of squamous cell carcinoma, adeno-carcinomas of the oesophagus are usually short, frequently ulcerative in type and have a poorer prognosis than squamous tumours.[38] However, tumours of the cardia are significantly larger than oesophageal adenocarcinomas, although they appear to have a better prognosis[55] than the latter. Both subgroups of adenocarcinoma had a poorer prognosis than squamous cancers in the series reported by Lund et al.[56] Oesophageal resection is the treatment most commonly selected for both palliation and cure because it is felt that chemo-therapy or radiotherapy does not have a significant place in the management of these tumours.[13,24] Resection is usually advised for the rare adenocarci-noma arising from congenital patches of ectopic columnar epithelium or from the oesophageal mu-cous glands remote from the cardia, although

radiotherapy has occasionally resulted in worth-while palliation for the inoperable case.[25]

When oesophagogastric resection is undertaken, the tumour must be removed with adequate margins of normal tissue to prevent local recurrence for both curative or palliative procedures. Bozzetti et al.[9] found that a distal margin of 8 cm was necessary to ensure complete tumour removal and a proximal margin of 10 cm is advised by Skinner.[99]

The extent of the gastric resection varies. Papa-christou and Fortner[85] showed that extended total gastrectomy (ETG), which includes removal of the distal pancreas and the coeliac lymph nodes, resulted in a significantly improved 5-year survival rate compared to proximal subtotal gastrectomy (PSG). The survival advantage for ETG may be as much related to the extent of lymphadenectomy as to the amount of stomach excised. However, in patients with stage III or IV disease, it is appropriate to perform the simplest type of gastrectomy compat-ible with adequate margins to prevent local recur-rence; depending on the tumour size this may necessitate ETG.

Where the adenocarcinoma has arisen in a Barrett's oesophagus, total removal of the columnar-lined segment is necessary because adenocarcinoma has been reported in residual columnar epithelium following resection.[40]

When total gastrectomy plus partial oesophagec-tomy is performed, gastrointestinal continuity can be restored using a Roux-en-Y jejunal loop. In the patients undergoing PSG and partial oesophagec-tomy, an oesophagogastrostomy is the simplest method of reconstruction. For adenocarcinoma aris-ing in a Barrett's oesophagus, the operative method selected will depend on the length of the columnar segment, the degree of shortening and the site of the adenocarcinoma; carcinomas arising in the middle third of the oesophagus will necessitate near-total oesophagectomy using either a transthoracic or a transhiatal approach and gastric reconstruction.[82,10]

It is not usually necessary to perform near-total oesophagectomy in addition to ETC.[13] In these patients an isolated bowel segment, commonly an isoperistaltic colonic segment, is used to reconstruct the alimentary tract.

Survival

Survival after curative resection for adenocarci-noma is dependent on the stage of the disease. In one series of 128 patients with adenocarcinoma undergoing resection, the 5-year survival rate was 18%,[42] although all but one of the long-term sur-vivors had stage I disease. Lund et al.[56] reviewed the results of resection in 339 Danish patients with adenocarcinoma and reported a 36% 5-year survival in those with stage I disease; this fell to 14% for stage II, 5% for stage III and a 3% 5-year survival rate for stage IV cancers.

Some workers have found no difference in survival after resection of squamous and adenocarcinomas;[18,42] but it appears that site of the adenocarcinoma has a significant influence on survival. Lund et al.[56] noted a 5-year survival of 9% for carcinoma of the cardia, which is similar to the 5-year survival after resection of 9.5% reported by Wang and Chien.[106]

The depressing long-term results of patients undergoing incomplete palliative resections for adenocarcinoma were confirmed by Couraud et al.[18] In this group of patients, 91.5% died within the first year and only 4.9% were alive after 2 years.

Bypass procedures have been advocated for palliation of dysphagia in patients with unresectable or metastatic disease. The extrathoracic reversed gastric bypass technique described by Giraud and Berzin[37] may be appropriate for cases without extensive gastric invasion. Intrathoracic bypass procedures and extrathoracic colon bypass are associated with prohibitively high morbidity and mortality rates,[66,79] and are not recommended. Many of the patients with unresectable adenocarcinoma of the oesophagus and cardia are frail and elderly; non-surgical methods of palliation may be most appropriate for these cases, including oesophageal intubation, fibreoptic laser therapy and electrofulguration.

Oesophageal intubation may be performed using the flexible fibreoptic endoscope and a peroral technique as described above. However, intubation of cancers in the distal oesophageal and cardial sites is more difficult than for those higher in the oesophagus because of angulation and distortion of the oesophageal axis at the oesophagogastric junction. Atkinson and Ferguson[4] have advised a two-stage procedure in which gradual oesophageal dilatation is performed before intubation. However, the risk of perforation is still high, with these authors reporting a perforation rate of 8–12.5%. The traction type of intubation necessitating laparotomy has a high mortality, but this may be required if the stricture cannot be dilated from above or if perforation occurs during an attempt at dilatation. Regardless of the technique of intubation, once the gastro-oesophageal junction has been rendered incompetent by a tube passing across it, oesophagogastric reflux is inevitable. Antireflux measures are mandatory in the management of patients undergoing intubation.

Fibreoptic laser therapy (FLT) has been used with encouraging results in palliation of adenocarcinoma at the oesophagogastric junction. Technical difficulties, similar to those experienced during peroral intubation, have been reported for non-contact FLT, and *non-contact laser* and *electrofulguration* are promising alternative methods of palliation. Where adenocarcinoma of the oesophagus and cardia cannot be resected completely, bypass procedures do not prolong survival more significantly than treatment modalities simply aimed at restoring luminal patency. In those patients with unresectable adenocarcinomas, the principal goal of treatment is the relief of dysphagia for the remaining months of life.

Horizons in oesophageal cancer

Treatment

It is unlikely that further refinements in surgical resection or radiotherapy will significantly alter the cure rates of oesophageal cancer. Modifications of the standard methods of oesophagectomy, such as en-bloc resection and extensive lymphadenectomy, or the addition of intracavitary to external beam radiotherapy, have not had any impact on 5-year survival rates once lymphatic spread has occurred. Nodal metastases, present in the majority of patients by the time of diagnosis, are an index of disseminated disease in 85–90% of these cases.

The available cytotoxic drugs have only limited activity in oesophageal cancer. When new potent chemotherapeutic agents are developed, chemoradiation therapy may allow the safe and complete resection of locally advanced tumours and cure patients with disseminated disease.

On the horizon is the development of monoclonal antibodies specific to oesophageal carcinoma antigens. With radioactive labelling of specific monoclonal antibodies, accurate determination of disease would be possible and radio-immunotherapy may become a new therapeutic modality for treatment of oesophageal cancer.

When significant advances in therapy are made, bypass surgery and endoscopic techniques to restore luminal patency will become outmoded methods of palliation. Until that time, technological progress in ultrasonic endoscopy, video-endoscopy, development of new photosensitizing agents to label malignant tissue and spectroscopic analysis could help to define and isolate the pathological process. With this information fed into a computer, a 'smart' laser system for laser aiming and dosimetry delivered selectively to cancer tissue would be a real advance in palliative management. Such 'smart' laser systems are already in use for the non-operative treatment of atherosclerotic obstruction of the coronary arteries and peripheral vasculature.

Detection

The importance of early detection is emphasized by the influence of stage of disease on treatment outcome. The 5-year survival after oesophagectomy for carcinoma in situ is over 90%, that for cancer localized to the oesophagus is 60% but only 10–15% of patients have any hope of cure once lymphatic metastases are present.

Cytological screening can detect early oesophageal cancer in asymptomatic individuals and identify those with dysplastic epithelium. Flow cytometric analysis of malignant tissue has shown that tumours composed of cells with a grossly abnormal DNA content are biologically aggressive. The marriage of cytological screening with flow cytometric DNA analysis offers the potential to detect the precancerous dysplasias and distinguish these from dysplasia of inflammatory origin. A combination of these techniques for cellular analysis will be relevant to screening both high-risk individuals and those in endemic areas.

Tumour markers of sufficient sensitivity and specificity to screen for oesophageal cancer do not exist. However, radiolabelled monoclonal antibodies to oesophageal carcinoma antigens could make serological screening for asymptomatic oesophageal cancer a reality.

Prevention

The cause of oesophageal cancer is unknown, although many risk factors in different areas of the world have been postulated. Avoidance of these risk factors and improvement in nutrition may reduce the incidence of oesophageal cancer. Use of gene mapping to define the subtle differences in genetic material that make an individual vulnerable to the development of oesophageal cancer and identification of the precipitating event – be it exposure to an environmental toxin or an oncogenic virus – offers the hope of prevention. It is in this area that the greatest potential for progress lies.

REFERENCES

1. Anderson, L. and Lad, T. (1982) Autopsy findings in squamous cell carcinoma of the esophagus. *Cancer*, **50**, 1587–1590.
2. Angorn, I.B. (1981) Intubation in the treatment of carcinoma of the esophagus. *World Journal of Surgery*, **5**, 535–541.
3. Asakawu, H., Watanari, J. and Hoshino, T. (1984) Clinical evaluation of hypoxic cell sensitivizor (misonidazole). *Gan to Kagaku Ryoho*, **11**, 1225–1230.
4. Atkinson, M. and Ferguson, R. (1977) Fibreoptic endoscopic palliative intubation of inoperable oesophagogastric neoplasms. *British Medical Journal*, **1**, 266–267.
5. Attah, Z. and Hadja, S. (1968) Benign and malignant tumours of the oesophagus at autopsy. *Journal of Thoracic and Cardiovascular Surgery*, **55**, 396–404.
6. Bader, M., Dittler, M.J., Ultsch, B. *et al.* (1986) Palliative treatment of malignant stenoses of the upper gastrointestinal tract using a combination of laser and after loading therapy. *Endoscopy*, **18**, 27–31.
7. Barr, H., Krasner, N., Raouf, A. and Walker, P.J. (1900) Prospective randomized trial of laser therapy only and laser therapy followed by endoscopic intubation for palliation of malignant dysphagia. *Gut*, **31**, 252–258.
8. Beatty, J.D., De Boer, G. and Rider, W.D. (1979) Carcinoma of the esophagus: pretreatment assessment, correlation of radiation treatment parameter with survival and identification of management of radiation treatment failure. *Cancer*, **43**, 2254–2267.
9. Bozzetti, F., Bonfanti, O., Bufalino, R. *et al.* (1982) Adequacy of margins of resection in gastrectomy for cancer. *Annals of Surgery*, **196**, 685–690.
10. Broe, P.J., Toung, T.J.K. and Cameron, J.L. (1980) Aspiration pneumonia. *Surgical Clinics of North America*, **60**, 155–164.
11. Bryer, J.V., Haffejee, A.A. and Jordan, J.P.L. (1990) Palliative selection therapy in patients with oesophageal carcinoma (Meeting Abstract). *South African Journal of Surgery*, **28**, 118.
12. Buset, B.M., Baise, M., Bourgeous, N. *et al.* (1987) Palliative endoscopic management of obstructive esophageal cancer: Laser or prosthesis? *Gastrointestinal Endoscopy*, **33**, 357–361.
13. Carter, A.D.C. and Anderson, J.R. (1988) Surgery for adenocarcinoma of the cardia – an overview. In: *Surgery of the Oesophagus*, pp. 597–604 (Ed.) Jamieson, G.G. Edinburgh: Churchill-Livingstone.
14. Castro, J.R., Chen, G.T., Pitluck, S. and Phillip, T.L. (1983) Helium charged particle radiotherapy of locally advanced carcinoma of the esophagus, stomach and biliary tract. *American Journal of Clinical Oncology*, **6**, 629–637.
15. Chavy, A.L., Rougier, M., Pieddeloup, C. *et al.* (1986) Esophageal prosthesis for neoplastic stenosis. A prognostic study of 77 cases. *Cancer*, **57**, 1426–1431.
16. Coonley, C.J., Bains, M., Holaris, B., Chapman, R. and Kilsen, D.P. (1984) Cisplatin and bleomycin in the treatment of esophageal carcinoma. *Cancer*, **54**, 2551–2555.
17. Cotton, M.H. and Sammon, A.M. (1989) Carcinoma of the oesophagus in Transkei: treatment by intubation. *Thorax*, **44**, 42–47.
18. Courand, L., Velly, J.F., Clerc, P. and Martigne,

C. (1989) Experience of partial oesophagectomy in surgical therapy of lower and middle thoracic oesophageal cancer: from a follow up of 366 cases. *European Journal of Cardiothoracic Surgery*, **3**, 99–103.

19. Desai, P.B., Advani, S.H., Dinshaw, K.A. *et al.* (1980) The long-term impact of front loading chemotherapy in inoperable esophageal cancer. *Oncology*, **37**(1), 78–82.

20. Diamantes, T. and Mannell, A. (1983) Oesophageal intubation for advanced oesophageal cancer: the Baragwanath experience 1977–1981. *British Journal of Surgery*, **70**, 555–557.

21. Dzienewski, G.P., Gamstatter, G., Klotter, H.J. and Rothmund, M. (1984) Palliative surgical therapy of incurable esophagus cancer by stomach bypass and endotube. *Zentralblatt für Chirurgie*, **109**(24), 1550–1554.

22. Earlam, R.J. and Cunha-Melo, J.R. (1980) Oesophageal squamous cell carcinoma I. A critical review of surgery. *British Journal of Surgery*, **67**, 381–390.

23. Earlam, R.J. and Cunha-Melo, J.R. (1980) Oesophageal squamous cell carcinoma II. A critical review of radiotherapy. *British Journal of Surgery*, **67**, 457–461.

24. Earlam, R.J. (1984) Oesophageal cancer treatment in North East Thames Region, 1981. Medical audit using Hospital activity analysis data. *British Medical Journal*, **288**, 1892–1894.

25. Earlam, R. (1988) Radiotherapy in the management of oesophageal cancer – an overview. In: *Surgery of the Oesophagus*, pp. 579–583 (Ed.) Jamieson, G.G. Edinburgh: Churchill-Livingstone.

26. Eastman, M.C. and Sali, A. (1980) Modern treatment of oesophageal strictures. *Medical Journal of Australia*, **1**, 129–301.

27. Ellis, F.H. (1988) Surgical palliation: esophageal resection – a surgeon's opinion. In: *International Trends in Thoracic Surgery*, Vol. 4, pp. 375–381 (Eds) Delarue, N.C., Wilkins, E.W. and Wong, J. St Louis: C.V. Mosby.

28. Ellis, F.A., Gibb, S.P. and Watkins, S.J. (1985) Overview of the current management of carcinoma of the esophagus and cardia. *Canadian Journal of Surgery*, **28**, 493–501.

29. Fan, S.T., Lau, W.Y., Yip, W.C. and Poon, G.P. (1987) Prediction of postoperative pulmonary complications in oesophagogastric surgery. *British Journal of Surgery*, **74**, 408–410.

30. Fleischer, D. (1989) Endoscopic laser therapy for esophageal cancer: present status with emphasis on past and future. *Lasers in Surgery and Medicine*, **9**, 6–16.

31. Fleischer, D., Kessler, F. and Haye, O. (1982) Endoscopic Nd:YAG laser therapy for carcinoma of the esophagus. A new palliative approach. *American Journal of Surgery*, **143**, 280–283.

32. Fok, M., Siu, K.F. and Wong, J. (1989) A comparison of transhiatal and transthoracic resection for carcinoma of the thoracic esophagus. *American Journal of Surgery*, **158**, 414–419.

33. Franklin, R., Steiger, Z., Vaishampayan, G. *et al.* (1983) Combined modality therapy for esophageal squamous cell carinoma. *Cancer*, **51**, 1062–1071.

34. Game, P.A. and Devitt, P.G. (1988) Intubation for carcinoma of the oesophagus. In: *Surgery of the Oesophagus*, pp. 805–811 (Ed.) Jamieson, G.G. Edinburgh: Churchill-Livingstone.

35. Gignoux, M., Roussel, A., Paillot, B. and Giller, M. (1987) The value of preoperative radiotherapy in esophageal cancer. Results of a study of the EORTC. *World Journal of Surgery*, **11**, 426–432.

36. Gill, P.G. (1988) Chemotherapy in the management of oesophageal cancer – an overview. In: *Surgery of the Oesophagus*, pp. 571–577 (Ed.) Jamieson, G.G. Edinburgh: Churchill-Livingstone.

37. Giraud, R.M. and Berzin, S. (1987) The reversed gastric esophagoplasty in palliation of carcinoma of the esophagus. *Surgery, Gynecology and Obstetrics*, **165**, 111–115.

38. Griffith, J.L. and Davis, J.T. (1980) A twenty year experience with surgical management of carcinoma of the esophagus and gastric cardia. *Journal of Thoracic and Cardiovascular Surgery*, **79**, 447–452.

39. Hagenmuller, F., Sander, C., Sander, R. *et al.* (1987) Laser and endothelium 192-Iridium radiation. *Endoscopy*, **19**, 16–18.

40. Hamilton, S.R., Hutcheon, D.F., Ravich, M.J., Cameron, J.L. and Paubon, M. (1984) Adenocarcinoma in Barrett's esophagus after elimination of gastroesophageal reflux. *Gastroenterology*, **86**, 356–360.

41. Hartley, L. Strong, R., Fielding, G. and Evans, E. (1985) Morbidity and mortality of operative intubation for malignant oesophageal obstruction. *Australian and New Zealand Journal of Surgery*, **55**, 555–557.

42. Hennessy, T.P. and Keeling, P. (1987) Adenocarcinoma of the esophagus and cardia. *Journal of Thoracic and Cardiovascular Surgery*, **94**, 64–68.

43. Hishikawa, Y., Taniguchi, M., Kamikongu, N., Tanaka, S. and Murra, T. (1988) External beam radiotherapy alone or combined with high dose rate intracavitary irradiation in the treatment of cancer of the esophagus in autopsy findings in 35 cases. *Radiotherapy and Oncology*, **11**, 223–227.

44. Huang, G.J., Wang, L.J., Liu, J.S. and Chang, G.Y. (1985) Surgery of esophageal carcinoma. *Seminars in Surgical Oncology*, **1**, 74–83.

45. Hurley, J.P. and Keeling, P. (1990) Transhiatal oesophagectomy – its role for tumours of the middle third of the intrathoracic oesophagus. *Irish Medical Journal*, **83**, 23–25.

46. Husemann, B. (1984) Preoperative radiotherapy or chemotherapy. In: *Cancer of the Esophagus in 1984*, pp. 55–58 (Ed.) Ciuli, R. Paris: Maloine SA Editeur.

47. Jensen, D.M., Machicado, G., Raindall, G.,

Tung, L.A. and English-Zych, S. (1988) Comparison of low-power YAG laser and BICAP tumor proble for palliation of esophageal cancer structures. **94**, 1263–1270.

48. Johnston, J., Quint, R., Petruzzi, C. and Namihira, Y. (1985) Development and experimental testing of a large BICAP probe for palliative treatment of obstructing esophageal and rectal malignancy. *Gastrointestinal Endoscopy*, **31**, 56–60.

49. Kasai, M., Mori, S. and Watanabe, T. (1978) Follow up results after resection of thoracic esophageal cancer. *World Journal of Surgery*, **2**, 543–551.

50. Kouzu, T., Konno, H., Sakuma, Y. *et al.* (1989) The present condition and future of PDT for esophageal cancer in Japan (Meeting Abstract). *Sixth World Congress of Bronchoesophagology* October 15–19, 1989, Tokyo, Japan, p.10.

51. Kukla, L., Lad, T., McGuire, W. and Thomas, P. (1981) Multimodal therapy of squamous carcinoma of the oesophagus (Meeting Abstract). *Proceedings of the ASCO and AACR*, **22**, 449.

52. Langer, M., Choi, N.C. Orlow, E. *et al.* (1986) Radiation therapy alone or in combination with surgery in the treatment of carcinoma of the esophagus. *Cancer*, **58**, 1208–1213.

53. Laramore, G.E., Davis, R.B., Olson, M.H., Cohen, L. and Raghaven, V. (1983) RTOG Phase I study on fast neutron teletherapy for squamous cell carcinoma of the esophagus. *International Journal of Radiation Oncology Biology and Physics*, **9**, 465–473.

54. Launois, B., Delarue, D., Campoin, J.P. and Kerbaol, M. (1984) Preoperative radiotherapy for carcinoma of the esophagus. *Surgery, Gynecology and Obstetrics*, **153**, 690–692.

55. Leichman, L. Steiger, Z., Seyde, H.G. *et al.* (1984). Preoperative chemotherapy and radiation therapy for patients with cancer of the oesophagus: a potentially curative approach. *Journal of Clinical Oncology*, **2**, 75–79.

56. Lund, O., Haserikam, J.M., Aagaard, M.T. and Kimose, H.H. (1989) Time-related changes in characteristics of prognostic significance in carcinoma of the oesophagus and cardia. *British Journal of Surgery*, **76**, 1301–1307.

57. Lundell, L., Leth, R., Lund, T. *et al.* (1989) Palliative endoscopic dilatation in carcinoma of the esophagus and esophagogastric junction. *Acta Chirugia Scandanavia*, **155**, 179–184.

58. Maeta, M., Koga, S., Kanayama, H. and Murakami, A. (1986) Does preoperative radiation for thoracic esophageal cancer promote intramural lymph invasion? *Japanese Journal of Surgery*, **2**, 84–90.

59. Mannell, A. and Plant, M.E. (1988) Lung function and thoracotomy. In: *Surgery of the Oesophagus*, pp. 125–128 (Ed.) Jamieson, G.G. Edinburgh: Churchill-Livingstone.

60. Mannell, A., Lambrechts, H., Becker, P.J. and Oosthuizen, M.M.J. (1990) The effect of intraoperative blood loss transfusion on healing of the oesophageal anastomosis. *Research in Surgery*, **2**, in press.

61. Mannell, A. and Becker, P.J. (1991) Evaluation of the results of oesophagectomy for oesophageal cancer. *British Journal of Surgery*, **78**, in press.

62. Mannell, A. (1988) Update of experience with esophageal cancer: now and tomorrow. *International Trends in General Thoracic Surgery*, **4**, 425–439.

63. Mannell, A. (1987) Resection for oesophageal cancer 1978–1984. Experience at Baragwanath Hospital, Johannesburg. *South African Medical Journal* (Suppl.), 27–29.

64. Mannell, A., Becker, P.J., Melissas, J. and Diamantes, T. (1986) Intubation vs dilatation plus bleomycin in the treatment of advanced oesophageal cancer. *South African Journal of Surgery*, **24**, 15–19.

65. Mannell, A., Becker, P.J., Melissas, J. and Sheils, R. (1988) Palliative treatment of oesophageal cancer with bleomycin and radiation therapy. *South African Journal of Surgery*, **26**, 55–59.

66. Mannell, A., Becker, P.J. and Nissenbaum, M. (1988) Bypass surgery for oesophageal cancer: early and late results in 124 cases. *British Journal of Surgery*, **75**, 283–286.

67. Marcial, V., Velez-Garcia, E., Cintron, J. and Yorach, A.A. (1980) Radiotherapy preceded by multi-drug chemotherapy for carcinoma of the oesophagus: a pilot study of the Radiation Therapy Oncology Group. *Cancer Clinical Trials*, **3**, 127–130.

68. Mathews, H.R., Powell, D.J. and McConkey, C.C. (1986) Effect of surgical experience in the results of resection for oesophageal carcinoma. *British Journal of Surgery*, **73**, 621–623.

69. Mellow, M.H. and Pinkas, H. (1985) Endoscopic laser therapy for malignancies affecting the esophagus and gastroesophageal junction. *Archives of Internal Medicine*, **145**, 1443–1446.

70. McIntyre, A.S., Morris, D.L., Sloan, R.L. *et al.* (1989) Palliative therapy of malignant esophageal strictures with the bipolar tumour probe and prosthetic tubes. *Gastrointestinal Endoscopy*, **35**, 531–535.

71. McManus, K.G., Ritchie, A.J., McGurgan, J., Stevenson, H.M. and Gibbons, J.R. (1990) Sutures, staples, leaks and strictures. A review of anastomosis in oesophageal resection at the Royal Victoria Hospital, Belfast 1977–86. *European Journal of Cardiothoracic Surgery*, **4**, 97–100.

72. Morita, K., Takago, I., Watanabe, M. *et al.* (1985) Relationships between the radiological features of esophageal cancer and the local control by radiation therapy. *Cancer*, **55**, 2668–2676.

73. Muller, J.M., Dienst, C., Brenner, U. and Pichmaier, H. (1982) Preoperative feeding in patients with gastrointestinal carcinoma. *Lancet*, **1**, 68–71.

74. Muller, J.M., Erasmi, H., Stelzner, M., Zieren, U. and Pichlmaier, H. (1990) Surgical therapy of oesophageal carcinoma. *British Journal of Surgery*, **77**, 845–857.

75. Murray, E.F., Powers, G.J., Birkett, D.H. and Care, D.R. (1988) Palliative laser therapy of advanced esophageal carcinoma: an alternative perspective. *American Journal of Gastroenterology*, **83**, 816–819.

76. Nava, H.R., Schuh, M.Z., Nambisan, R., Clark, J.L. and Douglas, H.O. (1989) Endoscopic ablation of esophageal malignancies with the Neodumium–YAG Laser and electrofulguration. *Archives of Surgery*, **124**, 225–228.

77. Newaishy, G.A., Read, G.A., Duncan, W. and Kerr, G.E. (1982) Results of radical radiotherapy of squamous cell carcinoma of the oesophagus. *Clinical Radiology*, **53**, 347–352.

78. Noberto, L., Ruol, A., Cusumano, A. *et al.* (1989) Results after Nd:YAG laser therapy and PDT (photodynamic therapy) of inoperable esophageal and cardial cancers (Meeting Abstract). *Sixth World Congress of Bronchoesophagology* 15–18 October, 1989, Tokyo, Japan, p. 25.

79. Orel, J.J., Vidmar, S.S. and Hrabar, B.A. (1982) Intrathoracic gastric and jejunal bypass for palliation of nonresectable esophageal carcinoma. *International Surgery*, **67**, 147–151.

80. Ong, G.B., Lam, K.H., Wong, J. and Lim, T.K. (1980) Jejunal esophagoplasty for carcinoma of the esophagus. *Japanese Journal of Surgery*, **10**, 15–26.

81. Oliver, S.E., Robertson, C.S., Logan, R.F. *et al.* (1990) What does radiotherapy add to survival over endoscopic intubation alone in inoperable squamous cell oesophageal cancer? *Gut*, **31**, 750–752.

82. Orringer, M.B. (1984) Transhiatal esophagectomy without thoracotomy for carcinoma of the thoracic esophagus. *Annals of Surgery*, **200**, 282–287.

83. Overgaard, J. and Khan, A.R. (1981) Selective enhancement of radiation response in a C_3H mammary carcinoma by Cis-platin. *Cancer Treatment Reports*, **65**, 501–503.

84. Pagliero, K.M. and Rowland, C.G. (1988) Brachy therapy for inoperable cancer of the esophagus and cardia. In: *International trends in General Thoracic Surgery*, Vol. 4, pp. 361–367 (Eds) Delarue, N.C., Wilkins, E.W. and Wong, J. St Louis: C.V. Mosby.

85. Papachristou, D.N. and Fortner, J.B. (1980) Adenocarcinoma of the gastric cardia: the choice of gastrectomy. *Annals of Surgery*, **192**, 58–64.

86. Parker, E.T., Marks, R.D., Kratz, J.M. and Chalhouni, A. (1985) Chemoradiation therapy and resection or carcinoma of the esophagus: short-term results. *Annals of Thoracic Surgery*, **2**, 121–125.

87. Paterson, I.M. and Wong, J. (1989) Anastomotic leakage: an avoidable complication of Lewis–Tanner oesophagectomy. *British Journal of Surgery*, **76**, 127–129.

88. Payne-James, J.J., Spiller, R.C., Misiewicz, J.J. and Silk, D.B. (1990) Use of ethanol induced tumour necrosis to palliate dysphagia in patients with esophagogastric cancer. *Gastrointestinal Endoscopy*, **36**, 43–46.

89. Pearson, J.G. (1966) The radiotherapy of carcinoma of the oesophagus and postcricoid region in South East Scotland. *Clinical Radiology*, **17**, 242–257.

90. Pearson, J.G. (1969) The value of radiotherapy in the management of oesophageal cancer. *American Journal of Roentgenology*, **105**, 500–513.

91. Pearson, J.G. (1983) Radiation therapy for carcinoma of the esophagus. In: *Thoracic Oncology*, pp. 303–325 (Eds) Choi, N.G. and Grillo, H.C. New York: Raven Press.

92. Poplin, E., Flemming, T., Leichman, L. and Seydel, G. (1987) Combined therapy for squamous cell carcinoma of the esophagus: a South West Oncology Group Study. *Journal of Clinical Oncology*, **5**, 622–628.

93. Proctor, D.S.C. (1980) Esophageal intubation for carcinoma of the esophagus. *World Journal of Surgery*, **4**, 451–461.

94. Quist, N., Rytton, N. and Laisen, K.E. (1987) Inoperable oesophageal and cardia cancer. Benefits from Celestin intubation. *Scandinavian Journal of Thoracic and Cardiovascular Surgery*, **21**, 61–63.

95. Richter, J.M., Hilgenberg, A.D., Christiensen, M.R. *et al.* (1988) Endoscopic palliation of obstructive esophagogastric malignancy. *Gastrointestinal Endoscopy*, **34**, 454–458.

96. Rothmund, M., Gamstatter, G. and Seitz, M. (1981) Retrosternal gastric bypass in the treatment of unresectable carcinoma of the esophagus (Meeting Abstract). *Ninety-eighth Congress of the German Society for Surgery*, April 1981, Münich, FRG Deutsch Gezellschaft für Chirurgie, p. A131.

97. Shahian, D.M., Neptune, W.D., Ellis, F.H. Jr and Watkins, E. Jr (1986) Transthoracic versus extrathoracic esophagectomy: mortality, morbidity and long-term survival. *Annals of Thoracic Surgery*, **4**, 237–246.

98. Simko, V. and Esseesse, I. (1990) Esophageal cancer: disease course and role of Nd:YAG laser, chemoradiation therapy and surgery. *Meeting of the American Society of Clinical Oncology*, **9**, A486.

99. Skinner, D.B. (1983) En bloc resection for neoplasms of the esophagus and cardia. *Journal of Thoracic and Cardiovascular Surgery*, **85**, 59–71.

100. Skinner, D.B., Little, A.G., Ferguson, M.K., Sorcano, A. and Staszak, V.M. (1986) Selection of operation for esophageal cancer based on staging. *Annals of Surgery*, **204**, 391–401.

101. Slevin, N.J. and Stout, R. (1989) Carcinoma of the oesophagus – a review of 108 cases treated by radical radiotherapy. *Clinical Radiology*, **40**, 200–203.

102. Sugimachi, K., Inokuchi, K., Kai, H., Hotta, T.,

Kawai, Y. and Shirakami, T. (1984) Newly designed endotract antenna for hyperthermo-chemo-radiotherapy for carcinoma of the esophagus (Meeting Abstract). *Hyperthermic Oncology*, 4th International Symposium, July 2–6, 1984, Aathus, Denmark, Abstract V14.

103. Sugimachi, K., Matsufuji, H. and Kai, H. (1988) Hyperthermia treatment effective for patients with carcinoma of the esophagus. In: *International Trends in General Thoracic Surgery*, Vol. 4, pp. 337–339 (Eds) Delarue, N.C., Wilkins, E.W. and Wong, J. St Louis: C.V. Mosby.

104. Tam, P.C., Siu, K.F., Cheung, H.C., Ma, L. and Wong, J. (1987) Local recurrences after subtotal oesophagectomy for squamous cell carcinoma. *Annals of Surgery*, **205**, 189–194.

105. Thomas, R.J.S. and Morstyn, G. (1988) Laser therapy for oesophageal cancer (1) photodynamic therapy. In: *Surgery of the Oesophagus*, pp. 819–822 (Ed.) Jamieson, G.G. Edinburgh: Churchill-Livingstone.

106. Wang, P.Y. and Chien, K.Y. (1983) Surgical treatment of carcinoma of the esophagus and cardia among the Chinese. *Annals of Thoracic Surgery*, **35**, 143–151.

107. Werner, I.D. (1978) The palliative management of squamous carcinoma of the intrathoracic and intraabdominal oesophagus. In: *Carcinoma of the Oesophagus*, pp. 445–448 (Ed.) Silber, W. Cape Town: A.A. Balkema.

108. Werner, I.D. (1979) The multidisciplinary approach in the management of squamous carcinoma of the oesophagus: The Groote Schuur Hospital experience. *Frontiers in Gastrointestinal Research*, **5**, 130–105.

109. Wong, J., Lam, K.H., Wei, W.I. and Ong, G.B. (1981) Results of the Kirschner operation. *World Journal of Surgery*, **5**, 547–552.

110. Wong, J., Siu, K.F. (1988) Squamous cell carcinoma of the esophagus. In: *International Trends in General Thoracic Surgery*, Vol. 4, pp. 164–180 (Eds) Delarue, N.C., Wilkins, E.W. and Wong, J. St Louis: C.V. Mosby.

111. Ydrach, A.A., Marcial, V.A., Parsons, J. *et al.* (1982) Misonidazole and unconventional radiation in advanced squamous cell carcinoma of the esophagus. A phase II study of the Radiation Therapy Oncology Group. *International Journal of Radiation Oncology Biology and Physics*, **8**, 357–359.

112. Yokoyama, Y., Sakamoto, K., Arai, M. and Akagi, M. (1989) Radiation and Surgical Stress induce significant impairment in cellular immunity in patients with esophageal cancer. *Japanese Journal of Surgery*, **19**, 535–543.

OTHER CONDITIONS

C.G. Bremner

DIVERTICULA OF THE PHARYNX AND OESOPHAGUS

Diverticula may be pharyngeal, midoesophageal or epiphrenic.

PHARYNGEAL POUCH (ZENKER'S DIVERTICULUM)

This is a pulsion diverticulum which starts in the midline posteriorly, through a potentially weak area which lies between the circular fibres of the crico-pharyngeal muscle below, and the oblique fibres of the inferior constrictor fibres above (Killian's dehiscence). The enlarging diverticulum is restricted by the rigid cervical spine, resulting in a deviation to one or other side (usually the left). Further enlargement causes pressure on the oesophagus and eventual obstruction (*Figure 1.78*).

Pathogenesis

It is assumed that the primary abnormality is related to cricopharyngeal muscle dysfunction, but, because the neck of the diverticulum is always above the cricopharyngeal muscle, the nature of the abnormal cricopharyngeal muscle dysfunction is uncertain. Premature contraction, delayed relaxation and spasm are abnormalities found in different series. Of 15 patients with pouches in the author's series, motility studies revealed either a high resting pressure (4), low resting pressure (4), failure of relaxation (1) or prolonged contraction on swallowing. Catheter orientation in the sphincter may explain the inconclusive results reported in most series. Knuff *et al.*[32] oriented the catheter assembly tips and found that the mean pressure in the cricopharyngeal sphincter zone was significantly lower in three of four positions. Complete relaxation occurred on swallowing in all patients in their series, and they therefore question the concept of sphincter in-

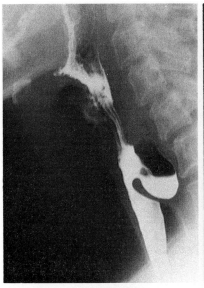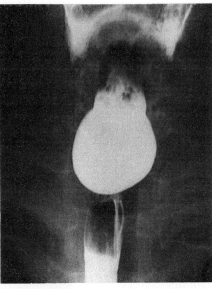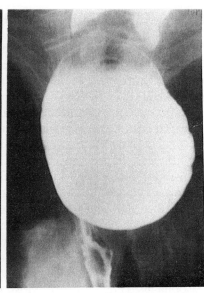

Figure 1.78 Cricopharyngeal (Zenker's) diverticulum: small pouch demonstrating the cricopharyngeal indentation posteriorly (left); medium-sized pouch suitable for myotomy and pexy (middle); large pouch, which required myotomy and excision (right).

coordination in patients with Zenker's diverticulum.

The cause of the cricopharyngeal abnormality is also incompletely understood. An associated hiatus hernia ranging from 22% to more than 90% has been reported[20] and Gage-White[23] found that this incidence was statistically relevant (39% hiatus hernias in 104 patients). Neuromuscular incoordination due to ageing or irritation from cervical osteophytes is another unproven theory of origin.

Clinical features

Most patients are elderly and present with increasing dysphagia, aspiration and weight loss. Diagnosis is best made on barium swallow examination. Cineradiology is a useful investigation especially in early cases. Fibreoptic endoscopy should be cautiously performed. Radiological and endoscopic assessment to exclude an associated hiatus hernia is also necessary. There is a small risk of developing squamous carcinoma, but less than 30 cases have been reported world-wide.[16]

Treatment

There are six methods of treatment:

1. Dilatation with Maloney mercury bougies will give only temporary relief.
2. Surgical cricopharyngeal myotomy: a 3–5 cm myotomy to include the upper oesophagus gives excellent results in diverticula of diameter 2 cm or less.
3. Surgical myotomy plus diverticulopexy to the prevertebral fascia is the preferred treatment in many centres for diverticula of 2–5 cm diameter, because of its safety.[20]
4. Excision and cricopharyngeal myotomy for large diverticula (+5 cm diameter).
5. Surgical inversion: Bowdler and Stell[8] compared excision plus myotomy with inversion and myotomy, and they believe that inversion is the treatment of choice because of a lower complication rate. The author has not used this method.
6. Internal pharyngo-oesophagotomy (Dohlman's technique):[15] the common wall between the diverticulum and the oesophagus is divided endoscopically. A revision of the technique using laser division has given reported success in 91.5% of 211 patients.[56] The disadvantage of this technique is a small risk of mediastinitis, and recurrence is more common.

Despite the failure to reach consensus on the physiological abnormality of the cricopharyngeal sphincter in Zenker's diverticulum, most authors advocate the addition of a cricopharyngeal myotomy. Radiological recurrence is more common after excision without myotomy, but few of the radiological recurrences are symptomatic. The recurrence rate at the Mayo Clinic after diverticulectomy alone was 3.6% (888 operations).[27] Myotomy should be avoided in the presence of a hiatus hernia with severe gastro-oesophageal reflux in order to avoid the risk of aspiration.

MID-OESOPHAGEAL DIVERTICULUM

Traction mid-oesophageal diverticula due to tuberculous mediastinal glands are uncommon and are usually symptom free. Pulsion mid-oesophageal diverticula are frequently associated with disordered oesophageal motility. In one series motor abnormalities were found on manometric studies in 16 of 28 patients tested without provocation.[47] Reflux oesophagitis may be associated with oesophageal dysmotility in some patients.

Symptoms are usually related to the underlying motor disorder, and not to the diverticulum. Dysphagia, chest pain and reflux symptoms may be present. Regurgitation may occur when the diverticulum reaches a large size and when the diverticulum fills with food before spilling over into the distal oesophagus (*Figure 1.79*). Most patients can be managed conservatively by treating the associated reflux or spasm. Surgery is indicated when medical therapy proves to be unsatisfactory. A long oesophagomyotomy distal to the excised diverticulum is performed via a right thoracotomy. Recurrence has been recorded when excision was performed without myotomy.[47]

EPIPHRENIC DIVERTICULUM (*Figure 1.79*)

Most patients with epiphrenic diverticula have associated disease of the distal oesophagus. Oesophageal muscle hypertrophy, spasm and achalasia have been reported to be associated with these diverticula.[13,47] Motor abnormalities related to gastro-oesophageal reflux may also be present. Dysphagia and chest pain are the common associated symptoms. A barium swallow will demonstrate the diverticulum and assess the size of the pouch, whilst motility studies may detect the motor abnormality. Provocative studies may be necessary if routine manometry is negative.

If achalasia is the primary disorder, surgical intervention will be necessary. A modified Heller-type myotomy with or without excision of the diverticulum is indicated. Small diverticula (<3 cm) do not require excision.

OESOPHAGEAL WEBS

A web is a mucosal abnormality which protrudes into the oesophageal lumen. It may be found at any level of the oesophagus, and may be congenital or acquired. Congenital webs are usually situated in the mid- or lower oesophagus and are rarely double. Acquired lesions are either idiopathic or associated

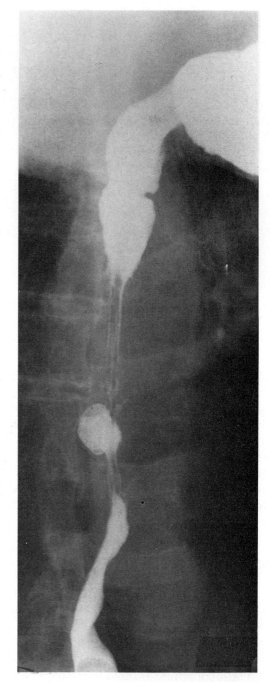

Figure 1.79 Mid-oesophageal diverticulum: a hiatus hernia and Schatzki's ring are also present.

with epidermolysis bullosa, chronic graft-vs-host disease following allogeneic bone marrow transplantation[37] or iron-deficiency anaemia. Acquired webs are usually situated in the postcricoid region (*Figure 1.80*). Only 60% of patients with postcricoid webs have anaemia[12].

A possible relationship to gastro-oesophageal reflux has been reported.[35] A mechanically defective lower oesophageal sphincter was found in 11 of 15 patients with webs who had been tested manometrically. Seven of these 15 patients also had hypo-motile responses to swallowing in the body of the oesophagus. Khosla[31] studied the association of iron-deficiency anaemia with cervical webs in an Indian population of 2840 patients. Of the 117 patients with iron-deficient anaemia, 15 (13%) had dysphagia and 6 of these had webs. Many webs are asymptomatic and are reported after barium swallow examinations. (*Figure 1.80*) Cervical dysphagia develops when the ring occludes the lumen. The lesion may be missed if a routine barium swallow is performed; endoscopy may also miss the lesion or even unknowingly rupture a thin web. Cine-radiology is the most useful investigation in this condition.[19]

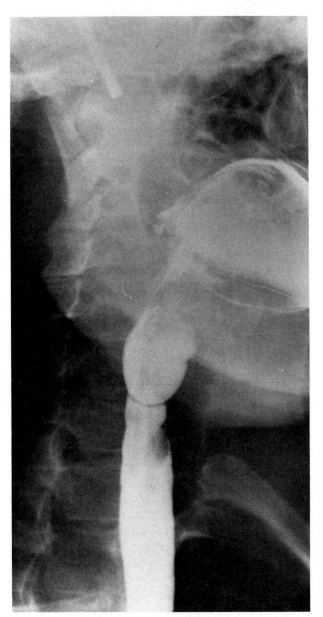

Figure 1.80 Oesophageal web.

The 15 patients in the author's series have all been managed by dilatation. A Maloney mercury bougie dilatation was adequate treatment in most patients. In two patients with a pin-hole opening in the web a guide-wire was passed through the opening and a Celestin bougie used for dilatation.[9] Occasionally repeated dilatation is necessary. Surgical excision via a right thoracotomy has been used on patients resistant to dilatation,[28] and this is an uncommon necessity.

OESOPHAGEAL RINGS

Ring-like defects in the lower oesophagus may be one of the following:

1. Mucosal rings.
2. Muscular or contractile rings.
3. Ring-like peptic strictures.
4. Neoplastic (leiomyoma) ring.
5. Vascular rings.

PATHOLOGY

The most common ring is the mucosal or Schatzki's (see *Figure 1.79*) ring which is a thin submucosal circumferential scar at the squamocolumnar junction which probably develops in response to gastro-oesophageal reflux.[18,59] They may be seen in 6–14% of routine barium meal examinations.[26] Microscopic examination of excised specimens of the ring contain stratified squamous epithelium on the upper surface and columnar epithelium on the lower surface. There may be hyperkeratosis of the squamous epithelium. A cellular infiltrate of lymphocytes, plasma cells and, rarely, polymorphonuclear leukocytes is seen in the lamina propria, attesting to a chronic and sometimes an acute inflammatory reaction.

The pathology of symptomatic muscular rings has been rarely described. Hypertrophic muscular bundles have been documented proximal to the squamocolumnar junction, and appear radiologically as a broader constriction than seen with mucosal rings. A ring-like peptic stricture presents with marked inflammation and submucosal fibrosis.

Uncommonly a leiomyoma may present as a ring. Vascular rings are more commonly associated with aberrant subclavian vessels in the upper oesophagus, but have been described in association with an aberrant intercostal artery.[57]

CLINICAL FEATURES

Many patients with radiological rings have no symptoms. Dysphagia and reflux symptoms may present the patient to the clinician. Dysphagia rarely develops until the lumen is less than 20 mm in diameter.

The 'steak-house syndrome'[42] is the classic presentation in which intermittent complete oesophageal obstruction, often during rapid eating of meat and bread, may occur at a steak dinner. Radiology, endoscopy and ambulatory pH studies will help to confirm the presence of reflux and the cause (see page 86).

TREATMENT

Dilatation with Maloney bougies and medical antireflux therapy will relieve most patients. However, if serious gastro-oesophageal reflux is documented, antireflux surgery should be considered. Leiomyomas will require surgical removal. Very occasionally surgical excision of a ring may be necessary.[39]

INFECTIONS OF THE OESOPHAGUS

Infective oesophagitis may be bacterial, viral or fungal, and of an acute or chronic nature. Acute streptococcal or diphtheritic oesophagitis may be secondary to upper respiratory tract infection. Tuberculosis and syphilis have been uncommon causes of chronic oesophagitis, but oesophageal tuberculosis has recently become more commonly associated with AIDS. Deep oesophageal ulceration and fistulation in a patient with AIDS strongly suggests tuberculosis.[14] Candida oesophagitis is the most common infective oesophagitis, and other less common mycotic infections are actinomycosis, mucormycosis, histoplasmosis and blastomycosis.

CANDIDA OESOPHAGITIS

Candida oesophagitis is caused by *Candida albicans*, which is a commensal organism found in the mouth and pharynx. Infection usually occurs in immunologically compromised people. Fibreoptic endoscopic biopsies were positive for candidiasis in 27% of patients with oesophageal cancer and 15% of patients with oesophagitis in the Scott and Jenkins study.[50] Blind brushing of the oesophagus is an economical and safe way to diagnose candidal oesophagitis in patients with AIDS.[6]

Patients present with dysphagia, retrosternal pain, vomiting or gastro-intestinal bleeding. Ulcer-

ation, perforation, fistulation into the aorta and stricture are complications.

Treatment

Antibiotics, steroids and immunosuppressive agents should be withdrawn and every effort made to improve the nutritional status of the patient. Drug therapy with nystatin (500 000 U 6-hourly, orally), amphotericin B (100–200 mg orally 6-hourly), imidazole and triazole derivatives are effective. The imidazole group includes clotrimazole, econazole, ketoconazole and miconazole. Econazole is used for local treatment as can miconazole. Ketoconazole is better absorbed and may cause fatal hepatotoxicity. Fluconazole is an oral triazole effective for candidiasis in a dose of 50 mg daily for 7–14 days.

VIRAL OESOPHAGITIS

The herpes simplex virus is the usual organism; herpes zoster infection is uncommon. Cytomegalovirus has been reported with increasing frequency. Human papilloma virus can cause papillomatosis[2,61] in the oesophagus. These infections are usually seen in debilitated and immunosuppressed patients, particularly those with leukaemia, but may occur with debilitating non-malignant disease. Patients may be symptom free or complain of dysphagia or chest pain. Ulceration, vesiculation and erosions are seen on endoscopy, and typical ground-glass intranuclear inclusion bodies can be seen on cytology.

Herpetic oesophagitis is usually self-limiting in healthy patients. In immunocompromised patients chemotherapy and antibiotics should be withheld. Acyclovir (200–400-mg orally five times daily for 5 days) can limit the duration of the illness.

IRRADIATION AND CHEMOTHERAPY OESOPHAGITIS

Irradiation to the cervical region or mediastinum may cause abnormal motility, ulceration and stricture[24] formation. Radiation injury is usually self-limiting and strictures that occur 3–18 months later are exceptional. Most strictures respond well to dilatation, and hydrocortisone injection into the area of a stricture may be successful.[41]

When combined with chemotherapy (especially doxorubicin or actinomycin D), even low doses of radiotherapy (less than 20-Gy) can cause oesophagitis with strictures. Recurrent episodes of oesophagitis may result from each dose of chemotherapy.[5]

FOREIGN BODIES IN THE OESOPHAGUS

Obstruction of the oesophagus by foreign bodies occurs in young children who accidentally swallow coins and other objects, and in middle-aged adults who obstruct with a food bolus resulting from a pre-existing stricture or a motility disorder of the oesophagus (*Figure 1.81*).

Meat and fish bones, marbles, dentures, thermometers, pins, needles, screws, nails, button batteries and even razor blades are other items that impact. Most foreign bodies impact at the points of physiological narrowing such as the pharyngo-oesophageal junction, aortic arch and diaphragmatic hiatus. A foreign body may also abrade the oesophagus and pass into the stomach leaving a sensation of discomfort. If left unattended, a foreign body may ulcerate through the wall and form a pouch in the posterior oesophageal wall. Postero-anterior and lateral radiographs of the chest and the lateral cervical spine should be taken in all cases to define the site and nature of the foreign body. Air seen in the prevertebral space indicates a perforation. Not all foreign bodies are opaque and a Dionosil swallow may be useful. Gastrografin is potentially dangerous because aspiration causes pulmonary oedema. A metal detector has been used to locate the site of a swallowed razor blade when chest radiographs and gastrografin swallows are negative.[30]

TREATMENT

Until recently, rigid oesophagoscopy under general anaesthesia was the method of choice for the removal of foreign bodies in the oesophagus. The following additional methods have been reported:

1. Fibreoptic removal.[3]
2. Bougienage technique[7] to push the foreign body into the stomach.
3. Foley catheter removal.[33]
4. Glucagon, effervescent agent and water[29] for food impaction.
5. Digestion of foodstuff with proteolytic enzyme.

All of these techniques have been performed without general anaesthesia and are also used in children. Removal may be difficult if presentation is with long-standing obstruction. Fibreoptic endoscopic removal has also been successful for fish and chicken bones. Objects with a sharp cutting edge

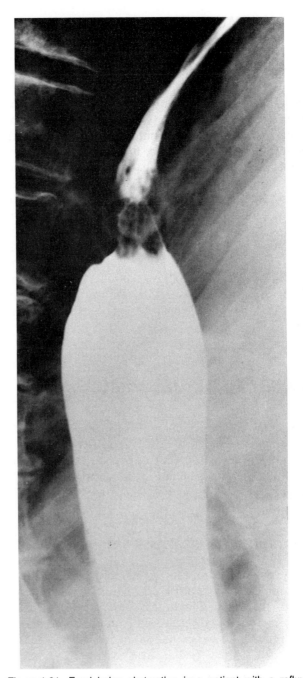

Figure 1.81 Food bolus obstruction in a patient with a reflux oesophageal stricture.

such as razor blades must only be removed if a sheath can be attached to the fibreoptic endoscope to advance over the object. Alternatively, a rigid scope will be necessary so as to pull the object into the scope for extraction. Fibreoptic removal is preferable in patients who have severe cervical spondylosis. Proteolytic digestion with papaine is contraindicated if there is any suspicion of mucosal erosion, and should preferably be avoided.

BUTTON BATTERIES

Impacted button batteries have a special significance. When lodged in the oesophagus button batteries may leak a caustic solution of 26–45% sodium
or potassium hydroxide which can cause serious
damage to the oesophagus.[36] Heavy metal poisoning is another potential hazard.[52] When viewed in an
anteroposterior projection, these batteries demonstrate a double density shadow due to their bi-
laminar structure. On lateral view the edges of most
disc batteries are rounded, unlike a coin. Despite
the potential hazards, current management is variable, and many practitioners have not been particularly concerned about them,[52] and have only acted if
the battery has not progressed on repeated radiographs. Swallowed dentures, large foreign bodies or
hooks may require surgical removal via either a
cervical or a thoracic route.

INJURY TO THE OESOPHAGUS

Oesophageal injury may be instrumental, spontaneous (emetogenic syndrome) or traumatic. Of 69
patients treated in 1 year in one series,[22] the perforation was iatrogenic in 33 (48%), spontaneous in
8 (12%) and the result of external trauma in 23
(33%).

INSTRUMENTAL PERFORATION

Any diagnostic or therapeutic procedure on the
oesophagus carries a risk of perforation. Flexible or
rigid endoscopy, dilatation of strictures and achalasia, sclerotherapy for varices, intubation prosthesis
and intracavitary irradiation are the usual causes.
Anterior spinal fusion also carries a risk of
perforation.

The most common causes are by rigid oesophagoscopy and dilatation of strictures. Oesophageal
perforation is a highly lethal condition unless it is
diagnosed early and treated vigorously. The clinician must always be alerted to the possibility of such
a disaster when performing these investigations and
treatments.

Clinical features

Chest pain following any procedure is highly suggestive of oesophageal damage. The pain is initially
fairly well localized to the neck, chest or epigastrium, and is severe. The patient is usually febrile.

Subcutaneous emphysema, pneumomediastinum,
dyspnoea and a tension pneumothorax may occur.

Investigations

A plain radiograph of the neck and chest will usually
reveal subcutaneous emphysema. A widened retropharyngeal space on lateral cervical films, air in the
prevertebral tissue planes and loss of the cervical
spine curvature are signs that the clinician must be
aware of. A Dionosil or Lipiodal swallow should be
the first contrast study. However, small leaks may-
be missed by water-soluble compounds. Careful
endoscopic visualization may be necessary if the
diagnosis is in doubt.

Treatment

Treatment may be conservative or surgical, and
should be individualized for each patient.

Conservative treatment

This is generally reserved for perforations that are
small, extrathoracic, and unassociated with pleural
effusions or underlying oesophageal disease. Non-
surgical management of oesophageal perforation
from pneumatic dilatation has been satisfactory in a
few reported instances.[53] Initial non-operative
treatment is usually the choice in patients who have
a diagnosis made only after 24 hours. Treatment
consists of antibiotics and intravenous feeding,
nasogastric drainage and intercostal drainage for
effusions or pneumothorax.

Primary surgical closure

This gives excellent results (92% survival) in early
cases, and is the treatment of choice at the Mayo
Clinic.[49] Intraoperative strengthening of the closed
perforation using a flap of pleura or pericardium
(Grillo technique) provides extra security.[25] If the
closure is at all in doubt, a controlled fistula technique using a T-tube is a safer alternative.[40]

Should mediastinitis develop, continuous oral
transoesophageal irrigation and drainage of the irri-
gating fluid by accurately positioned chest tubes
connected to suction may salvage a life-threatening
situation.[48] There is also a place for oesophageal
diversion for large perforations with extensive contamination, particularly when perforations are in
the lower thoracic oesophagus. A cervical oesophagostomy and closure of the gastro-oesophageal junction with gastric or colon interposition at a later date
may be necessary.

Immediate resection is a wise alternative when
resectable cancers have been perforated. The results

in two patients in their early seventies were excellent in the author's experience and Yeo *et al.*[63] have successfully treated four perforated cancers by transhiatal oesophagectomy.

EMETOGENIC SYNDROMES

Vomiting may cause a mucosal tear (Mallory–Weiss syndrome), oesophageal rupture (Boerhaave's syndrome) or an intramural rupture with haematoma formation.

Mucosal tears usually settle spontaneously, and rarely require sclerotherapy, laser therapy or operative intervention (see 'Gastrointestinal bleeding'). Oesophageal rupture (spontaneous rupture) is an extremely serious condition and has a high mortality rate unless the condition is recognized early and treated vigorously by surgical-closure and drainage.

Sudden severe pain after vomiting may mimic a heart attack or perforated peptic ulcer. Urgent chest radiographs and contrast swallows will usually confirm the diagnosis.

The management is similar to that described for instrumental perforation, but there is no place for conservatism and urgent surgical closure is mandatory. Late cases are managed as for late instrumental perforation. Intramucosal haematomas cause dysphagia, and contrast studies are usually diagnostic. Treatment is conservative.

EXTERNAL TRAUMA

Damage to the oesophagus by blunt trauma is exceptionally uncommon. Traumatic rupture by gunshot wounds and stabs require urgent surgical intervention.

CHEMICAL AND PHYSICAL OESOPHAGEAL DAMAGE

CORROSIVE POISONS

Accidental ingestion or suicidal attempts by young adults still occur fairly frequently because of the easy availability of corrosive poisons. They are usually either strong alkalis such as lye containing sodium or potassium hydroxide, or strong acids such as battery acid (sulphuric), pool acid (hydrochloric) and phosphoric acid. Other caustic agents include ammonia (oven cleaners), potassium permanganate, iodine, creosote, Lysol, paint remover and dry ice. Strong alkali is odourless and therefore the agent is com-

monly taken accidentally by children. Alkalis cause a liquefaction necrosis whereas acid agents cause a coagulation necrosis with eschar formation. Acids are more likely to cause gastric burns than are alkalis, and also result in a more severe systemic reaction. Up to 87% of acid ingestion cases have severe oesophageal damage and 38% develop strictures.[64] Involvement of all layers of the oesophagus may lead to perforation, mediastinitis, tracheo-oesophageal fistula and even erosion into the aorta. The ulcerating surface of a deep burn may be secondarily infected with *Escherichia coli*, *Klebsiella* sp., staphylococci and *Candida* sp.

Any strictures that develop may be localized, generalized, single or multiple. Pyloroantral obstruction is more likely with acid ingestion (*Figures 1.82* and *1.83*). In Tucker and Yarington's series of 3000 lye ingestions,[55] 4% resulted in strictures and 2% died compared to 33% strictures and an 18% mortality in 366 acid ingestions. In the author's own series of 59 corrosive burns 20 developed serious strictures and 1 patient died.[10]

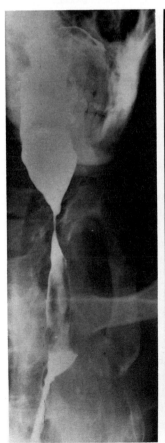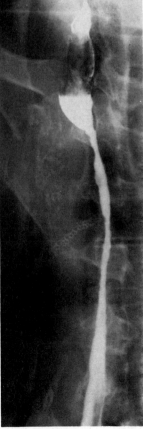

Figure 1.82 Corrosive stricture of the oesophagus: cervical stricture (left); long stricture in mid-oesophagus (right). This patient was suitable for a colon interposition.

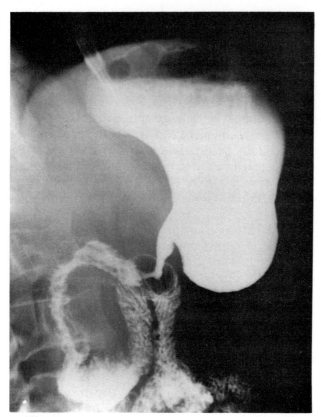

Figure 1.83 Acid-induced antral stricture which required antrectomy.

Clinical features

Signs and symptoms are unreliable indicators of severe injury; indicators are chest and epigastric pain, inability to swallow saliva, fever, tachycardia, shock, peritonitis, haematemesis, confusion, acidosis or evidence of coagulopathy. A late stricture can develop in a patient who was previously symptom free. Acute supraglottic oedema may necessitate urgent tracheotomy, and aspiration can cause acute pulmonary oedema. Dubost and Celerier[17] found tracheobronchial involvement in 9 of 100 severe caustic burns, and this complication carries a high mortality rate.

Treatment

Residual crystals of solid corrosives should be wiped out of the mouth as a first-aid measure. Emetics must not be given. Early management is supportive, for treating shock and pain. Fibreoptic endoscopy is a safe procedure and is performed within 36 hours to establish the extent and severity of damage. It has been the rule to pass the endoscope only to the site of the burn to avoid the risk of perforation, but this risk is minimal if a paediatric fibreoptic endoscope is used. In severe necrotizing lesions, the instrument should not be passed through the damaged area. Early chest and abdominal radiography may give evidence of mediastinitis, peritonitis or gastric perforation. If the patient can swallow, a contrast study (Dionosil) is useful to exclude perforation. Gastrografin may cause pulmonary oedema if aspirated, and is contraindicated in these patients. An atonic dilated oesophagus with gas trapping suggests muscle necrosis and impending perforation.

Antibiotics (ampicillin or a cephalosporin) are given for 10 days and nystatin for 5 days. Several studies have questioned the use of steroids,[21] and recently Anderson *et al.*[1] showed no benefit from their use in 60 patients (median age 2 years) studied over an 18-year period. Stricture developed in 10 of 31 children treated with corticosteroids and in 11 of 29 controls. The author's group no longer uses corticosteroids with patients.

Intraluminal stenting using a tailored length of Silastic tubing to prevent stricturing has been described by Reyes and Hill,[46] but this method has not gained popularity. The author has used the technique on six serious burns with complete failure in three.

There is also controversy over the optimal time to begin dilatation. Some authors have stressed the importance of maintaining the patency of the oesophageal lumen using a Ryle's or Levin's tube which is inserted on admission. The first dilatation may begin as early as 3–4 days using mercury-filled bougies. The author's practice is to wait for re-epithelialization and to begin dilatation with Maloney bougies at 3 weeks.[9]

Established strictures may require guided bougienage using Celestin or Savary dilators[9] or balloon dilators (Wilson-Cooks Medical Inc., Ontario). Attempts to control stricture formation by reducing collagen precursor transport or by interfering with collagen cross-linking have been successful in the experimental animal, but the drugs used (penicillamine, aminoproprionitrile) are too toxic for human use.[44]

Emergency resection of the stomach or oesophagus may be necessary in about 2% of patients. Severe strictures may require gastric or colon interposition. The author's preference is to use colon for young patients or when there is any gastric damage.

Further controversy has arisen concerning whether the oesophagus should be resected or bypassed because of the risk of developing carcinoma. The risk of developing carcinoma is less than 5% and the interval from injury to cancer change is 24–45 years.[4] This low incidence must be measured against the increased risk of resectional surgery. Perioesophageal fibrosis makes the resection more difficult. Ti[54] and others, however, have not found excision to be a hazardous procedure if performed soon after the injury.

DRUG-INDUCED OESOPHAGEAL DAMAGE

Oesophageal injury may result from tablet-induced oesophagitis, sclerotherapy, chemotherapy and irradiation.

Tablet-induced oesophagitis is likely to occur in elderly patients who have poor peristaltic activity in the oesophagus, and when tablets are swallowed without the aid of an adequate fluid bolus. Thirty-two different types of tablets have been reported to cause ulceration or stricture formation in the oesophagus, and every tablet should be regarded as having potential corrosive properties, in particular, doxycycline, tetracycline, emepromium bromide, potassium chloride, anti-inflammatory drugs and ferrous sulphate.[11] It is therefore very important when prescribing tablets or capsules to instruct patients to swallow them with the aid of a drink of water, and only to take tablets when in the upright position.

Sclerotherapy for control of oesophageal varices can cause ulceration and stricturing which is usually self-limiting, or easily controlled with gentle bougienage.

OESOPHAGEAL INVOLVEMENT BY SYSTEMIC DISEASE

The pharyngeal phase of swallowing may be affected by systemic disease and these are dealt with earlier under 'Cricopharyngeal disorders' (page 43). Systemic diseases affecting the oesophagus and lower sphincter are given in *Table 1.22*.

PROGRESSIVE SYSTEMIC SCLEROSIS (PSS)

This is the most common collagen disorder to affect the oesophagus. It occurs in the third to fifth decade and affects females more frequently than males. The 5-year survival is 33–70%.[58]

Pathology

The oesophagus is affected in up to 80% of patients with PSS. The small bowel, colon and stomach are also affected in this order of frequency. Oesophageal involvement may precede other systemic symptoms. The striated muscle is unaffected in contradistinction to polymyositis which affects the

Table 1.22 Systemic diseases that may affect the oesophagus

Collagen diseases
    Progressive systemic sclerosis ('scleroderma')
    Dermatomyositis
    Polymyositis
    Mixed connective tissue disease
    Lupus erythematosus
    Polyarteritis nodosa

Autoimmune disease
    Sjögren's disease

Neuropathy
    Diabetes mellitus
    Chronic alcoholism

Skin diseases
    Epidermolysis bullosa dystrophica
    Pemphigus
    Behçet's disease
    Steven–Johnson syndrome

smooth and striated muscle components of the oesophagus. The disease is characterized by a progressive weakening of the oesophageal muscle and the lower sphincter. Reflux therefore occurs through a mechanically defective lower sphincter and oesophageal clearance is markedly compromised because of the absence of motor power.

The main complication of scleroderma of the oesophagus is therefore serious reflux oesophagitis and stricture formation. A barium meal in the upright position shows rapid transit into the stomach (in contradistinction to achalasia where there is hold-up). In the supine position, however, there is no progression of barium into the stomach. Once a stricture develops, the radiological features may mimic achalasia, and endoscopy is necessary to confirm the presence of a reflux stricture. Because of the continued reflux a columnar-lining, Barrett's oesophagus may develop[51] (see 'Gastro-oesophageal reflux disease' page 82).

The presence of anticentromere antibodies in early scleroderma helps to predict the pattern of scleroderma which will evolve.[45] If antibodies are absent, a rapidly advancing or diffuse scleroderma is likely, whereas if antibodies are present, limited scleroderma or the CREST syndrome (calcinosis, Raynaud's syndrome, oesophageal dysfunction, sclerodactyly and telangiectasia) is more likely to develop.

Treatment

Therapy is aimed to prevent complications of reflux, and double doses of H_2-receptor antagonists or omeprazole should be used. There is some evidence that pro-kinetics may be of value in half of these patients.[60] In some series surgery was necessary in up to one-third of patients.[43] The presence of systemic disease must be carefully evaluated before embarking on surgery. In the author's own practice surgery has only been necessary in one of more than 40 patients. Dilatation and vigorous anti reflux therapy has been a reasonable compromise in these unfortunate patients.

Antireflux procedures performed for these patients will fail because of the poor motility,[34] and oesophageal replacement should be considered as the initial step in resistant cases. Resectional surgery has given excellent results.[43]

POLYMYOSITIS

This is similar to scleroderma but involves the striated segment as well. The clinician may be alerted to this possibility by motility changes throughout the oesophagus, and a muscle biopsy will be necessary to confirm the diagnosis.

SYSTEMIC LUPUS ERYTHEMATOSUS AND POLYARTERITIS NODOSA

Oesophageal involvement is not as common in systemic lupus erythematosus and polyarteritis nodosa, but the disorder is similar to that found in scleroderma.

SKIN DISEASES

Patients with epidermolysis bullosa dystrophica (recessive type) may present with oesophageal strictures. These are best treated by balloon dilatation to minimize further damage and repeated bullous formation in the oesophagus.

Behçet's disease may also result in stricture formation. Tylosis is a Mendelian dominant disorder characterized by keratosis of the soles and palms, and is associated with oesophageal ulceration, stricture and squamous cell carcinoma.

OBESITY

Oesophageal transit is significantly prolonged in obese patients[38] who also may have a raised lower gastro-oesophageal sphincter pressure gradient presumably caused by increased intra-abdominal pressure.

REFERENCES

1. Anderson, K.D., Rouse, T.M. and Randolph, J.G. (1990) A controlled trial of corticosteroids in children with corrosive injury of the oesophagus. *New England Medical Journal*, **323**, 637–640.
2. Balthazar, E.J., Megibow, A.J., Hulnick, D., Chao, K.C. and Beranbaum, E. (1987) Cytomegalovirus oesophagitis in AIDS radiographic features on 16 patients. *American Journal of Roentgenology*, **149**, 919–923.
3. Bendig, D.W. (1986) Removal of blunt esophageal foreign bodies with flexible endoscopy without general anaesthesia. *American Journal of Diseases of Children*, **140**, 789–790.
4. Bigelow, N.H. (1953) Carcinoma of the esophagus developing at the site of stricture. *Cancer*, **6**, 1159–1164.
5. Boak, D.K.B., Neuberger, P.E. and Teele, R.L. (1979) Esophagitis induced by combined radiation and adriamycin. *American Journal of Roentgenelogy*, **132**, 567–576.
6. Bonacini, M., Laine, L., Gal, A.A., Lee, A.A., Martin, M.M. and Strigle, S. (1990) Prospective evaluation of brushing of the esophagus for candida oesophagitis in patients with human immunodeficiency virus infection. *Gastroenterology*, **85**, 385–389.
7. Bonadio, W.A., Jona, J.Z., Glicklich, M. and Cohen, R. (1988) Esophageal bougienage technique for coin ingestion in children. *Journal of Pediatric Surgery*, **23**, 917–918.
8. Bowdler, D.A. and Stell, P.M. (1987) Surgical management of posterior pharyngeal diverticula: inversion versus one-stage excision. *British Journal of Surgery*, **74**, 988–990.
9. Bremner, C.G. (1982) Benign strictures of the esophagus. *Current Problems in Surgery*, **19**, 402–492.
10. Bremner, C.G. and Wright, N. (1991) Corrosive and non-reflux oesophagitis. In *Surgery of the Oesophagus*, Eds T.P.J. Hennessy and A. Cuschieri. Butterworths (in press).
11. Carlborg, B., Densert, O. and Lindqist, C. (1980) Esophageal lesions caused by orally administered drugs. An experimental study in the cat. *European Surgical Research*, **12**, 270–272.
12. Chisholm, M., Ardran, G., Callender, S.T. and Wright, R. (1971) A follow-up study of patients with post-cricoid webs. 1971. *Quarterly Journal of Medicine*, **159**, 409–420.
13. Debas, H.T., Payne, W.S., Cameron, A.J. and Carlson, H.C. (1980) Pathophysiology of the lower esophageal diverticulum and its implications for treatment. *Surgery, Gynecology and Obstetrics*, **151**, 593–600.
14. De Silva, R., Stoopack, P.M. and Raufman, J.P. (1990) Oesophageal fistulas associated wtih mycobacterial infection in patients at risk for AIDS. *Radiology*, **175**, 449–453.

15. Dohlman, G. and Mattsson, O. (1960) The endoscopic operation for hypopharyngeal diverticula: a roentgencinematographic study. *Archives of Otolaryngology*, **71**, 744–752.

16. Donald, P.J. and Huffman, D.I. (1979) Carcinoma in a Zenker's diverticulum. *Head and Neck Surgery*, **2**, 71–75.

17. Dubost, C. and Celerier, M. (1984) Severe tracheobronchial complication of the ingestion of caustics in adults. A case of perforation healed with a pulmonary patch. *Journal e Chirurgie (Paris)*, **121**, 1–6.

18. Eastridge, C.E., Pate, J.N. and Mann, J.A. (1984) Lower esophageal ring: experiences in treatment of 88 patients. *Annals of Thoracic Surgery*, **37**, 103–107.

19. Ekberg, O. and Nylander, G. (1983) Webs and web-like formations in the pharynx and cervical esophagus. *Diagnostic Imaging*, **52**, 10–18.

20. Ellis, F.H. Jr., Schlegel, J.F., Lynch, V.P. and Payne, W.S. (1969) Cricopharyngeal myotomy for pharyngo-esophageal diverticulum. *Annals of Surgery*, **170**, 340–349.

21. Ferguson, M.K., Migliore, M., Staszak, V.M. and Little, A.G. (1989) Early evaluation and therapy for caustic oesophageal injury. *American Journal of Surgery*, **157**, 116–120.

22. Flynn, A.E. Verrier, E.D., Way, L.W., Thomas, A.N. and Pellegrini, C.A. (1989) Esophageal perforation. *Archives of Surgery*, **124**, 1211–1215.

23. Gage-White, L. (1988) Incidence of Zenker's diverticulum with hiatus hernia. *The Laryngoscope*, **98**, 527–530.

24. Goldstein, H.M., Rogers, L.F., Fletcher, G.H. and Dodd, G.D. (1975) Radiological manifestations of radiation induced injury in the normal upper gastro-intestinal tract. *Radiology*, **117**, 135–140.

25. Gouge, T.H., Depan, H.J. and Spencer, F.C. (1989) Experience with the Grillo pleural wrap procedure in 18 patients with perforation of the thoracic esophagus. *Annals of Surgery*, **209**, 612–619.

26. Goyal, R.K., Glancy, J.J. and Spiro, H. (1970) Lower esophageal ring. *New England Journal of Medicine*, **282**, 1298–1305; 1355–1362.

27. Huang, B., Payne, W.S. and Cameron, A.J. (1984) Surgical management for recurrent pharyngo-oesophageal (Zenker's) diverticulum. *Annals of Thoracic Surgery*, **37**, 189–191.

28. Ikard, R.W. and Rosen, H.E. (1977) Midoesophageal webs in adults. *Annals of Thoracic Surgery*, **24**, 355–358.

29. Kaszar-Seibert, D.J., Korn, W.T., Bindman, D.J. and Shortsleeve, M.J. (1990) Treatment of acute esophageal food impaction with a combination of glucagon, effervescent agent and water. *American Journal of Roentgenology*, **154**, 533–534.

30. Kessler, A., Yellin, A. and Kronenberg, J. (1990) Use of a metal detector in the location of a swallowed razor blade in the oesophagus. *Journal of Laryngology and Otology*, **104**, 435–436.

31. Khosla, S.N. (1984) Cricoid webs – incidence and follow-up study in Indian patients. *Postgraduate Medical Journal*, **60**, 346–348.

32. Knuff, T.E., Benjamin, S.B. and Castell, D.D. (1982) Pharyngo-esophageal (Zenker's) diverticulum: a re-appraisal. *Gastroenterologoy*, **82**, 734–736.

33. Kooi, G.H. and Sakijan, A.S. (1989) Foley catheter removal of blunt oesophageal foreign bodies in children. *Medical Journal of Malaysia*, **44**, 156–159.

34. Mansour, K.A. and Malone, C.E. (1988) Surgery for scleroderma of the esophagus: a 12 year experience. *Annals of Thoracic Surgery*, **46**, 513–514.

35. Mason, R.J. and Bremner, C.G. (1990) Pharyngo-oesophageal webs: a complication of gastro-oesophageal reflux (abstract). *South African Journal of Surgery*, **28**, 117.

36. Maves, M.D., Lloyd, T.Y. and Carithers, J.S. (1986) Radiographic identification of ingested disc batteries. *Pediatric Radiology*, **16**, 154–156.

37. McDonald, G.B., Sullivan, K.M. and Plumley, T.F. (1984) Radiographic features of esophageal involvement in chronic graft-vs-host disease. *American Journal of Roentgenology*, **142**, 501–506.

38. Mercer, C.D., Rue, C., Hanelin, L. and Hill, L.D. (1985) Effect of obesity on esophageal transit. *American Journal of Surgery*, **149**, 177–181.

39. Molins, T., Payne, W.S., Cameron, A.J. and Mac Carty, R. (1988) An unusually intractable Schatzki ring. *Annals of Thoracic Surgery*, **45**, 327–329.

40. Naylor, A.R., Walker, W.S., Dark, J. and Cameron, J. (1990) T-Tube intubation in the management of seriously ill patients with oesophagopleural fistulae. *British Journal of Surgery*, **77**, 40–42.

41. Nelson, R.S., Hernandez, A.J., Goldstein H.M. and Saca. A. (1979) Treatment of irradiation esophagitis: value of hydrocortisone injection. *American Journal of Gastroenterology*, **71**, 17–23.

42. Norton, R.A. and King, G.D. (1963) 'Steakhouse Syndrome'. The symptomatic lower esophageal ring. *Lahey Clinic Bulletin*, **13**, 55–59.

43. Orringer, M.B. (1985) Transhiatal esophagectomy for benign disease. *Journal of Thoracic and Cardiovascular Surgery*, **90**, 649–655.

44. Peacock, E.E. (1981) Control of wound healing and scar formation in surgical patients. *Archives of Surgery*, **116**, 1325–1329.

45. Powell, F.C., Winkelmann, R.K. Venecie-Lemarchand, F., Spurbeck, J.L. and Schroeder, A.L. (1984) The anticentromere antibody: disease specificity and clinical significance. *Mayo Clinic Proceedings*, **59**, 700–706.

46. Reyes, H.M. and Hill, J.L. (1976) Modifications of the experimental stent technic for esophageal burns. *Journal of Surgical Research*, **20**, 65–70.

47. Rivkin, L., Bremner, C.G. and Bremner, C.H. (1984) Pathophysiology of mid-oesophageal and epiphrenic diverticula of the oesophagus. *South African Medical Journal*, **66**, 127–129.

48. Santos, G.H. and Frater, R.W. (1986) Transesophageal irrigation for the treatment of mediastinitis produced by esophageal rupture. *Journal of Thoracic and Cardiovascular Surgery*, **91**, 57–62.

49. Sarr, M.G., Pemberton, J.H. and Payne, W.S. (1982) Management of instrumental perforations of the esophagus. *Journal of Thoracic and Cardivascular Surgery*, **84**, 211–218.

50. Scott, B.B. and Jenkins, D. (1982) Gastro-intestinal candidiasis. *Gut*, **23**, 137–139.

51. Sprung, D.J. and Gibb, S.P. (1985) Dyplastic Barrett's esophagus in scleroderma. *American Journal of Gastroenterology*, **80**, 518–522.

52. Studley, J.G., Linehan, I.P., Oglivie, A.L. and Dowling, B.L. (1990) Swallowed button batteries: is there a consensus on management. *Gut*, **31**, 867–870.

53. Swedlund, A., Traube, M., Siskind, B.N. and McCallum, R.W. (1989) Nonsurgical management of esophageal perforation from pneumatic dilatation. *Digestive Diseases and Sciences*, **34**, 379–384.

54. Ti, T.K. (1980) Esophageal resection with pharyngogastrostomy for corrosive strictures of the pharynx and oesophagus. *British Journal of Surgery*, **67**, 798–800.

55. Tucker, J.A. and Yarington, C.T. (1979) The treatment of caustic ingestion. *Otolaryngology Clinics of North America*, **12**, 343–350.

56. Van Overbeek, J.J.M., Hoeksema, P.E. and Edens, E.T. (1984) Microendoscopic surgery of the hypopharyngeal diverticulum using electro-coagulation of carbon dioxide laser. *Annals of Otolaryngorhinolaryngology*, **93**, 34–36.

57. Warden, H.D. (1961) Esophageal obstruction due to aberrant intercostal artery: report of case. *Archives of Surgery*, **83**, 749–751.

58. Waters, P.F. and DeMeester, T.R. (1981) Foregut motor disorders and their surgical management. *Medical Clinics of North America*, **65**, 1235–1238.

59. Weaver, J.W. Kaude, J.V. and Hamlin, D.J. (1984) Webs of the lower esophagus: a complication of gastroesophageal reflux? *American Journal of Roentgenology*, **142**, 289–292.

60. Wermann, T. and Caspary, W.F. (1990) Effect of Cisapride on esophageal motility in healthy probands and patients with progressive systemic sclerosis. *Klinische Wochenschrifte*, **68**, 602–607.

61. Winkler, B., Capo, V., Reumann, N., Ma, A. and Porto, R. *et al.* (1985) Human papilloma virus infection of the oesophagus. *Cancer*, **55**, 149–155.

62. Worman, L.W. (1980) Pharyngo-esophageal diverticulum–excision or incision. *Surgery*, **87**, 236–237.

63. Yeo, C.J., Lillemoe, K.D., Klein, A.S. and Zinner, M.J. (1988) Treatment of instrumental perforation of the esophagus. *Archives of Surgery*, **123**, 1016–1018.

64. Zagar, S.A., Kochkar, R., Naqi, B., Metha, S., and Mehta, S.K. (1989) Ingestion of corrosive acids. Spectrum of injury to upper gastrointestinal tract and natural history. *Gastroenterology*, **97**, 720–727.

CHAPTER 2

STOMACH AND DUODENUM

EMBRYOLOGY AND ANATOMY

Caroline Doig

EMBRYOLOGY

The foregut elongates into the oesophagus and, by the end of the fourth gestational week, the stomach is recognizable as a fusiform dilatation. Beyond this, the gut merges into the yolk sac. This connection is initially wide but, by the fifth week, it is narrower and longer forming the vitelline-intestinal duct, which normally absorbs so that this connection is lost.

The stomach is in the median plane, separated ventrally from the pericardium by the septum transversum, although distally it is closely related to the dorsal aorta via a short dorsal mesogastrium. The liver develops as a hollow diverticulum in the ventral aspect of the foregut distal to the stomach dilatation, and grows headwards into the substance of the septum transversum, giving a ventral mesogastrium. By the 10-mm embryo stage, the curvatures of the stomach are beginning to be defined by more active growth of the dorsal border and the developing rudimentary fundus. This rapid growth brings the pylorus ventrally so that the stomach now has right and left surfaces.

During this time the rest of the gut increases in length, but with the dorsal aspect at a more rapid rate than the ventral so that a U-shaped loop is formed with a dorsal mesentery. This loop projects into the peritoneal cavity and, by virtue of its size, outside into the umbilical cord. This remains from the sixth week until the third month, i.e. from the 10–40 mm stage of the embryo, before returning to the abdomen having rotated through 270° in an anticlockwise fashion.

With growth of the fundus, the stomach is displaced to the left and rotates to the right, so that the right side becomes the dorsal and the left the ventral surface. This rotation leads to a space in the dorsal mesogastrium which becomes the lesser sac. It also means that the duodenum moves dorsally and to the right, its dorsal mesentery being absorbed due to the approximation of the bowel to the posterior abdominal wall; consequently, the duodenum becomes a retroperitoneal structure.

Early in the sixth week a small diverticulum, destined to become the caecum and appendix, develops in the caudal limb of the U-shaped loop. Although this conical-shaped diverticulum means that the large and the small bowel are distinguishable, it is not until the fifth month that it becomes

more distinguishable as a caecum and a rudimentary appendix.

When the U-shaped loop entered the umbilical cord, it had already rotated through 90°, the proximal (stomach) side to the right and the distal to the left. While outside the foetus, the gut elongates and becomes coiled, the mesentery adapting to these changes. The large bowel (colon) does not coil or grow as much. Once the 40-mm stage has been reached, the abdominal cavity has enlarged sufficiently to allow return of the gut. During the process of return, the bowel again rotates so that the small bowel moves to the right. The distal colon lies to the left with obliteration of the descending colon mesentery, allowing the left colic vessels to lie anterior to the left ureter. The adult relationship of the third part of the duodenum to the superior mesenteric artery is thus established. The caecum is the last to return to the abdomen, lying initially on top of the coils of small bowel, before passing to the right and distally. Its dorsal mesentery also absorbs into the posterior abdominal wall, so that it lies retroperitoneally. This should have been completed by the end of the third month.

The pancreas develops in two parts. The dorsal portion appears in the latter half of the fourth week, as a diverticulum in the dorsal wall proximal to the liver diverticulum. Growing into the dorsal meso-duodenum, it will become the neck, body and tail of the pancreas. Although some of the head comes from this portion, most originates from the ventral portion, which develops from the area around the primitive bile duct. Thus, the pancreas fuses, growing round the gut by the seventh week. The ducts also fuse so that the main duct consists of the ventral portion and part of the dorsal duct.

ANATOMY

The stomach is the most dilated portion of the gut, consisting of fundus, body, antrum and pylorus. The cardia lies to the left of the median plane behind the seventh costal cartilage at the level of the eleventh vertebral body. The pylorus lies just to the right of the median plane at the lower border of the first lumbar vertebral body. The lesser curvature gives attachment for the lesser omentum, which contains the right and left gastric vessels supplying this area of the stomach. The deepest part of the lesser curvature is the incisura or angular notch, which can vary in position. In the upper portion of the fundus, the greater curvature gives attachment to the gastrosplenic ligament with the short gastric vessels. In continuity, lower down, the greater omentum is attached, with the gastroepiploic vessels supplying the rest of the stomach. Lymphatic drainage follows the blood supply, draining to the glands in the lesser and greater omentum. The sympathetic nerve supply is mainly from the coeliac plexus. In addition to branches from the left phrenic nerve, inconsistent branches can come from the left splanchnic nerves, and the thoracic and lumbar sympathetic trunks. Parasympathetic supply is from the vagus nerve. The anterior nerve supplies the cardia before dividing into gastric and pyloric branches: the gastric branch via the greater anterior gastric nerve in the lesser omentum supplying the anterior surface of the stomach and the fundus; the two pyloric branches supplying the pylorus and antrum. The posterior vagus nerve has gastric branches supplying the posterior surface of the stomach and coeliac branches passing to the coeliac plexus. Anteriorly, the stomach lies in contact with the sixth, seventh, eighth and ninth ribs, and with the diaphragm. The left and quadrate lobes of the liver lie to the right and the transverse colon may lie anteriorly. The lesser sac, posteriorly, separates it from the diaphragm, left adrenal, upper portion of the left kidney, splenic artery, pancreas, left colic flexure and transverse mesocolon. The spleen is separated from the stomach by the greater sac.

The stomach consists of four coats: peritoneal or serosal surface; muscular layers of longitudinal, circular and oblique unstriped fibres; a submucosal or areolar layer; and a mucosal layer of honey-combed appearance with the openings of the gastric glands. In the cardia these glands are either simple, tubular or compound, racemose glands: the fundal glands are simple tubes the epithelium of which consists of (1) columnar chief cells producing pepsin and (2) oval parietal or oxyntic cells secreting acid; the pyloric glands are short and convoluted with some parietal cells.

PHYSIOLOGY

The acid state of the neonatal or premature stomach has yet to be clearly defined. Basal acid output is low at birth and thought to be even lower in the preterm infant,[2–4] but increases to the adult level at 1 month.[5] In association with other host defence mechanisms, this acid acts as a barrier in the stomach to the entry of unwanted substances. Levels of gastrin in newborn infants[7,9] or the very sick preterm infant[6] are uncertain. In the very pre-term baby, delay in gastric emptying can lead to abdominal distension with difficulty in feeding.[8] Such problems decrease with increasing gestational age, which also gives an increase in gastric antral pressure helping antral activity.[9]

References

1. Bissett,W.M., Watt, J.B., Rivers, R.P.A. and Milla, P.J. (1986) The ontogeny of small intestinal motor activity. *Pediatric Research*, **20**, 692–697.
2. Euler, A.R., Byrne, W.J., Cousins, J.M., Ament, M.E., Leake, R.D. and Walsh, J.H. (1977) Increased serum gastrin concentrations and gastric acid hyposecretion in the immediate newborn period. *Gastroenterology*, **72**, 1271–1276.
3. Euler, A.R., Byrne, W.J., Meis, P.J., Leake, R.D. and Ament, M.E. (1979) Basal and pentagastrin-stimulated acid secretion in newborn infants. *Pediatric Research*, **13**, 36–39.
4. Hyman, P.E., Clarke, D.D., Everett, S.L. *et al.* (1985) Gastric acid secretory function in preterm infants. *Journal of Pediatrics*, **106**, 467–469.
5. Kopel, F.B. and Barbero, G.J. (1967) Gastric acid secretion in infancy and childhood. *Gastroenterology*, **52**, 1101–1104.
6. Marchini, G., Lagercrantz, H., Milerad, J., Winberg, J. and Ulnas-Moberg, K. (1988) Plasma levels of somatostatin and gastrin in sick infants and small for gestational age infants. *Journal of Pediatric Gastroenterology and Nutrition*, **7**, 641–647.
7. Salmenperea, L., Perheentupa, J., Siimes, M.A., Adrian, T.E., Bloom, S.R. and Aynsley-Green, A. (1988) Effects of feeding regimen on blood glucose levels and plasma concentrations of pancreatic hormones and gut regulatory peptides at 9 months of age: comparison between infants fed with milk formula and infants exclusively breast fed from birth. *Journal of Pediatric Gastroenterology and Nutrition*, **7**, 651–658.
8. Siegal, M. (1983) Gastric emptying time in premature and compromised infants. *Journal of Pediatric Gastroenterology and Nutrition*, **2** (suppl. 1), S136.
9. Widstrom, A.M., Christensson, K., Ransjo Arvidson, A.B., Matthiesen, A.S., Winberg, J. and Uvnas Moberg, K. (1988) Gastric aspirates of newborn infants: pH volume and levels of gastrin- and somatostatin-like immunoreactivity. *Acta Paediatrica Scandinavica*, **77**, 502–504.

CONGENITAL ABNORMALITIES

Caroline Doig

PYLORIC ATRESIA

This uncommon congenital abnormality,[8,56] presents in the newborn period with gross distension of the stomach and no distal gas (*Figure 2.1*). Commonly associated with other abnormalities, especially of the skin[17,77] (*Figure 2.2*), it is almost uniformly fatal. Possible treatment involves anastomosis between bowel, duodenum and stomach in a partial gastrectomy-type operation.

MICROGASTRIA

An unusual impairment of normal development of the foregut can lead to microgastria (*Figure 2.3*),

often associated with other defects such as malrotation, asplenia and pulmonary abnormalities. Although usually fatal due to malnutrition, attempts at creating an artificial reservoir by means of a double-lumen Roux-en-Y loop (Hunt–Lawrence pouch)[86] have given some hope of survival. This abnormality must not be mistaken for a small stomach resulting from a hiatus hernia with stomach in the chest.

Other rarities are double pylorus[46,95] and antral webs,[11,83] the latter presenting as a possible pyloric stenosis. If partial, there may be delay in the diagnosis, even into adult life.[54] Treatment is by pyloroplasty and gastrostomy. A gastric duplication may present with signs of obstruction and an acute abdomen.[34,67]

Gastric volvulus, with a distended stomach as the predisposing cause, leads to collapse. The stomach

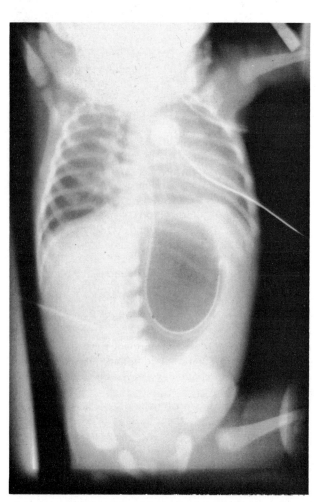

Figure 2.1 Plain radiograph of pyloric atresia showing only a large distended stomach and no distal gas. (Reproduced by permission of Manchester University Department of Medical Illustration.)

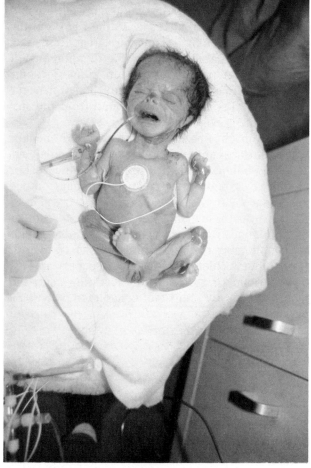

Figure 2.2 Associated skin lesion of congenital cutis dysplasia. (Reproduced by permission of Manchester University Department of Medical Illustration.)

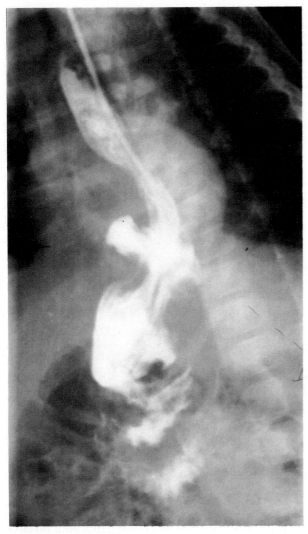

Figure 2.3 Radiograph taken after barium meal, showing microgastria.

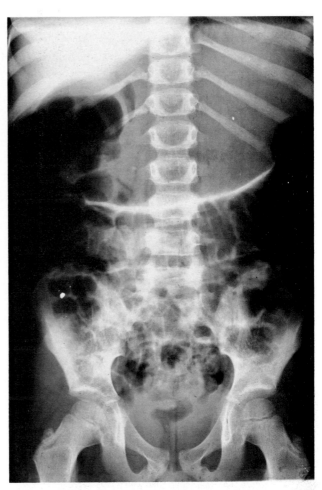

Figure 2.4 Radiograph showing acute dilatation of stomach, post-trauma.

either rotates rather like a spit on its cardiopyloric axis (organoaxial) or on the mesentery as on a skewer (mesenteroaxial). The inability to pass a gastric tube leads to suspicion of the diagnosis[16] confirmed by barium studies showing an abnormal stomach bubble. Fixation of the stomach with an associated gastrostomy should prevent further problems. The addition of a Nissen fundoplication will stop reflux.[42] Misdiagnosis with the more common acute dilatation of the stomach occurring after trauma is possible (*Figure 2.4*).

Abnormal motility causing delay in gastric emptying presents with vomiting associated with oesophageal reflux. Children with this impairment, e.g. those with familial dysautonomia,[88] benefit from fundoplication but not from surgery on the gastric outlet.

CONGENITAL HYPERTROPHIC PYLORIC STENOSIS

The thickened circular pyloric muscle obstructs the outlet of the stomach leading to projectile vomiting and failure to thrive. The exact aetiology is unknown. A neuropathic abnormality[30] or abnormal gastrin response[63] has been implicated but there is no conclusive proof.[37,55,92] The role of prostaglandins,[50] basal acid secretion[62] and immunochemistry[79] is also inconclusive.

The incidence is generally reported as 5 per 1000 live births with an increased incidence in siblings of up to 12 times, suggesting a possible environmental or genetic cause.[18] Thus, classically it occurs in the first male child born to parents who have themselves had the problem in infancy, especially if the mother has had the disease. Associated abnormalities of the genitourinary tract occur in 20% of such children,[6] not necessarily requiring treatment. There is an

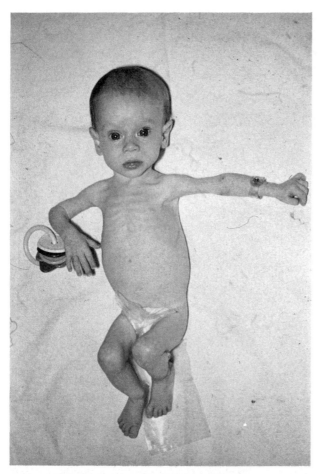

Figure 2.5 Marasmic child with pyloric stenosis.

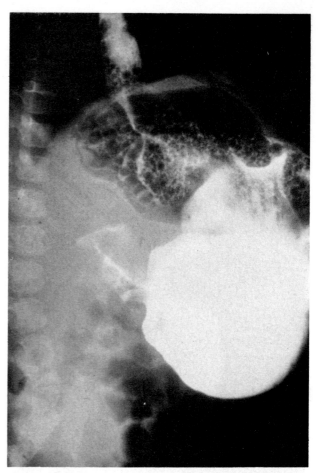

Figure 2.6 Radiograph taken after barium meal, showing pyloric stenosis.

association with other gastrointestinal abnormalities,[2] including diaphragmatic hernia,[4] and in children surviving oesophageal atresia surgery.[32]

CLINICAL FEATURES

The usual presentation is with forceful projectile vomiting often landing some feet away from the mother and child. Although it may be blood stained due to gastritis,[72] it will not be bile stained. The baby will be keen to feed despite the vomiting. If undiagnosed, the baby becomes marasmic (*Figure 2.5*) with metabolic alkalosis and hypochloraemia.[14]

By observing peristaltic waves in the upper abdomen and test feeding to confirm the pyloric 'tumour' by palpation, a clinical diagnosis can be made. However, if the tumour is small and under the liver it may be impossible to palpate.

INVESTIGATIONS

Ultrasonography[45,84] and/or a barium meal (*Figure 2.6*) will confirm diagnosis. Investigations should be performed in all vomiting children in whom no clear diagnosis has been made,[28] in order to exclude other surgical causes of vomiting such as oesophageal reflux duodenal stenosis and malrotation.

MANAGEMENT

Preoperative

Preoperative management involves rehydration and correction of the electrolyte imbalance by treating the alkalosis. Replacement of sodium and chloride to aid the excretion of bicarbonate, and the addition of potassium, will improve the alkalosis.[68] Oral feeds are stopped and the gastritis should be treated by washing out the stomach until clear of food debris. Once the blood chemistry has improved, surgery should be performed.

Operative

With modern paediatric anaesthesia, there is no place for local anaesthesia when operating on a baby

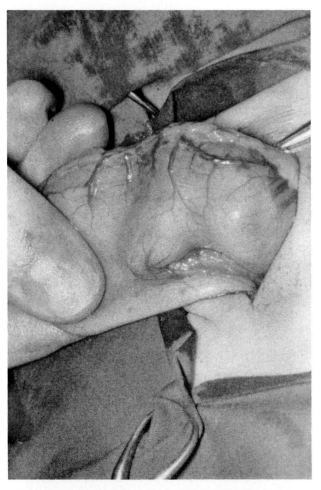

Figure 2.7 Operative photograph of the hypertrophied tumour.

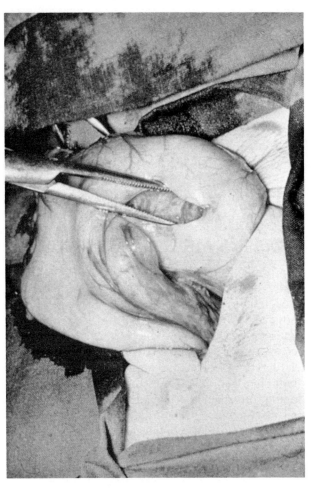

Figure 2.8 Operative detail of myotomy.

with pyloric stenosis.[60] Pyloromyotomy (Ramstedt's operation) involves cutting the circular muscle of the pylorus. A right upper transverse incision in the pyloric plane will lead to the rectus muscles, the fibres of which are separated. On opening the peritoneum, the liver must be reflected upwards and, by pulling on the omentum and transverse colon, the stomach becomes visible and can be held. Once the pylorus has been delivered (*Figure 2.7*), by grasping it between the thumb and index finger of the left hand, the muscle can be divided transversely, in the avascular area with a knife (*Figure 2.8*), without damaging the duodenum. Separation of all the fibres by a Spencer–Wells forceps allows the mucosa to bulge. Care should be taken to divide the tumour completely but not to perforate the duodenum. Such a perforation must be checked for by insufflating the stomach with air via the nasogastric tube.

There is no correlation between the duration or severity of symptoms and the size of the tumour.[85] Another approach through the umbilical region

gives a good cosmetic scar,[26,81] but also perhaps a potential risk of infection.

Although the baby can be fed within 6 hours with increasing amounts if the duodenum has not been perforated, it is probably better to wait 24 hours to allow the gastritis to settle.[29] Recurrent vomiting rarely indicates an incomplete myotomy, but rather a residual gastritis which will be cleared with further stomach wash-outs.[71] Occasionally, oesophagitis caused by reflux can be helped by sitting the baby up at a 60° angle.[73] Most postoperative vomiting improves over a 2-week period.

Because of prolonged preoperative dehydration and malnutrition, wound infection and dehiscence can be a problem. Although the results of this operation are generally satisfactory with normal feeding, there is a 20% risk of complication.[15,35] Problems with duodenal reflux may occur later,[80] but whether this leads to dyspepsia in adult life is uncertain. The use of endoscopic balloons to treat adult pyloric stenosis may suggest a future development for the treatment of congenital hypertrophic pyloric stenosis.[36,39]

Although most infants can be treated satisfactorily in a district general hospital, in the very small pre-term infant or one with respiratory problems referral to a paediatric surgeon will result in a better prognosis,[9,52,66] with the added advantage of paediatric anaesthesia. Although laparoscopic pyloromyotomy has been suggested, the small incision and short time involved in the usual approach means that the laparoscopic method is of little advantage.

DUODENAL ATRESIA AND STENOSIS

If the duodenum fails to recanalize completely, duodenal atresia results, with a diaphragm either at, above or below the ampulla of Vater.[13] Sometimes a windsock forms so that the stretched diaphragm becomes floppy; it appears to obstruct more distally, leading to problems at surgery. An incomplete diaphragm will give a stenosis. In the atretic duodenum, the pancreas frequently develops abnormally, enveloping the duodenum as an annular pancreas – an embryological anomaly[51] – merely indicating the internal problem. As with prepyloric portal veins,[12,23] this does not cause an obstruction.

CLINICAL FEATURES

The diagnosis of duodenal obstruction – possible duodenal atresia – can be made antenatally[38] (*Figure 2.9*). Maternal hydramnios also suggests the possible diagnosis. The incidence of the anomaly is 1 in 3000 live births.

The baby presents with vomiting which may or may not be bile stained, depending on the site of the obstruction. Abdominal distension is not marked because the blockage is high, although a fullness in the epigastrium due to the dilated stomach may be noted. Chromosomal abnormalities, e.g. trisomy 21 (Down's syndrome) are commonly associated in 40–50% of duodenal obstructions.[98] Other anomalies can be associated with this chromosomal abnormality, e.g. cardiac as well as skeletal anomalies.[5] The triad of oesophageal atresia, cardiac anomalies and duodenal atresia is usually fatal.[44]

INVESTIGATIONS

Plain abdominal radiographs will show a large stomach (*Figure 2.10a*) and the erect film classically shows that of a 'double bubble' appearance of the

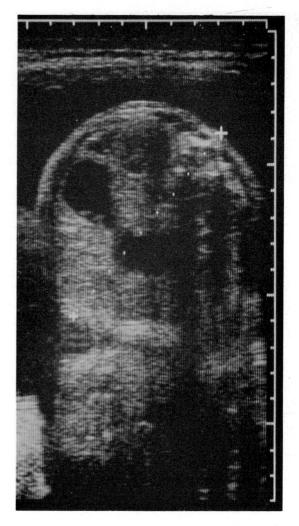

Figure 2.9 Antenatal ultrasound showing duodenal atresia. (Reproduced by permission of Manchester University Department of Medical Illustration.)

fluid levels in distended stomach and duodenum (*Figure 2.10b*). This only indicates a duodenal obstruction and may also be present with malrotation and volvulus. No gas is seen distally. If a nasogastric tube has been passed, it may be necessary to instil further air into the stomach to confirm the diagnosis. In infants with stenosis only, the diagnosis may be delayed and a misdiagnosis of pyloric stenosis made. Radiological appearances will show distal gas (*Figure 2.11*) as well as the dilated stomach and duodenum, a barium study indicating site of the diaphragm (*Figure 2.12*).

MANAGEMENT

Resuscitation is necessary before surgery in view of the gross disturbance in electrolytes following ex-

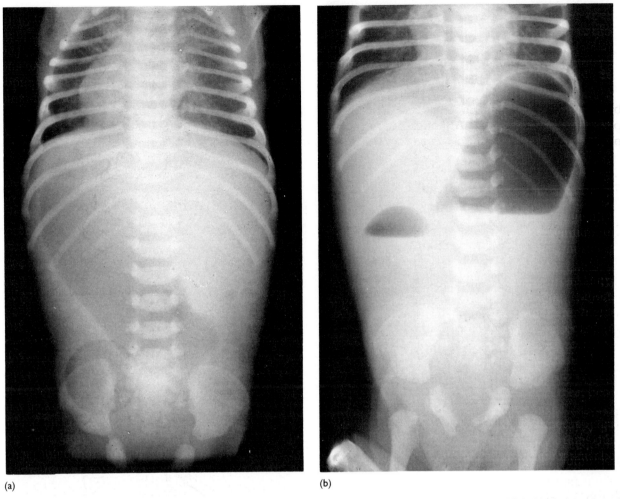

(a)   (b)

Figure 2.10   (a) Plain abdominal radiograph showing distended stomach. (b) On the erect film, there is a 'double bubble' of gastric and duodenal fluid levels of duodenal atresia.

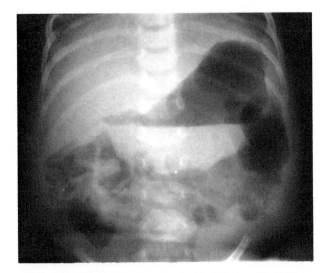

Figure 2.11   Radiograph showing double bubble with distal gas suggesting duodenal stenosis.

cessive vomiting or loss of fluid lying in the stomach and duodenum.

The treatment is the same whether dealing with a complete atresia or a stenosis: to bypass the obstruction as near as possible so as not to leave a blind loop. Through a transverse upper abdominal incision, the duodenum is mobilized; the upper jejunum and third part of the duodenum are then freed and brought through the transverse mesocolon to lie close to the proximal dilated duodenum and stomach. No attempt should be made to dissect the annular pancreas if present. After anastomosing these two parts of the duodenum together posteriorly in a transverse plane, the proximal bowel is opened and confirmation of the site and type of obstruction made by means of a probe. When the distal bowel is opened further, confirmation is obtained to check on the position of the windsock. If care is not taken, it is possible to anastomose the bowel above the diaphragm.[61,64] The anterior wall is closed in a single layer after a trans-anastomotic

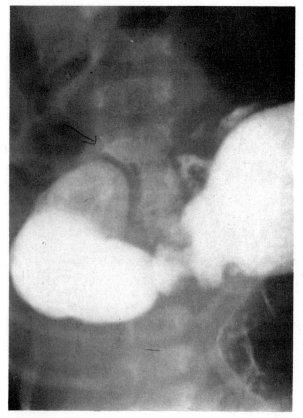

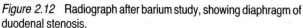

Figure 2.12 Radiograph after barium study, showing diaphragm of duodenal stenosis.

tube is passed via either the nose or a gastrostomy through the anastomosis into the upper jejunum (*Figure 2.13*). These trans-anastomotic tubes tend to spring back into the upper bowel so that a long enough portion should be threaded into the distal bowel. A gastrostomy or nasogastric tube must be

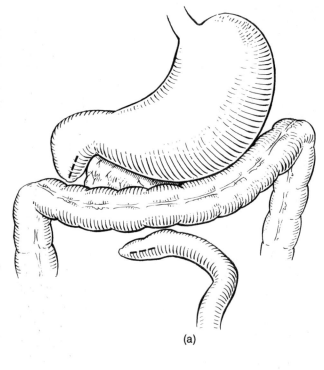

(a)

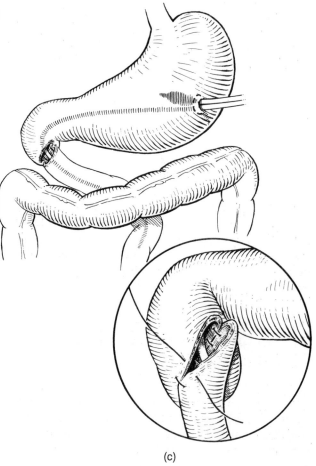

(c)

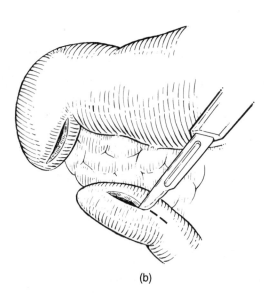

(b)

Figure 2.13 Operative details of duodenoduodenostomy: (a–c) different stages.

left in situ for some weeks until the gross distension of the stomach and duodenum has reduced, and normal peristalsis returns. The gastrostomy must be carefully fixed to the anterior abdominal wall because intraperitoneal feeds prove fatal. Although feeds through the trans-anastomotic tube can commence within 24–48 hours, oral feeding will be delayed until the gastric aspirate reduces. Such early milk feeds help avoid metabolic disturbances and dehydration.[20,94] The position of the end of the tube must first be checked by introduction of a small amount of contrast medium down the tube. Duodenoduodenostomy[31] has been shown to give better results than a duodenojejunostomy,[97] which has a longer loop that is liable to stagnation.

To try and obviate such surgery, both open and closed methods (by endoscopy)[57] of disrupting the diaphragm have been attempted with varying success. Open duodenoplasty to remove the diaphragm would appear to allow earlier feeding.[90] However, late obstruction of the duodenoduodenostomy suggests that trimming of the proximally dilated first section of the duodenum[22] should be part of the initial operation. If performed with a diamond-shaped duodenoplasty,[47] this reduces the problem of functional obstruction.[69]

Postoperatively, further loss of fluids can lead to electrolyte imbalance, requiring large amounts of intravenous fluids for correction. Although those diagnosed antenatally undergo surgery earlier, with less severe fluid disturbance as a result, there is little difference in the long-term results.[38]

The association with Down's syndrome may affect short-term results[3] but long-term results in any group are excellent.[75] Certainly, if a Down's syndrome baby is vomiting, early active measures should be taken to exclude the diagnosis and to treat them. Bile reflux may lead to late sequelae[48] and there may be a need for re-exploration because of this complication. More than a third of patients have prolonged jaundice[27] of unknown aetiology. Survival is likely in over 70% of children, with death due to other congenital abnormalities[58] and low birth weight.[7]

OTHER CAUSES OF DUODENAL OBSTRUCTION

Less common causes of obstruction of the duodenum in the older child are duplication cysts[96] (discussed later), tumours – usually malignant[53] – or intramural haematomas,[87] caused by trauma or bleeding disorder, e.g. associated with Henoch–Schönlein purpura.[19] Such haematomas only re-quire surgery if there is a tender enlarging mass or signs of peritonitis;[82] conservative management of nasogastric suction and parenteral nutrition is monitored by ultrasound.

MALROTATION

Malrotation of the bowel is an important form of duodenal obstruction presenting at any age and may lead on to volvulus and ischaemia of the small bowel. Malrotation and volvulus in utero may lead to intestinal atresia.[24]

Various forms of malrotation[78] (*Figure 2.14*) can occur, the most common being (1) non-rotation of all the intestine and (2) non-rotation of the right colon with normal rotation of the duodenum – both predisposing easily to volvulus of the small bowel; occasionally malposition of the duodenum, caecum, hepatic flexure or superior mesenteric vessels lead to other forms of malrotation with associated problems, e.g. a paraduodenal hernia.[21]

CLINICAL FEATURES

In view of the abnormal development, most children with malrotation will present early in the newborn period. Classically, the main problem is bile-stained vomiting due to the obstruction of the second part of the duodenum with bands. Colicky abdominal pain may suggest intermittent twisting of the bowel. Infants with failure to thrive should be investigated for malrotation, as many have an associated protein malnutrition.[41] A potential for serious problems exists because, in the usual form, the duodenojejuneal flexure now lies on the right as does the base of the mesentery. This narrow base allows the midgut to rotate around the superior mesenteric vessels. Volvulus occurs in over half of the children, leading to ischaemia and infarction of the whole of the small bowel. If ischaemia occurs, the passage of blood per rectum is associated with circulatory failure and death. These problems occur regardless of age at presentation,[59] even in the older child or adult,[33,89] so the diagnosis should be considered before such a catastrophe occurs. Bile-stained vomiting or recurrent colicky abdominal pain of unknown origin[54] necessitates urgent investigation and may require intervention.

INVESTIGATIONS

If volvulus has occurred, plain abdominal radiographs will show a duodenal obstruction with little or no distal gas in the small bowel, i.e. similar to the

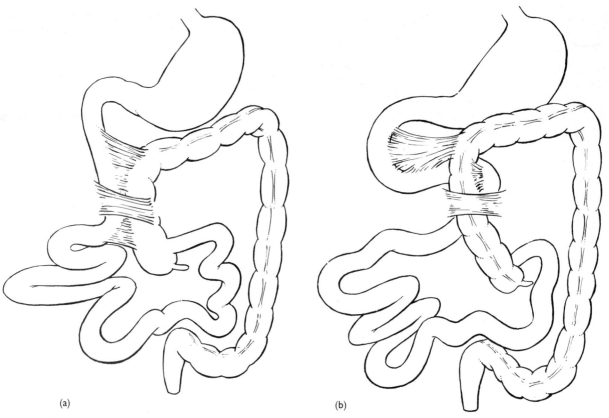

(a)   (b)

Figure 2.14   Different types of non-fixation and non-rotation: (a) non-rotation; (b) non-rotation of right colon. Both situations allow volvulus.

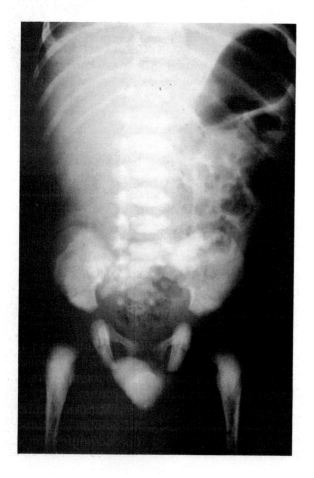

'double bubble' described in duodenal atresia. In the malrotated bowel without volvulus, the radiograph may be singularly unimpressive (*Figure 2.15*), although sometimes the gas shadows will lie to one side. Barium studies should not be delayed if the possibility of malrotation is seriously considered, because volvulus can occur at any time.[40] A barium meal and follow-through will delineate the position of the duodenojejunal flexure, which should lie at the level of the lesser curvature of the stomach to the left of the vertebral column; the position of the small bowel can be demonstrated (*Figure 2.16*). The bands obstructing the duodenum may be visualized (*Figure 2.17*). Minor degrees of malrotation can be difficult to demonstrate by radiological means.[25] Barium enema will show the position of the caecum and, if it is on the left side, indicates malrotation (*Figure 2.18*). If the caecum is mobile this may only show up on a delayed film (*Figure 2.19*). Associated abnormalities, especially in the newborn, are common, e.g. with diaphragmatic hernia, abdominal wall defects,[76] gastrointestinal atresia and stenosis as well as Hirschsprung's disease and intussusception.[24]

Figure 2.15   Plain radiograph of a neonate with malrotation.

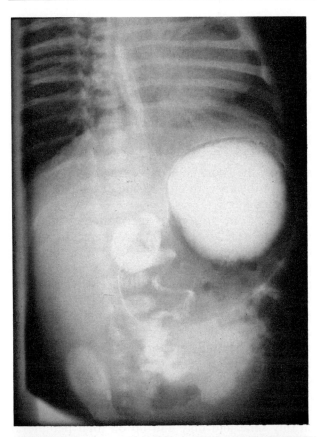

Figure 2.16 (left) Radiograph after barium meal, showing low and right-sided duodenojejunal flexure and abnormal position of small bowel.

Figure 2.17 (bottom left) Radiograph after barium meal, showing obstruction of duodenum with Ladd's bands.

Figure 2.18 (below) Radiograph showing abnormal position of caecum on barium enema.

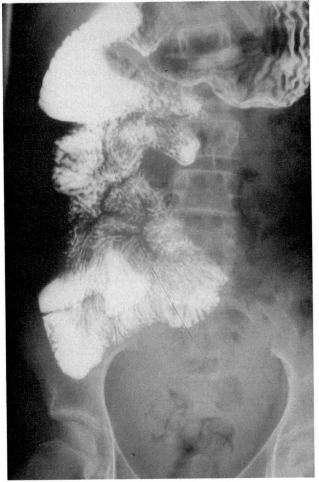

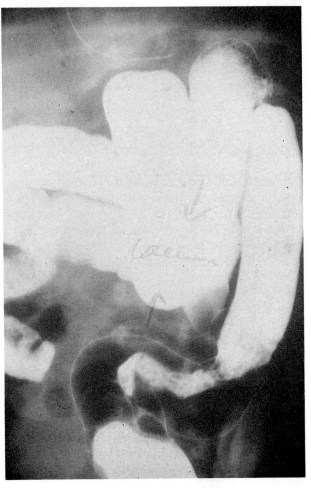

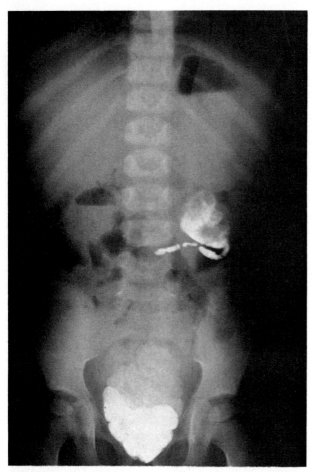

Figure 2.19 Plain abdominal radiograph after normal barium enema showing barium-filled appendix on left side.

MANAGEMENT

If malrotation alone is present, laparotomy performed to open up the base of the mesentery will prevent further volvulus. This operation also helps to fix the bowel so that recurrence is uncommon and the bowel rarely requires to be sutured in each iliac fossa.[10,74] No attempt should be made to return the bowel to the anatomically correct position, because the bowel will become ischaemic when normal development has not occurred. This leaves the caecum and the appendix (which may or may not be removed) on the left side of the abdomen.

If the bowel is twisted around the base of the mesentery, it is imperative that the bowel is untwisted in a clockwise direction. If volvulus has occurred or there have been recurrent problems over many years, it may be very difficult to undo these loops of bowel. However, if not carried out, the child will be prone to further problems and may later lose some of his or her bowel. If the bowel is already ischaemic, it may or may not recover by undoing the twist; if it remains ischaemic, resection of the bowel will be necessary. However, if the entire small bowel is ischaemic – which is likely in view of the blood supply – it may be wiser to undo the volvulus and return the infarcted bowel to the abdominal cavity. If the child survives, a second-look laparotomy 24 hours later will reveal rather less necrotic bowel to be resected. Even so, if the child survives, the short inadequate length of bowel will cause problems with growth and development – as discussed later.

Results from surgery for malrotation without volvulus are excellent. The chance of recurrent problems is low despite the bowel being in an abnormal position. Unfortunately, over 70% of malrotations presenting in the neonatal period are associated with volvulus, and the results are poor.[91] Older children may also die because the diagnosis has not been considered. Even if asymptomatic, malrotation should be operated on to prevent later problems.[70] Delay in gastric emptying may mean that some children still vomit due to the continuation of gastro-oesophageal reflux for some time.[43] When the entire bowel is necrotic most children die. Survivors have a stormy time and may end up on total parenteral nutrition for life.

Volvulus without malposition of the bowel may complicate intestinal atresias, meconium ileus or duplication cysts, which, by virtue of their size, allow the twist to occur. A similar situation occurs in midgut volvulus associated with dilatation of the ileum or in children with intestinal ascariasis.[93]

Situs inversus does not, of itself, require treatment but neonatal obstruction is more likely and there may be associated biliary atresia, annular pancreas or a preduodenal portal vein.[1,65]

REFERENCES

1. Adeyemi, S.D. (1988) Combination of annular pancreas and partial situs inversus: a multiple organ malrotation syndrome associated with duodenal obstruction. *Journal of Pediatric Surgery*, **23**, 188–189.
2. Ahmed, S. (1970) Infantile pyloric stenosis associated with major anomalies of the alimentary tract. *Journal of Pediatric Surgery*, **5**, 660–663.
3. Al-Salem, A.H., Khwaja, S., Grant, C. and Dawodu, A. (1989) Congenital intrinsic duodenal obstruction: problems in the diagnosis and management. *Journal of Pediatric Surgery*, **24**, 1247–1249.
4. Al-Salem, M.H., Grant, C. and Kwaja, S. (1990) Infantile hypertrophic pyloric stenosis and congenital diaphragmatic hernia. *Journal of Pediatric Surgery*, **25**, 607–611.

5. Atwell, J.D. and Klidjan, A.M. (1982) Vertebral anomalies and duodenal atresia. *Journal of Pediatric Surgery*, **17**, 237–245.

6. Atwell, J.D. and Levick, P. (1981) Congenital hypertrophic pyloric stenosis and associated anomalies in the genito-urinary tract. *Journal of Pediatric Surgery*, **16**, 1029–1034.

7. Baardson, A. and Knutrud, O. (1971) Mortality in neonatal duodenal obstruction. *Zeitschrift für Klinische Chirurgie*, **9**, 325–327.

8. Bar-Maor, J.A., Nissan, S. and Nevo, S. (1972) Pyloric atresia. A hereditary congenital anomaly with autosomal recessive transmission. *Journal of Medical Genetics*, **9**, 70–73.

9. Beynon, J., Brown, R., James, C. and Fernando, R. (1987) Pyloromyotomy: can the morbidity be improved? *Journal of the Royal College of Surgeons of Edinburgh*, **32**, 291–294.

10. Bill, A.H. and Graumam, D. (1966) Rational and technique for stabilization of the mesentery in cases of non-rotation of the mid-gut. *Journal of Pediatric Surgery*, **1**, 27–31.

11. Blazek, F.D. and Boeckman, C.R. (1987) Prepyloric antral diaphragm: delay in treatment. *Journal of Pediatric Surgery*, **22**, 948–951.

12. Bower, R.J. and Ternberg, J.L. (1972) Preduodenal portal vein. *Journal of Pediatric Surgery*, **7**, 579.

13. Boyden, E.A., Cope, J.C. and Bill, A.G. (1967) Anatomy and embryology of congenital intrinsic obstruction of the duodenum. *American Journal of Surgery*, **114**, 190–194.

14. Breaux, C.W., Hood, J.S. and Georgeson, K.E. (1989) The significance of alkalosis and hypochloremia in hypertrophic pyloric stenosis. *Journal of Pediatric Surgery*, **12**, 1250–1254.

15. Bristol, J.B. and Bolton, R.A. (1981) The results of Ramstedt's operation in a district general hospital. *British Journal of Surgery*, **68**, 590–593.

16. Cameron, A.E.P. and Howard, E.R. (1987) Gastric volvulus in childhood. *Journal of Pediatric Surgery*, **22**, 944–947.

17. Carmi, R., Sofer, S., Karplus, M. *et al.* (1982) Aplasia cutis congenita in two sibs discordant for pyloric atresia. *American Journal of Medical Genetics*, **11**, 319–324.

18. Carter, C.O. and Evans, K.A. (1969) Inheritance of congenital pyloric stenosis. *Journal of Medical Genetics*, **6**, 233–237.

19. Chittmittrapap, S., Chandrakamol, B. and Chomdej, S. (1988) Intramural haematoma of the alimentary tract in children. *British Journal of Surgery*, **75**, 754–757.

20. Curet-Scott, M.J., Meller, J.L. and Shermeta, D.W. (1987) Transduodenal feedings: a superior route of enteral nutrition. *Journal of Pediatric Surgery*, **22**, 516–519.

21. Dengler, W.C. and Reddy, P.P. (1989) Right paraduodenal hernia in childhood: a case report. *Journal of Pediatric Surgery*, **24**, 1153–1158.

22. Ein, S.H. and Shandling, B. (1986) The late nonfunctioning duodenal atresia repair. *Journal of Pediatric Surgery*, **21**, 798–801.

23. Esscher, T. (1980) Preduodenal portal vein – a cause of intestinal obstruction. *Journal of Pediatric Surgery*, **15**, 609–614.

24. Filstron, H.C. and Kirks, D.R. (1981) Malrotation – the ubiquitous anomaly. *Journal of Pediatric Surgery*, **16**, 614–619.

25. Firor, H.V. and Harris, V.J. (1974) Rotational anomalies of the gut: recognition of a neglected facet – isolated incomplete rotation of the duodenum. *American Journal of Radiology*, **120**, 315–319.

26. Fitzgerald, P.G., Lau, G.Y.P., Langer, J.C. and Cameron, G.A. (1990) Umbilical fold incision for pyloromyotomy. *Journal of Pediatric Surgery*, **25**, 1117–1119.

27. Fonkalsrud, E.W., de Lorimer, A.A. and Hayes, D.M. (1969) Congenital atresia and stenosis of the duodenum: a review compiled from the membership of the Surgical Section of the American Academy of Pediatrics. *Pediatrics*, **43**, 79–84.

28. Forman, H.P., Leonidas, J.C. and Kronfeld, G.D. (1990) A rational approach to the diagnosis of hypertrophic pyloric stenosis: do the results match the claims? *Journal of Pediatric Surgery*, **25**, 262–266.

29. Foster, M.E. and Lewis, W.G. (1989) Early postoperative feeding – a continuing controversy in pyloric stenosis. *Journal of the Royal Society of Medicine*, **82**, 532–539.

30. Freisen, S.R. and Pearse, A.S.E. (1963) Pathogenesis of congenital pyloric stenosis: histochemical analysis of pyloric ganglion cells. *Surgery*, **53**, 604–609.

31. Girvan, D.P. and Stephens, C.A. (1974) Congenital duodenal obstruction: a twenty-year review of its surgical management and consequences. *Journal of Pediatric Surgery*, **9**, 833–834.

32. Glasson, M.J., Bandrevics, V. and Cohen, D.H. (1973) Hypertrophic pyloric stenosis complicating esophageal atresia. *Surgery*, **74**, 530–534.

33. Gohl, M.L. and DeMeester, W.R. (1975) Midgut nonrotation in adults: an aggressive approach. *American Journal of Surgery*, **129**, 319–326.

34. Gonzales, O.R., Hardin, W.D., Issacs, H., Lally, K.P. and Brennan, L.P. (1988) Duplication of the hepatopancreatic bud presenting as pyloric stenosis. *Journal of Pediatric Surgery*, **23**, 1053.

35. Gray, D.W., Gear, M.W. and Stevens, D.W. (1984) The results of Ramstedt's operation: room for complacency? *Annals of the Royal College of Surgeons of England*, **66**, 280–281.

36. Griffin, S.M., Chung, S.C.S., Leung, J.W.C. and Li, A.K.C. (1989) Peptic pyloric stenosis treated by endoscopic balloon dilatation. *British Journal of Surgery*, **76**, 1147–1152.

37. Hamburg, M.A., Miguon, M., Ricoor, G., Accary, J. and Pellerin, D. (1979) Serum gastrin levels in hypertrophic pyloric stenosis of infancy. Response

to a gastrin secretion test. *Archives of Diseases of Childhood*, **54**, 208–214.

38. Hancock, B.J. and Wiseman, N.E. (1989) Congenital duodenal obstruction: the impact of an antenatal diagnosis. *Journal of Pediatric Surgery*, **24**, 1027–1031.

39. Heymans, H.S.A., Bartelsman, W.F.M. and Herweijer, T.J. (1988) Endoscopic balloon dilatation as treatment of gastric outlet obstruction in infancy and childhood. *Journal of Pediatric Surgery*, **23**, 139–141.

40. Houston, C.S. and Wittenborg, M.H. (1965) Roentgen evaluation of anomalies of rotation and fixation of the bowel in children. *Radiology*, **84**, 1–16.

41. Howell, C.G. Vozza, F., Shaw, S. *et al.* (1982) Malrotation, malnutrition and ischemic bowel disease. *Journal of Pediatric Surgery*, **17**, 469–476.

42. Idowa, J., Aitken, D.K. and Georgeson, K.E. (1980) Gastric volvulus in newborns. *Archives of Surgery*, **115**, 1046–1054.

43. Jolley, S.G., Tunnell, W.P., Thomas, S., Young, J. and Smith, E.I. (1985) The significance of gastric emptying in children with intestinal malrotation. *Journal of Pediatric Surgery*, **20**, 627–629.

44. Kawana, T., Ikeda, K., Nakagawara, A., Kajiwara, M., Fukazawa, M. and Hara, K. (1989) A case of VACTEL syndrome with antenatally diagnosed duodenal atresia. *Journal of Pediatric Surgery*, **24**, 1158–1162.

45. Keller, H., Waldmann, D. and Greiner, P. (1987) Comparison of preoperative sonography with intraoperative findings in congenital hypertrophic pyloric stenosis. *Journal of Pediatric Surgery*, **22**, 950–954.

46. Kelly, M.E., Mohtashemi, H., Patel, S. and Gupta, R.C. (1979) Report of a case of double pylorus. *Digestive Diseases and Sciences*, **24**, 807–812.

47. Kimura, K., Tsugawa, C., Ogawa, K. *et al.* (1977) Diamond shaped anastomosis for congenital duodenal obstruction. *Archives of Surgery*, **112**, 1262–1268.

48. Kokkonen, M.-L., Kalima, T., Jaaskelainen, J. and Louhimo, I. (1988) Duodenal atresia: late follow-up. *Journal of Pediatric Surgery*, **23**, 216–221.

49. Kullendorf, C.M., Mikaelsson, C. and Ivancev, K. (1985) Malrotation in children with symptoms of gastrointestinal allergy and psychosomatic abdominal pain. *Acta Paediatrica Scandinavica*, **74**, 296–299.

50. La Ferla, G., Watson, J., Fyfe, A.H.B. and Drainer, I.K. (1986) The role of prostaglandins E2 and F2 alpha in infantile hypertrophic pyloric stenosis. *Journal of Pediatric Surgery*, **21**, 410–414.

51. Lynn, H.B. (1979) Duodenal obstruction: atresia, stenosis and annular pancreas. In *Pediatric Surgery* (Ed.) Ravitch, M.M., Welch, K.J., Benson, C.D., Aberdeen, E. and Randolph, J.G., pp. 902–910. Chicago: Chicago Year Book.

52. McDonald, P.J. (1986) Ramstedt's operation in district hospitals – is it safe? *Journal of the Royal Society of Medicine*, **79**, 17–24.

53. Marshal, D.G. and Kim, F. (1987) Leiomyosarcoma of the duodenum. *Journal of Pediatric Surgery*, **22**, 1007.

54. Mitchell, K.G., McGowan, A., Smith, D.C. and Gillespie, G. (1979) Pyloric diaphragm, antral web, congenital antral membrane – a surgical rarity? *British Journal of Surgery*, **66**, 572–573.

55. Moazam, F., Rodgers, B.M., Talbert, J.L. and McGuigon, J.E. (1978) Fasting and post prandial serum gastrin levels in infants with hypertrophic pyloric stenosis. *Annals of Surgery*, **188**, 623–628.

56. Moore, C.C.M. (1989) Congenital gastric outlet obstruction. *Journal of Pediatric Surgery*, **24**, 1241.

57. Okamatsu, T., Arai, K., Yatsuzuka, M. *et al.* (1989) Endoscopic membranectomy for congenital duodenal stenosis in an infant. *Journal of Pediatric Surgery*, **24**, 367–368.

58. Perrelli, L. and Wilkinson, A.W.W. (1975) Mortality in neonatal duodenal obstruction: a review of 76 cases compared with a previous review of 142 cases. *Journal of the Royal college of Surgeons of Edinburgh*, **20**, 365–368.

59. Powell, D.M., Biemann, H.O. and Smith, C.D. (1989) Malrotation of the intestines in children: the effect of age on presentation and therapy. *Journal of Pediatric Surgery*, **24**, 777–781.

60. Rasmussen, L., Hansen, L.P. and Pedersen, S.A. (1987) Infantile hypertrophic pyloric stenosis: the changing trend in treatment in a Danish County. *Journal of Pediatric Surgery*, **22**, 953–961.

61. Richardson, W.R. and Martin, I.W. (1969) Pitfalls in the surgical management of the incomplete duodenal diaphragm. *Journal of Pediatric Surgery*, **4**, 303–309.

62. Rogers, I.M., Drainer, I.K., Dougal, A.J., Black, J. and Logan, R. (1979) Serum cholecystokinin in basal acid secretion and infantile pyloric stenosis. *Archives of Diseases of Childhood*, **54**, 773–774.

63. Rogers, I.M., Macgillan, F. and Drainer, I.K. (1976) Congenital hypertrophic pyloric stenosis: a gastrin hypothesis pursued. *Journal of Pediatric Surgery*, **11**, 173–176.

64. Rowe, M.B., Bichler, D. and Clatworthy, H.W. (1968) Windsock of the duodenum. *Annals of Surgery*, **116**, 444–445.

65. Ruben, G.D., Templeton, J.M. and Ziegler, M.M. (1983) Situs inversus: the complex inducing neonatal intestinal obstruction. *Journal of Pediatric Surgery*, **18**, 751–756.

66. Saunders, M.P. and Williams, C.R. (1990) Infantile hypertrophic pyloric stenosis: experience in a district general hospital. *Journal of the Royal College of Surgeons of Edinburgh*, **35**, 36–37.

67. Sieunarine, K. and Manmohansingh, E. (1989) Gastric duplication cyst presenting as an acute abdomen in a child. *Journal of Pediatric Surgery*, **24**, 1152.

68. Spicer, R.D. (1982) Infantile hypertrophic pyloric

stenosis: a review. *British Journal of Surgery*, **69**, 128–131.

69. Spigland, N. and Yazbeck, S. (1990) complications associated with surgical treatment of congenital intrinsic duodenal obstruction. *Journal of Pediatric Surgery*, **25**, 1127–1131.

70. Spigland, N., Brand, M.L. and Yazbeck, S. (1990) Malrotation presenting beyond the neonatal period. *Journal of Pediatric Surgery*, **25**, 1139–1142.

71. Spitz, L. (1979) Vomiting after pyloromyotomy for infantile hypertrophic pyloric stenosis. *Archives of the Diseases of Childhood*, **54**, 886–887.

72. Spitz, L. and Batcup, G. (1979) Haematemesis in infantile hypertrophic pyloric stenosis: the source of the bleeding. *British Journal of Surgery*, **66**, 827–829.

73. Spitz, L. and MacKinnon, A.E. (1984) Posture in the postoperative management of infantile pyloric stenosis. *British Journal of Surgery*, **71**, 643–644.

74. Stauffer, U.G. and Herrmann, P. (1980) Comparison of late results in patients with corrected intestinal malrotation with and without fixation of the mesentery. *Journal of Pediatric Surgery*, **15**, 9–13.

75. Stauffer, U.G. and Irving, I. (1977) Duodenal atresia and stenosis – long term results. *Progress in Pediatric Surgery*, **10**, 49–59.

76. Stewart, D.R., Colodny, A.L. and Daggett, W.C. (1976) Malrotation of the bowel in infants and children: a 15 year old review. *Surgery*, **79**, 716–719.

77. Swinburne, L. and Kohler, H.G. (1979) Familial pyloric atresia associated with EB. *Journal of Pediatrics*, **94**, 162–164.

78. Synder, W.H. and Chaffin, L. (1954) Embryology and pathology of the intestinal tract: Presentation of 40 cases of malrotation. *Annals of Surgery*, **140**, 368–372.

79. Tam, P.K. (1985) Observations and perspectives of the pathology and possible aetiology of infantile hypertrophic pyloric stenosis. A histological, biochemical, histochemical and immunocytochemical study. *Annals of the Academy of Medicine*, **14**, 523–528.

80. Tam, P.K.H., Saing, H., Koo, J., Wong, J. and Ong, G.B. (1985) Pyloric function five to eleven years after Ramstedt's pyloromyotomy. *Journal of Pediatric Surgery*, **20**, 236–238.

81. Tan, K.C. and Bianchi, A. (1986) Circumumbilical incision for pyloromyotomy. *British Journal of Surgery*, **73**, 399.

82. Touloukian, R.J. (1983) Protocol for nonoperative treatment of obstructing intramural duodenal hematoma during childhood. *American Journal of Surgery*, **145**, 330–334.

83. Tunell, W.P. and Smith, E.I. (1980) Antral web in infancy. *Journal of Pediatric Surgery*, **15**, 152–153.

84. Tunell, W.P. and Wilson, D.A. (1984) Pyloric stenosis: diagnosis by real time sonography: the pyloric muscle length method. *Journal of Pediatric Surgery*, **19**, 795–797.

85. Ukabiala, O. and Lister, J. (1987) The extent of muscle hypertrophy in infantile hypertrophic pyloric stenosis does not depend on age and duration of symptoms. *Journal of Pediatric Surgery*, **22**, 200–204.

86. Velasco, A.K.L., Holcomb, G.W. Templeton, J.M. and Ziegler, M.M. (1990) Management of congenital microgastria. *Journal of Pediatric Surgery*, **25**, 192–194.

87. Vellacott, K.D. (1980) Intramural haematoma of the duodenum. *British Journal of Surgery*, **67**, 36.

88. Vinograd, I., Udassin, R., Beilin, B., Neuman, A., Maayan, C. and Nissan, S. (1985) The surgical management of children with familial dysautonia. *Journal of Pediatric Surgery*, **20**, 632–636.

89. Wang, C.A. and Welch, C.E. (1963) Anomalies of intestinal rotation in adolescents and adults. *Surgery*, **54**, 839–844.

90. Weber, T.R., Lewis, J.E., Mooney, D. and Connors, R. (1986) Duodenal atresia: a comparison of techniques of repair. *Journal of Pediatric Surgery*, **21**, 1133–1136.

91. Welch, G.H., Azmy, A.F. and Ziervogel, M.A. (1983) The surgery of malrotation and midgut volvulus: a nine year experience in neonates. *Annals of the Royal College of Surgeons of England*, **65**, 244–248.

92. Werlin, S.L., Grand, R.J. and Drug, D.E. (1978) Congenital hypertrophic pyloric stenosis – the role of gastrin re-evaluated. *Pediatrics*, **61**, 883–884.

93. Wiersma, R. and Hadley, G.P. (1988) Small bowel volvulus complicating intestinal ascariasis in children. *British Journal of Surgery*, **75**, 86–87.

94. Wilkinson, A.W.W., Hughes, E.A. and Stevens, L.H. (1965) Neonatal duodenal obstruction: the influence of treatment on the metabolic effects of operation. *British Journal of Surgery*, **52**, 410–412.

95. Williams, R.S., Gilmore, I.T. and Johnson, A.G. (1981) Congenital double pylorus: a case report. *British Journal of Surgery*, **68**, 65.

96. Wold, M., Callery, M. and White, J.J. (1988) Ectopic gastric-like duplication of the pancreas. *Journal of Pediatric Surgery*, **23**, 1051–1052.

97. Young, D.G. and Wilkinson, A.W.W. (1966) Mortality in neonatal duodenal obstruction. *The Lancet*, **ii**, 18–22.

98. Young, D.G. and Wilkinson, A.W.W. (1968) Abnormalities associated with neonatal duodenal atresia. *Surgery*, **6**, 832–836.

GASTRODUODENAL SECRETION IN HEALTH AND DISEASE

C.M. Brown and W.D.W. Rees

GASTRIC ACID SECRETION

CELLULAR MECHANISMS[31,71]

The parietal cell secretes hydrochloric acid in mammals, and is situated in gastric glands present in the fundus and corpus. There are at least four endogenous substances which stimulate the parietal cell to secrete acid: calcium, histamine, gastrin and acetylcholine. Histamine type 2, gastrin and muscarinic cholinergic receptors are present on the basolateral membrane of the parietal cell.

Ligand–receptor binding at the membrane requires a secondary intracellular signal to stimulate acid secretion (*Figure 2.20*). Activation of the H_2-receptor by histamine produces a transmembrane signal which activates adenylate cyclase. This results in raised intracellular levels of cAMP. Protein kinases are activated which, in turn, results in phosphorylation of target proteins. AMP, phosphodiesterase inhibitors and forskolin (direct activator of adenylate cyclase) all increase parietal cell function. Cholinergic stimulation is thought to require intracellular Ca^{2+} as a second messenger. The calmodulin system is recruited with subsequent protein activation. A third mechanism involves activation of phospholipase C by muscarinic receptors.[55] Membrane lipids act as substrate and inositol triphosphate is released. This is linked to calcium mobilization from intracellular stores.

The resting parietal cell has a complex system of tubulovesicular membranes situated within the apical cytoplasm. In the resting state most of the enzyme necessary for acid secretion is stored in this system. During cellular activation, the tubulovesicular membranes fuse with the apical membrane of the parietal cell, conveying the enzyme to its active site. The so-called 'proton pump' is a H^+/K^+-dependent ATPase which secretes H^+ in exchange for extracellular K^+. This is an active process and accounts for most of the oxidative metabolism by the parietal cell.[20] There are two separate conductance channels for K^+ and CL^- in the apical membrane which facilitate hydrochloric acid secretion (*Figure 2.21*). Hydroxide ions are generated within the cell and converted to bicarbonate ions via carbonic anhydrase. An HCO_3^-/Cl^- exchanger is present on the basolateral membrane. This provides Cl^- for hydrochloric acid secretion and extrudes HCO_3^- in order to maintain intracellular pH.[86] Blood, which actively drains acid-secreting gastric tissue, carries more HCO_3^-: the so-called 'alkaline tide'.

CONTROL MECHANISMS

Central control

Cerebral control of gastric acid secretion was first recognized by William Beaumont in 1833. Fear and anger were noted to reduce gastric secretion in Alexis St Martin, a patient with a traumatic gastric fistula.[3] The 'cephalic phase' of gastric acid secretion was first investigated by Pavlov in 1910. He described gastric acid and pepsin output increasing in dogs with oesophageal fistulas, in response to sham feeding.[53] Sight and smell of food increased acid output, and anticipation of feeding in conditioned dogs, produced the same response. Recently, hypnosis has been shown to modulate gastric acid secretion in healthy human subjects.[36] Acid output increased in hypnotized subjects in response to suggestions about eating delicious food. In contrast, acid output declined in response to deep relaxation and thoughts directed away from hunger. These responses are clearly mediated through the central nervous system.

Electrophysiological studies have demonstrated stimulation of afferent nerve fibres in the vagus nerve, resulting from gastric distension. Microelectrode techniques have established the importance of the hypothalamus and dorsal motor nucleus of the

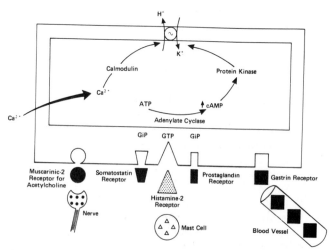

Figure 2.20 Model demonstrating receptors on the parietal cell basolateral membrane. H_2-receptor agonists cause activation of GTP regulatory protein which subsequently activates adenylate cyclase. Somatostatin and prostaglandin E_2 inhibit adenylate cyclase via G-inhibitory peptide. (Adapted, with permission, from Feldman, M. (1989) In: *Gastrointestinal Disease. Pathophysiology, Diagnosis, Management*, (Ed.) Sleisenger, M.H. and Fordtran, J.S., pp. 713–734. Philadelphia: W.B. Saunders.)

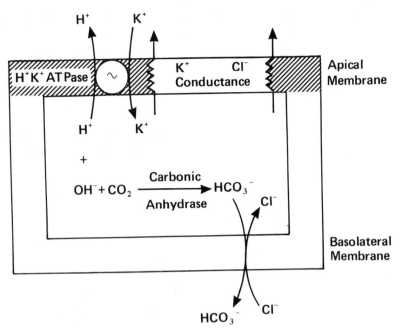

Figure 2.21 Model of ionic movements within the parietal cell essential for hydrochloric acid secretion. (Adapted, with permission, from Feldman, M. (1989) In: *Gastrointestinal Disease. Pathophysiology, Diagnosis, Management* (Ed.) Sleisenger, M.H. and Fordtran, J.S., pp. 713–734. Philadelphia: W.B. Saunders.)

vagal nerve, in regulating gastric acid secretion. The majority of motor neurons originating in the dorsal motor nucleus project to the stomach, as defined by axonoplasmic tracing techniques. Neurotransmitters and peptides injected intracerebrally into animals influence gastric acid secretion. Cholinergic excitation (acetylcholine, carbachol) increases acid secretion, an effect which is blocked by atropine and pirenzepine. γ-Aminobutyric acid (GABA) agonists (baclofen), gastrin and thyrotrophin-releasing hormone all stimulate gastric acid secretion[77] whilst prostaglandins E_2 and F_2, calcitonin-related peptides, adrenergic agonists, bombesin and gastrin-releasing peptide all inhibit gastric acid secretion. The last two peptides induce a similar response following intrathecal injection around the spinal cord – an inhibitory response thought to be mediated via the sympathoadrenal axis.[41,87]

Local control

The 'gastric phase' of acid secretion occurs when food is presented to the gastric lumen. Distension by food, saline or balloons stimulates gastric acid secretion by long, vagally mediated as well as local intragastric reflexes. These responses are thought to be mediated via acetylcholine and GABA in local neurons,[79] and are attenuated by atropine or H_2 receptor antagonists.

The protein content of meals provides a major stimulus to gastric acid secretion, especially the response to smaller digested peptides and amino acids. G cells present in the gastric antrum are stimulated to release gastrin, possibly in response to bombesin or gastrin-releasing peptide.[7] The human stomach secretes predominantly little gastrin (G17), and this acts as a local endocrine hormone, being transported to the corpus and fundus in the bloodstream. Here it binds to specific receptors on the parietal cell to stimulate acid secretion. Gastrin 17 also binds to local mast cells, causing degranulation and local histamine release. The histamine diffuses and by its 'paracrine effect' stimulates the H_2-receptors on parietal cells. There is some evidence that the type of protein is important in determining the acid secretory response and soy protein stimulates less gastrin and acid secretion in humans, compared with beef protein.[46] Gastrin-antibody neutralizing studies in dogs have confirmed the importance of gastrin in mediating the gastric phase of acid secretion.[40] Histamine also plays a central role in acid secretion as determined by studies on mast cell-deficient mice. Basal and stimulated levels of acid secretion is low in these animals, and correlates with low tissue levels of histamine.[76]

Gastric acid secretion is inhibited by low intraluminal pH, providing a negative-feedback mechanism. Low pH values in the gastric antrum inhibit gastrin release and this may occur via somatostatin inhibition. Somatostatin is released from S cells in response to luminal acid,[45,64] cholinergic stimulation[63] and other humoral factors such as calcitonin gene-related peptide.[6,27] Somatostatin also inhibits histamine release in response to gastrin,[62] and direct inhibition of parietal cells is possible by binding to specific somatostatin receptors on basolateral membrane. As a result a transmembrane signal is passed via G-inhibitory protein and adenylate cyclase is inhibited. The E prostaglandins are also potential inhibitors of acid secretion in many species. Parietal cells bear prostaglandin receptors, which when stimulated cause inhibition of adenylate cyclase via G-inhibitory protein.[30] The physiological role of such receptors remains to be clarified.

The 'intestinal phase' of gastric secretion occurs as a result of distension of the upper small intestine or the presence of peptides or amino acids. This stimulatory response is not abolished by denervating the bowel, and is therefore partially mediated by a humoral factor as yet not identified. An inhibitory 'intestinal phase' of gastric acid secretion occurs via three main stimuli: mechanical stimulation of the distal small bowel and colon inhibits acid secretion; acidic contents entering the duodenum stimulate release of secretin, which inhibits acid secretion;[8] and fatty foods entering the small intestine stimulate the release of two other peptides which have an inhibitory effect on acid secretion – neurotensin and peptide YY.[24]

MEASURING HUMAN GASTRIC ACID SECRETION

Acid secretion is measured in fasted patients by intubating the stomach and continually aspirating juice from the most dependent part. Volume, pH and titratable acidity of aspirated samples are measured over 1 hour to assess basal acid output. Maximal acid output is similarly measured over 1

hour following a maximal dose of pentagastrin (6 μg/kg by intramuscular injection).

An alternative method is to infuse a homogenized meal at a known pH into the stomach. Samples of gastric contents are aspirated at intervals and the pH measured. If the pH falls, alkali is added incrementally to raise the pH to baseline. Over a given period of time, the number of millimoles of base added equals the number of millimoles of acid secreted by the stomach. This is always an underestimate and corrections are applied for duodenal loss and reflux.[2,29]

DISORDERS OF ACID SECRETION

Hypersecretion

Peptic ulcer disease

Patients with benign gastric ulcer secrete gastric acid in similar quantities to normal controls (*Table 2.1*). Increased acid secretion occurs in one-third of patients with duodenal ulcer, and is associated with an increased parietal cell mass, although there is a large overlap with the normal range.

A circadian rhythm of acid secretion occurs in both normal subjects,[48] and patients with duodenal ulcer.[48,49] However, postprandial peaks and nocturnal levels of acid secretion are higher in patients with duodenal ulcer.[93] Cigarette smoking is associated with raised acid output in both normal subjects and duodenal ulcer patients.[10,83] *Helicobacter pylori* is increasingly recognized as a pathogenic organism causing gastritis and duodenal ulcer. Hypergastrinaemia, in response to this antral infection,[73] can cause an increased parietal cell mass, known to be associated with duodenal ulcer.

Zollinger–Ellison syndrome

Gastrin-secreting tumours may cause hypergastrinaemia leading to marked elevation in gastric acid secretion. These tumours are usually present in the pancreas, or occasionally the duodenal wall, and are multiple in 50% of cases. Rarely, tumours of the ovary or parathyroid glands can secrete gastrin.

Table 2.1 The mean and range of basal and maximal acid output (mmol/h) in normal subjects and patients with peptic ulcer

	Normal		Duodenal ulcer		Gastric ulcer	
	Basal	Peak	Basal	Peak	Basal	Peak
Men	1 (0–5+)	22 (<1–45)	4 (0–15+)	42 (15–100+)	1 (0–5+)	23 (3–40)
Women	1 (0–5+)	12 (<1–30)	2 (0–5+)	32 (15–100+)	1 (0–5+)	10 (1–30)

From Baron.[2]

Two-thirds of such lesions are malignant and may metastasize to liver, spleen, regional lymph nodes and peritoneum. A quarter of patients also have tumours or hyperplasia of the pituitary and parathyroid glands: the multiple endocrine neoplasia type 1 syndrome (MEN1). The secreted gastrin has trophic effects on gastric parietal cells which may enlarge to three to six times the normal size.

Ninety to ninety-five per cent of patients with Zollinger–Ellison syndrome present with recurrent or multiple peptic ulceration. Reflux oesophagitis is more common than previously thought, and one-third of patients complain of diarrhoea. Steatorrhoea is much less common, but can occur as a result of acidic inactivation of bile salts and lipases.

The diagnosis is established from a raised gastric acid output (15–100 mEq/h) associated with hypergastrinaemia. Normal levels of gastrin are less than 60 pg/ml and patients with gastrinoma often have gastrin levels in excess of 1000 pg/ml. Pernicious anaemia can also cause hypergastrinaemia in the Zollinger–Ellison range. In cases where the gastrin is only modestly raised, this can be greatly enhanced following intravenous secretin. In normal patients the gastrin response to secretin is minimal or absent.

Tumours are localized initially with a computed tomography (CT) scan, which has a 70% detection rate.[81] In patients with a negative CT scan, selective angiography will detect a further 16–28% of gastrinomas.[47] Recent studies suggest that the use of an endoscopic ultrasound probe may also enhance diagnostic yield. In some patients it is necessary to proceed to laparotomy, with careful palpation of the pancreas, in order to localize the tumour.

Medical treatment is indicated for patients before surgery, for those unfit for surgery or for those with metastatic disease. Omeprazole, a recently introduced proton pump inhibitor, has now superseded othe H_2 receptor antagonists, and blocks acid secretion in doses of 60–120 mg/day in most cases. Surgical resection is possible in 25% of cases, and these patients can expect a normal life expectancy free of acid-related disease. Average survival in patients with hepatic metastases is 2 years, whilst those with MEN1 have the worst outlook.

Miscellaneous

Gastric acid hypersecretion occurs in the retained antrum following partial gastrectomy. Residual gastrin cells are bathed in alkaline secretions from the afferent loop resulting in a high gastrin output. Acid hypersecretion also occurs in G-cell hyperplasia, systemic mastocytosis, extensive small bowel resection, severe gastro-oesophageal reflux disease[9] and Barrett's oesophagus,[50] and following portocaval shunting.[78]

Hyposecretion

Gastric acid secretion diminishes with age in both animals[35] and humans. Gastric acid hyposecretion occurs in achlorhydric patients with pernicious anaemia, although acid secretion studies are rarely required for diagnosis. Extensive intestinal metaplasia and gastric carcinoma can also be associated with low levels of acid secretion. Reduced acid output occurs in malnourished children[22] and experimental evidence suggests that acute gastrointestinal bleeding may inhibit acid and pepsin secretion. Intraduodenal infusions of autologous blood in healthy volunteers increases gastric inhibitory peptide levels and reduces gastric acid secretion. This may constitute a protective mechanism.[21]

PEPSINOGENS

PHYSIOLOGICAL ROLE

Pepsinogens are proteolytic enzyme precursors synthesized and secreted by gastroduodenal mucosa. There are similarities with other proteases such as renin. The oxyntic cell in lower vertebrates secretes both pepsinogens and hydrochloric acid, whereas in mammals the parietal cell solely secretes hydrochloric acid. Pepsinogens are secreted predominantly by chief cells present in the lower part of gastric glands, although there is a small contribution from mucous neck cells.

In the presence of acid, pepsinogens are activated to form active pepsins. Smaller peptides are cleaved from ingested proteins and these stimulate secretion of several gastrointestinal hormones including gastrin and cholecystokinin.

There are at least eight pepsinogens with different patterns of electrophoresis. Immunological studies put these into three distinct groups, with pepsinogens 1–5 belonging to group I, pepsinogens 6 and 7 to group II, and the eighth being an immunologically distinct, slow-moving protease. Recent studies suggest that there may be several other proteolytic factors in gastric mucosal extracts besides the eight already described. The gastric corpus and fundus secrete pepsinogens in both groups I and II. The gastric antrum and duodenal Brunner's glands secrete only group II pepsinogens. The physical properties of both groups are different. Optimum activity of group I pepsin occurs at pH 1.5–2.0, whereas pH 3.2 represents the most favourable pH for group II pepsin activity. Those in the latter group are also more resistant to alkaline denaturation.

Slow-moving protease is produced by superficial epithelial cells rather than in gastric glands, and accounts for less than 5% of total proteolytic activity of gastric mucosal extracts.

Pepsinogens can be detected in serum by radio-immunoassay. Group I pepsinogens are detected in urine whereas group II pepsinogens are found in semen, although the relevance of these findings is unclear.

SECRETORY MECHANISMS

A number of stimuli are known to increase pepsinogen secretion. Acetylcholine and carbachol mediate cholinergic stimulation of pepsinogen secretion. This probably occurs via stimulation of adenylate cyclase and cAMP production.[14] cAMP, forskolin, vasoactive intestinal polypeptide and cholecystokinin all stimulate pepsinogen secretion. Response to cholecystokinin is blocked by specific antagonists.[59] Prostaglandins of the E class also stimulate pepsinogen secretion, and similarities with forskolin-stimulated synthesis suggests a cAMP-mediated response. Luminal acid has no effect on pepsinogen secretion in chief cell monolayers, but higher concentrations of pepsin have an inhibitory effect.[15] De novo pepsinogen synthesis is also stimulated by carbachol, cholecystokinin, vasoactive intestinal polypeptide, forskolin and cAMP, but this is dependent on prior depletion of preformed pepsinogens.[14] Histamine and gastrin both stimulate pepsinogen secretion in vivo, although the response to gastrin is probably indirect as atropine and H_2 receptor antagonists are inhibitory.

Microscopic studies suggest that intracellular secretory granules initially fuse with each other, and then with the apical membrane. A biphasic pattern of secretion probably reflects rapid secretion of preformed pepsinogen, as detected by a rapid loss of secretory granules and a later phase involving secretion of newly synthesized pepsinogen.

Pathophysiology of pepsinogens

Basal and stimulated levels of group I pepsinogens are modestly elevated in duodenal ulcer patients. It was hoped that these could be used as markers or predictors of duodenal ulcer, but unfortunately they have not been found to be of clinical value. Pepsins are implicated in the pathogenesis of duodenal ulcer, but it is difficult to differentiate the relative importance of acid and pepsins. Many secretory stimuli that are common to both, and H_2 receptor antagonists, inhibit secretion of acid and pepsinogens.

Pepsin 3 is the major pepsin in humans with pepsin 1 accounting for only 3.6% of total pepsin activity in healthy volunteers. However, in gastric and duodenal ulcer patients, pepsin 1 accounts for 23 and 16.5%, respectively, of the total pepsin activity present. The pathogenic significance of these observations is that pepsin 1 has been shown to digest mucus more readily then pepsin 3, both at the optimum pH of 2 (twice as active) and at the higher pH of 4 (six times as active). Further confirmation of the relevance of these findings has been obtained by examining the mucolytic activity of gastric juice from duodenal ulcer patients at pH values of 2 and 4. The results showed that gastric juice from duodenal ulcer patients had significantly greater mucolytic activity than that from healthy controls. Such enhanced mucus digestion may impair the protective barrier afforded by gastroduodenal mucus gel and may therefore play a role in ulcer pathogenesis.[66]

MUCUS SECRETION

COMPOSITION AND SECRETION

Mucus is a complex material secreted by cells throughout the gastrointestinal tract. It consists of glycoproteins, called mucins, lipids, electrolytes and sloughed cells, although more than 70% is water.

Mucus is secreted by surface epithelial cells, mucous neck cells within gastric glands and Brunner's glands in the duodenum. The glycoprotein component consists of a protein with many carbohydrate side chains attached to the serine and threonine residues of the core, like the bristles of a test tube brush. The carbohydrate side chains are approximately 15 sugar residues long, the major sugars being galactose, fucose, N-acetylgalactosamine, and N-acetylglucosamine. The molecular weight of each subunit is around 500 000 and the terminal sugars of the carbohydrate side chains express antigenic determinants such as the ABO blood group system.[66]

Under normal conditions in vivo, the glycoprotein subunits are linked by disulphide bonds between non-glycosylated parts of the protein core. If such bonds are destroyed by agents such as N-acetyl-L-cysteine, or by proteolysis with pepsin, the polymeric structure is lost and mucus loses its gel-forming and viscous properties, becoming soluble mucus. This occurs under normal conditions with the surface mucus gel being continually eroded by pepsin and replaced by newly secreted mucin from the underlying epithelium. The precise nature of the

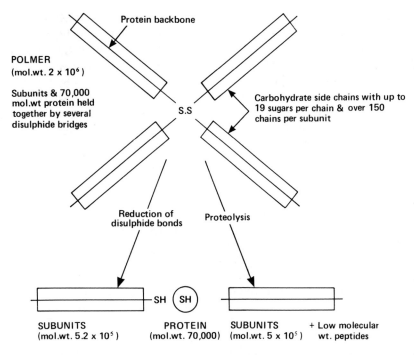

POLMER
(mol.wt. 2 x 10^6)

Subunits & 70,000
mol.wt protein held
together by several
disulphide bridges

Protein backbone

Carbohydrate side chains with up to
19 sugars per chain & over 150
chains per subunit

S.S

Reduction of
disulphide bonds

Proteolysis

SH (SH)

SUBUNITS
(mol.wt. 5.2 x 10^5)

PROTEIN
(mol.wt. 70,000)

SUBUNITS
(mol.wt. 5 x 10^5)

+ Low molecular
wt. peptides

Figure 2.22 The 'windmill model' for the structure of gastric mucus. (Reproduced, with permission, from Allen, A. (1981) In: *Physiology of the Gastrointestinal Tract* (Ed.) Johnson, L.R., pp. 617–639. New York: Raven Press.)

polymeric structure of mucus gel remains uncertain. One model proposes a tetrameric structure with four subunits linked together by disulphide bonds (*Figure 2.22*), whilst more recent data envisage a much longer or coiled structure (*Figure 2.23*).

MEASUREMENT OF MUCUS SECRETION

Methodological difficulties in quantifying the functional unit of mucus has hampered research into its nature and regulation. Radioactively labelled sugar residues and the measurement of soluble glycoprotein in gastric aspirate were used initially, but failed to provide information about the unstirred mucous gel layer.[26] Such indirect indices could not distinguish between increased glycoprotein synthesis and enhanced breakdown of the surface gel, and the early results were therefore difficult to interpret. However, two methods have now been described which measure thickness of the surface unstirred gel layer. One of these uses a slit-lamp and pachymeter system similar to that used by ophthalmologists to measure corneal thickness, whilst the

A)

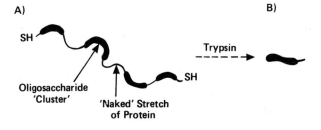

B)

SH

Oligosaccharide
'Cluster'

'Naked' Stretch
of Protein

SH

Trypsin

C)

D)

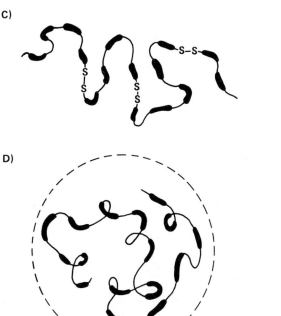

Figure 2.23 The 'coiled thread' model for the structure of gastric mucus. (Reproduced, with permission, from Carlstedt, I. and Sheehan, J.K. (1984) In: *Mucus and Mucosa (Ciba Foundations Symposium 109)*, pp. 157–166. London: Pitman.)

second involves phase contrast microscopy. These techniques have confirmed the existence of a continuous and dynamic gel layer overlying gastric epithelial cells, with a thickness of 0.2–0.6 mm in humans. As anticipated, the thickness of this layer is reduced by topical *N*-acetyl-L-cysteine and is enhanced by topical prostaglandin E_2. Of clinical significance are the observations that gel thickness may be reduced by aspirin and enhanced by carbenoxolone.

REGULATION OF MUCUS PRODUCTION

There appear to be at least two intracellular signals involved in mucus secretion. Cholinergic stimulation, which has been shown to enhance glycoprotein synthesis in a number of experimental models, is dependent on mobilization of intracellular calcium. This pathway is inhibited by atropine, depletion of intracellular calcium and inhibition of calmodulin. However, stimulation of mucus production by prostaglandin E_2 and forskolin is calcium-independent and probably dependent on cAMP.[65]

Apart from cholinergic stimulation, a variety of other neurohormonal agents have been shown to increase the formation of soluble glycoprotein, but the physiological significance of such findings remains in doubt. Studies on the mucus gel layer itself are limited to in vitro systems, and further evaluation must await the development of more sophisticated methodology.

FUNCTIONAL SIGNIFICANCE OF MUCUS GEL

Theories on the physiological role of mucus gel have ranged from those regarding it as a mere lubricant to those considering the gel layer as an important component of mucosal protection. The viscoelastic properties of the glycoprotein polymer help create an adherent unstirred layer that is adjacent to surface epithelial cells in the stomach and duodenum. With the discovery of bicarbonate transport across surface epithelium, the mucus gel layer became an essential component of a 'mucus–bicarbonate barrier' (see Bicarbonate secretion, p. 203), confining acid neutralization by bicarbonate to the unstirred layer. In this way, the surface epithelial cells were protected against direct exposure to damaging acid and pepsin. Recent studies have also shown that the mucus gel layer has hydrophobic properties largely due to its phospholipid content. Hydrophobicity was originally attributed to a mono- or bimolecular layer

of surface-active phospholipids lying between the mucus gel layer and the epithelial cell membrane. However, such hydrophobicity, which repels water containing hydrogen ions, is now also thought to lie within and on the luminal surface of mucus gel.[23] This surfactant-like property may be increased by topical prostaglandin E_2 and reduced by aspirin.[34] Study of this hydrophobic property has been enhanced by developing a method that allows its measurement in endoscopic biopsies from humans.[74]

MUCUS IN PEPTIC ULCER DISEASE

There is evidence that the polymeric structure of mucus gel may be defective in peptic ulcer disease, especially gastric ulcer, leading to a weaker and more easily digested gel structure. Furthermore, there is also evidence that the gastric juice of both gastric and duodenal ulcer patients, has greater proteolytic activity than normal (see Pepsinogen, p. 200). Non-steroidal anti-inflammatory drugs have been implicated in peptic ulcer pathogenesis, and it is of interest that these drugs reduce mucus production and the thickness of the gel layer. Surface hydrophobicity has recently been shown to be significantly reduced in both duodenal and gastric ulcer patients.[75] Hydrophobicity was also reduced in patients with antral gastritis due to infection with *H. pylori*. It is conceivable therefore that the organism damages mucous gel by either reducing the rate of mucus polymerization or increasing polymer destruction.[69] Although unlikely, it has been suggested that these effects may be related to increased ammonia production from the urease activity of *Helicobacter pylori*. The organism also releases enzymes such as lipases and proteases which directly damage glycoprotein structure and stability.[60,72] Interestingly, neither the *H. pylori* infection nor the associated reduced hydrophobicity is altered by histamine H_2 receptor antagonists.

MUCUS GLYCOPROTEIN IN GASTRIC CANCER

As mentioned, the ABO blood group is expressed in mucus glycoprotein of certain 'secretor' subjects. It has been shown that these antigens disappear from mucus gel, conferring 'non-secretor' status, following the development of gastric adenocarcinoma. Occasionally other antigens are expressed. The pathophysiological significance of these changes remains unknown and unfortunately such changes cannot serve as tumour markers.

GASTRODUODENAL BICARBONATE SECRETION

HISTORY

Gastric bicarbonate secretion was first postulated 100 years ago by Schierbeck, who noticed a high pCO_2 in the gastric lumen. Hollander demonstrated bicarbonate secretion in 1954 using fundic pouches after antrectomy and vagotomy. A protective mucus–bicarbonate layer was suggested by Heatley in 1959,[25] although experimental evidence was lacking until much later. Flemström performed pioneering experiments in 1977, demonstrating bicarbonate secretion by amphibian gastric mucosa mounted in Ussing chambers.[18] Since then, HCO_3^- secretion has been documented in mammalian stomach and duodenum in vitro and in vivo. Alkali secretion by the normal human stomach was first reported by Rees *et al*. in 1982.[58] An intubation and perfusion technique was employed with acid secretion suppressed by H_2 receptor antagonists. pH and pCO_2 of aspirated samples allows calculation of the HCO_3^- concentration via the Henderson–Hasselbach equation, and normal secretion is approximately $400\,\mu Eq/h$, i.e. 5–10% of the rate of acid secretion. A second later method involved measurements of osmolality.[17] Changes in osmolality occur when H^+ combines with HCO_3^-, and bicarbonate secretion by the normal stomach was calculated by this method to be $2300\,\mu Eq/h$, although this is probably an overestimate.[17] Recently, duodenal bicarbonate secretion has been demonstrated by Isenberg and colleagues, in an occluded 4 cm segment of human proximal duodenum.[51]

SECRETORY MECHANISMS

Stomach

Fundic epithelium secretes HCO_3^- almost exclusively by a metabolically active transcellular mechanism. This is in contrast to secretion by gastric antrum (and duodenum), where 30% of HCO_3^- secretion occurs by a paracellular passive mechanism. Calcium, carbachol, cyclic GMP and prostaglandins all stimulate HCO_3^- transport in amphibian fundic mucosa. Secretion is dependent on luminal Cl^-, suggesting a HCO_3^- exchange mechanism on the apical membrane. There are no changes in potential difference observed during secretion which supports an electroneutral transport process (*Figure 2.24*).

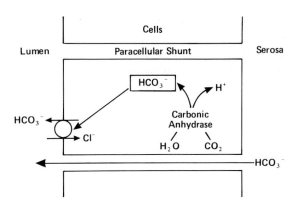

Figure 2.24 Transport mechanisms for bicarbonate ions across gastric epithelium.

Duodenum

The duodenal mucosa, Brunner's glands and pancreaticobiliary secretions may all contribute alkali to the duodenal lumen, although *in vivo* rat experiments suggest that Brunner's glands probably do not contribute significant quantities of bicarbonate.[85] Distal duodenal loops devoid of Brunner's glands secrete similar quantities of HCO_3^- compared to proximal duodenal loops in which these glands are present.

In contrast to fundic mucosa, the duodenum in rats secrete significant quantities of HCO_3^- by a passive paracellular shunt pathway[84] and extracellular HCO_3^- appears to be a major source of transported alkali. Luminal acid stimulates alkali secretion and this is associated with an increased transmucosal flux of radioactively labelled urea. This indicates that increased HCO_3^- secretion occurs via increased paracellular diffusion. There is conflicting evidence concerning the mechanism of prostaglandin E_2-stimulated duodenal alkali secretion in the rat. Some data show no increase in mucosal permeability indicating a transcellular pathway,[84] whereas other results suggest a passive paracellular route because prostaglandin-stimulated

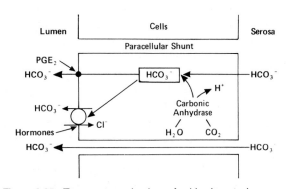

Figure 2.25 Transport mechanisms for bicarbonate ions across duodenal epithelium.

alkali secretion requires a blood:lumen alkali gradient.[28] Human perfusion studies suggest an active transport mechanism for HCO_3^- in the normal duodenum[51] with alkali secretion unaltered even in the absence of a blood:lumen gradient. Studies on rat duodenal enterocytes demonstrate that the Cl^-/HCO_3^- exchange in the duodenum is present in apical membrane[4] (*Figure 2.25*).

CONTROL MECHANISMS

Evidence is accumulating that the brain exerts central control over gastroduodenal HCO_3^- secretion, in a manner similar to gastric acid secretion. Electrical stimulation of the nucleus ambiguus in cats increases gastric alkalinity. Stimulation of cut vagus nerves enhances gastric and duodenal HCO_3^- secretion, whereas sham feeding increases the gastric HCO_3^- level in humans (a response negated by atropine). Thyrotrophin-releasing hormone injected into cerebral ventricles of rats increase duodenal HCO_3^- secretion[19,43] and this response is abolished by vagotomy or intravenous vasoactive intestinal polypeptide antagonist. This suggests that thyrotrophin-releasing hormone stimulates vagal fibres to release vasoactive intestinal polypeptide. Similar injection of somatostatin 28 also stimulates duodenal HCO_3^- secretion and this response is prevented by ganglion-blocking agents or truncal vagotomy.[42]

Local cholinergic neurons are also important in the regulation of duodenal HCO_3^- secretion. Electrical field stimulation in amphibian tissue increases HCO_3^- secretion, a response blocked by atropine and neurotoxins.[12] Splanchnic nerves mediate sympathetic inhibition of duodenal HCO_3^- secretion. The cut end of splanchnic nerves, when electrically stimulated, causes inhibition of duodenal alkalinization : a response blocked by guanethidine and yohimbine (α_2 adrenoreceptor antagonist).[32] Splanchnic nerve inhibition of duodenal HCO_3^- secretion also occurs in response to bleeding and hypotension,[32,33,70] and perfusion studies in humans have shown inhibitory effects of clonidine (α_2 agonist) on duodenal alkalinization.[37]

Gastric and duodenal bicarbonate secretion may be altered by a variety of neurohormonal agents, but as yet the physiological significance of such changes remains unknown. However, the stimulation of gastric and duodenal alkali secretion by topical acid is likely to represent a protective mechanism. Such acid 'autoregulation' of gastroduodenal alkali secretion was initially demonstrated in animals, but has recently been shown to exist in the human stomach and proximal duodenum.[1,11,80] Although early studies suggested that release of local prosta-

glandins may mediate this response, recent experiments have implicated vasoactive intestinal polypeptide.

PHYSIOLOGICAL RELEVANCE OF BICARBONATE SECRETION

In isolation, bicarbonate secretion would probably confer little protection and would be overwhelmed by intraluminal acid. Delivery of alkali into the unstirred layer provided by mucus gel confines such neutralization of acid to the cell surface, and has been shown to result in a significant pH gradient across mucus.[85] A similar 'mucus–bicarbonate' barrier has been demonstrated in the duodenal cap.

The relative importance of this barrier to overall protection still remains uncertain[57] and it can be overwhelmed by physiological levels of acid in the stomach (pH less than 1.5). It now seems likely that this barrier in the stomach is a weak 'first-line' defence against acid–pepsin attack. In the duodenum, however, the magnitude of alkali secretion is greater and studies have shown a correlation between inhibition of alkalinization and the development of villous injury.[82] Exogenous prostaglandins protect against acid-induced injury in the duodenum, and enhanced bicarbonate secretion may well mediate this response.[44] In contrast, acidification of the duodenum impairs healing of damaged epithelium where restitution is optimum at an alkaline pH.[16]

Although alkali secretion may be important in preserving the integrity of gastroduodenal mucosa, and in the re-epithelialization of superficial injury, there is little evidence that it plays a role in chronic ulcer healing where more complex processes, involving angiogenesis, chronic inflammatory cell infiltration and connective tissue deposition, appear essential to tissue healing.

BICARBONATE SECRETION IN PEPTIC ULCER DISEASE

Abnormalities of gastric and duodenal bicarbonate secretion have been described in gastric and duodenal ulcer disease, respectively. Using an indirect technique for calculating bicarbonate output, from changes in osmolality of gastric juice, reduced alkali production by the stomach has been demonstrated in patients with gastric ulcer. Similarly, reduced basal bicarbonate secretion and a blunted response to topical acid have been demonstrated in an isolated segment from patients with duodenal ulcer.[5] Vagal stimulation has been shown to increase gastric alkali secretion in humans and this response appears normal in patients with duodenal ulcer.[38] The functional significance of decreased duodenal alkalinization in duodenal ulcer patients has been studied by measuring juxtamucosal pH in the duodenal cap by an endoscopic pH probe.[56] In such patients, the duodenal epithelial cells were exposed to a more acidic environment than healthy controls, confirming that the abnormal rate of alkali secretion reduces the magnitude of the mucus pH gradient in the duodenal cap.

Whilst of interest, the importance of these changes in alkali secretion to ulcer pathogenesis remains unknown. A number of ulcer-healing drugs, such as sucralfate and colloidal bismuth subcitrate, have been shown to increase gastroduodenal alkali secretion both in vitro and in vivo.[13,39,67,68] However, such drugs have other effects on mucosal defence mechanisms and potential aggressors, such as *H. pylori*, and the relevance of the increased alkali secretion to their ulcer-healing actions remains unknown.

REFERENCES

1. Algazi, M.C., Chen, H.-S., Koss, M.A. *et al.* (1989) Effect of VIP antagonist on VIP-, PGE_2-, and acid-stimulated duodenal bicarbonate secretion. *American Journal of Physiology*, **256**, G833–G836.
2. Baron, J.H. (1978) *Clinical Tests of Gastric Secretion: History, Methodology and Interpretation*. London: Macmillan.
3. Beaumont, W. (1833) *Experiments and Observations on the Gastric Juice and the Physiology of Digestion*, pp. 9–23. Platsburgh: F.P Allen.
4. Brown, C.D.A., Dunk, C.R. and Turnberg, L.A. (1989) $Cl–HCO_3$ exchange and anion conductance in rat duodenal apical membrane vesicles. *American Journal of Physiology*, **257**, G661–G667.
5. Bukhave, K., Rask-Madsen, J., Hogan, D.L., Koss, M.A. and Isenberg, J.I. (1990) Proximal duodenal prostaglandin E_3 release and mucosal bicarbonate secretion are altered in patients with duodenal ulcer. *Gastroenterology*, **99**, 951–955.
6. Bunnett, N.W., Hellon, W.S., Debas, H.T. and Ensinck, J.W. (1990) CGRP stimulates the release of pro-somatostatin-derived peptides from the gastric fundus. *American Journal of Physiology*, **258**, G316–G319.
7. Campos, R.V., Buchan, A.M.J., Meloche, R.M., Pederson, R.A., Kwok, Y.N. and Coy, D.H. (1990) Gastrin secretion from human antral G-cells in culture. *Gastroenterology*, **99**, 36–44.
8. Christianson, J., Hansen, B., Hilstead, L. and Schaffalitzky De Muckadell, O.B. (1988) Effect of low-dose exogenous secretin on pentagastrin- and meal-stimulated gastric acid secretion in humans. *Digestive Diseases and Sciences*, **33**, 1277–1281.
9. Collen, M.J., Lewis, J.H. and Benjamin, S.B. (1990) Gastric acid hypersecretion in refractory gastroesophageal reflux disease. *Gastroenterology*, **98**, 654–661.
10. Corinaldesi, R., Stanghellini, V., Paparo, G.F., Paternico, A., Rusticali, A.G. and Barbara, L. (1989) Gastric acid secretion and gastric emptying of liquids in 99 male duodenal ulcer patients. *Digestive Diseases and Sciences*, **34**, 251–256.
11. Crampton, J.R., Gibbons, L.C. and Rees, W.D.W. (1987) Effect of luminal pH on the output of bicarbonate and PGE_2 by the normal human stomach. *Gut*, **28**, 1291–1295.
12. Crampton, J.R., Gibbons, L.C. and Rees, W.D.W. (1988) Neural regulation of duodenal alkali secretion: effects of electrical field stimulation. *American Journal of Physiology*, **254**, G162–G167.
13. Crampton, J.R., Gibbons, L.C. and Rees, W.D.W. (1988) Stimulation of amphibian gastroduodenal bicarbonate secretion by sucralfate and aluminium: role of local prostaglandin metabolism. *Gut*, **29**, 903–908.
14. Defize, J. and Hunt, R.H. (1988) Control of pepsinogen synthesis and secretion in primary monolayer cultures of canine gastric chief cells. *Digestive Diseases and Sciences*, **33**, 1583–1591.
15. Defize, D. and Hunt, R.H. (1989) Effect of hydrochloric acid and prostaglandins on pepsinogen synthesis and secretion in canine gastric chief cell monolayer cultures. *Gut*, **30**, 774–781.
16. Feil, W., Klimesch, S., Karner, P. *et al.* (1989) Importance of an alkaline microenvironment for rapid restitution of the rabbit duodenal mucosal in vitro. *Gastroenterology*, **97**, 112–122.
17. Feldman, M. and Barnett, C.C. (1983) Gastric bicarbonate secretion in humans. Effects of pentagastrin, bethanechol and 11,16,16-trimethyl prostaglandin E_2. *Journal of Clinical Investigation*, **72**, 295–303.
18. Flemström, G. (1977) Active alkalinisation by amphibian gastric fundic mucosa *in vitro*. *American Journal of Physiology*, **233**, E1–12.
19. Flemström, G. and Jedstedt, G. (1989) Stimulation of duodenal mucosal bicarbonate secretion in the rat by brain peptides. *Gastroenterology*, **97**, 412–420.
20. Frykhund, J., Gedda, K., Scott, D., Sachs, G. and Wallmark, B. (1990) Coupling of $H^+–K^+$-ATPase activity and glucose oxidation in gastric glands. *American Journal of Physiology*, **258**, G719–G727.
21. Fullarton, G.M., Boyd, E.J.S., Crean, G.P., Buchanon, K. and McColl, K.E.L. (1989) Inhibition of gastric secretion and motility by simulated upper gastrointestinal haemorrhage: a response to facilitate haemostasis? *Gut*, **30**, 156–160.
22. Gilman, R.H., Partanen, R., Brown, K.H. *et al.*

(1988) Decreased gastric acid secretion and bacterial colonisation of the stomach in severely malnourished Bangladeshi children. *Gastroenterology*, **94**, 1308–1314.

23. Goddard, P.J., Kao, Y.-C.J. and Lichtenberger, L.M. (1990) Luminal surface hydrophobicity of canine gastric mucosa is dependent on a surface mucus gel. *Gastroenterology*, **98**, 361–370.

24. Guo, Y.-S., Fujimura, M., Lluis, F., Tsong, Y., Greeley, G.H., Jr and Thompson, J.C. (1987) Inhibitory action of peptide YY on gastric acid secretion. *American Journal of Physiology*, **253**, G298–G302.

25. Heatley, N.G. (1959) Mucosubstance and a barrier to diffusion. *Gastroenterology*, **37**, 313–317.

26. Heim, H.-K., Oestmann, A. and Sewing, K.-Fr. (1990) Stimulation of glycoprotein and protein synthesis in isolated pit gastric mucosal cells by prostaglandins. *Gut*, **31**, 412–416.

27. Helton, W.S., Mulholland, M.M., Bunnett, N.W. and Debas, H.T. (1989) Inhibition of gastric and pancreatic secretion in dogs by CGRP: role of somatostatin. *American Journal of Physiology*, **256**, G715–G720.

28. Heylings, J.R. and Feldman, M. (1988) Basal and PGE_2-stimulated duodenal bicarbonate secretion in the rat in vivo. *American Journal of Physiology*, **255**, G470–G475.

29. Hobsley, M. (1988) Tests of gastric secretory function. In *Scientific Foundation of Gastroenterology* (Ed.) Sircus, W. and Smith, A.N. pp. 316–332. London: Heinemann.

30. Jaramillo, E., Mardh, S., Green, K., Persson, B., Rubio, C. and Aly, A. (1989) the effect of arachidonic acid and its metabolites on acid production in isolated human parietal cells. *Scandinavian Journal of Gastroenterology*, **24**, 1231–1237.

31. Johnson, L.R., Christensen, J., Jackson, M.J., Jacobson, E.D. and Walsh, J.H. (1987) *Physiology of the Gastrointestinal Tract*. New York: Raven Press.

32. Jönson, C. and Fändriks, L. (1989) Splanchnic nerve stimulation inhibits duodenal HCO_3^- secretion in the rat. *American Journal of Physiology*, **255**, G709–G712.

33. Jönson, C., Tunbäck-Hanson, P. and Fändriks, L. (1989) Splanchnic nerve activation inhibits the increase in duodenal HCO_3^- secretion induced by luminal acidification in the rat. *Gastroenterology*, **96**, 45–49.

34. Kao, Y.-C.J., Goddard, P.J. and Lichtenberger, L.M. (1990) Morphological effects of aspirin and prostaglandin on a canine gastric mucosal surface. Analysis with a phospholipid-selective cytochemical stain. *Gastroenterology*, **98**, 592–606.

35. Khalil, T., Singh, P., Fujimura, M., Townsend, M.D., Jr, Greeley, G.H. and Thompson, J.C. (1988) Effect of ageing on gastric acid secretion, serum gastrin and antral gastrin content in rats. *Digestive Diseases and Sciences*, **33**, 1544–1548.

36. Klein, K.B. and Spiegel, D. (1989) Modulation of gastric acid secretion by hypnosis. *Gastroenterology*, **96**, 1383–1387.

37. Knutson, L. and Flemström, G. (1989) Duodenal mucosal bicarbonate secretion in man. Stimulation of acid and inhibition by the alpha 2-adrenoreceptor agonist clonidine. *Gut*, **30**, 1708–1715.

38. Konturek, S.J., Kwiecen, N., Obtulowicz, W. *et al*. (1987) Vagal cholinergic control of gastric alkaline secretion in normal subjects and duodenal ulcer patients. *Gut*, **28**, 739–744.

39. Konturek, S.J., Bilski, J., Kwiecen, N., Obtulowicz, W., Kopp, B. and Oleksy, J. (1987) De-Nol stimulates gastric and duodenal alkaline secretion through prostaglandin dependent mechanism. *Gut*, **28**, 1557–1563.

40. Kovacs, T.O.G., Walsh, J.H., Maxwell, V., Wong, H.C., Azuma, T. and Katt, E. (1989) Gastrin is a major mediator of the gastric phase of acid secretion in dogs: proof by monoclonal antibody neutralisation. *Gastroenterology*, **97**, 1406–1413.

41. Lenz, H.J. (1988) CNS regulation of gastric and autonomic function in dogs by gastrin-releasing peptide. *American Journal of Physiology*, **255**, G298–G303.

42. Lenz, H.J. and Forquignon, I. (1990) Stimulation of duodenal bicarbonate secretion in conscious rats by cerebral somatostatin-28. Role of neurohumoral pathways. *Gastroenterology*, **99**, 340–344.

43. Lenz, H.J., Vale, W.W. and Rivier, J.E. (1989) TRH-induced vagal stimulation of duodenal HCO_3^- mediated by VIP and muscarinic pathways. *American Journal of Physiology*, **257**, G677–G682.

44. Leung, F.W., Miller, J.C., Reedy, T.J. and Guth, P.H. (1989) Exogenous prostaglandin protects against acid-induced deep mucosal injury by stimulating alkaline secretion in rat duodenum. *Digestive Diseases and Sciences*, **34**, 1686–1691.

45. Lucey, M.R., Wass, J.A.H., Rees, L.H., Dawson, A.M. and Fairclough, P.D. (1989) Relationship between gastric acid and elevated plasma somatostatin-like immunoreactivity after a mixed meal. *Gastroenterology*, **97**, 867–872.

46. McArthur, K.E., Walsh, J.H. and Richardson, C.T. (1988) Soy protein meals stimulate less gastric secretion and gastrin release than beef meals. *Gastroenterology*, **95**, 920–926.

47. Maton, P.N., Miller, D.L. Doppman, J.L. *et al*. (1987) Role of selective angiography in the management of patients with Zollinger–Ellison syndrome. *Gastroenterology*, **92**, 913–918.

48. Merki, H.S., Fimmel, C.J., Walt, R.P., Harre, K., Röhmel, J. and Witzel, L. (1988) Pattern of 24 hour intragastric acidity in active duodenal ulcer disease and in healthy controls. *Gut*, **29**, 1583–1587.

49. Moore, J.G. and Halberg, F. (1986) Circadian rhythm of gastric acid secretion in men with active

duodenal ulcer. *Digestive Diseases and Sciences*, **31**, 1185–1191.

50. Mulholland, M.W., Reid, B.J., Levine, D.S. and Rubin, C.E. (1989) Elevated gastric acid secretion in patients with Barrett's metaplastic epithelium. *Digestive Diseases and Sciences*, **34**, 1329–1335.

51. Odes, H.S., Hogan, D.L., Ballesteros, M.A., Wolosin, J.D., Koss, M.A. and Isenberg, J.I. (1990) Human duodenal mucosal bicarbonate secretion. Evidence suggesting active transport under basal and stimulated conditions. *Gastroenterology*, **98**, 867–872.

52. Ohe, K., Miura, Y., Taoka, Y., Okada, Y. and Miyoshi, A. (1988) Cysteamine-induced inhibition of mucosal and pancreatic alkaline secretion in rat duodenum. *Digestive Diseases and Sciences*, **33**, 330–337.

53. Pavlov, I. (1910) *The work of digestive glands* (translated by W.H. Thompson). London: C. Griffin.

54. Peeters, T., Motthifs, G., Depoortere, I., Cachet, T., Hoogmartens, J. and Vantrappen, G. (1989) Erythromycin is a motilin receptor agonist. *American Journal of Physiology*, **257**, G470–G474.

55. Pfeiffer, A., Rochlitz, H., Herz, A. and Paumgartner, G. (1988) Stimulation of acid secretion and phosphoinositol production by rat parietal cell muscarinic M_2 receptors. *American Journal of Physiology*, **254**, G622–G629.

56. Quigley, E.M.M. and Turnberg, L.A. (1987) pH of the microclimate lining human gastric and duodenal mucosa in vivo. Studies in control subjects and in duodenal ulcer patients. *Gastroenterology*, **92**, 1876–1884.

57. Rees, W.D.W. (1987) Mucus–bicarbonate barrier – shield or sieve. *Gut*, **28**, 1553–1556.

58. Rees, W.D.W., Botham, D. and Turnberg, L.A. (1982) A demonstration of bicarbonate production by the normal human stomach in vivo. *Digestive Diseases and Sciences*, **27**, 961–966.

59. Sakamoto, C., Matozaki, T., Nishisaki, H., Konda, Y., Nagao, M. and Nakano, O. (1990) Effects of CCK-receptor antagonists on CCK-stimulated pepsinogen secretion and calcium increase in isolated guinea pig gastric chief cells. *Digestive Diseases and Sciences*, **35**, 873–878.

60. Sarosiek, J., Bilski, J., Murty, V.L.N., Slomiany, A. and Slomiany, B.L. (1989) Colloidal bismuth subcitrate (De-Nol) inhibits degradation of gastric mucus by *Campylobacter pylori* protease. *American Journal of Gastroenterology*, **84**, 506–510.

61. Savarino, V., Mela, G.S., Scalabrini, P., Sumberaz, A., Fera, G. and Celle, G. (1988) 24 hour study of intragastric acidity in duodenal ulcer patients and normal subjects using continuous intraluminal pH-metry. *Digestive Diseases and Sciences*, **33**, 1077–1080.

62. Schubert, M.L. and Hightower, J. (1989) Inhibition of acid secretion by bombesin is partly mediated by release of fundic somatostatin. *Gastroenterology*, **97**, 561–567.

63. Schubert, M.L. and Hightower, J. (1990) Functionally distinct muscarinic receptors on gastrin somatostatin cells. *American Journal of Physiology*, **258**, G982–G987.

64. Schubert, M.L., Edwards, N.F. and Makhlouf, G.M. (1988) Regulation of gastric somatostatin secretion in the mouse by luminal acidity: A local feedback mechanism. *Gastroenterology*, **94**, 317–322.

65. Seidler, U. and Sewing, K.-Fr. (1989) Ca^{2+}-dependent and -independent secretagogue action on gastric mucus secretion in rabbit mucosal explants. *American Journal of Physiology*, **256**, G739–G746.

66. Sellers, L.A. and Allen, A. (1988) Mucus and gastroduodenal protection. In *Advances in Ulcer Pathogenesis* (Ed.) Rees, W.D.W. pp. 121–144. Lancaster: MTP Press.

67. Shorrock, C.J., Crampton, J.R., Gibbons, L.C. and Rees, W.D.W. (1989) Effect of bismuth subcitrate on amphibian gastroduodenal bicarbonate secretion. *Gut*, **30**, 917–921.

68. Shorrock, C.J., Garner, A., Hunter, A.H., Crampton, J.R. and Rees, W.D.W. (1990) Effect of bismuth subcitrate and sucralfate on rat duodenal and human gastric bicarbonate secretion in vivo. *Gut*, **31**, 26–31.

69. Sidebotham, R.L. and Baron, J.H. (1990) Hypothesis: *Helicobacter pylori*, urease, mucus and gastric ulcer. *The Lancet*, **335**, 193–194.

70. Sjövall, H., Forsell, H., Häggenbal, J. and Olbe, L. (1988) Reflex sympathetic activation in humans is accompanied by inhibition of gastric HCO_3^- secretion. *American Journal of Physiology*, **255**, G752–G758.

71. Sleizenger, M.H. and Fordtran, J.S. (1989) *Gastrointestinal Disease. Pathophysiology Diagnosis Management*. Philadelphia: W.B. Saunders.

72. Slomiany, B.L., Kasinathan, C. and Slomiany, A. (1989) Lipolytic activity of *Campylobacter pylori*: effect of colloidal bismuth subcitrate (De-Nol). *American Journal of Gastroenterology*, **84**, 1273–1277.

73. Smith, J.T.L., Pounder, R.E., Nwokolo, C.U. *et al.* (1990) Inappropriate hypergastrinaemia in asymptomatic healthy subjects infected with *Helicobacter pylori*. *Gut*, **31**, 522–525.

74. Spychal, R.T., Marrero, J.M., Saverymuttu, S.H. and Northfield, T.C. (1989) Measurement of the surface hydrophobicity of human gastrointestinal mucosa. *Gastroenterology*, **97**, 104–111.

75. Spychal, R.T., Goggin, P.M., Marrero, J.M. *et al.* (1990) Surface hydrophobicity of gastric mucosa in peptic ulcer disease. Relationship to gastritis and *Campylobacter pylori* infection. *Gastroenterology*, **98**, 1250–1254.

76. Stechschulte, D.J., Jr, Morris, D.C., Jilke, R.L., Stechschulte, D.J. and Dileepan, K.N. (1990)

Impaired gastric acid secretion in mast cell-deficient mice. *American Journal of Physiology*, **259**, G41–G47.

77. Stephens, R.L., Ishikawa Weiner, H., Novin, D. and Tache, Y. (1988) TRH analogue, RX 77368, injected into dorsal vagal complex stimulates gastric acid secretion in rats. *American Journal of Physiology*, **254**, G639–G643.

78. Sweeting, J. (1987) Gastric acid output after portocaval shunt. *Gastroenterology*, **93**, 905–906.

79. Tsai, L.H., Taniyama, K. and Tanaka, C. (1987) γ-Aminobutyric acid stimulates acid secretion from the isolated guinea pig stomach. *American Journal of Physiology*, **253**, G601–G606.

80. Vattay, P., Feil, W., Klimesch, S., Wenzl, E., Starlinger, M. and Schiessel, R. (1988) Acid stimulated alkaline secretion in the rabbit duodenum is passive and correlates with mucosal damage. *Gut*, **29**, 284–290.

81. Wawk, S.A., Doppman, J.L., Miller, D.L. *et al.* (1987) Prospective study of the ability of computed axial tomography to localize gastrinomas in patients with Zollinger–Ellison syndrome. *Gastroenterology*, **92**, 905–912.

82. Wenzl, E., Feil, W., Starlinger, M. and Schiessel, R. (1987) Alkaline secretion. A protective mechanism against acid injury in rabbit duodenum. *Gastroenterology*, **92**, 709–715.

83. Whitfield, P.F. and Hobsley, M. (1987) Comparison of maximal gastric secretion in smokers and non-smokers with and without duodenal ulcer. *Gut*, **28**, 557–580.

84. Wilkes, J.M., Garner, A. and Peters, T.J. (1988) Mechanisms of acid disposal and acid-mediated alkaline secretion by gastroduodenal mucosa. *Digestive Diseases and Sciences*, **33**, 362–367.

85. Williams, S.E. and Turnberg, L.A. (1981) The demonstration of a pH gradient across mucus adherent to rabbit gastric mucosa: evidence for a 'mucus–bicarbonate barrier'. *Gut*, **22**, 94–96.

86. Yanaka, A., Carter, K.J., Lee, H.-H. and Silen, W. (1990) Influence of Cl⁻ on pHi in oxynticopeptic cells of in vitro frog gastric mucosa. *American Journal of Physiology*, **258**, G815–G824.

87. Yang, H., Cuttitta, F., Raybould, H. and Tache, Y. (1989) Intrathecal injection of bombesin inhibits gastric acid secretion in the rat. *Gastroenterology*, **96**, 1403–1409.

GASTRODUODENAL MOTILITY IN HEALTH AND DISEASE

C.M. Brown and W.D.W. Rees

During the last decade, considerable advances in technology have enabled detailed study of gastroduodenal motor function in the stomach and duodenum. Not only have such studies explored local regulatory mechanisms, they have also defined complex relationships between the central nervous system and proximal gut function. Until recently, gastroduodenal epithelial disease, such as peptic ulceration, was considered a result of either abnormal secretory function or reduced mucosal resistance. However, there is now evidence that abnormal gastroduodenal motility may also be important in ulcer pathogenesis and in the genesis of non-ulcer dyspepsia. The following sections will address recent advances in the definition of gastroduodenal motor activity and its regulatory mechanisms, and the abnormalities of motility encountered in diseases of the stomach and duodenum.

GASTRODUODENAL MOTOR ACTIVITY

The principal function of the gastrointestinal tract is the digestion of ingested food and the subsequent absorption of such nutrients, together with fluid, electrolytes, minerals and vitamins. This is achieved by coordination and integration of secretory activity, intestinal motor activity and epithelial transport. Having acted as a receptacle for ingested food, the stomach then delivers its contents in a form, and at a rate, that are conducive to optimal duodenal digestion and subsequent duodenojejunal absorption. The importance of such activity to normal function is well illustrated by the devastating symptoms that may occur following gastric surgery or with diseases that cause gastroparesis.

The upper gut, in most non-ruminants, has a typical pattern of motor activity consisting of a cyclic pattern during fasting, termed the 'migrating motor complex', and a non-cyclic and less well-defined 'fed' pattern after oral feeding. The migrating motor complex is thought to act as a 'housekeeper', sweeping debris from the upper gut to the caecum in between meals. The fed pattern is believed to facilitate the mixing of nutrients with digestive juices and subsequently to expose the products of digestion to the absorptive surface of the small bowel.[36]

Interdigestive motor activity and its regulation

The migrating motor complex consists of a cyclic pattern of electrical and contractile activity that extends from the gastro-oesophageal junction to the ileocaecal junction during fasting (*Figure 2.26*). Each cycle lasts 90–120 minutes and consists of a period of quiescence (phase 1), progressing to intermittent contractile activity (phase 2), which terminates in an intense, but short, burst of contractions (phase 3). Some workers recognize the transition between phase 3 and the subsequent phase 1 as phase 4. This type of motor activity may be studied by measuring electrical activity of intestinal smooth muscle, measuring contractile activity either directly by implanted strain gauges or indirectly by recording intraluminal pressure, or more crudely by radiological screening of intraluminal contrast material. The precise function of interdigestive motor activity remains speculative, but an attractive and rather simple hypothesis suggests that it acts as an intestinal 'housekeeper', with each burst of phase 3 activity 'sweeping' intraluminal debris and secretions distally into the colon. This would serve to minimize luminal stasis and associated bacterial overgrowth. In support of such a role is the finding that small intestinal interdigestive activity is severely disrupted in diseases associated with intestinal stasis and bacterial overgrowth, such as diabetic autonomic neuropathy and progressive systemic sclerosis.[17,37,52]

The regulation of migrating motor activity during fasting remains controversial. Migrating motor complex-like activity can be induced by a number of agents, including motilin, somatostatin, morphine, trimebutine and erythromycin.[45] Motilin, a 22 amino acid residue peptide isolated from duodenal mucosa, has attracted considerable attention and may be important in inducing gastroduodenal phase 3 activity. Plasma motilin levels fluctuate in accordance with gastroduodenal phase 3 contractions. Motilin has direct action on gastric and duodenal smooth muscle, and motilin receptors have now been identified in these tissues.[9,28,35] Exogenous motilin induces gastroduodenal phase 3 activity and trimebutine probably acts by releasing motilin whereas erythromycin acts as a motilin receptor agonist. Suppression of endogenous motilin release by somatostatin or pancreatic polypeptide prevents phase 3 activity from occurring in the stomach. This information provides strong evidence that motilin is important in initiating phase 3 activity of the migrating motor complex in the gastroduodenal region. Subsequent propagation of phase 3 activity along the small intestine is probably dependent on both intrinsic and extrinsic neural mechanisms.

'Fed' pattern of motor activity and its regulation

In carnivores and omnivores, interdigestive motor activity is replaced by a 'fed' pattern after ingestion of nutrients.[51] The induction and maintenance of this motor activity depends upon either the presence of luminal nutrients in the stomach or the existence of gastric distension. The duration of the fed pattern is influenced by the nutrient contents of the stomach, being prolonged with lipid and relatively short with saline, carbohydrate and protein.[25,34,45] Non-nutrient gel such as polycarbophil and cellulose

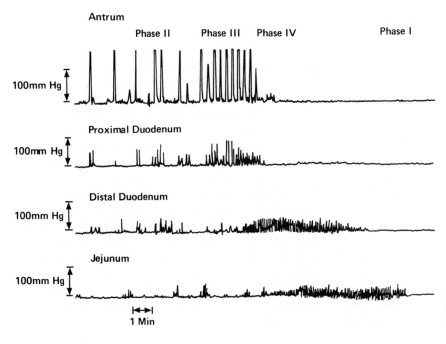

Figure 2.26 Pattern of interdigestive motor activity in the stomach and duodenum.

can maintain a fed pattern for several hours, as a result of gastric distension. Finally, conversion to a fed pattern can even be induced by the sight and smell of food.[57]

The fed pattern is non-cyclic and resembles phase 2 of the interdigestive motor complex. It extends from the proximal stomach to terminal ileum and persists for as long as food remains in the stomach. Although the duration of the fed pattern is influenced by the composition of a meal, the pattern of contractile activity in the stomach and small bowel is fairly consistent. Postprandial antral motility, however, does appear to be influenced by the physical nature of food. Homogenized meals induce a fed pattern with low amplitude and infrequent antral contractions, whereas a similar meal containing solid particles induced an intense and high amplitude antral response lasting around 60 minutes. It is conceivable that this response plays an important role in the grinding and filtering of solids prior to their delivery into the duodenum.

The precise regulation of the fed pattern remains uncertain but its function is to optimize the mixing and absorption of ingested nutrients. In the stomach, postprandial motility is also essential in regulating the delivery of nutrients at a rate and in a form that optimizes duodenal digestion and absorption. The induction and maintenance of a fed pattern depends upon a number of factors, including extrinsic nerve supply, local neural reflexes and released enteric hormones.[20,55] The extrinsic nerve supply is probably vital for the 'cephalic and enteric phases' of postprandial gastric motility. The cephalic–vagal gastric myoelectric responses to eating have been studied in animals and humans. Both sham feeding and eating increase the amplitude of gastric slow wave activity, although the response to eating lasts longer. In vagotomized patients, this response to sham feeding was absent. Further evidence for central nervous system regulation of the postprandial gastric response has been provided by studies on subjects during sleep. In such subjects, disruption of the nocturnal interdigestive pattern by food resembles that in the vagally denervated gut and implies diminished vagal influence on gut function during sleep.[1] Mediation of the enteric phase of postprandial gastric motility is more controversial. Support for neural regulation comes from studies where acute reversible vagal blockade, extrinsic denervation or complete autotransplantation prevent postprandial inhibition of gastric fasting activity by jejunal nutrient infusion. However, a recent study using complete extrinsic denervation of the stomach or transection of both extrinsic and intrinsic neural continuity, except for vagal innervation, in dogs has shown that jejunal nutrients

inhibit fasting cyclic motility in both stomach and small bowel. This study therefore suggests that hormonal factors play a major role in the enteric disruption of the gastric interdigestive motor complex.[20]

When infused intravenously, many peptide hormones such as cholecystokinin, gastrin, secretin, neurotensin, gastric inhibitory polypeptide, insulin, pancreatic polypeptide and somatostatin disrupt the gastric and intestinal interdigestive motor complex, producing a non-cyclic fed pattern of motor activity.[36,42] The precise physiological role of these hormones remains uncertain because pharmacological experiments fail to reproduce the dynamic plasma and mucosal changes in gastrointestinal hormones which occur after eating.

ELECTROPHYSIOLOGY OF GASTRODUODENAL MOTOR ACTIVITY

Although anatomists divide the stomach into three regions – fundus (portion above the gastro-oesophageal junction), corpus (between the gastro-oesophageal junction and the incisura angularis) and antrum (between the incisura and duodenal cap) – the physiologist usually distinguishes two functionally distinct regions. The proximal one-third of the stomach is electrically stable and does not undergo intensive phasic contractions. In contrast, the distal two-thirds undergo repeated electrical discharges and intensive phasic contractions. These differences have led to suggestions that the proximal region acts mainly as a reservoir, and the distal stomach plays an important role in the grinding of solids and regulating emptying (see Gastric emptying, p. 211).

Smooth muscle maintains a negative transmembrane potential and fluctuations in this potential trigger calcium influx, which, in turn, initiates muscle contraction. Fluctuations in membrane potential may be propagated along the gastric muscle leading to aborally propagated rings of contractions or peristalsis. Muscle cells from the proximal one-third of the stomach have lower resting negative membrane potentials which show little fluctuation. Cells from the distal two-thirds possess increasingly negative resting potential with increasing distance from the proximal region. These muscle cells also exhibit episodes of spontaneous depolarization. Regardless of site, all cells from the distal stomach show an abrupt discharge, called a pacesetter potential, once membrane potential has decayed to a certain value.[22] All cells may exhibit a sustained, more positive potential, called a plateau or action potential, which probably represents a calcium current and is associated with muscle contraction. The amplitude and duration of the contraction is pro-

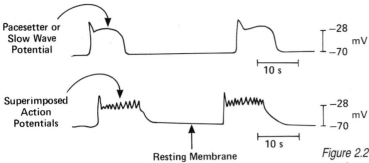

Pacesetter or
Slow Wave
Potential

−28
mV
−70

10 s

Superimposed
Action
Potentials

−28
mV
−70

10 s

Resting Membrane
Potential

Figure 2.27 Intracellular membrane potentials from antral smooth muscle.

portional to those of the plateau potential (*Figure 2.27*).

Pacesetter potentials originate along the greater curvature at the junction of the proximal stomach and middle third of the stomach. The frequency of discharges at this site exceeds that from more distal sites and as a result this zone becomes the dominant pacemaker. Pacesetter potentials from this site are propagated downwards and circumferentially along the longitudinal muscle at 3/min. Under certain neurohormonal conditions, action potentials develop on a pacesetter potential leading to muscle contraction which parallels the spread of the pacesetter potential. Therefore contractions move for a variable length along the distal stomach in an aboral direction and at a maximum frequency of 3/min.

The contractile activity of the proximal stomach is quite different. There are no pacesetter or action potentials at this site and muscle activity consists of prolonged tonic contractions, lasting 1–6 minutes, of low amplitude.[3] Unlike the large amplitude phasic contractions of the distal stomach, those of the proximal stomach are difficult to record and are not usually visible at fluoroscopy or endoscopy.

Neurohormonal agents usually modify gastric contractile activity by influencing the amplitude and duration of plateau potentials. Gastrin, cholecystokinin and acetylcholine increase the duration and amplitude of the plateau potential and resulting muscle contraction. In contrast, noradrenaline and neurotensin decrease the duration and amplitude of the plateau potential.

The electrophysiology of the proximal duodenum is very similar to that of the distal stomach, except that the frequency of pacesetter potentials is 11/min. Although the pacesetter potentials of the distal antrum are insulated from those of the proximal duodenum, there is some conduction of gastric signals across smooth muscle bundles – myogenic conduction. Therefore, some electrical recordings from the proximal duodenum show pacesetter potentials at the frequency of the antrum on which duodenal pacesetter potentials are superimposed. Ultrasonic

studies have also confirmed the existence of antroduodenal coordination, though the duodenum also contracts between antral cycles.

GASTRIC EMPTYING AND ITS CONTROL

The availability of more sophisticated and less invasive techniques for studying gastric emptying has helped improve understanding of the dynamics of how the stomach regulates the delivery of solids and liquids into the duodenum (*Figure 2.28*).

Early theories proposed that solids and liquids were propelled from the stomach by antral peristalsis after being stored in the proximal stomach.[42] Stored material was gently pushed towards the antrum and the greater inertia of solid particles led to their slower pattern of emptying compared with liquids. However, a number of observations suggested that the emptying of solids and liquids occurred by quite different and distinct mechanisms. First, liquid emptying may occur in the absence of recordable antral contractions. Surgical resection of the fundus increases liquid emptying without altering that of solids, whereas antrectomy had the opposite effect of increasing solid emptying without altering liquid emptying. Selective vagal denervation of the fundus increases intragastric pressure after a meal, while accelerating only liquid emptying. In contrast, vagal denervation of the antrum delays solid emptying without altering that of liquids. Recent theories therefore support a 'two-component' stomach with the tonic proximal region providing the driving force for liquid emptying and the peristaltic antrum controlling solid emptying. It seems likely that this hypothesis is too simplistic and that multiple mechanisms are responsible for regulating the emptying of nutrients, such as: proximal gastric tone, antral contractility, pyloric resistance, gastroduodenal coordination and duodenal resistance[4,8,10,33] (*Figure 2.29*). The viscosity of gastric contents and gravitational forces may also influence the pattern of gastric emptying. The 'two-component' system re-

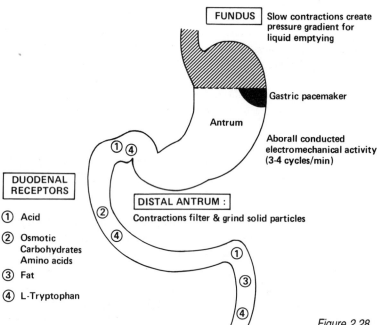

Figure 2.28 Factors regulating gastric emptying of food.

gards the antrum as the filtering, grinding and propulsion unit for solid particles. However, there is evidence that such functions are not unique to the antrum, and that the sorting of solid particles according to size is a property of both proximal and distal stomach. The emptying of solid food after antrectomy remains an active process and even in the absence of an antrum from 60 to 70% of emptied particles are smaller than 1 mm.

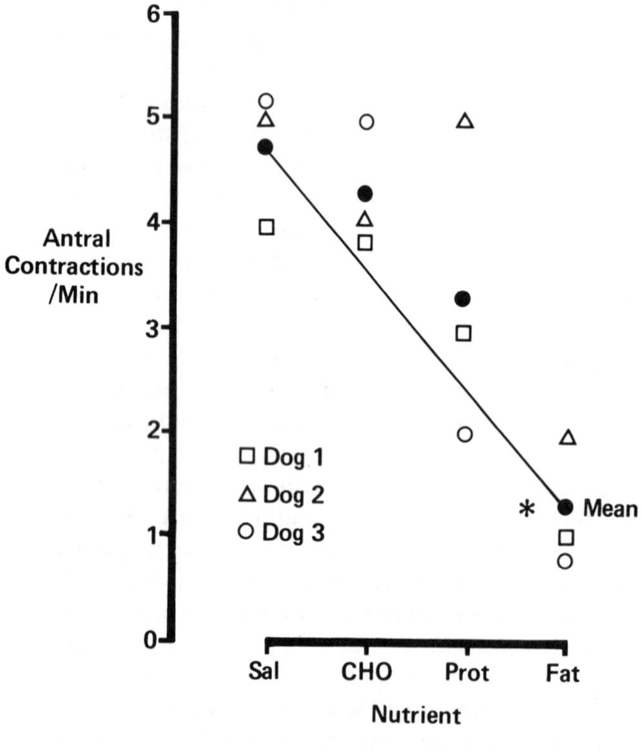

Patterns of gastric emptying

Gastric emptying of liquids is usually described as 'a simple exponential', implying a semilogarithmic decrease in intragastric volume with time. Recent computer analysis suggests that liquid emptying is not simply volume dependent and exhibits an initial rapid linear component followed by a slower component which is linear. Increasing the gastric concentration of nutrients, salts or acidity slows gastric emptying, although the nutrient load or titratable acidity entering the duodenum remains constant.[2,13,25,27,34,55] The pattern of solid emptying tends to be sigmoid in nature with a long initial phase, during which no solid is emptied, followed by a prolonged linear phase. Solid food enters the duodenum as particles smaller than 1 mm in diameter. Therefore, the initial delay in solid emptying may reflect the time taken for the stomach to reduce solid particles to this small size. This idea is supported by observations that food preground to 0.25 mm empties very rapidly, and easily fragmented solids empty faster than less easily fragmented particles. Studies using indigestible plastic spheres suggest that other factors such as changing gastric viscosity may also influence the rate of solid emptying.

The emptying of fat remains controversial. Unlike other solids, fat is often liquid at body temperature and may be easily fragmented to tiny particles.

Figure 2.29 Comparison of number of antral contractions per minute during perfusion of saline or different nutrients in upper small intestine: (Reproduced, with permission, from Kumar *et al.*[33])

Although quite variable, the emptying of triglyceride is similar to that of solid food with an initial lag phase followed by a slow linear phase. A number of mechanisms may be responsible for this pattern of emptying including the 'layering' of less dense lipid on the top of gastric contents and the adherence of fat to the hydrophobic surface of solid particles.

Regulation of gastric emptying

The rate of gastric emptying plays a crucial role in maintaining the optimal digestive activity and in the regulation of certain metabolic processes, such as glucose homoeostasis. There is evidence that the stomach itself has limited ability in 'sensing' its contents and relies on feedback mechanisms triggered by receptors within the proximal small bowel to control rate of emptying.[4,14,49,56] Much of the experimental data on regulation of gastric emptying has been derived using liquid meals, although information is now accumulating on the control of solid or mixed solid–liquid emptying.

Liquid emptying is particularly influenced by the osmolality, pH and fat content of the proximal intestinal lumen. Salts and poorly absorbed carbohydrates reduce gastric emptying as their osmolalities increase. Acid, carbohydrates, peptides, amino acids and fatty acids have effects on gastric emptying over and above their osmotic actions. Acid delays gastric emptying in proportion to the rate of delivery of titratable acid into the duodenum.[2] This means that weak acids are very effective in slowing emptying, even at pH 3–5 whereas strong acids may require very low pH values of 1–2 in order to generate significant titratable acid. Fatty acids are potent inhibitors of emptying, even at pH 7, and medium-chain fatty acids are more effective than long-chain ones. Monosaccharides reduce gastric emptying depending on their structure, with glucose and xylose being more potent than fructose. However, disaccharides and polysaccharides are equipotent to their monosaccharide components. Similarly, oligopeptides are equipotent to equivalent mixtures of their component amino acids. Some amino acids (tryptophan, phenylalanine, glutamate, cystein and arginine) slow gastric emptying directly whereas others do so by virtue of the osmolality produced. Other factors shown to influence gastric emptying include: the caloric content of a meal, duodenal distension, smoking, alcohol, exercise and the steroid sex hormones.[8,26,39,41,61] Although the data are few, similar mechanisms also appear to influence solid food emptying. Therefore, adding acid, glucose or triglycerides to solid food delays its emptying.

The nature of the sensory receptors and regulatory pathways that mediate intestinal modulation of gastric emptying remains uncertain. Osmoreceptors to saline are limited to the duodenum whereas receptors to acid, fat and glucose are present along considerable lengths of upper small bowel. Most nutrients delay gastric emptying in proportion to the amount entering the bowel per minute, suggesting recruitment of increasing numbers of receptors as larger loads of nutrients escape proximal absorption to reach distal locations.[34,55] It has been suggested that the inhibitory signal originates from shrinkage of the lateral intercellular space between enterocytes. Such shrinkage could be induced by hypertonic solutions in the lumen or by damage to the tight intercellular junctions by fatty acids (which chelate calcium ions) or by hydrogen ions (which displace calcium ions). The precise transmission of these signals to the stomach remains controversial, and it seems likely that both hormonal and neural mechanisms are important. Cholecystokinin is a strong candidate for hormonal regulation of gastric emptying but its action is complex.[14,48,49] It may be produced by endocrine cells within the upper small intestine but is also found within the central nervous system and in peripheral neurons. This and other evidence suggests that cholecystokinin may be involved in a combined neuroendocrine control mechanism of gastric emptying. The initial site of action of cholecystokinin is on primary afferent neurons which activate an inhibitory vagovagal reflex pathway leading to relaxation of proximal gastric smooth muscle.[49] Subsequently, cholecystokinin may increase resistance to flow at the pylorus by direct action on smooth muscle or indirectly via presynaptic stimulation of noradrenaline release.[14] The control of peptone and lipid emptying may therefore depend on activation of these mechanisms by released cholecystokinin. Studies suggest that cholecystokinin of endocrine origin is more important than neurally released cholecystokinin in modifying gastric emptying. Although intraduodenal acid releases hormones such as secretin and motilin, there is evidence that the delay in gastric emptying produced is mediated by a cholinergic reflex increasing pyloric motor activity. A similar mechanism may also control the gastric emptying of carbohydrates, such as glucose. Most carbohydrate is absorbed by the jejunum but substantial quantities of starch and vegetable carbohydrates may enter the ileum, and there is evidence that these may delay gastric emptying by release of peptide YY or non-vagally mediated neural mechanisms.[27] Duodenal distension may also be important in reducing gastric emptying. Balloon distension of the duodenum produces relaxation of the proximal stomach, and there is evidence that this response is mediated by non-adrenergic, non-cholinergic vagal fibres.[8]

It is therefore clear from the above discussion that the regulation of gastric emptying is a complex process dictated by the physical and chemical composition of food, receptor stimulation within the small intestine by emptied material from the stomach, and a variety of neurohormonal pathways which relay signals from the small bowel to gastric muscle.

DUODENOGASTRIC REFLUX

Retrograde flow of duodenal contents into the stomach is a normal occurrence and has been observed in up to 60% of healthy subjects. Abnormal patterns of duodenogastric reflux have been described in gastric ulcer, gall-bladder disease and reflux oesophagitis, but the role of such reflux in the manifestations and pathogenesis of such disorders remains uncertain.[12] The relationships between duodenogastric reflux and gastric ulcer have in particular been examined, but there is still a lack of convincing information that reflux of duodenal content is excessive or gastric clearance of such material is defective in gastric ulcer. Although bile acids, pancreatic enzymes and duodenal lysolecithin are capable of damaging gastric mucosa, there is little direct evidence that any of these factors are responsible for chronic gastric ulcers.

The magnitude of reflux is probably dependent on the coordination of antral and duodenal contractions, the existence of a high-pressure zone at the pylorus, and the frequency and direction of propagation of isolated duodenal contractions. There is little evidence that lack of antroduodenal coordination plays a significant role in producing duodenogastric reflux.[12] Although abnormalities in pyloric sphincter tone have been described in gastric ulcer, the existence of such a sphincter is hotly disputed and therefore the validity of such observations is questionable. Retrograde duodenal peristalsis may well be important in inducing reflux into the stomach, but there is little evidence to incriminate excess of such activity in gastric ulcer pathogenesis. On current evidence, the relevance of duodenogastric reflux to gastroduodenal disease seems insignificant. (Refer also to pages 236, 250, 293.)

RELATIONSHIP BETWEEN GASTRODUODENAL MOTILITY AND SECRETION

Traditionally, gastric secretion and motility are usually discussed separately but in health both functions occur simultaneously and there is some evidence that both activities are coordinated in the stomach as well as in the small intestine.[16]

During interdigestive motor activity, there is increased secretion of acid and pepsin during phase 3 activity in the gastroduodenal region. In animal models, gastric distension has been found to increase both motility and acid output whereas feeding decreases both motility and pepsin output in Heidenhain's pouches. The precise nature of the relationship between motility and gastric secretion remains controversial. It is conceivable that the relationship is coincidental due to the existence of parallel control mechanisms. The vagus nerves, for example, contain both motor and secretomotor fibres, whereas certain hormones, such as gastrin, stimulate motor activity and gastric secretion. A second explanation is that motor and secretory activities are directly linked. Experiments using gastric distension provide the strongest support for such a direct link. Distension-sensitive endings are mechanoreceptors and, when stimulated, involve vagovagal pathways and phasic modulation of vagal efferent activity. It is therefore conceivable that normal phasic motility stimulates vagal efferents, enhancing gastric secretion.

At present there is inadequate information to confirm the precise nature of the association between gastroduodenal motor activity and gastric secretion.

MOTILITY AND GASTRODUODENAL DISEASE

Satiety and eating disorders

There are a number of complex and interrelated mechanisms involved in the satiation process (*Figure 2.30*). Volume and distension of the stomach are involved in limiting larger meals by stimulating mechanoreceptors, which, in turn, activate vagal afferent fibres. In a recent animal study, it was found that the magnitude of gastric distension, which occurred normally after meal ingestion, was similar to that required to induce satiety in sham-fed dogs.[46] It was concluded that gastric distension required to produce satiety was triggered by a peripheral signal and conveyed by a non-cholinergic mechanism. Chemoreceptors may also be important, and may simultaneously control gastric emptying and satiety. Release of cholecystokinin by duodenal nutrients has been regarded as important in producing satiation and has been regarded by some as a putative 'satiety hormone'. However, experience with cholecystokinin antagonism suggests that it plays only a minor role in inducing satiety. There is more impressive evidence linking insulin to this physiologi-

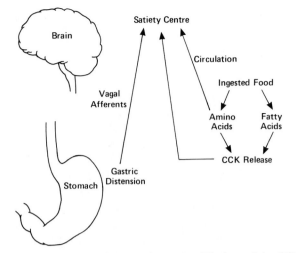

Figure 2.30 Factors that may be responsible for satiety. CCK, cholecystokinin.

cal function. Inhibition of prandial release of insulin by mannoheptulose has been shown to impair meal-induced satiety.

Most research on eating disorders, such as primary anorexia nervosa and bulimia nervosa, has focused on psychosocial and therapeutic aspects of

such disorders. However, there is evidence that abnormal gastric motility may be important in producing some of the symptoms, such as easy satiety, postprandial fullness, bloating and epigastric discomfort, encountered in these two diseases.[31] Delayed gastric emptying of a mixed meal has been described in both disorders (*Figure 2.31*) and may be associated with antral hypomotility. In bulimia nervosa, marked disturbance of oesophageal motility, including diffuse oesophageal spasm and achalasia, has been documented. It seems probable that these abnormalities of gastrointestinal function may be relevant to the development of abdominal symptoms but are unlikely to explain the aetiology of either disease. The mechanisms of disturbed gastrointestinal function in these disorders remain uncertain. In one study, delayed gastric emptying was associated with hypokalaemia and abnormal autonomic function is another possible cause of abnormal gastric motor activity.

Nausea and vomiting

These symptoms may be produced by a variety of clinical disorders, including gastric diseases such as peptic ulcer, gastric outlet obstruction and previous gastric surgery. Similar symptoms may, however, occur in the absence of a recognized cause and are termed 'idiopathic nausea and vomiting'. In a recent study, the contractile activity of the stomach and small bowel of 20 such patients was examined. Postprandial antral hypomotility was identified as a major abnormality in 14 of these patients.[30] Similar abnormalities have been described during fasting in patients with gastroparesis secondary to diabetes, previous gastric surgery or progressive systemic sclerosis. The cause of antral motor dysfunction in such patients remains unknown, and whether the abnormal motor pattern is responsible for the symptoms also remains to be established.

Nausea and vomiting are also common during the first trimester of pregnancy, with 50–80% of pregnant women complaining of nausea and just over 50% with daily episodes of vomiting. As with idiopathic nausea and vomiting, the pathophysiology of these symptoms in pregnancy also remains uncertain. However, in a study of 32 pregnant women, gastric dysrhythmias were found in 26.[32] Seventeen of these had tachygastria, with a pacesetter potential frequency of 4–9 cycles/min, and four had flat line patterns. In the six women with normal motor activity, their nausea scores were significantly lower than those with tachygastria and flat line rhythms. These abnormalities in gastric electrical activity reverted to normal and the nausea disappeared after

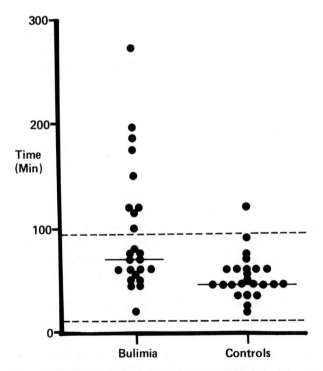

Figure 2.31 Gastric half-emptying time, in minutes, of a labelled test meal in 24 patients with bulimia nervosa and 24 healthy controls. [The solid lines represent median times. The area between the two broken lines represents 2 standard deviations of the mean half-emptying time in 24 healthy controls. (Reproduced, with permission, from Kiss *et al.*[31])

delivery. Gastric dysrhythmias have also been recorded in idiopathic nausea and vomiting, chronic dyspepsia, anorexia nervosa and diabetic gastroparesis, and may play an important role in causing upper abdominal symptoms. Further evidence that dysrhythmias may cause nausea is derived from vection-induced motion sickness which, in addition to producing intense nausea, also produces transient and chaotic gastric dysrhythmia.

Stress and gastroduodenal motor activity

An association between various emotions and symptoms arising from the gastrointestinal tract has been recognized for centuries, although definitive proof of such a link is still lacking. Two major reasons for such paucity of information are the lack of standardized methodology for applying stress and the invasive nature of techniques employed to quantify gastrointestinal motor function.[5]

However, both physical and mental stress have recently been shown to alter gastroduodenal motor activity in healthy subjects.[24,43] In one study on 12 healthy volunteers, the mental stress of solving anagrams and mental arithmetic significantly increased the duration of duodenal migrating motor complexes by 60%. Gastric secretion and flow rate were not altered but pancreatic enzyme output increased. In animals, acoustic stress prolonged gastric emptying and delayed the recovery of the interdigestive pattern of motor activity. In this study, the postprandial release of gastrin and pancreatic polypeptide was also enhanced.[19] Physical stress, such as cold water immersion, has been shown to reduce antroduodenal motor activity after eating in healthy subjects (*Figure 2.32*). This stimulus also prolonged orocaecal transit and this effect was partially prevented by a β-adrenergic blocker.[11] Transcutaneous electrical nerve stimulation has also been shown to reduce postprandial antral motility while simultaneously increasing circulating levels of β-endorphin.

The precise clinical relevance of these findings remains uncertain, but abnormalities of gastroduodenal motility may be responsible for certain stress-related symptoms in dyspeptic patients and those with the irritable bowel syndrome.

Peptic ulcer disease and antroduodenal motor activity

In over 40% of cases with dyspepsia, there is no detectable organic cause for the symptoms and the disorder is termed 'functional or non-ulcer dyspepsia'. It has been suggested that the symptoms in such

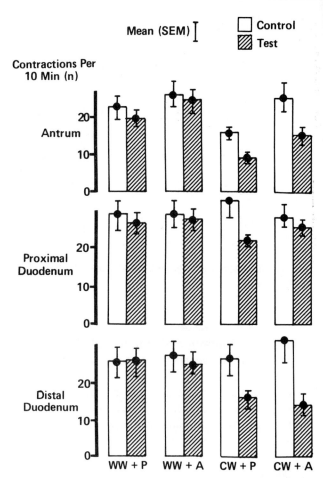

Figure 2.32 Effect of cold water stimulation on antral and duodenal motor activity: (a) antrum; (b) proximal duodenum; (c) distal duodenum. WW, warm water stimulation; CW, cold water; P, placebo; A, antenolol. (Reproduced, with permission, from O'Brien et al.[43])

patients are caused by abnormal motor activity in the upper gastrointestinal tract and certain observations are consistent with this hypothesis.[50] In one study, about 50% of patients with non-ulcer dyspepsia had delayed solid emptying, while in a further report, delayed solid emptying and reduced antral motor activity were described in a patient with intractable dyspepsia. Abnormal interdigestive motility in the gastroduodenal region has been associated with increased duodenogastric reflux, impaired gastric emptying and bile stasis. In a recent study, the prokinetic drug, cisapride, significantly increased fasting antral motility activity and decreased biliary reflux in a group of patients with severe dyspepsia and biliary reflux.[53] Cisapride has also been shown to increase the frequency of antral interdigestive motor complexes and the magnitude of antroduodenal contractile activity, while reducing the severity of symptoms in functional dyspep-

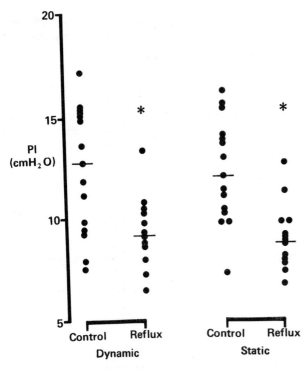

Figure 2.33 Dynamic and static gastric corpus–fundus pressure indices in patients with gastro-oesophageal reflux and in healthy controls. Each dot represents the mean of four observations per subject and horizontal bars indicate median values. *P < 0.01 compared with controls. (Reproduced, with permission, from Hartley et al.[21])

sia.[59] Such observations suggest that, in a significant proportion of subjects with functional dyspepsia, an abnormality of gastroduodenal motor activity may delay gastric emptying and increase biliary reflux which, in turn, cause upper abdominal symptoms. It is unlikely that such patients would respond to conventional ulcer therapy although they may well respond to prokinetic drugs.

Abnormal gastric motility may also play a role in the pathogenesis of gastro-oesophageal reflux disease (*Figure 2.33*). Studies of gastric function have demonstrated delayed gastric emptying and decrease antral motor activity in some patients with gastro-oesophageal reflux. A recent study of 12 patients with gastro-oesophageal reflux has demonstrated lower gastric pressure responses to distension compared with normal controls.[21] This abnormality of gastric adaptive relaxation may be due to a defect of the vagovagal inhibitory pathway, and may explain previously reported delayed emptying of solids and liquids in reflux patients. Because the lower oesophageal sphincter and the gastric fundus/corpus relax as an integrated unit, the pathophysiology of gastro-oesophageal reflux may be characterized by low-pressure responses throughout

this unit which favour reflux of gastric contents into the oesophagus.

The relevance of abnormal gastroduodenal motility to the pathogenesis and symptom pattern of peptic ulcers remains controversial. Reduced antral motor activity and delayed gastric emptying has been described in type 1 gastric ulcer, but may be the result rather than the cause of ulceration. Such results are, however, inconsistent with other studies demonstrating normal emptying in type 1 gastric ulcer and delayed emptying in prepyloric ulcers (type 3), and combined gastric and duodenal ulcers (type 2). Similarly, the importance of disturbed gastric motility in the genesis of gastritis is equally uncertain. Some authors have shown delayed gastric emptying in fundal gastritis,[58] whilst others have demonstrated a poor correlation between antroduodenal motor activity and antral gastritis in patients with bile reflux.[60] Clearly, these issues await further clarification and there is at present little evidence that abnormal motor activity is important in either the aetiology or manifestations of gastric ulcer and gastritis. Acid hypersecretion or rapid emptying of acid into the duodenum are often regarded as important factors in the pathogenesis of duodenal ulcer. Studies have shown that increased gastric emptying may account for an abnormally high postprandial acid load in the duodenum of duodenal ulcer patients. However, such abnormalities of emptying have been inconsistent and in a recent study on 99 consecutive male patients with endoscopically proven duodenal ulcer, the pattern of emptying of a solid–liquid meal was identical to that in healthy subjects[7] (*Figure 2.34*). As this is one of the largest studies of its kind, it seems very unlikely that disturbed gastric emptying plays a role in duodenal ulcer pathogenesis. This is supported by another recent study which failed to detect any major abnormalities of duodenal bulb clearance or duodenal transit in patients with active duodenal ulcer.[47] The importance of abnormal gastroduodenal motility in producing duodenal ulcer pain has also been investigated. Although such studies are plagued by methodological difficulties, the consensus opinion appears to be that 'spasm' of the antroduodenal muscle is unlikely to explain the development of ulcer pain, and that antispasmodic treatment plays little role in the prevention of duodenal ulcer symptoms.[29]

Gastroduodenal motor activity following gastric surgery

The vagus provides extrinsic cholinergic input to gastroduodenal smooth muscle cells to cause con-

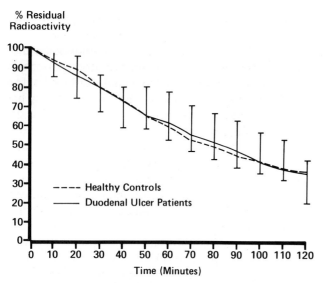

% Residual Radioactivity

Figure 2.34 Gastric emptying curves in 99 duodenal ulcer patients (solid lines) and in 23 healthy controls (dashed lines). Bars are standard deviations. (From Corinaldesi *et al.*[7])

traction. The vagus also provides pathways for receptive relaxation of the fundus allowing accommodation to a meal without a significant increase in intraluminal pressure.[18] Following truncal vagotomy, there is a loss of receptive relaxation which tends to enhance liquid emptying, but this is countered by reduced antral motility which delays solid emptying. The end-result is gastric stasis in a proportion of patients and hence truncal vagotomy is usually coupled with a pyloroplasty. Proximal or highly selective vagotomy alters receptive relaxation, increasing liquid emptying, but does not affect antral motor function. A similar increase in liquid emptying is observed after antrectomy, but when this is combined with truncal vagotomy there is, in addition, an increase in solid emptying.[6] In the majority of patients, the pattern of both liquid and solid emptying returns to normal within 6 months of surgery. However, in around 5% of patients who have undergone truncal vagotomy, with or without antral resection, abnormality of gastric emptying persists. In some patients, symptoms are produced by too rapid gastric emptying of nutrients and this syndrome is termed 'dumping'. In others, gastric stasis or gastroparesis may ensue leading to recurrent or intractable vomiting. Vagotomy also influences the fasting pattern of motor activity and the conversion of such cyclic activity to a fed pattern after eating. Whether these subtle and usually transient alterations in gastroduodenal motor activity have any clinical significance remains to be established.[23,40,54]

The mechanism whereby vagal transection alters gastroduodenal motility are likely to be complex and dependent on both the loss of sensory fibres in vagovagal reflex arcs and the direct motor supply to smooth muscle cells. Vagotomy produces abnormal gastric myoelectrical patterns with episodes of tachygastria.[15] As muscle contraction is controlled by the prevailing myoelectrical pattern, it seems likely that such dysrhythmias contribute to the deranged gastric function after vagotomy. However, this is likely to be an oversimplification as there appears to be a poor relationship between the occurrence of tachygastria and upper abdominal symptoms.

Idiopathic gastric dysrhythmias and gastroparesis

In addition to vagotomy, gastric dysrhythmia has also been described in diabetes mellitus and in some cases with anorexia nervosa, postoperative gastric stasis and gastric ulcer.[36] Cases of idiopathic gastric dysrhythmia have also been described where the symptoms are directly related to the abnormal myoelectrical activity. The first documented report, from the Mayo Clinic, described an abnormally fast pacesetter potential (5–20 cycles/min) in a 5-month-old infant with severe and intractable vomiting. The muscle from this patient also failed to generate plateau potentials and therefore contractions in response to the usual stimulants. Similar severe abnormalities of gastric myoelectrical activity have subsequently been described in a number of young patients with nausea and vomiting. Although rare, such cases provide valuable insight into the important role that disturbed myoelectrical activity in the stomach may play a role in the causation of unexplained upper gastrointestinal symptoms. Transient and less severe gastric dysrhythmias are, however, more common and may well play a role in producing unexplained dyspepsia.

Gastroparesis, characterized by intractable nausea and vomiting, bezoar formation and radiological/endoscopic evidence of the gastric stasis may be idiopathic or secondary to gastric surgery involving vagotomy, diabetes mellitus and collagen vascular diseases, such as systemic sclerosis and mixed connective tissue disease.[17,37,38,52] Diabetic gastroparesis was first described in 1958 and was thought to represent a vagal neuropathy. Such patients have abnormal antral motility characterized by disturbed or absent myoelectrical and contractile activity during phase 3 of the interdigestive cycle. Abnormality of pyloric 'tone' may also contribute to the delayed solid emptying, which is a sensitive indicator of gastric dysfunction in diabetics. The precise pathogenesis of the disorders still remains uncertain. Gastric smooth muscle is morphologically normal, although electrophysiological studies have demonstrated dysrhythmia. It seems likely that abnormal gastric motility in this disorder is, in part, related to autonomic neuropathy and, in part, to the metabolic consequences of glucose intolerance. A similar disorder has been described in patients with progressive systemic sclerosis and mixed connective tissue disease. These patients also have reduced antral motor activity and prolonged gastric emptying of solids. In the initial stages of these disorders, there is evidence that the abnormal motor activity is due to a neuropathic lesion that interferes with acetylcholine release. However, in end-stage progressive systemic sclerosis, there is an undoubted myopathic component where the muscle mass is replaced by connective tissue. During the initial 'neuropathic' phase, gastric motor activity may be restored by prokinetic agents such as bethanechol, metoclopramide, domperidone and cisapride. However, with the development of muscle atrophy and fibrosis the patients become unresponsive to such treatment.

REFERENCES

1. Accarino, A. and Malagelada, J.-R. (1990) Control of gastrointestinal motility. In: *Current Opinion in Gastroenterology* (Ed.) Holt, S. and Rees, W.D.W., **6**, 873–876. London: Science Press.

2. Allescher, H.D., Daniel, E.E., Dent, J., Fox, J.E.T. and Kostolanska, F. (1989) Neural reflex of the canine pylorus to intraduodenal acid infusion. *Gastroenterology*, **96**, 18–28.

3. Azpiroz, F. and Malagelada, J.R. (1987) Gastric tone measured by an electronic barostat in health and postsurgical gastroparesis. *Gastroenterology*, **92**, 934–943.

4. Azpiroz, F. and Malagelada, J.R. (1990) Perception and reflex relaxation of the stomach in response to gut distension. *Gastroenterology*, **98**, 1193–1198.

5. Camilleri, M. and Neri, M. (1989) Motility disorders and stress. *Digestive Diseases and Sciences*, **34**, 1777–1786.

6. Condon, R.E. and Sarna, S.K. (1982) Motility after abdominal surgery. *Clinics in Gastroenterology*, **11**(3), 609–620.

7. Corinaldesi, R., Stanghellini, V., Paparo, G.F., Paternico, A., Rusticali, A.G. and Barbara, L. (1989) Gastric acid secretion and gastric emptying of liquids in 99 male duodenal ulcer patients. *Digestive Diseases and Sciences*, **34**, 251–256.

8. De Ponti, F., Azpiroz, F. and Malagelada, J.R. (1987) Reflex gastric relaxation in response to distension of the duodenum. *American Journal of Physiology*, **252**, G595–G601.

9. Depoortere, I., Peeters, T.L. and Vantrappen, G. (1990) Development of motilin receptors and of motilin- and erythromycin-induced contractility in rabbits. *Gastroenterology*, **99**, 652–658.

10. Dooley, C.P. and Valenzuela, J.E. (1988) Antropyloroduodenal activity during gastric emptying of liquid meals in humans. *American Journal of Physiology*, **255**, G93–G98.

11. Enck, P., Merlin, V., Erckenbrecht, J.F. and Weinbeck, M. (1989) Stress effects on gastrointestinal transit in the rat. *Gut*, **30**, 455–459.

12. Eyre-Brook, I.A. and Johnson, A.G. (1988) Duodenogastric reflux and other motility disorders in gastric ulcer disease. In *Advances in Peptic Ulcer Pathogenesis* (Ed.) Rees, W.D.W. pp. 51–79. Lancaster: MTP Press.

13. Fone, D.R., Horowitz, M., Dent, J., Read, N.W. and Heddle, R. (1989) Pyloric motor response to intraduodenal dextrose involves muscarinic mechanisms. *Gastroenterology*, **97**, 83–90.

14. Forster, E.R., Green, T., Elliot, M., Bremner, A. and Dockray, G.J. (1990) Gastric emptying in rats: role of afferent neurons and cholecystokinin. *American Journal of Physiology*, **258**, G552–G556.

15. Geldof, H., Van der Schee, E.J., Blankenstein, M.V., Smout, A.J.P.M. and Akkermans, L.M.A. (1990) Effects of highly selective vagotomy on gastric myoelectrical activity. An electrogastrographic study. *Digestive Diseases and Sciences*, **35**, 969–975.

16. Greenwood, B. and Davison, J.S. (1987) The relationship between gastrointestinal motility and secretion. *American Journal of Physiology*, **252**, G1–G7.

17. Greydanus, M.P. and Camilleri, M. (1989) Abnormal postprandial antral and small bowel motility due to neuropathy or myopathy in systemic sclerosis. *Gastroenterology*, **96**, 110–115.

18. Grundy, D. (1988) Vagal control of gastrointestinal function. In *Clinical Gastroenterology*, Vol. 2 (1), (Ed.) Grundy, D. and Read, N.W. pp. 23–43. London: Bailliére Tindall.

19. Gue, M., Peeters, T., Depoortere, I., Vantrappen, G. and Bueno, L. (1989) Stress induced changes in gastric emptying, postprandial motility, and plasma gut hormone levels in dogs. *Gastroenterology*, **97**, 1101–1107.

20. Hakim, N.S., Sarr, M.G. and Spencer, M. (1989) Postprandial disruption of migrating myoelectric complex in dogs. Hormonal versus extrinsic nervous factors. *Digestive Diseases and Sciences*, **34**, 257–263.

21. Hartley, M.N., Walker, S.J. and Mackie, C.R. (1990) Abnormal gastric adaptive relaxation in patients with gastro-oesophageal reflux. *Gut*, **31**, 500–503.

22. Hinder, R.A. and Kelly, K.A. (1977) Human gastric pacesetter potential: site of origin, spread and response to gastric transection and proximal gastric vagotomy. *American Journal of Surgery*, **133**, 29–33.

23. Hocking, M.P., Harrison, W.D. and Sinisky, C.A. (1990) Gastric dysrhythmias following pylorus-preserving pancreaticoduodenectomy. Possible mechanism for early delayed gastric emptying. *Digestive Diseases and Sciences*, **35**, 1226–1230.

24. Holtmann, G., Singer, M.V., Kriebel, R., Stacker, K.H. and Goebell, H. (1989) Differential effects of acute mental stress on interdigestive secretion of gastric acid, pancreatic enzymes, and gastroduodenal motility. *Digestive Diseases and Sciences*, **34**, 1701–1707.

25. Houghton, L.A., Mangnall, Y.F. and Read, N.W. (1990) Effect of incorporating fat into a liquid test meal on the relationship between intragastric distribution and gastric emptying in human volunteers. *Gut*, **31**, 1226–1229.

26. Hutson, W.R., Roehrkasse, R.L. and Wald, A. (1989) Influence of gender and menopause on gastric emptying and motility. *Gastroenterology*, **96**, 11–17.

27. Jain, N.K., Boivin, M., Zinsmeister, A.R., Brown, M.L., Malagelada, J.R. and DiMagno, E.P. (1989) Effect of ileal perfusion of carbohydrates and amylase inhibitor on gastrointestinal hormones and emptying. *Gastroenterology*, **96**, 377–387.

28. Janssens, J., Peeters, T.L. and Vantrappen, G. (1990) Improvement of gastric emptying in diabetic gastroparesis by erythromycin. *New England Journal of Medicine*, **322**, 1029–1031.

29. Kang, J.Y., Yap, I., Guan, R., Tay, H.H. and Math, M.V. (1989) Acid induced duodenal ulcer pain: the influence of symptom status and the effect of an antispasmodic. *Gut*, **30**, 166–170.

30. Kerlin, P. (1989) Postprandial antral hypomotility in patients with idiopathic nausea and vomiting. *Gut*, **30**, 54–59.

31. Kiss, A., Bergmann, H., Abatzi, Th.-A. *et al.* (1990) Oesophageal and gastric motor activity in patients with bulimia nervosa. *Gut*, **31**, 259–265.

32. Koch, K.L., Stern, R.M., Vasey, M., Botti, J.J., Creasy, G.W. and Dwyer, A. (1990) Gastric dysrhythmias and nausea of pregnancy. *Digestive Diseases and Sciences*, **35**, 961–968.

33. Kumar, D., Ritman, E.L. and Malagelada, J.-R. (1987) Three dimensional imaging of the stomach: role of pylorus in the emptying of liquids. *American Journal of Physiology*, **253**, G79–G85.

34. Lin, H.C., Doty, J.E., Reedy, *et al.* (1989) Inhibition of gastric emptying by glucose depends on length of intestine exposed to nutrients. *American Journal of Physiology*, **256**, G404–G411.

35. Louie, D.S. and Owyang, C. (1988) Motilin receptors on isolated gastric smooth muscle cells. *American Journal of Physiology*, **254**, G210–G216.

36. McCallum, R.W. (1989) Motor function of the stomach in health and disease. In *Gastrointestinal Disease. Pathophysiology, Diagnosis, Management* (Ed.) Sleisenger, M.H. and Fordtran, J.S. pp. 675–713. Philadelphia: W.B. Saunders.

37. Malagelada, J.R., Rees, W.D.W., Miller, L.J. and Go, V.L.W. (1980) Gastric motor abnormalities in diabetic and postvagotomy gastroparesis: effect of metoclopramide and bethanechol. *Gastroenterology*, **78**, 286–293.

38. Marshall, J.B., Kretschmar, J.M., Gerhardt, D.C. *et al.* (1990) Gastrointestinal manifestations of mixed connective tissue disease. *Gastroenterology*, **98**, 1232–1238.

39. Miller, G., Palmer, K.R., Smith, B., Ferrington, C. and Merrick, M.V. (1989) Smoking delays gastric emptying of solids. *Gut*, **30**, 50–53.

40. Mistiaen, W., Van Hee, R., Blockx, P. and Hukens, A. (1990) Gastric emptying of solids in patients with duodenal ulcer before and after highly selective vagotomy. *Digestive Diseases and Sciences*, **35**, 310–316.

41. Moore, J.G., Datz, F.L. and Christian, P.E. (1990) Exercise increases solid meal gastric emptying rates in man. *Digestive Diseases and Sciences*, **35**, 428–432.

42. Myer, J.H. (1987) Motility of the stomach and gastrointestinal junction. In *Physiology of the Gastrointestinal Tract* (Ed.) Johnson, L.R. pp. 613–629. New York: Raven Press.

43. O'Brien, J.D., Thompson, D.G., Day, S.J., Burnham, W.R. and Walker, E. (1989) Perturbation of upper gastrointestinal transit and antroduodenal motility by experimentally applied stress: the role of beta-adrenoreceptor mediated pathways. *Gut*, **30**, 1530–1539.

44. Otterson, M.F. and Sarna, S.K. (1990) Gastrointestinal motor effects of erythromycin. *American Journal of Physiology*, **259**, G355–G363.

45. Ouyang, A., Sunshine, A.G. and Reynolds, J.C. (1989) Caloric content of a meal affects duration but not contractile pattern of duodenal motility in man. *Digestive Diseases and Sciences*, **34**, 528–536.

46. Pappas, T.N., Melendez, R.L. and Debas, H.T. (1989) Gastric distension in a physiologic satiety signal in the dog. *Digestive Diseases and Sciences*, **34**, 1489–1493.

47. Quon, M.G., Mena, I. and Valenzuela, J.E. (1989) Abnormalities in the duodenal transit and motility in duodenal ulcer patients: studies with a new isotopic technique. *Gut*, **30**, 579–585.

48. Raybould, H.E., Roberts, M.E. and Dockray, G.J. (1987) Reflex decreases in intragastric pressure in response to cholecystokinin in rats. *American Journal of Physiology*, **253**, G165–G170.

49. Raybould, H.E. and Tache, Y. (1988) Cholecystokinin inhibits gastric motility and emptying via a capsaicin-sensitive vagal pathway in rats. *American Journal of Physiology*, **255**, G242–G246.

50. Rees, W.D.W., Miller, L.J. and Malagelada, J.R. (1980) Dyspepsia, antral motor dysfunction and gastric stasis of solids. *Gastroenterology*, **78**, 360–365.

51. Rees, W.D.W., Malagelada, J.R., Miller, L.J. and Go, V.L.W. (1982) Human interdigestive and postprandial gastrointestinal motor and gastrointestinal hormone patterns. *Digestive Diseases and Sciences*, **27**, 321–329.

52. Rees, W.D.W., Leigh, R.J., Christofides, N.D., Bloom, S.R. and Turnberg, L.A. (1982) Interdigestive motor activity in patients with systemic sclerosis. *Gastroenterology*, **83**, 575–580.

53. Rezende-filho, J., DiLorenzo, C., Dooley, C.P. and Valenzuela, J.E. (1989) Cisapride stimulates antral motility and decreases biliary reflux in patients with severe dyspepsia. *Digestive Diseases and Sciences*, **34**, 1057–1062.

54. Schaap, H.M., Smout, A.J.P.M. and Akkermans, L.M.A. (1990) Myoelectrical activity of the Billroth II gastric remnant. *Gut*, **31**, 984–988.

55. Schulze-Delrieu, K. (1990) The load-to-length principle in the inhibition of gastric emptying by intestinal feedback. *Gastroenterology*, **98**, 1387–1388.

56. Spencer, M.P., Sarr, M.G., Soper, N.J. and Hakim, N.S. (1990) Jejunal regulation of gastric motility patterns: effect of extrinsic neural continuity to stomach. *American Journal of Physiology*, **258**, G32–G37.

57. Stern, R.M., Crawford, H.E., Stewart, W.R., Vasey, M.W. and Koch, K.L. (1989) Sham feeding. Cephalic–vagal influences on gastric myoelectric activity. *Digestive Diseases and Sciences*, **34**, 521–527.

58. Tatsuta, M., Ishi, H. and Okuda, S. (1990) Gastric emptying in patients with fundal gastritis and gastric cancer. *Gut*, **31**, 767–769.

59. Testoni, P.A., Bagnoli, F., Fanti, L. *et al.* (1990) Long-term oral cisapride improves interdigestive antro-duodenal motility in dyspeptic patients. *Gut*, **31**, 286–290.

60. Testoni, P.A., Fanti, L., Bagnolo, F. *et al.* (1989) Manometric evaluation of the interdigestive antroduodenal motility in subjects with fasting bile reflux, with and without antral gastritis. *Gut*, **30**, 443–448.

61. Willson, C.A., Bushnell, D. and Keshavarzian, A. (1990) The effect of acute and chronic ethanol administration on gastric emptying in cats. *Digestive Diseases and Sciences*, **35**, 444–448.

GASTRITIS

G.N.J. Tytgat

Acute gastritis, acute ulcer and acute mucosal damage are considered together because they represent the gastric mucosal responses to acute injury. Depending on the cause, they represent varying degrees of mucosal necrosis with subsequent inflammation. Acute gastritis has well-established and consistent clinical associations, such as a recent history of drug ingestion, alcohol excess leading to haemorrhagic erosions, shock, sepsis, multiorgan failure etc.

ACUTE GASTRITIS

AETIOLOGY

The causes are several and include the following:

1. The ingestion of large amounts of alcohol, large doses of analgesic drugs or non-steroidal anti-inflammatory drugs and cytotoxic drugs.

2. Gastric irradiation and freezing: irradiation may result in the appearance of prominent gastric folds with diminished pliancy, along with varying degrees of gastric erythema and friability. The mucosal erythema at close range is actually found to consist of multiple red islands (areae gastricae) with inner connecting pale linear areas (lineae gastricae). Along with this, telangiectasia may be evident. Radiation damage may be characterized further by antral narrowing, where the mucosal folds appear thickened, and covered with a remarkably friable and erythematous mucosa. Usually ulceration is superficial. Occasionally deep ulceration may be seen which heals slowly and is associated with scar deformity, obstruction or perforation.

3. Accidental or suicidal ingestion of corrosive substances, including acids, alkalis, fixatives such as formaldehyde and softeners such as lye (corrosive gastritis). Common corrosive agents are acids such as sulphuric acid, acetic acid and hydrochloric acid. Less common are nitric acid, formic acid and chromic acid. Common alkali or lye burns include caustic soda and bleach.[1]

4. Staphylococcal food poisoning.

5. Acute *Helicobacter pylori* gastritis.[13]

6. Severe bacterial infection of the gastric wall (acute phlegmonous or suppurative gastritis), involving the whole thickness of the stomach wall, due to bacterial invasion, usually by Gram-

positive cocci or *Escherichia coli*, in a patient with a pre-existing mucosal lesion such as cancer, ulcer or a postoperative gastritis.

CLINICAL FEATURES

After exposure to the aetiological agent, there is a rapid onset of abdominal discomfort, anorexia, nausea and vomiting. The clinical disease state is usually limited to a few hours or days, and in general recovery is complete.

In *acute corrosive gastritis*, the condition is more serious, with severe epigastric pain, retching and vomiting (often bloody). Shock may develop in the acute phase and survivors may develop gastric outlet obstruction.

In *acute phlegmonous gastritis*, the patient presents with evidence of an acute bacterial infection, with chills, fever, malaise, severe toxaemia and leukocytosis. There are also gastrointestinal symptoms, including nausea, vomiting (occasionally purulent), severe epigastric pain and tenderness.

INVESTIGATIONS

The diagnosis of acute gastritis first involves the exclusion of other diseases that may be accompanied by anorexia, nausea, vomiting and abdominal pain. Endoscopy in caustic or corrosive damage of the upper gastrointestinal tract is now regarded as a safe procedure providing information regarding the extent and severity of the injury, which ultimately has a bearing on the treatment and prognosis of this condition. Mucosal damage may be graded arbitrarily into three grades: mild (grade I), consisting mainly of mucosal hyperaemia and slight oedema; moderate (grade II), when there are, in addition, erosions or superficial ulcerations; and severe (grade III), when there are extensive and deep ulcerations.[1,14] Isolated gastric damage may occur in a substantial percentage of patients, especially after swallowing concentrated bleach or concentrated acids. Maximum involvement of the stomach is usually along the lesser curvature and in the region of the antrum. Often, but not always, the duodenum is spared, probably because of pyloric spasm and/or neutralization of acid by the alkaline contents of the duodenum. The most important complications are oesophageal stricture, gastric perforation and gastric outlet obstruction.

TREATMENT

In most patients the management of acute gastritis is expectant, with monitoring of body functions and replacement of any fluid or electrolyte loss.

Gastritis resulting from ingestion of a corrosive substance is more serious. Nasogastric suction with a silicone double-lumen tube, large doses of antacids (60 ml of aluminium magnesium hydroxide gel every 2 hours), H_2 receptor antagonists or proton pump inhibitors, and fluid replacement are advised. If at endoscopy necrotic blackened mucosa is seen, gastric resection is usually advised.[1,4,9] Survival after heavy corrosive ingestion will probably only be achieved by such aggressive measures.

The treatment of acute phlegmonous gastritis requires broad-spectrum antibiotics, acid suppression, rehydration and parenteral nutrition.

ACUTE GASTRIC ULCER

An ulcer is a circumscribed defect in the wall of the stomach or duodenum. Such lesions may penetrate varying distances through the stomach or duodenal wall; if focal mucosal necrosis does not extend deep into the muscularis mucosae, the term 'erosion' is to be preferred. An acute ulcer is a disease of abrupt or rapid onset and short duration. A focal mucosal defect superficial to the muscularis mucosae heals by epithelial regeneration without scar formation. In a deeper lesion, the amount of fibrosis produced is a reflection of the depth and duration of the lesion. Most acute ulcers therefore heal leaving little fibrotic reaction. Acute ulcers may be single or multiple; if multiple they are often termed 'areas of acute erosive gastritis' and occur predominantly in the gastric corpus.

AETIOLOGY

The aetiological factors to be considered are drugs, necrotizing agents, extreme physical stress, haemodynamic shock, severe burn, severe cerebral trauma, sepsis and multiorgan failure. There may be other, so far unidentified, factors.

Focal superficial necrosis may occur after administration of necrotizing agents, hypertonic fluids, ethanol, spices etc. Sheets of degenerated superficial epithelial cells exfoliate, creating a mucoid layer or cap over the damaged area. Resolution occurs by migration of mucous cells within the foveolae and upper gland area to form a new epithelial barrier. Bicarbonate-rich 'plasma shedding', through increased capillary permeability, enhances epithelial migration even in the presence of pronounced luminal acidity. Epithelial 'squamous-type' transformation of migrating cells is restricted to mucous cells. The free border of those cells is projected into long tongue-like lamellopodia, extending over denuded basal lamina. Once resolution starts, the proliferation of stem cells deeper within the mucosa is stimulated adding new cells to the epithelium.[5]

Focal necrosis, extending into the deeper glandular area without breaching the muscularis mucosae, heals by additional proliferation of gastric glands and surface epithelium cells. If the damage extends beyond the muscularis mucosae, the necrotic zone is eventually removed by macrophages and subsequently replaced by granulation tissue.[5]

Stress ulceration

The association of acute ulcer with serious injury and hypovolaemic shock is now well recognized. The introduction of rapid fluid and blood replacement and antibiotic therapy, in patients who would otherwise have died of hypovolaemic shock, was often complicated by acute stress ulceration in the second or third week after injury.[8] Acute stress ulcers are multifactorial in origin and those that perforate or bleed represent only a small fraction of the total number of cases. Factors that are of major aetiological significance include:[8,12]

1. Hypovolaemic shock
2. Sepsis
3. Renal, hepatic and pulmonary failure
4. Severe injuries (predominantly involving intra-abdominal or thoracoabdominal trauma)
5. Neurological injury, especially intracranial disease, trauma or operations (Cushing's ulcer)
6. Major burns (Curling's ulcers)
7. Severe bile reflux.

Acute stress ulceration is usually preceded by an episode of shock and decreased gastric mucosal blood flow.

Haemorrhagic gastritis simply defines the background gastric mucosal abnormality upon which erosions and superficial ulcers may develop. As acute erosions may progress into the submucosa to become true ulcers, especially after trauma and sepsis, there seems little point in attempting to differentiate these because they are pathogenically and clinically similar. Extension of the necrotic process into the submucosal layer where larger blood vessels are present is more likely to be associated with haemorrhage.

Usually, acute stress ulcers begin as multiple shallow erosions which are located preferentially in the corpus–fundus region of the stomach.[14] These lesions occur within minutes to hours of an acute episode of trauma or other serious illness. Within 24 hours of injury, petechiae and multiple shallow, red-based erosions may be observed. By 48 hours, the erosions become deeper, frequently with swelling at the margin. In some patients, the erosions spread to involve the entire corpus. Hypovolaemia is successfully treated, mucosal regeneration usually occurs and the integrity of the gastric mucosa is restored.

Drug-induced ulceration

Analgesic and anti-inflammatory drugs may evoke acute mucosal damage and ulceration accompanied by bleeding.[2,6,7] Bleeding usually results from rupture of small blood vessels just below the surface epithelium.[10]

Acute mucosal lesions can be produced by aspirin ingestion.[16] Despite numerous studies, there is no conclusive epidemiological evidence of an association between aspirin ingestion and overt bleeding.[11] Furthermore, those patients who do bleed following ingestion of aspirin do not rebleed on challenge.

Aspirin-induced gastric mucosal injury, which may occur in any area of the stomach, is initially characterized by focal intramural haemorrhage, appearing within 2 hours of the ingestion, followed after 8 or more hours by the appearance of focal mucosal erosions (*Figure 2.35*). Characteristically, the latter consist of multiple, small ($\leq$5 mm), shallow, white lesions, which lack depth. They are called ulcerations when they are deeper, sharply circumscribed and three-dimensional.

Gastric mucosal healing may take several days. Surprisingly, acute mucosal injury often resolves

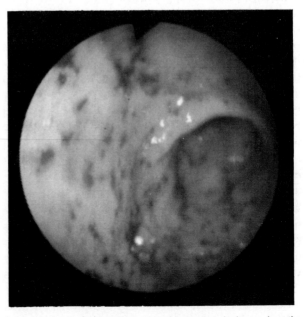

Figure 2.35 Aspirin-induced haemorrhagic lesions in the stomach.

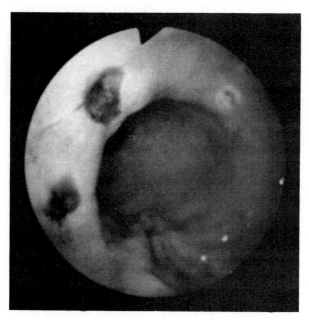

Figure 2.36 NSAID-induced mucosal damage.

despite continued aspirin therapy. The mechanism by which the injury appears localized remains unclear.

Multiple erosions or small shallow ulcers of the prepyloric antrum is the most common appearance for lesions caused by non-steroidal anti-inflammatory drugs (NSAIDs). White-based erosions and ulcers and focal erythema are often seen in conjunction (*Figure 2.36*).

A less common appearance is of one or more larger ulcers (>1.5 cm) often in the absence of erosions. Large ulcers are often found in the absence of surrounding endoscopic erythema or of gastritis histologically. The finding of multiple (generally three or more) small gastric ulcers constitutes an appearance highly suspicious of damage by NSAIDs. Despite their size, large ulcers associated with NSAID therapy may heal completely in due course once the offending drug is stopped.

CLINICAL FEATURES

Uncomplicated acute ulcers rarely produce symptoms. The diagnosis of an acute ulcer, when it is complicated by haemorrhage or perforation, is usually straightforward. By contrast, in the acute stress ulcer syndrome, diagnosis may be difficult. As the patient is ill and often confused, shock may be attributed to other causes, and symptoms such as pain may be distorted by analgesics given for other reasons, or by organic disease of the nervous system.

INVESTIGATIONS

The diagnosis[2,3,14] depends upon the following:

1. The recognition of the patients at risk.
2. The admission of such patients to an intensive care ward.
3. The initiation of measures that will detect bleeding or perforation at an early stage. This includes gastric aspiration in the search for hemorrhage and careful observation of patients in the search for perforation; if doubt exists, repeated ultrasonography and radiographs of the abdomen may be indicated.

When bleeding occurs, endoscopy should be performed as soon as the patient has been resuscitated.[6,7]

TREATMENT

Correction of hypovolaemia, sepsis and multiorgan failure is essential. Many therapeutic approaches have been used and include high-dose antacids, H_2 receptor antagonists, proton pump inhibitors and sucralfate. Sucralfate is associated with a reduced frequency of nosocomial infections.[15]

Frequently, broad-spectrum antibiotics need to be administered. Total parenteral nutrition must also be considered in debilitated, wasted and infected patients. Management in an intensive care ward is essential, if the development of stress-related acute ulceration is complicated by bleeding.

In the case of drug-induced ulceration the offensive agent should be discontinued. When this is impossible, administration of prostaglandins, H_2 receptor antagonists or sucralfate may be helpful.

REFERENCES

1. Bartelsman, J.F.W.M. and Tytgat, G.N.J. (1990) Caustic upper intestinal damage. In *Current Topics in Gastroenterology and Hepatology* (Ed.) Tytgat, G.N.J. and van Blankenstein, M. pp. 76–80. Stuttgart: Georg Thième Verlag.
2. Boyce, H.W. Jr. (1990) Drug-induced esophageal and gastric damage. In *Current Topics in Gastroenterology and Hepatology* (Ed.) Tytgat, G.N.J. and van Blankenstein, M. pp. 170–195. Stuttgart: Georg Thième Verlag.
3. Caruso, I. and Bianchi Porro, G. (1980) Gastroscopic evaluation of anti-inflammatory agents. *British Medical Journal*, **1**, 75.
4. Chung, R. and Den Besten, L. (1975) Fibreoptic endoscopy in the treatment of corrosive injury of the stomach. *Archives of Surgery*, **110**, 725.
5. Lacy, E.R. (1990) Gastric epithelial and membrane

restitution. *European Journal of Gastroenterology and Hepatology*, **2**, 178–181.

6. Lanza, F.L., Royer, G.L. and Nelson, R.S. (1980) Endoscopic evaluation of the effects of aspirin, buffered aspirin, and enteric-coated aspirin on gastric and duodenal mucosa. *New England Journal of Medicine*, **303**, 136–138.

7. Kimmey, M.B. (1989) Gastroduodenal effects of nonsteroidal anti-inflammatory drugs. *Postgraduate Medicine*, **85**, 67–73.

8. Lucas, C.E. (1981) Stress ulceration: the clinical problem. *World Journal of Surgery*, **5**, 139–151.

9. Nicosia, J., Thornton, J., Folk, F. and Saletta, J. (1974) Surgical management of corrosive gastric injuries. *Annals of Surgery*, **180**, 138.

10. Pfeiffer, C.J., Harding, R.K. and Morris, G.P. (1990) Ultrastructural aspects of salicylate-induced damage to the gastric mucosa. In *Drugs and Peptic Ulcer*. Vol. 2, *Pathogenesis of Ulcer Induction Revealed by Drug Studies in Humans and Animals* (Ed.) Pfeiffer, C. pp. 110–126. Boca Raton: CRC Press.

11. Piper, D.W., Gellatly, R. and McIntosh, J. (1982) Analgesic drugs and peptic ulcer. Human studies. In *Drugs and Peptic Ulcer*. Vol. 2, *Pathogenesis of Ulcer Induction Revealed by Drug Studies in Humans and Animals* (Ed.) Pfeiffer, C. pp. 76–94. Boca Raton: CRC Press.

12. Ritchie, W.P. (1981) Role of bile acid reflux in acute haemorrhage gastritis. *World Journal of Surgery*, **5**, 189–198.

13. Salmeron, M., Desplaces, N., Lavergne, A. and Houdart, R. (1986) Campylobacter-like organisms and acute purulent gastritis. *The Lancet*, **ii**, 975–976.

14. Silverstein, F.E. and Tytgat, G.N.J. (1987) *Atlas of Gastrointestinal Endoscopy*. Philadelphia, Toronto: Gower

15. Tryba, M. (1990) Stress bleeding prophylaxis with Sucralfate. *Scandinavian Journal of Gastroenterology*, **25**, (Suppl. 173), 22–33.

16. Weiss, A., Pitman, E.R. and Graham, E.C. (1961) Aspirin and gastric bleeding. Gastroscopic observations with a review of the literature. *American Journal of Medicine*, **31**, 266–278.

CHRONIC GASTRITIS

There is currently a resurgence of interest in gastritis. Knowledge about gastritis commenced when a link between the immune system and diffuse gastric mucosal disease was established. A further milestone followed the introduction of endoscopy, enabling the dual capabilities of gross visualization and targeted biopsy. The recent rediscovery of a Gram-negative spiral bacterium, *Helicobacter pylori*, which exclusively colonizes gastric-type epithelium, and the mounting evidence of its causal relationship

to gastritis, has further emphasized the marked heterogeneity of this disorder.

Chronic gastritis is a heterogeneous group of gastric mucosal disorders characterized by widespread injury, usually associated with a chronic or mixed acute or chronic inflammatory response. The clinical features of chronic gastritis are rather nebulous. The finding of chronic gastritis in asymptomatic subjects and in random population surveys has led some to conclude that the condition is a normal ageing process of no clinical consequence. Even those who believe chronic gastritis to be a genuine pathological process have difficulty in recognizing at which point the density of the inflammatory cell infiltration becomes 'abnormal'.

DEFINITION AND CLASSIFICATION

Chronic gastritis can be defined as any diffuse chronic inflammatory process involving the mucosal lining of the stomach. This definition encompasses both specific and non-specific subvariants of chronic gastritis. Specific forms of chronic gastritis are associated with distinct disease processes and include various entities such as established infections, granulomatous inflammation, eosinophilic infiltrative disorders and Ménétrièr's disease. A widely used classification was based on pathological observations of the gastric mucosa, which was described by Whitehead *et al.*[98] This classification includes the *grade* of gastritis (superficial or atrophic), its activity (quiescent or acute or chronic inflammation), the *mucosal type* affected (pyloric, body, cardiac, junctional or intermediate), and the presence and type of *metaplasia* (intestinal or pseudopyloric). Strickland and McKay[91] introduced the concept of type A (involving the corpus and associated with pernicious anaemia) and type B gastritis (antral atrophic gastritis). This was further refined by Glass and Pitchumoni,[27] who termed patchy gastritis of the whole stomach 'AB gastritis'. Correa's[9,11] classification links antral gastritis with *H. pylori* and duodenal ulcer, atrophic gastritis of the corpus with pernicious anaemia and multifocal gastritis with gastric ulcer and carcinoma. Types A (autoimmune), B (bacterial) and C (chemical) were advocated by Wyatt and Dixon,[103] whilst other variations on these themes were published by Stolte and Heilmann[90] and by Paull and Yardley.[71]

This brief survey emphasizes the multiplicity of classifications that have been advocated with consequent confusion and attendant difficulties in comparing data between various centres. Because of this, and because of the pivotal role that infection with *H. pylori* is now known to play in the pathogenesis of gastritis, a new system for the classifi-

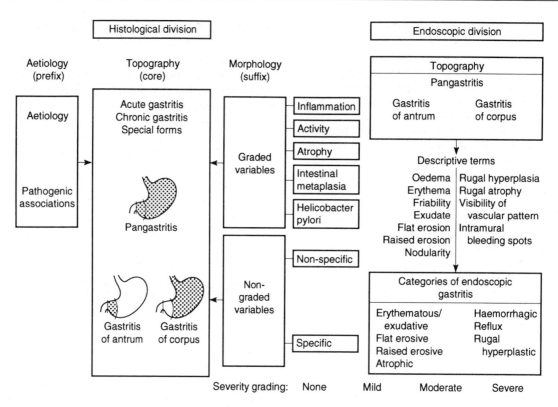

Figure 2.37 The Sydney system – a new classification.

cation of the responses of the gastric mucosa to injury was proposed in 1990, the Sydney system. The Sydney system aimed to produce a simple and comprehensive classification which would be flexible and capable of correlation with pre-existing classification systems.[60] This system has an endoscopic and histological division (*Figure 2.37*).[95]

PREVALENCE OF CHRONIC GASTRITIS

A number of recent biopsy studies in randomly selected population samples from different parts of Europe all indicate that chronic gastritis is common. These studies have also confirmed the increasing prevalence of gastritis in both corpus and antrum with advancing age. It should be emphasized, however, that most subjects in these studies displayed the milder grades of gastritis. Chronic gastritis with severe atrophy was observed in less than 5%. Siurala et al.[87] have applied a stochastic mathematical model to cross-sectional data obtained from such defined populations, in order to describe the progression of gastritis. The results suggest that, on a population level, chronic gastritis is a progressive disease and that chronic gastritis evolves into atrophic gastritis over many years. Recent application of this model by Villako et al.[96] suggests that antrum and corpus gastritis behave differently. Antrum-

predominant gastritis, once established, progresses more rapidly. This analysis, if correct, would support the concept proposed by Strickland and Mackay[91] of the existence of fundamentally different disease subsets within the spectrum of chronic gastritis.

AETIOLOGY AND NOSOLOGICAL ENTITIES

The views on the aetiology of chronic gastritis have undergone a dramatic reappraisal since 1983, when Marshall and Warren[55] rediscovered curved bacilli on the surface of gastric biopsies. Sufficient evidence has accumulated to suggest that most cases of non-autoimmune chronic gastritis can be considered to be a consequence of *H. pylori* infection. In clinical practice, *H. pylori* infection is causally responsible for about 80% of patients with chronic gastritis.[104] The next largest group is still unknown and termed 'idiopathic'. This accounts for some 10–15% of patients. Autoimmune-associated disease represents approximately 5%.[48] Other rarer aetiologies and special forms make up the remainder.

Special types of gastritis refer essentially to those with a specific pathology. Most of these types of gastritis are rare and include granulomatous gastritis (Crohn's disease, sarcoidosis, idiopathic), eosinophilic gastritis and the various forms of rugal hyperplastic gastritis (Ménétrièr's disease/hypertrophic hypersecretory gastritis).

SPECIFIC MICROBIAL CHRONIC GASTRITIS

The role of micro-organisms in gastritis, and thus a correct classification of the biopsy specimen, cannot be established if the patient has received any anti-microbial agent, including bismuth compounds, within the 4 weeks before biopsy. The primary consideration in the classification of gastritis is the presence, or absence, of *H. pylori* or, to a much smaller extent, of 'Gastrospirillum hominis'. Transient oral flora, such as *Streptococcus viridans* are found only incidentally and in small numbers.

Gastrospirillum hominis is present in 0.3% of Western subjects undergoing gastroscopy, but is more prevalent in animals. In half the subjects the organisms resides deep in the gastric tissue and does not provoke gastritis.

Cytomegolovirus occasionally causes gastritis. Widespread infection can occur in patients with human immunodeficiency virus (HIV). Cytomegalovirus involvement may appear as multiple white-based erosions or as large ulcers surrounded by multiple erosions. Biopsies taken from the base and edges may reveal intranuclear inclusions typical of cytomegalovirus.

Herpes simplex very rarely causes gastritis. The typical appearance of herpes simplex is that of diffuse, tiny, papular, ulcerating lesions. Biopsies may demonstrate 'ground-glass' nuclei and eosinophilic intranuclear inclusion bodies.

Candida albicans and other yeasts and fungi rarely cause gastritis.

H. pylori[30] *infection* (*Figures 2.38 and 2.39*)

This has a distribution which is world-wide and related to socioeconomic status. *H. pylori* colonizes the antrum in 95% of patients; half of these will also have the organism in the corpus. *H. pylori* inhabits exclusively gastric-type epithelium, including gastric metaplasia in the duodenum.[73] It does not colonize intestinal-type epithelium nor does it colonize severely dysplastic epithelium.[16] The distribution may be patchy. *H. pylori* is more numerous in active inflammation, and both neutrophil and eosinophil polymorphs are significantly increased in positive cases. Ultrastructurally, the organisms are found

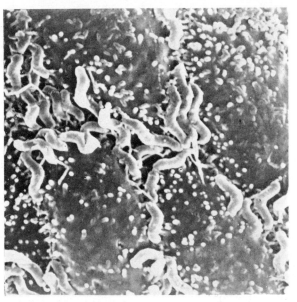

Figure 2.38 Scanning electron micrograph of *H. pylori* covering the gastric antrum.

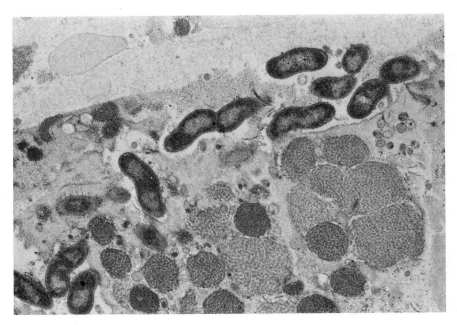

Figure 2.39 Ultrastructural appearance of *H. pylori* covering the surface epithelial cells embedded in the mucus layer.

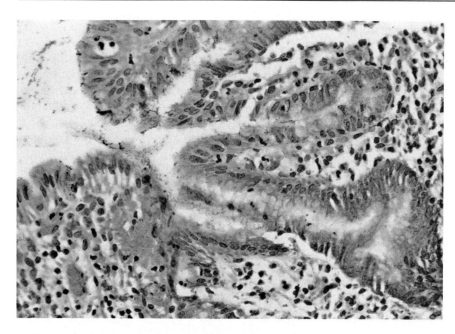

Figure 2.40 Warthin–Starry silver stain of *H. pylori* organisms covering the gastric mucosa.

very closely apposed to the epithelial plasma membrane where there is loss of microvilli and formation of shallow cup-like attachment sites. The infected epithelium shows degenerative changes comprising intracellular oedema, detachment from the basal lamina and cell necrosis. Further abnormalities consist of degeneration of intercellular junctions between the mucus-secreting epithelial cells, allowing the organism to enter the interepithelial spaces. Partly digested organisms may be seen in vacuoles within epithelial cells. Organisms may also be identified in phagocytic vacuoles inside polymorphs.

A remarkable feature of *H. pylori* is its urea-splitting capacity and the generation of ammonia in its immediate microenvironment. Whether or not

ammonia production is a pathogenic mechanism is controversial. Other potential mechanisms by which the organism may cause mucosal damage are: back-diffusion of hydrogen ions; proteolytic degradation of mucus; and the production of toxins.[3] The organisms may be detected histologically (*Figure 2.40*), on culture, serologically or by appropriate breath tests. Patients with *H. pylori* have raised levels of specific antibody in their serum,[61,72] of sufficient magnitude to permit serological diagnosis. Specific IgA and IgM antibodies can be detected in gastric juice, and secretion of IgA antibody is likely to interfere with bacterial adhesion. Coating of organisms by IgM and IgG, which have complement-fixing and opsonizing properties, would be likely to enhance neu-

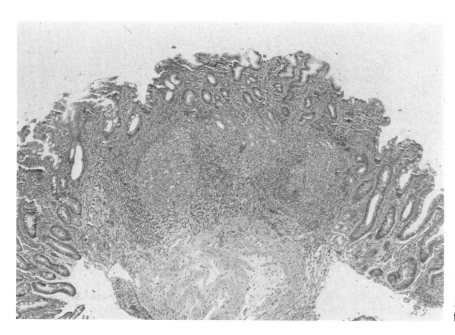

Figure 2.41 Abundance of lymphoid follicles in chronic *H. pylori* infection.

trophil activity against *H. pylori*, and may explain the association between colonization and polymorph activity. Enhanced production of the chemotatic factor leukotriene C4 (LTC4) has also been demonstrated. It has been shown that the number of CD4-positive lymphocytes (helper–inducer T cells) increases relative to CD8 suppressor cells.[75] These changes are paralleled by the acquisition of lymphoid follicles with germinal centres[16] (*Figure 2.41*).

Epidemiology

H. pylori-associated chronic gastritis is a common finding in dyspeptic patients referred for upper gastrointestinal endoscopy.[50,76] Studies from Europe,[6] North America and Colombia have shown that the prevalence of chronic gastritis increases with age,[3,34,57,63] and shows large geographical differences[3,34,57,63] (*Figure 2.42*). This association is observed in children,[19] in asymptomatic adult individuals (20%);[2,52] in patients with chronic dyspepsia (60–90%),[76,78] gastric ulcer (50–90%)[3,76] or duodenal ulcer (70–100%).[51,76]

The prevalence of *H. pylori* infection and of chronic gastritis rises with age, in parallel with the age-related increase in the prevalence of gastritis. Populations with a different ethnic background manifest significantly different gastric infection rates, but, whenever *H. pylori* is present, histological gastritis is always present. Differences in family structure, living standards and diet may provide epidemiological pointers towards identifying the source and mode of transmission of *H. pylori*, of which currently the human stomach appears to be the only known reservoir in nature.

Characteristics and natural history of *H. pylori*-related chronic gastritis

In *H. pylori* infection, the degree and activity of gastritis is usually more pronounced in the antrum (*Figure 2.43*). The inflammatory reaction in the corpus is often less marked.[65] *H. pylori*-induced gastritis is associated, not merely with a characteristic mixture of lymphocytes, plasma cells and neutrophilic granulocytes with leukodiapedesis into the foveolae, but also with basal lymphoid aggregates and lymphoid follicles in the mucosa.[16,90,103] Severe *H. pylori* infection in the corpus can probably induce erosions and giant folds (endoscopic rugal hyperplastic gastritis).

Siurala and co-workers[47,86] have demonstrated that chronic gastritis with variable degree of activity is a dynamic but slowly progressive process. In long-term follow-up studies performed in Finnish and Estonian individuals, it has become clear that chronic gastritis may sometimes present in childhood. Most commonly the prevalence and severity rise substantially in young adults and middle-aged individuals, sometimes leading to mild atrophic changes. During more prolonged follow-up, and usually in those over 60 years of age, atrophic changes are more prevalent either in the corpus, or in the antrum, or in both anatomical areas. Chronic

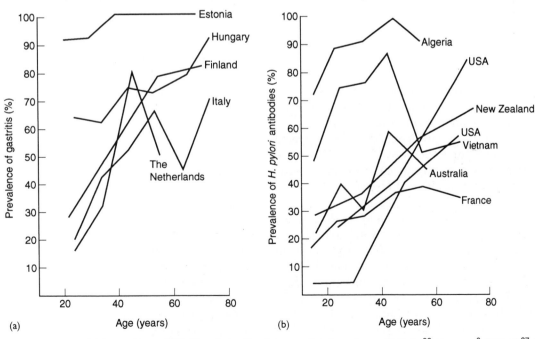

Figure 2.42 Prevalence of (a) gastritis and (b) *H. pylori* antibodies as a function of age: Estonia,[96] Hungary,[6] Finland,[87] Italy,[6] the Netherlands,[50] Algeria,[57] Vietnam,[57] USA,[34] Australia,[61] France.[34]

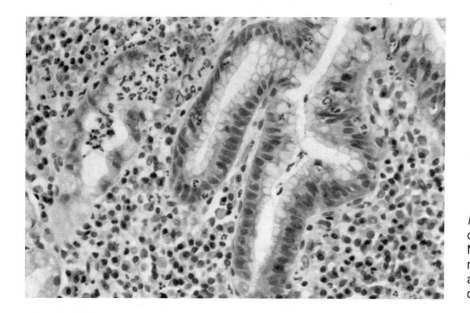

Figure 2.43 H. pylori infection with chronic gastritis with severe activity. Note the abundance of polymorphonuclear leukocytes in the lamina propria and permeating between the epithelial cells.

gastritis may heal spontaneously at any time, but this is rather rare. Ihamäki[42] reported the results of 27 years of follow-up of patients with normal mucosa and those with chronic gastritis. Of the 78 subjects with a normal corpus mucosa on initial examination, 58% developed chronic gastritis and 14% chronic gastritis with atrophy. Of 50 subjects who initially had chronic gastritis, 42% developed atrophic changes, whereas 18% showed a decrease in severity. Chronic gastritis can therefore improve during follow-up, but is usually a progressive dynamic process which ultimately leads to variable degrees of glandular atrophy. The frequency of intestinal metaplasia increases with the degree and duration of *H. pylori* gastritis. In case of advanced corpus atrophy with hypochlorhydria *H. pylori* may apparently be displaced by other opportunistic organisms.

Consequences of *H. pylori* infection

Information about the consequences of acute *H. pylori* infection comes from volunteer studies[56,64] and accidental *H. pylori* inoculation during acid secretory studies, or endoscopy.[28,53,74,100] In both volunteer studies, the subjects had a normal gastric mucosa before they swallowed *H. pylori*.

The first volunteer[56] developed acute symptoms, including epigastric pain, nausea and vomiting a few days after ingestion of *H. pylori*. Antral biopsies on the 10th day after ingestion of *H. pylori* revealed chronic gastritis with activity; spiral-shaped bacilli were seen adhering to the surface epithelium. Two weeks later, another antral biopsy was taken, by which time *H. pylori* was not found and the inflammatory reaction had subsided spontaneously.

The other volunteer[64] swallowed *H. pylori* and 2 days later developed epigastric pain, nausea and

cramps lasting for 10 days. On the fifth day, antrum and corpus biopsies were again taken. Antral mucosal histology showed chronic gastritis, but corpus biopsies were normal. On day 11 the corpus biopsies showed a mixed inflammatory infiltrate whereas the antrum biopsies revealed a more chronic inflammatory infiltrate. *H. pylori* was isolated from the corpus as well as from the antrum, during the following 2 months.

H. pylori inoculation can therefore lead to a bout of dyspepsia, of short duration, associated either with self-limiting colonization and acute gastritis, or with persisting infection and non-resolving chronic gastritis with variable degrees of activity but without symptoms.

In naturally acquired *H. pylori* infection, the source and mode of transmission remain unknown. Why some individuals have transient acute dyspepsia, whereas others remain symptom free, is unknown. Nor is it known why some infected subjects appear to recover spontaneously whereas others remain colonized for months or years, with or without symptoms, but almost always with ongoing chronic gastritis. Whether, and how often, spontaneous clearance of *H. pylori*-associated gastritis occurs in naturally acquired cases remain elusive.

Chronic *H. pylori* infection ultimately may lead to glandular atrophic changes in both antrum and corpus. Often polymorphs appear to congregate specifically around the pit–isthmic region which corresponds to the proliferative compartment. Damage of the stem cells at this site may be a factor in producing such glandular atrophy.[16] In *H. pylori*-positive chronic gastritis, the density of colonization by *H. pylori* appears to decrease with the development of atrophy. This suggests that other factors, such as genetic, macro- or microenvironmental influences, may also be important. The development of atrophy appears to evolve into three distinct phenotypes: atrophy limited to the antrum, atrophy limited to the corpus or atrophy involving both regions of the stomach. The final stage of severe gastric atrophy takes several decades to develop.[48,87]

Chronic atrophic gastritis with or without intestinal metaplasia is the most prevalent precursor for gastric cancer.[10,11,66] Three subtypes of intestinal metaplasia may be distinguished:

1. Type I or complete intestinal metaplasia has the histological appearance of small bowel mucosa and is characterized by the presence of goblet cells secreting acid sialomucins with a high proportion of N-acylated and occasionally O-acylated derivatives, Paneth cells and mature non-secretory absorptive cells with distinctive brush borders.
2. Type II or incomplete intestinal metaplasia is characterized by goblet cells between columnar surface epithelial cells, secreting N-acylated sialomucin and sometimes sulphomucins but no O-acylated sialomucin; there is almost always absence of Paneth cells and replacement of absorptive cells by secretory columnar mucous cells in various stages of differentiation. These secrete predominantly neutral mucin and/or a small amount of N-acylated but no O-acylated sialomucin.
3. Type III or incomplete metaplasia of the colonic or enterocolonic type resembles type II in most respects but the columnar mucous cells secrete mostly sulphomucin. A high iron–diamine–alcian blue staining is to be recommended to stain the colon-like crypts lined with sulphomucin-producing goblet cells.[23] A relationship between type III intestinal metaplasia and intestinal-type gastric cancer is highly likely.[12]

Functional consequences and associated diseases

Gastric function can be profoundly affected by progressive chronic gastritis. Stimulated acid secretion, fasting serum concentrations of pepsinogen I and output of intrinsic factor all decline. Gastrin levels increase in the presence of corpus atrophy, whilst the output of gastrin is diminished in antral atrophy.

Peptic ulcer disease is associated with chronic gastritis and *H. pylori*, but the relationships are complex.[16,29,31] Case–control studies suggest a 10-fold increase, especially of duodenal ulcer, in subjects with chronic gastritis.[84,85] The risk is affected by gender, age, and the distribution and severity of the gastritis. Thus, men with chronic gastritis, antral

or pangastritis have a six-fold to 16-fold increase in risk of duodenal ulcer, whereas antral gastritis and severe atrophy increase the risk of gastric ulcer.[26] In contrast, chronic gastritis of the corpus with atrophy decreases the risk of gastric ulcer. These considerations do not apply to duodenal ulcer, where corpus atrophy virtually never occurs.

Gastric polyps and gastric carcinoid tumours are also associated with chronic gastritis. Carcinoid tumours in the presence of chronic atrophic gastritis of the corpus may develop as a consequence of persistent hypergastrinaemia caused by falling gastric secretory capacity.

Gastric cancer may be related to the presence and progression of chronic gastritis. The risk of gastric carcinoma of the intestinal type is estimated to be three to four times higher in subjects with chronic atrophic gastritis of the corpus. The risk may be even higher in chronic pangastritis with severe atrophy. Although gastric carcinoma could be considered a late result of *H. pylori* infection, the sequence is multifactorial. It is usually postulated that cancers arise in areas of intestinal metaplasia. However, the specificity of intestinal metaplasia as an indicator of gastric cancer risk is rather poor because it may occur in up to 20% of the population.[43,44] The specificity may be enhanced by recognizing the 'colonic-type' of metaplasia.[12,83] Neoplastic transformation appears to involve a process of de-differentation from intestinal metaplasia to epithelial dysplasia and then to early carcinoma.[98] The initiating factors in the process of neoplastic transformation are poorly understood. Enhanced gastric epithelial cell proliferation often accompanies chronic gastritis.[101] In addition, the milieu of the stomach in patients with atrophic gastritis favours bacterial overgrowth and intragastric N-nitrosylation from bacterial reduction of nitrate-containing food.[79]

Treatment

If *H. pylori* is the principal aetiological factor in chronic gastritis, then eradication of the organism should result in symptomatic and histological improvement. Studies using colloidal bismuth subcitrate alone, or using combinations of bismuth compounds with antibiotics, have consistently shown that eradication of the organisms is accompanied by symptomatic improvement and a significant reduction or resolution in histological gastritis (*Figure 2.44*). Eradication of *H. pylori* is difficult and often requires triple therapy, consisting of a combination of a bismuth salt (either colloidal bismuth subcitrate or subsalicylate), metronidazole or tinidazole and either amoxycilline or tetracycline for a period of 1–2 weeks.[76,95] Such therapy, which has

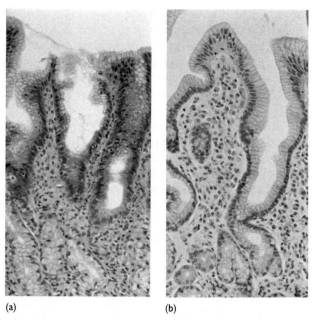

(a)   (b)

Figure 2.44   H. pylori chronic gastritis with activity before (left) and after (right) *H. pylori* eradication. Note reappearance of fully mature mucus-secreting foveolar cells and absence of neutrophils after successful therapy.

inherent side-effects, should be limited to patients with long-standing, rather severe dyspepsia that is resistant to the usual symptomatic measures. The latter include avoidance of offending foods, alcohol, excessive coffee, and the intermittent use of acid-neutralizing or antisecretory agents.

AUTOIMMUNE CHRONIC GASTRITIS

The link between the immune system and chronic gastritis was established with the identification of circulating autoantibodies to gastric intrinsic factor (intrinsic factor antibody – blocking type in 70%, binding type in 30%), and gastric parietal cells[14,15] (parietal cell antibody – present in 80–90%) in patients with pernicious anaemia.[91] Intrinsic factor antibody is restricted to evolving, or established pernicious anaemia, but parietal cell antibody is not so restricted and is associated with gastritis of variable severity. Parietal cell antibody–positive gastritis is more prevalent in relatives of patients with pernicious anaemia and in several endocrine disorders and vitiligo. Parietal cell antibody is absent in most patients with gastritis associated with *H. pylori*. Parietal cell antibody–positive gastritis merges into fully developed pernicious anaemia, characterized by antral sparing, corpus-predominant chronic gastritis with severe atrophy and hypergastrinaemia.

Autoimmune disturbance

The role of parietal cell antibody and intrinsic factor antibody, and of cellular immune reactions to gastric antigens, in the actual causation of chronic gastritis remains somewhat conjectural. Recent studies have uncovered additional heterogeneity of gastric autoantibodies beyond parietal cell antibody and intrinsic factor antibody, as originally defined. Thus, a parietal cell surface-reactive antibody (PCSA) has been described, which seems distinct from parietal cell microsomal (cytoplasmic) antibody (PCMA), and which is thought to contribute to parietal cell destruction by an antibody-dependent cytotoxic reaction. Recent work strongly indicates that canalicular membrane H^+/K^+ ATPase, the proton pump of the gastric parietal cell, is the major parietal cell microsomal antigen.[5,46] A gastrin receptor autoantibody has also been proposed, but at present its existence is uncertain. Immunopathological studies of the gastric mucosa in pernicious anaemia suggested a predominantly B-cell response and local production of both intrinsic factor antibody and parietal cell antibody.

Animal model

The most promising animal model of this disease is the inbred, thymectomized,[25,62] cyclosporin-treated mouse,[80] in which autoantibodies to the thyroid, stomach, adrenal cortex, testes, prostate, ovaries and pancreatic islets develop. Variable patterns of susceptibility and organ involvement reflect the existence of a genetic component in this model. Gastritis displays a remarkable resemblance to human autoimmune gastritis; 50% of susceptible animals show atrophic gastritis confined to the corpus, impaired intrinsic factor secretion and vitamin B_{12} malabsorption. The parietal cell microsomal antigenic target is similar in murine and human autoimmune gastritis. Experimental data indicate that the T cell is central to the initiation of the disease in this model. Neonatal thymectomy, or cyclosporin, may deplete organ-specific suppressor T cells, which normally restrain autoreactive effector T cells.[22] However, loss of organ-specific T-suppressor cells, or organ-specific autoreactive T-effector mechanisms, have not yet been identified in human autoimmune gastritis.

Histological and functional consequences

Most studies of human autoimmune gastritis have focused on the fully expressed advanced stage of this disorder. This is because autoimmune gastritis is clinically silent until vitamin B_{12} deficiency becomes manifest, unless relevant associations (pernicious anaemia relative, endocrinopathy) alert the clinician. Knowledge of the induction phase is scanty. In its classic appearance, the corpus mucosa is thinned and there is virtually complete loss of specialized cells, with apparent replacement of glands by downward extension of the proliferative compartment. Widespread intestinal metaplasia may give an appearance of villi and elongated pits. Chronic inflammatory cells are generally scanty and polymorphs are absent. The antral mucosa may be normal or may reveal less gastritis than in the corpus. Where the antrum is uninvolved there is G-cell hyperplasia and hypergastrinaemia as a consequence of hypochlorhydria. Raised gastrin levels may lead to proliferation of enterochromaffin-like cells in the corpus, causing diffuse enterochromaffin-like cell hyperplasia or carcinoid tumours.

Immunoreactive pepsinogen I is secreted by chief cells of the gastric corpus. Pepsinogen II, however, is present in chief cells, antral glands and mucous neck cells throughout the gastric mucosa. Atrophic gastritis of the corpus mucosa leads to low circulating pepsinogen I levels because the gastric lesion includes chief cell destruction. Pepsinogen II levels are unchanged, perhaps related to pyloric metaplasia of the corpus mucosa.[81,82] It has been proposed that a low pepsinogen I:II ratio, together with an absolute decrease in pepsinogen I, is indicative of atrophic gastritis, whereas a low ratio with a normal or elevated pepsinogen I level reflects the presence of less advanced gastritis.[81,82]

Patients with advanced autoimmune gastritis or pernicious anaemia are less frequently colonized by *H. pylori* than the general population.[24] It thus appears that advanced autoimmune gastritis presents an unfavourable environment to *H. pylori*. However, such data do not entirely eliminate a possible initiating role for *H. pylori* in a disease that has a natural history measured in decades before reaching its advanced stage. In addition, patients with autoimmune gastritis also have a low prevalence of positive serological response to *H. pylori*, suggesting lack of previous exposure to this organism.

Genetic factors

Autoimmune chronic gastritic is significantly more common in relatives with pernicious anaemia than in control subjects. The nature of the inherited factor(s) and the mode of inheritance are not established. There is evidence in families with pernicious anaemia that there may be an inherited susceptibility to gastric autoimmunity as defined by the presence of parietal cell antibodies. An association between established pernicious anaemia and a number of HLA-A, -B and -DR antigens does not extend to patients who have autoimmune gastritis but not pernicious anaemia.[99]

Clinical significance of autoimmune gastritis

Autoimmune gastritis is an uncommon cause of gastritis in humans. The prevalence of parietal cell antibody is 2–4% of adults in developed countries, rising to 10% in the seventh or eighth decade. Fully expressed autoimmune gastritis represents only a small fraction of all subjects with gastritis. Only 15–20% of subjects with parietal cell antibodies will progress to pernicious anaemia. One risk factor in the transition to pernicious anaemia is the development of autoantibodies to intrinsic factor. In contrast to this natural history of autoimmune gastritis, *H. pylori* gastritis rarely evolves to pernicious anaemia.[69] There is said to be a three- to fourfold increase of risk of gastric cancer in pernicious anaemia,[21,67] and the incidence of adenomatous polyps and severe epithelial dysplasia is also reported to be high.

Because of the relative rarity of autoimmune gastritis, its overall contribution as a risk factor for gastric carcinoma is low.[92] However, multiple polypoid carcinoid tumours of the stomach appear to be particularly associated with autoimmune gastritis.[4,38] These carcinoids may develop under the stimulus of sustained and marked hypergastrinaemia which provides a trophic stimulus to enterochromaffin-like cells.[20,54] More common than mini-carcinoids are multiple small sessile polyps, which may represent residual islands of relatively normal mucosa thrown into relief by the surrounding mucosal atrophy.[45]

Clinical features

The onset of symptoms in pernicious anaemia is usually insidious and the symptom pattern vague, thus delaying diagnosis. In the full-blown disease, patients may have symptoms caused by anaemia (fatigue, shortness of breath etc.), vague nonspecific dyspepsia, anorexia, soreness of tongue and mouth, paraesthesia, depression, impaired memory, and even cardiac failure. Subacute combined degeneration of the spinal cord is less common, but symptoms may antedate the macrocytic anaemia.

Examination may show anaemia and mild icterus. There may be brownish pigmentation of the skin and patches of vitiligo. Glossitis occurs in about half the patients. The spleen may be palpable. Neurological signs consistent with damage to the dorsal and lateral columns of the spinal cord may be present.

Investigations

Symptomatic patients have megaloblastic anaemia. Oval macrocytes with a wide variety of cell body inclusions are characteristic. Iron deficiency anaemia may also be present. Occult gastrointestinal bleeding, hypochlorhydria with malabsorption of food iron, and enhanced iron loss through increased gastric epithelial cell turnover all contribute to the development of iron deficiency. Erythrocyte survival is shortened. Leukocytes are normal or low in number. The number of hypersegmented neutrophils is increased. Thrombocytopenia may occur.

Serum vitamin B_{12} is low ($<100\,\mu g/ml$) because of malabsorption. Less than 10% of the ingested dose of ^{58}Co-labelled vitamin B_{12} is excreted in 48 hour urine collections (Schilling's test) because of the lack of gastric intrinsic factor secretion ($<200\,\mu g/h$). Improvement in absorption of labelled vitamin B_{12} occurs after the addition of intrinsic factor to the ingested vitamin B_{12}.

As a consequence of the severe corpus/fundus atrophic changes, gastric acid secretion ceases and anacidity develops, leading to a quite substantial rise of fasting serum gastrin, often exceeding 500 pmol/l. The gastrin rise is due to the removal of the inhibitory effect of gastric acid upon the antral G cells.[49] Only in patients with concomitant severe antral atrophic gastritis is serum gastrin in the normal range.

Parietal cell antibodies are almost always present but they lack specificity. Intrinsic factor antibodies are more specific but less sensitive.

Patients with pernicious anaemia are anacidic and unresponsive to stimulation with pentagastrin.

Treatment

Standard therapy is parenteral administration of vitamin B_{12}. The maintenance dose of intramuscular vitamin B_{12} is 1000 μg of cyanocobalamin every 1–2 months. Endoscopic monitoring for dysplasia and malignancy is controversial.[90]

IDIOPATHIC CHRONIC GASTRITIS

A variety of exogenous and endogenous agents can cause chronic gastric mucosal injury by a number of mechanisms mediated within the lumen of the stomach.[27] Suggested mechanisms include direct and repeated mucosal injury by drugs, nicotine, alcohol, hot beverages, hot chillies, pickles and spices, certain foods, IgE-mediated allergic reactions (to foodstuffs and drugs) and perhaps mucosal invasion by micro-organisms. The evidence that alcohol causes chronic gastritis is based on studies of the gastric mucosa in chronic alcohol populations where the prevalence of chronic gastritis may be as high as 80%. Similar, though less well-studied, associations are recorded in other populations, such as cigarette smokers or those ingesting hot beverages or foods for prolonged periods.

Many patients, even those with advanced gastritis, are asymptomatic. In others, presumably those with active inflammation in the presence of acid, various dyspeptic symptoms may be present. The therapy is symptomatic.

RUGAL HYPERPLASTIC GASTRITIS

Various rather ill-defined disease entities belong to the spectrum of rugal hyperplastic gastritis, sometimes also called gastropathy because of the paucity of inflammatory cells. Genuinely enlarged or giant folds do not flatten during maximal insufflation. In addition the rugae may reveal calibre changes or polypoid irregularities. Giant folds may be spread out over the whole stomach but usually they are present only in the corpus. Biopsy, either with a large-calibre biopsy forceps or with the snare rugectomy technique, is essential to make a proper histological diagnosis. The depth of a biopsy taken with a standard biopsy forceps is approximately 1 mm and barely samples muscularis mucosae, which is insufficiently deep to demonstrate foveolar, glandular or combined hyperplasia. Macroparticle biopsy taken with a polypectomy diathermy snare allows material with a diameter of 1–3 mm, extending into the submucosal layer and averaging 10 mm in width, to be studied.

There are multiple aetiologies for gastric fold enlargement; the more common ones include: Ménétrièr's disease, Zollinger–Ellison syndrome, lymphoma, carcinoma, peptic ulcer disease, postoperative stomach, granulomatous disease and gastric varices.

Ménétrièr's disease

Ménétrièr's disease,[58] described in 1888, is characterized by giant enlargement of strikingly convoluted gastric rugae, especially in the corpus, rarely in the antrum (*Figure 2.45*). Characteristic additional features are hypoproteinaemia and low normal or decreased acid secretion.[8] The condition is rare and

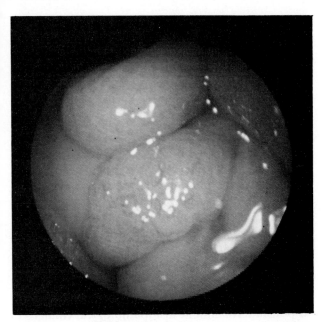

Figure 2.45 Severe fold enlargement as seen in Ménétrièr's disease.

may occur at any age. A description of Ménétrièr's disease follows on page 345.

Hyperplastic hypersecretory gastritis

This variant is characterized by severe inflammation predominantly of the gastric corpus mucosa. The mucosa is markedly widened with conspicuous enlargement of the foveolar area. Many polymorphonuclear leukocytes are present in the lamina propria and permeating between the epithelial cells which are focally degenerating. The aetiology remains unknown. Whether severe *H. pylori* infection may be responsible for this entity, at least in part, is a matter of current interest. Usually such patients complain of ulcer-like symptoms or non-specific dyspepsia. Whether this entity may ultimately evolve into a Ménétrièr-type picture is unknown. Therapy is symptomatic.

Zollinger-Ellison syndrome

The Zollinger–Ellison syndrome or gastrinoma is characterized by glandular hyperplasia because of the trophic action of gastrin. The mucosal thickness may be enlarged up to 2–3 mm. In most patients the folds are mildly enlarged and covered with copious amounts of clear acid fluid. Rarely, the folds are slightly irregular or nodular due to excessive accentuation of the areae gastricae pattern. Gastric ulceration is rare except when there is stasis due to

impaired gastric emptying because of ulcer disease or scarring in the bulb or duodenum. Diffuse inflammation with erosions may be present in the bulb. Large deep ulcers in the bulb or in the postbulbar duodenum up to the duodenojejunal flexure are common.

GRANULOMATOUS GASTRITIS

A granuloma is an accumulation of epithelioid cells (histiocytes) and multinucleated giant cells surrounded by lymphocytes. Often there is additional chronic inflammation with variable activity. Granulomata can be found in various inflammatory diseases, usually together with evidence of systemic involvement, such as sarcoidosis, Crohn's disease, syphilis, tuberculosis, histoplasmosis, leprosy and parasitic infestations. Large confluent granulomata with evidence of peripheral fibrosis might suggest sarcoidosis. Patchy gastritis with small basal epithelioid cell granulomata might suggest Crohn's disease. Granulomata can also be caused by food particles and foreign bodies that are thought to enter through breaks in the mucosa. Granulomatous gastritis can also be found incidentally in routine biopsies, or in resection specimens. It is impossible to distinguish the different causes on histopathological grounds alone unless tuberculous caseation is present. The ultimate diagnosis usually depends on the systemic manifestations of the underlying disease. A few patients with granulomatous gastritis have no other detectable site of granulomatous inflammation and are classified as idiopathic.

The endoscopic appearance of idiopathic granulomatous gastritis is non-specific. Idiopathic granulomatous gastritis usually involves the proximal stomach and occurs mainly in elderly patients.

Crohn's disease of the stomach and of the upper intestinal tract seldom occurs in the absence of involvement elsewhere.

Roughly 1% of patients with Crohn's disease may have gastric involvement. The prepyloric antrum is a predilection site giving rise to obstructive symptoms. Typically aphthoid erosions or superficial ulcers are seen in the prepyloric antrum with normal intervening mucosa. In some cases the mucosa between the ulcerations becomes nodular or polypoid, often referred to as a cobblestone appearance.

EOSINOPHILIC GASTRITIS

Eosinophilic gastritis usually occurs in the antrum and pyloric area, and is usually characterized by a dense infiltrate of eosinophils and polymorphonuclear leukocytes in the mucosa, submucosa and even the serosa.[68] The more proximal part of the stomach is usually not involved. Antral mucosal biopsies show acute inflammation with infiltration of eosinophils. However, a large number of eosinophils can also be found in case of chronic granulomatous diseases, amyloidosis, polyarteritis nodosa or carcinoma, but usually these conditions can readily be recognized. The cause of eosinophilic gastritis is unknown, but local allergic reaction has been suggested. To clarify the diagnosis further, clinical and biochemical investigations are necessary: peripheral eosinophilia, serum IgE levels, underlying allergic disorders and gastrointestinal parasitosis.

The most common endoscopic abnormality of diffuse eosinophic gastritis is stiffening and stenosis of the gastric antrum. Focal eosinophilic gastritis presents as a polypoid structure, usually located in the antrum. The mucosa covering the lesion looks similar to that of the adjacent gastric wall. Occasionally an erosive defect may be present at the top of the lesion.

Patients with eosinophilic gastritis often complain of nausea, abdominal pain and sometimes vomiting caused by pyloric (sub)obstruction. Anaemia due to blood loss and high numbers of eosinophils in the peripheral blood are common findings.

There is no specific treatment.

ENTEROGASTRIC REFLUX GASTRITIS

Enterogastric reflux gastritis is regarded by some authorities as a distinct syndrome usually occurring following gastric surgery.[17] Although duodenogastric bile reflux is a normal event in which, under physiological circumstances, no damage occurs to the gastric mucosa, an increase in amount and duration of duodenogastric biliary reflux may lead to characteristic changes of the gastric mucosal morphology and architecture.[77]

Reflux leads to chemical injury. The injurious refluxate contains pancreatic and duodenal secretions, bile salts and lysolecithin. Bile salts evoke initial mucus release followed by cell exfoliation after disruption of the mucous barrier.[77] Accelerated exfoliation of surface epithelial cells and a histamine-mediated vascular response become manifest as oedema and hyperaemia. Foveolar hyperplasia may be a response to excessive cell exfoliation from the surface epithelium.[17] When the injury is particularly severe, erosions may develop.

Dixon and colleagues[17] recently focused attention on the characteristic histopathology of postoperative alkaline gastritis. Histopathology shows elongation, tortuosity and hypercellularity of the gastric pits (foveolar hyperplasia), often giving the mucosa a villus-like appearance. Cell kinetic investigations reveal increased proliferation. Parietal and chief cells are usually replaced by mucous cells, but sometimes by intestinal-type cells. This loss of parietal and chief cells reduces the acid and pepsin secretion. In addition there is conspicuous vasodilatation and oedema in the lamina propria.

Endoscopic mucosal hyperaemia is an important feature of enterogastric reflux gastritis. Erythema and oedema sometimes regress following the creation of a Roux-en-Y limb.

O'Connor et al.[70] found a highly significant association between the severity of reflux gastritis and both hypochlorhydria and high bile acid concentrations. Wyatt[103] also observed reflux gastritis in 17% of non-surgical chronic dyspepsia patients and suggested that duodenogastric reflux might be responsible for similar histopathological changes in non-operated patients. It is thought that this type of gastritis may be caused by the damaging effect of bile acids, lysolecithin and pancreatic enzymes and, after partial gastrectomy, by the lack of the trophic effect of gastrin. Spontaneous enterogastric reflux in the intact stomach is much less common compared to that following gastric surgery. It may occur in gastric ulcer patients,[70] in patients with cholelithiasis, postcholecystectomy[94] or in patients with a gastroduodenal motor disorder.

Patients may complain of epigastric pain, bile vomiting and weight loss. These symptoms may start immediately after surgery or start years later. There is a poor correlation between the symptoms and the histological or endoscopic features. Diffuse hyperaemia and friability of the mucosa may be found in symptomatic as well as in asymptomatic patients. (Refer also to page 214.)

Treatment

Patients with epigastric pain and vomiting sometimes benefit from frequent, small meals. Cholestyramine, which binds bile acids, is not effective.[59] Antacids and sucralfate seem to help some patients. Prokinetic drugs such as cisapride or metoclopramide may be tried and are empirically occasionally helpful. Symptomatic improvement may also be obtained in some patients from administration of ursodeoxycholic acid.[88] Presumably this approach alters the quantity or quality of endogenous bile salts reaching the gastric mucosa. In desperate cases, surgical therapy aimed at diverting duodenal contents away from the stomach by Roux-en-Y reconstruction or jejunal loop interposition of at least 40 cm may be tried with variable success.[36]

LYMPHOCYTIC GASTRITIS

Lymphocytic gastritis is characterized by the presence of a large number of lymphocytes invading the surface and foveolar epithelium, with variable grades of polymorphs, plasma cells and lymphocytes in the lamina propria.[18,37,102] Endoscopically, gastric folds are thickened and studded with small nodules, bearing aphthoid or erupting erosions. Histologically, the epithelium is crowded with mature-looking lymphocytes, which are exclusively of the T-cell type, many of which are surrounded by a clear halo.

The pathogenesis of lymphocytic gastritis is unknown. An abnormal response to an as yet unknown antigen has been suggested. *H. pylori* infection may be demonstrable in a minority of the patients. The large number of T lymphocytes infiltrating the surface epithelium is reminiscent of coeliac disease.

COLLAGENOUS GASTRITIS

Collagenous gastritis is a rare type of chronic gastritis and only a few case reports have been published.[7] Endoscopically, erythema and nodularity are prominent in the corpus. Mucosal biopsies show patchy chronic gastritis, with predominant plasma cells and lymphocytes. The most remarkable feature is a focal band of collagen present immediately beneath the surface epithelial layer. The band does not extend into the deeper parts of the lamina propria. The cause of collagenous gastritis is unknown, but in parallel with collagenous sprue and collagenous colitis, an unknown agent, possibly food, stimulates the subepithelial fibroblasts to produce an excessive amount of collagen. The patients usually complain of recurrent abdominal pain. There is no specific treatment.

RAISED EROSIVE GASTRITIS (VARIOLIFORM GASTRITIS)

Raised erosive gastritis is characterized by the presence of variable numbers of discrete 5–10 mm nodular elevations, or raised erosions, mainly in the corpus/fundus area.[35] The most common endoscopic appearance is that of prominent folds in the corpus. Characteristically, there is a discrete nodular bulge to the fold with an erosion in the centre, usually covered with some exudate. The defect is often surrounded by a rim of erythema. Biopsies may show evidence of lymphocytic gastritis in some, but not all, patients. Other features are foveolar hyperplasia, variable numbers of inflammatory cells, some eosinophils between distended glands

and various degrees of fibrosis of the lamina propria. The aetiology remains elusive. An allergic cause has been suggested,[1] but never confirmed as is also the case for excessive enterogastric reflux. During prolonged follow-up, the number of raised erosions may increase, remain unchanged or regress for unknown reasons. Upon healing of the erosive lesions, polypoid unevenness of the gastric contour may remain, supporting the transition from raised erosive gastritis to hyperplastic polyposis of the stomach.

Raised (or varioliform) erosions may occasionally be found in asymptomatic individuals. Usually, however, such patients complain of dyspepsia with chronic nausea, anorexia and vague abdominal discomfort.

Treatment is usually symptomatic. For the rare patient with severe *H. pylori* infection, anti-*H. pylori* therapy may be attempted.

ACUTE HAEMORRHAGIC GASTRITIS

This type of gastritis is characterized endoscopically by focal or widespread bleeding erosions. Usually petechiae are seen between these erosions. The petechiae represent bleeding spots in the mucosa without loss of the overlying epithelium.

Mucosal biopsies may show destruction of the mucosal lining, usually limited by the muscularis mucosae, but sometimes extending through the muscularis mucosae. There may be conspicuous accumulation of erythrocytes in the lamina propria, usually without marked inflammatory reaction.

Acute haemorrhagic gastritis is a frequent finding in patients presenting with intestinal bleeding, particularly in those with a history of excessive alcohol intake or taking aspirin or non-steroidal anti-inflammatory drugs (NSAIDs). The pathogenesis of NSAID-induced mucosal damage is complex and not fully understood.[13,40] NSAIDs impair the mucosal defence by reducing the bicarbonate and mucus secretion, and reduce the mucosal blood flow. These effects are related to inhibition of gastric prostaglandin synthesis and can be prevented by the concomitant use of synthetic prostaglandins.[32,33]

Bleeding from these erosions usually stops spontaneously and the lesions tend to heal rapidly after alcohol abuse or NSAID usage is stopped.

IMMUNODEFICIENCY-ASSOCIATED CHRONIC GASTRITIS

Approximately 40% of patients with the common variable form of primary immunodeficiency display chronic gastritis.[39] Pan-hypogammaglobulinaemia and repeated bacterial infections are consistent features in this disorder. The gastric lesion is usually a severe pangastritis with equivalent involvement of both antral and corpus mucosa. Plasma cells are conspicuously absent from the inflammatory infiltrate and circulating gastric antibodies are not detected. The pathogenesis of this uncommon form of chronic gastritis is not established. Normogastrinaemia and achlorhydria are common. Absence of gastrin elevation is due to destruction of G cells by severe antral gastritis.[41] Patients with common variable immunodeficiency have a high incidence of gastric carcinoma.[39]

REFERENCES

1. André, C., André, R. and Truchot, R. (1982) La gastrite varioliforme: problèmes immunologiques et thérapeutiques. *Acta Endoscopica*, **12**, 137.

2. Barthel, J.S., Westblom, T.U., Havey, A.D. *et al.* (1988) Gastritis and *Campylobacter pylori* in healthy, asymptomatic volunteers. *Archives of Internal Medicine*, **148**, 1149–1151.

3. Blaser, M.J. (1988) Type B Gastritis, aging and *Campylobacter pylori*. *Archives of Internal Medicine*, **148**, 1021–1022.

4. Borch, K., Renvall, H. and Liedberg, G. (1985) Gastric endocrine cell hyperplasia and carcinoid tumours in pernicious anaemia. *Gastroenterology*, **88**, 638–648.

5. Burman, P., Mardh, S., Norberg, L. *et al.* (1989) Parietal cell antibodies in pernicious anaemia inhibit H^+, K^+-adenosine triphosphatase, the proton pump of the stomach. *Gastroenterology*, **96**, 1434.

6. Cheli, R., Simon, L., Aste, H. *et al.* (1980) Atrophic gastritis and intestinal metaplasia in asymptomatic Hungarian and Italian population. *Endoscopy*, **12**, 105–108.

7. Colletti, R.B. and Trainer, T.D. (1989) Collagenous gastritis. *Gastroenterology*, **97**, 1552–1555.

8. Cooper, B.T. and Chadwick, V.S. (1981) Ménétrièr's disease. In J.H. Moody (Ed.) Baron, F.P. pp. 141–191, *Butterworths International Medical Reviews*. London: Butterworth.

9. Correa, P. (1980) The epidemiology and pathogenesis of chronic gastritis. Three etiologic entities. *Frontiers of Gastroenterology Research*, **6**, 98–108.

10. Correa, P. (1982) Precursors of gastric and esophageal cancer. *Cancer*, **50**, 2554–2565.

11. Correa, P. (1988) Chronic gastritis: A clinico-pathological classification. *American Journal Gastroenterology*, **83**, 504–509.

12. Craanen, M.E., Blok, P., Dekker, W., Ferweda, J. and Tytgat, G.N.J. (1992) Early gastric cancer and intestinal metaplasia: Possible use of type III IM as a marker for intestinal-type EGC.

13. Davenport, H.W., Warner, H.A. and Code, C.F. (1964) Functional significance of gastric mucosal barrier to sodium. *Gastroenterology*, **47**, 142–152.

14. De Aizpurua, H.J., Cosgrave, L.J., Ungar, B. *et al.* (1983) Autoantibodies cyotoxic to gastric parietal cells in serum of patients with pernicious anemia. *New England Journal of Medicine*, **309**, 625.

15. De Aizpura, H.J., Ungar, B. and Toh, B.H. (1985) Autoantibody to the gastrin receptor in pernicious anemia. *New England Journal of Medicine*, **313**, 479.

16. Dixon, M.F. (1990) Progress in the pathology of gastritis and duodenitis. *Current Topics in Pathology*, **81**, 1–40.

17. Dixon, M.F., O'Connor, H.J., Axon, A.T.R., King, R.F.J.G. and Johnston, D. (1986) Reflux gastritis: distinct histopathological entity? *Journal of Clinical Pathology*, **39**, 524–530.

18. Dixon, M.F., Wyatt, J.L., Burke, D.A. and Rathbone, B.J. (1988) Lymphocytic gastritis – relationship to *Campylobacter pylori* infection. *Journal of Pathology*, **154**, 125–132.

19. Drumm, B., Sherman, P., Cutz, E. and Kamali, M. (1987) Association of *Campylobacter pylori* on the gastric mucosa with antral gastritis in children. *New England Journal of Medicine*, **316**, 1557–1561.

20. Eason, C.T., Spencer, A.J., Pattison, A. *et al.* (1989) The trophic effects of gastrin on fundic neuroendocrine cells of the rat stomach. *Alimentary Pharmacology and Therapeutics*, **3**, 245–251.

21. Elsborg, L. and Mosbech, J. (1979) Pernicious anaemia as a risk factor in gastric cancer. *Acta Medica Scandinavica*, **206**, 215–318.

22. Elson, C.O. (1990) Do organ-specific suppressor T cells prevent autoimmune gastritis. *Gastroenterology*, **98**, 226.

23. Filipe, M.I. (1989) Histochemistry of intestinal mucins. In *Gastrointestinal and Oesophageal Pathology* (Ed.) Whitehead, R. p. 71. Edinburgh: Churchill Livingstone.

24. Flejou, J.F., Bahame, P., Smith, A.C. *et al.* (1989) Pernicious anaemia and Campylobacter-like organisms: is the gastric antrum resistent to colonization? *Gut*, **30**, 60–64.

25. Fukuma, K., Sakaguchi, S., Kuribayash, K. *et al.* (1988) Immunologic and clinical studies on murine experimental autoimmune gastritis induced by neonatal thymectomy. *Gastroenterology*, **94**, 274.

26. Gear, M.W.L., Truelove, S.C. and Whitehead, R. (1971) Gastric ulcer and gastritis. *Gut*, **12**, 639–645.

27. Glass, G.B.J. and Pitchumoni, C.S. (1975) Atrophic gastritis. *Human Pathology*, **6**, 219–250.

28. Gledhill, T., Leicester, R.J., Addis, B. *et al.* (1985) Epidemic hypochlorhydria. *British Medical Journal*, **290**, 1383–1386.

29. Goodwin, C.S., Armstrong, J.A. and Marshall, B.J. (1986) *Campylobacter pyloridis*, gastritis and peptic ulceration. *Journal of Clinical Pathology*, **39**, 153–165.

30. Goodwin, C.S., Armstrong, J.A., Chilvers, T. *et al.* (1989) Transfer of *Campylobacter pylori* and *Campylobacter mustelae* to *Helicobacter* gen. nov as *Helicobacter pylori* comb. nov. and *Helicobacter mustelae* comb. nov., respectively. *International Journal of Systematic Bacteriology* 4 (39), 397–405.

31. Graham, D.Y. (1989) *Campylobacter pylori* and peptic ulcer disease. *Gastroenterology*, **96**, 615–625.

32. Graham, D.Y. (1989) Prevention of gastroduodenal injury induced by chronic nonsteroidal antiinflammatory drug therapy. *Gastroenterology*, **96** (suppl.), 675–681.

33. Graham, D.Y., Agrawal, N. and Roth, S.H. (1988) Prevention of NSAID-induced gastric ulcer with the synthetic prostaglandin misoprostol – a multicentre, double-blind, placebo-controlled trial. *The Lancet*, **ii**, 1277–1280.

34. Graham, D.Y., Klein, P.D., Opekun, A.R. and Boutton, T.W. (1988) Effect on age of the frequency of active *Campylobacter pylori* infection diagnosed by the urea breath test in normal subjects and patients with peptic ulcer. *Journal of Infectious Diseases*, **157**, 777–780.

35. Green, P.H.R., Gold, R.P., Marboe, C.C. *et al.* (1982) Chronic erosive gastritis: clinical, diagnostic and pathological features in nine patients. *American Journal of Gastroenterology*, **77**, 543–547.

36. Halpern, N.B., Hirschowitz, B.L. and Moody, F.G. (1973) Failure to achieve success with corrective gastric surgery. *American Journal of Surgery*, **124**, 108–115.

37. Haot, J., Hamichi, L., Wallez, L. and Mainguet, P. (1988) Lymphocytic gastritis: a newly described entity: a retrospective endoscopic and histological study. *Gut*, **29**, 1258–1264.

38. Harvey, R.F., Bradshaw, M.J., Davidson, C.M., Wilkinson, S.P. and Davies, P.S. (1985) Multifocal gastric carcinoid tumours, achlorhydria and hypergastrinaemia. *The Lancet*, **i**, 951–954.

39. Hermans, P.E., Diaz-Buxo, J.A. and Stobo, J.D. (1976) Idiopathic late-onset immunoglobulin deficiency: clinical observations in 50 patients. *American Journal of Medicine*, **61**, 221–237.

40. Hills, B.A., Butler, B.D. and Lichtenbergen, L.M. (1983) Gastric mucosal barrier: hydrophilic lining to the lumen of the stomach. *American Journal of Physiology*, **244**, G561–G568.

41. Hughes, W.S., Brooks, F.P. and Conn, H.O. (1972) Serum gastrin levels in primary hypogammaglobulinaemia and pernicious anaemia – studies in adults. *Annals of Internal Medicine*, **77**, 746–750.

42. Ihamäki, T., Saukkonen, M. and Siurala, M. (1978) Long-term observation of subjects with normal mucosa and with superficial gastritis. Results of 23–27 years follow-up examination. *Scandinavian Journal of Gastroenterology*, **13**, 771–776.

43. Ihamäki, T., Varis, K. and Siurala, M. (1979) Morphological, functional and immunological state of the gastric mucosa in gastric carcinoma families. *Scandinavian Journal of Gastroenterology*, **14**, 801–812.

44. Ihamäki, T., Kekki, M., Sipponen, P. and Siurala, M. (1985) The sequelae and course of chronic gastritis during a 30–40 year bioptic follow-up study. *Scandinavian Journal of gastroenterology*, **20**, 485–491.

45. Ikeda, T., Sennoue, I., Hara, M., Tsutsumi, Y., Harasawa, S. and Miwa, T. (1985) Gastric pseudopolyposis: a new clinical manifestion of type A gastritis. *American Journal of Gastroenterology*, **80**, 82–90.

46. Karlsson, F.A., Burman, P., Loof, L. *et al.* (1988) Major parietal cell antigen in autoimmune gastritis with pernicious anemia is the acid-producing H^+, K^+-adenosine triphosphatase of the stomach. *Journal of Clinical Investigation*, **81**, 475.

47. Kekki, M., Villako, K., Tamm, A. *et al.* (1977) Dynamics of antral and fundal gastritis in an Estonian rural population sample. *Scandinavian Journal of Gastroenterology*, **12**, 321–324.

48. Kekki, M., Siurala, M., Varis, K., Sipponen, P., Sistonen, P. and Nevanlinna, H.R. (1987) Classification principles and genetics of chronic gastritis. *Scandinavian Journal of Gastroenterology*, **22**(suppl. 141), 1–28.

49. Korman, M.G., Strickland, R.G. and Hansky, J. (1972) The functional 'G' cell mass in atrophic gastritis. *Gut*, **13**, 349–351.

50. Kreuning, J., Bosman, F.T., Kuiper, G., Wal, A.M. and Lindeman, J. (1978) Gastric and duodenal mucosa in 'healthy' individuals. *Journal of Clinical Pathology*, **31**.

51. Lambert, J.R., Dunn, K.L., Eaves, E.R. *et al.* (1985) Pyloric CLO in the human stomach. *Medical Journal of Australia*, **143**, 174.

52. Langenberg, M.L., Tytgat, G.N.J., Schipper, M.E.I. *et al.* (1984) Campylobacter-like organisms in the stomach of patients and healthy individuals. *The Lancet*, **i**, 1348.

53. Langenberg, W., Rauws, E.A.J., Oudbier, J.H. and Tytgat, G.N.J. (1990) Patient-to-patient transmission of *Campylobacter pylori* infection by fiberoptic gastroduodenoscopy and biopsy. *Journal of Infectious Diseases*, **161**, 507–511.

54. Lanzon-Miller, S., Pounder, R.E., Hamilton, M.R. *et al.* (1987) Twenty-four hour intragastric acidity and plasma gastrin concentration in healthy subjects and patients with duodenal or gastric ulcer, or pernicious anaemia. *Alimentary Pharmacology and Therapeutics*, **1**, 225–237.

55. Marshall, B.J. and Warren, J.R. (1984) Unidentified curved bacilli in the stomach of patients with gastritis and peptic ulceration. *The Lancet*, **i**, 1311–1315.

56. Marshall, B.J., Armstrong, J.A., McGechie, D.B. and Glancy, R.J. (1985) Attempt to fulfil Koch's postulates for pyloric campylobacter. *Medical Journal of Australia*, **142**, 436–439.

57. Mégraud, T., Brassens Rabbe, M.P., Denis, F., Berbouri, A. and Hoa, D.O. (1989) Seroepidemiology of *Campylobacter pylori* infection in various populations. *Journal of Clinical Microbiology*, **27**, 1870–1873.

58. Ménétrièr, P. (1888) Des polyadenomes gastriques et leurs rapports avec le cancer de l'estomac. *Arch. Physiol. Nrm. Pathol.*, **1**, 32.

59. Meskinpour, H., Elashoff, J., Steward, H. and Sturdevant, R.A.L. (1977) Effect of cholestyramine on the symptoms of reflux gastritis – a double-blind, crossover study. *Gastroenterology*, **73**, 441–443.

60. Misiewicz, J.J., Tytgat, G.N.J., Goodwin, C.S. *et al.* (1990) The Sydney system: a new classification of gastritis. In *Working Party Reports, World Congresses of Gastroenterology 1990*. Sydney: Blackwell Scientific Publications 1–10.

61. Mitchell, H.M., Lee, A., Berkowicz, J. and Borody, T. (1988) The use of serology to diagnose active *Campylobacter pylori* infection. *Medical Journal of Australia*, **149**, 604–609.

62. Mori, Y., Fukuma, K., Adachi, F. *et al.* (1989) Parietal cell autoantigens involved in neonatal thymectomy-induced murine autoimmune gastritis. Studies using monoclonal autoantibodies. *Gastroenterology*, **97**, 364.

63. Morris, A., Nicholson, G., Lloyd, G., Haines, D., Rogers, A. and Taylor, D. (1986) Seroepidemiology of *Campylobacter pyloridis*. *New Zealand Medical Journal*, **99**, 657–659.

64. Morris, A. and Nicholson, G. (1987) Ingestion of *Campylobacter pyloridis* causes gastritis and raised fasting gastric pH. *American Journal of Gastroenterology*, **82**, 192–199.

65. Morris, A., Maher, K., Thomson, *et al.* (1988) Distribution of *campylobacter pylori* in the human stomach obtained at postmortem. *Scandinavian Journal of Gastroenterology*, **23**, 257–264.

66. Morson, B.C., Sobin, L.H., Grundmann, E., Johansen, A., Nagayo, T. and Serck-Hansen, A. (1980) Precancerous conditions and epithelial dysplasia in the stomach. *Journal of Clinical Pathology*, **33**, 711–721.

67. Mosbech, J. and Vidabaeck, A. (1950) Mortality from and risk of gastric carcinoma among patients with pernicious anaemia. *British Journal of Medicine*, **2**, 390.

68. Nishikado, H., Kumada, H., Okuhira, M. *et al.* (1985) Diffuse eosinophilic gastritis (allergic granulomatosis): report of a case. *Gastrointestinal Endoscopy*, **27**, 111.

69. O'Connor, H.J., Axon, A.T.R. and Dixon, M.F. (1984) Campylobacter-like organisms unusual in Type A (pernicious anaemia) gastritis. *The Lancet*, **ii**, 1091.

70. O'Connor, H.J., Wyatt, J.L., Dixon, M.F. and Axon, A.T.R. (1986) Campylobacter-like organisms and reflux gastritis. *Journal of Clinical Pathology*, **39**, 531–533.

71. Paull, G. and Yardley, J.M. (1989) Pathology of *C. pylori*-associated gastric and esophageal lesions. In *Campylobacter pylori in Gastritis and Peptic Ulcer Disease* (Ed.) Blaser, M.J. pp. 73–97. New York: Igaku-Shoin.

72. Perez-Perez, G., Dworkin, B.M., Chodes, J.E. and Blaser, M.J. (1988) *Campylobacter pylori* antibodies in humans. *Annals of Internal Medicine*, **109**, 11–17.

73. Price, A.B. (1991) The Sydney system: a new classification of gastritis. *Journal of Gastroenterology and Hepatology*.

74. Ramsey, E.J., Carey, K.V., Peterson, W.L. *et al.* (1979) epidemic gastritis with hypochlorhydria. *Gastroenterology*, **76**, 1449–1457.

75. Rathbone, B.J., Trejosiewicz, L.K., Heatley, R.V. and Losowsky, M.S. (1989) Mucosal T-cell subjects in normal gastric antrum and *C. pylori* associated chronic gastritis. *Gut*, **29**, A1348.

76. Rauws, E.A.J., Langenberg, W., Houthoff, H.J., Zanen, H.C. and Tytgat, G.N.J. (1988) *Campylobacter pylori*-associated chronic active gastritis. A prospective study of its prevalence and the effects of antibacterial and antiulcer treatment. *Gastroenterology*, **94**, 33–40.

77. Rees, W. and Rhodes, J. (1977) Bile reflux in gastro-oesophageal disease. *Clinical Gastroenterology*, **6**, 179–200.

78. Rokkas, T., Pursey, C., Uzoechina, E. *et al.* (1990) *Campylobacter pylori* and non-ulcer dyspepsia. *American Journal of Gastroenterology*, **82**, 1149–1152.

79. Ruddell, W.S., Bone, E.S., Hill, M.J. *et al.* (1976) Gastric-juice nitrite: a risk factor for cancer in the hypochlorhydric stomach? *The Lancet*, **ii**, 1037–1039.

80. Sakaguchi, S. and Sakaguchi, N. (1989) Organ-specific autoimmune disease induced by elimination of T cell subset. V. Neonatal administration of cyclosporin A causes autoimmune disease. *Journal of Immunology*, **142**, 471.

81. Samloff, I.M. (1982) Pepsinogens I and II: purification from gastric mucosa and radioimmunoassay in serum. *Gastroenterology*, **82**, 26–33.

82. Samloff, I.M., Varis, K., Ihamäki, T. *et al.* (1982) Relationships among serum pepsinogen I, serum pepsinogen II, and gastric mucosal histology. *Gastroenterology*, **83**, 204–209.

83. Sipponen, P. (1981) Intestinal metaplasia and gastric carcinoma. *Annals of Clinical Research*, **13**, 139–143.

84. Sipponen, P., Seppälä, K., Äärynen, M., Helske, T. and Kettunen, P. (1989) Chronic gastritis and gastroduodenal ulcer: a case control study on risk of coexisting duodenal or gastric ulcer in patients with gastritis. *Gut*, **30**, 922–929.

85. Sipponen, P., Varis, K., Fräki, O., Korri, U.M., Seppälä, K. and Siurala, M. (1990) Cumulative 10-year risk of symptomatic duodenal and gastric ulcer in patients with or without chronic gastritis.

A clinical follow-up study of 454 outpatients. *Scandinavian Journal of Gastroenterology*, **25**, 966–973.

86. Siurala, M., Varis, K. and Wiljasalo, M. (1966) Studies of patients with atrophic gastritis: a 10–15 year follow-up. *Scandinavian Journal of Gastroenterology*, **1**, 40–48.

87. Siurala, M., Varis, K. and Kekki, M. (1980) New aspects on epidemiology, genetics, and dynamics of chronic gastritis. *Front Gastrointestinal Research*, **6**, 148–166.

88. Stefaniwsky, A.B., Tint, G.S., Speck, J. and Salen, G. (1982) Ursodeoxycholic acid (UDCA) reduces pain, nausea and vomiting in patients with bile acid reflux gastritis (abstract). *Gastroenterology*, **82**, 1188.

89. Stockbrügger, R.W., Menon, G.G., Beilby, J.O.W. *et al.* (1983) Gastroscopic screening in 80 patients with pernicious anaemia. *Gut*, **24**, 1141.

90. Stolte, M. and Heilmann, K.L. (1989) Neue Klassifikation und Graduierung der Gastritis. *Leber, Magen, Darm* (Baden-Baden), **19**, 220–226.

91. Strickland, R.G. and Mackay, I.R. (1973) A reappraisal of the nature and significance of chronic atropic gastritis. *American Journal of Digestive Diseases*, **18**, 426–440.

92. Strickland, R.G. (1975) Gastritis. In *Frontiers of Gastrointestinal Research* (Ed.) Van der Reis, L. pp. 12–48. Basel: Karger.

93. Svensson, J.O., Gelin, J. and Svanvik, J. (1986) Gallstones, cholecystectomy and duodenogastric reflux of bile acid. *Scandinavian Journal of Gastroenterology*, **21**, 181–187.

94. Tytgat, G.N.J. (1991) Endoscopic appearances in gastritis/duodenitis. *Journal of Gastroenterology and Hepatology*, **61**, 223–224.

95. Tytgat, G.N.J., Axon, A.T.R., Dixon, M.F., Graham, D.Y., Lee, A. and Marshall, B.J. (1990) *Helicobacter pylori*: Causal agent in peptic ulcer disease. In *Working Party Reports World Congresses of Gastroenterology*, pp. 36–45. Sydney: Blackwell Scientific.

96. Villako, K., Kekki, M., Tamm, A. *et al.* (1982) Epidemiology and dynamics of gastritis in a representative sample of an Estonian urban population. *Scandinavian Journal of Gastroenterology*, **17**, 601–607.

97. Whitehead, R. (1979) Mucosal biopsy of the gastrointestinal tract. In *Major Problems in Pathology*, vol. 3 (Ed.) Bennington, J.L. pp. 36–50. Philadelphia: W.B. Saunders.

98. Whitehead, R., Truelove, S.C. and Gear, M.W. (1972) The histologic diagnosis of chronic gastritis in fibroeptic gastroscope biopsy specimens. *Journal of Clinical Pathology*, **25**, 1–11.

99. Whittingham, S., Youngchaiyud, U., Mackay, I.R. *et al.* (1975) Thyrogastric autoimmune disease: Studies on the cell-mediated immune system and histocompatibility antigens. *Clinical Explanatory Immunology*, **19**, 289–299.

100. Wiersinga, W.M. and Tytgat, G.N.J. (1977) Clinical recovery owing to target parietal cell failure in a patient with Zollinger–Ellison syndrome. *Gastroenterology*, **73**, 1413–1417.

101. Winawer, S.J. and Lipkin, M. (1969) Cell proliferation kinetics in the gastrointestinal tract of man. IV. Cell renewal in the intestinalized gastric mucosa. *Journal of the National Cancer Institute*, **42**, 9–17.

102. Wolber, R., Owen, D., DelBuono, L. *et al.* (1990) Lymphocytic gastritis in patients with celiac sprue or spruelike intestinal disease. *Gastroenterology*, **98**, 310–315.

103. Wyatt, J.I. and Dixon, M.F. (1988) Chronic gastritis – a pathogenetic approach. *Journal of Pathology*, **154**, 113–124.

104. Yardley, J.H. and Paull, G. (1988) *Campylobacter pylori*: A new recognized infectious agent in the gastrointestinal tract. *American Journal of Surgical Pathology*, **12**(suppl. 1), 89–99.

DUODENITIS

G.N.J. Tytgat

Duodenitis is defined as an inflammatory condition of the proximal duodenum, usually with maximal involvement of the bulb, and often but not invariably associated with dyspeptic symptoms occurring in the absence of a chronic duodenal ulcer. The clinical importance of duodenal inflammation in the absence of chronic ulceration remains unclear. The entity previously called non-specific chronic duodenitis in particular remains controversial, and so is the relationship to duodenal ulcer.[18] In all probability, *H. pylori* infection is a major cause of chronic duodenitis.

AETIOLOGY

Most commonly, duodenitis is caused by *Helicobacter pylori* infection,[34] and by the exposure of the proximal duodenum to the potentially damaging effects of gastric acid and pepsin. Inflammatory changes are also known to be present in the mucosa surrounding peptic ulcers in the duodenum. The changes found in the proximal duodenum of patients with severe dyspepsia in the absence of frank duodenal ulceration are similar. These changes may therefore represent a stage in the development or regression of chronic duodenal ulceration.

Duodenal inflammation may also occur in specific conditions such as tuberculosis, Crohn's disease, coeliac disease, septicaemia, giardiasis and ankylostomiasis.[3,10] Inflammation has also been associated with duodenal diverticulosis, fistula, brünneroma, biliary, hepatic and pancreatic disease and chronic renal failure.

CLINICAL FEATURES

It is common to encounter patients with symptoms suggestive of peptic ulceration in whom no definite ulcer is revealed.[5] Symptoms are usually non-specific, but may have the periodicity and chronicity seen in patients with duodenal ulceration (ulcer-like dyspepsia). Epigastric bloating is common. Smoking, alcohol and spices often aggravate the pain and antacids sometimes, but not invariably, relieve it. Clinical examination is usually unremarkable.

INVESTIGATIONS

ENDOSCOPY

Endoscopy is routinely required to diagnose duodenitis and to exclude the presence of a duodenal ulcer.[2,4,12,15,21,30,31]

NORMAL APPEARANCE OF THE DUODENAL BULB

The normal duodenal bulb is pear-shaped and shows a uniform smooth lining of even colour and lustre. Upon close inspection, minute unevenness may be appreciated owing to the presence of villi, which give a velvety appearance to the mucosa.

Not uncommonly, islands of heterotropic gastric mucosa may be present, seen as small raised foci with a more opalescent or frosted appearance.

CLASSIFICATION OF ENDOSCOPIC APPEARANCES OF BULBAR INFLAMMATION[29]

Endoscopic erythematous/exudative/duodenitis

This is the most common endoscopic inflammatory condition in the bulb. The main abnormality is patchy erythema,[31] often combined with loss of lustre and occasionally with a few punctate spots of

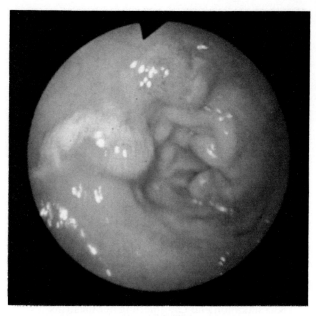

Figure 2.46   Endoscopic erosive duodenitis.

exudate. There may be mild friability. This form of duodenitis may be mild, moderate or severe.[17] Signs of prior ulcer disease may be seen as linear or circular scars.

Endoscopic erosive bulbitis/duodenitis

This is diagnosed when the dominant abnormality is of multiple erosions, often covered with whitish–yellow–greyish exudate (*Figure 2.46*). Erosions may be present in crops, coalesce and spread over large parts of the bulb. There always is evidence of concomitant erythema, friability and variable degrees of oedema, sometimes causing luminal narrowing.

Endoscopic haemorrhagic duodenitis

This is diagnosed when there is evidence of punctate or ecchymotic bleeding, in addition to the usual characteristics of inflammation.

Endoscopic nodular duodenitis

This is considered as a separate entity because it is nearly always seen in patients with renal insufficiency or on chronic dialysis. The dominant abnormality is diffuse nodularity of the bulb. The mucosa may be strikingly erythematous and covered with small erosions and punctate or confluent exudate[35] (*Figure 2.47*).

Duodenogastric reflux may be found in the presence of duodenitis, especially in those patients with

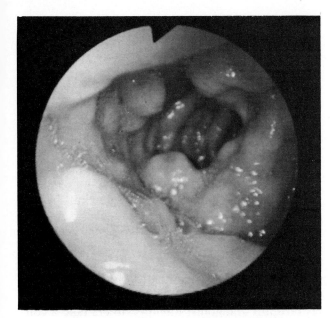

Figure 2.47 Endoscopic nodular duodenitis.

atrophic gastritis and duodenal ulcers.[20] Not infrequently, a concomitant duodenal ulcer with a wide surrounding area of inflammation is observed.

Endoscopic assessment alone is inadequate for diagnosing and grading the severity of duodenitis; multiple target biopsies are required for histological examinations.[9] Endoscopic trauma must be avoided.

HISTOLOGY

There is a wide range of appearances of the duodenal mucosa which may be found in asymptomatic individuals. Kreuning *et al.*[21,22] reported the histological and immunohistochemical changes found in 50 healthy volunteers. This study revealed abnormalities in 64% of individuals, with chronic inflammation in 12%. Changes ranged from an increase in the cellularity of the lamina propria, through variations in the size and shape of the villi, and gastric metaplasia with exclusion of Brünner's glands above the muscularis mucosae. Several studies have correlated endoscopic appearances, histological changes and clinical symptoms. Neutrophil infiltration, indicating active duodenitis, and increased round cell infiltration, indicating chronic duodenitis, are regularly found in symptomatic patients. Villous atrophy and gastric metaplasia are common. There seems to be a good correlation between more severe endoscopic duodenitis and histological duodenitis. On the contrary, in patients with mild duodenitis there is poor correlation between the endoscopic appearances and histology.[18]

Whitehead[32] defined grades of duodenitis using inflammatory cell infiltration together with villous and surface epithelial changes, distinguishing mild, moderate and severe categories with separate consideration of polymorph infiltration.

According to Jenkins *et al.*,[16] mild duodenitis exhibits increased numbers of plasma cells and oedema, and usually some polymorph response and increased gastric metaplasia. Severe duodenitis shows a large number of intraepithelial and lamina propria polymorphs but decreased plasma cells, together with severe villous atrophy. Gastric metaplasia is common in duodenitis. Gastric metaplasia presumably represents a non-specific response to continued injury and healing. Excessive acidity is a possible cause of injury in the proximal duodenum.[33] Although gastric metaplasia can be found in otherwise normal duodenal mucosa,[21,22,34] its relationship, in particular to active duodenitis, is well established. It seems likely that the polymorph response is directed towards *H. pylori* on the metaplastic epithelium.[19,33] In severe duodenitis, either alone or associated with duodenal ulceration, mucosal cell proliferation is increased.[1]

RADIOLOGY

As the inflammatory changes almost exclusively affect the mucosa, radiological features are not diagnostic. An irritable duodenal bulb with rapid emptying, and/or a comb or star appearance due to mucosal thickening, have been described.[27] Other features may include the presence of erosions or small superficial ulcers in the duodenal bulb. These changes are only found in advanced disease.[23] Chronic pancreatitis or carcinoma, or an adjacent ulcer, may also be associated with such changes. Comparison of conventional barium meal with endoscopy shows that the barium meal may be normal in half the patients diagnosed with duodenitis by endoscopy.

ROLE OF THE *H. PYLORI* IN THE AETIOLOGY OF CHRONIC DUODENITIS

The role of *H. pylori* in the aetiology of chronic duodenitis has been more difficult to establish than in gastritis. The presence of gastric metaplasia would allow *H. pylori* colonization to occur in the duodenum. Johnston *et al.*[19] found that *H. pylori* could be seen in areas of gastric metaplasia, in the duodenum of virtually all patients with duodenitis, but not in those with normal findings or inactive inflammation. Also, Wyatt et al.[33] studied the gastric and duodenal histology in a large group of dyspeptics. Those with active duodenitis had both H. pylori in the gastric antrum and significant metaplasia in the duodenum. It would appear therefore that active chronic duodenitis might result from spread of H. pylori infection from the antrum to areas of gastric metaplasia in the proximal duodenum, and that dyspeptic symptoms may be linked to the presence of active duodenitis.

DYSPEPSIA, DUODENITIS AND DUODENAL ULCERATION

Opinion is divided as to whether duodenitis on its own can cause dyspeptic symptoms.[11,30] The number of individuals with solitary duodenitis in the absence of gastritis is small. Usually duodenitis is linked to antral gastritis. Kreuning et al.[22] found that 83% of patients with ulcer-like dyspepsia had duodenitis, which the authors considered to be part of the duodenal ulcer spectrum. Whether the presence of a neutrophilic component is causal in the generation of dyspeptic symptoms, as suggested by some investigators, needs further evaluation. Dyspepsia is a common symptom and peptic ulceration, gastroduodenitis and functional dyspepsia can all present in a similar manner.[7] In addition to gastric and duodenal ulceration, reflux oesophagitis and pancreaticobiliary disorders, including cholelithiasis, may be responsible for dyspeptic symptoms. Duodenitis with gastric metaplasia is frequently found in patients with alcohol-associated chronic pancreatitis.[26]

The pathological sequence of hyperchlorhydria, duodenitis and duodenal ulcer was proposed long ago.[28] Many investigators consider that non-erosive and erosive duodenitis as well as duodenal ulcer represent a different response to the same peptic process. The majority of patients with duodenitis display a spectrum of endoscopic appearances reflecting different stages of activity of the inflammatory process and usually develop duodenal ulcers sooner or later. Erosive duodenitis with or without a duodenal ulcer is associated with increased gastric acid secretion. Thomson et al.[30] found that half of their patients presenting with endoscopic and symptomatic duodenitis subsequently developed duodenal ulcers and underwent surgery.

Not all investigators agree with this hypothesis;[2] some feel that, on the basis of acid secretory data and basal gastrin levels, duodenitis may not be a variant of duodenal ulcer disease.[8]

On balance, the majority would feel at present that duodenitis is part of the duodenal ulcer spectrum, rather than being a separate entity.

There is indeed a close association between chronic duodenitis with activity and the subsequent development of an ulcer crater.[14] Gastric metaplasia is a consistent histological finding in duodenitis, with patches of gastric-type mucous cells interspersed between the absorptive and goblet cells. Metaplasia probably results from a modulation of cellular differentiation from stem cells under the influence of altered environmental factors. Infection by H. pylori is restricted to gastric-type cells.[34] A close interrelation between gastric metaplasia/chronic duodenitis with activity and H. pylori-positive gastritis has been established.[33,34] Because many patients with erosive and non-erosive duodenitis do not have hyperchlorhydria and do not respond to the H_2 receptor antagonist therapy, others take a contrary view and feel that some patients suffer from autonomous erosive duodenitis where gastric acidity plays only a minor pathogenic role.[13]

TREATMENT

Chronic duodenitis is difficult to treat as the underlying aetiological factors remain unknown. When there is a specific factor causing the inflammation, this primary cause must be treated. Cessation of smoking, avoidance of salicylates and non-steroidal anti-inflammatory drugs, and abstinence from alcohol are usually recommended. Anticholinergics, antispasmodics and sedatives have a minor role to play in therapy. During an acute exacerbation of pain, use of antacids or an H_2 receptor antagonist is generally advised.

H_2 receptor antagonist therapy, besides healing the chronic duodenal ulcers, may improve symptoms and endoscopic duodenitis.[5] A double-blind study on dyspeptic patients with endoscopically proven duodenitis, but without chronic ulceration, revealed that cimetidine for 6 weeks caused a significant improvement in symptoms and in the endoscopic appearance when compared with the placebo group; however, was not associated with any change in the histological grading of the duodenitis.[24] The newer H_2 receptor antagonists will have a similar beneficial effect.

Pirenzepine therapy produces healing of endoscopically diagnosed gastroduodenitis with improvement in clinical symptomatology without side effects.[25] Insufficient information is available as yet with respect to the efficacy of anti-H. pylori therapy in duodenitis; however, based upon empirical experience, some patients with long-standing, rather severe dyspepsia do improve after successful eradication of the organism, with healing of the endoscopic and histological duodenitis. Information relating to the effect of vagotomy in duodenitis is fragmentary, and the wisdom of operative intervention is questionable.

REFERENCES

1. Branson, C.J., Boxer, M.E., Palmer, K.P. *et al.* (1981) Mucosal cell proliferation in duodenal ulcer and duodenitis. *Gut*, **22**, 277–282.
2. Classen, M., Koch, H. and Demling, L. (1970) Duodenitis: significance and frequency. In *Inflammation in Gut* (Ed.) Maratka, Z. and Ottenjann, R. *Bibliotheca Gastroenterologica*, Vol. 9. pp. 48–49. Basel: Karger.
3. Corachan, M., Oomen, H.A. and Sutorius, F.J. (1981) Parasitic duodenitis. *Transactions of the Royal Society of Tropical Medicine and Hygiene*, **75**, 385–389.
4. Cotton, P.B., Price, A.B., Tighe, J.R. and Beales, J.S.M. (1973) Preliminary evaluation of 'duodenitis' by endoscopy and biopsy. *British Medical Journal*, **3**, 430–433.
5. Danielsson, A., Ek, B., Nyhilin, H. and Steen, L. (1983) The relationship between active peptic ulcer, endoscopic duodenitis and symptomatic state after treatment with cimetidine. *Annals of Clinical Research*, **12**, 4–12.
6. DeLuca, V.A. (1989) No acid, polys, no 'active' gastritis, no dyspepsia – a proposal. *Journal of Clinical Gastroenterology*, **11**, 127–131.
7. DeLuca, V.A., Winnan, G.G., Sheahan, D.G. *et al.* (1981) Is gastroduodenitis part of the spectrum of peptic ulcer disease? *Journal of Clinical Gastroenterology*, **3**, 17–22.
8. Donovan, I.A., Green, G., Dykes, P.W. *et al.* (1975) The pathophysiology of duodenitis (abstract). *Gut*, **16**, 395.
9. Forrester, A.W., Joffe, S.N. and Lee, F.D. (1979) The endoscopic and histological features of peptic duodenitis. *Scandinavian Journal of Gastroenterology*, **14**(suppl.), 18–22.
10. Frandsen, P.J., Jarnum, S. and Malmstrum, J. (1980) Crohn's disease of the duodenum. *Scandinavian Journal of Gastroenterology*, **15**, 633–638.
11. Greenlaw, R., Sheahan, D.G., DeLuca, V., Miller, D., Myerson, D. and Myerson, P. (1988) Gastroduodenitis, a broader concept of peptic ulcer disease. *Digestive Diseases and Sciences*, **25**, 660–672.
12. Gregg, J.A. and Garabedian, M. (1974) Duodenitis. *American Journal of Gastroenterology*, **61**, 177–184.
13. Guslandi, M. (1985) Duodenitis. *The Lancet*, **2**, 1437.
14. Hasan, M., Ferguson, A. and Sircus, W. (1981) Duodenal mucosal architecture in non-specific and ulcer-associated duodenitis. *Gut*, **22**, 637–641.
15. Hirschowitz, B.J. (1962) Gastroduodenal endoscopy with the fibrescope. In *Current Gastroenterology* (Ed.) MacHardy, P. p. 158. New York: Harper & Row.
16. Jenkins, D., Goodall, A., Gillet, F.R. and Scott, B.B. (1985) Defining duodenitis: Quantitative histological study of mucosal responses and their correlations. *Journal of Clinical Pathology*, **38**, 1119–1126.
17. Joffe, S.N. (1982) Relevance of duodenitis to non-ulcer dyspepsia and peptic ulcerations. *Scandinavian Journal of Gastroenterology*, **17**(suppl. 79), 80–97.
18. Joffe, S.N., Lee, F.D. and Blumgart, L.H. (1978) Duodenitis. *Clinics in Gastroenterology*, **7**, 635–650.
19. Johnston, B.J., Reed, P.I. and Ali, M.A. (1986) Campylobacter-like organisms in duodenal and antral endoscopic biopsies: relationship to inflammation. *Gut*, **27**, 1132–1137.
20. Koelsch, K.A., Herms, G. and Kuhne, C. (1981) Duodenogastric-reflux-favouring behaviour of the pylorus in patients with gastritis and duodenitis. *Deutsche Zeitschrift für Verdauungs- und Stoffwechselkrankheiten*, **41**, 18–20.
21. Kreuning, J., Bosman, F.T., Kuiper, G. *et al.* (1978) Gastric and duodenal mucosa in 'healthy' individuals. *Journal of Clinical Pathology*, **31**, 69–77.
22. Kreuning, J., Wal vd, A.M., Kuiper, G. and Lindeman, J. (1989) Chronic non-specific duodenitis – a multiple biopsy study of the duodenal bulb in health and disease. *Scandinavian Journal of Gastroenterology*, **24**(suppl. 67), 16–20.
23. Kunstlinger, F.C., Theoni, R.F., Grendell, J.F. *et al.* (1980) The radiographic appearance of erosive duodenitis. *Journal of Clinical Gastroenterology*, **2**, 205–211.
24. MacKinnon, M., Willing, R.L. and Whitehead, R. (1982) Cimetidine in the management of symptomatic patients with duodenitis: a double-blind controlled trial. *Digestive Diseases and Sciences*, **27**, 217–219.
25. Morelli, A., Narducci, F., Pelli, M.A. and Spadacini, A. (1979) A double-blind short-term clinical trial of pirenzepine in duodenal ulcer. *Scandinavian Journal of Gastroenterology*, **14**(suppl.), 45–49.
26. Piubello, W., Vantini, I., Souro, L.A. *et al.* (1982) Gastric secretion, gastroduodenal histological changes and serum gastrin in chronic alcoholic pancreatitis. *American Journal of Gastroenterology*, **77**, 105–110.
27. Rhodes, J., Evans, K.T., Lawrie, J.H. and Forrest, A.P.M. (1968) Coarse mucosal folds in the duodenum. *Quarterly Journal of Medicine*, **37**, 151–169.
28. Rivers, A.B. (1931) Clinical study of gastritis and gastro-jejunitis. *Annals of Internal Medicine*, **4**, 1265–1281.

29. Sircus, W. (1985) Duodenitis: a clinical, endoscopic and histopathological study. *Quarterly Journal of Medicine*, **56**, 593–600.
30. Thomson, W.O., Joffe, S.N., Robertson, A.G., Lee, F.D., Imric, C.W. and Blumgart, L.H. (1977) Is duodenitis a dyspeptic myth? *The Lancet*, **i**, 1197–1198.
31. Venables, C.W. (1985) Duodenitis. *Scandinavian Journal of Gastroenterology*, **20**(suppl. 109), 91–97.
32. Whitehead, R. (1982) Morphologic aspects of duodenitis. *Scandinavian Journal of Gastroenterology*, **17**(suppl. 79), 80–83.
33. Wyatt, J.I., Rathbone, B.J., Dixon, M.F. and Heatley, R.V. (1987) *Campylobacter pyloridis* and

34. acid-induced metaplasia in the pathogenesis of duodenitis. *Journal of Clinical Pathology*, **40**, 841–848.
34. Wyatt, J.I., Rathbone, B.J., Sobala, G. *et al.* (1990) Gastric epithelium in the duodenum: its association with *Helicobacter pylori* and inflammation. *Journal of Clinical Pathology*, **43**, 981–986.
35. Zukerman, G.R., Mills, B.A., Koehler, R.E., Siegel, A., Harter, H.R. and De Schrijver-Kecskemeti, K. (1983) Nodular duodenitis. Pathologic and clinical characteristic in patients with end-stage renal disease. *Digestive Diseases and Sciences*, **28**, 1018–1024.

CHRONIC PEPTIC ULCER

EPIDEMIOLOGY AND AETIOLOGY

(J. Calam and S.F. Moss)

Chronic duodenal and gastric ulcers are epithelial breaches associated with both acute and chronic inflammatory responses. They are best considered as separate diseases and both are the common end results of several different processes. The isolation of *Helicobacter pylori* and emerging evidence for its role in duodenal ulceration has greatly increased interest in duodenal and gastric ulcer diseases. The epidemiology of duodenal and gastric ulcers is first considered, then their aetiology, and finally why some patients develop duodenal ulcers whereas others develop gastric ulcers.

EPIDEMIOLOGY

Epidemiological data can usefully help direct more precise approaches to the understanding of aetiology. The absolute numbers obtained depend on the diagnostic criteria which are applied to the population of interest. In addition, few studies discriminate between acute and chronic ulceration. Usually it is the trends and differences observed which are of the most interest. They presumably reflect a host of environmental factors, including ingested or inhaled substances as well as hygiene and bacteriology and, perhaps, psychological factors.

Prevalence

Prevalence is the proportion of the population affected at any one time. A Finnish endoscopic survey found that 1.4% of the population had an active duodenal ulcer and 0.3% a gastric ulcer.[27] The lifetime prevalence of duodenal ulcer is probably about 10% in males and 4% in females, and the prevalence of gastric ulcer 4 and 3%, respectively.[25,35,76]

Incidence

Incidence is the number of new cases per year. The figure for duodenal ulcer is about 0.15% in males and 0.03% in females.[5] Corresponding figures for gastric ulcer are 0.02% for each sex.[4]

Geographical differences

In most parts of the world duodenal ulcers are about three times as common as gastric ulcers whereas in some areas gastric ulcers are more common. These include Japan, Sri Lanka, The Andes, Turkey and some islands off northern Norway. In the UK, duodenal ulcer but not gastric ulcer is more common in the North[35] and in an urban environment.[53] The available evidence suggests that these differences reflect environmental and socioeconomic rather than racial differences.

Sex

Gastric ulcer shows an approximately equal sex incidence, or a slight male preponderance. According to different surveys duodenal ulcer disease is 1.5–3 times more common in males than females.[4,5,25,53]

Age

The incidence of duodenal and gastric ulcers appears to increase progressively with age and peaks at about 60 years. The prevalence of gastric ulcers is particularly low before the age of 40 years.

Changes with time

Changes in apparent incidence may be due to differences in diagnostic methods over the years but some comparable data is available from rates of perforation or death from peptic ulcer disease. The survey by William Brinton from the late 19th century indicates that gastric ulcer was then a disease of young women and was considerably more prevalent than duodenal ulcer.[7] From the turn of the century until about 1960 the duodenal ulcer prevalence rose to become several times more common than gastric ulcer, and gastric ulceration was predominantly a disease of the elderly. The incidence of duodenal ulcer appears to have stopped rising or may have even declined since about 1960.[35] Susser and Stein suggested that the depression of the 1930s put a cohort of individuals at risk of duodenal ulcer[65] and as colonization with *H. pylori* is strongly associated with social deprivation it is tempting to propose that this bacterium might have been responsible.

Socioeconomic group

Currently, duodenal ulcers are more prevalent in those of lower social status though 50 years ago they were less common in the poor. This difference may be partially explained by the change in smoking habits. Gastric ulcers remain more prevalent in social classes IV and V.

Epidemiological studies have enabled specific risk factors within populations to be identified.

Risk factors

Diet
It is important to distinguish between the foods, beverages and spices which cause dyspepsia and those which affect duodenal ulcer disease. It has been suggested that a rice-based diet is responsible for the higher incidence of duodenal ulcer in southern India compared with the north, where unrefined wheat is eaten.[44] Individuals from the south had a 5-year recurrence rate of 14% when their diet changed to wheat in the form of chapattis, compared with 84% when they remained on rice. A study from Norway also showed diminished recurrence of duodenal ulcer on a high-fibre diet.[60]

Coffee, even de[caffeinated?] acid secretion and can[ ] appear to predispose t[ ] Male college students wh[ ] developed less duodenal u[lcer] drinking counterparts,[50] bu[t] bland diets remains uncertain.[ ] causes acute mucosal damage,[ ] to be an important cause of[ ] ulcers.[20] In one survey, moder[ate consumptio]n of alcohol appeared to protect, perha[ps b]y inducing adaptive cytoprotection.[63] Both cirrhosis and chronic pancreatitis predispose to duodenal ulcer disease, perhaps by diminishing the secretion of alkali into the duodenum.

Drugs
Aspirin and other non-steroidal anti-inflammatory drugs (NSAIDS) cause acute damage to the gastroduodenal mucosa and ingestion of NSAIDS is associated with a greater incidence of hospital admissions with bleeding or perforation.[12,36,62,74] Corticosteroid drugs appear to increase the incidence of peptic ulcers but only at doses equivalent to 20 mg of prednisolone per day or more.[13]

Cigarette smoking
Epidemiological studies show that smoking increases the risk of duodenal ulcer disease in a dose-dependent manner independent of socioeconomic group.[20,40] The results of controlled trials also indicate that cigarette smoking impairs ulcer healing and increases the risk of recurrence.[40]

Helicobacter pylori
About 90% of duodenal ulcer and about 70% of gastric ulcer patients have gastric colonization with *H. pylori*, compared with about 40 and 50% of matched controls (see below).[17]

AETIOLOGY

Duodenal ulcer

Duodenal ulcer disease used to be perceived to be the common end-result of a number of abnormalities of gastroduodenal physiology such as excessive acid secretion, rapid gastric emptying and diminished duodenal prostaglandin synthesis. Now there is strong evidence that recurrences of duodenal ulcer disease are caused by *H. pylori*. This and the discovery that *H. pylori* increases gastrin release illustrates the need for an integrated approach in which the bacteriological, physiological, immunological and histological changes are considered together.

...at duodenal ulcer disease is inherited ...ted initially from studies showing familial ...ggregation and, more recently, from the discovery that certain associated abnormalities, such as a raised serum pepsinogen I level, ran in ulcer-predisposed families.[59] These findings may eventually prove to be due to intrafamilial spread of *H. pylori*, which is now known to cause both ulcers and hyperpepsinogenaemia I. However, the concordance of peptic ulcer is higher in monozygotic than dizygotic twins,[57] suggesting that genetic factors are involved. It may well be that genetic factors determine whether *H. pylori* colonization causes duodenal ulcer disease or not. Despite extensive investigation associations of duodenal ulcer disease with blood group O non-secretors and HLA antigens have not been found consistently.

Psychological aspects of duodenal ulcer disease

Folklore implicates 'stress' as a cause of peptic ulcer disease and some studies do provide evidence that duodenal ulcer disease is associated with psychological factors. Stress was presumably responsible for the increase in perforated duodenal ulcers during the Blitz of London.[64] Alexander believed that patients with duodenal ulcer have a subconscious conflict between a child-like desire to be dependent and the need to be an independent adult.[1] Such individuals display exaggerated self-sufficiency, driving ambition or aggression. These findings might operate through the known effects of psychological factors on the gastrointestinal and immune systems.

Helicobacter pylori

The existence of spiral organisms in the human stomach has been recognized since the last century. In 1983 Warren and Marshall first isolated *H. pylori* (previously *Campylobacter pyloridis*) from the human stomach.[75] This Gram-negative, flagellated, S-shaped or curved, microaerophilic organism has been found to colonize the gastric-type epithelia of humans and other primates, and is of increasing relevance in chronic peptic ulcer disease.[17]

PATHOGENETIC MECHANISMS RELATED TO *H. PYLORI*

It was rapidly established that *H. pylori* causes gastritis, and its pathogenic mechanisms are now gradually being unravelled. *H. pylori* lives in the juxtamucosal mucus layer, attached by specific adhesins to the gastric epithelial cell wall. It is capable of secreting a number of proteins capable of altering gastric pH, including the enzyme urease and a factor which inhibits acid secretion from parietal cells,[9] enabling it to colonize a normally highly acidic niche. It may also release a cytotoxin.[37]

Though it elicits a humoral and cell-mediated immune response, infection tends to persist; the reasons for this are unclear.

EVIDENCE THAT *H. PYLORI* IS AN IMPORTANT CAUSE OF DUODENAL ULCER DISEASE

There is now strong evidence that *H. pylori* causes relapse of duodenal ulcer disease. First, *H. pylori* is present in the stomach of 90% or more of patients with duodenal ulcer disease compared with a minority of matched controls.[17,45] Secondly, remission of duodenal ulcer disease is prolonged by regimes which eradicate *H. pylori*, to an extent which depends on the percentage of patients in whom *H. pylori* is eradicated. Finally, recurrence after eradication is rare, unless the patient becomes reinfected with *H. pylori*.[10,46,54]

To consider the aetiology of chronic duodenal ulcer disease it is now necessary to review the various abnormalities that have been described in this condition in relation to current knowledge of *H. pylori*. We will consider known abnormalities of the gastric fundus and body, the gastric antrum, the duodenum itself and of gastroduodenal motility, together with some observations whose basis is still insufficiently well defined to fit into this classification.

How important is a particular abnormality?

A general problem when considering abnormalities in duodenal ulcer disease is that the results of most measurements in patients overlap with the normal range. In this situation it is difficult to know whether the factor in question is highly important in a discrete minority of patients, or slightly important in most patients.

The gastric body and fundus in duodenal ulcer disease

MICROANATOMY

The gastric glands in these regions contain chief cells and parietal cells which secrete pepsin and acid, respectively. They are stimulated by acetylcholine, gastrin and histamine. In addition, there are endocrine cells, of which the most abundant are enterochromaffin-like cells. The isthmus of the gland contains mucous neck cells, which secrete mucus and pepsin, and the more superficial foveolus is lined with surface mucous cells which secrete bicarbonate as well as mucus. Towards the cardia, parietal and chief cells are replaced by mucous neck cells.

PATHOPHYSIOLOGY

Acid and pepsin

Patients with duodenal ulcer disease tend to secrete more acid and more pepsin than normal individuals.[3,31] Their increased secretion of acid and pepsin during maximal stimulation with pentagastrin or histamine probably reflects a greater mass of parietal and chief cells.[31] Three main theories have been put forward to explain the increased cell masses. First, there might be an increased trophic drive. For example, antral *H. pylori* infection increased the release of gastrin,[38] which has been shown to be trophic under experimental conditions and in the Zollinger–Ellison syndrome.[72] Also, peak acid output is greater in duodenal ulcer patients with *H. pylori* infection compared to those without.[38] However, although gastrin levels fall when *H. pylori* is eradicated,[23,39,41] maximally stimulated gastric secretion rates have not yet been shown to do so. Secondly, the expanded cell masses observed in duodenal ulcer disease might be due to an inherited trait. Rotter *et al.*[59] showed that plasma concentrations of group I pepsinogens correlate strongly with maximal acid output and that high levels run in ulcer-predisposed families, with more ulcers in individuals with elevated levels. However, these data may need to be reinterpreted because it has been found that serum group I pepsinogens diminish after eradication of *H. pylori*.[49] Thirdly duodenal ulcer patients may have more parietal and chief cells because they do not have a disease which destroys them. Fundal atrophy is indeed remarkably absent from patients with duodenal ulcer disease,[29] in contrast to the *H. pylori*-associated antral gastritis which is almost invariably present.[17]

Not only do duodenal ulcer patients have a greater mass of parietal and peptic cells but these cells are more strongly stimulated to secrete in these patients. Both basal and meal-stimulated rates of secretion tend to be greater, relative to their maximal acid secretory capacity, than in normal individuals.[3,18,30,31] This has been attributed to increased vagal stimulation of acid secretion under basal conditions[18] and increased postprandial gastrin release.[67] Also, some duodenal ulcer patients appear to have parietal cells which are more sensitive to gastrin[32,33] and a few have increased basal gastrin levels.[3] The discovery of *H. pylori* raises the possibility that this organism contributes to increased secretion by stimulating gastrin release.[38] It is also possible that *H. pylori*-related inflammation in the body of the stomach affects the physiology of parietal and peptic cells through increased concentrations of inflammatory mediators.[42,69]

Abnormalities of the gastric antrum in patients with duodenal ulcer disease

MICROANATOMY

The main cell type of the gastric antrum is a mucus-secreting cell similar to the mucous neck cell of the corpus. Antral glands also contain a few parietal cells. The most abundant endocrine cell type is the gastrin cell, which has microvilli extending into the lumen and is in intimate contact with and under the influence of adjacent somatostatin cells. Gastrin cells are innervated by nerve endings containing acetylcholine and gastrin-releasing peptide.

PATHOPHYSIOLOGY

Inflammation and *H. pylori* colonization of the gastric antrum is almost invariably present in patients with duodenal ulcer disease, and has been shown to be strongly associated with colonization with *H. pylori*.[17] *H. pylori* is present in about 90% of patients and its eradication leads to resolution of the inflammation.[55]

Walsh *et al.*[73] provided evidence that the normal inhibition of gastrin release by a low intragastric pH value is impaired in duodenal ulcer disease. Local release of somatostatin may be involved in this reflex.[6] The idea that defective inhibition might be due to alkalinization of the antral microenvironment by urease-derived ammonia[38] prompted studies which showed that *H. pylori* colonization is associated with increased basal and meal-stimulated gastrin release and that gastrin levels return to normal when *H. pylori* is eradicated.[23,39,41] Another possible explanation for these findings is that local inflammation might increase gastrin release. Leukocytes attracted to the antrum and activated by the presence of *H. pylori* would be expected to release a host of bioactive factors. In vitro, *H. pylori* increases the release of interleukins-1 and -6 and tumour necrosis factor by leukocytes and can itself secrete platelet-activating factor.[15,16,42] Interestingly, the related factors γ-interferon and interleukin-2 both release gastrin from the canine antrum.[69] A minority of duodenal ulcer patients have a greatly increased antral gastrin release which is familial and is associated with a high acid output and elevated serum pepsinogen I levels. In these patients the antrum was abnormally sensitive to a weak stimulant of gastrin release, possibly due to increased fasting duodenogastric reflux.[8,14,68]

Abnormalities of the duodenum in duodenal ulcer disease

MICROANATOMY

In the duodenum the majority of cells are absorptive epithelial cells, but mucus-secreting goblet cells are numerous. There are also scattered endocrine cells secreting gastrin, cholecystokinin and somatostatin. The base of the crypts contains undifferentiated and Paneth cells which secrete a variety of proteolytic enzymes as well as immunoglobulin A. Brunner's glands empty an alkaline, mucus-rich juice into the base of some of the crypts.

PATHOPHYSIOLOGY

Prostaglandins

In the duodenum, as in the stomach, prostaglandins protect the mucosa against the effects of acid and pepsin. They may do this partly by stimulating the secretion of bicarbonate into a mucus layer. The mucosal synthesis of both prostaglandins and bicarbonate has been shown to be diminished in duodenal ulcer disease.[26,28] NSAIDS, which decrease prostaglandin production, are more closely linked to gastric than duodenal ulceration (see below).

Gastric metaplasia

The duodenum of patients with duodenal ulcer disease contains areas of gastric epithelial metaplasia.[22,66] This is probably secondary to acid hypersecretion because it may be induced in experimental animals by chronic stimulation of gastric acid secretion.[22,66,79] It appears to be a non-specific response to injury. Gastric metaplasia is of particular interest because it allows *H. pylori*, which adheres only to gastric-type epithelium, to colonize the duodenum,[22] where it probably initiates local ulcerogenic mechanisms. How *H. pylori* in the duodenum causes ulcers there remains open to speculation. Some strains of *H. pylori* produce a toxin which produces vacuoles in cell culture lines.[37] Toxin-producing strains appear to be more prevalent in patients with duodenal ulcer disease than in patients with *H. pylori* but no ulcer.[19] It is also possible that *H. pylori*-related inflammation leads to local damage.

Gastroduodenal motility

Patients with duodenal ulcer disease tend to empty their stomachs more rapidly than normal individuals.[34,43,77] This might lead to a lower intraduodenal pH during emptying, but this has not yet been demonstrated.

Other causes of duodenal ulceration

Though the pathophysiological mechanisms above have been proposed to explain the vast majority of duodenal ulcers, there are a small number of well-defined syndromes which also produce duodenal ulcers. These include the Zollinger–Ellison syndrome associated with gastrin-secreting tumours, and parathormone-secreting tumours which may stimulate gastrin release and acid secretion by causing hypercalcaemia. Some patients have both parathyroid and pancreatic endocrine tumours as part of familial multiple endocrine neoplasia type I. In systemic mastocytosis, histamine is probably responsible for acid hypersecretion leading to duodenal ulceration. Duodenal ulcer disease is also associated with tremor and nystagmus in a rare

syndrome.[58] The association between duodenal ulcer and chronic lung diseases might be related to cigarette smoking. Associations between hepatic cirrhosis and chronic pancreatitis and duodenal ulcer disease might be due to diminished secretion of alkali into the duodenum. Duodenal ulceration in renal failure is probably due to a number of factors, which may include hypercalcaemia, diminished renal breakdown of gastrin and impaired removal of unidentified toxins. Finally, not all duodenal ulceration is due to the effects of acid and pepsin; it may rarely be caused by infections such as by herpes simplex, by ischaemia or by inflammatory conditions such as in Crohn's disease.

Gastric ulcer

Location

A high proportion of chronic gastric ulcers are located on the lesser curve, at or close to the junction between body and antral-type mucosa.[70] The mucosa of this junctional region appears more susceptible than either the body or the antrum.

Pathophysiology

ACID AND PEPSIN IN GASTRIC ULCER DISEASE

The secretion of acid and pepsin tends to be lower in patients with gastric ulcer disease then in matched normal individuals.[2,78] This probably reflects the loss of parietal and chief cells, due to atrophic gastritis, which is common in this condition.[21]

GASTRITIS IN GASTRIC ULCER DISEASE

Gastritis is almost invariably present in patients with gastric ulcer disease[21] and is probably due to *H. pylori* infection in about 60% of patients.[17] Treatment with bismuth chelate (De-Nol) and/or antibiotics may prolong remissions of gastric ulcer disease,[71] suggesting that *H. pylori* plays a role in ulcerogenesis, but evidence for this is scanty. The gastritis in gastric ulcer patients who are not infected with *H. pylori* is probably due to chemical injury from NSAIDS or duodenogastric reflux.[48]

Chronic ingestion of NSAIDS leads to gastric ulcers more often than duodenal ulcers.[24,62] They are believed to cause ulcers by inhibiting cyclooxygenase and thus the synthesis of prostaglandins.[56] Prostaglandins have many cytoprotective effects on the gastric mucosa, including the stimulation of secretion of mucus and bicarbonate, strengthening of intercellular tight junctions, stabilization of lysosomes, vasodilation and stimulation of epithelial growth.

Duodenogastric reflux is increased in patients with gastric ulcer disease. In an isotopic study it was present in 81% of patients compared with 42% of controls.[47] Bile salts can damage the gastric epithelium as well as the protective mucus layer. Reflux also exposes the gastric epithelium to pancreatic enzymes. The gastric epithelium, particularly in the antrum, secretes pancreatic secretory trypsin inhibitor, a potent inhibitor of trypsin and chymotrypsin which reflux from the duodenum. Gastric mucosal concentrations of pancreatic secretory trypsin inhibitor are diminished in gastric ulcer disease[51] but its secretion is increased by the prostaglandin E_1 analogue misoprostol.[52]

There is an increased proportion of damaged gastric mucus in gastric ulcer disease.[81] Damage could be due to H. pylori,[61] but trypsin can also degrade mucus unless sufficient pancreatic secretory trypsin inhibitor is present.[52] It has been suggested that gastric ulcers are due to ischaemia of the gastric epithelium. In support of this, ulcers are most commonly observed on the lesser curve, which appears to be supplied by end-arteries. However, no direct measurements of the local oxygen tensions have been made.

Conclusions

Current evidence points to the close involvement of H. pylori in the aetiology of chronic peptic disorders. There is a strong association between gastric H. pylori infection and both duodenal ulcer disease and chronic non-autoimmune (type B) gastritis. The association is much weaker for gastric ulcer and further research in this area is needed. Much of the earlier data now needs to be re-examined and the influence of H. pylori considered at all stages.

It is not known why H. pylori only causes gastritis in some individuals but ulcers in others. Clearly this could be due to differences in the 'seed' or 'soil'. In support of the former there is some evidence that different genomic sequences in H. pylori are associated with different diseases[80] and that duodenal ulcer disease is associated with strains which produce a vacuolating toxin.[19] Whether ulcers develop or not might also depend on whether the patient responds to H. pylori and other insults by developing changes such as atrophic gastritis, which diminishes acid secretion and is usually not present in patients with duodenal ulcer disease, and gastric metaplasia in the duodenum, which allows duodenal colonization with H. pylori and is typically present in these patients. Similarly, the development of gastric ulcer disease might reflect a different strain of H. pylori or the individual's susceptibility to a particular form of gastric damage. The individual's response may in turn be determined by as yet unidentified environmental factors, including eating habits and the age at which H. pylori is acquired, together with inherited factors, resulting in the observed geographical and temporal differences in peptic ulcer disease.

References

1. Alexander, F. (1950) *Psychosomatic Medicine*. New York: Norton.
2. Baron, J.H. (1978) *Clinical Tests of Gastric Secretion*. Oxford: Oxford University Press.
3. Blair, A.J. III, Feldman, M., Barnett, C. *et al.* (1987) Detailed comparison of basal and food-stimulated gastric acid secretion rates and serum gastrin concentrations in duodenal ulcer patients and normal subjects. *Journal of Clinical Investigation*, **79**, 582–587.
4. Bonnevie, O. (1975) The incidence of gastric ulcer in Copenhagen county. *Scandinavian Journal of Gastroenterology*, **10**, 231–239.
5. Bonnevie, O. (1975) The incidence of duodenal ulcer in Copenhagen county. *Scandinavian Journal of Gastroenterology*, **10**, 385–393.
6. Brand S.J. and Stone D. (1988) Reciprocal regulation of antral gastrin and somatostatin gene expression by omeprazole-induced achlorhydria. *Journal of Clinical Investigation*, **82**, 1059–1066.
7. Brinton W. (1867) *On the Pathology, Symptoms and Treatment of Ulcer of the Stomach*. London: Churchill.
8. Calam, J. and Tracy, H.J. (1980) Pyloric reflux and gastrin cell hyperfunction. *The Lancet*, **ii**, 918.
9. Cave, D.R. and Vargas, M. (1989) Effect of a *Campylobacter pylori* protein on acid secretion by parietal cells. *The Lancet*, **ii**, 187–189.
10. Coghlan, J.G., Gilligan, D., Humphreys, H., McKenna, D. *et al.* (1987) *Campylobacter pylori* and recurrence of duodenal ulcers – a 12 months follow-up study. *The Lancet*, **ii**, 1109–1111.
11. Cohen, S. and Booth, G.H. Jr (1975) Gastric acid secretion and lower-oesophageal-sphincter pressure in response to coffee and caffeine. *New England Journal of Medicine*, **293**, 897–899.
12. Collier, D.S. and Pain, J.A. (1985) Non-steroidal anti-inflammatory drugs and peptic ulcer perforation. *Gut*, **26**, 359–363.
13. Conn, H.D. and Blitzer, B.L. (1976) Non-association of adrenocorticosteroid therapy and peptic ulcer. *New England Journal of Medicine*, **294**, 473–479.
14. Cooper, R.G, Dockray, G.J., Calam, J. *et al.* (1985) Acid and gastrin responses during intragastric titration in normal subjects and duodenal ulcer patients with G-cell hyperfunction. *Gut*, **26**, 232–236.
15. Crabtree, J.E., Shallcross, T.M., Wyatt, J.I. *et al.* (1990) Tumour necrosis factor alpha secretion by *Helicobacter pylori* colonised gastric mucosa. *Gut*, **31**, A600–601.

16. Denizot, Y., Sobhani, I., Rambaud, J.-C. *et al.* (1990) Paf-acether synthesis by *Helicobacter pylori*. *Gut*, **31**, 1242–1245.

17. Dooley, C.P. and Cohen, H. (1988) The clinical significance of *Campylobacter pylori*. *Annals of Internal Medicine*, **108**, 70–79.

18. Feldman, M., Richardson, C.T. and Fordtran, J.S. (1980) Effect of sham feeding on gastric acid secretion in healthy subjects and duodenal ulcer patients. Evidence for increased vagal tone in some ulcer patients. *Gastroenterology*, **79**, 796–800.

19. Figura, N., Guglielmetti, P., Rossolini, A. *et al.* (1989) Cytotoxin production by *Campylobacter pylori* strains isolated from patients with peptic ulcers and from patients with gastritis only. *Journal of Clinical Microbiology*, **27**, 225–226.

20. Friedman, G.D., Siegelaab, A.B. and Seltzer, C.C. (1974) Cigarettes, alcohol, coffee and peptic ulcer. *New England Journal of Medicine*, **290**, 469–473.

21. Gear, M.W.L., Truelove, S.C. and Whitehead, R. (1971) Gastric ulcer and gastritis. *Gut*, **12**, 639–645.

22. Goodwin, C.S. (1988) Duodenal ulcer, *Campylobacter pylori*, and the 'leaking roof' concept. *The Lancet*, **ii**, 1467–1469.

23. Graham, D.Y., Opekun, A., Lew, G.M. *et al.* (1990) Ablation of exaggerated meal-stimulated gastrin release in duodenal ulcer patients after clearance of *Helicobacter (Campylobacter) pylori* infection. *American Journal of Gastroenterology*, **85**, 394–398.

24. Griffin, M.R., Ray, W.A. and Schaffner, W. (1988) Non-steroidal anti-inflammatory drug use and death from peptic ulcer in elderly persons. *Annals of Internal Medicine*, **109**, 359–363.

25. Grossman, M.I. (1980) Peptic ulcer: definition and epidemiology. In *The Genetics and Heterogeneity of Common Gastrointestinal Disorders* (Ed.) Rotter, J., Samloff, I.M. and Rimoin, D.L., pp. 21–30. New York: Academic Press.

26. Hawkey, C.J.. and Rampton, D.S. (1985) Prostaglandins and the gastrointestinal mucosa: are they important in its function disease or treatment? *Gastroenterology*, **89**, 1162–1188.

27. Ihamaki, T., Varis, K. and Siurala, M. (1979) Morphological, functional and immunological state of the gastric mucosa in gastric carcinoma families. Comparison with a computer-matched family sample. *Scandinavian Journal of Gastroenterology*, **14**, 801–812.

28. Isenberg, J.K., Selling, J.A., Hogan, D.L. *et al.* (1987) Impaired proximal duodenal mucosal bicarbonate secretion in patients with duodenal ulcer. *New England Journal of Medicine*, **361**, 374–379.

29. Kekki, M., Sipponen, P. and Siurula, M. (1984) Progression of antral and body gastritis in active and healed duodenal ulcer and duodenitis. *Scandinavian Journal of Gastroenterology*, **19**, 382–388.

30. Kirkpatrick, P.M. Jr and Hirschowitz, B.I. (1980) Duodenal ulcer with unexplained marked basal gastric acid hypersecretion. *Gastroenterology*, **79**, 4–10.

31. Lam, S.K. (1984) Pathogenesis and pathophysiology of duodenal ulcer. *Clinics in Gastroenterology*, **13**, 447–472.

32. Lam, S.K. and Koo, J. (1985) Gastrin sensitivity in duodenal ulcer. *Gut*, **26**, 485–490.

33. Lam, S.K., Isenberg, J.I., Grossman, M.I. *et al.* (1980) Gastric acid secretion is abnormally sensitive to exogenous gastrin released after peptone test meals in duodenal ulcer patients. *Journal of Clinical Investigation*, **65**, 555–562.

34. Lam, S.K., Isenberg, J.I., Grossman, M.I. *et al.* (1982) Rapid gastric emptying in duodenal ulcer patients. *Digestive Diseases and Sciences*, **27**, 598–604.

35. Langman, M.J.S. (1979) *The Epidemiology of Chronic Digestive Disease.* London: Arnold.

36. Langman, M.J.S. (1989) Epidemiological evidence on the association between peptic ulceration and anti-inflammatory drug use. *Gastroenterology*, **96**, 640–646.

37. Leunk, R.D., Johnson, P.T., David, B.C. *et al.* (1988) Cytotoxic activity in broth-culture filtrates of *Campylobacter pylori*. *Journal of Medical Microbiology*, **26**, 93–99.

38. Levi, S., Beardshall, K., Playford, R. *et al.* (1989) *Campylobacter pylori* and duodenal ulcers: the gastrin link. *The Lancet*, **i**, 1167–1168.

39. Levi, S., Beardshall, K., Swift, I. *et al.* (1989) Antral Campylobacter pylori, hypergastrinaemia, and duodenal ulcers: effect of eradicating the organism. *British Medical Journal*, **299**, 1504–1505.

40. McCarthy, D.M. (1984) Smoking and ulcers – time to quit. *New England Journal of Medicine*, **311**, 726–728.

41. McColl, K.E., Fullarton, G.M., ElNujumi, A.M. *et al.* (1989) Lowered gastrin and gastric acidity after eradication of *Campylobacter pylori* in duodenal ulcer. *The Lancet*, **ii**, 499–500.

42. Mai, U.E.H., Perez-Perez, G.I., Wahl, L.M. *et al.* (1990) Inflammatory and cytoprotective responses by human monocytes are induced by *Helicobacter pylori*: Possible role in the pathogenesis of type B gastritis (abstract). *Gastroenterology*, **98**, A662.

43. Malagelada, J.R., Longstreth, G.F., Deering, T.B. *et al.* (1977) Gastric secretion and emptying after ordinary meals in duodenal ulcer. *Gastroenterology*, **73**, 989–993.

44. Malhotra, S.L. (1978) A comparison of unrefined wheat and rice diets in the management of duodenal ulcer. *Postgraduate Medical Journal*, **54**, 6–9.

45. Marshall, B.J. and Warren, J.R. (1984) Unidentified curved bacilli in the stomach of patients with gastritis and peptic ulceration. *The Lancet*, **i**, 1311–1314.

46. Marshall, B.J., Goodwin, C.S., Warren, J.R. *et al.* (1988) Prospective double-blind trial of duodenal ulcer relapse after eradication of *Campylobacter pylori*. *The Lancet*, **ii**, 1439–1441.

47. Niemala, S., Heikkila, J. and Lehtola, J. (1984)

Duodenogastric bile reflux in patients with gastric ulcer. *Scandinavian Journal of Gastroenterology*, **19**, 896–898.

48. O'Connor, H.J., Dixon, M.F., Wyatt, J.I. *et al.* (1987) *Campylobacter pylori* and peptic ulcer disease. *The Lancet*, **ii**, 633–634.

49. Oderda, G., Vaira, D., Holton, J. *et al.* (1990) Combined amoxycillin and tinidazole for eradication of *Campylobacter pylori* associated gastritis in children. Effect of serum pepsinogen I, gastrin and IgG antibody titres (abstract). *Gut*, **30**, A733.

50. Paffenbarger, R.S. Jr, Wing, A.L. and Hyde, R.T. (1974) Chronic disease in former college students. XIII. Early precursors of peptic ulcer. *American Journal of Epidemiology*, **100**, 307–315.

51. Playford, R.J., Freeman, T.C., Quinn, C. *et al.* (1990) Diminished gastric mucosal pancreatic secretory trypsin inhibitor in chronic gastric ulcer and pernicious anaemia (abstract). *Gut*, **31**, A597–598.

52. Playford, R.J., Batten, J.J., Freeman, T.C. *et al.* (1991) Gastric output of pancreatic secretory trypsin inhibitor is increased by misoprostol. *Gut*, **32**, 1396–1400.

53. Pulvertaft, C.N. (1959) Peptic ulcer in town and country. *British Journal of Preventive and Social Medicine*, **13**, 131–138.

54. Rauws, E.A.J. and Tytgat, G.N.J. (1990) Cure of duodenal ulcer associated with eradication of *Helicobacter pylori*. *The Lancet*, **335**, 1233–1235.

55. Rauws, E.A.J., Langenberg, W., Houthoff, H.J. *et al.* (1988) *Campylobacter pylori* associated chronic active gastritis. A prospective study of its prevalence and the effects of antibacterial and antiulcer therapy. *Gastroenterology*, **94**, 33–40.

56. Redfern, J.S. and Feldman, M. (1989) Role of endogenous prostaglandins in preventing gastrointestinal ulceration: induction of ulcers by antibodies to prostaglandins. *Gastroenterology*, **96**, 595–605.

57. Rotter, J.I. (1980) The genetics of peptic ulcer: more than one gene, more than one disease. In *Progress in Medical Genetics*. Vol. 4, (Eds) Steinberg, A.G., Bearn, A.G., Motulsky, A.G. *et al.* pp. 1–58. Philadelphia: Saunders.

58. Rotter, J.I. (1983) Peptic ulcer. In *The Principles and Practice of Medical Genetics* (Eds) Emery, A.E.H. and Rimoin, D.L. pp. 863–879. New York: Churchill Livingstone.

59. Rotter, J.I., Sones, J.Q., Samloff, I.M. *et al.* (1979) Duodenal ulcer disease associated with elevated serum pepsinogen 1. An inherited autosomal dominant disorder. *New England Journal of Medicine*, **300**, 63–66.

60. Rydning, A., Berstad, A., Aadland, E. *et al.* (1982) Prophylactic effect of dietary fibre in duodenal ulcer disease. *The Lancet*, **ii**, 736–738.

61. Sidebotham, R.L. and Baron, J.H. (1990) Hypothesis: *Helicobacter pylori*, urease, mucus, and gastric ulcer. *The Lancet*, **335**, 193–195.

62. Sommerville, K., Faulkner, G., Langman, M. *et al.* (1986) Non-steroidal anti-inflammatory drugs and bleeding peptic ulcer. *The Lancet*, **i**, 462–466.

63. Sonnenberg, A., Muller-Lissner, S.A., Vogel, E. *et al.* (1981) Predictors of duodenal ulcer healing and relapse. *Gastroenterology*, **81**, 1061–1067.

64. Stewart, D.N. and Winser, D.M. (1942) Incidence of perforated peptic ulcer: effect of heavy air-raids. *The Lancet*, **i**, 259–261.

65. Susser, S. and Stein, Z. (1962) Civilisation and peptic ulcer. *The Lancet*, **i**, 115–118.

66. Tatsuta, M., Iishi, H., Yamamura, H. *et al.* (1989) Enhancement by tetragastrin of experimental induction of gastric epithelium in the duodenum. *Gut*, **30**, 311–315.

67. Taylor, I.L., Dockray, G.J., Calam, J. *et al.* (1979) Big and little gastrin responses to food in normal and ulcer subjects. *Gut*, **20**, 957–962.

68. Taylor, I.L., Calam, J., Rotter, J.I. *et al.* (1981) Family studies of hypergastrinaemic, hyperpepsinogenemic I duodenal ulcer disease. *Annals of Internal Medicine*, **95**, 421–425.

69. Teichmann, R.K., Grab, P.J., Hammer, C. *et al.* (1986) Gastrin release by interleukin-2 and gamma-interferon in vitro. *Canadian Journal of Physiology and Pharmacology*, **64**(suppl), 62.

70. Thomas, J., Greig, M., McIntosh, J. *et al.* (1980) The location of chronic gastric ulcer: A study of the relevance of ulcer size, age, sex, alcohol, analgesic intake and smoking. *Digestion*, **20**, 79–84.

71. Wagstaff, A.J., Benfield, P. and Monk, J.P. (1988) Colloidal bismuth subcitrate. A review of its pharmacodynamic and pharmacokinetic properties and its therapeutic use in peptic ulcer. *Drugs*, **36**, 132–157.

72. Walsh, J.H. (1987) Gastrointestinal Hormones. In *Physiology of the Gastrointestinal Tract*, 2nd edn. (Ed.) Johnson, L.R. pp. 181–254. New York: Raven Press.

73. Walsh, J.H., Richardson, C.T. and Fordtran, J.S. (1975) pH dependence of acid secretion and gastrin release in normal and ulcer subjects. *Journal of Clinical Investigation*, **55**, 462–468.

74. Walt, R., Katchinsky, B., Logan, R. *et al.* (1986) Rising frequency of ulcer perforation in elderly people in the United Kingdom. *The Lancet*, **i**, 489–492.

75. Warren, J.R. and Marshall, B. (1983) Unidentified curved bacilli on gastric epithelium in active chronic gastritis. *The Lancet*, **i**, 1273–1275.

76. Watkinson, G. (1960) The incidence of chronic peptic ulcer found at necropsy. *Gut*, **1**, 14–30.

77. Williams, N.S., Elashoff, J. and Meyer, J.H. (1986) Gastric emptying of liquids in normal subjects and patients with healed duodenal ulcer disease. *Digestive Diseases and Sciences*, **31**, 943–952.

78. Wormsley, K.G. and Grossman, M.I. (1965) Maximal histalog test in control subjects and patients with peptic ulcer. *Gut*, **6**, 427–431.

79. Wyatt, J.I., Rathbone, B.J., Dixon, M.F. *et al.* (1987) Campylobacter pyloridis and acid induced

gastric metaplasia in the pathogenesis of duodenitis. *Journal of Clinical Pathology*, **40**, 841–848.

80. Yoshimura, H.H., Evans, D.G. and Graham, D.Y. (1990) *H. pylori* strains from duodenal ulcer patients differ at the genomic level from those patients with simple gastritis (abstract). *Revista Espanola de Enfermadades Digestivas*, **78**(suppl.I), 6.

81. Younan, F., Pearson, J., Allen, A. *et al.* (1982) Changes in the structure of the mucous gel on the mucosal surface of the stomach in association with peptic ulcer disease. *Gastroenterology*, **82**, 827–831.

CHRONIC GASTRIC ULCER

CLINICAL FEATURES *(A.G. Morgan)*

Gastric ulceration is a disease of late middle age with a median age of between 50 and 60 years. Traditionally, men with gastric ulcers have outnumbered women (1.27:1) but some studies suggest that there is a female preponderance in the elderly.

Symptoms

There has been renewed interest in the symptoms of peptic ulcer disease, particularly as physical examination does not usually help the physician to arrive at the correct diagnosis. However, it should be stressed that there are many patients with gastric ulcers who have no symptoms. Indeed, the presence of dyspepsia does not correlate with the development of complications, particularly perforation and bleeding. An analysis of dyspeptic symptoms indicated that the clinical features of peptic ulcer disease as presented in many textbooks do not stand up to critical review.[41] The following description of the clinical features of gastric ulceration is therefore based principally on a paper published by Edwards and Coghill[26] in which they carefully recorded and analysed the symptoms of 84 patients with gastric ulcers.

Pain

Epigastric pain is the most common symptom (90%) and is often more severe than in duodenal ulcer disease. In about a third of patients there is radiation of the pain to the back. Many patients describe the pain as a nagging or cramp-like discomfort (33%). Acute pain (18%) or a hunger-like pain (13%) is less common. Dyspepsia is often cyclical, lasting usually 8 weeks (85%) with periods of freedom varying from 1 to 3 months. Pain may be precipitated or aggravated by food but this association was evident in only 24% of the patients, and in 12% the pain was unrelated to meals. Many patients (43%) are woken regularly from sleep by pain.

Additional symptoms

Many gastric ulcer patients complain of flatulence (65%), abdominal distension (55%), nausea (54%), belching (48%), loss of appetite (46%), acid regurgitation (43%), vomiting (38%) or waterbrash (33%). Approximately a quarter suffer from constipation (29%) or weight loss (24%).

Diagnosis from analysis of symptoms

Differential diagnosis includes non-ulcer dyspepsia, duodenal ulcer, gastric carcinoma, hiatal hernia and gallstone disease. The overlap in symptoms from these different conditions are considerable and many studies have concluded that it is not possible by analysis of the patient's symptoms alone to separate gastric from duodenal ulcer disease. Horrocks and de Dombal[41] described the clinical presentation of 360 patients with dyspepsia. These findings are summarized in *Table 2.2*. No single symptom provided a satisfactory separation for the purpose of diagnosis.

It would therefore be of great benefit if, by simple analysis of the patient's symptoms, patients with either ulcers or a cancer could be separated from those with non-ulcer dyspepsia. An attempt was made to place dyspeptic patients into risk groups.[19] Just over 1000 patients were studied and the results are shown in *Table 2.3*. It can be seen that it was impossible to separate gastric from duodenal ulcer, hence all medium- and high-risk patients must be investigated by endoscopy. Furthermore, this system of scoring symptoms remains too complicated to be used routinely in a hospital outpatient clinic or in general practice. Talley and others[85] found that a diagnosis of non-ulcer dyspepsia was much more likely than peptic ulcer disease if symptoms included mild upper abdominal pain which was not aggravated by food, an absence of night pain or vomiting or weight loss of 2 kg or more.

Physical signs

Physical examination is largely non-contributory. Epigastric tenderness may be evident. Anaemia may result from chronic blood loss. A succussion splash suggests gastric outlet obstruction.

INVESTIGATIONS *(A.G. Morgan)*

As a diagnosis based upon symptoms alone is unreliable, a definitive diagnosis can only be established

Table 2.2 Pattern of symptoms [a] in 360 patients with gastric and duodenal ulcer, gastric cancer and non-ulcer dyspepsia[41]

	Gastric ulcer	Duodenal ulcer	Gastric cancer	Non-ulcer dyspepsia
Age: proportion over 50 years	62	28	90	45
Sex ratio (male:female)	1:0.47	1:0.25	1:0.74	1:1.7
Pain				
Site: epigastric	66	86	54	52
Radiation to: shoulder	8	3	4	8
back	34	26	**10**	28
Pattern: continuous pain	12	8	**27**	6
episodic pain[b]	16	56	**0**	35
continuing attacks[c]	64	34	72	56
Relationship to food: immediate	20	**0**	18	14
delayed more than 20 minutes	45	50	31	**19**
not related	35	50	51	**7**
Eased by: antacids	36	39	**9**	26
food	2	**20**	1	4
Nocturnal	32	**70**	16	32
Proportion with symptoms for less than 1 year	50	18	**90**	34
Symptoms				
Anorexia	57	36	**90**	36
Weight loss (>3.2 kg in 1 month)	61	44	**82**	32
Dysphagia	5	4	**19**	8
Nausea	70	59	77	60
Vomiting	73	57	66	**34**

[a]Apart from the sex ratios, the figures are percentages.
[b]Episodic pain: pain that comes on for a few weeks, with periods of freedom for weeks or months.
[c]Continuing attacks: attacks of pain occurring for an hour or two at frequent intervals.

Table 2.3 Computer prediction compared with the final diagnosis in 1041 patients with dyspepsia

Final diagnosis	Computer prediction			
	Low risk	Medium risk	High risk	Total
Normal results	219	232	169	620
Hiatal hernia	47	40	42	129
Duodenal ulcer	25	134	38	197
Gastric ulcer	6	22	23	51
Gastric cancer	1	2	24	27
Cancer – not gastric	—	—	7	7
Other findings	3	2	5	10
Total	301	432	308	1041

by radiology or, preferably, by endoscopy with biopsy.

Radiology

The high incidence of gastric cancer in Japan led, in the mid-1960s, to the development and widespread use of double-contrast barium meal in mass-screening programmes in that country. Radiology may still have a place for screening but endoscopy is generally preferred amongst patients with dyspepsia. As radiology may still be the first investigation amongst patients with dyspepsia, the radiological findings in gastric ulcer are described.

Acute and chronic ulcers

Most ulcers are round or oval in shape with clear-cut margins and project beyond the margin of the stomach wall. There is sometimes a collar of oedematous mucosa that projects into the lumen of the stomach which disappears as the ulcer heals. The floor of a chronic ulcer is often irregular in shape. The usual sites of gastric ulcer are shown in *Table 2.4*. Multiple gastric ulcers occur in between 2 and 5% of patients. In Japan, 30% of gastric ulcers are linear in shape. Linear ulcers are less common in the West and usually result from the coalescence of a group of small ulcers or occur during ulcer healing.

Table 2.4 Sites of gastric ulcers

Site	Percentage
Lesser curve proximal to the angulus	45
Prepyloric region	19
High anterior or posterior wall	12
Antral	8
Angulus	7
Greater curve	5
Other sites	4

Gastric ulcer – benign or malignant?

The site of an ulcer is of little assistance in excluding a cancer. Ulcer healing is also unreliable because many malignant ulcers can undergo transient healing, either spontaneously or as the result of drug therapy. A smooth, sharply defined ulcer crater that projects beyond the margin of the stomach wall with intact mucosal folds that radiate towards its base suggests that it is benign. If the ulcer is irregular with raised, rolled margins that project within the stomach lumen and is associated with rigidity or nodularity of the adjacent mucosa and a loss of peristalsis during screening, it is more likely to be malignant (*Figure 2.48*).

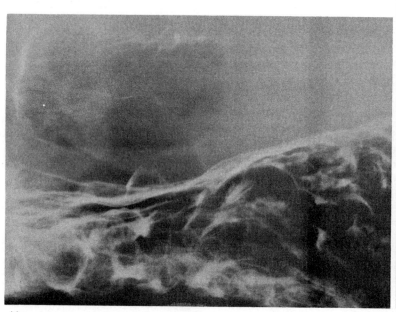
(a)

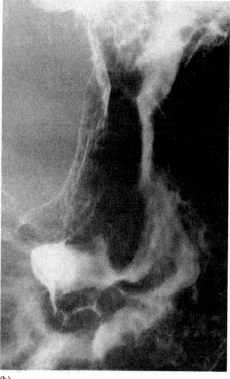
(b)

Figure 2.48 (a) Radiograph showing benign, cone-shaped penetrating ulcer on the posterior wall of the mid body of the stomach. (b) Radiograph showing malignant gastric ulcer on posterior wall with an irregular and raised margin.

In two separate studies,[78,67] standard radiological techniques failed to separate benign gastric ulcers from malignant ones in 31 and 40% patients, respectively.

In the British Society of Gastroenterology Early Gastric Cancer/Dysplasia Survey 1990[21], only 21% of the early gastric cancers were confidently diagnosed either with radiology or endoscopy alone, thus emphasizing the need to biopsy all gastric ulcers. It is therefore recommended that all patients with gastric ulcers are referred for endoscopy and biopsy.

Endoscopy

With the advent of slimmer, wider-angled instruments, endoscopy has had a further major impact on the investigation of gastric ulcers. In spite of these improvements endoscopy still remains an invasive technique although the risks are small, but this is more than outweighed by the ability to take biopsies and brush cytology of gastric lesions.

A benign ulcer should have a regular, punched out appearance with a smooth margin. The shape may vary, being round, oval or even linear. The base of the ulcer is covered with white fibrinoid material. The folds of the surrounding mucosa radiate towards the ulcer crater rather like the spokes of a wheel.

In contrast, an ulcerating gastric cancer usually has an irregular, nodular margin. On biopsy, the edge of the ulcer is often felt to be rigid and the biopsy site bleeds easily. The surrounding mucosal folds lose their stellate appearance, are often thickened and distorted and fail to reach the ulcer edge. Ulcers more than 2 cm in diameter have approximately four times the risk of being malignant than smaller ulcers but, as 95% of ulcers are benign, most large ulcers will still be benign.

Endoscopic biopsy

All ulcerating gastric lesions must be biopsied. Biopsies should be taken from the edge of the ulcer at all four quadrants as well as from the ulcer base. In practice it may be difficult to obtain biopsies from all four quadrants of an ulcer with a forward-viewing endoscope, and some endoscopists therefore suggest that a side-viewing instrument should also be used. However, provided at least six biopsies are taken from the ulcer edge, there appears to be little reduction in overall accuracy.[14]

Once the biopsies are taken, some endoscopists attempt to orient them with a dissecting microscope so that histological sections can be cut in the right plane. Usually serial sections through the biopsy are

taken if any suspicious changes are encountered. For the best results both the endoscopists and pathologists should review the histology together and in this way a correct diagnosis can be made in approximately 98% of all ulcers that are biopsied.

Cytology

Cytology complements both the visual appearance and the biopsy results. If all three parameters are used, a diagnostic accuracy rate of almost 100% can be obtained. Most endoscopists use a disposable brush to take cytological specimens, but it should be appreciated that the ulcer must be brushed vigorously enough to rub off cells rather than just the surface mucus.

TREATMENT: MEDICAL (A.G. Morgan)

Treatment of newly-diagnosed gastric ulcers

Non-specific measures

Doll and Pygott[23] first showed that a period of bed rest in hospital resulted in more rapid ulcer healing than outpatient therapy. However, with the advent of specific drug treatment, rapid healing can be achieved without bed rest or hospital admission. Doll also showed that the spread of ulcer healing could be further improved if smoking was discouraged. In the past, patients with gastric ulceration were advised to take small, frequent, bland meals but clinical trials have failed to show any relationship between diet and ulcer healing. Most gastric diets contained milk and it is now known that this is a strong stimulant of acid secretion and is not even a particularly good neutralizing agent. Likewise, small frequent meals have little buffering effect due, perhaps to the more continual stimulation of gastric acid secretion. Coffee and alcohol were likewise banned for ulcer patients. The stimulating effect of caffeine has, however, been shown to be small, and alcohol may even inhibit gastric acid output. Ulcer patients should, therefore, be allowed to choose their own diets and enjoy their meals.

Antacid therapy

Most clinical studies have shown little, if any, effect of antacid therapy on the healing rate of gastric ulcers. Isenberg and co-workers[45] performed a study in which cimetidine (1.2 g/day) was compared with low-dose antacid therapy and placebo. They found that cimetidine when compared with placebo at both the 8 and 12 week assessment period significantly hastened gastric ulcer healing, but low-dose antacid therapy had no such effect. In 1978 two

Table 2.5 Classification of histamine receptors

H_1 receptor functions	H_2 receptor functions
Contraction of smooth muscle within the gastrointestinal tract	Relaxation of contracted uterine smooth muscle
Contraction of smooth muscle in the respiratory tract	Increased rate of contraction of cardiac muscle
	Stimulation of gastric acid secretion

American studies were published in which cimetidine was compared with high-dose antacid therapy.[25,27] In one, an average of 228 mmol of in vitro buffing capacity per day was employed and in the other 279 mmol per day. Analysis of the healing rates for both studies showed a trend in favour of cimetidine when compared with this high-dose antacid therapy but in neither case did this reach statistical significance. Very high-dose antacid therapy may, therefore, hasten ulcer healing but the side-effects were common, with approximately 40% of the patients complaining of diarrhoea.

H₂ receptor antagonists

Histamine has a pivotal role as the final common mediator of gastric acid and pepsin secretion. Antihistamines block most of the other actions of histamine but have no effect on gastric acid secretion. It was, therefore, postulated that there were two receptor sites: H_1 receptors, being those blocked by the antihistamines; and H_2 receptors, which when blocked by specific receptor antagonists reduced gastric acid secretion (*Table 2.5*). Although gastric ulceration is usually associated with a normal or low acid output, further reduction in acid secretion from an H_2 receptor antagonist was capable of promoting ulcer healing.

CIMETIDINE

Cimetidine is an H_2 receptor antagonist which was first introduced in 1976, and by 1987 had been taken by over 50 million patients. It produces a dose-related inhibition of gastric acid secretion. As approximately 70% of the administered oral dose of cimetidine is excreted unchanged in the urine, patients with a creatinine clearance of less than 50 ml/min should receive a reduced dose.

In clinical practice, cimetidine appears to be extremely safe with a very low incidence of side-effects. Burland[12] published a review of the side-effects encountered in 2182 patients treated with cimetidine for a period of between 4 and 8 weeks and 884 patients on placebo therapy. The results are shown in *Table 2.6*.

Endocrine side-effects are very rare in patients given a normal therapeutic dose of cimetidine but, in high-dose therapy given to patients with Zollingen–Ellison syndrome, gynaecomastia is well documented. In a postmarketing study undertaken in the USA, 18 out of 9907 patients (0.18%) developed gynaecomastia which resolved spontaneously once therapy was discontinued.[31] Male impotence has also been associated with high-dose drug therapy but, in a double-blind placebo-controlled study of normal adult volunteers over 6 months, cimetidine had no effect either on spermatogenesis.

Reversible confusional states, agitation, hallucinations, irritability and somnolence have been reported, usually in the elderly or seriously ill patients. The incidence of mental confusion in 9928 patients taking cimetidine was 3.3% compared with 2.5% in 9351 control patients.[16]

H_2 receptors are present in the heart and blood vessels but oral therapy appears to have no effect on cardiovascular function, either at rest or during exercise. Rapid intravenous bolus injection of cimetidine can produce bradycardia, hypotension, cardiac arrhythmias and cardiac arrest in patients with serious underlying cardiovascular disease. It is therefore recommended that intravenous cimetidine is given slowly over 15–20 minutes.

Very rarely, reversible liver damage, interstitial nephritis, acute pancreatitis, thrombocytopenia, myalgia and arthralgia have been reported.

Cimetidine, due to its imidazole ring, binds reversibly to the hepatic cytochrome P-450 microsomal enzyme. Such binding reduces the clearance of certain drugs, including the benzodiazepines, propranolol, warfarin, phenytoin and theophyllin. Only the effect of warfarin, phenytoin and theophyllin appeared to be of clinical significance and, in co-prescribing, drug dosages may need to be reduced.

Table 2.6 Incidence of side-effects occurring in more than 1% of patients on short-term cimetidine therapy[12]

Symptom	Cimetidine (%)	Placebo (%)
Diarrhoea	1.8	1.0
Tiredness	1.7	1.6
Dizziness	1.3	1.0
Drowsiness	1.3	0.9
Rash	1.2	1.0

RANITIDINE

Ranitidine was first introduced into clinical practice in 1982 and is between five and 10 times more potent than cimetidine. The number of patient treatments has now exceeded 150 million. Ranitidine differs from cimetidine in that it has a furan and not an imidazole ring structure, and this is responsible for its independent pharmacology, Ranitidine has a slightly longer action than cimetidine in inhibiting histamine-stimulated gastric acid secretion. The absorption of oral ranitidine is not reduced by food. Between 20 and 30% of the administered oral dose of ranitidine is excreted unchanged in the urine and in patients with severe renal failure the elimination half-life rises from 2–3 hours to 4–9 hours. In patients with creatinine clearances of less than 50 ml/min the dosage of ranitidine should be halved.

Ranitidine is very well-tolerated, producing minor adverse effects such as headache, diarrhoea and constipation in less than 5% of patients – a rate similar to placebo-treated patients. In a study of 4532 patients treated with either ranitidine, cimetidine or placebo no significant difference was found in the incidence of side-effects (*Table 2.7*).[80] Serious and treatment-limiting adverse events occur rarely and are mainly, like cimetidine, in elderly or seriously ill patients or as idiosyncratic reaction.

Mental confusion, severe headaches, hallucinations and mania have been reported very rarely in seriously ill patients. In a survey of 9600 patients taking ranitidine the incidence of mental confusion was found in 1.9%.[44]

Very rarely, fever, rashes, bradycardia, heart block and gynaecomastia have been recorded. Likewise, thrombocytopenia, agranulocytosis and general myelosuppression. At therapeutic doses there is little binding of ranitidine with cytochrome P-450 and it therefore has little effect on the metabolism of such drugs as warfarin, diazepam, propranolol, phenytoin and theophyllin.

Table 2.7 Incidence of side-effects of ranitidine and cimetidine therapy[80]

Symptom	Ranitidine (n = 4532) (%)	Cimetidine (n = 908) (%)	Placebo (n = 1364) (%)
Headache	1.8	1.5	1.8
Tiredness	1.5	3.5	1.2
Diarrhoea	1.1	1.3	1.2
Constipation	0.8	1.4	0.7
Rash	0.5	0.6	0.2

NIZATIDINE

Nizatidine, an H_2 receptor antagonist, is an inhibitor of basal, nocturnal and stimulated gastric acid secretion whose potency lies between ranitidine and famotidine. Serum gastric concentrations are not significantly altered by oral nizatidine administration. Nizatidine has no anti-androgenic effect nor does it affect the hepatic metabolism of other drugs. Its absorption is unaffected by food ingestion but is reduced by concomitant antacid therapy. [^{14}C]Nizatidine has shown that over 90% of oral nizatidine is recovered in the urine and about 6% in the faeces. Unchanged nizatidine accounts for over 60% of the dose recovered from the urine. In patients with a serum creatinine clearance of less than 50 ml/min the oral dose should be reduced.

Nizatidine is well tolerated and the only side-effects seen more commonly than in placebo-treated patients are urticaria, somnolence and sweating. Adverse events occur in only 2% of patients and include headache, asthenia, chest pain, myalgia, abnormal dreams, rhinitis, pharyngitis, cough, pruritus and diarrhoea, but these adverse events are equally common in placebo-treated patients.

FAMOTIDINE

Famotidine is the most potent of the antisecretory H_2 receptor blockers and is 60 times more potent than cimetidine. Under normal conditions gastric acidity is inhibited by 70% during a 24-hour period by administration of famotidine 40 mg once at night. Comparable inhibition is seen with the administration of ranitidine 300 mg at night. There is no increase in serum gastrin levels. Famotidine has no anti-androgenic properties nor does it have any apparent effect on hepatic cytochrome P-450 enzyme activity and therefore no drug interactions are seen with therapeutic doses. Approximately 50% of an oral dose of famotidine is excreted unchanged in the urine. As with the other H_2 receptor antagonists the dose should be reduced in patients with a serum creatinine clearance of less than 50 ml/min or in elderly patients with renal impairment.

The usual side-effects of H_2 receptor blocker therapy, such as headaches, allergic rashes, constipation, diarrhoea and fatigue, have also been observed.

RESULTS OF TREATMENT

In a meta-analysis of the relationship between suppression of acidity and gastric ulcer healing, Howden and Hunt[42] have been able to show for the first time a significant correlation between ulcer healing rate after 2, 4 and 8 weeks of treatment, and suppression of 24 hour intragastric acidity. There was a weaker correlation between healing and sup-

Table 2.8 Meta-analysis of the relationship between suppression of acidity and gastric ulcer healing[42]

8 weeks of treatment	Healing rate	95% Confidence interval	Number of trials	Number of patients	Suppression of 24 hour acidity (%)
Omeprazole (40 mg)	95.9	92.4–98.3	1	171	98
Ranitidine (300 mg at night)	90.8	86.7–94.2	2	229	68
Nizatidine (150 mg twice daily)	90.0	82.5–95.6	1	80	—
Ranitidine (150 mg twice daily)	89.5	87.5–91.3	14	1010	68
Omeprazole (20 mg)	88.8	85.4–91.8	3	367	90
Nizatidine (300 mg at night)	86.5	78.7–92.8	1	89	—
Cimetidine (200 mg three times a day) + 400 mg at night	85.2	81.2–88.8	7	331	56
Cimetidine (300 mg four times a day)	83.7	72.2–92.6	2	49	65
Cimetidine (400 mg twice daily)	82.2	76.3–87.4	3	180	37
Famotidine (40 mg at night)	82.1	78.6–85.3	5	504	64
Enprostil (35 mg twice daily)	82.0	74.3–88.6	2	111	34
Placebo	53.4	49.5–57.3	8	638	—

pression of nocturnal acidity. As expected, the association between suppression of acidity and gastric ulcer healing rates was less marked than that described for duodenal ulcer.

The results of the meta-analysis, which is based on 74 trials since 1974 at 8 weeks, are shown in *Table 2.8*. This showed that healing rates depend on both the length of drug therapy and the degree of 24 hour acid suppression. After 2 weeks of therapy, healing rates of between 21 and 44% can be achieved compared with a placebo healing rate of 14%. After 4 weeks of therapy the healing rates range from 42 to 80% compared with a placebo healing rate of 33%. At the end of 8 weeks between 82 and 96% of gastric ulcers are healing compared with a placebo healing rate of 53%. Continued therapy for up to 12 weeks shows that almost all gastric ulcers can be healed. Factors influencing ulcer healing are size, age and smoking.

Proton pump inhibitors

The secretion of gastric hydrochloric acid depends on the passage of hydrogen ions across the secretory membrane of the parietal cell into the gastric lumen. This produces a steep hydrogen ion concentration gradient between the intracellular cytosol and the secretory canaliculi. The energy required for this process is generated by a highly specialized ATPase enzyme located in the secretory membrane of the parietal cell. The enzyme pumps H^+ ions from the cell into the lumen in exchange for K^+ ions and is termed the H^+/K^+-ATPase, or the proton pump.

Omeprazole, the first of this new class of drugs, is rapidly taken up and concentrated within the parietal cell. At low pH the drug is activated and forms a sulphonamide which is then unable to pass back across the cell membrane and this localizes the drug close to its site of action. The activated drug readily forms a disulphide link with the H^+/K^+-ATPase enzyme, thus inhibiting the proton pump mechanism. Omeprazole has a long-lasting, dose-dependent inhibition on both basal and stimulated gastric acid secretion. Therefore, a once-daily dosage provides effective 24 hour control of acid secretion. After a single dose the acid output returns to near pretreatment levels within 3–4 days. A daily 20 mg dosage decreases 24 hour intragastric acidity by between 80 and 85%. This compares with approximately 50% reduction for cimetidine (1.2 g daily), approximately 60% for ranitidine (150–300 mg daily) and 65% for famotidine (40 mg at night).

OMEPRAZOLE

Omeprazole is administered as enteric-coated granules within a gelatin capsule so as to prevent acid degradation within the stomach. Absorption is delayed with the enteric-coated formulation and the mean time to achieve peak plasma concentrations ranges from 2 to 5 hours. Omeprazole is metabolized on first pass through the liver and its systemic bioavailability increases over the first few days of treatment, eventually stabilizing at about 60%. The bioavailability is increased in patients with cirrhosis because of impaired liver metabolism. Intake of food or antacids does not influence the bioavailability of omeprazole (20 mg).

Omeprazole is rapidly distributed throughout the extracellular fluid but only crosses the blood–brain barrier to a limited extent. However, it rapidly disappears from all tissues except the gastric mucosa, where it is localized in the stomach wall and is confined to the tubulovesicles and secretory canaliculi of the parietal cells.

Omeprazole is eliminated almost entirely by

Table 2.9 A comparison of the side-effect profile of omeprazole and ranitidine

Adverse events	Omeprazole (n = 1032)(%)	Ranitidine (n = 787)(%)
Dyspepsia/pain	10.4	12.2
Nausea/vomiting	4.5	5.3
Headache/dizziness	4.2	3.6
Diarrhoea/constipation	2.7	2.8
Flatulence	2.7	1.8
Fatigue	1.2	0.5
Rash	0.5	3.0

metabolism and three main metabolites have been identified: the sulphone, sulphide and hydroxyomeprazole. None of these is considered to contribute to the antisecretory properties of omeprazole. About 60% of a radiolabelled dose is recovered as urinary metabolites within 6 hours and about 80% within 4 days. The remaining 20% is recovered in faeces, possibly following biliary secretion of unchanged drug metabolites. The pharmacokinetics of omeprazole has been especially studied in the elderly and those with chronic renal insufficiency, including dialysed patients. These studies show plasma drug concentrations and antisecretory effects within the same range as observed in healthy subjects. Although plasma clearances are reduced in patients with cirrhosis of the liver, there is no evidence of significant accumulation.

The reported adverse events in comparative trials of omeprazole and ranitidine show a very similar profile (Table 2.9). The fears that omeprazole might cause carcinoid tumours or gastric malignancy have so far not been substantiated from clinical studies; this issue is discussed later under Maintenance therapy (p. 265).

Omeprazole is metabolized within the liver. This occurs via the cytochrome P-450 system and therefore the pharmacokinetics of other drugs metabolized by this system have been evaluated during concomitant use of Losec. There is no alteration in the pharmacokinetics for theophylline or propranolol. There is an effect on the clearance of diazepam but this is less marked than with cimetidine and is unlikely to be of clinical significance. Omeprazole slightly reduces the total plasma clearance of oral phenytoin (22%). It is therefore advised that phenytoin plasma concentrations should be monitored in patients receiving omeprazole therapy. The same applies for warfarin where there is approximately a 10% increase in plasma warfarin concentration. Omeprazole is free of anti-androgenic effects and has not been found to cause mental confusion or a raised serum creatinine level.

RESULTS OF TREATMENT
So far studies using omeprazole suggest that it achieves rapid healing of gastric ulcers. At a dose of 20 mg, 40% of ulcers had healed at 2 weeks, 73% at 4 weeks and 89% at 8 weeks. When 40 mg/day was used the healing ratios were 80% at 4 weeks and 96% at 8 weeks (Table 2.8).

Anticholinergic drugs
Anticholinergic drugs have been used in the treatment of peptic ulcer disease in an attempt to achieve a medical vagotomy. At a dose necessary to produce a therapeutic inhibition of acid and pepsin secretion the side-effects on the anticholinergic action at receptor sites other than the stomach become troublesome.

PIRENZEPINE
Pirenzepine is claimed to be a selective antagonist acting only on the muscarinic receptors in the stomach and so reducing unwanted side-effects. At therapeutic doses some clinical studies have reported a dry mouth. Although it has little effect on the smooth muscle of the gut there is some inhibition of oesophageal peristalsis and occasional impairment of gastric emptying. Colonic motility is reduced and, in some studies, patients have reported constipation. As the drug is hydrophylic, it does not easily pass the blood-brain barrier and is therefore unlikely to cause mental confusion. Likewise, it has little effect on accommodation, pupil diameter and intraocular pressure. Unlike other anticholinergic drugs it may cause bradycardia and acute retention of urine.

Five trials have been published.[7,32,46,61,71] In three it was compared with carbenoxolone, in one against ranitidine and in the fifth against a placebo. There was no significant difference between pirenzepine, carbenoxolone or ranitidine therapy but it was significantly better than placebo in promoting ulcer healing. Pirenzepine produces significantly better results than gefarnate.[46] Pirenzepine is an effective drug for the treatment of gastric ulceration but because of its side-effects it is not used widely in gastric ulcer therapy.

Mucosal protective agents

The healing of an ulcer depends upon the balance between acid and pepsin and mucosal defence mechanisms. The main thrust of peptic ulcer treatment has been either to reduce acid and pepsin secretion or to protect the ulcer from attack by gastric contents (sucralfate and colloidal bismuth). Both carbenoxolone and deglycyrrhizinized liquorice (Caved-S) strengthen the mucosal defence mechanisms. Prostaglandins are naturally produced by the stomach and duodenum and stimulate the mucosal defence mechanisms. These include an increase in the proliferative activity of the mucosal epithelial cells, and a strengthening of the mucous bicarbonate barrier.

PROSTAGLANDINS

The cytoprotective effect of prostaglandins include their ability to protect microvascular integrity. Prostaglandins preserve the ability of the mucosa to re-epithelialize damaged tissue. They stimulate gastric mucous secretion as well as gastric and duodenal bicarbonate secretion. They inhibit gastric acid secretion and regulate mucosal blood flow.

MISOPROSTIL

Misoprostil is a synthetic prostaglandin E methyl ester analogue which has both potent antisecretory and cytoprotective actions on gastric and duodenal mucosa. Clinical trials have confirmed its efficacy in the treatment of both duodenal and gastric ulcers. It may also have an important role to play in the protection of the gastric and duodenal mucosa from non-steroidal anti-inflammatory drug-induced damage. Diarrhoea is the main side-effect and occurs in 3–15% of patients, but this may be self-limiting. More frequent administration at a lower dosage reduces the frequency of diarrhoea. Nausea, vomiting and abdominal pain have also been reported. No adverse ophthalmic or cardiovascular effects have been observed. As misoprostil does not affect the liver cytochrome P-450 activity, no direct interactions have been identified. Misoprostil, however, does have a uterotrophic effect and can induce an abortion and should therefore not be used in pregnancy or in those planning a pregnancy. It may also cause abnormal vaginal bleeding.[17]

Misoprostil has been shown to be as effective as cimetidine in the healing of gastric ulcers. Clinical trial data suggests that healing is related to the inhibition of acid secretion rather than an enhancement of mucosal defence by cytoprotective mechanisms.

ENPROSTIL

Enprostil is a synthetic dihydroprostaglandin E_2 and has a sufficiently long duration of antisecretory activity to allow twice daily dosage. Its mode of action and side-effects are similar to misoprostil.

Antimicrobial agents – colloidal bismuth subcitrate (De-Nol)

The active ingredient, colloidal bismuth subcitrate, is soluble in water but precipitates at a pH of less than 5.0. In gastric juice the optimum pH for precipitation is 3.5 and bismuth is deposited in an ulcer crater in preference to the surrounding mucosa. It forms a complex with the proteins on the ulcer base which may protect against the effect of gastric juice. Colloidal bismuth subcitrate also possesses some antipepsin activity, has no effect on gastric acid secretion but stimulates the production of prostaglandin E_2 and alkali secretion. Colloidal bismuth subcitrate has a specific role as an antimicrobial agent against *Helicobacter pylori*, both in vitro and in vivo. It has a direct action causing vacuolisation, loss of adherence to the epithelium, fragmented cell walls and condensation of cell contents.

Small amounts of bismuth are absorbed from the gastrointestinal tract and plasma concentrations plateau after about 4 weeks of therapy but rarely rise above 5 μg/l. The tissue distribution of colloidal bismuth subcitrate in humans is unknown. High doses of other bismuth salts administered for prolonged periods have produced encephalopathy in some patients. There has been one report of reversible central nervous symptoms in a man who received a high dose of colloidal bismuth subcitrate for 8 weeks followed by intermittent therapy with low doses for a total of 2 years. No such adverse effects have been reported during or after the use of De-Nol over 8 weeks.

The absorbed bismuth is excreted both in urine and faeces. Urinary excretion of bismuth continues for some weeks after stopping drug therapy, confirming some degree of tissue accumulation and a slow mobilization. It is thus recommended that colloidal bismuth subcitrate should be used with caution in patients with renal impairment. The newer tablet formation reduces the staining of the tongue and teeth seen with the liquid preparation although the stools are still blackened by the excretion of bismuth sulphide. Occasional side-effects are limited to reports of mild dizziness, headache and diarrhoea.

Table 2.10 Trials comparing colloidal bismuth subcitrate (CBS) with placebo in the treatment of gastric ulcer

Trial	Drug/dosage	Number of patients	Healing rate (%) at 4 weeks	
Boyes et al.[11]	CBS 120 mg four times a day	10	90	$P < 0.05$
	Placebo	10	30	
Lee and Nicholson[53]	CBS 240 mg four times a day	20	90	$P < 0.05$
	Placebo	17	35	
Poulantzas et al.[75]	CBS 120 mg four times a day	10	90	NS
	Placebo	6	33	
Lam et al.[52]	CBS	22	68	$P < 0.005$
	Placebo	25	20	
Morales et al.[60]	CBS 120 mg four times a day	15	87	$P < 0.05$
	Placebo	12	42	
Sutton et al.[82]	CBS	25	72	$P < 0.02$
	Placebo	25	36	
Glover et al.[34]	CBS 120 mg four times a day	16	63	$P < 0.05$
	Placebo	18	37	

NS, not significant.

CLINICAL RESULTS

Seven studies have compared colloidal bismuth subcitrate (120 mg four times a day) with placebo and all but one showed a statistically significant difference in favour of the drug (*Table 2.10*). Subsequently eight studies compared colloidal bismuth subcitrate with either cimetidine or ranitidine and showed that it was as effective as antisecretory drugs (*Table 2.11*). The healing rate at 4 weeks was 74%, at 6 weeks 76% and at 8 weeks 84%.

Sucralfate

Sucralfate is a basic aluminium salt of sucrose octasulphate and has little or no effect on blood coagulation. In the presence of acid, sucralfate becomes a highly condensed viscous adhesive substance with a low acid neutralizing capacity. Its reaction with acid is very slow but, since sucralfate adheres to the gastric mucosa, this acid-buffering capacity may still be important because the interaction occurs close to the mucosal surface. Sucralfate also combines with protein to create an adherent and protective barrier at the site of the ulcer. It therefore protects the ulcer from acid, pepsin and bile. The cytoprotective action of sucralfate is mediated by the stimulation of endogenous prostaglandins and their release from gastric mucosa. Gastric bicarbonate secretion is also increased and there is also decreased pepsin activity.

In a study involving 1663 patients who were treated with sucralfate, side-effects were noted in only 2.6%,[29] which included constipation and nausea. Drug interaction studies also indicate that sucralfate may interfere with the absorption of a number of drugs, including the tetracyclines, warfarin, phenytoin, cimetidine and digoxin. As sucralfate does not cause any systemic adverse effects it is thought to be a good alternative to H_2 receptor antagonist therapy.

CLINICAL RESULTS

Most of the clinical trials using sucralfate in the treatment of gastric ulcers involve very small numbers and few therefore demonstrate a significant difference either when compared with placebo or H_2 receptor antagonists.[20,30,35,39,40,48,51,55,58,70,74,76,77]
Combined results show healing rates that are identical to those achieved by antisecretory drugs, being 61% at 4 weeks, 67% at 6 weeks, 89% at 8 weeks and 96% at 12 weeks.

Carbenoxolone sodium

Carbenoxolone is derived from the hydrolysis of glycyrrhizic acid after extraction from liquorice root and was shown to be an effective drug for the treatment of gastric ulcers.[24] Carbenoxolone is absorbed through the gastric mucosa and is excreted in

Table 2.11 Trials comparing colloidal bismuth subcitrate (CBS) with H_2 receptor antagonist in the treatment of gastric ulcer

Trial	Drug/dosage	Number of patients	Healing rate (%) at 4 weeks	6 weeks	8 weeks	
Tanner et al.[86]	CBS liquid	33		66		NS
	Cimetidine	27		63		
Tytgat et al.[88]	CBS tablets	28	61		—	
	Cimetidine	30	43		NS	
	Placebo	22	18		P < 0.001	
Austad et al.[2]	CBS tablets			56		NS
	Cimetidine			69		
Gibinski et al.[33]	CBS liquid	47	68		81	NS
	Cimetidine	36	47		69	
Soltoft et al.[81]	CBS tablet	27	81			NS
	Cimetidine	77	74			
Shou-Po et al.[79]	CBS liquid	29	76			
	Cimetidine	26	54			
Cipollini et al.[13]	CBS tablets (480 mg)	26		89		NS
	Ranitidine (300 mg)	27		74		
Parente et al.[72]	CBS tablets (480 mg)	40	70		89	NS
	Ranitidine (300 mg)	40	63		79	
Cipollini et al.[13]	CBS tablets (480 mg)	26		89		NS
	Ranitidine (300 mg)	27		74		

NS, not significant.

the bile, then reabsorbed in the small intestine. It causes an increase in the life-span of the rapidly proliferating gastric epithelial cells, thus increasing mucus production, normalizing mucus composition and strengthening the mucus barrier.

Patients treated with carbenoxolone require careful follow-up to detect any clinical evidence of fluid retention, congestive heart failure, hypertension and hypokalaemia.

Many clinical trials have shown that carbenoxolene is more effective than placebo in healing gastric ulcers but, because of its side-effects, carbenoxolone no longer has a place in the treatment of gastric ulceration.

Deglycyrrhizinized liquorice

Deglycyrrhizinized liquorice contains less than 3% glycyrrhizinic acid and because of this does not have the fluid-retaining properties and risk of hypokalaemia which is seen with carbenoxolone. Deglycyrrhizinized liquorice is thought to have the same effect as carbenoxolone on the gastric mucosa. It stimulates and accelerates the differentiation to glandular cells in the gastric mucosa, thereby increasing mucus formation. Deglycyrrhizinized liquorice also increases gastric mucosal blood flow. It has no mineral corticoid-like action and may hence be safely used in the elderly patient. A few patients complain of its liquorice taste and mild laxative effect.

Only seven good studies[3,28,62,63,64,87,89] have evaluated treatment of gastric ulceration with deglycyrrhizinized liquorice. The total number of patients treated was small (196) and in only three was endoscopy rather than radiology used to check for ulcer healing. Combined results indicate that only 42% of gastric ulcers had healed by 4 weeks but more had healed at 8 weeks. Caved-S is seldom used because of its inconvenient dose regimen and tablet size.

Recommendations for initial treatment of gastric ulcers

If the ulcer is small (<2 cm) either full-dose H_2 receptor antagonist (taken twice daily or at night), colloidal bismuth subcitrate or sucralfate is recommended.

It is difficult to advise on the optimum antisecretory drug as there is little to choose between cimetidine 400 mg twice daily, ranitidine 300 mg at night, famotidine 40 mg at night and nizatidine 150 mg twice daily. Cimetidine and ranitidine are the most widely used; cimetidine should probably be avoided in patients on aminophylline or phenytoin.

For large ulcers (>2 cm) or ulcer complications, provided the initial biopsy of the gastric ulcer shows no evidence of malignancy, high-dosage H_2 receptor antagonist or omeprazole should be used.

H_2 receptor antagonists are preferred in *prepyloric ulcers* unless there is *H. pylori* infection.

In *recurrent ulcers* or ones associated with *H. pylori infection*, colloidal bismuth subcitrate is the drug of choice, possibly in combination with metronidazole and tetracycline. Endoscopy must be repeated after 8 weeks of therapy in all gastric ulcer patients to ensure that the ulcer has healed. In 10–20% of patients the ulcer persists despite medical therapy. If this is the case the ulcer must be rebiopsied, drug therapy should be continued and the endoscopy repeated after a total of 12 weeks of treatment. If the ulcer still remains unhealed, surgical treatment should be considered. If an operation is contraindicated, therapy for a further month with omeprazole at a dose of 40 mg in the morning is recommended but, if the ulcer persists despite these measures, the surgical option must be reassessed.

Ulcer recurrence and maintenance therapy

Almost two-thirds of gastric ulcers recur a year after healing; most recurrences occur within the first 6 months. Many studies indicate that it is the large ulcers which most frequently recur.

Role of maintenance therapy
Maintenance therapy may have to be considered if the ulcer recurs soon after initial healing. Maintenance therapy may be desirable if a recurrence occurs in a patient in whom surgical treatment might be contraindicated because of a high anaesthetic risk due to recent ischaemic heart disease or chronic obstructive airways disease. Maintenance therapy may be desirable if the ulcer has bled in the past or if non-steroidal anti-inflammatory drugs cannot be discontinued.

Maintenance therapy should be monitored endoscopically and, if an ulcer re-recurs or does not heal and *H. pylori* has been eliminated, surgical treatment must be offered. For maintenance therapy to be a viable alternative to surgery the drug therapy must be safe and effective. Compliance should be high and medication should be cheap.

Results of maintenance therapy
Many trials have been published on the results of maintenance therapy for gastric ulcers. There are few satisfactory double-blind studies since patient numbers are usually far too small. Of the 26 studies analysed,[1,5,6,8–10,15,18,20,37–39,43,47,49,50,54,56,57,64–66,68,69,3,84] 13 have a total of less than 50 patients, nine between 50 and 100 patients and only four have patient numbers greater than 100. This perhaps reflects the difficulties and expense of performing detailed long-term studies in a disease that usually occurs in the elderly. Okabe and others[69] showed that cimetidine was better than antacids for maintenance therapy but despite 253 patients the difference did not achieve statistical significance. Takemoto and colleagues[83] showed that cimetidine and sucralfate was significantly better than either agent alone. Two years later they reported[84] that ranitidine was more effective than sucralfate alone. Despite this, Humphreys and colleagues[43] showed that maintenance famotidine was no better than a placebo.

A summary of the results obtained from the maintenance trials are shown in *Table 2.12*. Maintenance H_2 receptor antagonist therapy has halved the recurrence rate during the first 6 months of therapy compared with placebo. The 6 month recurrence rate for sucralfate is almost identical to antisecretory therapy but the recurrence rate is higher by the end of a year's treatment. The combination of sucralfate and cimetidine was assessed in only one study but with outstanding results: 2.4% recurrence at 6 months. The combination of ranitidine and Caved-S is no more effective than ranitidine alone. Nevertheless, Caved-S as a single agent appears to be as effective as H_2 receptor antagonists.

Problems of maintenance therapy in these trials
Although all patients were endoscoped if they had symptoms, not all had a routine gastroscopy. When they did, asymptomatic ulcers were often found, the incidence varying from 11 to 87% (average 42%). The true recurrence rate on maintenance therapy is therefore dependent upon the frequency of routine endoscopy. We are still ignorant of the natural history of asymptomatic gastric ulcers and do not know if they remain asymptomatic and heal spontaneously or become symptomatic.

The placebo healing rate and the results of maintenance therapy for gastric ulcers is in part dependent upon the country of origin. For example, in Japan, gastric ulcers are more common than in Europe; they have a different distribution and are

Table 2.12 Summary of maintenance trials

Drug	Number of patients	Recurrence rate (%) at		
		6 months	12 months	24 months
Placebo	164	38	56	
H$_2$ receptor antagonist	657	22	24	24
Sucralfate	295	19	32	
Enprostil	43	28	40	
Caved-S	34		12	29
Carbenoxolane	15		47	
Cimetidine + sucralfate	40	2		
Ranitidine + Caved-S	48		20	30

more difficult to heal. This may explain some of the variance in the results of maintenance therapy.

Risk of ulcer recurrence is increased if the original ulcer is large, if the ulcer is prepyloric or if it is associated with increased acid secretion. Recurrent ulcers tend to recur more frequently than those with no previous history of ulceration.

All long-term studies are plagued by the problem of drug compliance. The returned drug count does not exclude a patient with poor compliance who has either hidden or destroyed his or her unused drugs. Compliance is improved with either daily or twice daily therapy.

Safety of maintenance therapy

No serious side-effects were encountered in any of the studies analysed earlier. No long-term side-effects have been found in the postmarket surveillance studies using H$_2$ receptor antagonists. Sucralfate has been in use in Japan for over 20 years without any reported serious side-effects, except for one case of encephalopathy in a patient with chronic renal failure which might have been associated with aluminium toxicity.

Profound and prolonged hypochlorhydria is now easily achievable by high-dose H$_2$ receptor antagonists or proton pump inhibitor therapy. Medical achlorhydria is associated with bacterial colonization of the stomach. Some bacterial species are capable of reducing dietary and salivary nitrate to nitrate. It has been postulated that nitrites react with nitrogen-containing groups, such as amines or amides, to produce nitroso compounds, which have a potential for local genotoxic reactions within the gastric mucosa. These compounds might theoretically increase the risk of gastric carcinoma in patients with achlorhydria. The risk might be minimized by single bedtime dosage of the drug, which will then allow a breakthrough of acid secretion for a part of the day.

In experimental animals, profound acid inhibition by several potent H$_2$ receptor antagonists has resulted in a range of changes from antral hyperplasia, dysplasia or adenocarcinoma. Furthermore, enterochromaffin-like hyperplasia of cells has been associated with the development of gastric carcinoids.

In 2 year toxicity studies in rats treated with omeprazole, an increase in the enterochromaffin-like cell density of the gastric mucosa was observed, resulting in non-metastasizing carcinoid tumours due to hypergastrinaemia. When omeprazole was given for 1 year only, the gastric mucosa rapidly returned to normal after therapy was discontinued. The dose of omeprazole used in these experiments was up to 400 times greater than the therapeutic range used in humans.

Results of long-term maintenance therapy

Bardan[4] described a group of 77 patients with gastric ulcers who were treated with cimetidine at a dose of 400 mg at night for a period of 6 years. Initially, endoscopy was performed at 6-monthly intervals and then at least yearly or if dyspeptic symptoms returned. Life table analysis shows that the cumulative symptomatic relapse rate during the first 5 years was 13, 19, 21, 21 and 26% respectively. Approximately the same proportion suffered from an asymptomatic ulcer recurrence found at routine endoscopy: 21% at 5 years. Of the 27 patients with ulcer recurrences, 20 (74%) rehealed within 12 weeks with full dose therapy. The average annual rate of symptomatic recurrence was 2%. No factors predicted patients who developed a recurrence. The authors were unable to ascertain if maintenance therapy reduces the risk of ulcer complications.

Penston and Wormsley[73] published a retrospective study based on 120 patients with gastric ulcers who received maintenance therapy with ranitidine (150–300 mg/day) for up to 7 years. The cumulative annual recurrence over 5 years was 3.5, 6.3, 9.4, 22.9 and 22.9%. They concluded that maintenance treatment with ranitidine for 5 years significantly reduces the risk of a symptomatic gastric ulcer recurrence. No complications were observed during therapy.

Recommendations for maintenance therapy

The use of maintenance therapy following the healing of a gastric ulcer has become widely accepted, particularly for large ulcers or ulcers that recur after a previous successful course of medical therapy. The argument in favour of maintenance treatment is that recurrence rates are high if no treatment is used and many recurrences are asymptomatic. There is a theoretical argument that maintenance therapy might reduce the risk of complications, but this has never been proven. H_2 receptor antagonists are the agents which have been most widely audited for maintenance therapy. Recurrence rates in the first year are almost halved compared with the rate in untreated patients. Long-term treatment with either cimetidine or ranitidine appear to be safe. Most ulcers that recur during maintenance therapy can be healed by reverting to full-dose therapy and, once healed, maintenance therapy can be continued. The addition of sucralfate may reduce the relapse rate but compliance using two agents is likely to be poor. Patients whose ulcer recurs despite maintenance therapy should be considered for surgical therapy.

References

1. Alstead, E.M., Ryan, F.P., Holdsworth, C.D., Ashton, M.G. and Moore, M. (1983) Ranitidine in the prevention of gastric and duodenal ulcer relapse. *Gut*, **24**, 418–420.
2. Austad, W.I., Hillman, L.C., Luey, K. *et al.* (1983) Gastric ulcer – a treatment comparison of colloidal bismuth with cimetidine, and 30 months follow up. *The New Zealand Society of Gastroenterology, Dunedin* (abstract).
3. Bardhan, K.D., Cumberland, D.C., Dixon, R.A. and Holdsworth, C.D. (1978) Clinical trial of deglycyrrhizinized liquorice in gastric ulcer. *Gut*, **19**, 799–782.
4. Bardhan, K.D. (1988) For the Anglo-Irish cimetidine long term study group. *Alimentary Pharmacology and Therapeutics*, pp. 395–405.
5. Barr, G.D., Kang, J.Y., Canalese, J. and Piper, D.W. (1983) A two-year prospective controlled study of maintenance cimetidine and gastric ulcer. *Gastroenterology*, **85**, 100–104.
6. Bianchi Porro, G.B. and Pietrillo, M. (1979) Short and long treatment of gastric ulcer – a controlled trial comparing cimetidine and carbenoxolone sodium. In *Second National Symposium on Cimetidine Brussels, 1979* (Ed.) Dresse, A. pp. 161–170. Amsterdam: Excerpta Medica.
7. Bianchi Porro, G. and Dal Monte, P.R. (1982) Pirenzepine for treatment of gastric ulcer. Results of two double-blind trial. *Symposium Advances in Gastroenterology with Selective Antimuscarinic Compound Pirenzepine, Stockholm, 1982* (abstracts), p. 48. Amsterdam: Excerpta Medica.
8. Bianchi Porro, G., Dal Monte, P.R., Lazzaaroni, M., Petrillo, M., D'Imperio, N. and Imbimbo, B.P. (1986) Pirenzepine and ranitidine for chronic gastric ulcer: a comparison in short-term and maintenance treatment. *Current Therapeutic Research*, **39**(1), 149–155.
9. Birger Jensen, K., Mollman, K.M., Rahbeck, I., Madsen, J.R., Rune, S.J. and Wulff, H.R. (1979) Prophylactic effects of cimetidine in gastric ulcer patients. *Scandinavian Journal of Gastroenterology*, **14**, 175–176.
10. Borsch, G. (1988) Roxatidine Acetate in the long-term maintenance of gastric ulcers. *Drugs*, **35**(suppl. 3), 134–138.
11. Boyes, B.E., Woolf, I.L., Wilson, R.Y., Cowley, D.J. and Dymock, I.W. (1975) Treatment of gastric ulceration with a bismuth preparation. *Postgraduate Medical Journal*, **51**(suppl. 5), 29–33.
12. Burland, W.L. (1982) *Worldwide TAGAMET Experience*, pp. 141–142. Smith, Kline and French.
13. Cipollini, F. and Altilia, F. (1987) Comparison of tri-potassium di-citrato bismuthate with ranitidine in healing and relapse of gastric ulcer. *British Journal of Clinical Practice*, **40**, 707–709.
14. Classen, M. and Roesch, W. (1974) Gastroscopy biopsy and cytology in early detection of stomach cancer. In *Early Gastric Cancer. Current States of Diagnosis* (Ed.) Grundmann, E., Grunze, H. and Witte, S. pp. 113–117. Berlin: Springer-Verlag.
15. Cockel, R., Dawson, J. and Jain, S. (1982) Ranitidine in the long-term treatment of gastric ulcers. In *The Clinical Use of Ranitidine* (Ed.) Misiewicz, J.J. and Wormsley, K.G. pp. 232–238. Medicine Publication Foundation.
16. Colin-Jones, D.G., Langman, M.J.S., Lawson, D.H. and Vessey, M.P. (1985) Post-marketing surveillance of the safety of Cimetidine: twelve-month morbidity report. *Quarterly Journal of Medicine New Series*, 54, 215, 253–268.
17. Committee on Safety of Medicines (1989) *Misoprostil Reports of Uterine Bleeding and Diarrhoea*, p. 27.
18. Da Silva, E.P. and Zaterka, S. (1981) Long-term treatment of gastric ulcer with cimetidine. *Clinical Therapeutics*, **4**(1), 24–31.
19. Davenport, P.M., Morgan, A.G. and Darnborough, A. (1985) Can preliminary screening of dyspeptic patients allow more effective use of investigational techniques. *British Medical Journal*, **290**, 217–220.
20. Dawson, J., Jain, S. and Cockel, R. (1984) Effect of ranitidine and cimetidine on gastric ulcer healing and recurrence. *Scandinavian Journal of Gastroenterology*, **19**, 665–668.
21. de Dombal, F.T., Price, A.B., Thompson, H. *et al.* (1990) The British Society of Gastroenterology,

early gastric/dysplasia survey: an interim report. *Gut*, **32**, 115–120.

22. DeLuca V.A. (1983) Sucralfate in the treatment of gastric ulcer diasese (abstract). *Gastroenterology* **84**(5, part 2), 1134.

23. Doll, R. and Pygott, F. (1952) Factors in rate of healing of gastric ulcers – admission to hospital, phenobarbitone and ascorbic acid. *The Lancet*, **ii**, 171–175.

24. Doll, R., Hill, I.D., Hutton, C. and Underwood, D.J. (1962) Clinical trial of a triterpenoid liquorice compound in gastric and duodenal ulcer. *The Lancet*, **ii**, 793–796.

25. Dyck, W.P., Belsito, A., Fleshler, B., Liebermann, T.R., Dickinson, P.B. and Wood, J. (1978) Cimetidine and placebo in the treatment of benign gastric ulcer. *Gastroenterology*, **74**(2), 410–415.

26. Edwards, F.C. and Coghill, N.F. (1968) Clinical manifestations in the patients with chronic atrophic gastritis, gastric ulcer and duodenal ulcer. *Quarterly Journal of Medicine*, **37**, 337–360.

27. Englert, E., Freston, J.W., Graham, D.Y. *et al.* (1978) Cimetidine, antacid and hospitalization in the treatment of benign gastric ulcer. *Gastroenterology*, **74**, 416–425.

28. Engqvist, A., Von Feilitzen, F., Pyk, E. and Reichard, H. (1973) Double-blind trial of deglycyrrhizinated liquorice in gastric ulcer. *Gut*, **14**, 711–715.

29. Fisher, S.S. (1981) Sucralfate. A review of drug tolerance and safety. *Journal of Clinical Gastroenterology*, **3**(suppl. 2), 181–184.

30. Fixa, B. and Komarkova, O. (1981) Aluminium sucrose sulphate in the treatment of gastric and duodenal ulcer. In *Duodenal Ulcer, Gastric Ulcer. Sucralfate, A New Therapeutic Concept* (Ed.) Caspary, W.F. pp. 80–84. Baltimore: Urban and Schwarzenberg.

31. Freston, J.W. (1987) Safety perspectives on parenteral H_2 receptor antagonists. *The American Journal of Medicine*, **83**(suppl. 6A), 58–67.

32. Gasbarrini, G., Giorgio-Conciato, M., D'Anchine, M. *et al.* (1978) Pirenzepine in the treatment of benign gastroduodenal diseases. *Scandinavian Journal of Gastroenterology*, **14**(suppl. 57), 25–31.

33. Gibinski, K., Nowak, A., Marlicz, K. *et al.* (1984) Dicytrynianobizmutan trojpotasowy w leczeniu wrzodu trawiennego i zapobieganiu nawrotowi wrzodu. *Polski Tygodnik Lekarski*, **39**, 1547–1550.

34. Glover, S.C., Cantlay, J.S., Weir, J. and Mowat, N.A.G. (1983) Oral tripotassium-dicitratobismuthate in gastric and duodenal ulceration: a double-blind controlled trial. *Digestive diseases and Sciences*, **28**, 13–17.

35. Hallerback, B., Anker-Hanven, O., Carling, L. *et al.* (1986) Short term treatment of gastric ulcer: a comparison of sucralfate and cimetidine. *Gut*, **27**, 778–783.

36. Hellier, M.D., Gent, A.E., Walker, J., Britten, D., Hutchison, C. and Gough, K.R. (1982) Ranitidine in the treatment of gastric ulcers: healing and maintenance (abstract). *Scandinavian Journal of Gastroenterology*, **17**(suppl. 79), 155.

37. Hellier, M.D., Gent, A.E., Walker, J., Britten, D., Hutchison, C. and Gough, K.R. (1982) Ranitidine in the treatment of gastric ulcers: healing and maintenance. *Scandinavian Journal of Gastroenterology*, suppl. 78, 155.

38. Hentschel, E., Schutze, K., Weiss, W. *et al.* (1983) Effect of cimetidine treatment in the prevention of gastric ulcer relapse: a one year double-blind multicentre study. *Gut*, **24**, 853–856.

39. Herrerias-Gutierrez, J.M., Pardo, L. and Segu, J.L. (1989) Sucralfate versus ranitidine in the treatment of gastric ulcer. *American Journal of Medicine*, **86**(suppl. 6A), 94–97.

40. Hjortrup, A., Svendsen, L.B., Beck, H., Hoffman, J. and Schroeder, M. (1989) Two daily doses of sucralfate or cimetidine in the healing of gastric ulcer – a comparative randomized study. *American Journal of Medicine*, **86**(suppl. 6A), 113–116.

41. Horrocks, J. C. and de Dombal, F.T. (1978) Clinical presentation of patients with dyspepsia. *Gut*, **19**, 19–26.

42. Howden, C.W. and Hunt, R.H. (1990) The relationship between suppression of acidity and gastric ulcer healing rates. *Alimentary Pharmacology and Therapeutics*, **4**, 25–33.

43. Humphries, T.J., Berlin, R.G., Fong, C., Berman, R.S. The Famotidine Gastric Ulcer Study Group and the Duke University Co-operative Study Group (1989) Are H_2-receptor antagonists effective in the maintenance of healing in benign gastric ulcer? *Gastroenterology* (suppl. 1), **96**(5(2)), A223.

44. Inman, W.H.W. (1983) Zantac. *PEM News*, Aug., pp. 9–13.

45. Isenberg, J., Elashoff, J., Sandersfield, M. and Peterson, W. (1982) Double-blind comparison of cimetidine and low-dose antacid versus placebo in the healing of benign gastric ulcer. *Gastroenterology*, **82**(5), 1090.

46. Ishimori, A. and Yamagata, S. (1982) Double-blind controlled study of pirenzepine on gastric ulcer and duodenal ulcer. *Abstracts of the Symposium on Advances in Gastroenterology with the Selective Antimuscarinic Compound Pirenzepine, Stockholme, 1982*, p. 46. Amsterdam: Excerpta Medica.

47. Jorde, R., Burhol, P.G. and Hansen, T. (1987) Ranitidine 150 mg at night in the prevention of gastric ulcer relapse. *Gut*, **28**, 460–463.

48. Kagevi, I., Anker-Hansen, O., Carling, L. *et al.* (1987) Swedish multicentre study on prepyloric and gastric ulcer. *Scandinavian Journal of Gastroenterology*, **22**(suppl. 127), 67–76.

49. Kinloch, J.D., Pearson, A.J.G., Woolf, I.L. and Young, P.H. (1984) The effect of cimetidine on the maintenance of healing of gastric ulceration. *Postgraduate Medical Journal*, **60**, 665–667.

50. La Brooy, S.J., Taylor, R.H., Ayrton, C. *et al.* (1980) Cimetidine in the maintenance treatment of gastric ulceration. *Hepatogastroenterology Suppl.*

II. International Congress of Gastroenterology, Hamburg (abstract E26:5).

51. Lahtinen, J., Aukee, S., Miettinen, P., Poikolainen, E., Paakkkonen, M. and Sandstrom, R. (1982) Sucralfate and cimetidine for gastric ulcer. A single-blind endoscopically controlled randomized study. 2nd International Sucralfate Symposium. *Abstracts of the 7th World Congress of Gastroenterology, Stockholm, 1982.*

52. Lam, S.K., Koo, J., Cheng, C.H., Ho, J. and Ong, G.B. (1981) Treatment of corpus and prepyloric gastric ulcers with tri-potassium dicitratobismuthate (De-Nol). *Gastroenterology*, **80**, 1202.

53. Lee, S.P. and Nicholson, G.I. (1977) Increased healing of gastric and duodenal ulcers in a controlled trial using tripotassium dicitrato-bismuthate. *Medical Journal of Australia*, **1**, 808–812.

54. Machell, R.J., Farthing, M.J.G., Ciclitira, P.J., Dick, A.P. and Hunter, J.O. (1979) Cimetidine in the prevention of gastric ulcer relapse. *Postgraduate Medical Journal*, **55**, 393–395.

55. Marks, I.N., Wright, J.P., Denyer, M., Garisch, J.A.M. and Lucke, W. (1980) Comparison of sucralfate with cimetidine in the short term treatment of chronic peptic ulcer. *South African Medical Journal*, **57**, 567–573.

56. Marks, I.N., Wright, J.P., Girdwood, A.H., Gilinsky, N.H. and Lucke, W. (1985) Maintenance therapy with sucralfate reduces rate of gastric ulcer recurrence. *The American Journal of Medicine,* **79**(suppl. 2C), 32–35.

57. Marks, I.N., Girwood, A.H., Wright, J.P. *et al.* (1987) Nocturnal dosage regimen of sucralfate in maintenance treatment of gastric ulcer. *American Journal of Medicine*, **83**(suppl. 3B), 95–99.

58. Martin, F., Farley, A., Gagnon, M. and Poitras, P. (1982) Comparative healing capacity of sucralfate and cimetidine in short term treatment of peptic ulcer. A double-blind randomized study (abstract). *Scandinavian Journal of Gastroenterology,* **17**(suppl. 78), 548.

59. Montgomery, R.D. and Cookson, J.B. (1972) The treatment of gastric ulcer. *Clinical Trials Journal,* **9**(1), 33–36.

60. Morales, A., Antezana, C., Roman, I. and Hurtado, C. (1982) Effecto de un derivado del bismuto (De-Nol) en la cicatrizacion de ulceras gastricas y duodenales. *Revista Medica de Chile,* **110**, 959–963.

61. Morelli, A., Pelli, A., Narducci, F. and Spadacini, A. (1979) Pirenzepine in the treatment of gastric ulcer. *Scandinavian Journal of Gastroenterology,* **14**(suppl. 57), 51–55.

62. Morgan, A.G., McAdam, W.A.F., Pacsoo, C., Walker, B.E. and Simmons, A.V. (1978) Cimetidine: an advance in gastric ulcer treatment? *British Medical Journal*, **ii**, 1323–1326.

63. Morgan, A.G., McAdam, W.A.F., Pacsoo, C. and Darnborough, A. (1982) Comparison between cimetidine and Caved-S in the treatment of gastric

ulceration, and subsequent maintenance therapy. *Gut*, **23**, 545–551.

64. Morgan, A.G., Pacsoo, C. and McAdam, W.A.F. (1985) Maintenance therapy: a two year comparison between Caved-S and cimetidine treatment in the prevention of symptomatic gastric ulcer recurrence. *Gut*, **26**(6), 599–602.

65. Morgan, A.G., Pacsoo, C., Taylor, P. and McAdam, W.A.F. (1987) Does Caved-S decrease the gastric ulcer relapse rate during maintenance therapy with ranitidine? *Alimentary, Pharmacology and Therapeutic*, **1**, 633–638.

66. Morgan, A.G., Pacsoo, C., Taylor, P. and McAdam, W.A.F. (1990) A comparison between enprostil and ranitidine in the management of gastric ulceration. *Alimentary, Pharmacology and Therapeutic.*

67. Mountford, R.A., Brown, P., Salmon, P.R., Alvarenga, C., Newman, C.S. and Read, A.E. (1980) Gastric cancer detection in gastric ulcer disease. *Gut*, **21**, 9–17.

68. Newton, K.A., Marks, I.N., Wright, J.P., Dent, D.M., Girdwood, A.H. and Lucke, W. (1986) Comparison of two different maintenance regimens of ranitidine in gastric ulcer disease. *South African Medical Journal*, **70**(part 1), 49.

69. Okabe, H., Inoue, K., Okabe, S. *et al.* (1987) A study of maintenance therapy with cimetidine on gastric ulcer relapse. *Current Therapeutic Research,* **41**(4), 478–491.

70. Orchard, R. and Elliot, C. (1981) A double-blind placebo controlled study of sucralfate in the treatment of gastric ulcer. In *Duodenal Ulcer, Gastric Ulcer. Sucralfate, A New Therapeutic Concept* (Ed.) Caspary, W.F. pp. 85–88. Baltimore: Urban and Schwarzenberg.

71. Osalladore, D., Chierichetti, S.M., Norberto, L. and Vibelli, C. (1979) Pirenzepine in severe duodenal ulcer and in gastric ulcer. *Scandinavian Journal of Gastroenterology*, **14**(suppl. 57), 33–39.

72. Parente, F., Lazzaroni, M., Petrillo, M. and Bianchi Porro, G. (1986) Colloidal bismuth subcitrate and ranitidine in the short-term treatment of benign gastric ulcer: an endoscopically controlled trial. *Scandinavian Journal of Gastroenterology,* **21**(suppl. 122), 42–45.

73. Penston, J.G. and Wormsley, K.G. (1990) Long-term maintenance treatment of gastric ulcers with ranitidine. *Alimentary, Pharmacology and Therapeutic.*

74. Pop, P., Nikkels, R.E., Dorrestein, G.C.M. *et al.* (1982) A study of the comparative healing rates of sucralfate and cimetidine in a short term treatment of duodenal and gastric ulcers. A single-blind randomized controlled Dutch–Belgian Multicentre Study. 2nd International Sucralfate Symposium. *7th World Congress of Gastroenterology, Stockholm, 1982.*

75. Poulantzas, J., Polymeropoulus, P.S. and Papasomatious, A. (1978) A double-blind evaluation of the effect of tri-potassium di-citrato

bismuthate in peptic ulcer. *British Journal of Clinical Practice*, **32**, 147–148.

76. Rey, J.-F. Legras, B., Verdier, A., Vicari, F. and Gorget, C. (1989) Comparative study of sucralfate versus cimetidine in the treatment of acute gastroduodenal ulcer: randomized trial with 667 patients. *American Journal of Medicine*, **86**(suppl. 6A), 116–122.

77. Rhodes, J., Mayberry, J.F., Williams, R.A. and Lowrie, B.W. (1981) Clinical trial of sucralfate in the treatment of gastric ulcer. In *Duodenal Ulcer, Gastric Ulcer. Sucralfate, A New Therapeutic Concept* (Ed.) Caspary, W.F. pp. 101–104. Baltimore: Urban and Schwarzenberg.

78. Schulman, A. and Simkins, K.C. (1975) The accuracy of radiological diagnosis of benign primary and secondary malignant ulcers and their correlation with three simplified radiological types. *Clinical Radiology*, **26**, 317–325.

79. Shou-Po, C. and Guo-Zong, P. (1986) Short-term treatment with colloidal bismuth subcitrate (De-Nol) and cimetidine in Chinese patients with gastric ulcer. *Clinical Trials Journal*, **23**, 215–219.

80. Simon, B., Muller, P. and Damman, H.G. (1982) Safety profile of ranitidine. *Scandinavian Journal of Gastroenterology*, **17**(suppl. 78) (abstract 359), 90.

81. Soltoft, J., Iversen, T.O., Linde, N.C., Rahbek, I. and Jacobsen, O. (1985) Kolloidal vismut subcitrat (De-Nol) labletter versus cimetidine ved behandling of ulcus ventriculi. *Ugeskrift für Laeger*, **147**, 1850–1851.

82. Sutton, D.R. (1982) Gastric ulcer healing with tripotassium dicitrato-bismuthate and subsequent relapse. *Gut*, **23**, 621–624.

83. Takemoto, T., Kimura, K., Okita, K. *et al.* (1987) Efficacy of sucralfate in the prevention of recurrence of peptic ulcer – double-blind multicentre study with cimetidine. *Scandinavian Journal of Gastroenterology*, **22**(suppl. 140), 49–60.

84. Takemoto, T., Namiki, M., Ishikawa, M. *et al.* (1989) Ranitidine and sucralfate as maintenance therapy for gastric ulcer disease: endoscopic control and assessment of scarring. *Gut*, **30**, 1692–1697.

85. Talley, N.J., McNeil, D. and Piper, D.W. (1987) Discriminant value of dyspeptic symptoms: a study of the clinical presentation of 221 patients with dyspepsia of unknown cause, peptic ulceration, and cholelithiasis. *Gut*, **28**, 40–46.

86. Tanner, A.R., Cowlishaw, J.L., Cowen, A.E. and Ward, M. (1979) Efficacy of cimetidine and tri-potassium dicitrato-bismuthate (De-Nol) in chronic gastric ulceration. *Medical Journal of Australia*, **1**, 1–2.

87. Turpie, A.G.G., Runcie, J. and Thompson, T.J. (1969) Clinical trial of deglycyrrhizinised liquorice in gastric ulcer. *Gut*, **10**, 199–302.

88. Tytgat, G.N.J., Van Bentem, N., Van Olffen, G. *et al.* (1982) Controlled trial comparing colloidal bismuth subcitrate tablets, cimetidine and placebo in the treatment of gastric ulceration. *Scandinavian Journal of Gastroenterology*, **17**(suppl. 80), 31–38.

89. Wilson, J.A.C. (1972) A comparison of carbenoxolone sodium and deglycyrrhizinated liquorice in the treatment of gastric ulcer in the ambulant patient. *The British Journal of Clinical Practice*, **26**(12), 563–566.

TREATMENT: SURGICAL *(C.W. Venables)*

While controversy still surrounds the best surgical procedure to perform for duodenal ulceration, Billroth I gastrectomy remains the most satisfactory operation for gastric ulceration. This is partly because of the reported results following gastrectomy[43] and partly because few surgeons deal with enough cases to evaluate any alternative procedure. In fact, our ability to evaluate alternative procedures has diminished even further in recent years with the advent of more effective medical treatments resulting in a diminished need for operative treatment.[35]

Johnston[22] suggested that gastric ulcers could be subdivided into three different types depending on the position of the ulcer within the stomach (*Figure 2.49*). These were:

- *Type I ulcer* – a chronic ulcer situated on or proximal to the gastric angulus (incisura) with no macroscopic evidence of duodenal, pyloric or prepyloric ulceration.
- *Type II ulcer* – a chronic gastric ulcer on or proximal to the angulus with an ulcer or scar in the duodenum or pyloric canal.
- *Type III ulcer* – a chronic ulcer occurring within 3 cm of the pylorus ('prepyloric ulcer') with or without duodenal ulceration, scarring or a type I ulcer.

Johnston demonstrated a difference between these three types of ulcer in respect to the patient's 12-hour and overnight basal acid secretion, blood group and physical characteristics.[23] He suggested that surgical treatment might differ with the type of ulcer present. However, his analyses were based on radiological examinations of the stomach, which are now known to underestimate the incidence of duodenal and prepyloric ulceration, and the author's studies on endoscopically confirmed ulcers (using a combined pentagastrin/insulin secretion test) have failed to confirm a consistent difference in stimulated secretion between these three types (*Figure 2.50*). It seems unlikely, therefore, that one can reliably decide the correct surgical approach to a gastric ulcer based entirely on its position. This is borne out by the poor results which have followed the treatment of type III ulcers by proximal gastric vagotomy.[1]

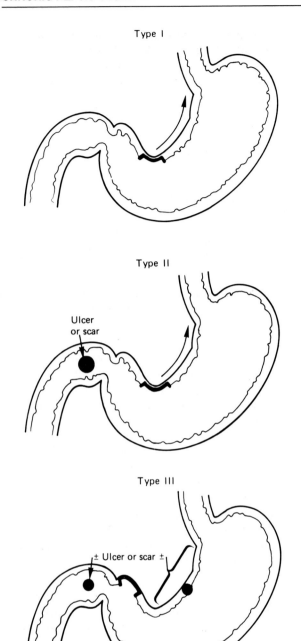

Figure 2.49 Types of gastric ulcer as described by Johnston (arrows indicate area where ulcer may occur).

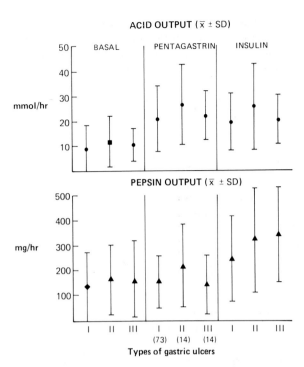

Figure 2.50 Mean basal, pentagastrin- and insulin-stimulated acid and pepsin outputs ($\pm$ standard deviation) recorded in 73 type I, 14 type II and 14 type III gastric ulcer patients studied in Newcastle (Freeman Hospital).

Indications for surgery

The indications for surgical treatment have been further refined by easy access to gastric endoscopic examination – which allows the exclusion of malignancy by biopsy and cytology – and by the introduction of more effective medical treatments.[36] They can now be defined as follows.

Failure to heal

This is now the main indication for surgical treatment. Healing is of particular importance in gastric ulceration. This is because such ulcers are much more likely to bleed, occur more commonly in the elderly – who withstand complications poorly – and may contain foci of malignancy undetected at the first biopsy. Furthermore, unhealed gastric ulcers can be asymptomatic – particularly when the patient is on a non-steroidal anti-inflammatory drug (NSAID), which also increases the risk of perforation or bleeding. For this reason it is the author's practice to always assess the healing of a gastric ulcer by repeat endoscopy and to recommend surgical treatment for an ulcer which remains unhealed after at least 3 months of effective medical treatment. This would now usually include treatment with bismuth subcitrate (De-Nol), a therapeutic course of an H_2 receptor antagonist and, most recently, omeprazole.

Failed long-term control

Gastric ulcers, like all chronic peptic ulcers, have a tendency to recur, although this is less common than with a duodenal ulcer unless the patient is on an ulcerogenic agent such as an NSAID. These recurrent ulcers are often asymptomatic and can only be detected by repeat endoscopy after healing. For this reason, and because such patients are often elderly, it is the author's practice to place all gastric ulcer patients on long-term maintenance therapy using a low dose of an H_2 receptor antagonist. Recent evidence suggests that if the presence of *Helicobacter pylori* is eliminated by a combined antibiotic and bismuth subcitrate treatment, one may be able to avoid the need for long-term maintenance therapy.[38] But this is still controversial and, for the moment, the author continues to use H_2 receptor antagonists to prevent recurrence.

Even with such therapy there are a few patients in whom the ulcer recurs. If this remains a problem it is the author's practice to recommend surgery. As these ulcers are often asymptomatic, endoscopic assessments to detect recurrence are repeated every 6 months in the first year and then annually. Such a regime has the additional advantage of allowing the detection of a malignancy missed during the healing period.

Side-effects or poor compliance

With the increased number of effective treatments available, 'side-effects' are now an extremely uncommon reason for recommending surgery.[3] However, there remain a few patients who for various reasons refuse to take regular treatment or find it impossible to do so. Whilst patients in this latter group often end up with poor results following an operation, a surgeon may find it extremely difficult to avoid operating under such circumstances.

Suspected malignancy/dysplasia

All gastric ulcers should be regarded as malignant until proved otherwise. For this reason, patients on medical treatment must have regular repeat endoscopies with biopsies from the ulcer edge and including brush cytology. If *severe* dysplasia is found in any of these biopsies, surgical treatment is now regarded as the correct treatment. This is because there is a high probability of a small focus of malignancy being present in the area of the ulcer or elsewhere within the stomach.

Social reasons

There are some patients for whom, because of their occupation or abode, it is safer to perform an operation than embarking on a long course of medical treatment.

Rationale of surgical treatment

The surgeon has only a limited range of options for the management of ulcer disease – either the physiological control of gastric secretion can be altered or varying amounts of gastric mucosa removed to reduce secretion and/or abnormal mucosa.

Gastric ulceration occurs when the balance between the erosive properties of the gastric juice and the intrinsic ability of the mucosa to resist digestion is disturbed. The surgeon can influence this balance either by altering the secretory mechanism or by removing diseased mucosa.

Alteration of physiological control

VAGOTOMY

Vagotomy will reduce the neural control of acid secretion by reducing the amount of acetylcholine released from the vagal nerve endings within the submucosa in response to nervous stimuli. In addition, it also reduces the sensitivity of the parietal and chief cells to other stimuli such as gastrin and histamine.

These changes are reflected in a reduction in 'basal' secretion and in the response of the stomach to food and other external stimuli. Division of the vagal trunks at the hiatus ('truncal vagotomy') also denervates the remainder of the intestinal tract and pancreaticobiliary systems with an incidence of side-effects such as dumping and diarrhoea. Antral denervation also impairs the 'antral pump' mechanism – responsible for controlling gastric emptying – leading to gastric retention. Proximal gastric vagotomy only divides the vagal branches to the secretory mucosa and thus results in fewer side-effects. Unfortunately, this latter form of vagotomy can be technically difficult or impossible when a gastric ulcer occurs on the lesser curve.

ANTRECTOMY

Gastrin is mainly produced within the antral mucosa, so removal of this area reduces hormonal stimulation of gastric secretion. Dragstedt[9] proposed that gastric ulceration was caused by impaired gastric emptying which resulted in an increased release of gastrin resulting in hypersecretion. Whilst this may explain the occasional gastric ulcer found in association with pyloric stenosis it has not been confirmed in the majority of patients with gastric ulcer disease.

Removal of diseased antral mucosa

There are several reasons for believing that the antral mucosa is abnormal in gastric ulceration. Severe atrophic chronic gastritis, often with intestinal metaplasia, is usually present in the antrum and extends up the lesser curve as far as the area of ulceration. These changes persist after ulcer healing and are therefore thought to be 'primary' rather than 'secondary' in type. A long-standing theory as to their cause is that of 'bile reflux'. Gastric ulceration has been shown to be associated with increased amounts of bile within the gastric lumen[10,39] and duodenal reflux can be observed during radiological examinations[5] and with BIDA (p-butyl-imido-diacetic acid) scans.

A more recent theory is that these changes are secondary to damage caused by infection of the stomach by *H. pylori*, which is usually present in chronic gastric ulcer patients (except those where the disease is caused by NSAIDs). This organism can induce an acute gastritis, which is reversed by eradication of the infection, but there is no convincing evidence that treatment of the organism will allow the antral mucosa to return to normal in patients with chronic gastric ulceration. The mechanism by which this damages the mucosa is unclear but is thought to be related to production of urea by the bacteria.

Whatever the exact mechanism there is no doubt that mucosa affected by chronic gastritis is more liable to ulceration.[40] Studies have shown that the mucus covering the antrum in such patients is mainly of an incomplete molecular form[46] which provides a poor defence against autodigestion by pepsin or traumatic damage. Measurements of electrical potential difference across the gastric mucosa have also suggested that there is an increased back-diffusion of hydrogen ions from the lumen and into the mucosa in such patients.

Types of operation (*Figure 2.51*)

Gastric resection alone

BILLROTH I GASTRECTOMY

This remains the most popular operation for gastric ulcer. Good results have been reported when only 3–4 cm of antrum have been removed[30] but most surgeons believe that all of the damaged antral mucosa and, if possible, the ulcer crater should be removed. Jensen *et al.*[18] suggested that the results of surgery were improved if intraoperative testing was used to determine the junction between the antral and body mucosa so that all of the antral mucosa were removed. Removal of the ulcer is relatively straightforward when it occurs in the area of the incisura but it can be extremely difficult when it occurs within a few centimetres of the oesophageal hiatus. In this latter situation the use of the 'Pauchet manoeuvre' – in which the ulcer is removed with a narrow tongue of the lesser curve – can be extremely helpful in avoiding removal of too much of the body of the stomach.[48] This should avoid some of the undesirable metabolic side-effects that occur from a near total gastrectomy.[15] After resection, a new

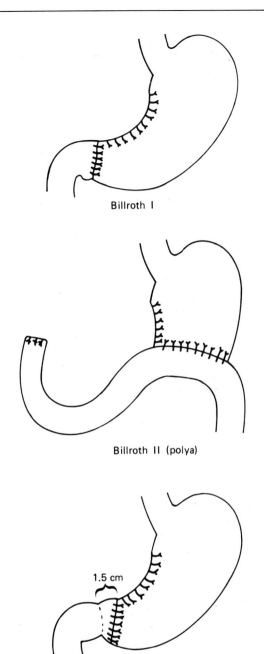

Figure 2.51 Diagrammatic representation of types of gastric resection used in gastric ulcer management.

lesser curve is constructed and an end-to-end anastomosis between the gastric remnant and the duodenum is performed.

BILLROTH II (POLYA) GASTRECTOMY

This operation is rarely used for gastric ulceration.[41] It is usually only performed when the gastric remnant is too small to easily reach the duodenum without tension or because the proximal duodenum is severely distorted or stenosed from previous duodenal ulceration or surgery. The major disadvantage of this procedure is that increased bile reflux is an inevitable consequence of the gastrojejunal anastomosis. This bile reflux can lead to 'bile vomiting' and may predispose to malignant change within the gastric remnant.

PYLORUS-PRESERVING GASTRECTOMY

This procedure was first described by Maki et al.[29] It is performed in a similar way to a Billroth I gastrectomy; the principal difference being that 1.5 cm of antrum is preserved proximal to the pylorus. It is clearly an inappropriate operation for type III gastric ulcers but has been used effectively for type I ulcers with good long-term results.[42]

Vagotomy and excision of the ulcer (*Figure 2.52*)

It is now widely accepted that if a vagotomy is to be used to treat a gastric ulcer it must be accompanied by excision of the ulcer itself to exclude malignancy. At one stage it was considered that a four quadrant biopsy from the ulcer was sufficient; however, follow-up studies have shown that there is still a risk of missing a focus of malignancy by this method. The ulcer can be excised either using a transgastric approach[6] or by an external excision, taking care

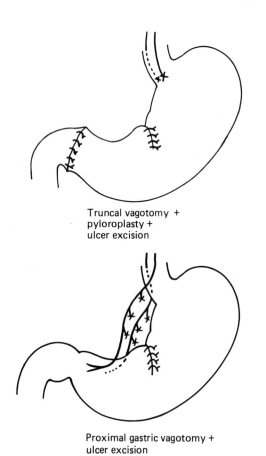

Truncal vagotomy +
pyloroplasty +
ulcer excision

Proximal gastric vagotomy +
ulcer excision

Figure 2.52 Diagrammatic representation of vagotomy procedures used in gastric ulcer management.

that the stomach closure does not result in a stenosis, particularly if the ulcer is near to the oesophageal hiatus.

TRUNCAL VAGOTOMY AND DRAINAGE

This is performed in an identical manner to that for a duodenal ulcer, the only addition being excision of the ulcer. On theoretical grounds a pyloroplasty is preferable to a gastroenterostomy as the drainage procedure, because the former is accompanied by less bile reflux.

PROXIMAL GASTRIC VAGOTOMY

This procedure is complicated by the scarring and oedema that occurs with an ulcer located along the lesser curve. It may be impossible under these circumstances to identify the 'nerve of Laterjet'. Johnston et al.[21] suggested that good results could be obtained if the division of the vagal nerve branches to the gastric body mucosa began just proximal to the ulcer. However, this procedure has not been widely accepted by others as there is a risk of inducing necrosis of the lesser curve.[13]

Results of operation

The ideal operation would be one that offered a certain 'cure' without any side-effects or operative mortality. Obviously no operation can meet these stringent criteria and it is for this reason that medical therapy is now commonly selected for most patients with gastric ulceration.

Type I gastric ulcer

This is the commonest type of gastric ulcer encountered in clinical practice. As a result the response to surgical treatment in such cases has been most studied. Such ulcers can be treated by Billroth I gastrectomy, truncal vagotomy and drainage, or by proximal gastric vagotomy alone (with ulcer excision).

Clearly, the ideal way to determine the best operation is by means of a 'surgical controlled trial'. Three such trials have been published (*Table 2.13*), two comparing gastrectomy against truncal vagotomy and pyloroplasty and one against proximal gastric vagotomy. Unfortunately, these trials include relatively small numbers of patients – which reflects the difficulty in recruiting large numbers of gastric ulcers – so it is necessary to examine other large series where only one type of operation has been performed.

These studies show that Billroth I gastrectomy provides the highest chance of cure but is associated with twice the mortality rate (4% overall). One of the problems in assessing these larger series is that

Table 2.13   Results of surgery for type I[a] gastric ulcer

	Number of patients	Mortality (%)	Recurrence (%)
Billroth I gastrectomy			
Salzer[41]	631	4	2
Hollender et al.[17]	228	3	0
Nielsen et al.[34]	97	6	5
Pichlmayr et al.[37]	109	0.7	5
Thomas et al.[43]	144	0.7	3.5
Madsen et al.[28]	20[b]	4	0
Duthie and Kwong[12]	50[b]	0	4
Duthie and Bransom[11]	30[b]	0	7
Total	1309	4	2
Truncal vagotomy and pyloroplasty			
Kronborg[26]	123	2	13
Draft et al.[25]	103	3	5
De Miguel[30]	73	0	19
Eastman and Gear[14]	58	0	8
Cade and Allen[4]	65	4	4.5
Madsen et al.[28]	23	0	13
Duthie and Kwong[12]	50	0	10
Proximal gastric vagotomy			
Duthie and Bransom[11]	26	0	15
Johnston and Axon[19]	104	1	5
Muller[33]	52	5	4
Total	677	2	9

[a] Johnston's classification: see text.[20]
[b] Randomized controlled trial.

they usually include 'all-comers' so that the mortality rate may be affected by some operations being performed as emergencies. This contrasts with controlled trials where only elective operations are performed.

Type II gastric ulcers

The incidence of this type of ulcer varies from 15 to 25% in different series. They tend to occur in a younger age group, have a higher male-to-female ratio and have many of the clinical features of duodenal ulcer disease.[8] For these reasons it has been suggested that they should be surgically treated as for duodenal ulcer (*Table 2.14*) although a recent review has concluded that proximal gastric vagotomy is no longer an acceptable operation as the recurrence rate is too high (33% at 10 years).[24]

Certainly, such an approach is supported by the fact that healing of both ulcers usually occurs during treatment with H_2 receptor antagonists, although

Table 2.14   Results of surgery for type II[a] gastric ulcer

	Number of patients	Type of operation	Recurrence (%)
Kronborg[26]	16	Truncal vagotomy and pyloroplasty	0
Johnston et al.[21]	25	Proximal gastric vagotomy	0
Pichlmayr et al.[37]	16	Billroth I gastrectomy	7
Pichlmayr et al.[37]	5	Proximal gastric vagotomy	20
Douglas and Duthrie[8]	39	Truncal vagotomy and pyloroplasty	0

[a] Johnston's classification: see text.[20]

Table 2.15   Results of surgery for type III[a] gastric ulcer

	Number of patients	Type of operation	Recurrence (%)
Anderson et al.[1]	59	Proximal gastric vagotomy	22
Becker and Siewert[2]	40	Proximal gastric vagotomy	20
Pichlmayr et al.[37]	15	Billroth I gastrectomy	0
Pichlmayr et al.[37]	32	Proximal gastric vagotomy	25
Kronborg[28]	78	Truncal vagotomy and pyloroplasty	6

[a]Johnston's classification: see text.[20]

the gastric ulcer may heal more slowly than the duodenal ulcer.

Type III gastric ulcers

It used to be considered that such ulcers could be treated as for a duodenal ulcer. However, there is now overwhelming evidence that prepyloric ulcers do not respond well either to proximal gastric vagotomy (*Table 2.15*) or to H_2 receptor antagonists. In addition, there is a relatively high incidence of malignancy in such ulcers. For this reason it is recommended that a Billroth I gastrectomy be performed with the addition of a vagotomy if either there is an active duodenal ulcer also present or the ulcer has failed to respond to prolonged medical therapy.

Side-effects of gastric surgery

Short-term effects

These usually become apparent within the first few months following operation. As far as the immediate period after operation is concerned, vagotomy procedures fair much better than gastrectomy. This is apparent in the controlled surgical trials, where postoperative bleeding, anastomotic dehiscence, gastric hold-up, intra-abdominal sepsis and pulmonary embolus are all more common after gastrectomy. As a result the mean length of hospital stay is longer for gastrectomy than for vagotomy procedures.

After hospital discharge, vagotomy-treated patients fair slightly worse, as temporary dysphagia and diarrhoea are more common than after gastrectomy. Gastrectomy is, however, associated with a slightly higher incidence of postoperative vomiting.

Medium-term side-effects

These include dumping, diarrhoea, vomiting and heartburn. Usually such symptoms are reported within the first year of follow-up but rarely, for some inexplicable reason, they can first appear several years later. All of these problems are encountered after all types of gastric surgery, so it is important to

determine whether they are more common after gastrectomy than after vagotomy.

In Newcastle the author has monitored the long-term sequelae of gastric operations. Patients were regularly reviewed in a gastric follow-up clinic and symptoms recorded in a standardized manner after all operations. As a result it has been possible to compare results after Billroth I gastrectomy for gastric ulcer (*Figure 2.53*) with those after truncal vagotomy and pyloroplasty for duodenal ulcer. These studies have shown that less than 15% of patients record any postoperative symptom at any follow-up interval after Billroth I gastrectomy; in addition, there is a tendency for the incidence of such symptoms to diminish with time. This contrasts with the author's results after truncal vagotomy and pyloroplasty, where the overall incidence of symptoms appeared to increase with time.[44] In addition, a detailed analysis reveals that even when postoperative symptoms are present they are usually only mild or moderate in severity and occur infrequently.

Comparing individual symptoms after gastrectomy versus vagotomy and pyloroplasty reveals that none is more common after gastrectomy and diarrhoea is much less common. These results are similar to those reported during controlled surgical trials where smaller numbers of patients were followed-up.[12,28]

It has not been the author's practice to use Visick grading in his studies as, like Hall et al.[16] he believes that such a grading system is too subjective and based upon a clinician's interpretation of results rather than a true reflection of the patient's views. However, it was the impression of all who worked in the author's follow-up clinic that patients were far happier after Billroth I gastrectomy than after truncal vagotomy – a view supported by Thomas et al.[43] who reported that 84% of their patients were in Visick grades I and 2 at a mean interval of 8.4 years after Billroth I gastrectomy.

Whilst a proximal gastric vagotomy may produce comparably good results, as far as postoperative symptoms are concerned, the increased recurrence rate and technical problems involved in performing

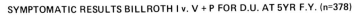

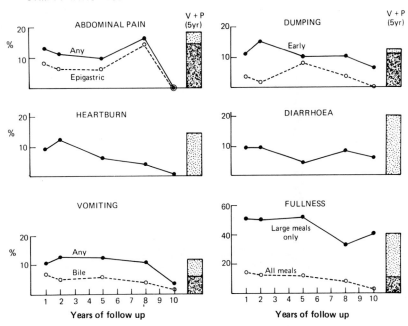

Figure 2.53 Prospective symptomatic results recorded in the author's gastric follow-up clinic in 99 patients treated by Billroth I gastrectomy for chronic gastric ulcer (28 followed up for at least 10 years). Results are compared with incidence of the same symptoms following vagotomy and pyloroplasty (V + P) at 5-year follow-up.

this operation make it unsuitable for the treatment of gastric ulcer.

Finally, a brief comment on the Maki operation is required. He has claimed excellent results but only a few other centres have used it[27,47] and there is insufficient information available to evaluate whether this offers any real advantage over the good results obtained by Billroth I gastrectomy.

Long-term side-effects

It is important to examine the long-term consequences of any gastric procedure, as patient's may live for over 30 years after their operation. It is well to remember that subtotal gastrectomy (as practised for many years for duodenal ulcer) was abandoned because of the serious long-term effects of this procedure. These included iron and vitamin B_{12} deficiency anaemia, malabsorption, metabolic bone disease and late carcinoma of the gastric remnant.

There are relatively few long-term reviews of gastric surgery for gastric ulceration. Thomas *et al.*[43] reviewed 144 patients treated by Billroth I gastrectomy after a mean interval of 9.4 years (range 3–15 years). They were unable to find evidence of significant metabolic side-effects after this operation. Their patients' weights had risen, on average, 4.4 kg, only 8% showed evidence of anaemia and there was no biochemical evidence of metabolic bone disease. Their results are supported by the author's own findings after the same operation (*Figures 2.54*

and *2.55*), where anaemia and iron deficiency were extremely uncommon and the small change in alkaline phosphatase level noted in the author's first analysis was later found to be due to changes in methodology.[45]

Finally, there is the question as to whether gastric carcinoma is a long-term consequence of operations for gastric ulcer.[6,7] Since the last edition of this book there have been a number of further publications on this question but, in spite of these, it remains an area of great controversy.[35] Overall, it seems that there is an increased risk of developing a stump carcinoma 15–20 years after gastric surgery and that this risk is greatest after operations for gastric ulcer rather than duodenal ulcer and after Billroth II (Polya) gastrectomy rather than Billroth I. Moller and Toftgaard[32] have recently claimed that at 25 years after gastric surgery the risk is 2.2 times that of a 'control' population but even their results have been questioned. Certainly the author has not encountered a case of 'stump cancer' in his long-term follow-up of gastric ulcer patients treated by Billroth I gastrectomy in Newcastle whilst he has seen carcinomas develop after vagotomy and pyloroplasty.

In conclusion, it would seem that Billroth I gastrectomy is not associated with any significant long-term side-effects which would militate against its use in the management of a gastric ulcer. If surgery is to be undertaken then this would appear to be the best operation to perform.

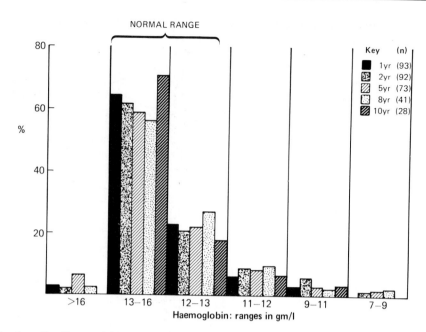

Figure 2.54 Analysis of results of haemoglobin measurements in the author's prospective studies of Billroth I gastrectomy. Results are expressed as the percentage of patients whose haemoglobin falls within the defined ranges at each follow-up interval.

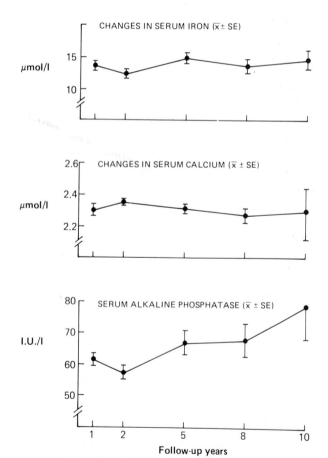

Figure 2.55 Mean ± standard error of serum iron, calcium and alkaline phosphatase levels at each follow-up interval in the author's prospective studies of Billroth I gastrectomy for gastric ulcer.

References

1. Andersen, D., Hostrup, H. and Amdrup E. (1978) Aarhus County Vagotomy Trials II: an interim report on reduction in acid secretion and ulcer recurrence following parietal cell vagotomy and selective vagotomy. *World Journal of Surgery*, **2**, 91–100.

2. Becker, H.D. and Siewart, J.R. (1980) Advances in ulcer disease. In *Excertia Medica* (Eds) Holtermuller, K.H. and Malagelada, J.R. pp. 516–526. Amsterdam: Elsevier.

3. Bloom, B.S. (1991) Cross-national changes in the effects of peptic ulcer disease. *Annals of Internal Medicine*, **114**, 558–562.

4. Cade, D. and Allan, D. (1979) Long term follow-up of patients with gastric ulcers treated by vagotomy, pyloroplasty and ulcerotomy. *British Journal of Surgery*, **66**, 46–47.

5. Capper, W.M., Airth, G.R. and Kilby, J.O. (1966) A test of pyloric regurgitation. *The Lancet*, **ii**, 621–623.

6. Chung, R.S. (1981) Transgastric approach to posterior juxta-esophageal gastric ulcer. *American Surgeon*, **47**, 247–250.

7. Domellof, L. and Janunger, K.G. (1977) The risk for gastric carcinoma after partial gastrectomy. *Journal of Surgery*, **134**, 581–584.

8. Douglas, M.C. and Duthie, H.L. (1971) Vagotomy for gastric ulcer combined with duodenal ulcer. *British Journal of Surgery*, **58**, 721–724.

9. Dragstedt, L.B. (1956) A concept of the aetiology of gastric and duodenal ulcers. *Gastroenterology*, **30**, 208–220.

10. Du Plessis, D.J. (1965) Pathogenesis of gastric ulceration. *The Lancet*, **i**, 974–978.

11. Duthie, H.L. and Bransom, C.J. (1979) Highly selective vagotomy with excision of the ulcer compared with gastrectomy for gastric ulcer in a randomised trial. *British Journal of Surgery*, **66**, 43–45.

12. Duthie, H.L. and Kwong, N.K. (1973) Vagotomy or gastrectomy for gastric ulcer. *British Medical Journal*, **iv**, 78–81.

13. DuToit, D.F. and Kemp, C.B. (1979) Lesser curve necrosis following PGV for GU. *South African Medical Journal*, **55**, 98–100.

14. Eastman, M.C. and Gera, M.W.L. (1979) Vagotomy and pyloroplasty for gastric ulcers. *British Journal of Surgery*, **66**, 238–241.

15. Gebhardt, C., Moschinski, D. and Usmiani, J. (1977) Die behandlung des kardianahen ulcus ventriculi. *Langgenbecks Archiv für Chirurgie*, **243**, 313–318.

16. Hall, R., Horrocks, H.C., Clamp, S.E. and DeDombal, F.T. (1976) Observer variation in assessment of results of surgery for peptic ulcer. *British Medical Journal*, **i**, 814–816.

17. Hollender, L.F., Bur, F., Peteghem, R.P. *et al.* (1978) Hat die Resektion nach Billroth I Beim Magengeschwur an Bedeutung verloren. *Zentrablatt fur Chirurgie*, **103**, 329.

18. Jensen, H.E., Badskaer, J., Andersen, B.N. and Johansen, A. (1979) Precise antrectomy. *World Journal of Surgery*, **3**, 765–773.

19. Johnston, D. and Axon, A.T.R. (1980) Long-term results of HSV in the treatment of benign gastric ulcer. *Gut*, **21**, A455.

20. Johnston, D., Humphrey, C.S., Smith, R.B. and Wilkinson, A.R. (1972) Treatment of gastric ulcer by highly selective vagotomy without a drainage procedure: an interim report. *British Journal of Surgery*, **59**, 787–792.

21. Johnston, D., MacDonald, R.C. and Axon, A.T.R. (1982) Highly selective vagotomy with ulcer excision. In *Vagotomy in Modern Surgical Practice* (Ed.) Baron, J.H. *et al.* pp. 197–201. London: Butterworth.

22. Johnston, H.D. (1975) The classification and principles of treatment of gastric ulcers. *The Lancet*, **ii**, 518–520.

23. Johnston, H.D., Love, A.H.G., Rogers, N.C. and Wyatt, A.P. (1964) Gastric ulcer, blood groups and acid secretion. *Gut*, **5**, 402–411.

24. Kelly, K.A. (1991) Operations for peptic ulcer (editorial). *Surgery*, **109**, 802–803.

25. Kraft, R.O., Myers, J., Overton, S. and Fry, W.J. (1971) Vagotomy and gastric ulcer. *American Journal of Surgery*, **121**, 122.

26. Kronberg, O. (1982) Truncal vagotomy and drainage for gastric ulcer. In *Vagotomy in Modern Surgical Practice* (Ed.) Baron, J.H. *et al.* pp. 195–197. London: Butterworth.

27. Liavag, I., Roland, M. and Broch, A. (1972) Gastric function after pylorus-preserving resection for gastric ulcer. *Acta Chirurgica Scandinavica*, **138**, 511–516.

28. Madsen, P., Kronborg, O., Hart-Hansen, O. and Pedersen, T. (1976) Billroth I gastric resection versus truncal vagotomy and pyloroplasty in the treatment of gastric ulcer. *Acta Chirurgica Scandinavica*, **142**, 151–153.

29. Maki, T., Shiratori, T., Hatafuku, T. and Sugawra, K. (1967) Pylorus-preserving gastrectomy as an improved operation. *Surgery*, **61**, 838–845.

30. Miguel, J. de (1975) Recurrence of gastric ulcer after selective vagotomy and pyloroplasty for chronic uncomplicated gastric ulcer. *British Journal of Surgery*, **62**, 875–878.

31. Miguel, J. de (1979) Pylorectomy and pre-pyloric antrectomy for gastric ulcer. *British Journal of Surgery*, **66**, 48–50.

32. Moller, H. and Toftgaard, C. (1991) Cancer occurrence in a cohort of patients surgically treated for peptic ulcer. *Gut*, **32**, 740–744.

33. Muller, C., Stadler, G.A. and Allgower, M. (1979) Die proximal selective vagotomie biem Ulcus Ventriculi selective proximale Vagotomie. In *Gastroenterologischer Symposium: Köln 1978*. Stuttgart: George Thieme.

34. Nielsen, J., Amdrup, E., Christiansen, P. *et al.* (1973) Gastric ulcer II: surgical treatment. *Acta Chirurgica Scandinavica*, **139**, 460–465.

35. Northfield, T.C. and Hall, C.N. (1990) Carcinoma of the gastric stump: risks and pathogenesis (editorial). *Gut*, **31**: 1217–1219.

36. Paimela, H., Tuompo, P.K., Perakyla, T., Saario, I., Hockerstedt, K. and Kivilaakso, E. (1991) Peptic ulcer surgery during the H2-receptor antagonist era: a population-based epidemiological study of ulcer surgery in Helsinki from 1972–1987. *British Journal of Surgery*, **78**, 28–31.

37. Pichlmayr, R., Lohlein, D. and Kujat, R. (1982) Vagotomy or partial gastric resection as elective treatment for gastric ulcer. In *Vagotomy in Modern Surgical Practice* (Ed.) Baron, J.H. *et al.* pp. 205–212. London: Butterworth.

38. Rauws, E.A.J. and Tytgat, G.N.J. (1990) Cure of duodenal ulcer associated with eradication of 'Helicobacter pylori'. *The Lancet*, **335**, 1233–1235.

39. Rhodes, J., Barnado, D.E., Phillips, S.F. *et al.* (1969) Increased reflux of bile into the stomach in patients with gastric ulcer. *Gastroenterology*, **57**, 241–252.

40. Ritchie, W.P. and Delaney, J.P. (1968) Pathogenesis of gastric ulcer: an experimental model. *Surgical Forum*, **19**, 312–313.

41. Salzer, G. (1967) Indikationen zur Resektion nach Billroth I und Billroth II Einschlieblich des Hochsitzenden ulcus. *Klinische Medsinische*, **22**, 13.

42. Sekine, T., Sato, T., Maki, T. and Shiratori, T. (1975) Pylorus-preserving gastrectomy for gastric ulcer: one to nine year follow-up study. *Surgery*, **77**, 92–99.

43. Thomas, W.G., Thompson, M.H. and Williamson, R.C.N. (1982) The long term outcome of Billroth I

partial gastrectomy for benign gastric ulceration. *Annals of Surgery*, **195**(2), 189–195.

44. Venables, C.W., Wheldon, E.J. and Cranage, J.D. (1980) Adverse effects of gastric surgery for peptic ulceration. *Journal of the Royal College of Physicians*, **14**, 173–177.

45. Venables, C.W., Wheldon, E.J. and Johnston, I.D.A. (1982) The long-term metabolic sequelae of truncal vagotomy and drainage. In *Vagotomy in Modern Surgical Practice* (Ed.) Baron, J.H. *et al.* pp. 288–293. London: Butterworth.

46. Younan, F., Pearson, J., Allen, A. and Venables, C.W. (1982) Changes in the structure of the mucous gel on the mucosal surface of the stomach in association with peptic ulcer disease. *Gastroenterology*, **82**, 827–831.

47. Zakrys, M. and Pawlowski, A. (1977) Pylorus preserving gastrectomy in the treatment of gastric ulcer. *Annales Universitatis Marie Curie-Sklodowsk*, **32**, 9–13.

48. Zhaoying, C., Weihan, L. and Qunying, C. (1980) Management of high-lying gastric ulcers. *Chinese Medical Journal*, **93**, 293–296.

CHRONIC DUODENAL ULCER

CLINICAL FEATURES   *(J. Calam and S.F. Moss)*

Symptoms

The principal symptom of duodenal ulcer disease is epigastric pain which wakes the patient at night, is altered by food, relieved by alkali and occurs in episodes. Patients also commonly complain of other symptoms, including heartburn, nausea, weight loss and abdominal distension,[5,7,9] and such atypical presentations and asymptomatic ulcers are relatively more common in the elderly and in patients taking non-steroidal anti-inflammatory drugs.[3,12,13] Much less frequently, patients present with symptoms of complications: haemorrhage, pyloric stenosis or perforation.

Pain

CHARACTER AND LOCATION

Descriptions of the character of the pain by the patient – 'sharp', 'dull', 'hunger', 'like a ball' and so on – are not particularly helpful. The pain is typically located in the epigastrium, but may be anywhere in the upper abdomen, particularly on the right. Pain below the umbilicus is very unlikely to be due to a duodenal ulcer. The pain tends to be localized and patients can often locate it by pointing: the 'pointing sign'. Radiation of the pain through to the back suggests that the ulcer is located posteriorly and penetrating towards the pancreas. Burning pain in the chest – heartburn – is associated with gastro-oesophageal reflux.

TEMPORAL ASPECTS

The pain very often wakes the patient at about 3 a.m. The patient then takes alkali, milk or food to gain relief. This is highly characteristic but must be distinguished from the exacerbations of gastro-duodenal reflux which occur on lying flat.

Pain due to duodenal ulceration tends to alter on ingestion of food. Usually it diminishes, but in some patients it gets worse. Patients who have received antacids or H_2 receptor antagonists usually describe a relief of symptoms, but response to such treatment may occur in dyspeptic patients whether or not they have a duodenal ulcer.[4] Very characteristically, the pain of duodenal ulcer disease occurs in exacerbations, which typically last for 1–4 weeks, interspersed with remissions which occur spontaneously and typically last for 1–6 months. Spontaneous healing and relapse of duodenal ulcer are observed during placebo-controlled trials; rates vary quite widely due to factors such as cigarette smoking and alkali ingestion.

PHYSIOLOGICAL ASPECTS OF PAIN

Although some aspects of the pain produced by duodenal ulcers is quite characteristic, our understanding of its physiological basis is rudimentary. It is not clear whether the pain is transmitted from the duodenum to the central nervous system via the afferent vagal fibres, by sympathetic connections including the coeliac plexus[2] or via intercostal innervation of the peritoneum. Some ideas are popular and may well be true. First that pain emanates from nerve endings at the edge of the ulcer crater which are stimulated by the inflammatory mediators released, such as bradykinin and prostaglandins. Secondly that diurnal exacerbations in the pain are largely due to low pH. Thus the postprandial elevation of intragastric pH, which is due to buffering by food, leads to relief of pain. Night pain may be related to basal hypersecretion for a long period without neutralisation by food. However, attempts to reproduce the pain by stimulating acid secretion with pentagastrin[1] or instilling acid into the duodenum of patients with duodenal ulcers[8,10,11] have met with variable results. In one of the studies pain was not reproduced reliably unless the ulcer was spontaneously symptomatic at the time.[1] It is not clear why some ulcers cause pain whereas others do not; it has been proposed that the pain originates in the oesophagus and is related to the incompetence of the lower oesophageal sphincter.[6]

Physical signs

Physical examination usually only reveals epigastric tenderness but is important in the exclusion of other conditions. The presence of a succussion splash after fasting suggests pyloric stenosis.

References

1. Bates, S., Sjoden, P.O., Fellenius, J. and Nyren, O. (1989) Blocked and non-blocked acid secretion and reported pain in ulcer, non-ulcer dyspepsia and normal subjects. *Gastroenterology*, **97**, 376–383.

2. Campbell, J.N., Raja, S.N., Cohen, R.H., Manning, D.C., Khan, A.A. and Meyer, R.A. (1989) Peripheral neural mechanisms of nociception. In *Textbook of Pain*, 2nd edn. (Eds) Wall, P.W. and Melzack, R.H. pp. 22–45. London: Churchill Livingstone.

3. Capurso, L., Dalmonte, P.R., Mazzeo, F. *et al.* (1984) Comparison of cimetidine 800 mg once daily and 400 mg twice daily in acute duodenal ulceration. *British Medical Journal*, **289**, 1418–1420.

4. Chatterji, A.N. (1980) A double blind and randomised placebo-controlled study of ranitidine in duodenal ulcer patients. *Hepatogastroenterology*, suppl. 299.

5. Earlam, R. (1976) A computerised questionnaire analysis of duodenal ulcer symptoms. *Gastroenterology*, **71**, 314–317.

6. Earlam, R. (1985) On the origin of duodenal ulcer pain. *The Lancet*, **i**, 973–974.

7. Edwards, F.C. and Coghill, N.F. (1968) Clinical manifestations in patients with chronic atrophic gastritis, gastric ulcer and duodenal ulcer. *Quarterly Journal of Medicine*, **37**, 337–360.

8. Harrison, A., Isenberg, J.I., Schapira, M. and Hagie, L. (1982) Most patients with active symptomatic duodenal ulcers fail to develop ulcer-type pain in response to gastroduodenal acidification. *Journal of Clinical Gastroenterology*, **4**, 105–108.

9. Horrocks, J.C. and de Dombal, F.T. (1978) Clinical presentation of patients with 'dyspepsia'. Detailed symptomatic study of 360 patients. *Gut*, **19**, 19–26.

10. Joffee, S.N. and Primrose, J.N. (1983) Pain provocation test in peptic duodenitis. *Gastrointestinal Endoscopy*, **29**, 282–284.

11. Kang, J.Y., Yap, I., Guan, R. and Tay, H.H. (1986) Acid perfusion of duodenal ulcer craters and ulcer pain: a controlled double blind study. *Gut*, **27**, 942–945.

12. Penston, J.G. and Wormsley, K.G. (1990) Asymptomatic duodenal ulcers – implications of heterogeneity (review). *Alimentary Pharmacology and Therapeutics*, **4**, 557–567.

13. Scapa, E., Horowitz, M., Waron, M. and Eshchar, J. (1989) Duodenal ulcer in the elderly. *Journal of Clinical Gastroenterology*, **11**, 502–506.

INVESTIGATIONS (J. Calam and S.F. Moss)

Because of the low sensitivity and specificity of symptoms and signs[6,7,14,19] the diagnosis of duodenal ulcer requires definitive investigation. Endoscopy is superior as regards sensitivity and specificity and allows biopsies to be obtained, but double-contrast barium radiology is generally satisfactory and better tolerated. Both investigations are operator dependent and the strategy chosen will depend on local resources but should probably include one of the methods for the diagnosis of *Helicobacter pylori* infection.

Barium meal

A duodenal ulcer is seen as a collection of barium in a crater on several films (*Figure 2.56*). Scarring of the duodenum, which is a feature of chronic duodenal ulcer disease, can either obscure an ulcer or create the illusion that one is present. In one study, only 60% of ulcers were detected and 20% of positive results were false.[9] Small ulcers, less than 5 mm in diameter, were even more difficult to diagnose. Comparison with endoscopy has shown that barium studies are not as accurate as endoscopy.[3,5,17]

Endoscopy

Modern endoscopes have made it possible to inspect all of the duodenal bulb mucosa directly, although some skill is required if there is pyloric stenosis and at the junction of the first and second parts of the duodenum. The ulcer craters and associated inflammation are readily seen (*Figure 2.57*). It should be borne in mind that the sedation used can cause respiratory depression and cardiac arrhythmias.[13] It has become usual in clinical trials to define duodenal ulcers as having a diameter of at least 5 mm although many duodenal ulcers are smaller. It is common to find many tiny 'salt and pepper' ulcers in the duodenum of dyspeptic patients who may at other times have larger ulcers.

Measurement of acid and gastrin

Patients with duodenal ulcer disease tend to secrete more gastric acid but there is considerable overlap with the normal population (see Epidemiology and aetiology, p. 246) and the measurement of acid secretion is not necessary in ordinary duodenal ulcer disease. The Zollinger–Ellison syndrome is too rare to justify routine gastrin measurement. However, if ulceration is atypical in location, unusually aggressive or relapses particularly promptly when therapy is

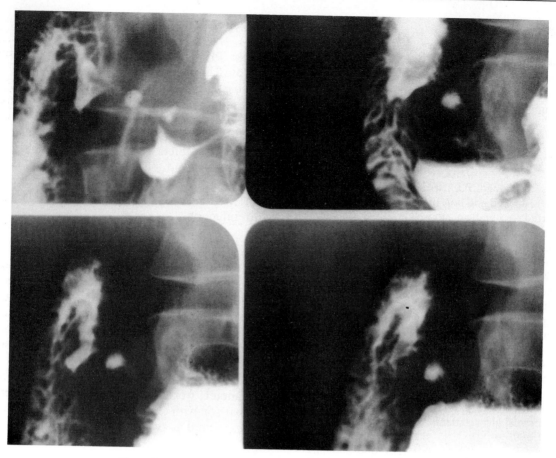

Figure 2.56 Barium meal demonstrating ulceration in the duodenal bulb.

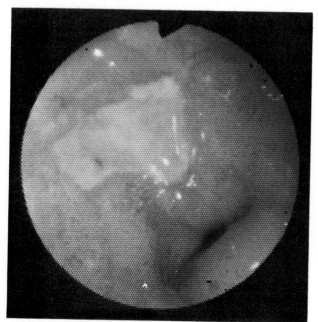

Figure 2.57 Endoscopic appearance of duodenal ulceration. (Reproduced, with permission, from Schiller *et al.* (1986) *A Colour Atlas of Gastrointestinal Endoscopy*, London: Chapman and Hall.)

stopped then fasting gastrin should be measured once the effects of acid-suppressing drugs have worn off.

Diagnosis of H. pylori

Investigation of duodenal ulcer disease should also involve determining whether *H. pylori* is present because the eradication of this organism greatly prolongs remissions of duodenal ulcer disease. Gastric *H. pylori* may be detected at endoscopy, by breath test or by serology.

Culture of *H. pylori* from endoscopic biopsies

The organism may be cultured from one or two biopsies.[4,10,11] Obviously, the biopsy forceps and endoscope should be free from organisms and antiseptics. For maximum sensitivity, biopsies should be placed in a transport medium such as cystine brucella broth. If there is to be any delay the specimen should be kept at 4°C until processing, which should in any case be within 4 hours. Microaerophilic incubation for several days on enriched medium is required for growth of the organism.

The biopsy urease test

A number of recipes and kits are available. All are based on the pH change which occurs when the organism's urease splits urea to release ammonia.[16] Two biopsies are taken 1–2 cm from the pylorus on the greater curve and placed in a solution containing urea, a pH indicator, a buffer and a bacteriostatic agent. The latter is added to make sure that only preformed urease is detected and to suppress extraneous urease-forming organisms that might spoil the medium before its use. The incubation time varies from test to test.[1] The time taken for the change to take place may reflect the number of organisms present.

Histological diagnosis of *H. pylori* infection

Handling should be kept to a minimum because it may remove the mucus layer which contains the organisms. Fixation in formalin is satisfactory. Silver staining using the Warthin–Starry method is excellent but expensive, and other stains, including modified Giemsa and haematoxylin and eosin, are suitable for routine work.[20] Immunological methods of staining are more specific for *H. pylori*, but are also more cumbersome and expensive, and generally unnecessary.

Non-invasive tests for *H. pylori*

UREASE BREATH TESTS

The subject ingests isotopic carbon-labelled urea and any carbon dioxide that is produced by urease can then be detected in the breath. [14]C emits a small amount of radiation but is inexpensive and conveniently counted in a β counter.[2] [13]C is not radioactive so that repeated studies are safe, but it is more expensive and requires a mass spectrometer for its detection.[12] The urea is given with a nutrient-dense meal in order to delay gastric emptying – this maximizes exposure of the organism to urea. These tests are becoming more convenient now that the duration of breath collection may be reduced to less than 1 hour.[15]

SEROLOGY

Early tests tended to cross-react with *Campylobacter jejuni*. Second-generation enzyme-linked immunosorbent assays that detect IgG antibodies to specific preparations of *H. pylori* proteins, including urease, appear to be both specific and sensitive.[8,18] Levels fall on eradication and rise again on reinfection. Serology is convenient but is slower than other tests to respond to changes in *H. pylori* status.

Practical aspects of testing for *H. pylori*

All of the various tests are satisfactory and the choice will usually depend upon the resources available. If endoscopy is to be performed then biopsies may conveniently be taken for histology, the urease test and culture. Tests based on only two biopsies occasionally give false negative results in patients with a few organisms because the bacteria are typically distributed in patches. The breath tests do not have this problem, and are probably best for showing that *H. pylori* is truly absent.

Differential diagnosis

Common conditions which need to be distinguished from duodenal ulcer disease include oesophagitis, gastric ulcer, gastritis and cancer, gallstones, pancreatitis, the irritable bowel syndrome, non-ulcer dyspepsia and symptoms due to alcohol or drugs.

Less common causes of peptic ulcers in the duodenum include mastocytosis, in which histamine is presumably responsible for gastric acid hypersecretion, the Zollinger–Ellison syndrome and pancreatic insufficiency, where relatively less alkali is secreted into the duodenum.

'Non-peptic' ulcers of the duodenum may be due to inflammatory conditions such as Crohn's disease and tuberculosis, vasculitides and tumours, particularly lymphoma.

References

1. Arvind, A.S., Cook, R.S., Tabaqchali, S. and Farthing, M.J. (1988) One-minute endoscopy room test for *Campylobacter pylori*. *The Lancet*, **i**, 704.
2. Bell, G.D., Weil, J., Harrison, G. *et al.* (1987) ^{14}C urea breath analysis, a non-invasive test for *Campylobacter pylori* in the stomach. *The Lancet*, **i**, 1367–1368.
3. Brown, P., Salmon, P.R., Burwood, R.J., Knox, A.J., Clendinnen, B.J. and Read, A.E. (1978) The endoscopic, radiological and surgical findings in chronic duodenal ulceration. *Scandinavian Journal of Gastroenterology*, **13**, 557–560.
4. Dent, J.C. and McNulty, C.A. (1988) Evaluation of a new selective medium for *Campylobacter pylori*. *European Journal of Clinical Microbiology and Infectious Diseases*, **7**, 555–558.
5. Dooley, C.P., Larson, A.W., Stace, N.H. *et al.* (1984) Double-contrast barium meal and upper gastrointestinal endoscopy: a comparative study. *Annals of Internal Medicine*, **101**, 538–545.
6. Earlam, R. (1976) A computerised questionnaire analysis of duodenal ulcer symptoms. *Gastroenterology*, **71**, 314–317.
7. Edwards, F.C. and Coghill, N.F. (1968) Clinical manifestations in patients with chronic atrophic gastritis, gastric ulcer and duodenal ulcer. *Quarterly Journal of Medicine*, **37**, 337–360.
8. Evans, D.J., Evans, D.G., Graham, D.Y. and

   Klein, P.D. (1989) A sensitive and specific
   serological test for *Campylobacter pylori* infection.
   Gastroenterology, **96**, 1004–1008.

9. Gelfand, D.W., Gale, W.J., Ott, D.J., Wu, W.C.
   and Meschan, I. (1985) The radiological detection
   of duodenal ulcers: effects of examiner variability,
   ulcer size and location, and technique. *American
   Journal of Roentgenology*, **145**, 551–553.

10. Goodwin, C.S. (1989) Campylobacter pylori:
    detection and culture. In Campylobacter pylori *and
    Gastroduodenal Disease* (Eds) Rathbone, B.J. and
    Heatley, R.V. pp. 60–62. Oxford: Blackwell.

11. Goodwin, C.S., Blincow, E.D., Warren, J.R. *et al.*
    (1985) Evaluation of culture techniques for
    Campylobacter pyloridis from endoscopic biopsies
    of gastric mucosa. *Journal of Clinical Pathology*, **38**,
    1127–1131.

12. Graham, D.Y., Evans, D.J., Alpert, L.C. *et al.*
    (1987) *Campylobacter pylori* detected non-
    invasively by the ^{13}C-urea breath test. *The Lancet*,
    i, 1174–1176.

13. Hart, R. and Classen, M. (1990) Complications of
    diagnostic gastrointestinal endoscopy. *Endoscopy*,
    22, 229–233.

14. Horrocks, J.C. and de Dombal, F.T. (1978) Clinical
    presentation of patients with 'dyspepsia'. Detailed
    symptomatic study of 360 patients. *Gut*, **19**, 19–26.

15. Logan, R., Dill, S., Walker, M. *et al.* (1990) The
    detection of H. pylori using a European standard 13
    carbon breath test (abstract). *Revista Espanola de
    Enfermedades Digestivas*, **78**(suppl. 1), 14.

16. McNulty, C.A., Dent, J.C., Uff, J.S., Gear, M.W.
    and Wilkinson, S.P. (1989) Detection of
    Campylobacter pylori by the biopsy urease test: an
    assessment in 1445 patients. *Gut*, **30**, 1058–1063.

17. Martin, T.R., Vennes, J.A., Silvis, S.E. and Ansel,
    H.J. (1980) A comparison of upper gastrointestinal
    endoscopy and radiography. *Journal of Clinical
    Gastroenterology*, **2**, 21–25.

18. Newell, D.G. and Stacey, A.R. (1989) Antigens for
    serodiagnosis of *Campylobacter pylori* infection.
    Gastroenterology Clinical Biology, **13**, 37B–41B.

19. Sjodin, I., Svedlund, J., Dotevall, G. and Gillberg,
    R. (1985) Symptom profiles in chronic peptic ulcer
    disease. A detailed study of abdominal disease and
    mental symptoms. *Scandinavian Journal of
    Gastroenterology*, **20**, 419–427.

20. Wyatt, J.I. and Gray, S.F. (1989) Detection of
    Campylobacter pylori by histology. In
    Campylobacter pylori *and Gastroduodenal Disease*
    (Eds) Rathbone, B.J. and Heatley, R.V. pp. 63–68.
    Oxford: Blackwell.

TREATMENT: MEDICAL *(J. Calam and S.F. Moss)*

As effective ulcer healing regimes have been developed the relative importance of general measures
has diminished. However, it has become apparent
during controlled trials that cigarette smoking both
delays ulcer healing and increases rates of relapse;[23,32,42,43] an effect most evident in the placebo-
treated group. Similarly, excessive alcohol ingestion
should be discouraged. It is associated with failure of
medical therapy,[15] though this may be due to the
known poor compliance rate in alcoholics. Interestingly, in one study, moderate drinkers had less
ulcers than teetotallers.[42] Non-steroidal anti-
inflammatory drugs should be avoided if possible
because their use is associated with further ulceration (see Epidemiology and aetiology, p. 246),
though they have not definitely been shown to
impair healing. Psychological stress can cause ulcers
but most patients cannot change their lifestyle and
this is in any case no longer necessary. Similarly,
although there is some evidence that wheat fibre
protects patients from ulcers,[28] the efficacy of current medical therapy has relegated the importance
of diet.

Healing the ulcer

General considerations
Duodenal ulcers are healed quite rapidly by a variety of regimes. H_2 receptor antagonists are currently by far the most widely used. One strange
aspect is that many quite different regimes have
appeared to produce similar healing rates. This is to
some extent explained by statistical considerations
which mean that huge studies are necessary to show
small differences. However, it is necessary to estimate whether small differences in efficacy justify
large differences in price. Also, although the initial
aim is to heal the ulcer the use of a regime which also
prolongs remission is clearly desirable. It is quite
clear that compliance is an important determinant of
the success of therapy. Factors which improve
compliance include simple regimes, explanation,
encouragement, and calendar packs.

Specific regimes
Broadly speaking, drugs used in the treatment of
chronic duodenal ulcer disease may work in four
different ways. They may buffer gastric acid (antacids), inhibit gastric acid secretion (H_2 receptor
antagonists and proton pump inhibitors), enhance
mucosal defence mechanisms or suppress *H. pylori*.
Some drugs have more than one effect.

ANTACIDS
Antacids predominantly act by buffering gastric
acidity, though a cytoprotective effect may also be
important.[18] Antacids cure ulcers and relieve symptoms but they have a large number of side-effects
when taken chronically and their use has declined

with the development of safer and more powerful agents.

H₂ RECEPTOR ANTAGONISTS
Mechanism of ulcer healing
These agents heal ulcers by inhibiting the stimulatory effect of histamine on peptic and parietal cells. By doing so they also effectively inhibit stimulation by gastrin, acetylcholine and the vagus nerve. Ulcers are believed to heal because the corrosive and proteolytic effects of acid and pepsin are withdrawn.

Doses, efficacy and side-effects
The characteristics of the different agents are given in *Table 2.16*. They have been shown to be equally effective when taken once daily or in divided doses.

Studies which compared the healing rates produced by the different agents have shown no appreciable differences between them.[10] The complete healing rates average 78% after 4 weeks and 92% after 8 weeks of treatment. Side-effects are rare[10] and include biochemical hepatitis and gynaecomastia. The latter is more common with cimetidine than ranitidine and has not been noted with the others. Numerous drug interactions have been reported, particularly with cimetidine, and are principally due to the competition between cimetidine and some other drugs for metabolism by the hepatic cytochrome P-450 enzyme system. These interactions become clinically important with warfarin, theophylline and phenytoin because their action is prolonged. An expected side-effect secondary to the inhibition of gastric acid secretion is an elevation of the plasma gastrin concentration. This is mild and of no clinical significance.

PROTON PUMP INHIBITORS – OMEPRAZOLE
Nature and mechanism of action
Omeprazole is a substituted benzimidazole. It acts by inhibiting the H^+/K^+-ATPase located on the luminal border of parietal cells which pumps hydrogen ions into the lumen in exchange for potassium ions. Omeprazole is a prodrug which is both concentrated and activated by the low pH within the acid canaliculus of the parietal cell[49] and its effect disappears over about 72 hours when all the proton pumps have been replaced by de novo synthesis. The elevation of luminal pH which is produced by omeprazole prevents the activation of pepsin. Doses of 20 mg daily produce more profound inhibition of gastric acid secretion than the usual doses of H₂ receptor antagonists; typically elevating the intragastric pH value above 4 for all but 3 hours of the day.[35] The rate of healing of duodenal ulcers by omeprazole 20 mg/day is consequently greater than that of ranitidine 300 mg daily.[20]

Side-effects
Omeprazole rarely produces side-effects, but has been reported to interact with cytochrome P-450, thereby affecting the metabolism of some other drugs. The administration of large doses of omeprazole to rats during toxicity testing led to massive hypergastrinaemia, which in turn caused growth of gastric enterochromaffin-like cells, leading in some cases to gastric carcinoid tumours. Similar changes occur very occasionally in patients who secrete no acid because they have atrophic gastritis. Though this initially caused some anxiety with regard to the safety of omeprazole it has been found that clinical doses only produce an approximately three-fold elevation of plasma gastrin concentrations in humans, and have no effect on enterochromaffin-like cells.[6]

MUCOSAL PROTECTION – SUCRALFATE
Nature and mechanism of action
This sucrose aluminium sulphate compound was initially developed as a pepsin inhibitor, based on the observation that certain sulphated carbohydrates could inhibit the actions of pepsin. Sucralfate has other potentially ulcer-healing cytoprotective effects. It increases mucosal blood flow and bicarbonate secretion, stimulates endogenous prostaglandin synthesis, enhances cellular proliferation and increases the binding of salivary epidermal growth factor to the ulcer base.[45]

Table 2.16 Comparison of H₂ receptor antagonists for the treatment of duodenal ulcer

| Drug | Daily healing dose (mg) | Serum half-life (hours) | % Excretion of oral drug | | Effect on cytochrome P-450 |
			Hepatic	Renal	
Cimetidine	800	2	60	40	Marked
Ranitidine	300	2	73	27	Mild
Nizatidine	300	1.5	22	78	Negligible
Famotidine	40	3	75	25	Negligible

Dose, efficacy and side-effects
The dose is 1 g four times per day, 1 hour before meals and at night. Constipation is the only common side-effect. Less than 2% of the dose is absorbed and although aluminium toxicity has not been reported it should be used cautiously in patients with renal impairment. In clinical trials sucralfate has generally produced healing of duodenal ulcer disease at a rate which is not significantly different from the H_2 receptor antagonists.[24]

ANTIMICROBIALS – BISMUTH SUBCITRATE (TRIPOTASSIUM DICITRATO BISMUTHATE, BISMUTH CHELATE)
Nature and mechanism of effect
Bismuth subcitrate contains bismuth in a chelated form which diminishes, but does not altogether prevent, its systemic absorption. It is still not altogether clear how bismuth subcitrate heals duodenal ulcers. Like sucralfate it has a number of useful actions: it combines with ulcer slough and might thus protect the crater,[21] increases prostaglandin synthesis,[22] decreases peptic activity[1] and increases mucus secretion. In addition, it has specific effects on *H. pylori*, which is now believed to play an important role in the aetiology of duodenal ulcers. Bismuth subcitrate accumulates on the surface of the bacterium[29] and has a bactericidal effect,[27] possibly by interacting with the organism's urease enzyme. At present it is not clear how bismuth subcitrate heals duodenal ulcers. It is probable that *H. pylori* causes tissue damage by releasing toxins or by inducing inflammation. Though the eradication of *H. pylori* is important in preventing ulcer relapse, rates of ulcer healing do not depend on whether *H. pylori* is eradicated or not. Treatment with bismuth subcitrate only completely eradicates *H. pylori* in about 20% of patients but invariably suppresses *H. pylori*.[36] There is no evidence that gastric secretion of acid or pepsin is directly altered by bismuth subcitrate.

Dose, efficacy and side-effects
Bismuth subcitrate is available in liquid and tablet forms and should be taken on an empty stomach. The dose is either 240 mg twice daily, 30 minutes before breakfast and the evening meal, or 120 mg four times daily taken 30 minutes before all three meals and 2 hours after the evening meal. Healing of duodenal ulcers occurs at a similar rate to healing on H_2 receptor antagonists.[26,50] There is some evidence that pain relief is slower on bismuth subcitrate than on H_2 receptor antagonists, but this has been disputed. Bismuth subcitrate blackens the stools, and the liquid may also blacken the tongue and teeth, but other side-effects are rare. Bismuth subcitrate is

contraindicated in renal failure; some bismuth is absorbed and bismuth is detectable in the urine up to 2 weeks after a course of bismuth subcitrate.[14] Bismuth encephalopathy has only occurred after overdose or in renal failure.

PROSTAGLANDINS – MISOPROSTOL
Nature and mechanism of action
Misoprostol is an analogue of the naturally occurring prostaglandin E_1. It inhibits gastric acid secretion but to a lesser extent than H_2 receptor antagonists.[33,51] It shares the ability of prostaglandins to prevent mucosal injury. Prostaglandins probably produce cytoprotection via several mechanisms, including the stimulation of secretion of bicarbonate and mucus and mucosal blood flow.[19] Prostaglandin synthesis is diminished in the duodenal mucosa of patients with duodenal ulcer disease[19] and non-steroidal anti-inflammatory drugs diminish prostaglandin synthesis by inhibiting the enzyme cyclo-oxygenase. Despite the theoretical advantages of prostaglandin analogues their ability to heal duodenal ulcers is predominantly due to their inhibition of acid secretion.[17]

Dose, efficacy and side-effects
To heal ulcers, $800 \mu g$ is taken daily in divided doses. Healing rates are comparable to those achieved by H_2 receptor antagonists after 4 weeks but pain relief was inferior with misoprostol.[34] Misoprostol effectively heal duodenal ulcers in patients taking non-steroidal anti-inflammatory drugs[40] but whether they are more effective than other agents in this respect is unknown. Misoprostol can cause uterine contractions and is contraindicated in pregnancy. It can also cause menorrhagia and hypotension. In practice, the most frequent side-effect is diarrhoea, which is self-limiting and dose-dependent.

LIQUORICE DERIVATIVES
The liquorice derivatives carbenoxolone and deglycyrrhizinized liquorice (Caved-S) have some ulcer-healing effect. In the case of carbenoxolone this may be due to the stimulation of mucus secretion. However, neither the mechanisms of action nor the efficacy of these preparations have been studied in sufficient detail to allow them to compete with more recent remedies. Carbenoxolone is probably not as effective as cimetidine in healing duodenal ulcers and can produce serious hypokalaemia and fluid retention through an aldosterone-like effect.

Duration of healing regimens
In practice, several different approaches are used to determine the duration of therapy. Drug manufacturers recommend treatment for set periods of any-

thing from 4 to 12 weeks (duogastrone) whilsts purists may treat until endoscopy has shown healing. This is mandatory for gastric ulceration, where there is a risk of malignancy, but not in duodenal ulcer disease. Alternatively, the doctor, and particularly the patient, may decide to treat until the symptoms disappear – though ulcer healing may be slower, this method is cheaper, with comparable symptom relief to conventional regimens.[46]

Treatment failures

If an ulcer fails to heal on an H_2 receptor antagonist then there is a choice of continuing the same dose for longer, increasing the dose or changing to a different drug. There is evidence to support all these approaches.[5,20,48]

Keeping the ulcer healed

It is relatively easy to heal most duodenal ulcers but control or prevention of recurrence is now the more important challenge. Until recently, discussion of this problem has centred on the use of H_2 receptor antagonists versus surgery but there is now exciting evidence that long remissions or even 'cure' of duodenal ulcer disease may be obtained by eradication of *H. pylori*.

Histamine H_2 receptor antagonists

These may be used in several ways.

MAINTENANCE THERAPY

Administration of half of the healing dose as a single dose at night is highly effective in preventing recurrence[2,44] and its complications.[3] The efficacy of the different agents has been compared by multicentre trials and show ranitidine to be superior to cimetidine at reducing recurrence rates over a year.[12,41] Patients appear to accept the need to take daily medication, but maintenance therapy is an expensive exercise, as cost per month is replaced by cost per year.

'ON DEMAND' THERAPY

Here, treatment is taken only when symptoms occur, with details of the regimen decided either by the patients or by the doctor. This is likely to lead to further courses of treatment being taken without delay for recurrences. The drug may also be taken for non-ulcer dyspepsia, for which H_2 receptor antagonists are effective – the relationship of dyspepsia to the presence of an ulcer being variable.

Regimens for eradication of *H. pylori*

In 1981, Martin *et al.* made the remarkable observation that duodenal ulcers remain healed for longer

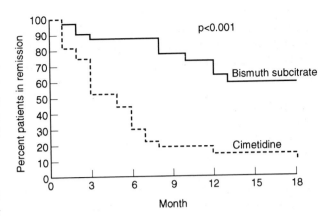

Figure 2.58 Relapse rates of duodenal ulcers after healing with cimetidine or colloidal bismuth subcitrate. (Reproduced, with permission, from Martin *et al.*[31])

after they have been healed with bismuth subcitrate compared with cimetidine[31] (*Figure 2.58*). This finding has since been confirmed by others[7] and may be explained by the discovery of *H. pylori*. It was found that the duration of remission of duodenal ulcer disease is greatly increased if *H. pylori* is eradicated[4,30,37] (*Figure 2.59*). It is rare for ulcers to recur unless the patient has been reinfected with *H. pylori*. It is therefore likely that *H. pylori* is a cause – perhaps the most important cause – of recurrence of duodenal ulcer disease.

Studies of the eradication of *H. pylori* have revealed a number of important points. Bismuth and many antibiotics kill *H. pylori in vitro* but, when patients are given bismuth subcitrate alone, *H. pylori* is generally only suppressed, reappearing within a few days in about 80% of cases when bismuth subcitrate is stopped. Eradication is now

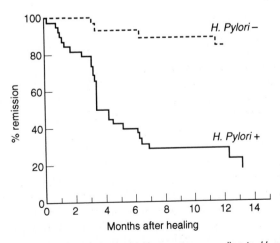

Figure 2.59 Duodenal ulcer relapse rates according to *H. pylori* status after initial ulcer healing. (Modified, with permission, from Marshall *et al.*[30])

defined as the absence of the organism 4 weeks after the cessation of therapy, as patients who are free of the organism at that time usually remain free after 1 year.[38] When patients are given single antibiotics without bismuth subcitrate, *H. pylori* rapidly develops resistance, so that more than one drug is required for successful eradication.

Effectiveness *in vivo* is highly dependent on whether the drug reaches and works in the microenvironment of *H. pylori*. The nitroimidazoles such as metronidazole are secreted in gastric juice and are active at a low pH and, consequently, they are included in most regimens. However, the use of metronidazole for the treatment of infections has led to the emergence of resistant strains of *H. pylori*. In the West, about 20% of strains are now resistant to metronidazole and the figure rises to 80% in parts of Africa.[11]

An international working party recently considered the optimum regimen and recommended bismuth subcitrate 120 mg 4 times daily, metronidazole 400 mg three times a day and tetracycline 500 mg 4 times daily, all to be given for 2 weeks for eradication[8] although bismuth subcitrate may be given for up to 8 weeks if ulcer healing is also required. Amoxycillin may be used as an alternative to tetracycline, but may be less well tolerated. The regime is quite complicated and success depends to a large extent on compliance but it typically achieves eradication rates of about 80%.

Sucralfate

Some studies have shown that remissions are longer after sucralfate compared with H_2 receptor antagonists[24,47] although this has not been consistently found. The reason for this is not clear and does not appear to be due to effects on *H. pylori*.

Misoprostol

Misoprostol is effective in the prevention of acute duodenal ulceration caused by non-steroidal anti-inflammatory drugs in healthy volunteers[25,40] but in patients taking these drugs a benefit was only shown for gastric and not for duodenal ulceration.[13] However, in placebo-controlled trials, ranitidine has been shown to be effective at preventing duodenal ulceration in such patients.[9,39]

Conclusions

Recently, attention has been attracted away from the acid suppression produced by H_2 receptor antagonists and omeprazole and on to the importance of *H. pylori* in duodenal ulcer recurrence. Better understanding of this organism and the develop-

ment of effective simple regimes for its eradication are likely to provide the major focus for research in the field of duodenal ulcer therapy.

References

1. Baron, J.H., Barr, J., Batten, J., Sidebotham, R. and Spencer, J. (1986) Acid, pepsin, and mucus secretion in patients with gastric and duodenal ulcer before and after colloidal bismuth subcitrate (De-Nol). *Gut*, **27**, 486–490.
2. Bianchi Porro, G. and Petrillo, M. (1986) The natural history of peptic ulcer disease: the influence of H_2-antagonist treatment. *Scandinavian Journal of Gastroenterology*, **21**(suppl. 121), 46–52.
3. Boyd, E.J., Wilson, J.A. and Wormsley, K.G. (1984) Safety of ranitidine maintenance treatment of duodenal ulcer. *Scandinavian Journal of Gastroenterology*, **19**, 394–400.
4. Coghlan, J.G., Gilligan, D.H., Humphries, H. *et al.* (1987) *Campylobacter pylori* and recurrence of duodenal ulcers – a 12 months follow-up study. *The Lancet*, **ii**, 1109–1111.
5. Collen, M.J., Stanczak, C.A. and Ciarleglio, C.A. (1987) Basal acid output in patients with refractory duodenal ulcer disease (abstract). *Gastroenterology*, **92**, 1351.
6. Creutzfeldt, W., Lamberts, R., Stockmann, F. and Brunner, G. (1989) Quantitative study of gastric endocrine cells in patients receiving long term treatment with omeprazole. *Scandinavian Journal of Gastroenterology*, **24**(suppl. 166), 122–128.
7. Dobrilla, G., Vallaperta, P. and Amplatz, S. (1988) Influence of ulcer healing agents on ulcer relapse after discontinuation of acute treatment: a pooled estimate of controlled clinical trials. *Gut*, **29**, 181–187.
8. Editorial (1990) Gastroenterologists in Sydney: histology and *Helicobacter*. *The Lancet*, **336**, 779–780.
9. Ehsanullah, R.S., Page, M.C. and Tildesley, G.W. (1988) Prevention of gastroduodenal damage induced by non-steroidal anti-inflammatory drugs: controlled trial of ranitidine. *British Medical Journal*, **297**, 1017–1021.
10. Feldman, M. and Burton, M.E. (1990) Histamine-2 receptor antagonists: standard therapy for acid-peptic disease. *New England Journal of Medicine*, **323**, 1672–1680, 1749–1755.
11. Glupczynski, Y., Burette, A., DeKoster, E. *et al.* (1990) Metronidazole resistance in *Helicobacter pylori*. *The Lancet*, **335**, 976–977.
12. Gough, K.R., Bardhan, K.D., Crowe, J.P. *et al.* (1984) Ranitidine and cimetidine in prevention of duodenal ulcer relapse: a double-blind randomised multicentre comparative trial. *The Lancet*, **ii**, 659–662.
13. Graham, D.Y., Agarwal, N.M. and Roth, S.H. (1988) Prevention of NSAID-induced gastric ulcers

with misoprostol: multicentre double blind placebo-controlled trial. *The Lancet*, **ii**, 1277–1280.

14. Hamilton, I., Worsley, B.W., O'Connor, H.J. and Axon, A.T. (1983) Effects of dipotassium dicitrato bismuthate (TDB) tablets or cimetidine in the treatment of duodenal ulcer. *Gut*, **24**, 1148–1151.

15. Hasan, M. and Sircus, W. (1981) The factors determining success or failure of cimetidine treatment of peptic ulcer. *Journal of Clinical Gastroenterology*, **3**, 225–229.

16. Hawkey, C.J. and Rampton, D.S. (1985) Prostaglandins and the gastrointestinal mucosa: are they important in its function disease or treatment? *Gastroenterology*, **89**, 1162–1188.

17. Hawkey, C.J. and Walt, R.P. (1986) Prostaglandins for peptic ulcer: a promise unfulfilled. *The Lancet*, **ii**, 1084–1085.

18. Hollander, D., Tarnawski, A. and Gergely, H. (1986) Protection against alcohol-induced gastric mucosal injury by aluminum containing compounds – sucralfate, antacids and aluminium sulfate. *Scandinavian Journal of Gastroenterology*, **21**(suppl. 125), 151–153.

19. Isenberg, J.K., Selling, J.A., Hogan, D.L. and Koss, M.A. (1987) Impaired proximal duodenal mucosal bicarbonate secretion in patients with duodenal ulcer. *New England Journal of Medicine*, **361**, 374–379.

20. Jones, D.B., Howden, C.W., Burget, D.W., Kerr, G.D. and Hunt, R.H. (1987) Acid suppression in duodenal ulcer: a meta-analysis to define optimal dosing with anti-secretory drugs. *Gut*, **28**, 1120–1127.

21. Koo, J., Ho, J., Lam, S.K., Wong, J. and Ong, G.B. (1982) Selective coating of gastric ulcer in tripotassium dicitrato bismuthate. *Gastroenterology*, **82**, 864–870.

22. Konturek, S.J., Radecki, T., Piastucki, I. and Drozdowicz, D. (1986) Advances in the understanding of the mechanisms of cytoprotective action by colloidal bismuth subcitrate. *Scandinavian Journal of Gastroenterology*, **21**(suppl. 122), 6–10.

23. Korman, M.G., Hansky, J., Merrett, A.C. and Schmidt, G.C. (1982) Ranitidine in duodenal ulcer: incidence of healing and effect of smoking. *Digestive Diseases and Sciences*, **27**, 712–725.

24. Lam, S.K. (1989) Implications of sucralfate-induced ulcer healing and relapse. *American Journal of Medicine*, **86**(suppl. 6A), 122–126.

25. Lanza, F.L., Fakouhi, D., Rubin, A. *et al.* (1989) a double-blind placebo-controlled comparison of the efficacy and safety of 50, 100 and 200 micrograms qid in the prevention of ibuprofen induced gastric and duodenal mucosal lesions and symptoms. *American Journal of Gastroenterology*, **84**, 633–636.

26. Lee, F.I., Samloff, I.M. and Hardman, L. (1985) Comparison of tri-potassium dicitrato bismuthate tablets with ranitidine in healing and relapse of duodenal ulcers. *The Lancet*, **i**, 1299–1302.

27. McNulty, C.A., Dent, J. and Wise, R. (1985) Susceptibility of clinical isolates of *Campylobacter pylori* to 11 anti-microbial agents. *Antimicrobial Agents and Chemotherapy*, **28**, 837–838.

28. Malhotra, S.L. (1978) A comparison of unrefined wheat and rice diets in the management of duodenal ulcer. *Postgraduate Medical Journal*, **54**, 6–9.

29. Marshall, B.J., Armstrong, J.A., Francis, G.J., Nokes, N.T. and Wee, S.H. (1989) Antibacterial action of bismuth in relation to *Campylobacter pyloridis* colonisation and gastritis. *Digestion*, **37**(suppl. 2), 16–30.

30. Marshall, B.J., Goodwin, C.S., Warren, J.R. *et al.* (1988) Prospective double-blind trial of duodenal ulcer relapse after eradication of *Campylobacter pylori*. *The Lancet*, **ii**, 1439–1441.

31. Martin, D., May, S., Tweedle, D., Hollanders, D., Ravenscroft, M. and Miller, J. (1981) Difference in relapse rates of duodenal ulcer after healing with cimetidine or tripotassium dicitrato bismuthate. *The Lancet*, **i**, 7–10.

32. Massarrat, S. and Eisenmann, A. (1981) Factors affecting the healing rate of duodenal and pyloric ulcers with low-dose antacid treatment. *Gut*, **22**, 97–102.

33. Monk, J.P. and Clissold, S.P. (1987) Misoprostol: a preliminary review of its pharmacodynamic and pharmacokinetic properties, and therapeutic efficacy in the treatment of peptic ulcer disease. *Drugs*, **33**, 1–30.

34. Nicholson, P.A. (1985) A multicentre comparison of 2 dosage regimes of misoprostol and cimetidine in the treatment of duodenal ulcer in out-patients. *Digestive Diseases and Sciences*, **30**(suppl.), 171S–177S.

35. Prichard, P.J., Yeomans, N.D., Mihaly, G.W. *et al.* (1985) Omeprazole: a study of its inhibition of gastric pH and oral pharmacokinetics after morning or evening dosage. *Gastroenterology*, **88**, 64–69.

36. Rauws, E.A. and Tytgat, G.N. (1989) *Campylobacter pylori*: treatment of gastritis. In Campylobacter pylori *and Gastroduodenal Disease* (Ed.) Rathbone, B.J. and Heatley, R.V. pp. 225–231. Oxford: Blackwell.

37. Rauws, E.A. and Tytgat, G.N. (1990) Cure of duodenal ulcer associated with eradication of *Helicobacter pylori*. *The Lancet*, **335**, 1233–1235.

38. Rauws, E.A., Langenberg, W., Houthoff, H.J., Zanen, H.C. and Tytgat, G.N. (1988) *Campylobacter pyloridis*-associated chronic active antral gastritis: a prospective study of its prevalence and the effects of antibacterial and antiulcer treatment. *Gastroenterology*, **94**, 33–40.

39. Robinson, M.G., Griffin, J.W., Bowers, J. *et al.* (1989) Effect of ranitidine on gastroduodenal mucosal damage induced by nonsteroidal anti-inflammatory drugs. *Digestive Diseases and Sciences*, **34**, 424–428.

40. Roth, S., Agrawal, N., Mahowald, M. *et al.* (1989) Misoprostol heals gastroduodenal injury in patients with rheumatoid arthritis receiving aspirin. *Archives in Internal Medicine*, **149**, 775–779.

41. Silvis, S.E. (1984) Results of the United States

maintenance trials. *American Journal of Medicine*, **77**(suppl. 5B), 33–38.

42. Sonnenberg, A., Muller-Lissner, S.A., Vogel, E. *et al.* (1981) Predictors of duodenal ulcer healing and relapse. *Gastroenterology*, **81**, 1061–1067.

43. Sontag, S., Graham, D.Y., Belsito, A. *et al.* (1984) Cimetidine, cigarette smoking and recurrence of duodenal ulcer. *New England Journal of Medicine*, **311**, 689–693.

44. Strum, W.B. (1986) Prevention of duodenal ulcer recurrence. *Annals of Internal Medicine*, **105**, 757–761.

45. Szabo, S. and Hollander, D. (1989) Pathways of gastrointestinal protection and repair: mechanism of action of sucralfate. *American Journal of Medicine*, **86**(suppl. 6A), 23–31.

46. Thorat, V.K., Misra, S.P. and Anand, B.S. (1990) Conventional versus on demand therapy for duodenal ulcer: results of a controlled therapeutic trial. *American Journal of Gastroenterology*, **85**, 243–248.

47. Tovey, F.I., Husband, E.M., Yiu, Y.C. *et al.* (1989) Comparison of relapse rates and of mucosal abnormalities after healing of duodenal ulceration after one year's maintenance with cimetidine or sucralfate: a light and electron microscopic study. *Gut*, **30**, 586–593.

48. Tytgat, G.N., Lamers, C.B., Hameeteman, W., Jansen, J.M. and Wilson, J.A. (1987) Omeprazole in peptic ulcers resistant to histamine H_2 receptor antagonists. *Alimentary Pharmacology and Therapeutics*, **1**, 31–38.

49. Wallmark, B. (1989) Omeprazole: mode of action and effect on acid secretion in animals. *Scandinavian Journal of Gastroenterology*, **24**(suppl. 166), 12–18.

50. Ward, M., Halliday, C. and Cowen, A.E. (1986) A comparison of colloidal bismuth subcitrate tablets and ranitidine in the treatment of chronic duodenal ulcers. *Digestion*, **34**, 173–177.

51. Wilson, D.E. (1986) Therapeutic aspects of prostaglandins in the treatment of peptic ulcer disease. *Digestive Diseases and Sciences*, **31**(suppl. 2), 42S–46S.

TREATMENT: SURGICAL

(D. Johnston and I. Martin)

Preservation of the integrity of the pyloric sphincter and the antral mill has been the major advance in the surgical treatment of peptic ulceration in the past 25 years. This has been made possible by the use of highly selective vagotomy (otherwise known as parietal cell or proximal gastric vagotomy), which confines the vagal denervation to the acid- and pepsin-secreting part of the stomach, leaving the gastric antrum innervated by the nerves of Latarget. There

is now wide agreement that highly selective vagotomy is the safest operation, produces the fewest side-effects such as dumping and diarrhoea and is followed by the fewest metabolic sequelae. Debate focuses on the incidence of recurrent ulceration, which in the hands of some surgeons is low but has been as high as 20% or even more in other series. This wide variation in recurrent ulceration is unrelated to preoperative factors such as acid output, age of the patient or length of ulcer history, but is related to the surgeon who operates, to the operative technique used and to incomplete vagotomy. Recent developments in laparoscopic technique have provided an opportunity to perform highly selective vagotomy without laparotomy.

Choice of treatment: medical or surgical?

In this era of effective medical therapy one might well ask if *any* patients need surgical treatment; many physicians are now suggesting that they do not. Most surgeons would still regard this view as a trifle extreme. It should be remembered that surgical treatment is more effective than medical treatment in curing peptic ulcers, and that highly selective vagotomy is more specific in its action than is medical treatment.

Effectiveness

When 100 patients with active duodenal ulceration are treated medically, about 10–15% of the ulcers remain unhealed.[102] After almost any form of surgical treatment the incidence of recurrent ulceration is only 1–2% in the first postoperative year. If we now consider 100 patients whose duodenal ulcers have been healed by a course of H_2 receptor antagonists or proton pump inhibitors who are not given maintenance treatment, the incidence of recurrent ulceration within 6 months is about 70%.[4,70] By contrast, vagotomy, once done, is always present, and could be regarded as being equivalent to life-long medical therapy. Hence, whereas the recurrence rate in the absence of maintenance therapy is 70% with medical treatment, it is still only 1–2% after vagotomy. Such comparisons, though to some extent artificial, have some validity, since most physicians prefer to treat their patients with intermittent courses of H_2 receptor antagonists in full dosage rather than giving them continuous maintenance therapy.

A minority of physicians, however, treat the ulcer by full-dosage therapy and then give maintenance therapy indefinitely, or at least for several years. Even with such aggressive medical therapy, however, about 10% of ulcers will fail to heal and a further 10% will recur within a year, so that the cumulative incidence of failure after one year is about 20%.[4] After vagotomy, the comparable figure is 2%.

These recurrences during medical therapy are not innocuous. Some recurrent ulcers cause pain and some are 'silent', but all of them are inevitably accompanied by progression of the pathological process: the ulcer continues to penetrate the wall of the stomach or duodenum, further fibrosis takes place, and life-threatening perforation, haemorrhage or gastric outlet obstruction are ever-present risks. Whilst it would be wrong to exaggerate the extent of such dangers, they must not be ignored and, now that the mortality of elective vagotomy for duodenal ulcer is as low as 0.2–0.3%, it is possible that medical treatment, prolonged over many years, may carry a greater risk to life than surgical treatment.

Specificity

H_2 receptor antagonists and proton pump inhibitors affect not only the stomach, but also other systems of the body. A highly selective vagotomy, on the other hand, is specific to the proximal three-quarters of the stomach and has no ill-effects on other parts of the body. Moreover, highly selective vagotomy has been with us for 25 years, whereas many modern drugs have only been widely used for 2 or 3 years, so the full extent of their side-effects and potential dangers is not yet known.

Other considerations

Peptic ulceration is a chronic disease characterized by remissions and exacerbations, and prolonged medical therapy implies that the patient must take pills for many years, which many find irksome. Hence, compliance with medical therapy leaves much to be desired, and this probably accounts for a proportion of the recurrences. Surgical treatment, in contrast, is permanent in its effect. Moreover, after surgical treatment there is no necessity to keep attending the doctor's office or the hospital, whereas with repeated courses of medical treatment or with long-term maintenance therapy the patient's life is more likely to be dominated and distorted by the presence of the ulcer and the fear that it may recur. In addition, some physicians evince unbounded zeal in checking on the healing of the ulcer by means of repeated endoscopies, which are unpleasant to the individual patient and expensive to the state, the patient or the insurance company. Hence, although in the short term a surgical operation is expensive, in the long run it may be cheaper than medical therapy.[80]

Despite the above remarks the authors believe most patients with duodenal ulcer should be treated medically in the first instance. The authors' only plea is that such medical therapy should not be continued for so long that the ulcer enlarges, to create pathological havoc and clinical danger. There will, of course, always be the category of elderly, unfit patients in whom prolonged maintenance therapy is entirely logical because of the risks of surgery. For the remainder, the authors feel that if, despite good medical treatment, the patient continues to be troubled by painful exacerbations of the ulcer that interfere with work, sleep or general enjoyment of life, he or she should be considered for surgical treatment.

In short, the indications for surgical intervention remain the traditional ones, namely failure of medical treatment or the occurrence of life-threatening complications such as perforation, obstruction or haemorrhage. What precisely constitutes 'failure of medical treatment' remains a matter for debate.

In selecting patients for surgical treatment, it is desirable to avoid or forestall surgical failure. There are three main causes of such failure: recurrent ulceration, side-effects of the operation and selection of unsuitable patients for surgical treatment. The last group should, if possible, be identified before operation and surgery withheld. The difficulty, of course, is that this group tend to do badly both with medical and with surgical treatments. Identification of such patients is difficult and controversial. The authors' practice is to avoid operating on patients who smoke and drink to excess and who ignore advice to moderate these habits. The authors believe that the postoperative 'albatross syndrome' – in other words, continuing to plague the surgeon with distressing abdominal complaints after the operation – can be predicted with some confidence in young-to-middle-aged people who smoke and drink heavily, are tattooed, and (taking into account the current difficulties with employment) show little interest in holding down a steady job. Such patients are frequently young, underweight males. A history of psychiatric upset is also a relative contraindication. The authors would not utterly deny such patients the potential benefits of surgery, but certainly try to avoid operating on them, being prepared instead to offer them prolonged maintenance treatment with a variety of the newer anti-ulcer drugs in the hope that they may obtain a cure or modify their lifestyle. These patients spoil any surgical series because, even if they do not develop recurrent ulceration, they complain of numerous symptoms at the gastric follow-up clinic and so end up being classed as Visick grade IV, the category of failure.

Choice of elective operation

This is, and always has been, a compromise – a kind of Odyssean steering between the Scylla of total gastrectomy, which would be 100% effective but crippling and dangerous, and the Charybdis of sham laparotomy, which is safe, with few side-effects, but ineffectual. Of course, in practice the spectrum of operations available is not so unethically wide, but it still varies greatly, between gastric resection with or without vagotomy at the one extreme and laparoscopic highly selective vagotomy at the other. Vagotomy combined with antrectomy is almost completely effective in curing peptic ulcers, because it removes both the vagal drive and the parietal cells and the principal source of gastrin, but by the same token it brings with it the side-effects and sequelae of both gastric resection and vagotomy. Highly selective vagotomy, on the other hand, is less effective, but considerably safer, produces few side-effects and has minimal metabolic sequelae.

Certain operative procedures, formerly widely used in the treatment of duodenal ulcer, can be virtually omitted from consideration. Partial gastrectomy, for example, is rapidly falling into disuse even in countries like Germany where it held sway for a century, because not only is the patient four times as likely to die as after highly selective vagotomy, but it also produces significantly more side-effects (such as dumping), more weight loss and anaemia in the long term, and possibly an increased risk that gastric carcinoma will develop 20–25 years later. Selective gastric vagotomy combined with a drainage procedure, while an important milestone in the historical development of surgery for peptic ulcer, has now been virtually abandoned, because it still involves vagal denervation of the gastric antrum together with a pyloroplasty or gastroenterostomy. Most surgeons feel that if they are going to take the trouble to perform a selective type of vagotomy, they might as well perform a highly selective vagotomy that keeps the antral mill innervated and the pyloric sphincter intact. Thus, in the UK today the choice lies between highly selective vagotomy and truncal vagotomy with a drainage procedure (truncal vagotomy and drainage), while in North America vagotomy combined with antrectomy still has its staunch adherents. Fortunately, the results of some excellent prospective trials that compare highly selective vagotomy with vagotomy and drainage and vagotomy and antrectomy are now available, and will be described later.

Highly selective vagotomy and truncal vagotomy: a 'physiological' comparison

When Dragstedt reintroduced truncal vagotomy in his classic paper in 1943,[24] he described truncal vagotomy alone, without a drainage procedure.

Later, however, it was found that 30–50% of the patients who were treated by truncal vagotomy developed gastric retention, so destruction of the pylorus by means of a pyloroplasty or its bypass by gastroenterostomy became an integral part of the operation. Truncal vagotomy was thought to heal the duodenal ulcer partly by abolishing the direct vagal drive to the parietal cell mass and partly by diminishing vagal release of gastrin from the antrum. The addition of a drainage procedure was regarded with equanimity, because it was believed that gastric reservoir function was still preserved after vagotomy with drainage, and that the sequelae of partial gastrectomy such as dumping and bilious vomiting could be avoided, especially when pyloroplasty was used as the drainage procedure. Finally, it was thought that severance of the vagal fibres to the liver, gallbladder, bile ducts, pancreas and small intestine – an integral part of truncal vagotomy – was of minor importance and would not produce side-effects. All these assumptions about truncal vagotomy are now known to be false. It is because truncal vagotomy is physiologically unsound that in controlled prospective trials its clinical results have been found to be somewhat inferior to those of gastric resection with or without vagotomy.[36,59,79]

Serum gastrin

Gastrin levels in humans are no higher when the gastric antrum is left innervated, as in highly selective vagotomy, than when it is vagally denervated, as in truncal vagotomy.[41] Both types of vagotomy lead to a significant increase in serum gastrin compared with preoperative levels. Since the stomach has been found to empty satisfactorily through the intact pylorus when the antrum is left innervated,[2,11,46] these findings are of great importance, because truncal vagotomy is clearly illogical and the performance of a pyloroplasty or gastroenterostomy is unnecessary. Hence, these well-known side-effects of gastric surgery – dumping, diarrhoea and bilious vomiting – which are attributable in large measure to loss of the pylorus, can now be virtually eliminated.

Lower oesophageal sphincter

The necessity of mobilizing the distal 5–6 cm of oesophagus and clearing it of all vagal fibres is common to both truncal and highly selective vagotomy. Both types of vagotomy are followed by symptoms of heartburn in 10–20% of patients. What is not often recognized, however, is that 60% of patients complain of heartburn before vagotomy and in most of them heartburn is either absent or greatly improved after operation. Neither truncal vagotomy and drainage nor highly selective vagotomy lowers pressure in the resting lower oesophageal sphincter,[95,96] so surgical manoeuvres designed to increase the competence of the lower oesophageal sphincter in the course of vagotomy for duodenal ulcer are probably unnecessary. On the other hand, if heartburn is a prominent preoperative symptom, and especially if it is accompanied by the presence of a large hiatal hernia or severe oesophagitis, it is probably advisable to add an antireflux procedure to the vagotomy.

Gastric secretion

Both truncal vagotomy and highly selective vagotomy diminish secretion of acid and pepsin to a similar extent. Basal acid output is reduced by an average of 70–80% and maximal acid output by about 60%.[39] After both types of vagotomy an increasing proportion of patients develop positive responses to the insulin test,[34,57,71] as time passes, but these positive responses show little correlation with recurrent ulceration. It seems likely that many patients have a highly incomplete, but still adequate, vagotomy. There is little rationale in performing routine preoperative acid secretion tests, which are disliked by patients. However, routine determination of basal serum gastrin levels before operation seems advisable, because the assay is easy to perform and permits the occasional case of Zollinger–Ellison syndrome to be detected before operation. After vagotomy, there again seems little point in routinely testing gastric function, unless a new type of vagotomy is being introduced, or some form of quality control is warranted to monitor the efficiency of the surgeon. Whether this 'quality control' should be intraoperative, in the form of the Burge electrical stimulation test[8] or the Grassi test,[37] or postoperative, in the form of a Hollander insulin test[43] or a modified sham-feeding test,[28,63,64,68] is still a matter for debate.

Gastric motility, intragastric pressure and gastric emptying

Both truncal vagotomy and highly selective vagotomy impair receptive relaxation and accommodation to distension by a meal, with the result that postprandial intragastric pressure is higher after vagotomy than before operation.[89] This rise in pressure produces a sensation of fullness or discomfort, which is experienced by 20–40% of patients after any type of vagotomy and causes them to reduce the size of their meals. The symptom is very mild in most patients and only a few are seriously inconvenienced. The elevation of intragastric pressure after both truncal vagotomy and highly selective vagotomy leads to accelerated gastric emptying of liquids, a feature that is more marked after truncal vagotomy and drainage than after highly selective vagotomy. Thus, while dumping can occur after both types of vagotomy, it is significantly more common after truncal vagotomy with a drainage procedure. It has been shown by several authors that the stomach behaves as an incontinent organ (for liquids) after truncal vagotomy and drainage, and that the fluid cascading out of the stomach in the early minutes after a meal gives rise not only to dumping but also to rapid intestinal transit and diarrhoea in susceptible individuals.[13,75] Gastric emptying of solid food is virtually normal after highly selective vagotomy,[7,14,16,44,45,68] whereas after truncal vagotomy it may be slow, excessively fast or normal. Myoelectrical activity in the stomach is disorganized after truncal vagotomy, whereas after highly selective vagotomy the regular three-per-minute rhythm of electrical activity in the antrum is maintained with a normal waveform.[92,93] As time passes, these abnormalities diminish, but even in the long term, gastric myoelectrical activity, motility and emptying are much closer to the normal after highly selective vagotomy than after truncal vagotomy.

When a hypertonic test meal of glucose solution is given orally to patients after highly selective vagotomy or truncal vagotomy and drainage, significantly more dumping, diarrhoea and hypotension are produced in the patients who had undergone truncal vagotomy and drainage than in those who have undergone highly selective vagotomy.[48] Clinically, too, episodic diarrhoea occurs in about 25% of patients after truncal vagotomy (2–4% being severely afflicted), whereas after highly selective vagotomy only about 4% of patients develop diarrhoea, and this is always mild.[56] While gastric incontinence followd by rapid intestinal transit of fluids is partly responsible for 'postvagotomy' diarrhoea, preservation of the hepatic and coeliac branches of the vagus, as in highly selective vagotomy, is also of value, because diarrhoea is significantly more common after truncal vagotomy and drainage than after selective vagotomy with a drainage procedure.[61,67]

Duodenogastric reflux

In normal people the pylorus provides a relatively effective barrier against reflux of what Silen has termed 'malevolent gall' into the stomach. Bile salts and perhaps other constituents of the duodenal contents such as lysolecithin damage the gastric mucosal barrier and so facilitate acid–peptic attack, for example in patients with gastric ulceration.[19,52] Dewar and his colleagues have shown that the stomach concentrations of bile acids before operation are significantly elevated both in patients with duodenal ulcer[20] and in patients with gastric ulcer.[21] As might be expected, these levels increase still further after both truncal vagotomy and drainage and partial gastrectomy. After highly selective vagotomy, however, duodenogastric reflux is found to be significantly diminished, presumably because the elevated intragastric pressure and the presence of an intact pylorus combine to minimize such reflux. These findings may be important, because duodenogastric reflux predisposes to the development of gastritis[9,25,29,60,69,82] and perhaps to gastric carcinoma.[22,86,90] The carcinoma of the gastric stump that develops after partial gastrectomy is not evenly distributed in the gastric mucosa, but appears near the stoma, where the concentration of bile salts is presumably highest. Again, in patients with benign gastric ulcer it seems illogical to employ an operation such as partial gastrectomy or vagotomy with drainage that increases duodenogastric reflux, when it is known that such reflux damages the gastric mucosa by rendering it more susceptible to the action of endogenous acid and pepsin.

Liver and biliary tract

After truncal vagotomy in dogs, bile flow diminishes and the bile becomes more lithogenic in composition.[15,30,33] In humans, the volume of the resting gallbladder increases significantly after truncal vagotomy,[51,83] whereas it does not change after selective or highly selective vagotomy.[49,78] Shields and colleagues[5] have shown that truncal vagotomy with pyloroplasty leads to significant delay in gallbladder emptying after a meal and to disturbance of the normal integration of gastric emptying and gallbladder emptying. Although in their review article in 1969, Fletcher and Clark concluded that the connection between truncal vagotomy and gallstones was 'not proven',[31] 15 years later papers by Clave and Gaspar,[12] Csendes et al.,[18] Tompkins et al.[97] and Sapala et al.[84] leave little doubt that the incidence of gallstones is significantly increased after truncal vagotomy. In fact, the mean incidence of gallstones seems to be about 20% within 5 years of truncal vagotomy. The authors have reviewed the incidence of gallstones in 100 patients who were followed up for a mean period of 9 years after highly selective vagotomy and found an incidence of 11%, which, as far as they could calculate, did not differ significantly from the expected incidence in their area in people of similar age and sex distribution. The question of a possible connection between vagotomy and the subsequent development of gallstones is important clinically for two reasons. First, it is obviously undesirable that an operation designed to cure one benign condition should give rise to another painful and potentially hazardous condition that often necessitates operative treatment. Secondly, severe episodic diarrhoea is a com-

plication of truncal vagotomy and drainage in only 2–4% of patients, but when cholecystectomy is added to truncal vagotomy and drainage the incidence of diarrhoea may be as high as 50%, and between 10 and 20% of patients experience severe diarrhoea.[94,99] It follows that when patients who have both duodenal ulceration and gallstones come to operation, truncal vagotomy should be avoided. Even in the absence of gallstones, the possibility that truncal vagotomy might predispose to the subsequent development of gallstones is a relative contraindication to the performance of this type of vagotomy.

Pancreas

It used to be taught that truncal vagotomy did not impair pancreatic function in man, but such statements were based on the results of unsophisticated tests of pancreatic function in which secretion was often stimulated by unphysiological amounts of secretin and pancreozymin, given intravenously. When a more physiological stimulus is used, such as a meal, or amino acids perfused through the duodenum, it becomes clear that pancreatic exocrine secretion is diminished by about 50% after truncal vagotomy,[74] whereas after highly selective vagotomy no such impairment is found.[68,81,88] We have also shown that pancreatic endocrine function is altered after truncal vagotomy.[47] In normal people and in patients who have undergone highly selective vagotomy, glucose given by mouth elicits a much greater secretion of insulin than the same amount of glucose given intravenously. After truncal vagotomy, however, insulin secretion after oral glucose is no greater than insulin secretion after intravenous glucose. Hence truncal vagotomy in humans seems to interfere with the entero-insulin axis, perhaps by modifying nervous reflexes or the release of some endocrine substance from the mucosa of the upper small intestine.

Faecal fat excretion and long-term effects on nutrition

After highly selective vagotomy, fat excretion is normal,[26] whereas after truncal vagotomy and drainage it is significantly increased and about 40% of patients develop steatorrhoea,[17,100] though the degree of steatorrhoea is mild and asymptomatic in the majority. However, in 10–20% of patients after truncal vagotomy and drainage, faecal fat output increases to 10 g/day or more (>30 mmol/day) and malabsorption may contribute to nutritional deficiency in the long term. Certainly, long-term studies by Wheldon and her colleagues in Newcastle, England,[98,101] suggest that there is significant weight loss and iron deficiency anaemia after truncal vagotomy with a drainage procedure. The authors have studied 100 patients for more than 10 years after highly selective vagotomy in Leeds and so far have found no evidence of iron-deficiency anaemia and no evidence of weight loss. Indeed, after highly selective vagotomy there was a significant gain in weight during the first postoperative year, after which body weight remains constant and does not differ significantly from the ideal body weight for height.

Clinical results of highly selective vagotomy for duodenal ulcer at Leeds General Infirmary

Follow-up of the many hundreds of patients who have undergone highly selective vagotomy has been undertaken in the gastric follow-up clinic by methods that have been described previously.[36] This clinic is also attended by many patients who have undergone operations other than highly selective vagotomy. Various modifications of highly selective vagotomy have been used in Leeds. Goligher, for example, in 1974[35] described a modification whereby 10–11 cm of prepyloric stomach was left innervated rather than the 5–7 cm described originally by Johnston in 1970.[55] Hill[42] also described an anterior highly selective, posterior truncal vagotomy, without pyloroplasty, but since the philosophy of this differs fundamentally from highly selective vagotomy, the results of Hill's operation are not recorded. Obesity of the patient was not a contraindication to the use of highly selective vagotomy, although it obviously made the procedure more difficut and prolonged. The mean age of the patients was 44 years, their mean weight 68 kg, and the mean length of ulcer history before operation was 9 years. All ulcers were treated by highly selective vagotomy alone unless the patient had clinical symptoms of gastric outlet obstruction before operation.

The preoperative acid-secretory characteristics of these patients did not differ from those of patients in similar series in Europe and North America. This series is therefore fairly typical of patients coming to elective surgery for duodenal ulcer in Britain during the 1970s, and the lessons derived from our experience are probably widely applicable.

Operative mortality
There was no mortality. Furthermore, there has been no ulcer-related mortality during follow-up.

Postoperative morbidity
Postoperative morbidity has been minimal. In fact, the patients' postoperative progress has been so smooth and their gastric emptying, in particular, so satisfactory, that the authors' custom is to nurse them with neither a nasogastric tube nor an intra-

venous drip from the time of operation. All patients over the age of 40 years received prophylactic subcutaneous heparin before operation and for at least 5 days after operation. Most patients were fit for discharge from hospital 5–7 days after operation.

Splenectomy for trauma was required at the time of highly selective vagotomy in 0.7% of patients. The incidence of non-fatal pulmonary embolism was 0.7%. Three per cent of patients developed wound infection and 2% an incisional hernia. Reoperation in the early postoperative period was required by 1% of patients for wound dehiscence, ileus, intestinal obstruction and, in one case, peritonitis. This case of peritonitis was of particular interest, because for the first 11 years after the introduction of highly selective vagotomy no case of lesser curve necrosis was encountered, but in the 12th year this patient was found at reoperation to have a perforation of the lesser curvature just proximal to the incisura.

Side-effects of operation
Highly selective vagotomy succeeded in its aim of significantly diminishing the incidences of dumping, diarrhoea and bilious vomiting. The virtual abolition of diarrhoea by the use of highly selective vagotomy and to the large reduction in dumping was first documented by us in 1972.[56] As the years have passed, the large differences that exist between vagotomy with drainage or gastric resection on the one hand and highly selective vagotomy on the other have persisted. Moreover, this advantage in favour of highly selective vagotomy has not been bought at the price of any corresponding increase in the incidence of other side-effects such as heartburn, vomiting or dysphagia (*Table 2.17*). Although the data shown in *Table 2.17* are not based on any prospective trial, they have been confirmed by randomized trials in other centres.

Recurrent ulceration
Recurrent ulceration is defined as any peptic ulcer causing symptoms that develop after highly selective vagotomy. However, recurrent ulceration may occur without producing symptoms, and in centres where patients have undergone routine endoscopy after highly selective vagotomy, the incidence of silent or asymptomatic recurrence was 30–50% of the incidence of symptomatic recurrence.[76]

After 5–14 years of follow-up in Leeds, 237 (82% of all patients) were reviewed. Approximately half of the missing patients had either died of causes unrelated to peptic ulceration or had emigrated, while half were lost to follow-up. The patients who were lost to follow-up did not differ significantly from those who attended for review.

Table 2.17 Percentage incidence of side-effects after different elective operations for duodenal ulcer

Symptom	Polya partial gastrectomy[a] (n = 107)	Truncal vagotomy with antrectomy[a] (n = 116)	Truncal vagotomy with gastro-jejunostomy[a] (n = 119)	Truncal vagotomy with pyloroplasty[a] (n = 161)	Selective vagotomy with drainage[b] (n = 85)	Highly selective vagotomy (n = 212)
Early dumping	22	9	18	12	20	2
Diarrhoea	7	23	26	22	16	5
Bilious vomiting	13	14	15	10	7	3
Epigastric fullness	37	36	40	37	38	23
Nausea	23	17	13	18	26	9
Food vomiting	6	10	4	4	—	2
Late dumping	1	4	6	2	—	2
Flatulence	20	23	18	20	—	9
Heartburn	8	16	20	13	14	18
Dysphagia	0	0	1	1	2	2

All patients were male except in the selective vagotomy with drainage group, of whom 24 were female. The inverviewing panel did not know which type of vagotomy had been performed.
[a] From Goligher *et al.*[36,36a]
[b] From Johnson and Goligher;[54] the drainage procedure was pyloroplasty in 68 and gastrojejunostomy in 17.

The *incidence* of recurrent ulceration after 5–14 years was 11.8%. Of the 40 patients who developed recurrence (after 0–14 years of follow-up), 22 (55%) presented within 3 years of operation and 29 (73%) within 5 years, but there were occasional recurrence up to 9 years after operation.

The *site* of recurrent ulceration was duodenal in 27 patients and pyloric or gastric in the remainder. The mean interval between operation and the diagnosis of recurrence was 3.8 years.

Six of the 40 patients presented as emergencies, one with perforation and five with haemorrhage. Thirty-four patients complained of recurrent pain. Four of the six emergency cases were treated by partial gastrectomy with good results, while the other two fared well with conservative management. Of the 34 patients who presented with pain, seven underwent reoperation and 27 have been treated medically, mainly with H_2 receptor antagonists. There was no mortality among these 40 patients, either from the reoperations or from the recurrent ulcers themselves. Approximately two-thirds of the patients treated with H_2 receptor antagonists have achieved good results and many of them are doing well at present without any treatment whatsoever. Thus, only 2% of patients who underwent highly selective vagotomy for duodenal ulcer in Leeds came to reoperation for recurrent peptic ulceration.

Long-term metabolic sequelae

BODY WEIGHT

The net effect in 140 patients who were followed up for a mean of 10 years after highly selective vago-

tomy was a small but significant weight gain during the first year after operation only. Weight loss of more than 3 kg was recorded in 34% of patients after truncal vagotomy with pyloroplasty (*Figure 2.60*), compared with 13% of patients after highly selective vagotomy (*Figure 2.61*); weight gain of more than 3 kg was recorded in 52% of patients after highly selective vagotomy but in only 25% of patients after truncal vagotomy with pyloroplasty (both these differences are statistically significant: $P < 0.01$).

ANAEMIA

Only one of 90 patients who were studied a mean of 9 years after highly selective vagotomy was found to be anaemic, and she had menorrhagia.

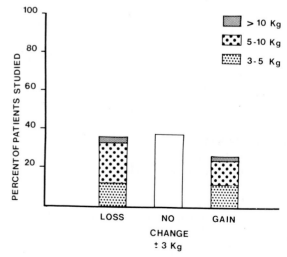

Figure 2.60 Change in body weight after truncal vagotomy and pyloroplasty for duodenal ulcer in 67 male patients.

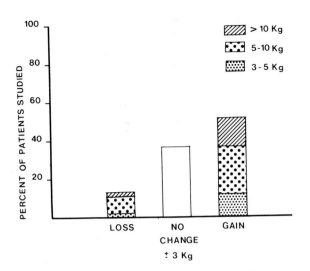

Figure 2.61 Change in body weight after highly selective vagotomy for duodenal ulcer in 103 male patients.

TUBERCULOSIS

Tuberculosis was diagnosed in only one patient after highly selective vagotomy.

CARCINOMA OF THE STOMACH

Carcinoma of the stomach has not been diagnosed in any patient after highly selective vagotomy for duodenal ulcer.

These results from the University Department of Surgery at Leeds General Infirmary show that over a 14-year period, elective highly selective vagotomy for duodenal ulcer had no operative mortality and little postoperative morbidity, produced few side-effects such as dumping, diarrhoea and bilious vomiting, and did not lead to metabolic deficiency of any kind in the long term. The incidence of recurrent ulceration after five to eight years of follow-up was

10%, which should be compared with a figure of 8% after truncal vagotomy with pyloroplasty and 11% after selective vagotomy and drainage in the same department.

Results of highly selective vagotomy worldwide and results of prospective controlled trials

The operative mortality, Visick grades and incidences of recurrent ulceration after highly selective vagotomy in a number of surgical centres are shown in *Table 2.18*. The operation is extremely safe, most centres recording no mortality whatsoever. In a survey of the operative mortality of elective highly selective vagotomy Johnston reported 17 deaths after 5257 operations, a mortality of 0.3%.[53] It can also be seen that 80 to 90% of patients were classified in Visick grades I and II. However, the incidence of recurrent ulceration ranged from 1.5 to 26%. The period of follow-up in several of these papers was fairly short, and in the Manchester study reported by Koffman *et al.*,[65] for example, the recurrence rate was 21%. The wide range of recurrence will be noted and cause speculation as to why it should be so.

Highly selective vagotomy compared with vagotomy and drainage

There have been several trials of highly selective vagotomy versus selective vagotomy and drainage,[3,62,72,85] the results of which have tended to favour highly selective vagotomy, mainly because the incidence of dumping after selective vagotomy and drainage ranged from 20 to 40%, whereas after highly selective vagotomy it was 3–8%. Diarrhoea and vomiting were also less common after highly selective vagotomy than after selective vagotomy and drainage. In Kronborg and Madsen's trial no

Table 2.18　Clinical results of highly selective vagotomy for duodenal ulcer (review of the literature)

	Number of patients	Operative mortality (%)	Length of follow-up (years)	Visick I + II (%)	Recurrent ulceration (%)
Dorricott *et al.*[23]	116	0	1	82	4.3
Makey *et al.*[73]	115	0	1–5	91	5.1
Stoddard *et al.*[92]	64	0	1–5	93	6.0
Kennedy *et al.*[62]	50	0	1–4	96	2.0
Christiansen *et al.*[10]	83	0	2–5	72	16.0
Sawyers *et al.*[85]	86	1.2	1–4	96	3.5
Grassi[38]	298	0	2–7	95	1.5
Koffman *et al.*[65]	77	0	2.5–5.5	72	21.0
Andersen *et al.*[3]	273	0.7	2–5	83	9.8
Jordan[58]	35	0	5	—	11.4
Madsen and Kronborg[72]	50	0	5–8	—	26.0

Table 2.19 Percentage incidence of side-effects in a prospective trial of highly selective vagotomy and truncal vagotomy and pyloroplasty

Symptom	Highly selective vagotomy (n = 56)	Truncal vagotomy with pyloroplasty (n = 55)	Significance of difference (P)
Early dumping	2	17	<0.01
Late dumping	4	17	<0.05
Flatulence	20	42	<0.01
Bile vomiting	4	18	<0.02
Postprandial distension	21	44	<0.02
Diarrhoea	7	13	NS
Nausea	13	24	NS
Heartburn	16	18	NS
Dysphagia	5	5	NS
Food vomiting	7	11	NS

NS, not significant.

From the prospective randomized trial in Sheffield by Stoddard et al.[91] Patients were male and were followed up for 6–66 months. The interviewer did not know which type of operation had been performed.

Table 2.20 Percentage incidence of side-effects in a prospective randomized trial of highly selective vagotomy and truncal vagotomy and pyloroplasty

Symptom	Truncal vagotomy with pyloroplasty (% of 68)	Highly selective vagotomy (% of 69)	Significance of difference (P)
Diarrhoea	39	7	<0.001
Severe diarrhoea	6	0	
Epigastric fullness	39	15	<0.01
Dumping	13	4	NS
Bile vomiting	17	7	NS
Heartburn	28	25	NS
Weight loss >2 kg	35	13	<0.001

NS, not significant.

From the prospective randomized trial in Aberdeen by Fraser et al.[32] Patients were followed up for 20–97 months (mean 61 months). Results assessed independently by two physicians who did not know which type of operation had been performed.

fewer than 22% of patients developed recurrent ulceration after highly selective vagotomy, and yet 78% of patients (all the others) were in Visick grades I or II after highly selective vagotomy, whereas only 68% of patients were placed in Visick grades I and II after selective vagotomy and drainage.

Truncal vagotomy and drainage compared with highly selective vagotomy

One of the earliest trials of this kind was conducted by Stoddard and colleagues in Sheffield.[91] The incidence of side-effects in the two groups is shown in Table 2.19. Side-effects were significantly more common after truncal vagotomy with pyloroplasty than after highly selective vagotomy. These authors concluded that highly selective vagotomy was superior to truncal vagotomy with pyloroplasty.

A large multicentre trial of highly selective vagotomy versus truncal vagotomy with pyloroplasty was carried out in Manchester by Koffman and his colleagues.[65] The results were much less favourable to highly selective vagotomy, the incidence of recurrent ulceration being 21%, compared with 8% after truncal vagotomy with pyloroplasty. However, no form of quality control, either intraoperative or postoperative, was used. The results serve as a warning of what may happen when a new operative technique such as highly selective vagotomy is introduced within a short space of time and employed by a large number of surgeons.

Undoubtedly the most elegant prospective trial of truncal vagotomy with pyloroplasty versus highly selective vagotomy has been carried out by Matheson and his colleagues in Aberdeen.[32] All 140 patients were operated upon by one experienced surgeon and subsequently reviewed by two independent physicians who were not aware of which operation had been performed. Follow-up was virtually 100% and the mean follow-up was 5 years. There were no deaths in either group of patients, but side-effects were significantly more common after truncal vagotomy with pyloroplasty than after highly selective vagotomy (Table 2.20). Four of 70 patients developed recurrent ulceration after truncal vagotomy with pyloroplasty, whereas only 1 of 69 patients developed recurrence after highly selective vagotomy. The overall clinical results were good to excellent in 87% of patients after highly selective vagotomy and in 70% of patients after truncal vagotomy with pyloroplasty. Matheson and his colleagues concluded that highly selective vagotomy, although technically more demanding than truncal vagotomy and drainage, yielded superior clinical results.

Highly selective vagotomy compared with vagotomy and antrectomy

Such trials are of particular interest because they compare the most conservative procedure with the most aggressive. Furthermore, even before the trial

Table 2.21 Overall clinical evaluation in a prospective trial of highly selective vagotomy versus truncal vagotomy with Billroth I antrectomy (truncal vagotomy with antrectomy) or selective vagotomy with pyloroplasty

Clinical grading	Highly selective vagotomy (n = 49)	vs	Billroth I antrectomy (n = 50)	Highly selective vagostomy (n = 37)	vs	Selective vagotomy with pyloroplasty (n = 37)
Visick I	86[a]		56	78		73
Visick II	10		38	16		11
Visick III	0		0	3		13
Visick IV	4		6	3		3

From the prospective randomized controlled trial of Sawyers *et al.*[85] Figures are the percentage of patients in each grade.
[a] Significant difference: $P < 0.01$.

Table 2.22 Postoperative sequelae in a prospective randomized trial of highly selective vagotomy versus truncal vagotomy with Billroth I antrectomy (truncal vagotomy with antrectomy) or selective vagotomy with pyloroplasty

Symptom	Highly selective vagostomy (n = 49)	vs	Billroth I antrectomy (n = 50)	Highly selective vagostomy (n = 37)	vs	Selective vagotomy with pyloroplasty (n = 37)
Dumping	0[a]		22	3		22
Diarrhoea	2[a]		18	0		3
Reflux gastritis	0		4	3		5
Epigastric fullness	8		0	8		8

From the study by Sawyers *et al.*[85] Figures are the percentage incidence of each symptom.
[a] Significant difference: $P < 0.05$

Table 2.23 Incidence of side-effects 1 year after operation in a prospective trial of highly selective vagotomy versus truncal vagotomy with antrectomy (Billroth I)

Symptom	Highly selective vagotomy (n = 82)	Truncal vagotomy with antrectomy (n = 78)	P
Dumping	2	9	NS
Diarrohea	5	14	<0.05
Vomiting	7	19	<0.05
Epigastric fullness	10	36	<0.0005
Heartburn	10	23	<0.05
Abdominal pain	11	12	NS
Dysphagia	0	4	NS

NS, not significant.
From a multicentre randomized trial of highly selective vagotomy and carried out in Birmingham, London and Rotterdam by Dorricott *et al.*[23] Figures are the percentage incidence of each symptom. The interviewer did not know which type of operation had been performed.

has begun it can be confidently predicted that vagotomy with antrectomy will emerge as superior with regard to recurrent ulceration, because surgical ablation of both the vagal and the gastrin influence on the parietal cells results in a recurrence rate of 1%. By contrast, when antrectomy is omitted, the incidence of recurrent ulceration after any type of vagotomy is usually between 5% and 15%. The question, then, is whether the predictable superiority of vagotomy with antrectomy with respect to recurrence is outweighed by the highly selective vagotomy advantages in terms of operative risk, side-effects and metabolic consequences.

Three excellent prospective trials of highly selective vagotomy and vagotomy with antrectomy have been performed, by Jordan in Houston, Texas,[58] by Sawyers *et al.* in Nashville, Tennessee,[85] and by Dorricott and his colleagues in a multicentre study in Birmingham, London and Rotterdam.[23] The incidences of side-effects of operation and the Visick grades in some of these studies are shown in *Tables 2.21, 2.22* and *2.23*. The results of the three trials are in close agreement: postoperative morbidity and gastric retention is significantly greater after vagotomy with antrectomy than after highly selective vagotomy. Dumping, diarrhoea and vomiting are significantly more common after vagotomy with antrectomy than after highly selective vagotomy, and loss of weight is significantly greater after vagotomy with antrectomy than after highly selective vagotomy. Fewer patients return to full-time work after vagotomy with antrectomy than after highly selective vagotomy. Recurrent ulceration is more common after highly selective vagotomy than after vagotomy with antrectomy, but the number of reoperations is about the same after either procedure, because more patients require reoperation for the relief of gastric stasis after vagotomy with antrectomy than after highly selective vagotomy. During the early years after operation, the overall clinical results (Visick grades) are better after highly selective vagotomy than after vagotomy and antrectomy.

Recurrent ulceration after highly selective vagotomy, and how to prevent it

Highly selective vagotomy is in many respects the ideal operation for duodenal ulcer – safe, with few side-effects or metabolic consequences. Its potential 'Achilles' heel', however, is the incidence of recurrent ulceration, which in the hands of some surgeons has been as low as 1–2% after 5 years of follow-up, whereas others have reported recurrence rates of 21–26% after shorter periods of follow-up.

It is possible that ulcer recurrence may be related to preoperative acid output, to stasis of food in the antrum after operation, or to factors such as completeness of the vagotomy. Should those patients who have gross hypersecretion of acid receive an antrectomy? Is there any test that could be used during operation to prove that the vagotomy is 'adequate'?

In Leeds, data on 40 patients with recurrent ulceration after highly selective vagotomy were compared with data on 399 patients who did not develop recurrence. Recurrence was unrelated to the patient's sex, age, length of ulcer history or previous history of perforation or haemorrhage. Postoperative gastric emptying of solid and liquid meals was the same in those with recurrence as in those without recurrence.

Preoperative basal and peak acid outputs were the same in patients who developed recurrence as in those who did not. Preoperative hypersecretors of acid were no more likely to develop recurrence after highly selective vagotomy than were normosecretors. This finding has been confirmed in the Aarhus County Vagotomy Trial.[1] Hence 'tailoring' the magnitude of the operation to preoperative acid output does not seem logical.

Postoperative acid outputs, in contrast, were significantly greater in patients who were destined to develop recurrent ulceration than in patients who did not develop recurrence (*Table 2.24*). Basal and insulin-stimulated acid outputs were significantly greater in those with recurrence than in those without, whereas 'maximal' acid response to pentagastrin differed only slightly between the two groups of patients. Hence the pentagastrin test is much less useful in predicting recurrence than is the insulin test (or perhaps, than the modified sham feeding test). The greatest percentage difference was in the basal acid output. When the insulin test 1 week after

Table 2.24 Acid outputs in patients with and without recurrent ulceration after highly selective vagotomy (HSV) for duodenal ulcer at Leeds General Infirmary

		Number of patients	Acid output (mmol/h)		
			Before HSV	*One week after HSV*	*More than 1 year after HSV*
Basal acid output	Recurrence	28	7.2	1.5	**4.3**[a]
	No recurrence	90	7.6	0.8	**1.4**
					(*n* = 44)
Pentagastrin stimulated peak acid output	Recurrence	28	49	24	27
	No recurrence	100V47	23	23	
					(*n* = 44)
Insulin stimulated peak acid output	Recurrence	28	—	**2.1**	**9.8**
	No recurrence	100	—	**0.6**	**4.7**
					(*n* = 44)

[a] Bold figures indicate a significant difference (*P* < 0.01) between patients with and without ulceration.

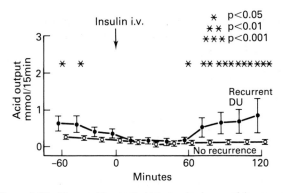

Figure 2.62 Mean acid outputs ($\pm$1 standard error of the mean) in response to insulin 1 week after highly selective vagotomy for duodenal ulcer in 17 patients who subsequently developed recurrent duodenal ulcer and in 100 patients who did not develop recurrence.

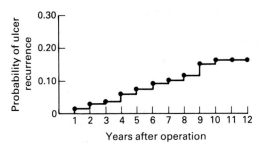

Figure 2.63 Probability of developing a recurrent ulcer during follow-up after highly selective vagotomy for duodenal ulcer.

highly selective vagotomy was 'positive' by Hollander's criteria the chances that recurrent ulceration would subsequently develop were 1 in 4 (25%); when the test was 'negative' the chances of recurrence were 1 in 16 (6.7%). In short, the cause of recurrent ulceration is to be sought at the time of operation. Before operation, patients who will develop recurrence and patients who will not are indistinguishable; after operation they differ significantly with respect to acid output (*Figure 2.62*). Thus, recurrence is usually caused by incomplete vagotomy and is due, presumably, to faulty operative technique.

The next question is whether highly selective vagotomy carries an inevitable recurrence rate or is recurrence variable, depending on the surgeon and the adequacy of the vagotomy performed. In *Figure 2.63* is shown the cumulative probability that a patient will develop recurrent ulceration after highly selective vagotomy in Leeds. However, the real answer to the question lies in the data shown in *Figure 2.64*, where it can be seen that the mean

incidence of recurrence (12%) after highly selective vagotomy is meaningless without the knowledge that one surgeon has an incidence of recurrence of 3%, while another has an incidence of recurrence of 28%.

How to achieve a 'complete' highly selective vagotomy and a low incidence of recurrent ulceration

Good exposure of the operative field with a 'head-up' tilt and the use of a special substernal retractor to expose the oesophagus are of prime importance. In patients with duodenal ulcer, the parietal cell mass is extensive, often reaching within 6 cm of the pylorus. Hence, vagal denervation must go far enough distally, to within 5–7 cm of the pylorus, if the distal portion of the acid-secreting mucosa is to be vagally denervated. Between incisura and cardia, the vagotomy is bound to be complete, because the lesser omentum with its neurovascular bundle is separated completely from the lesser curvature. It is important to spend about 20–30 minutes thoroughly mobilizing the oesophagus and clearing the distal 5–6 cm of all nerve fibres.[35,40] At the same time, the upper 3–4 cm of the greater curvature are mobilized. When performed in this way, highly selective vagotomy is usually complete, as shown by the insulin test 1 week

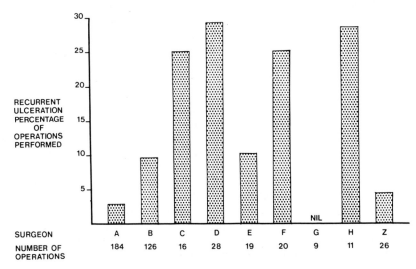

Figure 2.64 Incidence of recurrent ulceration after highly selective vagotomy for duodenal ulcer expressed as a percentage of the number of operations performed by individual surgeons.

later, and the incidence of recurrent ulceration is 2% at 5 years and 3–4% after 10 years.

We have conducted prospective controlled trials of the Burge electrical stimulation test and the Grassi test (both used at operation after highly selective vagotomy was completed) to see whether completeness of vagotomy was thereby improved, but no convincing evidence in favour of either test was found, compared with the results that were obtained in a 'control' group of patients whose highly selective vagotomy was performed in the usual way.[6,27,87] However, Johnson and Baxter,[50] and Allgöwer's group[77] have produced persuasive evidence in favour of the use of the Grassi and the Burge test, respectively, so the question of intraoperative testing remains open. Certainly some of the lowest recurrence rates after highly selective vagotomy have been reported by surgeons who do not use such tests: it remains to be seen whether the use of these tests helps surgeons with high recurrence rates to improve their results, or assists those learning to use the technique to achieve 'complete' vagotomy of the parietal cell mass regularly.

References

1. Amdrup, E., Andersen, D. and Høstrup, H. (1978) The Aarhus County Vagotomy Trial I. An interim report on primary results and incidence of sequelae following parietal cell vagotomy and selective gastric vagotomy in 748 patients. *World Journal of Surgery*, **2**, 85–90.

2. Amdrup, E., Jensen, H.-E., Johnston, D. *et al.* (1974) Clinical results of parietal cell vagotomy (highly selective vagotomy) two to four years after operation. *Annals of Surgery*, **180**, 279–284.

3. Andersen, S., Høstrup, H. and Amdrup, E. (1978) The Aarhus County Vagotomy Trial II. An interim report on reduction of acid secretion and ulcer recurrence rate following parietal cell vagotomy and selective gastric vagotomy. *World Journal of Surgery*, **2**, 91–100.

4. Bardhan, K.D. (1981) Long-term management of duodenal ulcer – a physician's view. In *Cimetidine in the 80s* (Ed.) Baron, J.H. pp. 95–112. Edinburgh: Churchill Livingstone.

5. Baxter, J.N., Grime, J.S., Critchley, M. and Shields, R. (1983) The effect of truncal vagotomy and pyloroplasty on the relationship between gastric emptying and gall bladder emptying. *British Journal of Surgery* (in press).

6. Blackett, R.L., Baltas, B., King, R.F.G.J. *et al.* (1983) Does the Grassi test lead to more complete vagotomies? A prospective randomized trial (PRT). *British Journal of Surgery*, **70**, 294.

7. Buckler, K.G. (1967) Effects of gastric surgery upon gastric emptying in cases of peptic ulceration. *Gut*, **8**, 137–147.

8. Burge, H. and Vane, J.R. (1958) Method of testing for complete nerve section during vagotomy. *British Medical Journal*, **i**, 615–618.

9. Capper, W.M., Airth, G.F. and Kilby, J.O. (1966) A test for pyloric regurgitation. *Lancet*, **ii**, 621–623.

10. Christiansen, J., Jensen, H.-E., Ejby-Poulsen, P. *et al.* (1981) Prospective controlled vagotomy trial for duodenal ulcer. Primary results, sequelae, acid secretion and recurrence rates. *Annals of Surgery*, **193**, 49–55.

11. Clarke, R.J. and Alexander-Williams, J. (1973) The effect of preserving antral innervation and of a pyloroplasty on gastric emptying after vagotomy in man. *Gut*, **14**, 300–307.

12. Clave, R.A. and Gaspar, M.R. (1969) Incidence of gall bladder disease after vagotomy. *American Journal of Surgery*, **118**, 169–174.

13. Cobb, J.S., Bank, S., Marks, I.N. and Louw, J.H. Gastric emptying after vagotomy and pyloroplasty. Relation to some post-operative sequelae. *American Journal of Digestive Diseases*, **16**, 207–215.

14. Colmer, M.R., Owen, G.M. and Shields, R. (1973) Pattern of gastric emptying after vagotomy and pyloroplasty. *British Medical Journal*, **ii**, 448–450.

15. Cowie, A.G.A. and Clark, C.G. (1972) The lithogenic effect of vagotomy. *British Journal of Surgery*, **59**, 363–367.

16. Cowley, D.J., Vernon, P., Jones, T. *et al.* (1972) Gastric emptying of solid meals after truncal vagotomy and pyloroplasty in human subjects. *Gut*, **13**, 176–181.

17. Cox, A.G., Bond, M.R., Podmore, D.A. and Rose, D.P. Aspects of nutrition after vagotomy and gastrojejunostomy. *British Medical Journal*, **i**, 465–469.

18. Csendes, A., Larach, J. and Godoy, M. (1978) Incidence of gallstone development after selective hepatic vagotomy. *Acta Chirurgica Scandinavica*, **144**, 289–291.

19. Davenport, H.W. (1969) Gastric mucosal haemorrhage in dogs. Effects of acid, aspirin and alcohol. *Gastroenterology*, **56**, 439–449.

20. Dewar, P., King, R. and Johnston, D. (1982) Bile acid and lysolecithin concentrations in the stomach in patients with duodenal ulcer before operation and after treatment by highly selective vagotomy, partial gastrectomy or truncal vagotomy and drainage. *Gut*, **23**, 569–577.

21. Dewar, E.P., King, R.F.G. and Johnston, D. (1983) Bile acid and lysolecithin concentrations in the stomach of patients with gastric ulcer before operation and after treatment by highly selective vagotomy, Billroth I partial gastrectomy and truncal vagotomy and pyloroplasty. *British Journal of Surgery*, **70**, 401–406.

22. Domellof, L., Eriksson, S. and Janunger, K.G. (1975) Late precancerous changes and carcinoma of the gastric stump after Billroth II resection. *Acta Chirurgica Scandinavica*, **141**, 292–297.

23. Dorricott, N.J., McNeish, A.R., Alexander-Williams, J. *et al.* (1978) Prospective randomised multicentre trial of proximal gastric vagotomy or truncal vagotomy and antrectomy for chronic duodenal ulcer: interim results. *British Journal of Surgery*, **65**, 152–154.

24. Dragstedt, L.R. and Owens, F.M. (1943) Supradiaphragmatic section of the vagus nerves in the treatment of duodenal ulcer. *Proceedings of the Society of Experimental Biology and Medicine*, **53**, 152–154.

25. Du Plessis, D.J. (1965) Pathogenesis of gastric ulceration. *The Lancet*, **i**, 974–978.

26. Edwards, J.P., Lyndon, P.J., Smith, R.B. and Johnston, D. (1974) Faecal fat excretion after truncal, selective and highly selective vagotomy for duodenal ulcer. *Gut*, **15**, 521–525.

27. Eltringham, W.K., Thompson, M.H., Davies, P.W. *et al.* (1982) The Grassi test and acid secretion. In: *Vagotomy in Modern Surgical Practice* (Eds) Baron, J.H., Alexander-Williams, J., Allgöwer M. *et al.* pp. 91–95. Sevenoaks: Butterworth.

28. Feldman, M., Richardson, C.T. and Fordtran, J.S. (1980) Experience with sham feeding as a test for vagotomy. *Gastroenterology*, **79**, 792–795.

29. Fisher, R. and Cohen, S. (1973) Pyloric-sphincter dysfunction in patients with gastric ulcer. *New England Journal of Medicine*, **288**, 273–276.

30. Fletcher, D.M. and Clark, C.G. (1969) Changes in canine bile-flow and composition after vagotomy. *British Journal of Surgery*, **56**, 103–106.

31. Fletcher, D.M. and Clark, C.G. (1968) Gall-stones and gastric surgery. A review. *British Journal of Surgery*, **55**, 895–899.

32. Fraser, A.G., Brunt, P.W. and Matheson, N.A. (1983) A comparison of highly selective vagotomy with truncal vagotomy and pyloroplasty – one surgeon's results after 5 years. *British Journal of Surgery*, **70**, 485–488.

33. Fritz, M.E. and Brooks, F.P. (1963) Control of bile flow in the cholecystectomized dog. *American Journal of Physiology*, **204**, 825–828.

34. Gillespie, G., Elder, J.B., Gillespie, I.E. *et al.* (1970) The long term stability of the insulin test. *Gastroenterology*, **58**, 625–632.

35. Goligher, J.C. (1974) A technique for highly selective (parietal cell or proximal gastric) vagotomy for duodenal ulcer. *British Journal of Surgery*, **61**, 337–345.

36. Goligher, J.C., Pulvertaft, C.N., DeDombal, F.T. *et al.* (1968) Five-to-eight-year results of Leeds/York controlled trial of elective surgery for duodenal ulcer. *British Medical Journal*, **ii**, 781–787.

36a. Goligher, J.C., Pulvertaft, C.N., Irvin, T.T. *et al.* (1972) Five-to-eight-year results of truncal vagotomy and pyloroplasty for duodenal ulcer. *British Medical Journal*, **i**, 7–13.

37. Grassi, G. (1971) A new test for complete nerve section during vagotomy. *British Journal of Surgery*, **58**, 187–189.

38. Grassi, G. (1977) The results of highly selective vagotomy in our experience (787) cases. *Chirurgia Gastroenterologica*, **11**, 51–58.

39. Greenall, M.J., Lyndon, P.J., Goligher, J.C. and Johnston, D. (1975) Longterm effect of highly selective vagotomy on basal and maximal acid output in man. *Gastroenterology*, **68**, 1421–1425.

40. Hallenbeck, G.A., Gleysteen, J.J., Aldrete, J.S. and Slaughter, R.L. (1976) Proximal gastric vagotomy: effects of two operative techniques on clinical and gastric secretory results. *Annals of Surgery*, **184**, 435–442.

41. Hansky, J. and Korman, M.G. (1973) Immunoassay studies in peptic ulcer. *Clinics in Gastroenterology*, **2**, 275–291.

42. Hill, G.L. and Barker, M.C.J. (1978) Anterior highly selective vagotomy with posterior truncal vagotomy: a simple technique for denervating the parietal cell mass. *British Journal of Surgery*, **65**, 702–705.

43. Hollander, F. (1948) Laboratory procedures in the study of vagotomy (with particular reference to the insulin test). *Gastroenterology*, **11**, 419–425.

44. Howlett, P.J., Ward, A.S. and Duthie, H.L. (1964) Gastric emptying after vagotomy. *Proceedings of the Royal Society of Medicine*, **67**, 836–838.

45. Howlett, P.J., Sheiner, H.J., Barber, D.C. *et al.* (1976) Gastric emptying in control subjects and patients with duodenal ulcer before and after vagotomy. *Gut*, **17**, 542–550.

46. Humphrey, C.S. and Wilkinson, A.R. (1972) The value of preserving the pylorus in the surgery of duodenal ulcer. *British Journal of Surgery*, **59**, 779–783.

47. Humphrey, C.S., Dykes, J.R.W. and Johnston, D. (1975) Effects of truncal, selective and highly selective vagotomy on glucose tolerance and insulin secretion in patients with duodenal ulcer. *British Medical Journal*, **ii**, 112–116.

48. Humphrey, C.S., Johnston, D., Walker, B.E. *et al.* (1972) Incidence of dumping after truncal and selective vagotomy and pyloroplasty and highly selective vagotomy without drainage procedure. *British Medical Journal*, **iii**, 785–788.

49. Inberg, M.V. and Vuorio, M. (1969) Human gallbladder function after selective gastric and total abdominal vagotomy. *Acta Chirurgica Scandinavica*, **135**, 625–633.

50. Johnson, A.G. and Baxter, H.K. (1977) Where is your vagotomy incomplete? Observations on operative technique. *British Journal of Surgery*, **64**, 583–586.

51. Johnson, F.E. and Boyden, E.A. (1952) The effect of double vagotomy on the motor activity of the human gall bladder. *Surgery*, **32**, 591–601.

52. Johnson, A.G. and McDermott, S.J. (1974) Lysolecithin: a factor in the pathogenesis of gastric ulceration. *Gut*, **15**, 710–713.

53. Johnston, D. (1975) Operative mortality and postoperative morbidity of highly selective vagotomy. *British Medical Journal*, **iv**, 545–547.

54. Johnston, D. and Goligher, J.C. (1976) Selective, highly selective or truncal vagotomy? *Surgical Clinics of North America*, **56**, 1313–1334.

55. Johnston, D. and Wilkinson, A.R. (1970) Highly selective vagotomy without a drainage procedure in the treatment of duodenal ulcer. *British Journal of Surgery*, **57**, 289–296.

56. Johnston, D., Humphrey, C.S., Walker, B.E. *et al.* (1972) Vagotomy without diarrhoea. *British Medical Journal*, **iii**, 788–790.

57. Johnston, D., Wilkinson, A.R., Humphrey, C.S. *et al.* (1973) Serial studies of gastric secretion in patients after highly selective (parietal cell) vagotomy without a drainage procedure for duodenal ulcer. II. The insulin test after highly selective vagotomy. *Gastroenterology*, **64**, 12–21.

58. Jordan, P.H. (1979) An interim report on parietal cell vagotomy versus selective vagotomy and antrectomy for treatment of duodenal ulcer. *Annals of Surgery*, **189**, 643–652.

59. Jordan, P.H. and Condon, R.E. (1970) A prospective evaluation of vagotomy-pyloroplasty and vagotomy-antrectomy for treatment of duodenal ulcer. *Annals of Surgery*, **172**, 547–563.

60. Keighley, M.R.B., Asquith, P. and Alexander-Williams, J. (1975) Duodenogastric reflux: a cause of gastric mucosal hyperaemia and symptoms after operations for peptic ulceration. *Gut*, **16**, 28–32.

61. Kennedy, T., Connell, A.M., Love, A.H.G. *et al.* (1973) Selective or truncal vagotomy? Five-year results of a double-blind prospective, randomised, controlled trial. *British Journal of Surgery*, **60**, 944–948.

62. Kennedy, T., Johnston, G.W., MacRae, K.D. and Spencer, E.F.A. (1975) Proximal gastric vagotomy: interim results of a randomised controlled trial. *British Medical Journal*, **ii**, 301–305.

63. Knutson, U. and Olbe, L. (1973) The gastric acid response to sham feeding in duodenal ulcer patients after proximal selective vagotomy. *Scandinavian Journal of Gastroenterology*, **20**(suppl.), 16.

64. Knutson, U. and Olbe, L. (1973) Gastric acid response to sham feeding in the duodenal ulcer patient. *Scandinavian Journal of Gastroenterology*, **8**, 513–522.

65. Koffman, C.G., Hay, D.J., Ganguli, P.C. *et al.* (1983) A prospective randomized trial of vagotomy in chronic duodenal ulceration: 4-year follow up. *British Journal of Surgery*, **70**, 342–345.

66. Kronborg, O. and Andersen, D. (1980) Acid response to sham feeding as a test for completeness of vagotomy. *Scandinavian Journal of Gastroenterology*, **15**, 119–121.

67. Kronborg, O., Malmstrom, J. and Christiansen, P.M. (1970) A comparison between the results of truncal and selective vagotomy in patients with duodenal ulcer. *Scandinavian Journal of Gastroenterology*, **5**, 519–524.

68. Lavigne, M.E., Wiley, Z.D., Martin, P. *et al.* (1979) Gastric, pancreatic and biliary secretion and the rate of gastric emptying after parietal cell vagotomy. *American Journal of Surgery*, **138**, 644–651.

69. Lawson, H.H. (1964) Effect of duodenal contents on the gastric mucosa under experimental conditions. *The Lancet*, **i**, 469–472.

70. Leading article (1978) Cimetidine for duodenal ulcer. *The Lancet*, **ii**, 1237–1238.

71. Lyndon, P.J., Greenall, M.J., Smith, R.B. *et al.* (1975) Serial insulin tests over a five-year period after highly selective vagotomy. *Gastroenterology*, **69**, 1188–1195.

72. Madsen, R. and Kronborg, O. (1980) Recurrent ulcer 5½–8 years after highly selective vagotomy without drainage and selective vagotomy with pyloroplasty. *Scandinavian Journal of Gastroenterology*, **15**, 193–199.

73. Makey, D.A., Tovey, F.I. and Heald, R.J. (1979) Results of proximal gastric vagotomy over 1–5 years in a district general hospital. *British Journal of Surgery*, **66**, 39–42.

74. Malagelada, J.R., Go, V.L.W. and Summerskill, W.H.S. (1974) Altered pancreatic and biliary function after vagotomy and pyloroplasty. *Gastroenterology*, **66**, 22–27.

75. McKelvey, S.T.D. (1970) Gastric incontinence and postvagotomy diarrhoea. *British Journal of Surgery*, **57**, 741–747.

76. Mühe, E., Muller, C., Martolini, S. *et al.* (1982) Five-years' results of a prospective multicentre trial of proximal gastric vagotomy. In *Vagotomy in Modern Surgical Practice* (Eds) Baron, J.H., Alexander-Williams, J., Allgöwer, M. *et al.* pp. 176–186. Sevenoaks: Butterworth.

77. Muller, C., Martolini, S. and Allgöwer, M. (1982) The vagometer electrotest (modified Burge test) for completeness of vagotomy. In *Vagotomy in Modern Surgical Practice* (Eds) Baron, J.H., Alexander-Williams, J., Allgöwer, M. *et al.* pp. 77–85. Sevenoaks: Butterworth.

78. Parkin, G.J.S., Smith, R.B. and Johnston, D. (1973) Gall bladder volume and contractility after truncal, selective and highly selective (parietal cell) vagotomy in man. *Annals of Surgery*, **178**, 581–586.

79. Postlethwait, R.W. (1973) Five year follow-up results of operations for duodenal ulcer. *Surgery, Gynecology and Obstetrics*, **137**, 387–392.

80. Pounder, R. (1981) Maintenance treatment, part 3 – cost effectiveness. In *Cimetidine in the 80s* (Ed.) Baron, J.H. pp. 89–94. Edinburgh: Churchill Livingstone.

81. Ramus, N.I., Williamson, R.C.N., Oliver, J.M. and Johnston, D. (1982) Effect of highly selective vagotomy on pancreatic exocrine function and on cholecystokinin and gastrin release. *Gut*, **23**, 553–557.

82. Rhodes, J., Barnardo, D.E., Phillips, S.F. *et al.* (1969) Increased reflux of bile into the stomach in patients with gastric ulcer. *Gastroenterology*, **57**, 241–252.

83. Rudick, J. and Hutchison, J.S.F. (1964) Effects of vagal nerve section on the biliary system. *The Lancet*, **i**, 579–581.

84. Sapala, M.A., Sapala, J.A., Resto Soto, A.D. and Bouwman, D.L. (1979) Cholelithiasis following subtotal gastric resection with truncal vagotomy. *Surgery, Gynecology and Obstetrics*, **148**, 36–38.

85. Sawyers, J.L., Herrington, J.L. and Burney, D.P. (1977) Proximal gastric vagotomy compared with vagotomy and antrectomy and selective gastric vagotomy and pyloroplasty. *Annals of Surgery*, **186**, 510–515.

86. Schrumpf, E., Stadaas, J., Myren, J. *et al.* (1977) Mucosal changes in the gastric stump 20–25 years after partial gastrectomy. *The Lancet*, **ii**, 467–469.

87. Shorey, B.A., Owens, C., Davies, P. *et al.* (1977) Which is the best test of completeness of vagotomy – the Burge, the Grassi or the insulin test. *British Journal of Surgery*, **64**, 298.

88. Smith, R.B., Edwards, J.P. and Johnston, D. (1981) Effect of vagotomy on exocrine pancreatic and biliary secretion in man. *American Journal of Surgery*, **141**, 40–46.

89. Stadaas, J. and Aune, S. (1970) Intragastric pressure/volume relationship before and after vagotomy. *Acta Chirurgica Scandinavica*, **136**, 611–612.

90. Stalsberg, H. and Taksdal, S. (1971) Stomach cancer following gastric surgery for benign conditions. *The Lancet*, **ii**, 1175–1177.

91. Stoddard, C.J., Vassilakis, J.S. and Duthie, H.L. (1978) Highly selective vagotomy or truncal vagotomy and pyloroplasty for chronic duodenal ulceration: a randomized prospective clinical study. *British Journal of Surgery*, **65**, 793–796.

92. Stoddard, C.J., Brown, B.H., Whittaker, G.B. *et al.* (1973) Effects of varying the extent of vagotomy on the myoelectrical and motor activity of the stomach in man. *British Journal of Surgery*, **60**, 307.

93. Stoddard, C.J., Smallwood, R., Brown, B.H. and Duthie, H.L. (1975) The immediate and delayed effects of different types of vagotomy on human gastric myeloelectric activity. *Gut*, **16**, 165–170.

94. Taylor, T.V., Lambert, M.E., Qureshi, S. and Torrance, B. (1978) Should cholecystectomy be combined with vagotomy and pyloroplasty. *The Lancet*, **i**, 295–298.

95. Temple, J.G., Goodall, R.J.R., Hay, D.J. and Miller, D. (1979) The effect of highly selective vagotomy and truncal vagotomy on the lower oesophageal sphincter. *British Journal of Surgery*, **66**, 360.

96. Thomas, P.A. and Earlam, R.J. (1973) The gastro-oesophageal junction before and after operations for duodenal ulcer. *British Journal of Surgery*, **60**, 717–719.

97. Tompkins, R.E., Kraft, A.R., Zimmerman, E. *et al.* (1972) Clinical and biochemical evidence of increased gallstone formation after complete vagotomy. *Surgery*, **71**, 196–200.

98. Venables, C.W., Wheldon, E.J. and Johnston, I.D.A. (1982) The long-term metabolic sequelae of truncal vagotomy and drainage. In *Vagotomy in Modern Surgical Practice* (Eds) Baron, J.H., Alexander-Williams, J., Allgöwer, M. *et al.* pp. 288–294. Sevenoaks: Butterworth.

99. Ward, M.W.N., Clark, C.G. and Karamanolis, D. (1982) Cholecystectomy and vagotomy – an unhappy combination. *Gut*, **23**, A900.

100. Wastell, C. and Ellis, H. (1966) Faecal fat excretion and stool colour after vagotomy and pyloroplasty. *British Medical Journal*, **i**, 1194–1197.

101. Wheldon, E.J., Venables, C.W. and Johnston, I.D.A. (1970) Late metabolic sequelae of vagotomy and gastroenterostomy. *The Lancet*, **i**, 437–440.

102. Wormsley, K.G. (1981) Short-term treatment of duodenal ulceration. In: *Cimetidine in the 80s* (Ed.) Baron, J.H. pp. 3–8. Edinburgh: Churchill Livingstone.

THE FUTURE OF PEPTIC ULCER SURGERY *(T.V. Taylor)*

There have been many changes of attitudes in the treatment of peptic ulcer in recent years. These have occurred due to the availability of more powerful antisecretory drugs, which are now virtually always able to heal the most resistant of ulcers, in the short term, and the recognition that *Helicobacter pylori* is important in ulcer pathogenesis. The aphorism of Schwartz, 'no acid, no ulcer', holds true but there is increasing evidence that the eradication of *H. pylori* from the stomach may result in long-term healing of the ulcer. The aetiological equation may thus read: duodenal ulcer = acid–pepsin ± *H. pylori* versus mucosal resistance. If it is shown in the next few years that eradication of this organism from the stomach results in long-term cure of ulcers, then treatment strategies may change radically, involving a 2-week course of triple therapy and a further reduction in elective ulcer surgery. Despite the decline in the prevalence of peptic ulcer there has been no corresponding reduction in mortality, which is steadily increasing, particularly in elderly females. The factors responsible for this rising mortality may be the increased use of non-steroidal anti-inflammatory drugs, for which 22 million prescriptions are given each year (in addition to over-the-counter sales) and possibly the declining use of definitive surgery rendering more people vulnerable to the potentially fatal complications of bleeding and perforation.

One indication for elective ulcer surgery, are those patients with an aggressive ulcer diathesis which repeatedly relapses on cessation of full-dose treatment with H_2 receptor antagonists or omeprazole who are approaching the age of 50 years. In these patients, long-term ulcer healing by vagotomy may reduce the potentially fatal risks of bleeding and perforation over their advancing years. Clearly, if operations could be made simpler, safer, less expensive and less traumatic, by employing laparoscopic techniques, there may be a resurgence of interest in surgical treatment.

The surgical option of choice for duodenal ulcer is some form of pylorus-preserving vagotomy. Although concern has been expressed at the recurrent ulcer rates after highly selective vagotomy, which may be as high as 30% at 18 years as in the Copenhagen study, this strategy can still be justified since: (1) recurrences can be readily treated by medication; (2) these ulcers tend to be less aggressive with a low risk of perforation or bleeding; and (3) much lower recurrence rates are reported by other groups. Pylorus-preserving vagotomy also remains free of the incapacitating and untreatable complications of dumping, diarrhoea and bilious vomiting. Furthermore, this form of surgery is very safe, the perioperative mortality for conventional highly selective vagotomy or anterior lesser curve seromyotomy and posterior truncal vagotomy being as low as 0.2–0.3%. The consistent report of late recurrences following highly selective vagotomy is perplexing. After all other forms of vagotomy the vast majority of recurrent ulcers occur within 2 years of the operation. Any nerve regeneration or hormonal changes would be expected to be complete by 2 years. The problem may relate to inadequate gastric motility following proximal gastric denervation. Holle, who first introduced highly selective vagotomy in humans in 1967, always used a drainage procedure. Although on physiological grounds division of the pylorus may seem heretical, the fact is that there is a lower incidence of recurrence in the series of over 1600 patients reported by Holle.

The wider adoption of laparoscopic techniques could restore some of the lost enthusiasm for surgical treatment. The procedure of highly selective vagotomy or alternatively of anterior highly selective vagotomy or anterior lesser curve seromyotomy combined with posterior truncal vagotomy is eminently feasible laparoscopically, particularly using diathermy or a laser to divide the gastric (parietal cell) branches of the nerve of Latarjet. Laparoscopic cholecystectomy is now widely employed, with 40% of gallbladders now being removed in this way in the

USA. Other intra-abdominal procedures are currently being investigated, including resection of the oesophagus and colon. Rapidly improving technology has facilitated the wider and safer use of laparoscopic surgery. Anterior lesser curve seromyotomy with posterior truncal vagotomy has been performed in Houston and in France. Highly selective vagotomy has also been performed in Europe. In performing the dissection along the lesser curvature, three anatomical considerations are pertinent. First, the gastric branches of the nerve of Latarjet have no particular predilection to run with the vessels along the wall of the stomach; secondly, these nerves always run superficial to the blood vessels; and, thirdly, the nerves do not tend to branch before entering the gastric musculature about one-third of the way along the stomach to innervate the gastric mucosa. Consideration of these anatomical criteria indicates that division of the serosa and blood vessels about 1 cm away from the lesser curvature will result in denervation of the parietal cell mass, a fact that has been confirmed by open surgical procedures. Laparoscopic seromyotomy, if this is preferred, should extend from the incisura angularis to the gastro-oesophageal junction. Postoperatively nasogastric decompression is unnecessary and the patient can be discharged on the following day. Consequently, morbidity and hospital stay are much less than with conventional surgical practice.

Such minimally invasive surgery, if proven to be safe and effective over the next few years, may well have a major impact on the management of chronic peptic ulcers, particularly as recurrence rates after discontinuing H_2 receptor antagonist therapy approach 90% at 1 year. Perhaps the major competitor to a conservative surgical approach would be the long-term efficacy of triple therapy in the eradication of *H. pylori* and maintenance of ulcer healing. Nevertheless, there will always be some patients who are non-compliant drug takers in whom minimally invasive surgery achieving complete vagotomy of the acid-secreting part of the stomach may offer real theraputic promise in the future.

ACUTE BLEEDING PEPTIC ULCER

AETIOLOGY   *(R.P. Walt and M.J.S. Langman)*

The frequency of peptic ulcer bleeding in the general population is uncertain. Haematemesis and melaena are conventionally considered as obligatory causes of hospital admission, and so hospital case series should provide useful information. However, mild episodes may present late, or not at all, whilst patients with abrupt and massive haemorrhage may die before admission is possible.[1,11] Errors can also arise from extrapolating data from case series to the population at large because patients may be admitted from outside the catchment population of a hospital (because of particular expertise), or because elderly patients remain uncounted as they are preferentially admitted to geriatric rather than acute services. This point may be particularly important as the proportion of older patients with ulcer complications has been increasing, and at a greater rate than might be expected from the increased number of elderly in the general population.

Data from the Hospital In-patient Enquiry (HIPE), which collects discharge or death diagnoses from a 10% sample of all admissions in England and Wales, and a similar set from the Scottish Hospital In-patient Statistics (SHIPS) give reasonable information for the UK. Diseases are classified using the International Classification of Disease (ICD) code which has itself changed over the past 20 years. Codings for ulcer bleeding were omitted for approximately a 25-year period before being reinstated with the ninth revision. It has therefore been difficult to explore the patterns of change and hence to seek causal relationships for variations detected. Despite the deficiencies, HIPE data are valuable as a broad representation of what is happening in the community.

The frequency of various other conditions leading to haematemesis or melaena varies from country to country and other causes are discussed elsewhere. Peptic ulcer bleeding represents about 50% of all causes of upper gastrointestinal haemorrhage in the UK (*Table 2.25*).

Table 2.25 Diagnostic categories observed in patients admitted with haematemesis and melaena in the UK

Category	Oxford 1963–1967 (n = 688) (%)[a]	Nottingham 1975–1979 (n = 526) (%)[b]
Duodenal ulcer	30.1	23.2
Gastric ulcer	14.1	25.5
Gastric cancer	2.6	3.0
Acute gastric lesions	N	6.7
Oesophagitis and ulcer	N	12.2
Mallory Weiss syndrome	N	N
Oesophageal varices	3.1	1.9
Other known categories	31.0	
Diagnosis unclear	19.2	27.4

N, not stated.
[a] From Schiller *et al.*[12]
[b] From Dronfield *et al.*[3]

Classic teaching has been that gastric ulcer is more serious and likely to cause death than duodenal ulcer. It has been emphasized that duodenal ulcer is much more likely to be the cause of bleeding in men than women. Such statements are not straightforward, and account of age distributions must be taken. HIPE data from 1984 show 521 deaths from 3705 episodes of gastric ulcer bleeding and 432 deaths in 4684 episodes of duodenal ulcer haemorrhage (14.1% against 9.8%). However, women are nearly three times as likely to die as men from duodenal ulcer bleeding (15.1% versus 5.9%). These figures fit well with the authors' previous observation of rising mortality from peptic ulcer in elderly women.[14] The reasons are unclear.

Genetics

Gastric and duodenal ulceration has a familial predisposition, with ulcers of the same type appearing in the same and successive generations. Hypersecretion of pepsinogen I is genetically determined but there is no evidence to suggest that this predisposes patients to bleeding. Blood group O is strongly associated with bleeding ulcer.[8] The basis is unclear though relatively high circulating levels of antihaemophiliac globulin in patients with the other blood groups may explain this association.[10]

Environmental factors

Common environmental exposure within families may be as important as or indeed explain familial disease occurrence. Thus, transmission of *Helicobacter pylori* within family contacts is a plausible explanation although only a minority of patients exposed to *H. pylori* develop peptic ulcer.

Drugs

Recent studies have clarified the risk of ulcer complications associated with use of aspirin and nonsteroidal anti-inflammatory drugs (NSAIDs). *Table 2.26* demonstrates that the risks of complications, including bleeding, are raised three to four times in aspirin or NSAID takers. For gastric ulcer, a similar risk for ulcer occurrence has been identified. This indicates that it is the frequency of ulcer development which underlies outcome rather than any particular propensity for patients taking NSAIDs to die from ulcer complications. In contrast, duodenal ulcer occurrence may not be increased by NSAIDs while complications clearly are. This suggests that NSAID use may lead to bleeding from established ulcers at this site.

Table 2.26 Anti-inflammatory drug use and complications of peptic ulcer in the UK

	Relative risk	95% confidence interval	Reference
Non-aspirin NSAIDs			
Bleeding			
Gastric	2.8	1.5–5.4	13
Duodenal	2.7	1.3–5.8	13
Perforation			
Peptic	7.3	4.4–4.8	2
Ulcer death	2.9	1.4–6.3	11
Aspirin			
Bleeding			
Gastric	3.3	1.4–8.5	4
Duodenal	3.0	1.4–7.1	4

The assumption that the increasing mortality and frequency of ulcer complications in elderly women may be explained totally by the fact that this group also shows increasing use of NSAIDs is facile and almost certainly incorrect. Calculation of the population attributable risk shows that NSAIDs could account for up to 25% of all hospital admissions with ulcer bleeding and a further 10% could be due to aspirin use. The ulcer perforation rate in older women (as a measure of complications) has virtually trebled in recent years and cannot be explained by increasing use of NSAIDs which has occurred in all age groups equally.

Other factors

There is no evidence to suggest that cigarette smoking increases the risk of bleeding over and above that due to any increment in ulcer frequency. Alcohol consumption is also classically associated with ulcer bleeding but evidence to support this is non-existent. It has been suggested that ulcer bleeding tends to present in spring and winter[7] although a basis for this observation is unclear.

Dietary associations with peptic ulcer remain poorly substantiated though claims have been made for a protective effect of dietary fibre.[9] More recently, an association of duodenal ulcer with high refined carbohydrate intake has been described,[6] as has an association with low dietary linoleic acid intake.[5] No particular dietary constituent had been associated with bleeding.

References

1. Armstrong, C.P. and Blower, A.L. (1987) Non-steroidal anti-inflammatory drugs and life threatening complications of peptic ulcer. *Gut*, **28**, 527–532.
2. Collier, D.S. and Pain, J.A. (1985) Non-steroidal anti-inflammatory drugs and peptic ulcer perforation. *Gut*, **26**, 359–363.
3. Dronfield, M.W., Langman, M.J.S., Atkinson, M. *et al.* (1982) Outcome of endoscopy and barium radiography for acute upper gastrointestinal bleeding: controlled trial in 1037 patients. *British Medical Journal*, **284**, 545–548.
4. Faulkner, G., Prichard, P., Somerville, K.W. and Langman, M.J.S. (1988) Aspirin and bleeding peptic ulcers in the elderly. *British Medical Journal*, **297**, 1311–1313.
5. Grant, H.W., Palmer, K.R., Riesmesma, R.R. and Oliver, M.F. (1990) Duodenal ulcer is associated with low dietary linoleic acid intake. *Gut*, **31**, 997–998.
6. Katschinski, B.D., Logan, R.F.A., Edmond, M. and Langman, M.J.S. (1990) Duodenal ulcer and refined carbohydrate intake: a case control study assessing dietary fibre and refined sugar intake. *Gut*, **31**, 993–996.
7. Langman, M.J.S. (1964) The seasonal incidence of bleeding from the upper gastrointestinal tract. *Gut*, **5**, 142–144.
8. Langman, M.J.S. and Doll, R. (1965) ABO blood groups and secretor status in relation to clinical characteristics of peptic ulcer. *Gut*, **6**, 270–273.
9. Malhotra, S.L. (1964) Peptic ulcer in India and its aetiology. *Gut*, **5**, 412–416.
10. Preston, A.E. and Barr, A. (1964) The plasma concentration of factor VIII in the normal population. *British Journal of Haematology*, **10**, 238–245.
11. Quader, K. and Logan, R. (1988) Peptic ulcer deaths: how many occur at home after non-steroidal anti-inflammatory drug prescribing? *Gut*, **29**, A1443.
12. Schiller, K.F.R., Truelove, S.C. and Williams, D.G. (1970) Haematemesis and melaena with special reference to factors influencing outcome. *British Medical Journal*, **2**, 7–14.
13. Somerville, K., Faulkner, G. and Langman, M.J.S. (1986) Non-steroidal anti-inflammatory drugs and bleeding peptic ulcer. *The Lancet*, **i**, 462–464.
14. Walt, R.P. Katchinski, B., Logan, R. and Langman, M.J.S. (1986) Rising frequency of ulcer perforation in elderly people in the United Kingdom. *The Lancet*, **i**, 489–492.

DIAGNOSIS   *(R.P. Walt and M.J.S. Langman)*

Emergency endoscopy offers the ability to make a diagnosis and should therefore influence management. This has never been satisfactorily proven in clinical trials yet the logic seems sound and more benefit seems to come from early rather than delayed endoscopy.[2] Nevertheless, a summary of trials concluded that benefit was not great from emergency endoscopy.[1] Few would argue that contrast radiology is as effective in diagnosis as endoscopy following gastrointestinal haemorrhage. Selective angiography could identify the bleeding lesion but is of no significant clinical use in the management or diagnosis of peptic ulcer haemorrhage.

References

1. Erickson, R.A. and Glick, M.E. (1986) Why have controlled trials failed to demonstrate a benefit of oesophagogastroduodenoscopy in acute upper gastrointestinal bleeding. A probability model analysis. *Digestive Diseases and Sciences*, **31**, 760–768.
2. Forrest, J.A.H., Finlayson, N.D.C. and Shearman, D.J.C. (1974) Endoscopy in gastrointestinal bleeding. *The Lancet*, **ii**, 394–397.

TREATMENT *(R.P. Walt and M.J.S. Langman)*

Admission to hospital is recommended for patients with suspected or proven gastrointestinal haemorrhage. The importance of admission is to offer general support with resuscitation and close observation. Many argue that no change in mortality has followed technological advances but a trend of declining mortality from gastrointestinal haemorrhage seems apparent. The reasons for this are not clear. Nevertheless if mortality rates in hospitals with particular interests in the management of gastrointestinal bleeding are followed this reduction is demonstrable (*Table 2.27*). It has been argued that these changes are due to the development of combined medical and surgical specialist units but an exact relationship is not obvious. The data from Nottingham (which does not have such a unit) suggest that other factors may prevail. Mortality rates must be considered in the light of an increasingly elderly population who would be expected to fare badly. Thus, an increase in general fitness of the elderly may partly explain the changes in mortality. Changing referral patterns within an area because of improved geriatric services could also confound. Nevertheless, it remains probable that units which use internal guidelines for the management of gastrointestinal bleeding, for example criteria on when to intervene surgically,[24,39] serve their patients well.

The guidelines used in the Birmingham General Hospital appear to have stood the test of time and were introduced following a controlled trial of early or delayed surgery.[24,39] Compliance with these guidelines elsewhere should produce similar morbidity rates in other hospitals. Two broad groups of patients are considered separately. Surgery is used for exanguinating haemorrhage and spurting arterial bleeding seen at endoscopy. Surgical intervention in patients over 60 years old is triggered by one rebleed in hospital, the requirement for four units of blood or colloid to maintain haemodynamic stability, or the need for 8 units of blood over a 48-hour period. In younger patients, surgery is advised for two hospital rebleeds, 8 units of blood or colloid for initial volume replacement or 12 units of blood transfused over 48 hours. In Birmingham these guidelines have been associated with an overall mortality rate for peptic ulcer of 4%, with 8% in patients over 80 years of age.[39] Clinicians with particular interests in gastrointestinal bleeding probably help to encourage improvements in care.

Table 2.27 Results of studies of gastrointestinal bleeding

Trial	Years	n	Rebleeding (%)	Operation (%)	Death (%)
Results published from trials in Nottingham 1975–1990					
Dronfield *et al.*[9]	1975–1977	318	NS	24.5	9.6
Dronfield *et al.*[10]	1975–1979	1037	NS	18.1	8.0
Barer *et al.*[3]	1980–1982	775	24	18.4	10.6
Somerville *et al.*[33]	1982–1984	630	25	11.0	8.9
Daneshmend *et al.*[8]	1986–1989	1147	16	10.8	6.1
Results published from studies from The General Hospital, Birmingham 1970–1988					
Allan and Dykes[1]	1970–1973	300	15	34.0	9.6
Morris *et al.*[24]	1980–1983	142[a]	NS	40.1[b]	7.0
Wheatley and Dykes[39]	1984–1988	342[a]	NS	20.2	3.8

NS, not significant.
[a] Only peptic ulcer patients included.
[b] Surgery in 59% of patients over 60 years and 21% of those under 60 years.

Continual audit of practice and results is necessary to identify such change.

What remains uncertain is whether the actual advice offered in specific guidelines is important in aiding management or whether the existence of guidelines which are actually followed is the critical point. The declining operation rates shown in *Table 2.27* for peptic ulcer bleeding make the point that increasingly selective surgical policies are being employed. In terms of audit, particular attention should be paid to the deaths of patients under the age of 60 years because expected death rates are of the order of 1% or less in this group.

Pharmacological intervention

The management of gastrointestinal haemorrhage would be improved if a simple, safe, effective and generally applicable drug therapy were available. Such treatment could be started before formal diagnosis, when patients are first admitted to hospital. No particular expertise would be needed to prescribe. A logical approach would be to inhibit the natural tendency for blood clot to lyse in the gastric lumen thus exposing the naked vessel. Elevating gastric pH should inhibit intragastric fibrinolysis by inactivation of pepsin and a range of drugs have been used in an attempt to achieve this. Alternatively, systemic antifibrinolytic agents have been used. Assessment of the data from therapeutic trials is difficult but there is no strong support for the routine use of any drug.

The problems evaluating haemorrhage trials

The efficacy of any treatment is conventionally measured by comparing end-points such as recurrence of bleeding, operation and death rates, but each may have interpretational problems because they are difficult to define. Thus, transfusion requirements are doctor dependent, rebleeding rates are difficult to identify, and surgical intervention is doctor and patient dependent even if firm criteria are employed. Death rates, the last common measure, is an obviously hard observation of outcome yet, in order to demonstrate an important reduction of say 30%, large trials including at least 1000 patients are needed. This is because expected overall mortality is around 10% or less and with lower numbers it is possible to conclude that treatments are valueless when studies lack the power to detect a real and important effect. *Table 2.28* shows the numbers needed if a halving of mortality is to be demonstrated with any certainty. No published trial had included 1000 patients or more until 1990[8] and even that trial was barely large enough. Studies have lately tended to be planned on the premise that

Table 2.28 Power requirements of studies to demonstrate changes in death or operation rates

	Power	Total to be included in trial
Death rate reduced from 10 to 5%	0.5	504
	0.8	948
Operation rate reduced from 25 to 15%	0.5	284
	0.8	540

All figures based upon a significance level of $P = 0.05$.

expected death rates are about 10% but published data suggest that a figure of 6% is now more realistic.

Another difficulty relates to subgroup analyses. When no significant difference is found overall, investigators are inevitably tempted to look for positive findings which might have been obscured in the totality of the data. A prior hypothesis does not usually exist and such analyses should be accepted as methods for identifying a group for whom another trial could be designed on the basis of the new hypothesis. Conclusive statements are not validly obtainable from such analyses though they are often made.

The timing of pharmacological intervention is also of potential importance. If treatment is started on arrival in hospital the most severe cases and also the mildest are potentially offered it. A delay of 24 hours to identify a particular group of patients would tend to eliminate those who may already have undergone surgery or died as well as those thought clinically not to need treatment. Nevertheless, early entry is essentially pragmatic, the answer being one which is applicable to clinical practice. The later entry which may define a particular disease (for example peptic ulcer with stigmata of haemorrhage[38]) leads to an explanatory trial whereby it can be seen that a particular treatment affects outcome in a specific disease. These points are crucial since the ultimate need is to know who entered the trial and what happened to all of them. All too often it is not possible to determine how many patients were randomized into a particular trial and what was the overall outcome.

Death is the firmest end-point but use of this criterion can be misleading from the explanatory viewpoint. Many deaths arise through coincident, pre-existent disease. Surgery is often considered unethical or inappropriate in some. In others, surgery for bleeding identifies the underlying condition, for instance pancreatic cancer, and treatment of this is associated with a more major procedure and subsequent death. It is natural to discount such cases from analysis and thus bias results unconsciously. It is therefore important that all categorizations including deaths are completed before code breaking.

Antisecretory therapy

H₂ receptor antagonists

Conflicting results abound, but the consensus is that benefit has not been conclusively demonstrated.[7] *Table 2.29* summarizes data obtained in 27 trials using cimetidine and ranitidine. Meta-analysis was applied after an attempt to identify all series treated whether published or not (an important point because negative studies are less likely to see the light of day than positive ones). A modest trend towards a reduction in rebleeding and just significant trends for operation and death rates were shown. However, the data lack conviction because of their weak trend, and the marginal level of significance. When the subgroups of gastric and duodenal ulcer were analysed separately, a somewhat greater effect was seen in gastric rather than duodenal ulcer (*Table 2.30*). This observation is statistically significant, and could, in theory, arise because the drug regimens used in the trials would not have been

Table 2.29 Overall results of meta-analysis of trials of H₂ receptor antagonists (total studied 2670)[7]

All patients	Percentage change	95% confidence intervals
Rebleeding	−11	−27 to +8
Operation	−22	−39 to 0
Death	−30	−50 to −4

Table 2.30 Subgroup analysis in trials of H₂ receptor antagonists[9]

	Percentage change	95% confidence intervals
Gastric ulcer[a]		
Rebleeding	−32	−53 to −2[c]
Operation	−39	−61 to −5[c]
Death	−47	−70 to −4[c]
Duodenal ulcer[b]		
Rebleeding	−7	−32 to +27
Operation	−24	−48 to +10
Death	−21	−58 to +50

[a] Total studied 702.
[b] Total studied 971.
[c] Significant difference $P < 0.05$.

expected to raise gastric pH adequately, perhaps particularly in duodenal ulcer. Thus, 24-hour pH studies have shown that the standard regimens did not raise the pH above 4.0 consistently.[27] An argument for increasing doses or giving continuous infusions which render patients achlorhydric is prevalent[23] but initial results are not encouraging.[38] There now seems no justification for routine use of H₂ receptor antagonists in upper gastrointestinal tract bleeding.

Proton pump inhibitors

Omeprazole is the only drug which has been widely studied: one trial of adequate size in gastrointestinal bleeding has been reported. Oral therapy takes some time to become maximally effective so intravenous regimens were developed to rapidly produce sustained hypoacidity.[37] Results ultimately obtained in a randomized placebo-controlled trial using the best omeprazole regimen in 1147 patients were disappointing. The result suggested that an early diminution of stigmata of bleeding occurred, but rebleeding and mortality were not significantly altered.[8] The 95% confidence intervals for mortality, which was higher in the omeprazole group, still encompassed the possibility of benefit, because overall mortality rates in placebo- and drug-related individuals were very low.

Somatostatin

Evidence of benefit with the natural hormone or an analogue is also conflicting and conclusive recommendations cannot be made[5,32] but routine use cannot presently be condoned.

Antifibrinolytic therapy

Tranexamic acid has been tested in reasonable numbers of patients. Individual studies are again not large enough to give conclusive answers but a combined analysis has suggested possible benefit.[14] One trial substantially weights the results of the meta-analysis.[3] This aside, there is reason to believe that systemic anti-fibrinolytic therapy could reduce rebleeding, and hence operation and mortality rates. The size of these changes is similar to that found in the meta-analysis with H₂ receptor antagonists. As for the other drugs, on present evidence routine use cannot be justified.

Endoscopic intervention

Arguably the most important advantage of early endoscopy is that it provides the opportunity to apply haemostatic devices to bleeding lesions. The use of sclerotherapy for oesophageal varices is long-standing. There are few who now dispute the value of the technique either as an acute management option or in the long-term prevention of further haemorrhage. The use of mechanical, chemical or electrical methods of haemostasis in peptic ulcer bleeding has been more recent and is gaining acceptance. The techniques commonly employed are laser photocoagulation, heater probe coagulation, electrocoagulation and injection sclerotherapy. Other methods may become available with technological advances, including the use of microwaves. Most early trials employed laser photocoagulation but expense and technical difficulties make it less generally applicable.

The techniques require a learning phase and results from centres where the procedures are established may not be reproduced in other hospitals. Therefore, results of trials cannot necessarily be translated to ordinary practice. The responses of patients characteristically excluded from clinical trials cannot be predicted from current experience. As many as 75% of cases presenting with bleeding are excluded in some studies.[31] A meta-analysis of results with all methods of endoscopic haemostasis recently performed confirms the impression that laser photocoagulation is effective.[31] Comparisons of one treatment method with another are needed.

The complications of all the techniques are similar and predictable. Perforation or increasing ulcer size is reported in a small number of cases. However, in the relatively few reported series the techniques appear safe.

Laser photocoagulation

Laser light causes vaporization, and the heat so produced induces coagulation when lasers are applied to tissue. The argon laser is avidly absorbed by haemoglobin and has limited tissue penetration. The neodymium:yttrium aluminium garnet (Nd:YAG) laser has greater tissue penetration. Although a number of controlled trials have been published, many are too small to allow confident conclusions to be drawn (Table 2.31). The position of the ulcer in some patients makes it inaccessible for endoscopic therapy. Experience reduces the access problem but a proportion of patients still cannot receive treatment. However, where the ulcers have been photocoagulated, a small reduction in emergency surgery or mortality has often been demonstrated. This benefit is particularly apparent with those ulcers containing a visible vessel[34] or in those actively bleeding from an artery.[35,36] Where ulcer bleeding is brisk and the ulcer accessible, the role of laser photocoagulation is best demonstrated.[31] It might be argued that the results are not very impressive and the capital expense and technical difficulties associated with laser therapy should be considered before purchasing a unit. Nevertheless, it appears that useful reductions in mortality as well as surgical intervention are possible.

Heater probe coagulation

The major problem of coagulation by heat at the end of a probe is that subsequent movement of the probe may dislodge the adherent coagulum. 'Non-stick'

Table 2.31   Results of trials of laser treatment of upper gastrointestinal bleeding (percentages in parentheses)

Trial	Randomized		Rebleeding		Surgery		Death		Significance
	Laser	Control	Laser	Control	Laser	Control	Laser	Control	
Lawrence et al.[19] (argon)	60	—	5 (8)	—	13 (22)	—	5 (8)	—	
Vallon et al.[36] (argon)	68	68	20 (29)	23 (34)	17 (25)	19 (28)	5 (7)	10 (14)	NS[a]
Swain et al.[34] (argon)	36	40	11 (31)	17 (43)	8 (22)	14 (35)	0	7 (18)	$P < 0.02$ for death[b]
Krejs et al.[16] (Nd:YAG)	85	89	19 (22)	18 (20)	14 (16)	15 (17)	1 (1)	1 (1)	NS
Rutgeerts et al.[28] (Nd:YAG)	52	58	5 (10)	12 (21)	3 (6)	9 (16)	8 (15)	8 (14)	NS
Swain et al.[35] (Nd:YAG)	70	68	7 (10)	27 (40)	7 (10)	24 (35)	1 (1)	8 (12)	$P < 0.01$ for rebleeding, <0.05 for death
Mcleod et al.[21] (Nd:YAG)	21	24	6 (29)	8 (33)	5 (24)	8 (33)	1 (5)	2 (8)	NS[c]

NS, not significant.
[a] $P < 0.05$ if patients with spurting only are considered and two are excluded from laser group because of failure to apply the beam accurately.
[b] $P < 0.05$ for rebleeding if analysis confined to non-bleeding visible vessels or a combination of bleeding and non-bleeding visible vessels.
[c] $P < 0.01$ for rebleeding and operation in arterial spurters which received laser treatment (33% did not for technical reasons).

coatings and water jets have been developed to reduce this problem. Published experience is limited with the Teflon-covered heater probe although uncontrolled studies have suggested that the device can produce haemostasis. Access in duodenal ulcer bleeding is reputedly difficult. One positive controlled trial[11] is insufficient to recommend the widespread use of this technique.

Compared with Nd:YAG laser treatment the heater probe was less (but not significantly so) effective.[22] Comparison of the heater probe with pure alcohol injection or with controls has shown a significant reduction in surgical intervention with the heater probe.[20]

Electrocoagulation

Two general methods exist: multipolar or monopolar. With the latter, electric current flows from the tip through the patient to a ground plate. The simplest multipolar electrodes are bipolar, comprising two electrodes separated by 1–2 mm. Current flows between these electrode poles, coagulating tissues in contact. Many electrodes are now commonly arranged around the probe (multipolar). A water pump produces a jet which limits the tendency for the probes to stick. The results of controlled trials (*Table 2.32*) are similar to results obtained using other haemostatic methods. Where direct

Table 2.32 Controlled trials of bipolar electrocoagulation for upper gastrointestinal bleeding (percentages in parentheses)

Trial	Randomized		Rebleeding		Surgery		Death		Significance
	Electro-coagulation	Control	Electro-coagulation	Control	Electro-coagulation	Control	Electro-coagulation	Control	
Goudie *et al.*[13]	21	25	7 (33)	5 (20)	2 (10)	2 (8)	0	0	NS
Kernohan *et al.*[15]	21	24	9 (43)	7 (29)	3 (14)	5 (21)	0	1 (4)	NS
Laine[17]	21	23	—	—	3 (14)	13 (57)	3 (14)	0	$P < 0.03$ for surgery[a]
O'Brien *et al.*[25]	101	103	17 (17)	34 (33)	7 (7)	10 (10)	13 (13)	14 (14)	$P < 0.002$ for rebleeding
Brearley *et al.*[4]	21	21	6 (29)	8 (38)	5 (24)	4 (19)	0	0	NS
Laine[18]	31	29	6 (19)	12 (41)	3 (10)	8 (28)	1 (3)	0	NS

NS, not significant.
[a] Half the patients had Mallory–Weiss tears or vascular malformations. No significant difference between surgery rates in peptic ulcer bleeds.

Table 2.33 Controlled trials of injection sclerotherapy for upper gastrointestinal bleeding (percentages in parentheses)

Trial	Randomized		Rebleeding		Surgery		Death		Significance
	Schlerothpy	Control	Schlerothpy	Control	Schlerothpy	Control	Schlerothpy	Control	
Panes *et al.*[26] (P + A)	55	58	3 (6)	25 (43)	3 (6)	20 (34)	2 (4)	4 (7)	$P < 0.02$ for rebleeding or surgery
Balanzo *et al.*[2] (P + A)	36	36	7 (19)	7 (19)	7 (19)	12 (33)	1 (3)	1 (3)	NS
Chung *et al.*[6] (A)	34	34	—	—	5 (15)	14 (41)	3 (9)	2 (6)	$P < 0.02$ for surgery
Rutgeerts *et al.*[30] (P + A)	40	20	3 (8)	12 (60)	3 (8)	11 (55)	2 (5)	2 (10)	$P <$ for rebleeding
(A)	40		7 (18)		6 (15)		4 (10)		NS

NS, not significant.
P, polidocanol; A, adrenaline.
[a] Trial also compared laser photocoagulation and control group not strictly comparable. Polidocanol plus adrenaline injection was most effective but not significantly more so than laser plus adrenaline injection.

comparisons have been made, electrocoagulation is no more or less effective than laser photocoagulation.[12,29] Meta-analysis of further studies may clarify whether one method is better than another, but at the moment insufficient data precludes this approach.[31]

Injection sclerotherapy

One practical endoscopic intervention involves injection of sclerosant (polidocanol, alcohol) with or without adrenaline in and around the ulcer base. Most endoscopists are familiar with the equipment and technique, which is used for sclerotherapy of oesophageal varices. The problems of access are unlikely to be any different with this technique. Controlled experience is limited but endoscopic sclerosis appears effective (*Table 2.33*). Injection therapy provides similar results to laser photocoagulation, yet poorer initial haemostasis than the heater probe.[20,30] There is limited evidence that laser photocoagulation is aided by injection of adrenaline beforehand.

References

1. Allan, R.N. and Dykes, P.W. (1976) A study of factors influencing mortality rates from gastrointestinal haemorrhage. *Quarterly Journal of Medicine*, **54**, 533–550.
2. Balanzo, J., Sainz, S., Such, J. *et al.* (1988) Endoscopic haemostasis by local injection of epinephrine and polidocanol in bleeding ulcer. A prospective randomized trial. *Endoscopy*, **20**, 289–291.
3. Barer, D., Ogilvie, A., Henry, D. *et al.* (1983) Cimetidine and tranexamic acid in the treatment of acute upper-gastrointestinal tract bleeding. *New England Journal of Medicine*, **308**, 1571–1575.
4. Brearley, S., Hawker, P.C., Dykes, P.W. and Keighley, M.R.B. (1987) Perendoscopic bipolar diathermy coagulation of visible vessels using a 3.2 mm probe: a randomised trial. *Endoscopy*, **19**, 160–163.
5. Christiansen, J., Ottenjann, R. and Von-Arx, F. (1989) Placebo controlled trial with the somatostatin analogue SMS 201–995 in peptic ulcer bleeding. *Gastroenterology*, **97**, 568–574.
6. Chung, S.C.S., Leung, J.W.C., Steele, R.J.C., Crofts, T.J. and Li, A.J.C. (1988) Endoscopic adrenaline injection for actively bleeding ulcers: a randomised trial. *British Medical Journal*, **296**, 1631–1633.
7. Collins, R. and Langman, M. (1985) Treatment with histamine H2 receptor antagonists in acute upper gastrointestinal hemorrhage. *New England Journal of Medicine*, **313**, 660–666.
8. Daneshmend, T.K., Hawkey, C.J., Langman, M.J.S., Logan, R.F.A., Long, R.G. and Walt, R.P. (1990) Omeprazole versus placebo for acute upper gastrointestinal bleeding. *Gut*, **31**, A1206.
9. Dronfield, M.W., McIllmurray, M.B., Ferguson, R., Atkinson, M. and Langman, M.J.S. (1977) A prospective, randomised study of endoscopy and radiology in acute upper gastrointestinal tract bleeding. *The Lancet*, **i**, 1167–1169.
10. Dronfield, M.W., Langman, M.J.S., Atkinson, M. *et al.* (1982) Outcome of endoscopy and barium radiography for acute upper gastrointestinal bleeding: controlled trial in 1037 patients. *British Medical Journal*, **284**, 545–548.
11. Fullarton, G.M., Birnie, G.G., Macdonald, A. and Murray, W.R. (1989) Controlled trial of heater probe treatment in bleeding peptic ulcers. *British Journal of Surgery*, **76**, 541–544.
12. Goff, J.S. (1986) Bipolar electrocoagulation versus Nd–YAG laser photocoagulation for upper gastrointestinal bleeding lesions. *Digestive Diseases and Sciences*, **31**, 906–910.
13. Goudie, B.M., Mitchell, K.G., Birnie, G.G. and Mackay, C. (1984) Controlled trial of endoscopic bipolar electrocoagulation in the treatment of bleeding peptic ulcers. *Gut*, **25**, A1185.
14. Henry, D.A. and O'Connell, D.L. (1989) Effects of fibrinolytic inhibitors on mortality from upper gastrointestinal haemorrhage. *British Medical Journal*, **298**, 1142–1146.
15. Kernohan, R.M., Anderson, J.R., McKelvey, S.T.D. and Kennedy, T.L. (1984) A controlled trial of bipolar electrocoagulation in patients with upper gastrointestinal bleeding. *British Journal of Surgery*, **71**, 889–891.
16. Krejs, G.J., Little, K.H., Westergaard, H., Hamilton, J.K., Spady, D.K. and Polter, D.E. (1987) Laser photocoagulation for the treatment of acute peptic ulcer bleeding. *New England Journal of Medicine*, **316**, 1618–1621.
17. Laine, L. (1987) Multipolar electrocoagulation in the treatment of active upper gastrointestinal tract haemorrhage: a prospective controlled trial. *New England Journal of Medicine*, **26**, 1613–1617.
18. Laine, L. (1989) Multipolar electrocoagulation in the treatment of peptic ulcers with nonbleeding visible vessels: a prospective controlled trial. *Annals of Internal Medicine*, **110**, 510–514.
19. Laurence, B.H., Vallon, A.G., Cotton, P.B. *et al.* (1980) Endoscopic laser photocoagulation for bleeding peptic ulcers. *The Lancet*, **i**, 124–126.
20. Lin, H.J., Lee, F.Y., Kang, W.M., Tsai, Y.T., Lee, S.D. and Lee, C.H. (1990) Heat probe thermocoagulation and pure alcohol injection in massive peptic ulcer haemorrhage: a prospective, randomised controlled trial. *Gut*, **31**, 753–757.
21. Macleod, I.A., Mills, P.R., Mackenzie, J.F., Joffe, S.N., Russell, R.I. and Carter, D.C. (1983) Neodymium yttrium aluminium garnet laser photocoagulation for major haemorrhage from peptic ulcer and single vessels: a single blind

controlled study. *British Medical Journal*, **286**, 345–346.

22. Matthewson, K., Swain, C.P., Bland, M., Kirkham, J.S., Bown, S.G. and Northfield, T.C. (1990) Randomised comparison of Nd YAG laser, heater probe and no endoscopic therapy for bleeding peptic ulcer. *Gastroenterology*, **98**, 1239–1244.
23. Merki, H.S., Neumann, J., Kaufmann, D. *et al.* (1988) Continuous intravenous infusions of famotidine maintain high intragastric pH in duodenal ulcer. *Gut*, **29**, 453–457.
24. Morris, D.L., Hawker, P.C., Brearley, S., Simms, M., Dykes, P.W. and Keighley, M.R.B. (1984) Optimal timing of operation for bleeding peptic ulcer: prospective randomised trial. *British Medical Journal*, **288**, 1277–1281.
25. O'Brien, J.D., Day, S.J. and Burnham, W.R. (1986) Controlled trial of small bipolar probe in bleeding peptic ulcers. *The Lancet*, **i**, 464–467.
26. Panes, J., Viver, M., Forne, E., Garcia, E.O., Marco, C. and Garau, J. (1987) Controlled trial of endoscopic sclerosis in bleeding peptic ulcers. *The Lancet*, **ii**, 1292–1294.
27. Reynolds, J.R., Walt, R.P., Clark, A.G., Hardcastle, J.D. and Langman, M.J.S. (1987) Intragastric pH monitoring in acute upper gastrointestinal bleeding and the effect of intravenous cimetidine and ranitidine. *Alimentary Pharmacology and Therapeutics*, **1**, 23–30.
28. Rutgeerts, P., Vantrappen, G., Broeckaert, L. *et al.* (1982) Controlled trial of YAG laser treatment of upper digestive haemorrhage. *Gastroenterology*, **83**, 410–416.
29. Rutgeerts, P., Vantrappen, G., Van Hootgem, P.H. *et al.* (1987) Neodymium YAG laser photocoagulation versus multipolar electrocoagulation for the treatment of severely bleeding ulcers: a randomized comparison. *Gastrointestinal Endoscopy*, **33**, 199–202.
30. Rutgeerts, P., Vantrappen, G., Broeckaert, L., Coremans, G., Janssons, J. and Heile, M. (1989) Comparison of endoscopic polidocanol injection and YAG laser therapy for bleeding peptic ulcers. *The Lancet*, **i**, 1164–1166.
31. Sacks, H.S., Chalmers, T.C., Blum, A.L., Berrier, J. and Pagano, D. (1990) Endoscopic haemostasis. *Journal of the American Medical Association*, **264**, 494–499.
32. Somerville, K.W., Henry, D.A., Davies, J.G., Hine, K.R., Hawkey, C.J. and Langman, M.J.S. (1985) Somatostatin in treatment of haematemesis and melaena. *The Lancet*, **i**, 130–132.
33. Somerville, K., Faulkner, G. and Langman, M.J.S. (1986) Non-steroidal anti-inflammatory drugs and bleeding peptic ulcer. *The Lancet*, **i**, 462–464.
34. Swain, C.P., Bown, S.G., Storey, D.W., Kirkham, J.S., Northfield, T.C. and Salmon, P.R. (1981) Controlled trial of argon laser photocoagulation in bleeding peptic ulcers. *The Lancet*, **ii**, 1313–1316.
35. Swain, C.P., Kirkham, J.S., Salmon, P.R., Bown, S.G. and Northfield, T.C. (1986) Controlled trial of

Nd YAG laser photocoagulation in bleeding peptic ulcers. *The Lancet*, **ii**, 1113–1116.
36. Vallon, A.G., Cotton, P.B., Laurence, B.H., Miro, J.R.A. and Oses, J.C.S. (1981) Randomised trial of endoscopic argon laser photocoagulation in bleeding peptic ulcer. *Gut*, **22**, 228–233.
37. Walt, R.P., Reynolds, J.R., Langman, M.J.S. *et al.* (1985) Intravenous omeprazole rapidly raises intragastric pH. *Gut*, **26**, 902–906.
38. Walt, R.P., Cottrell, J., Mann, S., Freemantle, N. and Langman, M.J.S. (1991) A randomised double blind controlled trial of intravenous famotidine infusion in 1005 patients with peptic ulcer bleeding. *Gut*, **32A**.
39. Wheatley, K.E., Dykes, P.W. (1990) Upper gastrointestinal bleeding – when to operate. *Postgraduate Medical Journal*, **66**, 926–931.

SURGERY FOR BLEEDING PEPTIC ULCER *(D.L. Morris and A.V. Dilley)*

Surgery is an important aspect of the treatment of bleeding peptic ulcer. It is, however, only a part, and integration with resuscitation, diagnostic endoscopy, endoscopic therapy and medical therapy is of great importance. Such integration requires a collaborative effort from the physician and surgeon that is not widespread; not only must minds meet but it is important that adequate facilities, management procedures and dedicated staff exist. Emergency endoscopy facilities should be physically close to the operating theatre and ideally a specific area of a hospital ward should be dedicated to the care of gastrointestinal bleeds or, failing this, that serious bleeds be admitted to high-dependency or intensive-care areas.

When to operate

The '*timing*' of surgery for bleeding peptic ulcer influences mortality. Operations on patients after large-volume transfusions and prolonged hypotension results in high mortality, especially in the elderly. It is also clear that operating 'early' on well-resuscitated patients yields lower operative mortality, but such a policy carries a much higher operation rate and it is not clear that this will produce an *overall* fall in mortality. The results of a study at the General Hospital in Birmingham[32] did indicate that, in patients over 60 years of age, an aggressive early surgical approach produced an overall reduction in mortality, especially for gastric ulcer, where the mortality for a relatively conservative approach was 24% and an aggressive approach was 0%. In patients under 60 years of age, no such difference was seen, probably related to the ability of such patients to withstand hypotension at the time of rebleeding without detriment. The criteria used to indicate the need for surgery in this study for aggressive management were the presence of *any* of the following factors: four units of blood or plasma expander for volume replacement, any episode of rebleeding, endoscopic stigmata, or a previous upper gastrointestinal bleed and two years' dyspepsia. In the delayed or conservative group, the criteria for operation were: 8 units of blood or expander, second rebleed or persistent bleeding (12 units in 48 hours).

Endoscopy

The value of accurately locating the source of bleeding is now well accepted. If patients are found to have active arterial bleeding, two-thirds are likely to require surgery.

Visible vessel

The use of prognostic data in determining the need for surgery is less well established. It is clear that the visible vessel predicts rebleeding with its attendant risks, but it is not yet clear that 'prophylactic' surgery is justified. Certainly, surgery is not indicated for minor stigmata – a randomized study[34] showed a five-fold higher mortality in a group of patients over 59 years of age undergoing 'prophylactic' surgery for stigmata other than the visible vessel. It is not known whether surgery is indicated for a visible vessel, although this was one of the criteria in the Birmingham trial.

The role of therapeutic endoscopy is well established in the visible vessel and several different techniques are available which have been reviewed. It is important that enthusiastic endoscopic treatment should, however, not be allowed to worsen the outcome. In the bleeding patient, the endoscopist must know when to stop and it is certainly important in such cases that the surgeon be aware of the case and, preferably, that he or she be present, in the event that urgent surgery is required.

Upper gastrointestinal bleeding team

Several authors have provided support for the belief that an experienced and dedicated team can reduce mortality and morbidity – Hunt reported a reduction in mortality from 8 to 3.9% in two successive 5-year periods from 1972 to 1982,[21] a 12% mortality having been found in a retrospective study from 1961 to 1970.[20] Hellers and Ihre[17] reported a fall in mortality from 20 to 8% by a series of policy changes – admission to an intensive-care ward, early endo-

scopy and early surgery. Himal *et al.*[18] also achieved a reduction in mortality from bleeding peptic ulcer and attributed this to admission of patients to a surgery intensive-care unit and an aggressive surgical policy.

Choice of operation for upper gastrointestinal bleeding

There are no controlled trials comparing different operations for bleeding duodenal and gastric ulcers. The literature is also confused by the changing nature of bleeding ulcer (many more patients are now over 60 years of age) and differences between countries, such as age of patients and incidence of cardiovascular and other coexistent disease). *Tables 2.34–2.38* review the mortality of individual operations. It is clear that mortality rates vary quite considerably for all types of operation.

Undersewing

The role of oversewing alone is not yet clear. Whilst the available literature is small, there is some evidence that a low mortality can be achieved (10%).[33] The overall mortality in the literature (*Table 2.34*) is high at 31% but this is probably explained by its use in very ill, high-risk patients. This view is supported by the very small numbers reported by all other authors. The risk of rebleeding after this procedure does not seem to be excessive (1 in 20).[33] Whilst a prospective randomized trial is required, it is possible that this could be the procedure of choice, at least in high-risk patients with gastric ulcer. The experience of undersewing alone in duodenal ulcer is smaller but its role must not be dismissed for the old or very ill patient.

Table 2.34   Undersew alone for bleeding ulcer

	Ulcer type	Mortality	Rebleeding[a]
Kaplan *et al.*[27]	GU	3/3	
	DU	2/2	2.5
Kim *et al.*[29]		5/7	0/7
Hunt *et al.*[22]	GU	0/1	
Bekada *et al.*[1]		1/3	1/3
Rogers *et al.*[33]	GU	2/20	1/20
Schein and Gecelter[35]	GU	0/7	
Branicki *et al.*[4]	DU	1/1	
Total		14/44 (31%)	4/35 (11%)

GU, gastric ulcer; DU, duodenal ulcer.
[a]During acute admission.

Proximal gastric vagotomy

There is currently a small literature on the use of this procedure for bleeding duodenal ulcer (*Table 2.35*). The length of time required to do this operation probably mitigates against its use for emergency bleeding except in young, fit patients. Mortality in selected patients has been low but this reflects case selection, as rates of up to 15% have been reported. Other than for the possible long-term morbidity advantage over procedures denervating the entire stomach, there is little prospect of improving acute results.

Vagotomy and pyloroplasty

This is currently the standard operation used by most surgeons for bleeding duodenal ulcer. Mortality rates are summarized in *Table 2.36* and, where available, rebleeding is also noted. There is less experience of vagotomy and pyloroplasty in gastric ulcer; mortality appears to be considerably higher (33%) than for duodenal ulcer (8%). Rebleeding rates after vagotomy are relatively small (approximately 10%) but it is not established whether vagotomy reduces rebleeding rates compared with undersewing the bleeding vessel alone.

Billroth I gastrectomy

This operation is still the most common procedure for bleeding gastric ulcer with good results (*Table 2.37*), both in terms of a relatively low operative

Table 2.35 Proximal gastric vagotomy for bleeding ulcer

	Ulcer type	Mortality
Johnston et al.[26]	DU	0/10
Gorey et al.[15]	DU	0/25
Bekada et al.[1]	DU	0/5
Branicki et al.[4]	DU	0/21
Falk et al.[12]	DU	5/33
Total		5/94 (5.3%)

Table 2.36 Vagotomy and pyloroplasty for bleeding ulcer

	Ulcer type	Mortality	Rebleed
Farris and Smith[13]	DU	2/48	3/48
Weinberg[42]	DU	1/47	7/47
Farris and Smith[14]	DU	3/100	—
Klingensmith and Oles[30]	B	1/42	—
Schiller et al.[36]	DU	6/110	—
	GU	0/15	4/163
Jensen et al.[25]	GU	3/7	—
Vogel[41]	DU	3/45	—
Kaplan et al.[27]	DU	14/82	—
	GU	3/10	10/98
Buckingham and Remine[6]	DU	3/32	—
Brooks et al.[5]	DU	9/78	6/78
Chang et al.[8]	B	0/12	—
Heideman et al.[16]	B	6/39	3/20[a]
Kim et al.[29]	B	9/140	3/40
Stone et al.[38]	DU	1/18	0
Dronfield et al.[11]	DU	7/60	—
	GU	4/8	—
Inberg and Linna[23]	B	2/23	—
Hunt et al.[22]	GU	2/3	—
Hunt[20]	DU	5/62	—
Bekada et al.[1]	B	5/77	10/77
Rogers et al.[33]	GU	10/22	1/22
Schein and Gecelter[35]	DU	3/40	—
	GU	1/5	—
Branicki et al.[3]	GU	3/9	—
Branicki et al.[4]	DU	7/59	—
Total	DU	65/823 (8%)	43/404 (10.6%)
	GU	26/79 (33%)	

B, DU and GU.
[a]Fatalities only.

Table 2.37 Billroth I gastrectomy for bleeding ulcer

	Ulcer type	Mortality	Rebleeding
Kaplan et al.[27]	DU	2/7	⎫
	GU	1/14	⎬ 2/21
Cocks et al.[9]	DU	3/30	7/224[a]
	GU	28/194	—
Jensen et al.[25]	GU	3/33	—
Schiller et al.[36]	DU	2/12	⎫
	GU	8/81	⎬ 10/151
Inberg and Linna[23]	B	6/72	—
Heideman et al.[16]	B	12/180	2/83[a]
Chang et al.[8]	B	1/16	—
Kim et al.[29]	B	1/45	0/45
Buckingham and Remine[6]	B	4/29	
Dronfield et al.[11]	GU	7/33	—
Hunt et al.[22]	GU	4/27	—
Hunt[20]	DU	1/20	—
	GU	8/46	—
Bekada et al.[1]	B	1/9	0/9
Schein and Gecelter[35]	GU	11/84	—
Branicki et al.[3]	GU	8/37	—
Branicki et al.[4]	DU	0/15	—
Total	DU	8/88 (9.5%)	21/524 (4%)
	GU	78/649 (11.5%)	
	All	116/1084 (10.7%)	

B, DU and GU.
[a]Fatalities only.

mortality (11%) and a low rebleeding rate (4%). The trend to using less-invasive procedures is currently not yet well supported.

Billroth II gastrectomy

This used to be the operation of choice for bleeding duodenal ulcer. Published results (*Table 2.38*) must be interpreted with care, as recent results may reflect the increasing age of patients and the more selective use of this procedure. A Billroth II gastrectomy in the presence of a very scarred duodenum with a large ulcer can be a very difficult and dangerous operation. This may be especially relevant because many young surgeons will have little elective experience of gastric resection other than for gastric neoplasia, where closure of the normal duodenum is technically easy. Rebleeding after gastric resection is considered to be a smaller problem than lesser procedures, but bleeding from suture lines or erosions can occur.

Cause of postoperative death

Study of the cause of postoperative death may help to improve results, but the limitations of the litera-ture must be understood. The cause of death may be uncertain. For the sake of simplicity, a single cause of death is usually quoted but, this is probably an oversimplification of a multifactorial problem. *Table 2.39* is a digest of 27 papers which detail 482 deaths following surgery for bleeding peptic ulcer. The commonest cause of postoperative death was cardiovascular, accounting for 101, respiratory for 74 and 'cardiorespiratory' for another 37. Rebleeding was responsible for 82 deaths. Other causes include anastomotic leakage 34, renal failure 22, sepsis 56, cerebrovascular accident 16 and pulmonary embolus 12.

A number of postoperative deaths are due to the surgical complications of rebleeding (16%), leaks (11%) and sepsis (5%) but the incidence of these complications is variable, suggesting that surgical technique is still important.

It is all too easy to describe the medical causes of postoperative demise as 'unavoidable' or predetermined when this may be far from the case: postoperative cardiovascular complications are frequently related to timing of surgery – number and length of episodes of hypotension, quality of monitoring and speed and adequacy of resuscitation.

Table 2.38 Billroth II gastrectomy for bleeding ulcer

	Ulcer type	Mortality	Rebleeding
Schiller et al.[36]	GU	5/27	
	DU	8/56	11/146
	Other	18/64	
Jensen et al.[25]	GU	3/47	
Cocks et al.[9]	GU	0/32	
	DU	33/275	
Inberg and Linna[23]	B	6/72	—
Chang et al.[8]	B	0/7	
Heideman et al.[16]	B	12/33 + 4/22[a]	3/33[b]
Kim et al.[29]	B	0/10	1/10
Stone et al.[38]	DU	7/109	
Hunt et al.[22]	GU	1/8	
Bekada et al.[1]	B	3/11	2/11
Hunt[20]	DU	7/66	—
	GU	2/15	
Branicki et al.[4]	DU	0/4	—
Branicki et al.[3]	GU	1/10	—
Total	DU	55/510 (10.8%)	
	GU	12/139 (8.6%)	14/167 (8.4%)

B, DU and GU.   [a]Elective.   [b]Fatalities only.

Table 2.39 Cause of postoperative deaths

	n	Cardiovascular	Respiratory	Renal	CVA leak	Rebleeding	Sepsis	Other
Farris and Smith[13]	2							CVA 2
Weinberg[42]	2		1					
Kaplan et al.[27]	54	5	15		4	8	4	CVA 3
Farris and Smith[14]	3	1	1			1		CVA 1
Snyder et al.[37]	23	11	2			4	4	CVA 2
Boulos et al.[2]	8	2	1			2	1	CVA 1
Jensen et al.[25]	9	2	1	1	1	1	1	
Cocks et al.[9]	71	13	12	3	3	8	3	CVA 3
Kim et al.[28]	33	13	6	8	2	2	2	
Jensen and Guldberg[24]	7					4		
Inberg and Linna[23]	12		2	1	6	1	1	CVA 1
Brooks et al.[5]	11	2	2	1		4		CVA 2
Buckingham and Remine[6]	7				3	2	1	
Chang et al.[8]	1		1					
Heideman et al.[16]	39	—	17	—	11	10		
Kim et al.[29]	12	5		2		2	2	CVA 1
Dronfield et al.[11]	22	4	7	1	1	1	6	CVA 1
Wong et al.[44]	34	3	9	3			23	CVA 1
Vellacot et al.[40]	54	—	35	—	2	5	12	
Hunt[20]	25	5	5		5	7		
Hoffman et al.[19]	2		1			1		
Branicki et al.[3]	12	2	4				2	
Schein and Gecelter[35]	19	—	14	—	2	3		
Teenan and Murray[39]	2	—	2	—				
Branicki et al.[4]	8		4	2		1	1	
Falk et al.[12]	5		1					MOF 3
Total 482	101	37	74	22	34	82	56	CVA 16

MOF, multiorgan failure; CVA, cerebrovascular accident.

Postoperative renal failure is also influenced by preoperative management as well as the management of the renal failure. Respiratory deaths are an important cause of postoperative mortality and have received little attention. The possible effect of endoscopy in increasing risks of aspiration have not been addressed. The causes for postoperative respiratory deaths are undoubtedly multifactorial, including aspiration, atelectasis (collapse) and infection. Postoperative abdominal distension and over sedation are also important contributing factors.

Operation for erosive gastritis

The diagnosis of erosive gastritis must be accurate: our experience indicates that many patients labelled as having erosive gastritis in fact have undiagnosed ulcers or, occasionally, a calibre-persistent artery of the stomach (or Dieulafoy lesion or submucosal orbital malformation). The need for surgery in erosive gastritis has been reduced very considerably, possibly due to widespread use of H_2 receptor antagonists and other methods of pH control in the intensive-care unit. Endoscopic therapy should be used aggressively in such patients together with therapeutic control of gastric secretion before any thought is given to operation. If operation is essential, then the choice of operation is not easy. The literature would favour vagotomy and drainage but the mortality of this option at approximately 30% (vagotomy and pyloroplasty 38%,[10] 24%,[43] 35%[7]) and rebleeding rates are high (25, 47 and 39.3%, respectively). It is difficult to know if similar results would now be reported in patients who have not been controlled with H_2 receptor antagonists. The need for surgery for erosive gastritis is very rare, but, if bleeding persists, total gastric resection in the hands of an experienced surgeon may be the safest option.

Practical considerations

Endoscopy

If the surgeon did not perform the endoscopy, he or she should discuss the case with the endoscopist. If necessary, endoscopy is repeated in theatre to be sure that the site of bleeding is identified.

Anaesthesia

It is crucial that the anaesthetist is sufficiently experienced, and, if there is time, that the patient is adequately resuscitated. The ability to infuse large volumes rapidly is essential, and a large IV cannula should have been sited to secure venous access. Adequate amounts of blood and the ability to warm it rapidly are also important.

Operative procedure

Adequate exposure is essential. Rapid opening may be required in shocked, rapidly bleeding patients. The stomach and/or duodenum should be opened at an appropriate place. All the blood clot should be removed so that the source of bleeding can be seen. If there is an ulcer and it is actively bleeding, the index finger is placed over it, and the blood sucked out, so that the ulcer can be seen clearly. It is often useful to place a large nylon suture above and below the vessel without tying it for control of exposure. Once the bleeding is controlled, the artery is accurately oversewed with non-absorbable or long-lasting sutures.[31] Closure of the stomach or duodenum is not usually difficult. If the duodenum is very deformed and fixed, then a Finney pyloroplasty or simple closure and a gastrojejunostomy may be safer than a very tenuous Heineke–Mikulicz pyloroplasty. Generally, a gastrectomy is avoided for duodenal ulcer bleeding because it can be difficult to close the duodenal stump.

If there is a large posterior duodenal ulcer, a gastrectomy may be the only option and, if there is difficulty closing the duodenum, a Foley catheter duodenostomy in the second part acts as a useful safety valve. Many now take the view that vagotomy is largely irrelevant to the acute episode and is probably best avoided if the patient is ill. If the ulcer cannot be located, the gastroduodenostomy should be extended as far as is necessary: it may take patience to close it, but control of the bleeding is paramount.

Prophylactic measures

REBLEEDING

Postoperative haemorrhage may be due to failure to adequately control the original source of bleeding, anastomotic haemorrhage or erosive gastritis. The role of medical therapy in preventing or reducing the incidence of any of these three types of bleeding is *not* yet clear but most would now regard it as prudent to treat medically after vagotomy or resection and mandatory after undersewing alone. Choice of agent is relatively limited because luminal administration immediately following surgery is probably best avoided. H_2 receptor antagonists are probably the agents of choice. The value of proton pump inhibitors in this situation is not yet established.

THROMBOEMBOLISM

Pulmonary embolus is an important cause of postoperative death in these patients and the use of graduated compression stockings as well as subcutaneous heparin seems well justified. No excess in the rebleeding rate has been reported in patients undergoing surgery for gastrointestinal bleeding treated with low-dose heparin.

INFECTION

Sepsis may be responsible for morbidity and mortality and short-term antibiotic prophylaxis is advised.

References

1. Bekada, H., Charikhi, M., Haicheur, R., Yanes, Y. and Mentouri, B. (1984) Bleeding peptic ulcer. 10 years' experience. *American Journal of Surgery*, **147**, 375–377.

2. Boulos, P.B., Harris, J., Wyllie, J.H. and Clark, C.G. (1971) Conservative surgery in 100 patients with bleeding peptic ulcer. *British Journal of Surgery*, **58**(11), 817–819.

3. Branicki, F.J., Boey, J., Fok, P.J. *et al.* (1989) Bleeding gastric ulcer: a prospective evaluation of rebleeding and mortality. *Australian and New Zealand Journal of Surgery*, **59**, 551–562.

4. Branicki, F.J., Boey, J., Fok, P.J. *et al.* (1990) Bleeding duodenal ulcer. A prospective evaluation of risk factors for rebleeding and death. *Annals of Surgery*, **211**(4), 411–418.

5. Brooks, J.R., Kia, D. and Membreno, A.A. (1975) Truncal vagotomy and pyloroplasty for duodenal ulcer. *Archives of Surgery*, **110**, 822–825.

6. Buckingham, J.M. and Remine, W.H. (1975) Results of emergency surgical management of hemorrhagic duodenal ulcer. *Mayo Clinic Proceedings*, **50**, 223–226.

7. Byrne, J.J. and Guardione, V.A. (1973) Surgical treatment of stress ulcers. *American Journal of Surgery*, **125**, 464–467.

8. Chang, F.C., Drake, J.E. and Farha, G.J. (1977) Massive upper gastrointestinal hemorrhage in the elderly. *American Journal of Surgery*, **134**, 721–723.

9. Cocks, J.R., Desmond, A.M., Swynnerton, B.F. and Tanner, N.C. (1972) Partial gastrectomy for haemorrhage. *Gut*, **13**, 331–340.

10. Cody, H.S. III and Wichern, W.A. (1977) Choice of operation for acute gastric mucosal hemorrhage. Report of 36 cases and review of literature. *American Journal of Surgery*, **134**, 322–325.

11. Dronfield, M.W., Atkinson, M. and Langman, M.J.S. (1979) Effect of different operation policies on mortality from bleeding peptic ulcer. *The Lancet*, **26**, 1126–1128.

12. Falk, G.L., Hollinshead, J.W. and Gillet, D.J. (1990) Highly selective vagotomy in the treatment of complicated duodenal ulcer. *Medical Journal of Australia*, **152**, 574–576.

13. Farris, J.M. and Smith, G.K. (1960) Vagotomy and pyloroplasty. A solution to the management of bleeding duodenal ulcer. *Annals of Surgery*, **152**(3), 416–427.

14. Farris, J.M. and Smith, G.K. (1967) Appraisal of the long-term results of vagotomy and pyloroplasty

15. Gorey, T.F., Lennon, F. and Heffernan, S.J. (1984) Highly selective vagotomy in duodenal ulceration and its complications. A 12-year review. *Annals of Surgery*, **200**(2), 181–184.

16. Heideman, M., Larsson, I., Stenquist, B., Zederfeldt, B. and Darle, N. (1977) Surgical management of gastroduodenal haemorrhage. *Acta Chirurgica Scandinavica*, **143**, 307–312.

17. Hellers, G. and Ihre, T. (1975) Impact of changes to early diagnosis and surgery in major gastrointestinal bleeding. *The Lancet*, **ii**, 1250–1251.

18. Himal, H.S., Perrault, C. and Mzabi, R. (1978) Upper gastrointestinal haemorrhage: Aggressive management decreases mortality. *Surgery*, **84**, 448–452.

19. Hoffman, J., Devantier, A., Koelle, T. and Jensen, H.-E. (1987) Parietal cell vagotomy as an emergency procedure for bleeding peptic ulcer. *Annals of Surgery*, **206**(5), 583–585.

20. Hunt, P.S. (1984) Surgical management of bleeding chronic peptic ulcer. A 10 year prospective study. *Annals of Surgery*, **199**(1), 44–50.

21. Hunt, P.S. (1986) Bleeding ulcer: Timing and technique in surgical management. *Australian and New Zealand Journal of Surgery*, **56**, 25–30.

22. Hunt, P.S., Hansky, J., Korman, M.G., Francis, J.K., Marshall, R.D. and McCann, W. (1980) The management of bleeding gastric ulcer. A prospective study. *Australian and New Zealand Journal of Surgery*, **50**(1), 41–44.

23. Inberg, M.V. and Linna, M.I. (1975) Massive haemorrhage from gastroduodenal ulcer. A series of 149 cases operated on. *Acta Chirurgica Scandinavica*, **141**, 664–669.

24. Jensen, H.-E. and Guldberg, O. (1974) Selective vagotomy and drainage for bleeding duodenal ulcer. *Acta Chirurgica Scandinavica*, **140**, 406–409.

25. Jensen, H.-E., Amdrup, E., Christiansen, P. *et al.* (1972) Bleeding Gastric ulcer. Surgical and non-surgical treatment of 225 patients. *Scandinavian Journal of Gastroenterology*, **7**, 535–540.

26. Johnston, D., Lyndon, P.J., Smith, R.B. and Humphrey, C.S. (1973) Highly selective vagotomy without a drainage procedure in the treatment of haemorrhage perforation, and pyloric stenosis due to peptic ulcer. *British Journal of Surgery*, **60**(10), 790–797.

27. Kaplan, M.S., List, J.W., Stemmer, E.A. and Connolly, J.E. (1972) Surgical management of upper gastrointestinal bleeding in the aged patient. *American Journal of Gastroenterology*, **58**(2), 109–123.

28. Kim, U., Dreiling, D.A., Kark, A.E. and Rudick, J. (1974) Factors influencing mortality in surgical treatment for massive gastroduodenal hemorrhage. *American Journal of Gastroenterology*, **62**(1), 24–35.

29. Kim, U., Rudick, J. and Aufses, A.H. Jr (1978) Surgical management of acute upper

gastrointestinal bleeding. Value of early diagnosis and prompt surgical intervention. *Archives of Surgery*, **113**, 1444–1447.

30. Klingensmith, W. and Oles, P. (1968) Vagotomy and pyloroplasty for massively bleeding duodenal and gastric ulcers. *American Journal of Surgery*, **116**, 759–762.

31. McIntyre, R. and Hunt, P.S. (1984) Rebleeding after surgery for bleeding duodenal ulcer. *Digestive Surgery*, **1**, 77.

32. Morris, D.L., Hawker, P.C., Brearley, S., Simms, M., Dykes, P.W. and Keighley, M.R.B. (1984) Optimal timing of operation for bleeding peptic ulcer: prospective randomised trial. *British Medical Journal*, **288**, 1277–1280.

33. Rogers, P.N., Murray, W.R., Shaw, R. and Brar, S. (1988) Surgical management of bleeding gastric ulceration. *British Journal of Surgery*, **75**, 16–17.

34. Saperas, E., Perez Ayuso, R., Bordas, J.M., Teres, J. and Pera, C. (1987) Conservative management of bleeding duodenal ulcer without a visible vessel: prospective randomized trial. *British Journal of Surgery*, **74**, 784–786.

35. Schein, M. and Gecelter, G. (1989) APACHE II score in massive upper gastrointestinal haemorrhage from peptic ulcer: prognostic value and potential clinical applications. *British Journal of Surgery*, **76**, 733–736.

36. Schiller, K.F.R., Truelove, S.C. and Williams, D.G. (1970) Haematemesis and melaena, with special reference to factors influencing the outcome. *British Medical Journal*, **ii**, 7–14.

37. Snyder, E.N. Jr and Stellar, C.A. (1968) Results from emergency surgery for massively bleeding duodenal ulcer. *American Journal of Surgery*, **116**, 170–176.

38. Stone, A.M., Stein, T., McCarthy, K. and Wise, L. (1978) Surgery for bleeding duodenal ulcer. *American Journal of Surgery*, **136**, 306–308.

39. Teenan, R.P. and Murray, W.R. (1990) Late outcome of undersewing alone for gastric ulcer haemorrhage. *British Journal of Surgery*, **77**, 811–812.

40. Vellacott, K.D., Dronfield, M.W., Atkinson, M. and Langman, M.J.S. (1982) Comparison of surgical and medical management of bleeding peptic ulcers. *British Medical Journal*, **284**, 548–550.

41. Vogel, T.T. (1972) Critical issues in gastroduodenal hemorrhage. The role of vagotomy and pyloroplasty. *Annals of Surgery*, **176**(2), 144–148.

42. Weinberg, J.A. (1961) Treatment of the massively bleeding duodenal ulcer by ligation, pyloroplasty and vagotomy. *American Journal of Surgery*, **102**, 158–165.

43. Wilson, W.S., Gadacz, T., Olcott, C. III, and Blaisdell, F.W. (1973) Superficial gastric erosions. Response to surgical treatment. *American Journal of Surgery*, **126**, 133–140.

44. Wong, J., Lam, S.K., Lee, N.W., Lai, C.L., Lam, P. and Ong, G.B. (1980) Immediate operation for acute non-variceal gastrointestinal haemorrhage in patients aged 50 years and over. *Australian and New Zealand Journal of Surgery*, **50**(2), 150–154.

GASTRIC TUMOURS

BENIGN TUMOURS (INCLUDING GASTRIC POLYPS)

(M.D.A'C. Horton and D.L. Morris)

Gastric polyps are rare: autopsy series have reported incidences of 0.2–0.8%.[1] Benign tumours of the stomach are much less common than malignant growths. Benign gastric epithelial tumours are very important to the gastroenterologist because some are considered premalignant and can be cured by endoscopic biopsy while other benign tumours of the stomach serve as a marker of other premalignant gastric conditions.[21] Benign non-epithelial tumours of the stomach are uncommon and pose problems of diagnosis and management to the gastroenterologist.

'Gastric polyp' is a general term used to describe protruding benign epithelial tumours of the stomach. These tumours have been classified macroscopically as either sessile or pedunculated.[29] Histologically, the commonest polyps are of the neoplastic and hyperplastic types. The main neoplastic polyp is the adenoma. True hyperplastic polyps and hyperplastic polypoid lesions occur five times more frequently than gastric adenomas[10] and are usually multiple and sessile. Most pedunculated polyps are adenomas but sessile polyps may be of either histological type.

EPITHELIAL TUMOURS

Polypoid adenoma

This is the commonest benign gastric epithelial tumour. Its prevalence in the general population was assessed to be less than 1%[5] in a pathological study and 0.23% in an endoscopic study.[25] This is a true neoplasm showing unrestrained cell replication and incomplete differentiation. The histological appearance is similar to a colonic adenoma, with hyperchromatic elongated nuclei, frequent nuclear atypia and an abrupt transfer to normal gastric mucosa at its edge. Intestinal metaplasia is commonly seen in association with both types of epithelial polyp. Macroscopically these adenomas may be pedunculated or sessile, are usually single, and most commonly occur in the antrum. The sessile tumours may appear as a plaque surrounded by normal gastric epithelium or occasionally as a depressed lesion, perhaps mimicking an early gastric carcinoma.[12] These polyps are often an incidental finding at endoscopy, although very rarely they may be responsible for an intussusception.

In one series of 97 patients with gastric polyps, 35% were incidental findings in gastrectomy specimens for carcinoma, whereas only 5% were found in gastric resections for peptic ulcer.[24] Carcinoma in situ may occur in up to 50% of gastric adenomatous polyps,[21] either in the polyp itself or in the gastric remnant.

Treatment

The only means of obtaining an adequate biopsy is by examination of the entire polyp. This may be achieved by endoscopic polypectomy but may be complicated by bleeding and peptic ulcer at the excision site. These risks may be reduced by prophylactic anti-ulcer treatment.[7] A 40% recurrence rate was reported from a 23-centre follow-up study in Germany of over 6000 gastric polypectomies in 1177 patients.[18] Later development of carcinoma occurred in less than 2% of polyps but the rate was higher in adenomas than hyperplastic polyps.

Depressed gastric adenomas

These smaller depressions are filled with atypical columnar cells (intestinal type) with hyperchromatic nuclei. Their appearance is very similar to polypoid adenomas. Severe atypia or carcinoma in situ is frequently seen.[28] Malignant change is probably even more common than in polypoid adenomas.[12]

Hyperplastic polyps

Hyperplastic polyps (also called regenerative polyps or hyperplastic–adenomatous polyps) are not true neoplasms but are formed from overgrown normal gastric foveolar and glandular elements, with only minor loss of mitotic control and no loss of cellular differentiation. They account for over 70% of gastric polyps.[21] These polyps may be subdivided into true hyperplastic polyps (HPP) and polypoid lesions formed by foveolar hyperplasia (FH), fundic gland hyperplasia (FGH) and antral gland hyperplasia (AGH), of which the HPP and the FGH are the commonest.[21]

Hyperplastic polyps are usually multiple, sessile, less than 2 cm in diameter and are found typically in the fundus and body of the stomach. Intestinal metaplasia both in the polyp and adjacent mucosa is common. Atrophic gastritis and intestinal metaplasia was seen in adjacent mucosa in over 70% of Snover's series.[21] Simultaneous invasive carcinoma was seen in 12%, far more than would be expected by chance alone. Adenomatous polyps can occur with hyperplastic polyps[21] and some feel that they are different stages of the same disease.

Treatment

Malignant transformation in hyperplastic polyps is very rare and is perhaps more closely related to the underlying gastric epithelial change such as is seen in atrophic gastritis. Size is not a very good indication of risk.[20] Thus, even though endoscopic removal of these polyps is technically easy, careful, regular, endoscopic follow-up with multiple biopsies is advocated. The role of prophylactic gastrectomy is very controversial and probably not indicated.

Polyps formed by fundic gland hyperplasia probably have little, if any, malignant association.

Disorders associated with gastric polyps

Atrophic gastritis

In a follow-up of patients 10 years after partial gastrectomy, 9% were found to have gastric polyps,[6] the majority occurring around the stoma. Most of these polyps were of the hyperplastic type. In a study reviewing the histology of benign gastric polyps seen over 30 years in one hospital, *atrophic gastritis* with *intestinal metaplasia* was present in the adjacent mucosa of 72% of cases in which the adjacent mucosa was available for examination.[21] In a study from Greece, only 2.6% of non-operated stomachs were found to have hyperplastic polyps, compared with 12–15% following different types of gastric surgery. Patients with *pernicious anaemia* have an increased risk of hyperplastic polyps.[4]

Polyposis syndromes

Over 50% of patients with *familial adenomatous polyposis* and Gardner's syndrome[3,19,26] have gastric polyps.

Gastroduodenal polyps occur in 40% of patients with *Peutz–Jegher's syndrome* and endoscopic removal is advocated to prevent intussusception. The risk of malignancy is very small.[19,27]

Whilst *juvenile polyposis* produces principally colonic polyps, lesions may also occur in the stomach. In the *Cronkhite–Canada syndrome* (gastrointestinal polyposis, alopecia, onychodystrophy and hyperpigmentation), the gastric polyps are of the retention type and similar to the appearance in Ménétrièr's disease. *Cowden's disease* (multiple harmatoma syndrome) is associated with gastric hyperplastic polyps.

NON-EPITHELIAL TUMOURS

Leiomyoma

Although clinically rare, this is the commonest non-epithelial benign gastric tumour. Small nodular lesions may be found in almost 50% of autopsies.[9] Leiomyomas usually enlarge in their submucosal site to form intraluminal polypoid lesions, on the summit of which there are often multiple small ulcers. Less commonly they grow out from the serosal surface of the stomach.

Leiomyoma usually presents with haematemesis due to bleeding from central ulceration on the summit of the lesion.[8,19] Intussusception is rare but necrosis and calcification may occur. Microscopically, most leiomyomas show well differentiated smooth muscle and hyalinized connective tissue. However, some tumours are very cellular and may display hyperchromatic nuclei, with round rather than spindle-shaped cells. Differentiation from leiomyosarcoma in such cases can be difficult and should be based on the size of the tumour and the number of mitotic figures present.[15]

Treatment

Diagnosis of gastric leiomyoma is commonly made by double-contrast barium meal or endoscopy: histological confirmation can be difficult. Endoscopic biopsy is unlikely to be adequate unless the ulcerated area is sampled. Endoscopic removal of pedunculated lesions has been described but local surgical excision with a cuff of normal tissue is usually advised to prevent further bleeding and to obtain histological confirmation of the lesions.[19] Endoscopic ultrasonography or computed tomography scanning can provide information about staging where malignancy is suspected[23] and endoscopic ultrasonography is probably superior to computed axial tomography for both diagnosis and follow-up.[23]

Other benign gastric polyps

Other rare gastric polyps include *carcinoid tumours*, *inflammatory fibroid polyps* and *lipomas*. Whilst there does not appear to be any evidence of malignant change in inflammatory fibroid polyps, concomitant carcinoma has been seen.[11] Neurogenic tumours such as *schwannomas* and *neurofibromas* may be associated with von Reklinghausen's disease and these tumours usually present with abdominal pain or upper gastrointestinal tract bleeding; malignant change does occur.[2] *Gastric pseudolymphoma* is a benign condition seen as a response to chronic inflammation but may develop into a gastric lymphoma, or be associated with lymphoma.[17]

Benign duodenal tumours

Benign duodenal tumours are found in approximately 1% of duodenoscopic examinations.[14] Most tumours located in the first part of the duodenum are benign but the risk of malignancy increases as they become more distal.[22] *Adenoma* is the commonest tumour,[14] and gastrointestinal bleeding the most common presentation. Duodenal adenomas may be associated with familial adenomatous polyposis. The risk of malignant change is not as clear as in gastric adenomas but, with the exception of familial adenomatous polyposis associated adenomas, it is thought to be low. *Villous adenoma* is more rare, usually solitary, and the tendency to bleed or undergo malignant change is much greater. Obstruction of the duodenum or ampulla can occur with benign villous adenomas and they may grow up the common bile duct.

Brunner's gland adenomas are rare and are usually confined to the fourth part of the duodenum; malignant change probably does not occur. *Leiomyomas, lipomas, inflammatory fibroid polyps*[16] and *carcinoid tumours*[13] can also give rise to duodenal polypoid lesions.

References

1. Bone, G.E. and McClelland, R.N. (1976) Management of gastric polyps. *Surgery, Gynecology and Obstetrics*, **142**, 933–948.
2. Bruneton, J.N., Drouillard, J., Roux, P. *et al.* (1983) Neurogenic tumors of the stomach. Report of 18 cases and review of literature. *ROFO: Fortschritte auf dem Gebiete der Rontgenstrahlen und der Nuklearamedizin (Stuttgart)*, **139**(2), 192–198.
3. Eichenberger, P., Hammer, B., Gloor, F. *et al.*

(1980) Gardner's syndrome with glandular cysts of the fundic mucosa. *Endoscopy*, **12**, 63–67.

4. Elsborg, L., Andersen, D., Myhre-Jensen, O. *et al.* (1977) Gastric mucosal polyps in pernicious anaemia. *Scandinavian Journal of Gastroenterology*, **12**, 49.

5. Grafe, W., Thorbjarnason, B. and Pearce, J.M. (1960) Benign neoplasms of the stomach. *American Journal of Surgery*, **100**, 561–571.

6. Janunger, K.G. and Domellof, L. (1978) Gastric polyps and precancerous mucosal changes after partial gastrectomy. *Acta Chirurgica Scandinavica*, **144**, 293–298.

7. Lanza, F.L., Graham, D.Y., Nelson, R.S. *et al.* (1981) Endoscopic upper gastrointestinal polypectomy. *American Journal of Gastroenterology*, **75**(5), 345–348.

8. Lee, F.I. (1979) Gastric leiomyoma and leiomyosarcoma – five cases. *Postgraduate Medical Journal*, **55**, 575–578.

9. Meissner, W.A. (1944) Leiomyoma of the stomach. *Archives of Pathology*, **38**, 207–209.

10. Ming, S.C. and Goldman, H. (1969) Gastric polyp. A histological classification of its relation to carcinoma. *Cancer*, **18**, 721.

11. Mori, M., Tamura, S., Enjoji, M. *et al.* (1988) Concomitant presence of inflammatory fibroid polyp and carcinoma or adenoma in the stomach. *Archives of Pathology and Laboratory Medicine* (*Chicago*), **112**, 829–832.

12. Nakamura K., Sakaguchi, H. and Enjoji, M. (1988) Depressed adenoma of the stomach. *Cancer*, **62**(10), 2197–2202.

13. Ott, D.J., Wu, W.C., Shiflett, D.W. *et al.* (1980) Inflammatory fibroid polyp of the duodenum. *American Journal of Gastroenterology*, **73**, 62–64.

14. Reddy, R.R., Schuman, B.M. and Priest, L.R.J. (1981) Duodenal polyps: diagnosis and management. *Journal of Clinical Gastroenterology*, **3**, 139–145.

15. Rorchod, M. and Kempson, R.L. (1977) Smooth muscle tumours of the gastrointestinal tract and retroperitoneum. A pathologic analysis of 100 cases. *Cancer*, **39**, 255–262.

16. Saunders, R.J. and Axtell, H.K. (1964) Carcinoids of the gastrointestinal tract. *Surgery, Gynecology and Obstetrics*, **119**, 369–380.

17. Schwarz, M.S., Sherman, H., Smith, T. *et al.* (1989) Gastric pseudolymphoma and its relationship to malignant gastric lymphoma. *American Journal of Gastroenterology*, **84**(12), 1555–1559.

18. Seifert, E., Gail, K. and Weismuller, J. (1983) Gastric polypectomy. Long-term results (survey of 23 centres in Germany). *Endoscopy*, **15**, 8–11.

19. Senewiratne, S., Strong, R. and Reasbeck, P.G. (1987) Smooth muscle tumours of the upper gastrointestinal tract. *Australian and New Zealand Journal of Surgery*, **57**, 299–302.

20. Smith, H.J. and Lee, E.L. (1983) Large hyperplastic polyps of the stomach. *Gastrointestinal Radiology*, **8**, 19–23.

21. Snover, D.C. (1985) Benign epithelial polyps of the stomach. *Pathology Annual*, **20**, 303–329.

22. Stassa, G. and Klingensmith, W.C. (1969) 111 primary tumours of the duodenal bulb. *American Journal of Roentgenology*, **107**, 105–110.

23. Tio, T.L., Tytgat, G.N.J. and den Hartog Jager, F.C.A. (1990) Endoscopic ultrasonography for the evaluation of smooth muscle tumours in the upper gastrointestinal tract: an experience with 42 cases. *Gastrointestinal Endoscopy*, **36**, 342–350.

24. Tomasulo, J. (1971) Gastric polyps. Histologic types and their relationship to gastric carcinoma. *Cancer*, **27**, 1346–1355.

25. Ueno, K., Oshiba, S., Yamayata, S. *et al.* (1976) Histochemical classification and follow up study of gastric polyp. *Contemporary Topics in Immunobiology*, **5**, 23–38.

26. Ushio, K., Sasagawa, M., Doi, H. *et al.* (1976) Lesions associated with familial polyposis coli. Studies of lesions of the stomach, duodenum, bones and teeth. *Gastrointestinal Radiology*, **1**, 67.

27. William, C.B., Goldblatt, M. and Delaney, P.V. (1982) Top and tail endoscopy and follow up in Peutz–Jegher's syndrome. *Endoscopy*, **14**, 22–34.

28. Xuan, Z.X., Ambe, K. and Enjoji, M. (1991) Depressed adenoma of the stomach, revisited. *Cancer*, **67**(9), 2382–2389.

29. Yamada, T. (1966) Polypoid lesion in the stomach. *Stomach and Intestine* (*Tokyo*), **1**, 43.

GASTRIC CARCINOMA

EPIDEMIOLOGY *(T. Hirayama)*

The aetiology of cancer is still under intensive research. The most probable mechanism would be to postulate a two-stage mechanism of carcinogenesis. The first stage is the operation of 'initiators' on cell DNA, causing mutation (oncogene activation or inactivation of suppressor gene). The second phase is the exposure to 'promoters' causing dedifferentiation (perhaps due to oncogene amplification). The principal 'initiators' and 'promoters' have been searched for by intensive epidemiological studies.

Classification

Gastric cancer can be divided into two main types: 'diffuse' or undifferentiated and 'intestinal' or differentiated as described by Lauren.[12] The intestinal type usually arises from mucosa with intestinal metaplasia while the diffuse variety stems from proper gastric mucosa. Recent studies suggest that these two types are related to the amplification of two different oncogenes, c-erbB-2 and K-*sam* oncogene for the intestinal type and diffuse type, respectively.[16] These two types show distinct epidemiological features and are sharply contrasted. Distributions by sex and age were found to be quite different to each other.[6] The diffuse undifferentiated type is more predominant in females (42.3% of 3618 cases) than in males (29.1% of 6876 cases). It is also more frequent in younger age groups: under the age of 39 years the predominance was 51.8% (of 1535 cases) between 40–59 years, 35.6% (of 4336 cases), and over 60 years, 25.8% (of 4623 cases). It is also more predominant in certain occupations.

Mortality

According to the National Vital Statistics for 1988 in Japan, 30 009 males and 17 995 females died from gastric cancer, the mortality rate per 100 000 of the population being 50.0 and 29.0, respectively. The corresponding rates for the USA (1986) were 7.2 and 4.4, and for England and Wales (1985) 24.3 and 15.8, respectively. The relative frequency or the percentage of gastric cancer to cancer of all sites in Japan was 24.6 for males and 21.5 for females in 1982. The corresponding values for the USA were 3.4 and 2.5, and for England and Wales 8.1 and 6.1, respectively.

Incidence

Based on data of population-based cancer registries in Miyagi (Japan), in Japanese in Hawaii, in Connecticut (USA) and in Birmingham (UK) the adjusted (to world population) incidence rates of gastric cancer per 100 000 of the population in 1978–1982 were calculated in males as 79.6 for Japan, 28.4 for Japanese in Hawaii, 10.8 for the USA and 20.3 for the UK. In females the figures were 36.0 for Japan, 14.1 for Japanese in Hawaii, 4.3 for the USA and 8.4 for the UK.[10]

Risk factors

Exogenous factors
GEOGRAPHY
There are marked variations in the incidence of gastric cancer between and within various countries. The geographical pattern of incidence for gastric cancer is quite unique and entirely different (*Figure 2.65*) from the pattern for oesophageal cancer. Sometimes, even adjacent countries, prefectures or villages show striking differences as shown in cancer maps of the USA, China and Japan. Some of the

variation in incidence of gastric cancer may be due to differences in the nitrate content of the local water supply. High dietary nitrate may be converted to *N*-nitroso compounds in the presence of certain bacteria.[3,14]

TIME TRENDS
There is a uniform decline in the standardized stomach cancer death rate in almost all countries in the world, including Japan, Japanese in Hawaii and US Caucasians (*Figure 2.66*). This fall in mortality is believed to reflect certain essential changes in the factors governing the aetiology of the disease, in addition to the limited effect of nationwide mass-screening.[2,11,17] Changes in economic status and, in particular, changes in diet must be important factors. The introduction of electric refrigerators is believed to have played a major role in the falling frequency of stomach cancer since this method of food preservation replaced older methods (in particular, preservation by salting). Case–control studies conducted in Japan and in Hawaii showed that the frequency of gastric carcinoma was closely associated with the intake of highly salted foods.

SOIL TYPE
A close association was observed between gastric cancer and soil type, acidic soil being associated with a greater frequency of the disease. The association may be connected with the intake of trace metals such as zinc as they are easily absorbed into vegetables, grains and eventually in animals and humans if soil is acidic.

AIR POLLUTION
The association between gastric cancer and air pollution is also suspected but supporting evidence is limited.

SOCIOECONOMIC STUDIES
In those countries where socioeconomic studies have been conducted, the disease has a tendency to be more common in the lower socioeconomic strata.

OCCUPATION
There is a higher risk of gastric cancer in certain occupations such as in metal workers.[8]

SMOKING
In the current large-scale prospective population study in progress in Japan (1966–1982), the age-standardized death rate per 100 000 of the population for gastric cancer in males was 215.5 for daily smokers (1 291 645 person years) compared with 149.0 for non-smokers (310 506). In the case of females it was 98.3 for smokers (219 975) and 83.3

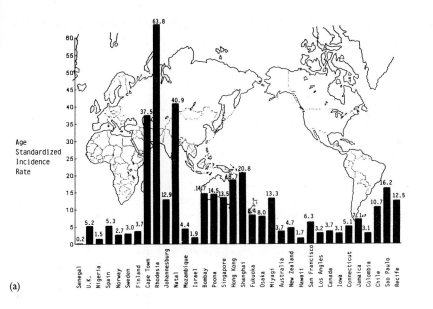

(a)

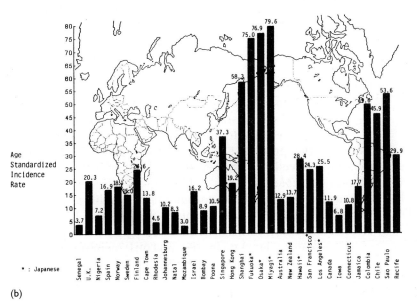

* : Japanese

(b)

Figure 2.65 (a) Incidence of cancer of the oesophagus in males. (b) Incidence of cancer of the stomach in males. (Source: IARC (1987) *Cancer Incidence in Five Continents*, Vol. V. Lyon: International Agency for Research on Cancer. Rates from previous publications were used when absent from Vol. V.)

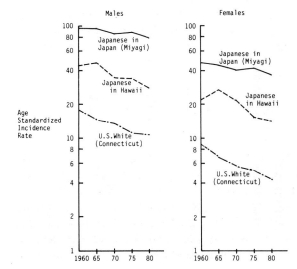

for non-smokers (1 816 199). The mortality ratio of smokers to non-smokers was 1.45 for males ($P <$ 0.01) and 1.18 for females ($P < 0.01$). The association with cigarette smoking was quite striking when the sex/age-standardized mortality rate ratio for gastric cancer was compared among selected lifestyle variables (*Figure 2.67*). No other lifestyle variable was observed to enhance the risk.

Figure 2.66 Age-standardized incident rate (100 000 of the population) for stomach cancer in Japanese in Japan (Miyagi), Japanese in Hawaii and US Caucasians in Connecticut 1960–1980. (Source: UICC/IACR (1966–1987) *Cancer Incidence in Five Continents*, Vols I–V. Geneva/Lyon: Union International Contra le Cancrum/International Agency for Research on Cancer.)

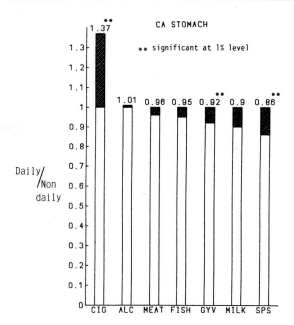

Figure 2.67 Sex/age-standardized mortality rate ratio by selected lifestyle variables. Cohort study 1966–1982, Japan. GIG, cigarettes; ALC, alcohol; GYV, green–yellow vegetables; SPS, soya bean paste soup.

Table 2.40 Effect of dietary factors on the risk of gastric cancer in studies in Japan

| | Relative risk[a] | |
	Males	Females
Highly salted food[b]	4.07	7.23
Dairy products[b]	0.22	0.29
Green–yellow vegetables[c]	0.65	0.59
5-year increased intake[d]	0.73	
Soya bean paste soup[e]	0.78	0.74

[a] Risk in group with daily intake of dietary factor relative to risk group with no intake of dietary factor.
[b] Matched case–control study: 300 males and 154 females in each group.
[c] Prospective study.[10] 16-year follow-up of 265, 118 people aged 40 years and above.
[d] Risk in those who increased their intake of yellow–green vegetables during the first 5 years of observation relative to risk in those who remained in the non-daily-intake group throughout the study.
[e] Cohort study.[9]

The association with cigarette smoking is most striking for cancer of the cardia.

ALCOHOL

No increased risk of stomach cancer was observed among daily drinkers of alcohol compared to non-daily drinkers in the author's prospective population study: 199.1 versus 197.5 in males and 83.9 versus 85.6 in females, respectively. The sex/age-standardized mortality rate ratio for daily alcohol drinkers was 1.01.

DIET

Dietary factors have long been suspected to be risk factors in gastric cancer. The promoting effect of highly salted foods (particularly pickles and fish) and the protective effect of dairy products were observed by case–control studies conducted in Japan (Table 2.40).

Among these, consumption of highly salted foods appeared to be of unique importance. In animals, sodium chloride administration was observed to cause damage in the mucous membrane of the

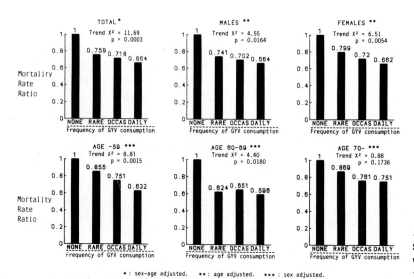

* : sex-age adjusted.   ** : age adjusted.   *** : sex adjusted.

Figure 2.68 Mortality rate ratio for cancer of the stomach by frequency of green–yellow vegetable (GYV) consumption. Cohort study 1966–1982, Japan.

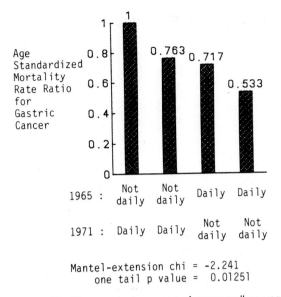

Mantel-extension chi = -2.241
one tail p value = 0.01251

Figure 2.69 Changes in frequency of green–yellow vegetable consumption and subsequent mortality rate ratio for gastric cancer (age standardized) in males. Cohort study 1971–1982, Japan.

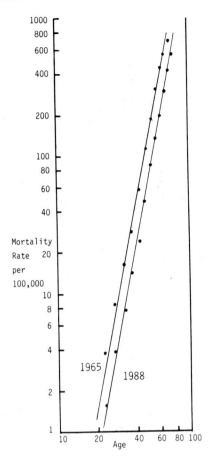

Figure 2.70 Age-specific mortality rate for gastric cancer in males in Japan in 1965 and 1988.

glandular stomach of rats. Carcinogenesis by MNNG (*N*-methyl-*N*'-nitro-*N*-nitrosoguanidine) was found to be enhanced by co- and postadministration of sodium chloride.

In addition, the intake of green–yellow vegetables rich in β-carotene and vitamine C was noted to lower the risk of stomach cancer significantly in the author's large-scale prospective study (*Table 2.40*). The sex/age-standardized mortality rate ratio for daily consumers of green–yellow vegetables compared to non-consumers was 0.66. The higher the frequency of consumption the lower the risk for gastric cancer, both in males and females and in any age group (*Figure 2.68*). In this study, those who increased their intake of green–yellow vegetables during the first 5 years of observation were found to show a lowered risk of gastric cancer in the course of a subsequent follow-up (*Figure 2.69*).[10] Thus, improvement of diet might reduce the risk of gastric cancer. Soya beans were also observed to lower the risk and daily intake of soya bean paste soup was noted to carry a significantly lower mortality rate for gastric cancer in the author's cohort study (*Table 2.40*).[9]

Endogenous factors

SEX

A prominent epidemiological characteristic of this disease is the almost constant male:female ratio in mortality and morbidity, which is almost always about 60% higher in males than in females. This relationship is true for most countries, suggesting common factors that affect the occurrence of gastric cancer, e.g. a smoking habit which until recently prevailed in males.

AGE

The linear rise in the rate of incidence when plotted on a logarithmic scale for age and death has long been discussed in testing models of carcinogenesis (*Figure 2.70*).

BLOOD GROUPS

A slightly higher risk of gastric cancer has been observed in people with blood group A.

HEREDITY

Studies on the familial aggregation of gastric cancer in the literature are in close agreement. There is a two- to three-fold excess risk of gastric cancer among near relatives of gastric cancer patients. In case–control studies in six Japanese prefectures in 1963 the father had died of gastric cancer in 15 out of 148 cases of gastric cancer compared with 4 out of 153 controls under the age of 49 years. Similar frequencies for mothers were 2 and 2, respectively.

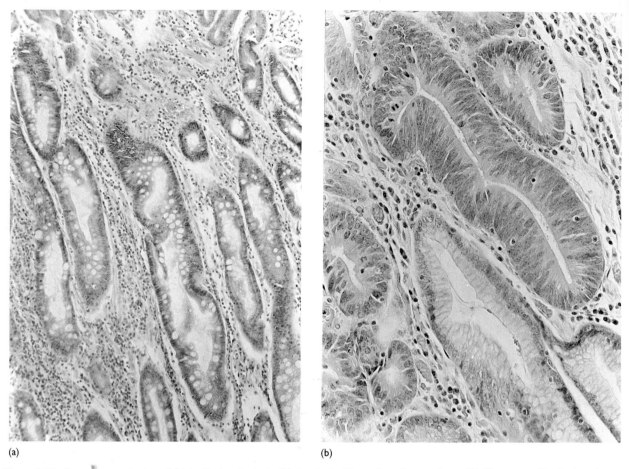

(a)   (b)

Figure 2.71   Precancerous lesions: (a) intestinal metaplasia; (b) dysplasia. (Reproduced by courtesy of H. Thompson, Birmingham.)

Thus, a four-fold increased risk was observed in fathers of patients with gastric cancer but not in mothers. By contrast, in patients aged over 50 years, the father had died of gastric cancer in 44 out of 763 cases of gastric cancer compared with 31 out of 771 controls. The frequencies for mothers were 16 and 22, respectively. Again, a significant risk was observed in fathers but not in mothers.[4]

PREDISPOSING CHANGES

Intestinal metaplasia (*Figure 2.71*) is the major predisposing factor in patients with the intestinal type of gastric cancer. Pernicious anaemia has been reported to coexist with the disease but this association is quite infrequent and is seldom observed as a factor. An association between gastric ulcers and the later development of cancer has often been postulated but supporting evidence is quite limited. There is evidence that persistent gastric hypochlorhydria and bile reflux may initiate areas of intestinal metaplasia and atrophic gastritis, which may be responsible for the increased risk of cancer after gastric resection.[13] The cocarginogens which have been

implicated in the postoperative stomach include *N*-nitroso compounds and free bile acids.[1,14,15] In summary, although many factors have been suspected and studied, one must recognize that dietary influence is apparently the most important factor in cancer of the stomach, in particular the risk-enhancing effect of consumption of highly salted food and the risk-reducing effect of consumption of green–yellow vegetables rich in β-carotene and vitamine C. The possibility of chemical carcinogens acting as both initiators and promoters is also high. Chemical factors have been suggested by animal experiments after feeding strong mutagens such as MNNG and also by the epidemiological observations of the associations of cancer with cigarette smoking and certain occupations.

References

1. Domellof, L., Reddy, B.S. and Weisburger, J.H. (1980) Microflora and deconjugation of bile acids in alkaline reflux after partial gastrectomy. *American Journal of Surgery*, **140**, 291–295.

2. Fukao, A., Hisamichi, S. and Sugawara, N. (1987) A case–control study on evaluating the effect of mass screening on decreasing advanced stomach cancer. *Journal of Gastroenterology Mass Survey*, **75**, 112–116 (in Japanese).

3. Hill, M.J., Hawksworth, G. and Tattersall, G. (1973) Bacteria, nitrosamines and cancer of the stomach. *British Journal of Cancer*, **28**, 256–262.

4. Hirayama, T. (1971) Epidemiology of stomach cancer. In *Early Gastric Cancer. Gann Monograph on Cancer Research*, Vol. 11 (Ed.) Murakami, T. pp. 3–19. Tokyo: University of Tokyo Press.

5. Hirayama, T. (1975) Epidemiology of cancer of the stomach with special reference to its recent decrease in Japan. *Cancer Research*, **35**, 3460–3463.

6. Hirayama, T. (1979) The Epidemiology of gastric cancer in Japan. In *Gastric Cancer* (Ed.) Pfeiffer, C.J. pp. 60–82. New York: Gerhard Witzstrick.

7. Hirayama, T. (1980) *Cancer Risks by Site. UICC Technical Report Series*, Vol. 41 (Ed.) Hirayami, T., Waterhouse, J. and Fraumeni, J. Geneva: Union International Contra le Cancrum.

8. Hirayama, T. (1981) Proportion of cancer attributable to occupation obtained from a census population-based large cohort study in Japan. In *Quantification of Occupational Cancer. Banbury Report*, Vol. 9 (Ed.) Peto, R. and Schneiderman, M. pp. 631–649. New York: Cold Spring Harbor Laboratory.

9. Hirayama, T. (1982) Relationship of soybean paste soup intake to gastric cancer risk. *Nutrition and Cancer*, **3**(4), 223–233.

10. Hirayama, T. (1982) Does daily intake of green–yellow vegetable lower the risk of cancer in man? An example of application of epidemiological methods to identify individuals at low risk. *Proceedings of the Symposium on Host Factors in Human Carcinogenesis. IARC Scientific Publications*, Vol. 39 (Ed.) Bartsch, H., Armstrong, B. and Davis, W. pp. 531–540. Lyon: International Agency for Research on Cancer.

11. Kuroishi, T., Hirose, K., Nakagawa, N. and Tominaga, S. (1983) Comparisons of trend in stomach cancer mortality between the model areas for stomach cancer screening and the control areas. *Journal of Gastroenterology Mass Survey*, **58**, 45–52 (in Japanese).

12. Lauren, P. (1965) The two main histological types of gastric carcinoma, diffuse and so-called intestinal type carcinoma. *Acta Pathologica et Microbiologica Scandinavica*, **64**, 31–49.

13. Nicholls, J.C. (1979) Stump cancer following gastric surgery. *World Journal of Surgery*, **3**, 731–736.

14. Reed, P.I., Smith, P.L.R., Haines, K. *et al.* (1981) Gastric juice *N*-nitrosamines in health and gastroduodenal disease. *The Lancet*, **ii**, 550–552.

15. Schlag, P., Bockler, R., Ulrich, H. *et al.* (1980) Are nitrite and *N*-nitroso compounds in gastric juice risk factors for carcinoma in the operated stomach? *The Lancet*, **i**, 727–729.

16. Terada, M. (1990) Molecular aspects of gastric cancer. Abstract of the 4th General Meeting of WHO–Collaborating Center for Primary Prevention. Tokyo. *Diagnosis and Treatment of Gastric Cancer*, 116–117.

17. Tsukuma, H., Mishima, T. and Oshima, A. (1983) Prospective study of 'early' gastric cancer. *International Journal of Cancer*, **31**, 421–426.

Screening *(T. Hirayama)*

Early detection programmes for gastric cancer by means of screening started in 1960 in Japan. A government study was introduced from 1966 and helped the rapid spread of the programme. About 5 million people have been screened annually by mass gastrography in Japan in recent years. The number examined by mass radiography for gastric cancer and the number detected in 1988 was 5 221 116 and 6 414, respectively. This programme is thought to have screened nearly 10% of persons between 40 and 69 years of age and achieved a detection rate of 1.2 per 1000 (*Table 2.41*).

The age-specific rates of annually screened persons per 1000 of the population are highest at 40–59 years of age in both men and women. The decline in deaths from gastric cancer is higher in the age groups where coverage by mass screening is most commonly performed.[2] When the extent of decline between the incidence rate and death rate was compared, the proportion of decline was much higher in death rate than in incidence rate (*Table 2.42*).[4] These data suggest the existence of the effect of screening on mortality decline in addition to the effect of change in risk factors such as the decrease in highly salted food consumption.

Nearly 90% of the mass screenings are conducted by a mobile radiography unit, and the photofluorographic methods are well standardized. The patient is asked to swallow effervescent granules before the examination and six gastrocamera pictures are taken in various positions. Roll film 70–100 mm in width is used. It takes only 3–4 minutes to examine one person by this method, and 50–60 persons can be screened each day. This method is used for the purpose of economy and as a means of minimizing radiograph hazards without sacrificing diagnostic efficiency. The radiographs thus taken are examined by specialists and the cases which require further detailed examinations, such as fibre-optic gastroduodenoscopy and biopsy, are selected. A much higher proportion of early gastric cancers are found by such methods than with conventional diagnostic radiographic methods in outpatient departments.[3] Of the cases of gastric cancer detected by screening in 1987, 64.1% were without lymph node metastasis.[4]

Table 2.41   Results of mass screening for gastric cancer in Japan (nationwide statistics) 1988

Total screened	5 221 116
Gastric cancer cases detected	6414 (gastric cancer cases ÷ total screened, 0.12%)
Percentage operated on	97.7
Percentage with early cancer[a]	
In detected cases	53.7
In resected cases	62.4

[a]Early cancer is defined as the presence of cancer cells located within the mucosa or submucosa of the stomach.

Table 2.42   Changes in the age-adjusted[a] incidence rate of gastric cancer and the age-adjusted death rate from this cancer in the Miyagi prefecture 1960–1980 for patients 40 years of age and older (per 100 000 of the population)

	Male		Female	
	Incidence rate	*Death rate*	*Incidence rate*	*Death rate*
1960	95.4	71.6	47.2	37.5
1965	91.2	74.6	43.9	35.2
1970	85.4	63.5	40.6	33.2
1975	90.3	56.1	42.2	29.0
1980	80.6	48.7	37.4	23.9
Change (%)[b]	−15.5	−31.9	−20.8	−36.3

From Hisamichi.[4]
[a]Standard population: Segi and Doll's world population (UICC world population).

$$^{b}\text{Change} = \frac{(\text{rate in 1980} - \text{rate in 1960})}{\text{rate in 1960}} \times 100 \ (\%)$$

The 5- and 10-year survival rates for gastric cancer cases detected by mass screening are significantly higher than in patients detected in outpatient clinics. The results of follow-up in screened persons clearly show a significantly lower gastric cancer-adjusted death rate compared to unscreened persons: in males, this was 61.9 out of 38 377.5 screened person years versus 137.2 out of 20 653.0 unscreened person years, and, in females, 28.1 out of 48 888.5 screened person years versus 53.8 out of 21 579.5 unscreened person years.[3] Similar results have been reported in other areas.

The change in the gastric cancer death rate from 1969–1972 to 1973–1977 in 14 municipalities having an average screening rate of 17.7% was compared with that of 28 randomly selected comparable control municipalities having an average screening rate of 7.7%. The death rate from gastric cancer decreased by 25.5% in high-screening areas (being 97.5 per 100 000 in 1969–1972 and 73.0 per 100 000 in 1973–1977) compared to 0.7% in the low-screening areas (P < 0.05) (death rates being 84.9 per 100 000 in 1969–1972 and 84.3 per 100 000 in 1973–1977).[3]

A significant effect of relative protection, 2.92 (95% confidence interval 2.09–4.08), was observed by a case–control study among examinees who were screened a year before with negative result (*Table 2.43*).[1] Annual screening is generally recommended as the relative protection is the highest in the group receiving the screening every year.

The following results of a natural history study of early gastric cancer also suggests the effectiveness of mass screening for prevention of deaths from gastric cancer. Forty-three cases in a total of 56 early gastric cancers detected in the Center for Adult Diseases in Osaka were followed up without performing surgical operations. Of the 43 cases, 27 progressed to clinical invasive cancer within 6–88 months (with a median of 27 months). It was also observed that 12 out of 34 early gastric cancer cases who did not receive surgical operation died from gastric cancer in the observation period, having a median survival of 77 months. These results suggested that detection and surgical resection of early gastric cancer would prevent death from gastric cancer.[4]

The observed effect of mass screening for gastric cancer may be influenced by lead-time or length bias. Furthermore, the influence of selection bias

Table 2.43 Effect of mass screening of gastric cancer (a case–control study)

	Number of cases (advanced) cancer	Number of controls	Relative risk[a]
Never screened	156	89	1.00
Negative by screening in previous year	132	220	2.92 $\begin{cases} 2.89 \\ 4.08 \end{cases}$

Modified from Fukao *et al.*[1]
[a]95% confidence limits

cannot be neglected in interpreting results, since none of the evaluations made so far has been based on a randomized trial.

It has also been suggested that certain haematological, immunological, bacteriological and gastric juice markers might be used for screening. Such potential markers include carcinoembryonic antigen, α-fetoprotein, lactic dehydrogenase and *Helicobacter pylori*. In combination these markers might detect patients suitable for more invasive screening procedures, but their use in this field has not been confirmed.

References

1. Fukao, A., Hisamichi, S. and Sugawara, N. (1987) A case–control study on evaluating the effect of mass screening on decreasing advanced stomach cancer. *Journal of Gastroenterology Mass Survey*, **75**, 112–116 (in Japanese).
2. Hirayama, T. (1978) Outline of stomach cancer screening in Japan. In *Screening in Cancer. UICC Technical Report Series*, Vol. 40 (Ed.) Miller, A.B. pp. 264–278. Geneva: Union International Contra le Cancrum.
3. Hisamichi, S. (1978) Prognosis of the patients with gastric cancer detected by mass survey. In *Principles and Practice in Gastric Mass Survey Examination*, pp. 91–96. Tokyo: Kanehara Shuppan (in Japanese).
4. Hisamichi, S. (1989) Screening for gastric cancer. *World Journal of Surgery*, **13**, 31–37.
5. Miki, K., Ichinose, M., Kawamura, N. *et al.* (1989) The significance of low serum pepsinogen levels to detect stomach cancer associated with extensive chronic gastritis in Japanese subjects. *Japan Journal of Cancer Research*, **80**, 111–114.

CLINICAL FEATURES, DIAGNOSIS AND TREATMENT *(J.W.L. Fielding)*

Cancer of the stomach is the most common neoplasm of the upper gastrointestinal tract. Although there is epidemiological evidence that the incidence of adenocarcinomas is declining, there are still more than 10 000 deaths a year from gastric cancer in the UK alone. There have been many advances in its management. The improvements of surgical and anaesthetic techniques have effectively reduced postoperative mortality from 50% in the last century to 5% in modern times. Similarly, developments in endoscopy and radiology have greatly facilitated diagnosis. The treatment remains primarily surgical and is stage-dependent. While most patients present with advanced disease, the identification of high-risk groups and improved clinical awareness of the disease should increase the number of patients diagnosed with the favourable 'early' lesion. Also, it is hoped that the cytotoxic effects of certain therapeutic agents might be translated into improvements in survival rates. The diagnosis and management of gastric cancer is multi-disciplinary, requiring the expertise of gastroenterologists, radiologists, surgeons and oncologists.

Adenocarcinomas comprise 95% of all malignant diseases of the stomach, so this section will be concerned predominantly with the clinical features, diagnosis and treatment of this disease, although the less common epithelial and non-epithelial tumours will also be described. These are squamous cell carcinomas, carcinoids, lymphomas and leiomyosarcomas.

Adenocarcinoma of the stomach

Clinical features

The classical symptoms of 'advanced' gastric cancer are abdominal pain, dyspepsia, anorexia, anaemia, vomiting and dysphagia. 'Early' gastric cancer is a lesion in which the depth of penetration of the primary tumour is limited histologically to the submucosa of the stomach, irrespective of the presence or absence of lymph node metastases.[33] Approximately 30% of all patients with early gastric cancer have a long history of dyspepsia which is indis-

Table 2.44 Incidence of symptoms of gastric cancer

| | First symptom | | Symptoms at presentation of 'early' gastric cancer. |
	UK : Radcliffe study[43]	Europe[28]	UK : West Midlands study[13]
Symptoms related to gastrointestinal tract[a]	310 (83.6%)	678 (75.2%)	71 (82.6%)
Constitutional[b]	51 (13.7%)	187 (20.8%)	11 (12.8%)
Other	10 (2.7%)	36 (4.0%)	4 (4.7%)

[a]Dyspepsia, vomiting, abdominal pain, epigastric pain, indigestion, dysphagia, haematemesis, melaena.
[b]Weight loss, anaemia, weakness, lassitude, fever.

tinguishable from chronic peptic ulcer disease. The 5-year survival following surgical resection of this lesion is 90% in Japan[20]. The difficulty for the physician is differentiating between the symptoms of benign upper gastrointestinal disorders and malignancy. It is important to identify the 'symptomatic at-risk' patients in whom it is essential to establish a precise diagnosis before initiating therapy.

Gastrointestinal bleeding occurs in about one-third of patients. It is usually occult, but occasionally massive. Acute perforation is rare.

Males develop gastric cancer more commonly than women in the ratio of 3:2. The highest incidence occurs between the ages of 55 and 65 years. Sex and age distributions are the same in both 'advanced' and 'early' gastric cancer.[13]

Particularly relevant is an analysis of the first symptoms of the disease. Detailed studies of the presenting symptoms[28,43] have demonstrated that the first symptom of patients who later presented with advanced disease was similar to that found in patients with 'early' gastric cancer (*Table 2.44*). There is no typical dyspeptic syndrome that is diagnostic of gastric cancer, the symptoms may be typical of an ulcer or vague, such as abdominal discomfort or belching (*Table 2.45*).

By the time the patient is admitted to hospital, the clinical picture will have changed from that of the

first symptom. The most striking feature is that 78% of patients have lost weight compared with only 18.9% of patients with 'early' gastric cancers. Similar findings have been reported by Green et al.,[17] who made direct comparisons between early and advanced lesions, weight loss being significantly less common in patients with 'early' gastric cancer. It should be stressed that dyspepsia is a symptom and not a diagnosis and that no patient over the age of 40 years complaining for the first time of dyspepsia should be treated until a definitive histological diagnosis has been established.

Physical examination is often unrewarding in gastric cancer, only 32% of patients having a palpable abdominal mass. However, there may be manifestations of metastatic disease, such as palpable lymph nodes, hepatic metastases or ascites. The presence of a palpable mass signifies advanced disease. Thus, the absence of physical signs in a symptomatic patient does not exclude gastric malignancy. However, the presence of a mass does not indicate inoperability.

Investigations

The diagnosis of gastric cancer is made by radiology and fibre-optic endoscopy. These are complementary investigations and should not be considered mutually exclusive.

The only type of barium meal[40] examination capable of diagnosing early gastric cancer (*Figure 2.72*) is a double-contrast study, preferably facilitated by inducing hypotonia and using compression. The fibre-optic endoscope allows a full macroscopic assessment of the gastric mucosa and enables biopsies and brush cytology to be obtained from a lesion. After macroscopic assessment of an abnormality at least six to eight biopsies should be taken. Repeated endoscopy and biopsy may be necessary to establish the diagnosis, especially if there is radiological or endoscopic suspicion of malignancy or if a benign appearing lesion fails to heal completely, or fails to remain healed. In addition, the healed area

Table 2.45 Nature of early dyspeptic symptoms evaluated in 251 patients in the Radcliffe study[43]

Symptom	Percentage
Mild[a]	21
Ulcer type	26.3
Pain after meals (unrelieved by food and alkalis)	14.7
Long history of vague dyspepsia	11.6
Continuous pain	18.7
Pyloric stenosis	7.6

[a]Vague abdominal discomfort, fullness, belching, regurgitation.

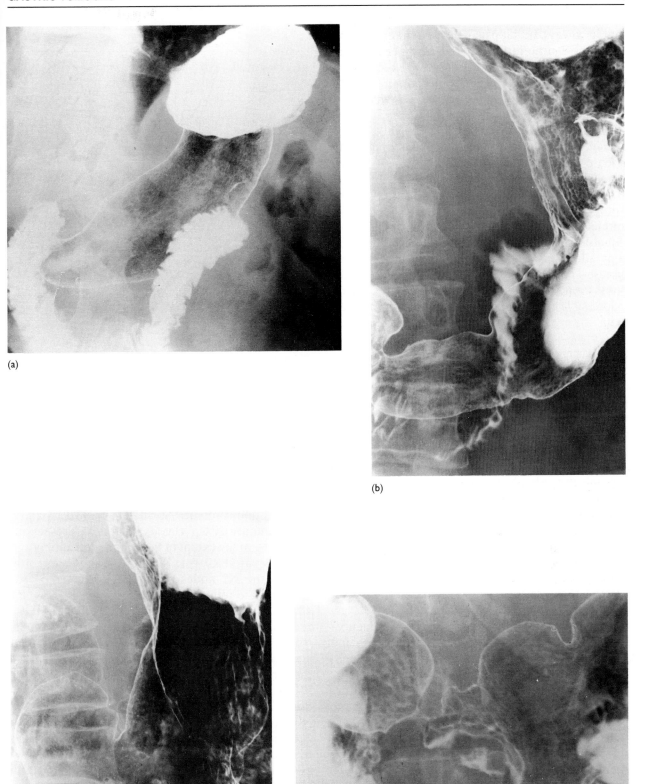

(a)

(b)

(c)

(d)

Figure 2.72 Double-contrast barium studies (a) demonstrating 'early' and (b–d) advanced gastric carcinomas.

should always be biopsied on review endoscopy. Accuracy can be further increased by brushing all suspicious lesions for cytological examination. Using radiology and endoscopy in combination, the accuracy of diagnosis of gastric cancer is 98%.[35]

PREOPERATIVE INVESTIGATIONS

Specific preoperative investigations to stage the disease or determine resectability usually prove unreliable.

Angiography, liver function tests and radio-isotope scans have all been evaluated and proven unreliable. Computed axial tomography has been valuable in the assessment of liver disease. Laparoscopy allows visualization and biopsy of metastatic disease, particularly the liver and peritoneal deposits, but is limited in its inability to visualize inaccessible areas (i.e. the lesser sac) and assess fixity.

Management

Surgery is the only effective treatment of adenocarcinoma of the stomach and none should be denied its possible benefit. Whilst investigations may give an indication of the stage of disease, most patients deserve a laparotomy unless prior laparoscopy has revealed extensive hepatic or peritoneal metastases or if the patient is otherwise unfit for operation. This general principle of operative assessment must be accepted for most patients because palliation is usually best achieved by surgery. The aim of the 'stage-appropriate' operation for gastric cancer must be to apply a treatment designed for maximal survival time while allowing patients to enjoy an optimal quality of life.

Surgical treatment must be related to the known pattern of spread and recurrence following resection, whether the extent of resection influences long-term survival, the postoperative mortality and the effect of the reconstructive procedure on long-term morbidity.

Gastric neoplasms may spread by: (1) direct extension; (2) lymphatic embolization; (3) lymphatic permeation; (4) bloodstream embolization; and (5) transplantation.[6] Direct extension may penetrate surrounding organs (particularly the pancreas or submucosally) and into the oesophagus and duodenum; it is not true that the pylorus limits spread.[46]

Lymph node metastasis is common. The International Union Against Cancer (UICC)[45] has classified lymph nodes as N1, N2 and N3 (*Figure 2.73*) and postoperative survival is related to the extent of node involvement. The Japanese, though using a more complicated system,[24] have reported a 5-year survival rate for N1 involvement of 38.5%, with an N2 involvement of 22.8%, an N3 involvement of

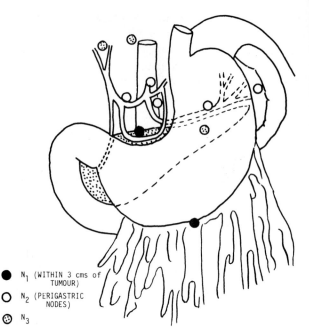

N1 (WITHIN 3 cms of TUMOUR)

N2 (PERIGASTRIC NODES)

N3

Figure 2.73 TNM classification of tiers of lymph nodes. N1: nodes within 3 cm of the neoplasm. N2: nodes on lesser or greater curvature further than 3 cm from primary and nodes on the common hepatic artery, coeliac axis, left gastric artery, splenic artery and splenic hilum. N3: nodes at porta hepatis and para-aortic and retropancreatic nodes.

11.1% and an N4 involvement of 8.5%. (The UICC classification combines N3 and N4 as N3.) Japanese gastroenterologists classify surgical resections according to the extent of the lymphadenectomy and are designated R0, R1, R2 and R3 (an R1 resection excises the N1 nodes etc.). The corrected 5-year survival rate following an R0 resection is 26%, R1 42.4%, R2 49.5% and R3 40%. In the light of these results, curative surgery is best reserved for patients whose extent of disease is limited to N2 involvement and the most appropriate resection would remove these nodes (R2).

The possible sites of recurrence of gastric carcinoma are in the gastric remnant, local residual lymph nodes and distant metastases. Remnant recurrence may occur in 10–15%, and this has been used as an argument for total gastrectomy.[36] However, there is no evidence that this significantly increases survival. The necessity of the lymphadenectomy in curative operations for gastric cancer is supported by the increased survival of R2 resections. Further support is gained from the report of 59 patients with apparently benign gastric ulcers removed surgically which subsequently proved to be carcinomas on histological examination.[11] Twenty-four had a further operation to achieve a radical lymphadenectomy and the 5-year survival rate in this group was 56% compared to 23% in the remainder. This supports the concept of wide surgical resection and lymphadenectomy as the treatment of choice for gastric cancer and suggests that surgical resection can influence the natural history of the disease.

The limiting factor to extensive resection is postoperative mortality. The overall mortality of total gastrectomy is 21%, which is considerably higher than that of 4% following partial gastrectomy.[27] Similarly, extensive lymphadenectomies have been reported to effectively reduce the 5-year survival rate from 28% to 17%.[16] Thus, the most appropriate curative resection is a subtotal gastrectomy with an N2 lymphadenectomy.

In considering the method of reconstruction, all the factors related to benign disease must be considered. The reconstructive procedure, if badly conceived or badly constructed, may produce more severe symptoms than does the cancer itself. The reconstruction of a partial gastrectomy should be a modified Billroth I, Billroth II (Polya) or Roux-en-Y technique (*Figure 2.74*). The incidence of postgastrectomy problems, such as vomiting, diarrhoea, dumping, haematological and nutritional effects, is similar for the three anastomoses, but the Billroth II and the Roux-en-Y techniques have the advantage of providing a wider stoma at a distance from the site of likely recurrence thus reducing the risk of postoperative obstruction due to recurrent disease. Furthermore, the Roux-en-Y reconstruction reduces the risk of troublesome bile reflux.

Total gastrectomy is occasionally associated with adverse long-term nutritional effects. Malabsorption of fat and protein occurs and the absorption of glucose usually shows a pattern of early hyperglycaemia and late hypoglycaemia. As a consequence many patients lose weight, which can be corrected by dietary supplementation. Megaloblastic and iron-deficiency anaemia commonly occur, warranting appropriate replacement therapy. The construction of a gastric pouch and the use of a jejunal segment to permit the passage of food through the duodenum have been used as reconstructive procedures,[29] but there is no evidence that they prevent the metabolic consequences. The most commonly employed reconstructions are the Roux-en-Y, Henley jejunal interpositions and the Omega loop (*Figure 2.75*). The incidence of postgastrectomy syndromes, such as distension, dumping and diarrhoea, is similar for all three methods, occurring in about 20% of all patients. In addition, bile reflux into the oesophagus is associated with significant morbidity and this can be prevented by constructing a 50 cm Roux-en-Y or 25 cm interposition.

At laparotomy, the first consideration is whether the tumour is resectable. Curative resection is impossible in the presence of peritoneal seedlings, distant metastases, extension to unresectable adjacent structures or involvement of N3 lymph nodes.

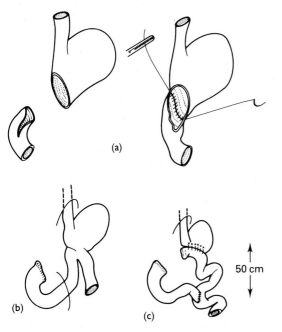

Figure 2.74 Reconstructive procedures for a partial gastrectomy: (a) modified Billroth I; (b) Billroth II (Polya); (c) Roux-en-Y gastrojejunostomy.

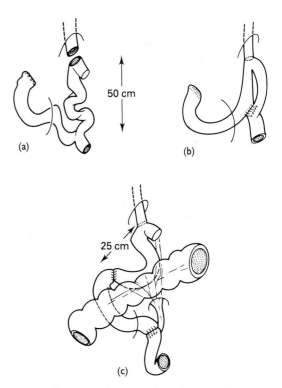

Figure 2.75 Reconstructive procedures for a total gastrectomy; (a) Roux-en-Y; (b) Omega gastrojejunostomy; (c) Henley jejunal interposition.

Macroscopic assessment as to the presence of lymphatic metastases is unreliable. Therefore, in the presence of an apparently curative adenocarcinoma, N3 nodes should be excised for immediate assessment of metastases, using either frozen section or imprint cytology.[32]

RADICAL GASTRECTOMY

The definitive radical surgical operation is an R2 resection and should be reserved for patients in whom lymph node involvement does not extend beyond the N2 nodes. The first step is to detach the greater omentum from the transverse colon and mesocolon (*Figure 2.76a*). The right gastroepiploic artery is then ligated flush with the gastroduodenal artery. The next step includes the detachment of the lesser omentum from the under surface of the left lobe of the liver upwards to the oesophageal hiatus, and then the separation of the anterior leaf of the

hepatoduodenal ligament downwards to the origin of the right gastric vessels. These vessels are divided and ligated, removing the appropriate lymph nodes.

The duodenum is divided and the distal stomach with the attached omentum is reflected over the left coastal margin (*Figure 2.76b*). A portion of the duodenal cuff is excised for frozen section examination. Thereafter the lymph nodes of the hepatoduodenal ligament and those behind the pancreas are dissected en bloc from right to left through Winslow's foramen and the dissection is continued to the nodes along the common hepatic artery, gastroduodenal artery and those at the root of the coeliac axis. The left gastric artery is isolated, divided and ligated with removal of appropriate nodes. Then the lymph nodes along the splenic artery are dissected towards the splenic hilus. If the presence of pancreatic nodal metastases demands it, resection of the pancreas and spleen can be performed for complete clearance. The attachments of the right cardia to the oesophageal hiatus are separated, both the vagal nerves are divided and the lymph nodes of

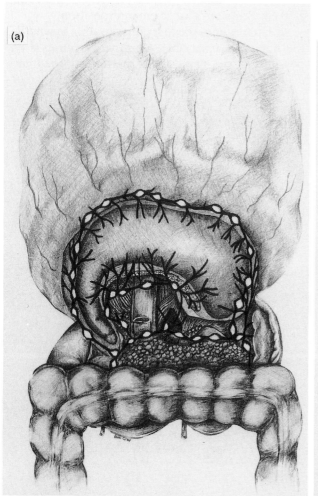
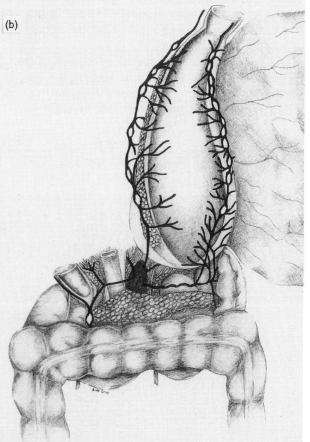

Figure 2.76   (a) Radical gastrectomy (R2): the omentum has been dissected off the transverse colon and the N2 lymph nodes exposed. (b) Radical gastrectomy (R2): the N2 nodes have been dissected off the gastroduodenal artery, common hepatic artery, coeliac axis, splenic artery, left gastric artery and splenic hilum prior to dividing the stomach.

the right cardia are removed. This completes the mobilization of the stomach and the lymphadenectomy; a partial or total gastrectomy is then performed to ensure a 6 cm clearance of the primary. In a total gastrectomy the spleen is mobilized by dividing the lienorenal ligament; the splenic artery and vein and then the oesophagus are divided and the stomach removed.

Gastrointestinal continuity should be restored after a partial gastrectomy by either a modified Billroth I or Billroth II anastomosis and after a total gastrectomy by either a Roux-en-Y or jejunal interposition.

PALLIATIVE SURGERY

The ideal form of palliative treatment must be considered individually for each patient, evaluating the symptoms to be palliated and the quality of life afforded by the procedure. The symptoms most commonly requiring palliation are obstruction, pain and haemorrhage, and the procedures available are bypass, intubation, excision and resection (*Figure 2.77*). Pyloric obstruction may be palliated by resection or gastroenterostomy. Obstruction at the cardia is relieved by resection if feasible; if not, non-operative endoscopic intubation is preferred to operative intubation. Haemorrhage must be controlled by resection.

Pain is a frequent symptom. It may be intermittent like peptic ulcer pain or constant and related to the extragastric spread of the neoplasm. Resection of the carcinoma usually controls ulcer-type pain but that related to extragastric extension or metastatic disease is seldom relieved by resection. Symptomatic relief can often only be achieved by analgesics, although occasionally radiotherapy or chemotherapy might help. The best palliation follows resection[37] and the surgeon should always attempt this even if macroscopic disease cannot be completely removed.

Clinicopathological features

STAGING

Clinicopathological features of gastric cancer are important for the accurate staging of tumours (*Table 2.46*). Clinically, the important factors are the extent of the disease, resectability and whether the resection is radical (curative) or palliative. Pathologically, the important microscopic factors are the depth of penetration of the primary lesion (*Figure 2.78*) and lymph node involvement (*Figure 2.73*).

Table 2.46 Staging system for gastric carcinoma

Stage	Clinical	Pathology
I	Radical resection (T1 N0 M0)	Muscularis propria − Serosa − Node − (T1 N0 M0)
II	Radical resection (T2–4 N0 M0)	Muscularis propria + Serosa ± Node − (T2–4 N0 M0)
III	Radical resection (TX–4 N1–3 M0)	Muscularis propria ± Serosa ± Node + (TX–4, N1–3, M0)
IVA	Palliative resection (TX–4 NX–3 M0–1)	Residual disease (TX–4 N0–3 M0–1)
IVB	Inoperable (TX–4 NX–3 M0–1)	Positive histology (T4 N0–3 M0–1)

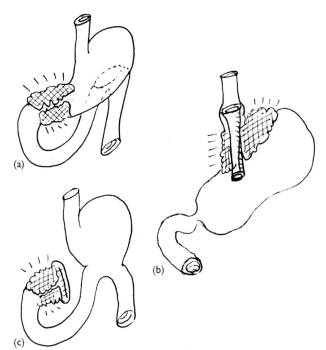

Figure 2.77 Palliative procedures: (a) gastroenterostomy; (b) intubation; (c) exclusion.

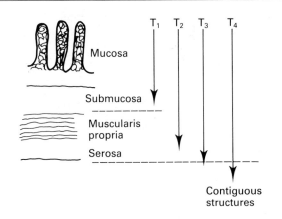

Figure 2.78 The TNM classification of depth of penetration of the primary tumours.

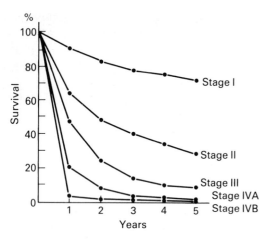

Figure 2.79 Five-year age-adjusted survival according to stage for gastric adenocarcinomas in the West Midlands (1960–1969).

The age-adjusted 5-year survival rates are 72.2, 29.4, 9.0, 1.8 and 0.8% for stages I, II, III, IVA and IVB, respectively (*Figure 2.79*).

PATHOLOGY
Gastric adenocarcinomas are most frequently found in the pyloric antrum: 49.8% of them are found here – 12.5% are found in the body, 18.4% in the lesser curvature, 10.4% in the cardia, 5.1% in the greater curvature, 0.1% on the anterior wall and 2.9% on the posterior wall.[4] Recent data shows that the incidence of lesions at the cardia is increasing. Macroscopically, lesions can be described as ulcera-

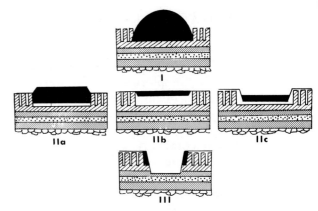

Figure 2.80 Classification of early gastric cancer. Type I (protruded): protrusion into the gastric lumen. Type II (superficial): the surface is slightly uneven. Type II can be subdivided into the following three subtypes: type IIa (elevated) – the surface is slightly elevated; type IIb (flat) – hardly any noticeable elevation from or depression in the surrounding mucosa; type IIc (depressed) – slightly depressed surface. Type III (excavated): marked excavation in the gastric wall.

tive, polypoidal, diffuse scirrhous (linitis plastica) and superficial. The proportion of carcinomas in each group varies in different series. Berkson had 75, 10 and 5% in each respective group.[3] More recently, particularly in Japan, the incidence of 'early' gastric cancers (superficial) has increased – to 30% in one report.[44] As a result of this, a macroscopic classification has been evolved for 'early' lesions (*Figure 2.80*).

Table 2.47 An international comparison of the surgical treatment of gastric cancer

		Laparotomy rate (%)	Resection rate (%)	Curative resection rate (%)	Overall and 5-year survival (%)
Europe					
Brookes *et al.*[4]	1950–1959	63.5	42.5	26.5	4.9
Desmond[10]	1944–1970	—	54.0	18.4	8.0
Svennevig and Nysted[42]	1959–1968	71.3	45.0	32.3	10.0
Inberg *et al.*[23]	1946–1955	53.9	21.1	17.1	3.7
	1956–1965	62.0	32.1	25.2	6.5
	1966–1972	69.3	45.1	23.6	10.8
USA					
Dupont *et al.*[12]	1948–1973	76.0	48.0	22.5	7.4
Cady *et al.*[5]	1940–1949	80.0	—	37.0	7.0
	1957–1966	94.0	58.0	44.0	11.0
Hoerr[21]	1950–1972	96.0	54.6	46.4	15.1
Adashek *et al.*[1]	1956–1965	71.0	39.0	24.0	8.0
	1966–1975	76.0	51.0	31.0	10.0
Japan					
Mine *et al.*[31]	1955–1963	93.2	63.2	52.3	14.4
Muto *et al.*[34]	1941–1961	98.7	79.4	—	19.0
Kajitani and Takagi[25]	1946–1970	97.7	—	67.0	33.3
Kajitani and Miwa[24]	1963–1966	94.3	63.4	44.7	16.4

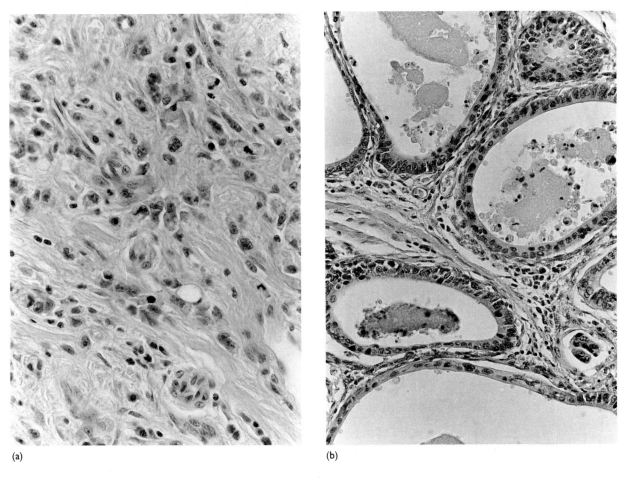

Figure 2.81   Adenocarcinoma: (a) diffuse; (b) intestinal. (Courtesy of H. Thompson, Birmingham.)

Gastric carcinomas may be multicentric: at presentation 2.2% have more than one primary and on histological examination 22% are multicentric. Microscopically, the degree of differentiation can be graded according to Broder's classification from grade 1 (well differentiated) to grade 4 (undifferentiated). A more valuable classification is that of Lauren, who described lesions as either intestinal or diffuse (*Figure 2.81*).[26] The prognosis is better for the intestinal type. Also, there are important associations with epidemiological findings. The intestinal type is common in areas of high incidence (such as Japan) and it is only the incidence of this lesion that has declined recently.

The earlier stage of disease and the higher incidence of intestinal cancer is probably the reason why the prognosis is apparently better in studies in Japan than in studies in other areas (*Table 2.47*).

Failure of surgery
Recurrent disease following radical resection is due to the progressive development of micrometastases. The sites of recurrence are both local and distant. The local recurrences may be in the gastric bed, gastric stump or residual local lymph nodes. Distant metastases may occur at many sites, but most commonly in the liver or peritoneal cavity and more rarely in the lungs and bones. In a postmortem study of 92 patients who had previously had subtotal gastrectomies, McNeer *et al.* found some form of local recurrence in 80.5% and recurrence at distant sites alone in 15.2%.[30] Gunderson analysed the Minnesota patients who had had reoperations.[2,18] There was evidence of recurrent cancer in 80.4%, and the recurrence was entirely local in 53.7% of the group (*Figure 2.82*). The high incidence of recurrent disease following surgery and the possibility that more extensive surgery might reduce this has already been explored. However, the inability of surgery to eradicate all disease and prevent the development of recurrence highlights the limitations of surgery as a single therapy in the management of gastric cancer. It is clear that adjuvant therapies must be evaluated in an attempt to improve control of this disease.

Chemotherapy
Cytotoxic agents have been evaluated in advanced disease and subsequently as an adjuvant to surgery. In advanced disease these agents have been used

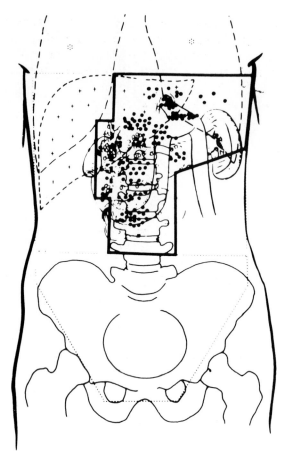

Figure 2.82 Sites of recurrence after curative resection.[18] *, lung metastasis; +, liver metastasis; △, wound implant; ●, local failures in surrounding organs or tissues; ○, lymph node failure.

singly and as combinations, the latter showing improved response rates (*Table 2.48*). A 'response' is defined here as a reduction of at least 50% in the size of a measurable lesion. Chemotherapy may improve early survival,[39] but there is no evidence for higher long-term survival.

Cytotoxic agents should be most effective when the tumour burden is small, as after curative surgical resection. The results of adjuvant studies are conflicting. Imanaga and Nakazoto reported a controlled study of 2636 patients using mitomycin and demonstrated overall improvement of 13.5% at 5 years and 10% at 10 years in the treated group.[22] However, the British Stomach Cancer Group's controlled study of adjuvant fluorouracil and mitomycin in 411 patients has failed to show improvement in survival.[14] Similarly, Franz and Cruz and Higgins failed to show any benefit from adjuvant chemotherapy.[15,19] However, the Gastro-Intestinal Tumour Study Group have reported a significant benefit from adjuvant chemotherapy.[9]

Whilst there is no convincing evidence from European and American studies to suggest that chemotherapy should be employed routinely, the fact that responses are obtained and that some studies have shown improved survival indicate that this type of treatment must continue to be evaluated in controlled prospective studies.

Radiotherapy

As many recurrences are local or regional and occur in an area that can be encompassed in a radiotherapy field, it is pertinent to consider the possible use of irradiation. The development of megavoltage radiotherapy has permitted radiation to be given without excessive damage to adjacent normal tissues. Robinson and Cohen demonstrated improved survival in patients receiving conventional postoperative irradiation, 40% surviving at 2 years compared to 20% in the group receiving no postoperative irradiation.[38] More work is now being done on the value of adjuvant radiotherapy after radical resections. Catterall *et al.* used fast-neutron irradiation in 29 unselected patients, and in the 19 with a palpable epigastric lesion produced resol-

Table 2.48   Cytotoxic agents in advanced gastric cancer[8,39,41]

Agent	Response rate (%)
Single agents	
Fluorouracil	22
Mitomycin	30
Carmustine (BCNU)	18
Doxorubicin (Adriamycin)	24
Combination chemotherapy	
Fluorouracil + semustine (methyl-CCNU) + doxorubicin	36
Fluorouracil + semustine	40
Fluorouracil + doxorubicin + mitomycin	43
Cisplatin + adriamycin + etoposide	60

ution in 16; 14 patients subsequently underwent a postmortem examination and 10 had no macroscopic evidence of tumour, although all but two had residual microscopic foci of malignant cells.[7] However, following neutron treatment, there was considerable damage to the stomach, and the authors recommended that gastrectomy should be performed routinely 4–6 months after irradiation. The British Stomach Cancer Group have reported a controlled study using postoperative radiotherapy. This trial has failed to show that radiotherapy conferred any survival benefit.

Squamous cell carcinoma and carcinoids

Squamous cell carcinomas are exceedingly rare (0.04–0.7% of all cancers), and four times as common in men as in women; their presentation is similar to that of adenocarcinoma. Similarly, argentaffinomas are not common, and the diagnosis is frequently only established at postmortem. They occur with equal frequency in men and women and the presenting symptoms are similar to adenocarcinomas, though they are often associated with a long preoperative history. Radiologically, carcinoids appear as polypoid neoplasms. If there is a small tumour with no evidence of metastasis it should be excised locally, but for neoplasms greater than 2 cm in diameter or with metastatic disease, the operation appropriate to the stage should be performed. The prognosis is good; among the 15 reported patients followed for more than 5 years, there have been 12 survivors. Amongst the 90 reported cases, six had the malignant carcinoid syndrome, producing large amounts of 5-hydroxytryptophan and histamine.

Non-epithelial tumours

The most frequently encountered non-epithelial tumours are lymphomas and leiomyosarcomas.

Lymphoma
These account for between 0.5 and 8% of gastric cancers and about 60% of all sarcomas involving the stomach. Often gastric lymphoma is a manifestation of a generalized disease: 50% of lymphosarcomas have a gastric element, but only 4–6% have primary gastric involvement. The stomach is, however, the most common site of extranodal involvement.

Most frequently these are non-Hodgkin's lymphomas (usually lymphosarcoma or reticulum cell lymphomas); between 5 and 10% are Hodgkin's disease. Macroscopically, these lesions are difficult to differentiate from adenocarcinomas, and the diagnosis is usually only established by their characteristic histological appearance. Initially, the tumour may metastasize to the regional nodes, further dissemination may occur to distant nodes and can involve the peritoneum and liver.

The sexes are equally affected and, though the mean age is in the 60s, it may occur in the young. The most common symptom is dyspepsia, which can have all the variable characteristics of symptoms associated with adenocarcinomas (*Tables 2.44* and *2.45*).

Preoperatively, the histological diagnosis is difficult to establish. Double-contrast radiology will be diagnostic of a gastric lesion, and the endoscopic findings are usually indistinguishable from those of adenocarcinoma. Because of the diffuse infiltration, endoscopic biopsy will only establish the diagnosis in 29% of patients.

Curative treatment is surgical, and for disease localized to the stomach without evidence of nodal metastasis resection has a 47% five-year survival rate. It is hoped that, in view of the efficacy of chemotherapy for non-Hodgkin's lymphomas, this survival may be further improved. Postoperative radiotherapy may be used as an adjuvant to surgical resection, but there is no evidence as yet that this improves survival.

Leiomyosarcoma
Leiomyosarcoma comprise 1–3% of all gastric tumours. The tumours are most commonly located on the anterior and posterior wall of the stomach. Macroscopically the tumours are bulky and vascular with multiple areas of ulceration. Microscopically, they originate from smooth muscle, and the frequency of mitotic figures is usually diagnostic. Direct spread is rare and lymph node involvement does not occur. At laparotomy, macroscopic dissemination is found in 10–45% of patients.

The incidence is approximately the same in men and women and the most frequent presenting symptom is bleeding, 75% having either haematemesis or melaena. There may also be associated epigastric symptoms, and on physical examination an abdominal mass is found in up to 60% of patients.

The diagnosis is established by a combination of endoscopy and radiology. Since they are usually located on the anterior or posterior wall, they can easily be missed if compression is not a routine part of the double-contrast study.

The curative treatment is surgical and involves a wide local excision without any lymphadenectomy. The prognosis is quite good, with a 5-year survival rate ranging from 37 to 54%. Neither palliative nor adjuvant chemotherapy or radiotherapy has been shown to be of benefit.

References

1. Adashek, K., Sangel, J. and Longmire, W.P. (1979) Cancer of the stomach. Review of ten year's intervals. *Annals of Surgery*, **189**, 6–10.
2. Aste, H., Amadori, D., Maltoni, G. *et al.* (1981) Early gastric cancer detection in four areas at different gastric cancer death rates. *Acta Endoscopica*. **11**, 123–132.
3. Berkson, J. (1964) Statistical summary. In *Cancer of the Stomach* (Ed.) Remine, W.H., Priestley, J.T. and Berkson, J. p. 207. Philadelphia: W.B. Saunders.
4. Brookes, V.S., Waterhouse, J.A.H. and Powell, D.J. (1965) Carcinoma of the stomach: 10 year survey of results and of factors affecting prognosis. *British Medical Journal*, **i**, 1577–1583.
5. Cady, B., Ramsden, D.A., Stein, A. and Haggitt, R.G. (1977) Gastric cancer. *American Journal of Surgery*, **133**, 423–429.
6. Carnett, J.B. and Howell, J.C. (1932) A case of coarctation of the aorta and gastric carcinoma with a discussion of the metastases. *Surgical Clinics of North America*, **12**, 1351–1362.
7. Catterall, M., Kingston, D., Lawrence, G. *et al.* (1975) The effects of fast neutrons on inoperable carcinoma of the stomach. *Gut*, **16**, 150–156.
8. Comis, R. and Carter, S. (1974) A review of chemotherapy in gastric cancer. *Cancer*, **34**, 1576–1586.
9. Gastrointestinal Tumour Study Group (1982) Controlled trial of adjuvant chemotherapy following curative results for gastric cancer. *Cancer*, **49**, 1116–1122.
10. Desmond, A. (1976) Radical surgery in treatment of carcinoma of stomach. *Proceedings of the Royal Society of Medicine*, **69**, 867–869.
11. Desmond, A., Nicholls, J. and Brown, C. (1975) Further surgical management of gastric ulcer with unsuspected malignant change. *Annals of the Royal College of Surgeons*, **57**, 101–104.
12. Dupont, J.B., Lee Rillens, J., Burton, G.R. and Cohen. I. (1978) Adenocarcinoma of the stomach: review of 1497 cases. *Cancer*, **41**, 941–947.
13. Fielding, J.W.L., Ellis, D.J., Jones, B.G. *et al.* (1980) Natural history of 'early' gastric cancer: results of a 10-year regional survey. *British Medical Journal*, **281**, 965–967.
14. Fielding, J.W.L., Fagg, S.L., Jones, B.G. *et al.* (1983) An interim report of a prospective, randomised, controlled study of adjuvant chemotherapy in operable gastric cancer. *World Journal of Surgery*, **7**, 390–399.
15. Franz, J.L. and Cruz, A.B. (1977) The treatment of gastric cancer with combined surgical dissection and chemotherapy. *Journal of Surgical Oncology*, **9**, 131–137.
16. Gilbertson, V.A. (1969) Results of treatment of stomach cancer. *Cancer*, **23**, 1305–1308.
17. Green, P., O'Toole, K., Weinberg, L. and Goldfarb, J. (1981) Early gastric cancer. *Gastroenterology*, **81**, 247–256.
18. Gunderson, L. (1976) Radiation therapy: results and future possibilities. *Clinics in Gastroenterology*, **5**, 743–776.
19. Higgins, G.A. (1976) Chemotherapy, adjuvant to surgery, for gastrointestinal surgery. *Clinics in Gastroenterology*, **5**, 795–808.
20. Hirayama, T. (1981) Methods and results (cost effectiveness) of gastric cancer screening. In *Gastric Cancer – Advances in the Biosciences*, Vol. 32 (Ed.) Fielding, J.W.L., Newman, C.E., Ford, C.H.J. and Jones, B.G. pp. 77–84. Oxford: Pergamon Press.
21. Hoerr, S.O. (1973) Prognosis for carcinoma of the stomach. *Surgery, Gynaecology and Obstetrics*, **137**, 204–209.
22. Imanaga, H. and Nakazoto, H. (1977) Results of surgery for gastric cancer and the effect of adjuvant mitomycin C in cancer recurrence. *World Journal of Surgery*, **1**, 213–227.
23. Inberg, M.V., Heinonen, R., Rantakokko, V. and Viikari, S.J. (1975) Surgical treatment of gastric carcinoma. *Archives of Surgery*, **110**, 703–707.
24. Kajitani, T. and Miwa, K. (1979) Treatment results of stomach cancer in Japan, 1963–1966. In *WHO cc Monograph, No. 2* (Ed.) Kajitani, T. and Miwa, K. Japan: WHO Collaborating Centre for Evaluation of Methods of Diagnosis and Treatment of Stomach Cancer.
25. Kajitani, T. and Takagi, K. (1979) Cancer of the stomach at Cancer Institute Hospital, Tokyo. *Gann Monograph on Cancer Research*, **22**, 77–87.
26. Lauren, P. (1965) The two main histological types of gastric carcinoma, diffuse and so-called intestinal type carcinoma. *Acta Pathologica et Microbiologica Scandinavica*, **64**, 31–49.
27. Longmire, W.P. (1980) Gastric carcinoma: is radical gastrectomy worth while? *Annals of the Royal College of Surgeons (England)*, **62**, 25–34.
28. Lundh, G., Burn, J.I., Kolig, G. *et al.* (1974) A co-operative international study of gastric cancer. *Annals of the Royal College of Surgeons (England)*, **54**, 219–228.
29. Lygidakis, N.J. (1981) Total gastrectomy for gastric carcinoma: a retrospective study of different procedures and assessment of a new technique of gastric reconstruction. *British Journal of Surgery*, **68**, 649–655.
30. McNeer, G., Vandenberg, H., Down, F.Y. and Boden, A. (1951) A critical evaluation of subtotal gastrectomy for cure of cancer of the stomach. *Annals of Surgery*, **134**, 2–7.
31. Mine, M., Majima, S., Harada, M. and Etani, S. (1970) End results of gastrectomy for gastric cancer. *Surgery*, **68**, 753–758.
32. Morris, D.L., Moore, J., Thompson, H. and Keighley, M.R.B. (1982) Accuracy of per-operative lymph node cytology in gastric carcinoma. *Clinical Oncology*, **8**, 219–221.

33. Murakami, T. (1979) Early cancer of the stomach. *World Journal of Surgery*, **3**, 685–692.
34. Muto, M., Maki, T., Majima, S. and Yamaguchi, I. (1968) Improvement in the end results of surgical treatment of gastric cancer. *Surgery*, **63**, 229–235.
35. Nagao, F. and Takahishi, M.D. (1979) Diagnosis of advanced gastric cancer. *World Journal of Surgery*, **3**, 693–700.
36. Pichlmayr, R. and Meyer, H.J. (1981) Patterns of recurrence in relation to therapeutic strategy. In *Gastric Cancer – Advances in the Biosciences*, Vol. 32 (Ed.) Fielding, J.W.L., Newman, C.E., Ford, C.H.J. and Jones, B.G. pp. 171–184. Oxford: Pergamon Press.
37. Remine, W.H. (1981) Preoperative assessment and palliative surgery. In *Gastric Cancer – Advances in the Biosciences*, Vol. 32 (Ed.) Fielding, J.W.L., Newman, C.E., Ford, C.H.J. and Jones, B.G. pp. 123–137. Oxford: Pergamon Press.
38. Robinson, E. and Cohen, Y. (1977) The combination of surgery, radiotherapy and chemotherapy in the treatment of gastric cancer. *Recent Results in Cancer Research*, **32**, 177–180.
39. Schien, R.S., Coffey, R. and Smith, F.P. (1981) Chemotherapy and combined modality treatment of gastric cancer. In *Gastric Cancer – Advances in the Biosciences*, Vol. 32 (Ed.) Fielding, J.W.L., Newman, C.E., Ford, C.H.J. and Jones, B.G. pp. 139–147. Oxford: Pergamon Press.
40. Sherman, R.S. and Snyder, R.E. (1960) Roentgenologic surveys for gastric neoplasms. *Journal of the American Medical Association*, **8**, 949–956.
41. Smith, F.P., Cambareri, R.J., Killen, J.Y. and Schein, P.S. (1980) Gastrointestinal Cancer. In *Cancer Chemotherapy: The EORTC Cancer Chemotherapy Annual*, Vol. 2 (Ed.) Pinedo, H. pp. 284–298. Amsterdam: Excerpta Medica.
42. Svennevig, J.L. and Nysted, A. (1976) Carcinoma of the stomach. *Acta Chirurgica Scandinavica*, **142**, 78–81.
43. Swynnerton R.F. and Truelove, S.C. (1952) Carcinoma of the stomach. *British Medical Journal*, **1**, 287–292.
44. Takagi, K. (1981) Stages of gastric cancer and reconstruction after surgery. In *Gastric Cancer – Advances in the Biosciences*, Vol. 32 (Ed.) Fielding, J.W.L., Newman, C.E., Ford, C.H.J. and Jones, B.G. pp. 91–122. Oxford: Pergamon Press.
45. UICC (1978) *TNM Classification of Malignant Tumours*, 3rd edn. Geneva: Union International Contra le Cancre.
46. Zinninger, M. and Collins, W. (1949) Extension of carcinoma of the stomach into the duodenum and oesophagus. *Annals of Surgery*, **130**, 557–566.

MÉNÉTRIÈR'S DISEASE

B.T. Cooper

Ménétrièr's disease was first described in 1888, but in spite of more than 300 reported cases in the literature, the disease is almost as mysterious now as when it was first described. Ménétrièr described two disorders – gastric polyposis and giant gastric rugae – but it is the latter which now bears his name. The eponymous name is more satisfactory than many other names given to the disorder as most are misleading pathologically.[5] The most satisfactory alternative would be hyperplastic gastropathy. The characteristic features of the disease are giant gastric rugae (folds), which are frequently associated with excessive gastric protein loss and hypoproteinaemia.

AETIOLOGY[6]

The aetiology of Ménétrièr's disease is unknown but, although familial incidence has been reported,[14] it is probably an acquired disorder. Cytomegalovirus has been isolated from the gastric mucosa of three children, *Helicobacter pylori* from two adults and both tuberculosis and histoplasmosis can cause giant rugae, but there is little evidence to support an infective aetiology for Ménétrièr's disease. The increased gastric epithelial cell turnover is similar to that seen in Zollinger–Ellison syndrome and has led to speculation that a hormonal stimulus to the gastric mucosa is responsible. However, there is no evidence for an abnormality of hormone secretion including gastrin although raised gastric mucosal prostaglandin E_2 levels have been reported in a case of transient Ménétrièr's disease associated with carcinoid syndrome.[2]

Reported immunological abnormalities include peripheral blood eosinophilia, increased IgM plasma cell numbers in gastric fundal mucosa, increased fractional catabolic rate of IgM and impaired delayed hypersensitivity responses to BCG vaccine and *Candida*. However, studies are few and no patient has been reported with all these abnormalities. The presence of food antibodies probably reflects increased gastric permeability.

There is increased gastric mucosal fibrinolysis,[15] *in vitro*, which can be inhibited by the antiplasmin drug tranexamic acid, with improved symptoms and mucosal appearances as well as decreased gastric protein loss. The theory that plasminogen activation is involved in aetiology is attractive because plasmin increases vascular permeability.

Trophic factors in saliva such as epidermal growth factor may stimulate large rugae in animals but there is no evidence for this in humans. In the veterinary literature, giant gastric rugae have been described in a number of species following different stimuli such as dithiothreitol in dogs, shale oil in monkeys, neonatal thymectomy in mice, and parasitic and fungal infections in snakes, monkeys and horses. The general view is that Ménétrièr's disease is the result of a hypersensitivity response to dietary or other antigens but the animal and limited human data suggest that Ménétrièr's disease might represent a common response to a number of different endogenous or exogenous stimuli.

PATHOLOGY[3,7,13]

The large gastric folds, which are so prominent macroscopically, have been likened to the contours of the brain.[7] The stomach feels boggy and heavy and when palpated from the serosal side feels like a 'bag of worms'.[7] The demarcation line between involved and normal areas is very sharp.

The most important histological feature is hyperplasia of the mucus-producing cells in the gastric glands, leading to cystic change in the middle and deep thirds of the glands and to elongation of the pits and glands resulting in mucosal thickening (*Figure 2.83*).[3,13] The cysts contain periodic acid–Schiff-positive material. The glands may be relatively straight or very branched and tortuous. There is often a relative or absolute deficiency of parietal and oxyntic cells. In some patients, there is diffuse or patchy inflammation of the epithelium and lamina propria with infiltration by neutrophils, eosinophils, plasma cells or lymphocytes. Mucosal erosions may be seen. Intestinal metaplasia can occur in inflamed areas. The lamina propria, muscularis mucosa and submucosa may be oedematous. Two features are virtually diagnostic of Ménétrièr's disease but they are not seen in every case: (1) smooth muscle fibres extending from the muscularis mucosa through the lamina propria to the apices of the gastric glands (*Figure 2.83*); (2) penetration of the muscularis mucosa by gastric glands which can balloon into the submucosal and may be misdiagnosed as carcinoma. On electron microscopy, the interepithelial cell spaces are dilated, there is intense micropinocytosis of the capillary endothelial cells beneath the mucus-producing cells[4] and tight junctions between gastric epithelial cells are widened.[12] These may be involved in the mechanism of protein loss.

PATHOPHYSIOLOGY

GASTRIC SECRETION

Achlorhydria or hypochlorhydria are common in Ménétrièr's disease, occurring in 50–70% of cases.[6,19] Serum gastrin is mildly elevated in approximately half the cases, probably reflecting a diminished parietal cell mass. Little is known about pepsin secretion. Gastric secretory studies help to separate Ménétrièr's disease from 'hypertrophic hypersecretory gastropathy',[21] in which thickened

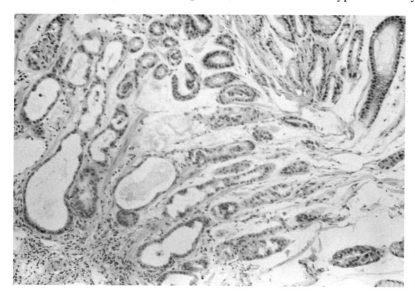

Figure 2.83 Endoscopic biopsy in a case of Ménétrièr's disease, showing elongated glands with cystic dilatation of the bases and smooth muscle fibres passing from the bases of the glands towards their apices.

rugae, mucosal hyperplasia and acid hypersecretion occur, although a few cases have been described with features of both disorders.

GASTRIC PROTEIN LOSS

This is a cardinal feature of the disease: 80% of patients have a low serum albumin level at presentation.[19] Protein loss has been confirmed by perfusion studies and it is completely abolished by total gastrectomy. Electrophoresis of gastric juice shows increases in both albumin and the globulins, indicating a non-selective loss.[11] The protein loss can be demonstrated by any test for gastrointestinal protein loss such as the intravenous ^{51}Cr-labelled albumin test. Protein turnover studies have shown increased fractional catabolic rates for plasma proteins and normal or increased synthesis rates of plasma proteins.[11] Gastric protein loss probably results from alteration in the passive permeability of the gastric epithelium (widened gastric epithelial tight junctions) and may be mediated by a cholinergic mechanism.[12] There is no evidence that protein loss is a result of lymphatic blockage, mucosal ulceration or excessive secretion of mucus.

LABORATORY TESTS

Iron deficiency anaemia is found in about 50% and peripheral blood eosinophilia in 12% of cases.[6] Intrinsic factor secretion is normal but development of atrophic gastritis leads to vitamin B_{12} malabsorption.[8]

CLINICAL FEATURES[6,19,20]

The disease can occur in adults of any age, with a peak in the fourth decade for females and in the sixth decade for males. The male-to-female ratio is 3:1. The disease has been described in Caucasians, American Negroes and Japanese, but this racial distribution probably reflects availability of advanced medical services rather than any racial predisposition. The onset is usually insidious but acute onset may follow apparent hypersensitivity to foods or drugs. Usually there are no obvious precipitating factors. The duration of symptoms can vary from 1 week to 20 years. The important symptoms are epigastric pain and dyspepsia (75%), weight loss (30–60%), vomiting (40%), peripheral oedema (40%) and diarrhoea (20%). The epigastric pain is variable in intensity and duration, may be cramp-like, burning or stabbing and is frequently dyspeptic

with relief from food and antacids. Anorexia and some evidence of gastric blood loss are common. Severe gastric haemorrhage is rare but can be the presenting complaint, as can chronic iron-deficiency anaemia. The commonest signs are localized epigastric tenderness and peripheral oedema. Ascites, pleural effusion and epigastric mass have been reported. Patients are at increased risk of severe or recurrent infections and thromboembolism.[19,20]

NATURAL HISTORY

The natural history of this disorder is largely unknown, but the disease can be very protracted, with reports of unrelieved symptoms for up to 20 years. In one review of 120 cases, two-thirds of patients had some form of gastric resection, but the majority of the remainder had continued symptoms.[19] Nevertheless, there are well documented cases of spontaneous recovery three months to five years after diagnosis. In some of these cases, the gastric mucosa changed to atrophic gastritis.[1,8]

CANCER RISK[5]

There have been many reports of patients with Ménétrièr's disease and coexistent carcinoma of the stomach. Whether or not Ménétrièr's disease predisposes to carcinoma has been disputed. Carcinoma can cause large gastric rugae and the diagnosis of Ménétrièr's disease in many of these cases was not based on histological criteria; however, patients with well-documented Ménétrièr's disease have developed carcinoma of the stomach during follow-up. The carcinoma risk seems to be about 10%.[19] Circumstantial evidence for the association is the change to atrophic gastritis, which itself has a carcinoma risk, and the increased gastric epithelial cell proliferation rate, which may predispose to malignant change.

MÉNÉTRIÈR'S DISEASE IN CHILDREN

An apparently identical disease has been described in about 20 children aged 2 months to 14 years.[6] Characteristic features are a short history (1–12 weeks), peripheral blood eosinophilia and, in most cases, a spontaneous and permanent remission anytime up to 6 months after presentation.

INVESTIGATIONS

The radiological and gastroscopic appearances suggest but do not confirm the diagnosis of Ménétrièr's disease, which can only be made if the typical histological appearances are found. To do this and to exclude other causes of large gastric rugae,[5] an adequate gastric biopsy which includes the muscularis mucosa is necessary. Where this is not possible with an endoscopic, snare or suction biopsy, a full-thickness biopsy at laparotomy is indicated.

RADIOLOGICAL FEATURES[6,18]

No radiological feature is pathognomonic of the disease. The most characteristic feature is the thick uneffaceable gastric rugae, 1–2 cm in height, which can sometimes appear as polyps or mucosal masses. Between the rugae are deep sulci, into which barium may run, giving a spiculated appearance, which may mimic gastric ulceration. Barium often mixes with mucus in the lumen to give a characteristic reticulated appearance. The mucosal abnormalities may occur anywhere in the stomach, including the antrum, but they are most prominent along the greater curve. The radiological differential diagnosis is large and includes carcinoma and lymphoma.[5]

ENDOSCOPIC APPEARANCES[6]

The most striking abnormalies are the thick, tortuous gastric rugae which do not flatten with intra-luminal air. The mucosa may be dull, reddened, oedematous, cobblestoned, nodular or even polypoid. There may be patchy hyperaemia, haemorrhage or erosions. Chronic gastric ulcer is an occasional associated finding. Mucus is prominent, coating the mucosa tenaciously or lying free in the lumen.

TREATMENT

Treatment may be medical or surgical. As spontaneous remission occurs and some patients do seem to respond to medication, the older view that Ménétrièr's disease must be treated by some form of gastric resection is no longer tenable. Medical treatment should always be tried first.

MEDICAL TREATMENT

A bland diet and antacids may help some, and nutritional support is important in most. Nutritional deficiency occurs because of anorexia and because the liver cannot synthesize enough protein to replace that lost from the stomach even though much of that protein is normally digested and reabsorbed. A high-energy, high-protein diet is indicated and enteral feeding may be required. Intravenous albumin is of only temporary value in relieving hypoproteinaemic oedema. The drug treatment of Ménétrièr's disease is confused because many favourable responses can be explained by spontaneous remission. The effects of withdrawal and readministration of apparently beneficial drugs have rarely been reported. A number of treatments may have helped some cases: tranexamic acid,[15] anticholinergics,[10] corticosteroids,[22] cimetidine[16,20] and elimination of *H. pylori* infection.[17] Gastric irradiation has been tried but is not recommended. If a patient responds to treatment or remits spontaneously, life-long follow-up is mandatory because of the risk of carcinoma.

SURGICAL TREATMENT

A full-thickness biopsy at laparotomy is necessary if endoscopic or suction biopsies fail to provide a definite histological diagnosis. Indications for gastric resection are intractable symptoms, severe or persistent hypoproteinaemic oedema, gastric bleeding or the presence of or high risk of carcinoma. Total gastrectomy leads to complete and permanent relief of symptoms[19] and is now less of a problem with modern surgical techniques and nutritional support. In the past partial gastrectomy with removal of all the diseased mucosa was favoured. This is not always technically possible and anastomoses involving diseased mucosa frequently break down. Moreover, recurrence in previously normal gastric mucosa is well documented after partial gastrectomy.[9] The results of vagotomy alone are conflicting.[5] If an operation is indicated, the procedure of choice is probably total gastrectomy. Perioperative subcutaneous heparin is recommended because of the risk of venous thromboembolism.[19,20]

REFERENCES

1. Berenson, M.M., Sannella, J. and Freston, J.W. (1976) Ménétrièr's disease. Serial morphological, secretory and serological observations. *Gastroenterology*, **70**, 257–263.
2. Boyd, E.J.S., Hulks, G., Thomas, J.S. and McColl, K.E.L. (1988) Hypertrophic gastritis associated with increased gastric mucosal PGE$_2$ concentration in a patient with carcinoid syndrome. *Gut*, **29**, 1270–1276.
3. Butz, W.C. (1960) Giant hypertrophic gastritis. A report of 14 cases. *Gastroenterology*, **39**, 183–190.

4. Chambourlier, P., Pin, G., Treffot, M.J. *et al.* (1979) Syndromes oedémateux rélévateurs d'une maladie de Ménétrièr. *Semaine des hopitaux de Paris*, **55**, 684–688.

5. Cooper, B.T. (1987) Ménétrièr's disease. *Digestive Diseases*, **5**, 33–40.

6. Cooper, B.T. and Chadwick, V.S. (1981) Ménétrièr's disease. In *Butterworths International Medical Reviews: Foregut* (Eds) Baron, J.H. and Moody, F.G. pp. 141–191. London: Butterworth.

7. Feiber, S.S. (1955) Hypertrophic gastritis. Report of 2 cases and analysis of 50 pathologically verified cases from the literature. *Gastroenterology*, **28**, 39–69.

8. Frank, B.W. and Kern, F. (1967) Ménétrièr's disease. Spontaneous metamorphosis of giant hypertrophy of the gastric mucosa to atrophic gastritis. *Gastroenterology*, **53**, 953–960.

9. Gold, B.M. and Meyers, M.A. (1977) Progression of Ménétrièr's disease with postoperative gastrojejunal intussception. *Gastroenterology*, **73**, 583–586.

10. Gordon, M.N., Schaefer, E.J. and Finkel, M. (1976) Treatment of protein losing gastropathy with atropine. *American Journal of Gastroenterology*, **56**, 535–539.

11. Jarnum, S. and Jensen, K.B. (1972) Plasma protein turnover (albumin, transferrin, IgG, IgM) in Ménétrièr's disease (giant hypertrophic gastritis): evidence of non-selective protein loss. *Gut*, **13**, 128–137.

12. Kelly, D.G., Miller, L.J., Malagelada, J.R. *et al.* (1982) Giant hypertrophic gastropathy (Ménétrièr's disease): pharmacologic effects on protein leakage and mucosal ultrastructure. *Gastroenterology*, **83**, 581–589.

13. Kenney, F.D., Dockerty, M.B. and Waugh, J.M. (1954) Giant hypertrophy of gastric mucosa: a clinical and pathologic study. *Cancer*, **7**, 671–681.

14. Klein, O., Colombel, J.F., Maunory, V. *et al.* (1989) Familial Ménétrièr's disease. *American Journal of Gastroenterology*, **84**, 575–576.

15. Kondo, M., Ikezaki, M., Katu, H. and Masuda, M. (1978) Anti-fibrinolytic therapy of giant hypertrophic gastritis (Ménétrièr's disease). *Scandinavian Journal of Gastroenterology*, **13**, 851–856.

16. Krag, E., Frederiksen, H.J., Olsen, N. and Henriksen, J.H. (1978) Cimetidine treatment of protein-losing gastropathy (Ménétrièr's disease). A clinical and pathophysiological study. *Scandinavian Journal of Gastroenterology*, **13**, 636–639.

17. Lepore, M.J., Smith, F.B. and Bonanno, C.A. (1988) Campylobacter like organisms in patients with Ménétrièr's disease. *The Lancet*, **i**, 466.

18. Reese, D.F., Hodgson, J.R. and Dockerty, M.B. (1962) Giant hypertrophy of the gastric mucosa (Ménétrièr's disease): a correlation of the roentgenologic, pathologic and clinical findings. *American Journal of Roentgenology*, **88**, 619–626.

19. Scharschmidt, B.F. (1977) The natural history of hypertrophic gastropathy (Ménétrièr's disease). *American Journal of Medicine*, **63**, 644–652.

20. Searcy, R.M. and Malagelada, J.R. (1984) Ménétrièr's disease and idiopathic hypertrophic gastropathy. *Annals of Internal Medicine*, **100**, 565–570.

21. Stempien, S.J., Dagradi, A.E. and Reingold, I.M. *et al.* (1964) Hypertrophic hypersecretory gastropathy. *American Journal of Digestive Diseases*, **9**, 471–493.

22. Winney, R.J., Gilmour, H.M. and Matthews, J.D. (1976) Prednisolone in giant hypertrophic gastritis (Ménétrièr's disease). *American Journal of Digestive Diseases*, **21**, 337–339.

OTHER GASTRODUODENAL DISORDERS

B.T. Cooper

GASTRIC BEZOARS

A bezoar is a solid, compacted mass of food or foreign matter that has undergone some digestive change in the gut. Bezoars can be classified into three main groups: phytobezoars, trichobezoars and concretions.[9]

Clinical features and diagnosis

Bezoars in the stomach can cause nausea, vomiting, anorexia, weight loss and upper abdominal pain, discomfort and fullness.[9] The commonest symptoms are epigastric pain (74%) and episodic nausea and vomiting (64%). An epigastric mass may be palpable in 57% of phytobezoars and 88% of trichobezoars. Bezoars can cause gastritis, peptic ulceration and iron deficiency and have been associated with gastric carcinoma.[35] Peptic ulceration is commoner with phytobezoars (24%) than with trichobezoars (10%).[9] Gastric outlet and intestinal obstruction sometimes occur.[5,9]

A full blood count may show iron deficiency anaemia or a mild leukocytosis.[9] Hypoproteinaemia has been described with trichobezoar.[14]

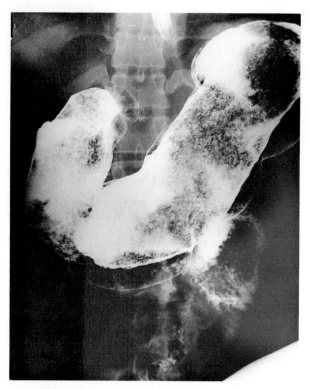

Figure 2.84 Barium meal examination of a 20-year-old girl showing a large trichobezoar.

Bezoars can be seen on an erect plain abdominal film but diagnosis is usually made either at barium meal (*Figure 2.84*) or upper gastrointestinal endoscopy. The latter is probably the best diagnostic technique and direct visualization allows classification of its type.

PHYTOBEZOAR

These may be composed of almost any plant material such as fibres, leaves, roots or skins. Bezoars composed of plant material and hair (trichophytobezoar) can occur. Phytobezoars tend to be more abrasive than hair bezoars, which probably explains why gastritis and peptic ulcer frequently occur. Phytobezoars are commoner than trichobezoars and occur most frequently in males over 30 years of age.[5] Factors which predispose to their development are hypochlorhydria, diminished antral motility and poor mastication of plant material in the diet.[6] Thus, bezoars may be seen after partial gastrectomy, after truncal vagotomy, in disorders such as gastroparesis diabeticorum,[3] and have been described in patients taking H_2 receptor antagonists.[28] Their prevalence is related to the number of partial gastrectomies in the population.[5,6] Postgastrectomy bezoars follow Billroth I and Billroth II gastrectomies, especially if there has

also been a vagotomy.[32] Bezoars can follow any drainage procedure with truncal vagotomy[7] but seem to be a particular problem after antrectomy, when gastric emptying of solids is impaired.[3,7]

In the USA, the commonest type of phytobezoar (70%) is the persimmon bezoar (diospyrobezoar), which is often unrelated to any recognizable predisposing factor.[9] They are particularly likely to cause gastric ulceration. The persimmon fruit, especially if unripe, has astringent properties attributed to a substance called phlobotannin which coagulates on contact with dilute acid.

Phytobezoars can be treated non-surgically. Initially, a liquid diet is administered followed by gastric lavage and suction associated with attempts at manual external disruption. If this is unsuccessful, the bezoar can be fragmented using a biopsy forceps,[21] polypectomy snare or laser[27] at endoscopy. Instillation into the stomach of proteolytic enzymes such as papain,[6] acetylcysteine[33] and cellulase[30,35] have been helpful in breaking up phytobezoars. If non-surgical methods fail, surgical removal is necessary because the mortality for untreated phytobezoar is very high.[9] It is necessary to educate patients at risk about the importance of good dentition and proper chewing of fruits.[5] Patients with impaired antral motility may require treatment with a prokinetic drug, e.g. metoclopramide, to prevent bezoar formation.[3,28]

TRICHOBEZOAR

These are hairballs composed of decaying foodstuff enmeshed in enormous amounts of hair.[9] They may be present for many years before causing symptoms. Eventually they grow to such a size as to form a J-shaped cast of the stomach and are nearly always black (*Figure 2.85*). They result from chronic ingestion of hair and are commonest in females less than 30 years of age. Most patients give a history of trichophagia although only a small minority of patients have psychiatric disorders. The only treatment is surgical removal. Because the hairball is full of bacteria, there is a risk of peritonitis resulting from soilage of the peritoneum during removal.

CONCRETIONS

A whole variety of other substances may aggregate in the stomach to form a compact, hard mass, particularly milk protein (lactobezoar) and various drugs (medication bezoars) including theophylline, sucralfate, ion exchange resins and antacid tablets or gel. Aluminium hydroxide gel concretions are described in patients with chronic renal failure and can pass into the small intestine causing obstruction.[18]

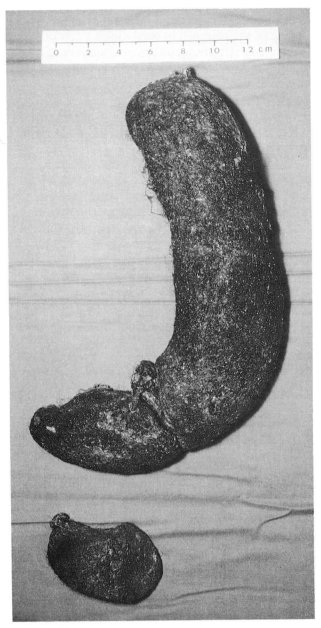

Figure 2.85 Trichobezoar from *Figure 2.84*.

ACUTE DILATATION OF THE STOMACH

Acute dilatation of the stomach is now rare because of the better management of severely ill and post-operative patients. In most cases, it results from an impairment of gastric motility leading to a localized paralytic ileus associated with excessive gastric secretion. It can be seen in a variety of situations: following upper abdominal surgery, prolonged immobilization, severe trauma, severe pain at any site, septicaemia, intra-abdominal acute inflammation (peritonitis, pancreatitis, appendicitis, cholecysti-

tis), metabolic disorders (diabetic ketoacidosis, hepatic encephalopathy, hypercalcaemia, hypocalcaemia, hypothyroidism), refeeding following starvation, e.g. in anorexia nervosa.[15] It may also follow strangulation of a paraoesophageal hiatal hernia or gastric volvulus.

CLINICAL FEATURES

The main symptoms are severe abdominal pain, vomiting, hypotension and shock. An epigastric mass may be palpable. Complications include aspiration of vomit and spontaneous rupture of the stomach[10] or postoperative abdominal evisceration. The diagnosis is usually suspected on clinical grounds and confirmed by a plain abdominal radiograph.

TREATMENT

Treatment involves vigorous resuscitation with intravenous replacement of fluid and electrolytes, and aspiration of the stomach with a wide-bore nasogastric tube, which is necessary to decompress the stomach and must be continued until gastric emptying returns to normal. If acute dilatation results from a strangulated paraoesophageal hernia or volvulus, emergency surgery is necessary to prevent gastric necrosis and rupture.

PHLEGMONOUS AND EMPHYSEMATOUS GASTRITIS

PHLEGMONOUS GASTRITIS

Aetiology

This is purulent bacterial infection of the stomach involving the muscularis mucosa and the submucosa.[24] The inflammation does not directly affect the epithelium although it may slough off as the infection progresses. The inflammation may also extend through to the serosa from which pus can be expressed at laparotomy, but does not extend into the oesophagus or duodenum. The condition is extremely rare and may follow a bacterial infection at a site remote from the stomach and/or septicaemia. Causative organisms include staphylococci, streptococci, pneumococci, *Escherichia coli* and *Klebsiella* species.[24] There is no convincing evidence that factors such as achlorhydria or gastric ulcer predispose to the condition.

Clinical features

Patients usually present with the features of an acute abdomen and are ill, often febrile and rapidly deteriorate. Typically, the patient vomits pus, blood or a cast of the stomach. In some patients, the abdominal features are relatively unimpressive in the context of severe coexisting disease. Such cases may only be diagnosed at autopsy.

An even rarer chronic form of phlegmonous gastritis is reported which presents with gastric outflow obstruction, persistent low-grade fever or haematemesis.[24]

Investigations

The diagnosis of phlegmonous gastritis is suggested by evidence of gross mucosal thickening of the stomach on plain abdominal radiography or barium meal. Gastric dilatation can be seen. Gas in the stomach wall will be seen in emphysematous gastritis. There are very few reports of the endoscopic appearances of phlegmonous gastritis but the main findings are large swollen, spongy, red or purple mucosal folds.[4] As the disease is subepithelial, endoscopic biopsy does not necessarily reveal the diagnosis.

Treatment

The patient requires vigorous resuscitation with intravenous fluid and electrolytes. Antibiotic therapy appropriate for sepsis without a known organism must be started as soon as the diagnosis is suspected. Virtually all cases that have been treated conservatively have died. Therefore, laparotomy is essential. In most cases, a total gastrectomy is required although if the disease is localized to the antrum, a partial gastrectomy may be sufficient. Surgical mortality is about 20%.[24] A case of phlegmonous gastritis localized to the antrum has been reported which was diagnosed by snare biopsy at endoscopy and was treated vigorously with antibiotics but without surgery.[4] The authors speculated that the pus was allowed to drain through the snare biopsy site.

EMPHYSEMATOUS GASTRITIS

This is an extremely rare form of phlegmonous gastritis caused by gas-forming organisms such as *Clostridium welchii*.[11] The diagnosis is made by the appearance of gas in the stomach wall on plain abdominal radiography or at barium meal. Most patients die despite surgical therapy but survival after medical treatment alone is reported.[11] Cicatrization of the stomach in survivors is a complication which may require reconstructive surgery at a later date.

THE SUPERIOR MESENTERIC ARTERY SYNDROME

The superior mesenteric artery syndrome is a controversial disorder in which the superior mesenteric artery leaves the aorta at an acute angle and, as it travels through the root of the mesentery, it crosses over the duodenum just to the right of the midline, thus compressing and obstructing the duodenum.[1,17,22] A majority of patients affected are young adults although individuals aged from 1 to 81 years have been reported[17] and there is a female preponderance (60%).[1]

CLINICAL FEATURES

The disorder may occasionally be acute in onset with the features of acute proximal small intestinal obstruction, but more typically the disorder is chronic with recurring attacks.[1] Typical symptoms are epigastric fullness and bloating after meals, vomiting and central abdominal colic. Relief of the symptoms by lying on the left side or by adopting a knee-chest position is common and has some diagnostic significance.[1] It has been described in association with pancreatitis and peptic ulcer. Suggested predisposing factors include prolonged bed rest, severe weight loss, previous abdominal surgery and loss of abdominal muscle tone. It can occur acutely after placement in a body cast or spica (cast syndrome).[1]

INVESTIGATIONS

Barium meal examination shows duodenal obstruction just to the right of the midline with dilatation of the stomach and proximal duodenum.

TREATMENT

Treatment involves intravenous replacement of fluid and electrolytes, and gastric decompression with a nasogastric tube. The most effective of the many surgical operations that have been performed for this disorder seems to be duodenojejunostomy.[1]

CARCINOMA OF THE DUODENUM

EPIDEMIOLOGY AND PATHOLOGY

Small intestinal carcinomas make up less than 1% of all intestinal carcinomas. Nevertheless, 33–48% of all small intestinal carcinomas occur in the duodenum[34,37] despite the fact that the duodenum constitutes only about 8% of the length of the small intestine.[34] Duodenal carcinomas are rare; 0.2 cases occurred per 100 000 of the population per year in one English city.[8] The commonest carcinomas found in the duodenum are those arising from the ampulla of Vater but, if only true duodenal carcinomas are considered, such carcinomas are commonest in the intra-ampullary duodenum (~50%) with the remainder in the periampullary (30–40%) and supra-ampullary regions.[16,34]

Macroscopically, duodenal carcinomas may be flat, stenosing, ulcerating, infiltrating or polypoid. Virtually all are adenocarcinomas although adenosquamous carcinomas can occur.[34] The adenocarcinomas are often papillary[2] and mostly well differentiated despite metastatic spread.[26] They are locally invasive and can spread to local and regional lymph nodes, pancreas, liver, peritoneum, ovaries and lungs. Distant metastases tend to occur late.[34]

Disorders predisposing to the development of duodenal carcinoma are familial adenomatous polyps[25] often associated with Gardner's syndrome,[29] Peutz–Jegher syndrome[31] and coeliac disease.[13] Although small intestinal carcinoma can complicate Crohn's disease, the majority of such cases occur in the ileum and duodenal carcinoma in Crohn's disease is extremely rare.[12] There is no evidence to suggest that chronic duodenal ulcer or duodenitis predispose to carcinoma.

CLINICAL FEATURES

Duodenal carcinoma may appear in adults of any age but the majority of cases occur in the sixth and seventh decades and the average age at presentation is 58 years.[34] The proportion of males to females is approximately equal.

Patients usually present with abdominal pain, gastrointestinal bleeding or jaundice.[20,34,37] Half to two-thirds of patients have epigastric pain which is aggravated by eating and, later, is associated with weight loss, vomiting and the features of small intestinal obstruction. Two-thirds have evidence of occult gastrointestinal bleeding and may have iron deficiency anaemia; overt bleeding with haematemesis and/or melaena is unusual. At presentation, 20–30% of patients are jaundiced.[16,34] These patients have periampullary tumours and may pass 'silver stools' if there has been overt bleeding from the lesion. A palpable mass is unusual but hepatomegaly and ascites may be present in advanced cases.

INVESTIGATIONS

The diagnosis can be suggested at barium meal (*Figure 2.86*) but it may be missed.[16,37] Accuracy is increased by hypotonic duodenography. Upper gastrointestinal endoscopy with biopsy and brush cytology is necessary to confirm the diagnosis. Even carcinomas in the third and fourth parts of the duodenum can be reached at endoscopy.

The differential diagnosis includes benign chronic duodenal ulcer, Crohn's disease, lymphoma, other causes of obstructive jaundice and direct spread of pancreatic or other tumours to involve the duodenum. Duodenal carcinoma should be considered in large non-healing duodenal ulcers in the elderly,

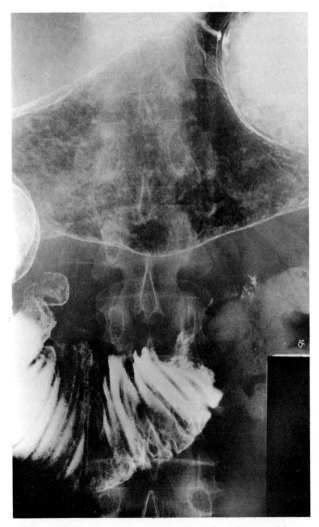

Figure 2.86 Barium meal examination of a 65-year-old man showing duodenal obstruction as a result of duodenal carcinoma.

especially if they are located beyond the cap; it is probably advisable that such ulcers are biopsied and brushed routinely.

TREATMENT

Curative resection can be attempted in 50–80% of cases.[16,19,37] For periampullary and supra-ampullary lesions, the surgical choice is pancreatico-duodenectomy, despite its significant operative mortality.[16,19,23,34,36,37] For distal lesions, opinion is divided between segmental resection[16,20,34] and pancreaticoduodenectomy.[19] Five-year survival after attempted curative resection is 15–20%[23,34,37] although a 5-year survival as high as 46% has been reported.[16] Prognosis is poor if there is transmural spread or local lymph node metastases.[16,19] Presentation with melaena is associated with a poor prognosis.

Bypass or segmental resection is performed for palliation. Survival in patients in whom curative resection is not possible is less than 6 months. Chemotherapy and radiotherapy have little place in current treatment.

REFERENCES

1. Barner, H.B. and Sherman M.D. (1963) Vascular compression of the duodenum. *Surgery, Obstetrics, Gynecology*, **117**, 103–118.
2. Blumgart, L.H. and Kennedy, A. (1973) Carcinoma of the ampulla of Vater and duodenum. *British Journal of Surgery*, **60**, 33–60.
3. Brady, P.G. (1978) Gastric phytobezoars consequent to delayed gastric emptying. *Gastrointestinal Endoscopy*, **24**, 159–161.
4. Bron, B.A., Deghle, P., Pellani, S., Krejs, G.J., Siebenmann, R. E. and Blum, A.L. (1977) Phlegmonous gastritis diagnosed by endoscopic snare biopsy. *American Journal of Digestive Diseases*, **22**, 729–733.
5. Bucholz, R.R. and Haisten, A.S. (1972) Phytobezoars following gastric surgery for duodenal ulcer. *Surgical Clinics of North America*, **52**, 341–352.
6. Cain, G.D., Moore, P. and Patterson, M. (1968) Bezoars – a complication of the post-gastrectomy state. *American Journal of Digestive Diseases*, **13**, 801–809.
7. Calabuig, R., Navarro, S., Cario, I., Artigas, V., Mores, J. and LaCalle, J.P. (1989) Gastric emptying and bezoars. *American Journal of Surgery*, **157**, 287–290.
8. Cooper, M.J. and Williamson, R.C.N. (1985) Enteric adenoma and carcinoma. *World Journal of Surgery*, **9**, 914–920.
9. DeBakey, M. and Ochsner, A. (1938/9) Bezoars and concretions. A comprehensive review of the literature with an analysis of 303 collected cases and a presentation of 8 additional cases. *Surgery*, **4**, 934–963, **5**, 132–160.
10. Evans, D.S. (1968) Acute dilatation and spontaneous rupture of the stomach. *British Journal of Surgery*, **55**, 940–942.
11. Gonzalez, L.L., Schowengerdt, C., Skinner, H.H. and Lynch, P. (1963) Emphysematous gastritis. *Surgery, Gynecology, Obstetrics*, **116**, 79–87.
12. Hawker, P.C., Gyde, S.N., Thompson, H. and Allan, R.N. (1982) Adenocarcinoma of the small intestine complicating Crohn's disease. *Gut*, **23**, 188–193.
13. Holmes, G.K.T., Dunn, G.I., Cockel, R. and Brookes, V.S. (1981) Adenocarcinoma of the upper small bowel complicating coeliac disease. *Gut*, **21**, 1010–1016.
14. Hossenbocus, A. and Colin-Jones, D.G. (1973) Trichobezoar, gastric polyposis, protein losing gastroenteropathy and steatorrhoea. *Gut*, **14**, 730–732.
15. Jennings, K.P. and Klidjian, A.M. (1974) Acute gastric dilatation in anorexia nervosa. *British Medical Journal*, **ii**, 477–478.
16. Joesting, D.R., Beart, R.W., van Heerden, J.A. and Wieland, L.H. (1981) Improving survival in adenocarcinoma of the duodenum. *American Journal of Surgery*, **141**, 228–231.
17. Kaiser, G.C., McKain, J.M. and Shumacher, H.B. (1960) The superior mesenteric artery syndrome. *Surgery, Gynecology, Obstetrics*, **110**, 133–140.
18. Korenman, M.D., Stubbs, M. and Fish, J.C. (1978) Intestinal obstruction from medication bezoars. *Journal of the American Medical Association*, **240**, 54–55.
19. Lai, E.C.S., Doty, J.E., Irving, C. and Tompkins, R.K. (1988) Primary adenocarcinoma of the duodenum: analysis of survival. *World Journal of Surgery*, **12**, 695–699.
20. Lillemoe, K. and Imbembo, A.L. (1980) Malignant neoplasms of the duodenum. *Surgery, Gynecology, Obstetrics*, **150**, 822–826.
21. McKechnie, J.C. (1972) Gastroscopic removal of a phytobezoar. *Gastroenterology*, **62**, 1047–1051.
22. Mansberger, A.R., Hearn, J.B., Byer, R.M., Fleisig, N. and Buxton, R.W. (1968) Vascular compression of the duodenum. *American Journal of Surgery*, **115**, 89–96.
23. Michelassi, F., Erroi, F., Dawson, P.J. *et al.* (1989) Experience of 647 consecutive tumours of the duodenum, ampulla, head of pancreas and distal common bile duct. *Annals of Surgery*, **210**, 544–554.
24. Miller, A.I., Smith, B. and Rogers, A.I. (1975) Phlegmonous gastritis. *Gastroenterology*, **68**, 231–238.
25. Mir-Madjilesse, S., Farmer, R.G. and Hawk, W.A. (1973) Villous tumours of the duodenum and jejunum. *American Journal of Digestive Diseases*, **18**, 467–472.
26. Morson, B.C. and Dawson, I.M.P. (1979)

Gastrointestinal Pathology, 2nd edn, pp. 408–411. Oxford: Blackwell.

27. Naveau, S. (1986) Gastric phytobezoar destruction by Nd:YAG laser therapy. *Gastrointestinal Endoscopy*, **32**, 430–431.

28. Nichols, T.W. (1981) Phytobezoar formation: a new complication of cimetidine therapy. *Annals of Internal Medicine*, **95**, 70.

29. Pauli, R.M., Pauli, M.E. and Hall, J.G. (1980) Gardner's syndrome and periampullary malignancy. *American Journal of Medical Genetics*, **6**, 205–219.

30. Pollard, H.B. and Block, G.E. (1968) Rapid dissolution of phytobezoars by cellulase enzyme. *American Journal of Surgery*, **115**, 933–936.

31. Reid, J.D. (1974) Intestinal carcinoma in the Peutz–Jegher syndrome. *Journal of the American Medical Association*, **229**, 833–834.

32. Rigler, R.G. and Grininger, D.R. (1970) Phytobezoars following partial gastrectomy. *Surgical Clinics of North America*, **50**, 381–386.

33. Schang, H.A. (1970) Acetylcysteine in the removal of bezoar. *Journal of the American Medical Association*, **214**, 1329.

34. Spira, I.A., Ghazi, A. and Wolff, W.I. (1977) Primary adenocarcinoma of the duodenum. *Cancer*, **39**, 1721–1726.

35. Van Thiel, D.H., DeBelle, R.C., Painter, T.D., McMillan, W.B. and Haradin, A.R. (1975) Phytobezoar occurring as a complication of gastric carcinoma. *Gastroenterology*, **68**, 1292–1296.

36. Warren, K.W., Choe, D.S., Plaza, J. and Betihan, M. (1977) Results of radical resection for periampullary carcinoma. *Annals of Surgery*, **181**, 534–539.

37. Williamson, R.C.N., Welch, C.E. and Malt, R.A. (1983) Adenocarcinoma and lymphoma of the small intestine. *Annals of Surgery*, **197**, 172–178.

CHAPTER 3

THE SMALL INTESTINE

ANATOMY AND CONGENITAL ABNORMALITIES

Caroline Doig

ANATOMY

The small intestine is a convoluted tube from the pylorus to the ileocaecal valve. Measured at autopsy it is about 6 m in length in adults, though maintained shorter in life by muscular tone. It consists of the duodenum lying retroperitoneally and a mesenteric-borne intraperitoneal portion, of which the proximal two-fifths are jejunum and the distal three-fifths are ileum. The duodenum is fixed in a curve around the pancreas and can be divided into four parts. The first passes backwards to the right of the spinal column, close to the gall-bladder. The common bile duct and the pancreatic duct join to the ampulla in the mid-second part. The third part passes across the mid-line over the inferior vena cava and the aorta and is crossed by the superior mesenteric vessels, and the root of the mesentery. The final part passes upwards to the left of the aorta towards the level of the lesser curvature of the stomach. The jejunum generally occupies the left upper quadrant of the abdomen and the ileum lies mainly over the right psoas towards the ileocaecal valve in the right iliac fossa. There is no definite point of transition between the jejunum and ileum but the jejunum is generally thicker and wider with more prominent transverse folds. The fan-shaped mesentery lies from the left upper quadrant to the right lower iliac area, being attached to the left of the L_2 vertebra, and caudally at the base of L_4/L_5, overlying the right sacroiliac joint. It contains fat, lymph nodes and lacteal and blood vessels. Proximally the blood vessels have a single arcade and distally there are 3–4 arcades.

The bowel in cross-section consists of serous peritoneal coat, two layers of muscle coats, longitudinal and circular, an areolar submucous layer and a mucous membrane consisting of circular folds and villi. Histological development starts with a single layer of cells changing at about 8–10 weeks of fetal life to a columnar pattern with villi. By 12 weeks the cells resemble mature enterocytes.[89]

The structure of the small intestine reflects its physiological role.[31] This is primarily its role in absorption but includes a major immunological role. For the latter, lymphoid aggregates are present throughout the small intestine but most prominently in the ileum as Peyer's patches.

To aid absorption, many anatomical features increase the surface area of the small intestine. The mucosa and submucosa are thrown into gross folds, the plicae semilunares, about 0.75 cm in height, more prominent proximally in duodenum and jejunum. The mucosa is then further amplified by being thrown into multiple microscopic projections, finger-like villi, 0.5–1.5 mm in length, which are covered with a single layer of absorptive enterocytes. The enterocytes themselves further amplify the absorptive area by a specialized microvillus zone on their luminal surface, each microvillus being about 1 μm long and 0.1 μm in diameter.

The villi have a central core containing vascular and lymphatic channels lying within the lamina propria. The main cellular elements of the villi surface are enterocytes, but this layer also contains some lymphocytes and some neuroendocrine cells, and lymphocytes and plasma cells feature in the lamina propria of the villus. Tight intercellular junctions bind the enterocytes together, although this layer is permeable to salt and water. The enterocytes themselves are tall columnar cells resting on a basal lamina and having a luminal glycocalix on the microvillus surface.

While the villi are, in a healthy Western population, typically finger-like in shape, there may be minor variations with leaf-shaped or ridge-shaped villi admixed. This aspect of small intestinal architecture is best defined by dissecting microscopic examination of biopsies, and the range of what is normal varies considerably geographically. In tropical or subtropical climates, flatter appearances with broader leaves, tongues and ridges are much more common. Convolutions, complex villous forms resembling the surface of the brain, may be accepted as normal in the tropical context, but more than a few are definitely abnormal in a Western environment. The shape of the villi normally tends to alter distally along the small intestine, with those of the ileum being stubbier and shorter than those more proximally.

The villous enterocytes are progressively replaced from the proliferative zone of the epithelium, the crypts of Lieberkühn, which form pits adjacent to the villi. Kinetic analysis has demonstrated a complex relationship between the rate of proliferation and the villous architecture, and paradoxically the 'flat' villous architecture of coeliac disease, for example, is associated with increased cell proliferation and crypt hyperplasia. Normally, it takes 48–72 hours for cells to migrate from crypts to the surface of the villus, and for extrusion from the end to occur. During this migration, cells mature, changing from shorter columnar cells with basal nuclei to taller cells with a central nucleus, gaining specific digestive enzymes, such as sucrase and lactase, and losing those relevant to cell proliferation, such as thymidine kinase. At the upper crypt level some cells begin to take on the appearance of goblet cells. The pathway of migration, from a crypt to the villous tip, is complex. A variety of morphometric methods have been described to provide a framework for analysis of crypt–villous architecture, and inflammatory cell infiltration in disease. They are complex but avoid the risks of simplistic interpretation of pathological change.

In addition to the enterocytes, other significant cell populations are the neuroendocrine cells scattered between normal enterocytes, and Paneth cells at the base of the crypts. The former have a role in paracrine control of absorption and secretion; the Paneth cells have a high lysozyme content and may have bactericidal functions but, in addition, may form a source of enzymes similar to those of the pancreas.[12]

CONGENITAL ABNORMALITIES

The complex embryological development of the intestine offers a background for a variety of congenital abnormalities. The central phenomenon is the process of rotation of the intestine. At about 6 weeks of embryonic life the midgut extends as a prolonged loop into the umbilical cord, whilst the superior mesenteric vessels form the axis of this loop. At approximately 3 months the loop of intestine begins to rotate around this arterial axis – counterclockwise as the abdomen of the fetus is viewed from the front. The lower limb thus passes upwards so that its future derivatives, the colon and ileum, come to lie above and in front of the upper limb, from which the duodenum and jejunum will derive. Subsequently, as the gut returns from the cord to within the abdomen, a further 90° rotation takes place, carrying the caecum to the right lower quadrant of the abdomen.

ROTATION

Incomplete rotation commonly leaves the caecum high on the right side of the abdomen beneath the liver; when more marked, the rotation of the jejunum *to* the left upper quadrant of the abdomen, or of the caecum and transverse colon *out of* the left side of the abdomen, may not have occurred. Whilst minor or even major degrees of incomplete rotation may be entirely asymptomatic, complications may occur either because the process is associated with persistence of developmental bands, which may initiate obstruction, because incomplete development of the mesentery predisposes to volvulus, or because internal hernias develop, usually paraduodenal or paracaecal. Precise classifications of rotatory anomalies encompass:

1. Non-rotation – with a right-sided small intestine and left-sided colon.
2. Reversed rotation – when a clockwise 90° rotation leaves the small bowel superficial to the transverse colon, which often passes through the small intestinal mesentery.
3. Malrotation – failure to complete the normal rotatory process.

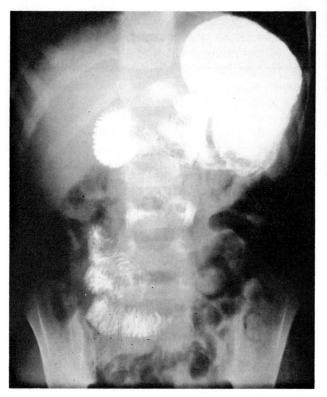

Figure 3.1 Barium study showing duodenal obstruction from Ladd's bands in malrotation.

Malrotation

Malrotation may have clinical consequences, usually as a result of either volvulus or band adhesions, or an associated abnormality such as a persistent omphalomesenteric duct or atresia.[26] Most anomalies present within the first few weeks of life, although older children[67,80] may have problems and, rarely, intermittent symptoms may present in adult life.[90,91] Malrotation is discussed more fully in chapter 2 (Stomach and Duodenum).

Although bile stained vomiting[85] or recurrent abdominal pain is a more usual presentation, the condition may be found unexpectedly during a barium series.[38]

When volvulus occurs, the small intestine and proximal colon volve around the superior mesenteric vessels, resulting in partial or total intestinal obstruction. The associated ischaemia may lead on to gastrointestinal bleeding; sepsis, perforation and peritonitis may all supervene.[41] Plain radiology shows the findings of proximal dilation. Definition of the presence of volvulus has been achieved *in utero* by ultrasound.[74] Malrotation and established volvulus requires surgical intervention, and in neonates the mortality of an episode of volvulus is of the order of 10–20% due to associated ischaemia.[7] In addition to correcting the volvulus and resection of ischaemic bowel, preventive measures such as fixing

the mesentery and division of associated bands must be performed.[9,82,94]

Duodenal obstruction may occur in malrotation from a combination of factors (*Figure 3.1*). Band adhesions (Ladd's bands) between the high-laced caecum and the posterior abdominal wall may compress the duodenum, or associated anomalies such as an annular pancreas, duodenal atresia and stenosis,[4] or paraduodenal herniation[19] may contribute. Plain radiography may show gastric and duodenal dilatation.

ATRESIAS

Atresias arise from incomplete canalization,[52] damage to the blood supply[47] during the bowel's return to the abdomen[53] or intussusception of bowel.[1] In familial cases,[69] other causes such as intrauterine inflammation[68] should be involved. Amniocentesis for intrauterine investigations has also been implicated.[84]

The atresia may be a complete or incomplete diaphragm within the lumen of the gut, a fibrous band in place of bowel, an area of gut missing or a gap in both the bowel and the mesentery.[56] All forms are caused by varying degrees of vascular damage from occlusion of a small end artery to infarction of the mesentery and associated bowel. These anomalies occur in 1/6000 live births. There is an equal distribution of atresias between the jejunum and the ileum.[33,86] Multiple atresias can be found in about 20%,[18,23,54] including colonic atresias.[45,92] Small bowel stenosis is found in only 5%.

At operation, the proximal bowel is grossly dilated while the distal remains small, especially if the damage occurs early. If damage happens later in development the distal bowel may contain meconium and be nearer normal size. The more distal of multiple atresias may be difficult to diagnose, especially if of the diaphragm type, as there will be no disparity in size.

If the blood supply to the small bowel is damaged at source the supply is taken over by distal vessels coming in a retrograde manner from the ileocolic artery. Such a blood supply is insufficient and the more proximal bowel becomes atretic and avascular – called 'apple peel',[21,97] because of how the bowel hangs on the distal blood supply, or 'Christmas tree,'[93] fir tree or barberpole.' The gut is frequently short in length and the proximal portion often has a very tenuous blood supply, making an anastomosis difficult.

Presentation and diagnosis

The mother may have had polyhydramnios. Small bowel atresias, especially of the apple peel or multiple type, can occur in families.[5,11,29,90] Antenatal diagnosis is possible (*Figure 3.2*). The newborn presents with bile-stained vomiting and failure to pass meconium, although the late type may pass some meconium from the distal gut. Distension depends on the site of obstruction.

Diagnosis is made by means of erect (or lateral decubitus) and supine abdominal radiographs showing a small bowel obstruction with fluid levels, the number indicating the level of the atresia (*Figure 3.3*) and no colonic gas. Care should be taken to differentiate this problem from that of meconium ileus, which also presents with a small bowel obstruction. The use of Gastrografin will not always help[22] and urgent laparotomy may be necessary to make the diagnosis.

Treatment

At operation the site of the first atresia is obvious (*Figure 3.4*). Resection of the proximal portion of the distal collapsed bowel allows for passage of a catheter and instillation of fluid to show any further atretic areas in the small and large bowel.

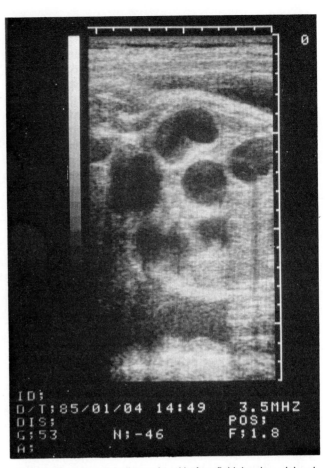

Figure 3.2 Antenatal diagnosis with few fluid levels – jejunal atresia. (By permission of Manchester University Department of Medical Illustration.)

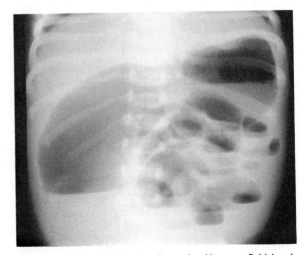

Figure 3.3 Plain abdominal radiograph with more fluid levels – ileal atresia.

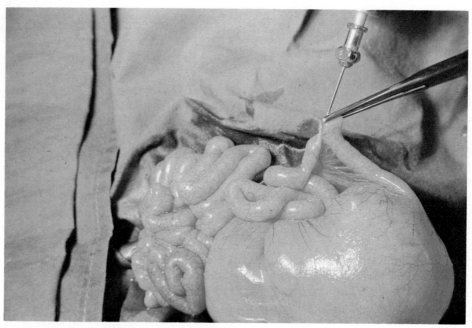

Figure 3.4 Findings at operation: grossly dilated proximal bowel and small collapsed bowel beyond diaphragm, and instillation of fluid distally to delineate further atresias.

In ileal atresias it is relatively easy to resect proximal dilated bowel until more normal peristaltic bowel is reached without compromising the length of bowel left. If the dilated portion is not removed it acts as a sump and causes an obstruction.[62,75] Fish-tailing of the distal bowel is usually necessary on the antimesenteric edge to allow for end-to-end anastomosis (*Figure 3.5*). End-to-side anastomosis should not be done as this leads later to enlargement of the end of the bowel and problems with bacterial overgrowth. With the more proximal atresias, such resection is more difficult, especially in high jejunal cases, as this would involve the duodenum. Since ischaemic damage is limited,[34] tailoring of the proximal bowel[39,87] may give a better anastomosis and is preferable to infolding (plication)[17] of the proximal bowel to equate the sizes of lumen. Such high atresias should not be treated with stomas as these would be of the high-output type. Lower down the bowel it may be better to form stomas side by side to allow the output from the proximal stoma to be instilled via a catheter into the distal stoma, to prevent fluid and electrolyte loss and promote an increase in the size of the narrow distal bowel.

In the ileal atresias, the results are excellent as the atresia usually occurred late and primary anastomosis is possible. Jejunal atresias occur in babies with low gestational age and birth weight, giving a higher mortality. Often the postoperative course is prolonged and complicated. In the high atresias or the apple peel type, the bowel is often already short, so that after surgery there may be insufficient length for normal development.

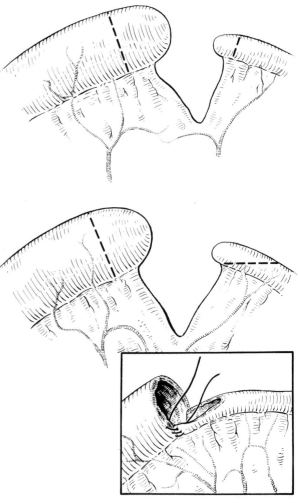

Figure 3.5 Fish-tailing to allow end-to-end anastomosis.

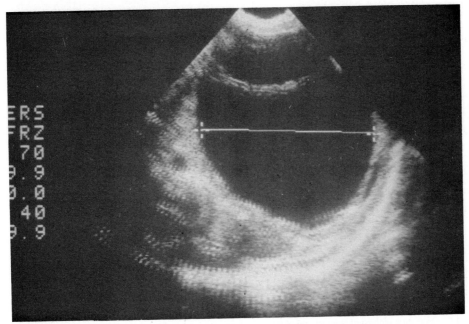

Figure 3.6 Antenatal ultrasound showing large mesenteric cyst.

In all cases, 85% survival can be expected. Surgery before perforation has occurred should ensure reasonable results,[3] even in the premature baby.

DUPLICATIONS

During development, any area of the bowel[40] from the oesophagus to the rectum can be duplicated by groups of cells separating off. One theory[24] suggests that adhesions between the notocord and the endoderm allows splitting off of some endoderm cells, leading to a duplication, and accounting for the associated vertebral anomalies. Such duplications have a complete muscular wall lying along the mesenteric border of the gut with the same blood supply as the adjacent bowel. It can be difficult to distinguish duplications of the gut from mesenteric cysts and they may coexist. In the foregut, above the diaphragm, the lining mucosa may be either respiratory or alimentary. If the lining of the cyst is that of the intestinal tract it is possible for this or ectopic gastric mucosa to ulcerate, leading to bleeding or perforation.[73]

Presentation is of a mass, antenatally found by ultrasound (*Figure 3.6*) or on palpation. The displacement of the bowel may be seen on a plain abdominal radiograph with flattening of the bowel (*Figure 3.7*), even obstructing the bowel. Small or large bowel barium enemas may also visualize this. If large, it may twist, leading to ischaemia of the intestine. Although usually presenting during childhood in the first year of life, problems may not arise

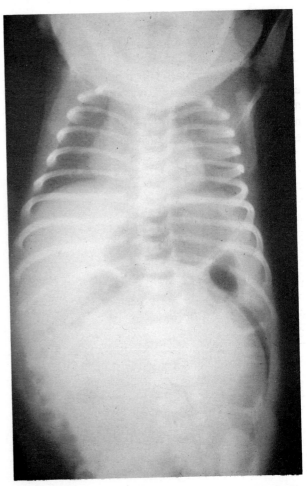

Figure 3.7 Plain radiograph showing flattening of loop of bowel by a duplication.

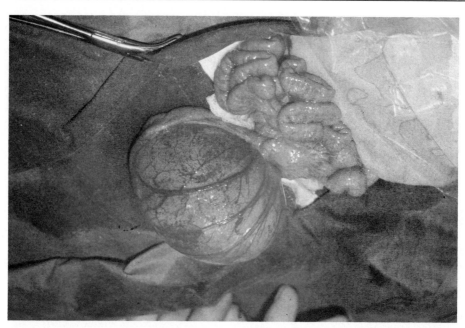

Figure 3.8 Operative picture of twisted bowel due to a mesenteric cyst. The flattening of the bowel is also seen.

until adult life.[95] The usual type is cystic, but tubular duplications[78] of the long areas of bowel can occur. Although the duodenum[70] can be involved, the small bowel is the most frequent site.[37] An association with vertebral anomalies may lead to the diagnosis.[24]

Treatment of small- or moderate-sized duplication is by resection and anastomosis. However, if a large or necessary part of bowel is involved this may not be possible. Mucosal stripping of the extra lumen to give a double-barrelled appearance[10] may

be the best that can be achieved but there is a risk of malignant change later.[64] Enucleation of the cyst[63] is rarely possible as the remaining bowel wall and blood supply are closely involved. Thoracic duplications,[81] either bronchogenic or enteric, are difficult to differentiate from hamartomatous malformations of the lung and may be associated with oesophageal atresia.[36] Other cysts, omental, mesenteric cysts or retroperitoneal[2] are not necessarily congenital but may be traumatic, neoplastic or infectious in origin.[88] Found anywhere along the bowel,

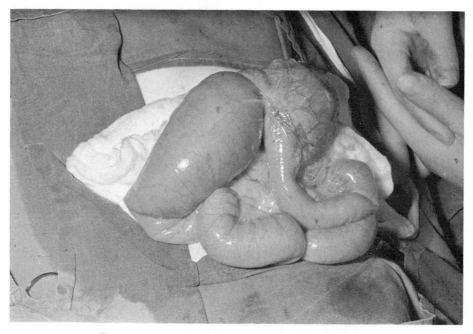

Figure 3.9 Loop of ileum involved in segmental dilatation.

they present as an acute abdomen in a child, sometimes undergoing volvulus (*Figure 3.8*).[59] An exact diagnosis preoperatively is unusual since there are no distinctive features, but ultrasound[28] can help improve preoperative diagnosis. Treatment is by resection and anastomosis. Aspiration or marsupialization is contraindicated.

A less severe maldevelopment gives a segmental dilatation of the intestine which, although uncommon, can occur throughout the gut, in the colon,[13] duodenum,[72] jejunum[71] and, more frequently, the ileum.[8,44] The cause of this obstruction is unknown but it is possible that it is a form of atresia; local deficiency of circular muscle with associated proximal dilatation has been described.[42] In the ileum the dysgenesis appears to be an intrinsic abnormality associated with the junction with the yolk sac. Although the bowel is patent, the infant presents with obstruction and on radiography has a dilated terminal ileum. Resection of the dilated portion (*Figure 3.9*) with anastomosis gives excellent results. However, long-term evaluation of vitamin B_{12} and folic acid absorption will be necessary.

VITELLOINTESTINAL ABNORMALITIES

When the embryonic mid-gut extends into the umbilical cord the apex of the loop is the vitellointestinal or omphalomesenteric duct communicating with the yolk sac. Persistence of this duct as a diverticulum gives rise to Meckel's diverticulum; this may on occasions be connected with the umbilicus by a fibrous cord, or else isolated cysts may lie along this pathway.

The actual duct can remain intact so that an opening at the umbilicus discharges gas and/or faeces.[77] Looking like an actual stoma, it more commonly presents as a discharging, slow to heal umbilical stump or polyp.[49] Although this is a rare anomaly (1 in 15 000 births),[46] an unusual appearance of the umbilicus should suggest this diagnosis. There is a danger of intussusception of bowel through the vitillene-intestinal duct at the umbilicus.[61,66]

Other problems arise if the duct only partially disappears, leaving a band (*Figure 3.10*) to cause an internal hernia. Such bands may also be found in association with Meckel's diverticulum. An enclosed cyst either at the umbilicus or along the connecting band may become infected, giving rise to an abscess.[32]

The commonest abnormality of the duct is partial absorption, leaving a Meckel's diverticulum which is usually situated 0.5 m from the ileocaecal valve. It can be of varying length and may be wide necked and may be found in association with other congenital abnormalities.[79] Commonly in adults the diverticulum becomes infected and mimics acute appendicitis. If associated with a band, internal herniation and obstruction may result.[20] Major gastrointestinal bleeding is the more usual presentation in infants. The bleeding is characteristically bright red or maroon coloured rather than melaena but bleeding may be occult[25] as a result of the acid produced in the ectopic gastric mucosa ulcerating the adjacent small bowel, which is unprotected by mucus. Pain is not necessarily a feature. Perforation, occurring in 15% is extremely dangerous

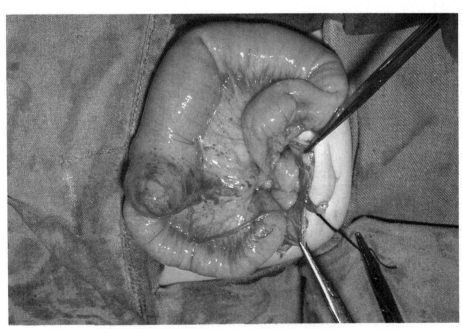

Figure 3.10 Internal band from intestine to umbilicus.

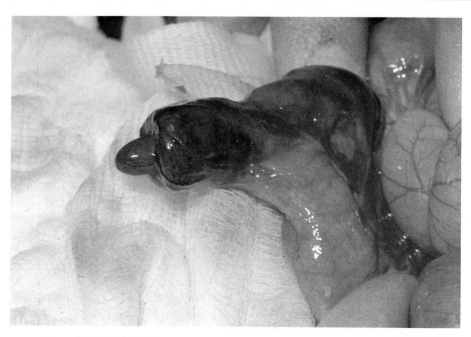

Figure 3.11   Meckel's diverticulum which has been involved in an intussusception.

and associated with foreign bodies impacted in the diverticulum. Infection with *Helicobacter pylori* may be present if gastric mucosa is found.[60] Fifty per cent of these complications occur in infants under 1 year of age.[57] Rarely, the diverticulum may be involved in a groin hernia – Littre's hernia.[65] If the actual diverticulum invaginates, bleeding may be the result of an intussusception (*Figure 3.11*).

The diagnosis may be difficult and only finally resolved at laparotomy as barium studies tend to be unhelpful. The neck requires to be wide and the diverticulum empty for it to fill with barium. Lateral views may show tethering and, despite the poor demonstration, should be part of the investigations.[15] The ectopic gastric mucosa filling the lumen may be visualized by means of a technetium scan using technetium-99m pertechnetate[14] if bleeding persists or ulceration has occurred.[16] The addition of pentagastrin and glucagon may enhance the uptake, giving increased sensitivity,[6] but often the results of this test are disproved. If the Meckel's diverticulum is complicated by bleeding or acute inflammation, resection is necessary. This should be done by means of a V-shaped incision to resect not only the diverticulum but also the area of small bowel adjacent,[96] since this is the site of ulceration. The more difficult decision is to know whether to resect a Meckel's diverticulum found by chance at surgery. The risk of complications in such diverticula is more than 25%.[43] If the diverticulum looks unlikely to give problems, i.e. wide necked, and the laparotomy is being performed in the presence of

infection, the diverticulum should be left *in situ*.[51] However, even in the presence of pus, if the diverticulum is deemed likely to give trouble in the future, it should be removed.[50] The outcome is excellent.[55]

REFERENCES

1. Adejuyigbe, O. and Odesanmi, W.O. (1990) Intrauterine intussusception causing intestinal atresia. *Journal of Pediatric Surgery*, **25**, 562.
2. Adejuyigbe, O., Lawal, O.O., Akinola, D.O. and Nwosu, S.O. (1990) Omental and mesenteric cysts in Nigerian children. *Journal of the Royal College of Surgeons, Edinburgh*, **35**, 181.
3. Adeyemi, S.D. (1988) Prognostic factors in neonatal intestinal obstruction: a prospective study of Nigerian newborns with bowel obstruction. *Journal of Pediatric Surgery*, **23**, 135.
4. Adeyemi, S.D. (1988) Combination of annular pancreas and partial situs inversus: a multiple organ malrotation syndrome associated with duodenal obstruction. *Journal of Pediatric Surgery*, **23**, 188.
5. Al-Awadi, S.A., Farag, T.I., Naguib, K., Cuschieri, A. and Issa, M. (1981) Familial jejunal atresia with 'apple-peel'. *Journal of the Royal Society of Medicine*, **74**, 499.
6. Anderson, G.F., Stakianakis, G., King D.R. and Boles, E.T. (1980) Hormonal enhancement of technetium-99m pertechnetate uptake in experimental Meckel's diverticulum. *Journal of Pediatric Surgery*, **15**, 900.
7. Andrassy, R.J. and Mahour, G.H. (1981)

Malrotation of the midgut in infants and children: a 25 year review. *Archives of Surgery*, **116**, 158.

8. Bell, M.J., Ternberg J.L. and Bower, R.J. (1982) Ileal dysgenesis in infants and children. *Journal of Pediatric Surgery*, **17**, 395.

9. Bill, A.H. and Graumam, D. (1966) Rational and technique for stabilization of the mesentery in cases of non-rotation of the mid-gut. *Journal of Pediatric Surgery*, **1**, 27.

10. Bishop, H.C. and Koop, C.E. (1964) Surgical management of duplications of the alimentary tract. *American Journal of Surgery*, **107**, 434.

11. Blyth, H.H. and Dickson, J.A.S. (1969) Apple peel syndrome (congenital intestinal atresia): a family study of seven index cases. *Journal of Medical Genetics*, **6**, 275.

12. Bohe, M., Lindström, C.G. and Ohlsson, K. (1987) Vamping occurrence of gastroduodenal immunoreactive pancreatic secretory trypsin inhibitor. *Journal of Clinical Pathology*, **40**, 1345–1348.

13. Brawner, J. and Shafer, A.D. (1973) Segmental dilatation of the colon. *Journal of Pediatric Surgery*, **8**, 957.

14. Cooney, D.R., Duszynski, D.O., Camboa, E., Karp, M.P. and Jewett, T.C. (1982) The abdominal technetium scan (a decade of experience). *Journal of Pediatric Surgery*, **17**, 611.

15. Craig, O. and Murfitt, J. (1980) Radiological demonstration of Meckel's diverticulum. *British Journal of Surgery*, **67**, 881.

16. Dawson, D.J., Khan, A.N., Nutall, P. and Shreeve, D.R. (1985) Technetium 99m-labelled-sucralfate isotope scanning in the detection of peptic ulceration. *Nuclear Medicine Communications*, **6**, 319.

17. de Lorimier, A.A. and Harrison, M.R. (1983) Intestinal plication in the treatment of atresia. *Journal of Pediatric Surgery*, **18**, 734.

18. de Lorimier, A.A., Fonkalsrud, E.W. and Hays, D.M. (1969) Congenital atresia and stenosis of the jejunum and ileum. *Surgery*, **65**, 819.

19. Dengler, W.C. and Reddy, P.P. (1989) Right paraduodenal hernia in childhood: a case report. *Journal of Pediatric Surgery*, **24**, 1153.

20. Diamond, T. and Russell, C.F.J. (1985) Meckel's diverticulum in the adult. *British Journal of Surgery*, **72**, 480.

21. Dickson, J.A.S. (1970) Apple peel small bowel: an uncommon variant of duodenal and jejunal atresia. *Journal of Pediatric Surgery*, **5**, 595.

22. Ein, S.H., Venugopal, S. and Mancer, K. (1985) Ileocaecal atresia. *Journal of Pediatric Surgery*, **20**, 525.

23. El Shafie, M. and Rickham, P.P. (1970) Multiple intestinal atresia. *Journal of Pediatric Surgery*, **5**, 655.

24. Fallon, M., Gordon, A.R.G. and Lendrum, A.C. (1954) Mediastinal cysts of the foregut origin associated with vertebral anomalies. *British Journal of Surgery*, **41**, 520.

25. Farthing, M.G., Griffiths, N.J., Thomas J.M. and Todd, I.P. (1981) Occult bleeding from Meckel's diverticulum. *British Journal of Surgery*, **68**, 176.

26. Filstron, H.C. and Kirks, D.R. (1981) Malrotation – the ubiquitous anomaly. *Journal of Pediatric Surgery*, **16**, 614.

27. Firor, H.V. and Harris, V.J. (1974) Rotational anomalies of the gut: recognition of a neglected facet – isolated incomplete rotation of the duodenum. *American Journal of Radiology*, **120**, 315.

28. Geer, L.L., Mittelstaedt, C.A., Staab, E.V. and Gaisie, G. (1984) Mesenteric cyst: sonographic appearance with CT correlation. *Pediatric Radiology*, **14**, 102.

29. Gibson, M.F. (1987) Familial multiple jejunal atresia with malrotation. *Journal of Pediatric Surgery*, **22**, 1013.

30. Gohl, M.L. and DeMeester, W.R. (1975) Midgut nonrotation in adults: an aggressive approach. *American Journal of Surgery*, **129**, 319.

31. Grand, R.J., Watkins, J.B. and Torti, F.M. (1976) Development of the human gastrointestinal tract: a review. *Gastroenterology*, **70**, 790.

32. Grosfeld, J.L. and Franken, E.A. (1974) Intestinal obstruction in the neonate due to vitelline duct cysts. *Surgery, Gynecology and Obstetrics*, **138**, 527.

33. Grosfeld, J.L., Ballantine, T.V.N. and Shoemaker, R. (1979) Operative management of intestinal atresia and stenosis based on pathologic findings. *Journal of Pediatric Surgery*, **14**, 368.

34. Hamdy, M.H., Man, D.W.K., Bain, D. and Kirkland, I.S. (1986) Histochemical changes in intestinal atresia and its implications on surgical management: a preliminary report. *Journal of Pediatric Surgery*, **21**, 17.

35. Heij, H.A., Moorman-Voestermans, C.G.M. and Vos, A. (1990) Atresia of jejunum and ileum: is it the same disease? *Journal of Pediatric Surgery*, **25**, 635.

36. Hemalatha, V., Batcup, G., Brereton, R.J. and Spitz, L. (1980) Intrathoracic foregut cyst (foregut duplication) associated with esophageal atresia. *Journal of Pediatric Surgery*, **15**, 178.

37. Hocking, M. and Young, D.G. (1981) Duplications of the alimentary tract. *British Journal of Surgery*, **68**, 92.

38. Houston, C.S. and Wittenborg, M.H. (1965) Roentgen evaluation of anomalies of rotation and fixation of the bowel in children. *Radiology*, **84**, 1.

39. Howard, E.R. and Othersen, H.B. (1973) Proximal jejunoplasty in the treatment of jejunal atresia. *Journal of Pediatric Surgery*, **8**, 685.

40. Howat, J.M. and Grant, J.C. (1970) Non-vitelline accessory enteric formations. *British Journal of Surgery*, **57**, 205.

41. Howell, C.G., Vozza, F., Shaw, S. *et al.* (1982) Malrotation, malnutrition and ischemic bowel disease. *Journal of Pediatric Surgery*, **17**, 469.

42. Humphrey, A., Mancer, K. and Stephens, C.A.

(1980) Obstructive circular-muscle defect in the small bowel in a one-year-old child. *Journal of Pediatric Surgery*, **15**, 197.

43. Hutchison, G.H. and Randall, P.E. (1981) Meckel's diverticulum: a study in the north Manchester area. *Journal of the Royal College of Surgeons, Edinburgh*, **26**, 86.

44. Irving, I.M. and Lister, J. (1977) Segmental dilatation of the ileum. *Journal of Pediatric Surgery*, **12**, 103.

45. Jackman, S. and Brereton, R.J. (1988) A lesson in intestinal atresias. *Journal of Pediatric Surgery*, **23**, 852.

46. Kadzombe, E. and Currie, A.B.M. (1988) Neonatal fistula from the appendix to the umbilicus. *Journal of Pediatric Surgery*, **23**, 1059.

47. Kaga, Y., Hayashida, Y., Ikeda, K., Inokuthi, K. and Hashimoto, N. (1975) Intestinal atresia in fetal dogs produced by localized ligation of mesenteric vessels. *Journal of Pediatric Surgery*, **10**, 949.

48. Kullendorf, C.M., Mikaelsson, C. and Ivancev, K. (1985) Malrotation in children with symptoms of gastrointestinal allergy and psychosomatic abdominal pain. *Acta Paediatrica Scandinavica*, **74**, 296.

49. Kutin, N.D., Allen, J.E. and Jewett, T.C. The umbilical polyp. *Journal of Pediatric Surgery*, **14**, 741.

50. Lang-Stevenson, A. (1983) Meckel's diverticulum: to look or not to look: to resect or not to resect. *Annals of the Royal College of Surgeons of England*, **65**, 218.

51. Leijonmarck, C.-E., Bonman-Sandelin, K., Frisell, J. and Raf, L. (1986) Meckel's diverticulum in the adult. *British Journal of Surgery*, **73**, 146.

52. Louw, J.H. (1952) Congenital intestinal atresia and stenosis in the newborn. *South African Journal of Clinical Science*, **3**, 109.

53. Louw, J.H. (1959) Congenital intestinal atresia and stenosis in the newborn: observations on its pathogenesis and treatment. *Annals of the Royal College of Surgeons of England*, **25**, 209.

54. Louw, J.H. (1966) Jejunoileal atresia and stenosis. *Journal of Pediatric Surgery*, **1**, 8.

55. Mackey, W.C. and Dineen, P. (1983) A fifty year experience with Meckel's diverticulum. *Surgery, Gynecology and Obstetrics*, **156**, 56.

56. Martin, L.W. and Zerella, J.T. (1976) Jejunoileal atresia: a proposed classification. *Journal of Pediatric Surgery*, **11**, 399.

57. Meguid, M., Canty, T. and Eraklis, A.J. (1974) Complications of Meckel's diverticulum. *Surgery, Gynecology and Obstetrics*, **139**, 541.

58. Milla, P.J. (1988) Gastrointestinal motility disorders in children. *Pediatric Clinics of North America*, **35**, 311.

59. Mollitt, D.L., Ballantine, T.V.N. and Grosfeld, J.L. (1978) Mesenteric cysts in infancy and childhood. *Surgery, Gynecology and Obstetrics*, **147**, 182.

60. Morris, A., Nicholson, G., Zwi, J. and Vanderwee, M. (1989) *Campylobacter pylori* infection in Meckel's diverticula containing gastric mucosa. *Gut*, **30**, 1233.

61. Mustafa, R. (1976) Double intussusception of the small bowel through a patent vitello-intestinal duct. *British Journal of Surgery*, **63**, 452.

62. Nixon, H.H. and Tawes, R. (1971) Etiology and treatment of small intestinal atresia: analysis of a series of 127 jejunoileal atresias and comparison with 62 duodenal atresias. *Surgery*, **69**, 41.

63. Norris, R.W., Brereton, R.J., Wright, V.M. and Cudmore, R.E. (1986) A new approach to duplications of the intestine. *Journal of Pediatric Surgery*, **21**, 167.

64. Orr, M.M. and Edwards, A.J. (1975) Neoplastic change in duplications of the alimentary tract. *British Journal of Surgery*, **62**, 269.

65. Perlman, J.A., Hoover, H.C. and Safer, P.K. (1980) Femoral hernia with strangulated Meckel's diverticulum (Littre's hernia): case report and review of the literature. *American Journal of Surgery*, **139**, 286.

66. Pinter, A., Schubert, W., Pilaszanovich, I. and Szemledy, F. (1978) Patent vitelline duct: a survey of 38 patients. *Zeitschrift für Kinderchirurgie*, **23**, 386.

67. Powell, D.M., Biemann, H.O. and Smith, C.D. (1989) Malrotation of the intestine in children: the effect of age on presentation and therapy. *Journal of Pediatric Surgery*, **24**, 777.

68. Puri, P. and Fujimoto, T. (1988) New observations on the pathogenesis of multiple atresias. *Journal of Pediatric Surgery*, **23**, 221.

69. Rickham, P.P. and Karplus, M. (1971) Familial and hereditary intestinal atresia. *Helvetica Paediatrica Acta*, **26**, 561.

70. Ross, E.R.S., Larkworthy, W. and Hutter, F.H.D. (1987) A cyst of the second part of the duodenum. *Journal of the Royal College of Surgeons, Edinburgh*, **32**, 170.

71. Rossi, R. and Giocomino, M.A. (1973) Segmental dilatation of the jejunum. *Journal of Pediatric Surgery*, **8**, 335.

72. Rovira, J., Morales, L., Parri, F.J., Julia, V. and Claret, I. (1989) Segmental dilatation of the duodenum. *Journal of Pediatric Surgery*, **24**, 1155.

73. Royle, S.G. and Doig, C.M. (1988) Perforation of the jejunum secondary to a duplication cyst lined with ectopic gastric mucosa. *Journal of Pediatric Surgery*, **23**, 1025.

74. Samuel, N., Dicker, D., Feldberg, D. and Goldman, J.A. (1984) Ultrasound diagnosis and management of fetal intestinal obstruction and volvulus *in utero*. *Journal of Perinatal Medicine*, **12**, 333.

75. Santulli, T.V., Chen, C. and Schullinger, J.N. (1970) Management of congenital atresia of the intestine. *American Journal of Surgery*, **119**, 542.

76. Sarre, R.G., Frost, A.G., Jagelman, D.G., Petras, R.E., Sivak, M.V. and McGannon, E. (1987)

Gastric and duodenal polyps in familial adenomatous polyposis: a prospective study of the nature and prevalence of upper gastrointestinal polyps. *Gut*, **28**, 314.

77. Scalettar, H.E., Mazarsky, M.M. and Rascoff, H. (1952) Congenital entero-umbilical fistula due to patent vitelline duct. *Journal of Pediatrics*, **40**, 310.

78. Schwartz, D.L., Becker, J.M., Schneider, K.M. and So, H.B. (1980) Tubular duplication with autonomous blood supply: resection with preservation of adjacent bowel. *Journal of Pediatric Surgery*, **15**, 341.

79. Simms, M.H. and Corkery, J.J. (1980) Meckel's diverticulum: its association with congenital malformation and the significance of atypical morphology. *British Journal of Surgery*, **67**, 216.

80. Spigland, N., Brandt, M.L. and Yazbeck, S. (1990) Malrotation presenting beyond the neonatal period. *Journal of Pediatric Surgery*, **25**, 1139.

81. Superina, R.A., Ein, S.H. and Humphreys, R.P. (1984) Cystic duplications of the esophagus and neurenteric cysts. *Journal of Pediatric Surgery*, **19**, 527.

82. Stauffer, U.G. and Herrmann, P. (1980) Comparison of late results in patients with corrected intestinal malrotation with and without fixation of the mesentery. *Journal of Pediatric Surgery*, **15**, 9.

83. Stewart, D.R., Colodny, A.L. and Daggett, W.C. (1976) Malrotation of the bowel in infants and children: a 15 year old review. *Surgery*, **79**, 716.

84. Swift, P.G.F., Driscoll, I.B. and Vowles, K.D.J. (1979) Neonatal small-bowel obstruction associated with amniocentesis. *British Medical Journal*, **i**, 720.

85. Synder, W.H. and Chaffin, L. (1954) Embryology and pathology of the intestinal tract: presentation of 40 cases of malrotation. *Annals of Surgery*, **140**, 368.

86. Tega, K., Schnatterly, P. and Shaw, A. (1981) Multiple intestinal atresias: pathology and pathogenesis. *Journal of Pediatric Surgery*, **16**, 194.

87. Thomas, C.G. (1969) Jejunoplasty in the correction of jejunal atresia. *Surgery, Gynecology and Obstetrics*, **129**, 545.

88. Vanek, V.W. and Phillips, A.K. (1984) Retroperitoneal, mesenteric and omental cysts. *Archives of Surgery*, **119**, 838.

89. Varkonyi, T., Gergely, G. and Varro, V. (1974) The ultrastructure of the small intestal mucosa in the developing human fetus. *Scandinavian Journal of Gastroenterology*, **9**, 495.

90. Young, I.D., Kennedy, R. and Ein, S.H. (1986) Familial small bowel atresia and stenosis. *Journal of Pediatric Surgery*, **21**, 792.

91. Wang, C.A. and Welch, C.E. (1963) Anomalies of intestinal rotation in adolescents and adults. *Surgery*, **54**, 839.

92. Weiss, R.R.G., Ryan, D.P., Ilstad, S.T., Noseworthy, J. and Martin, L.W. (1990) A complex case of jejunoileocolic atresias. *Journal of Pediatric Surgery*, **25**, 560.

93. Weitzman, J.J. and Vanderhoof, R.S. (1966) Jejunal atresia with agenesis of the dorsal mesentery with 'Christmas tree' deformity of the small intestine. *American Journal of Surgery*, **111**, 443.

94. Welch, G.H., Azmy, A.F. and Ziervogel, M.A. (1983) The surgery of malrotation and midgut volvulus: a nine year experience in neonates. *Annals of the Royal College of Surgeons of England*, **65**, 244.

95. Wig, J.D., Chowdhary, A., Suri, S. and Joshi, K. (1984) Left duplication in an adult. *British Journal of Surgery*, **71**, 20.

96. Williams, R.S. (1981) Management of Meckel's diverticulum. *British Journal of Surgery*, **68**, 477.

97. Zivkoric, S.M. and Milonsevic, V.R. (1979) Duodenal and jejunal atresia with agenesis of the dorsal mesentery: "apple-peel" small bowel. *American Journal of Surgery*, **137**, 767.

THE GUT RESPONSE TO A MEAL AND ITS HORMONAL CONTROL

J.R. Malagelada

THE NORMAL HUMAN DIET

The human diet is extraordinarily varied. Even if one only considers the dietary habits prevalent in the Western world, where some common standards are identifiable, the range of foods and beverages consumed by adults is very wide. Therefore, it is difficult to define a physiological meal or even establish its limits. Nevertheless, it is important to recognize that the human gastrointestinal tract handles ingested elements in different ways, adapting its response to the different characteristics of the foods consumed. Ordinary meals are physically and chemically heterogeneous; they are composed of both solid and liquid substances and contain more than one essential nutrient such as protein, fat or carbohydrate.[69,76]

Physiological meals usually contain, or decompose intragastrically into, different physical phases: aqueous, solid and oil (fats that are liquid at body temperature). Water constitutes the largest mass in the typical meal. It may be taken as plain water or in other liquid beverages. Water may also be released intragastrically from certain foods and, conversely, may be adsorbed by some elements of the meal, such as pectins and other fibre components.

Two classes of solid foods can be recognized – digestible and non-digestible solids. Digestible solids (e.g. cooked meat, liver, egg, starch-based tubers) tend to be broken down into fine particulate matter by gastric grinding contractions and largely hydrolysed by luminal gut enzymes as a prelude to their absorption. In contrast, non-digestible solids (typically dietary fibre derived from the cell wall of plants) are impervious to both the mechanical forces and enzymic action, and thus tend to progress along the upper gastrointestinal tract as solid particles; this progression is dependent on particular types of physiological motor activity.

Fat exists in different physicochemical forms. Ninety per cent of the fat in the American diet is composed of triglycerides containing fatty acids with 16–18 carbon molecules. Shorter-chain fatty acids are found in milk and vegetable oils. Some fats (e.g. butter) are liquefied at body temperature; others (e.g. olive oil) are ingested in liquid form. Animal fat that remains solid at body temperature is probably handled by the stomach in the same way as the meat which is usually intimately associated with it.

Carbohydrate can also be ingested in different physical forms; this may greatly influence its effect on gastric emptying and its absorption. Sucrose, which constitutes about a quarter of the total carbohydrate intake, and other soluble carbohydrates are partly dissolved in the intragastric aqueous phase, if they are not already ingested in solution. Starch, which constitutes about 50% of dietary carbohydrate, is largely found in grains and vegetables (particularly tubers and legumes), in association with pectins and other structural fibre. The extent to which such foods are susceptible to trituration and mixing varies a great deal. Some are soft, easily digestible solids, whereas others are so protected by structural fibre as to be virtually unavailable for hydrolysis.

Most dietary protein is animal protein that is ingested in solid form such as meat, fish and cooked egg. About one-third of dietary protein may be provided by vegetable protein in foods such as cereal grains, nuts and peanuts. Unlike fats and the majority of carbohydrates, protein is subjected not only to mechanical trituration in the stomach but also to chemical hydrolysis by pepsin. (Some hydrolysis of carbohydrate also occurs before the duodenum due to the action of salivary amylase.)

HORMONAL CONTROL OF GUT RESPONSES TO A MEAL: GENERAL CONCEPTS

The gastric, pancreatic, biliary and intestinal responses to a meal are carefully regulated by hormonal and neural mechanisms (*Figure 3.12*). The way in which these mechanisms regulate and integrate digestive functions to permit 'normal' handling of the meal is complex. It is important to recognize that every function of every digestive organ is affected, both positively and negatively, by neural input and by hormones. The net response of an organ at any point in time in the postprandial period is a summation of the many agonistic, antagonistic and potentiating effects of all the regulatory substances which affect it.

To gain insight into the role of hormones in this process, we must understand the location of the gastrointestinal endocrine cells and their stimuli for secretion. Each peptide is synthesized and secreted by a distinct cell type which is found in a characteristic area of gut. These have been very successfully mapped morphologically using immunocytochemistry, but our understanding of the physiology of these cells is more indirect because, as the endocrine cells are scattered amongst enterocytes which are of similar size and density, it is difficult to isolate them for *in vitro* study. Much of our understanding of these functions is, therefore, derived from 'black box'-type experiments, in which a particular luminal stimulus is given and peripheral blood levels of hormones are measured. The local events in the mucosa, with paracrine modulation of enterocytes by adjacent endocrine cells, are only now emerging in their complexity.

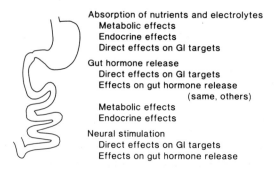

Figure 3.12   Regulation of digestive function. Major aspects of neurohormonal regulation and postabsorptive effects are listed.

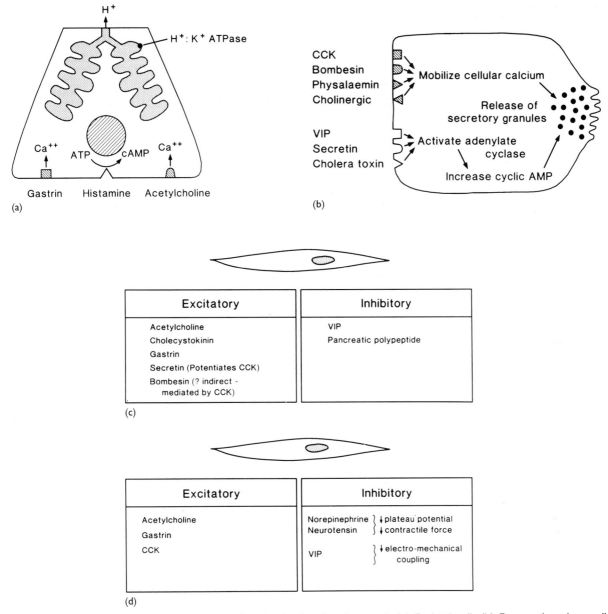

Figure 3.13 Prototypes of regulation of cellular function in the digestive tract. (a) Parietal cell. (b) Pancreatic acinar cell. (c) Gallbladder smooth muscle cell. (d) Antral smooth muscle cell.

The major regulator of secretion of most gastrointestinal hormones is the composition of the intestinal chyme at that level of the bowel associated with each particular endocrine cell type. This is complicated by a differential gastric emptying of liquids and solids and of different nutrients, non-uniformity of bowel transit, and differential nutrient absorption rates. All of this results in a constantly changing milieu in the bowel, with the composition of the chyme at any given level of the bowel constantly changing in the postprandial period. Combining an understanding of luminal events with an understanding of gastrointestinal endocrine cell location and function permits correlation of various events.

There are many gastrointestinal hormones, each of which affects multiple gastrointestinal target cells (*Figure 3.13*). They also directly or indirectly affect classical endocrine and metabolic functions. These effects may be mediated by the absorption of nutrients or fluid and electrolytes, as well as by direct interaction between gastrointestinal hormones and endocrine organs. Thus, there are many interactions going on at any point in time in the postprandial period. *Table 3.1* identifies the major hormones, their sites and major physiological roles; however, this is by no means an exhaustive list of potential relevant agents. To varying degrees these substances may act as classic endocrine agents, via the

Table 3.1 The major gastrointestinal hormones

Hormone	Main site of distribution	Major physiological roles
Gastrin	Gastric antrum – G cells	Stimulates gastric acid secretion ? Trophic to gastric mucosa
Motilin	Duodenal mucosa and more distally – M cells	Regulates interdigestive complex of intestinal motility
Cholecystokinin	Upper small intestinal mucosa – I cells	Stimulates pancreatic secretion Stimulates gall bladder contraction
Secretin	Upper small intestinal mucosa – S cells	Stimulates pancreatic secretion
GIP (gastric inhibitory polypeptide or glucose-dependent insulinotropic peptide)	Upper small intestinal mucosa – K cells	Stimulates insulin secretion Inhibits acid secretion
Vasoactive intestinal peptide (co-localizes with peptide–histidine–methionine in humans)	Nerve fibres of gastrointestinal tract	Regulator of blood flow and secretion
Enteroglucagon	Distal small intestinal colonic mucosa – L cells	? Trophic to intestine
Pancreatic polypeptide	Pancreas	? Feedback inhibition of pancreatic and biliary secretion
Peptide YY	Distal small intestinal and colonic mucosa – L cells	'Ileal brake'. Inhibition of gastric emptying, pancreatic secretion and intestinal transit
Neurotensin	Distal small intestinal and colonic mucosa – N cells	? 'Ileal brake'
Somatostatin	Mucosal D cells and nerves throughout gastrointestinal tract	Inhibits secretion and motility widely in gastrointestinal tract

bloodstream, as paracrine regulators of adjacent cells by diffusion, as autocrine stimulators of their cells of origin, or as neurotransmitters in peptodergic nerve fibres. A full discussion of this field lies outside the scope of this chapter.[83] For clarity, in this section, and *Table 3.1*, those areas where function has been clearly established are concentrated on.

GASTRIC SECRETION AFTER A MEAL

The gastric secretory response to a meal is characterized by a rapid increase in secretory rate which begins when a person starts eating (or even earlier if he or she psychically anticipates appetizing food). Peak rates are reached between 30 and 60 minutes after ingestion of the meal. Thereafter, gastric secretion rapidly decreases towards basal rates; a low plateau is frequently observed during the third to fifth hour after meals, with some food still remaining in the stomach (*Figure 3.14*).

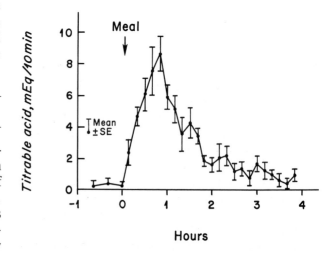

Figure 3.14 Postprandial gastric acid output in man. The biphasic profile of the normal secretory response to a meal is shown. (Reproduced, with permission, from Malagelada *et al.*[53])

The initial accelerating phase corresponds to a predominance of stimulatory forces over inhibitory forces; the converse is true for the decelerating phase. Peak acid output occurs at the transition point between these two phases. When many individuals with a wide range of secretory capacities are studied, a statistically significant correlation is observed between responses to exogenous secretagogues and luminal stimuli.[25,56] However, even during the period of peak secretion, a balance between stimulatory and inhibitory mechanisms is also likely to be occurring; therefore, the latter should not be assumed to be identical to 'maximal acid output' as measured after administration of high doses of exogenous secretagogues. In addition, gastric secretory capacity varies enormously, even among apparently healthy individuals. Extensive studies of gastric acid secretion during basal conditions and in response to secretagogues[3] show that 'maximal' acid secretion rates ranging from less than 5 to over 60 mEq/h are found in unselected populations. Although fewer individuals have been studied in response to meals, there is similar variation.

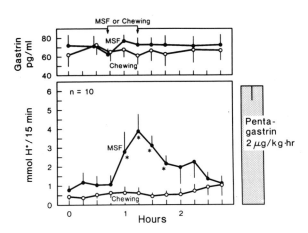

Figure 3.15 Gastrin and gastric acid responses to modified sham feeding in health. Modified sham feeding (MSF) provides a standardized measurement of cephalic stimulation of gastric acid secretion in man. Note the absence of a rise in serum gastrin. (Modified from Konturek, S.J. (1981). In: *Gastric Secretion, Basic and Clinical Aspects*, pp. 62–79 (Eds) Konturek, S.J. and Domschke, W. New York: Thieme Stratton.)

THE STIMULATORY PHASE OF POSTPRANDIAL GASTRIC SECRETION

There is little doubt about the importance of cephalic stimulation during the early period of postprandial gastric secretion. However, unlike in the dog, in which sham feeding stimulates gastric secretion to the same level achieved by injection of maxillary stimulating doses of exogenous histamine or gastrin,[71] sham feeding achieves only partial stimulation in humans (*Figure 3.15*) – experimentally, with modified sham feeding, about one-third of the maximal secretory capacity.[75,57] In patients with duodenal ulcer in whom a true sham-feeding technique was employed (that is, including actual swallowing of an appetizing meal), Knutson and Olbe[39] obtained about one-half the maximal acid response to pentagastrin. Cephalic stimulation of gastric acid secretion in humans is probably mediated by direct vagal stimulation of the parietal area and through vagal stimulation of gastrin release from the antrum,[87] but the contribution of other less classic neurotransmitters, such as peptidergic nerves, remains to be elucidated.[90] The relative contribution of thought, sight, taste etc. have been analysed.[23]

Another important part of the stimulus provided by a meal probably comes from gastric distension. The response to fundal or body distension is mediated by vagovagal and intramural cholinergic reflexes.[31] The human gastric response to distension

with inert aqueous solutions experimentally amounts to one-third of the maximal response, and it is probably responsible for about one-third of the response to a meal as well.[10,35,81] Gastric distension acts not only via vagal influences, but also in the antrum by reducing gastrin release.

The third component of the gastric sensory response is independent of distension and is largely attributed to gastrin release, although there may be some direct food-mediated stimulation of the oxyntic area.[14]

Gastrin is the classic hormone most responsible for stimulation of gastric acid secretion. It is rapidly released after a meal from G cells in the gastric antrum. The main stimuli for gastrin release seem to be amino acids and peptides; thus, protein meals give rise to larger increases in serum gastrin than do meals rich in carbohydrates or fats. The vagus also seems to play a role in the release of gastrin; its stimulatory effect occurs during the cephalic phase of gastric secretion. Calcium is another stimulant of gastrin release. In addition to the predominant role of gastrin as the hormonal mediator of gastric acid production, interactions as yet not fully elucidated occur involving other gastrointestinal hormones present in the stomach. Bombesin may enhance acid secretion.

Although the main effect of gastrin seems to be stimulation of gastric acid secretion, it also has effects on smooth muscle in the stomach and surrounding sphincters as well as a trophic influence on various gastrointestinal tissues. Its trophic effects on parietal cell mass may explain the reduction in gastric secretory response observed in individuals receiving total parenteral nutrition for prolonged periods of time.[40]

The quantitative importance of the intestinal phase of postprandial gastric secretion is less well defined. Unlike the cephalic and gastric phases, which early in the postprandial period are overwhelmingly stimulatory, during the intestinal phase net inhibition of net stimulation may occur, depending on a variety of factors.

Gastrin secretion can be stimulated at a level of the intestine where there is no gastrin to mediate this response. An ileal entero-oxyntin has been described but its status and cell of origin are contentious.[30,100]

A postabsorptive effect of amino acids and peptides in stimulating gastric acid secretion has also been described. This appears not to be mediated by gastrin, and may be a direct effect of the nutrient on the gastric parietal cells.[14]

THE INHIBITORY PHASE OF POSTPRANDIAL GASTRIC SECRETION

As indicated earlier, gastric secretion peaks around 1 hour after ingestion of food and declines rather rapidly afterwards, reflecting a predominance of inhibitory over stimulatory factors.[53] This occurs not only because of increasing inhibitory forces but also because the stimulatory forces are decreasing. First, the effects of cephalic stimulation are reduced because the visual and olfactory stimuli of the food

are gone, chewing and swallowing no longer occur, and a feeling of satiety develops. Second, gastric distension diminishes as the volume of the gastric contents begins to decline by the end of the first hour or earlier (*Figure 3.16*). The only stimulatory factors that remain are the chemical action of food in the stomach and, depending on the type of meal, perhaps some stimulation from the intestine.

The decline in stimulatory activity coincides with a strengthening of inhibitory forces, the most important of which appears to be acidification of gastric contents.[99] In most normal individuals, acidification of gastric contents proceeds until a pH of about 2.0 is reached; the secretory rate then markedly declines. This luminal pH is optimum for peptic activity and, therefore, it makes teleological sense that gastric secretion would be inhibited when it is reached. Probably gastric and duodenal pH-sensitive mechanisms are involved, but the neuro-hormonal mechanisms by which gastric and duodenal acidification inhibits postprandial gastric secretion are poorly understood. Diminution of antral and duodenal gastrin release by low pH may be important.[13,99] There is also the possibility of a paracrine effect of the vagal release of somatostatin at low antral pH.[94] Bulbogastrone,[2] a humoral agent released from the acidified duodenal bulb in experimental animals, has not been evaluated in humans to assess its physiological status. Secretin appears to be released after meals and probably plays a physiological role in stimulating the exocrine pancreas and hepatic secretion of bicarbonate.[7,80] Whether it plays a physiological role in regulating postprandial gastric acid secretion is unclear.

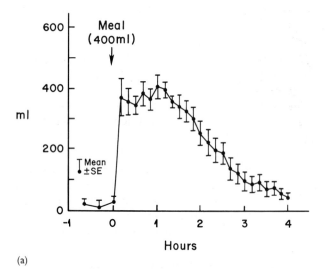

(a)

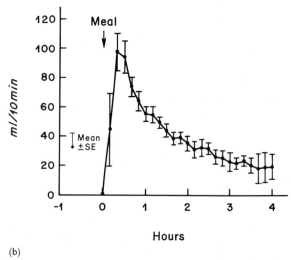

(b)

Figure 3.16 (a) Postprandial volume of gastric contents. (b) Volume of gastric contents emptied into the duodenum after meals in health. Intragastric volume during the first postprandial hour is relatively stable. During this period gastric secretory activity and emptying rates peak and offset each other. When secretory rates decline intragastric volume also falls. (Reproduced, with permission, from Malagelada *et al.*[53])

Other hormones in the small bowel seem to be primarily inhibitory to gastric acid secretion. In fact, lipid and carbohydrates infused into any part of the small intestine will inhibit acid secretion, and even protein will inhibit acid secretion when it is infused into the distal small bowel. Which hormones predominantly mediate these effects is not well understood.

Cholecystokinin is released in response to protein, fat, acid and calcium. Its main effects are in stimulating gallbladder contraction, stimulating pancreatic enzyme secretion, augmenting the action of secretin on pancreatic secretion, and decreasing the tone in the body of the stomach; it also has a trophic influence on the pancreas. More recently, this peptide has been postulated to play a role in augmenting satiety; however, this activity has not been fully characterized.

Gastric inhibitory polypeptide is secreted in response to protein, fat and carbohydrate. Its main physiological action seems to be as an incretin. Although this hormone received its name because of its activity in inhibiting gastric acid secretion in the rat, in humans it seems to have little or no activity to do this.

Neurotensin, peptide YY and enteroglucagon are hormonal markers for the distal small bowel. They each have potential roles in inhibiting gastric acid secretion but the physiological significance is unclear.

Motilin is released in response to intestinal acid. This peptide seems to have its major physiological effect during the interdigestive period in stimulating the initiation of the migrating myoelectric complex.

THE MOTOR RESPONSE OF THE UPPER GUT TO A MEAL

THE FASTING MOTOR PATTERN

Fasting gut motility is characterized by cyclic periods of activity alternating with quiescence. These cycles consist of three identifiable phases: motor quiescence (phase I), irregular but persistent contractions (phase II), and a short burst of rhythmic contractions (phase III).[8,89,97] In healthy volunteers the range of duration of each cycle (measured as the interval between two consecutive phase IIIs) varies from 53 to 136 minutes, depending on the individual studied. The duration of interdigestive cycles also varies considerably within each individual (in one healthy person, cycles varied in duration from 49 to 149 minutes).[74]

Cyclic electrical and motor activity usually originates in the stomach or upper small intestine and is propagated distally from the upper gut to the terminal ileum, taking approximately the same period of time as the intercycle interval. Motilin and pancreatic polypeptide increase just before or during the most intense motor activity (phase III) arrives at the level of the upper gut. On the other hand, gastrin, gastric inhibitory polypeptide, glucagon, insulin and enteroglucagon remain low and constant in the interdigestive period and do not vary at all with the interdigestive motor activity. Although gastrin and cholecystokinin have been shown to inhibit interdigestive motor activity, these hormones are not present at a level adequate to cause this effect during the interdigestive period. Ingestion of a meal abolishes the interdigestive activity and elevates the concentrations of these hormones.

POSTPRANDIAL MOTOR ACTIVITY

Ingestion of a meal modifies interdigestive motor activity in several ways. Assuming it is eaten at an ordinary pace, the volume of the meal (ranging from 400 to 800 ml for most meals), plus the volume of gastric secretion and swallowed saliva, far exceeds the gastric emptying rate (*Figure 3.16*). The expansion of intragastric volume during the early postprandial period with minimal increase in intragastric pressure is an expression of the 'reservoir' function of the stomach. Receptive relaxation and accommodation are largely a function of the proximal stomach and are partially mediated through vagal reflexes, perhaps in close association with those stimulating gastric secretion in response to fundal distension.[1,6,38,86] It is not surprising, therefore, that early satiety and postprandial epigastric fullness are a common complaint of patients after vagotomy. Relaxatory vagal fibres are probably non-adrenergic and non-cholinergic.[36]

The motor responses of the stomach to a meal are determined in part by the physicochemical composition of the meal. Studies in the author's laboratory have shown that ingestion of 400 ml of 0.15 mol/l saline (an inert, isotonic solution) does not usually disturb the on-going fasting motor activity.[73] In contrast, ingestion of a liquid meal containing nutrients inhibits the characteristic fasting cycle activity and replaces it with an irregular pattern of intestinal pressure activity termed the 'fed pattern'. In the antrum, very little phasic pressure activity occurs after a liquid meal. When most of the liquid has been emptied from the stomach, characteristic interdigestive migrating motor complexes reappear. Carbohydrate- or protein-containing meals inter-

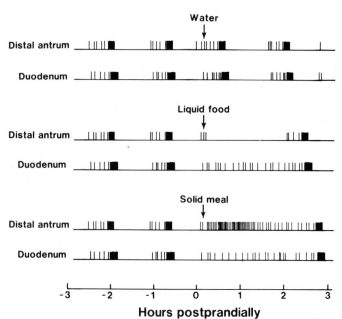

Water

Distal antrum

Duodenum

Liquid food

Distal antrum

Duodenum

Solid meal

Distal antrum

Duodenum

-3   -2   -1   0   1   2   3
Hours postprandially

Figure 3.17 Antral and duodenal motor responses to different types of meals in humans. The top tracings illustrate the typical response to ingestion of a small amount of water or saline, which cause no perceptible change in the interdigestive migrating motor pattern. The middle tracings illustrate the responses to liquid food. Antral phasic pressure activity disappears until the majority of the meal has been evacuated from the stomach. In the duodenum, irregular activity characteristic of the fed pattern is observed. The bottom tracings illustrate the response to a solid meal, which causes intense distal antral phasic pressure activity. The duodenal fed pattern is similar to that observed after liquid food. (Reproduced, with permission, from Malagelada, J.-R. (1981) In: *Physiology of the Gastrointestinal Tract*, Vol. 2, pp. 893–924 (Ed.) Johnson, L.R. New York: Raven Press.)

rupt the interdigestive motor pattern for a shorter time than lipid meals or mixed meals containing all essential nutrients; the duration of the interruption approximately coincides with the duration of gastric emptying for each meal.

Ingestion of a solid or solid and liquid meal is associated with a pattern of gastric motor activity different from that for inert and nutrient-containing liquid meals. Shortly after ingestion of solid food, vigorous contractions take place in the distal antrum, which cause phasic increases in pressure often reaching over 100 mmHg.[72] These contractions occur at or close to the maximal rate (established by the gastric pacemaker) of 3/min, and are most apparent in the terminal antrum. The antral pressure waves may persist for several hours, evolving later into a migrating phase III which signals the re-establishment of the interdigestive motor pattern. Therefore, meals of different physical characteristics and composition differ in the types of antral pressure response they elicit in the stomach, but the intestinal motor fed pattern shows no such differences on visual inspection (*Figure 3.17*).

The mechanism responsible for postprandial inhibition of interdigestive cyclic motility may be both neuronal and hormonal.[91,92,103] Vagotomy reduces the inhibitory effects of eating. Protein and mixed meals release gastrin, which has been shown to inhibit interdigestive motor activity in both the dog and human.[32,54,102] However, gastrin release is not responsible for the interruption of gastric motor activity after lipid and carbohydrate meals. Numerous other hormones, including cholecystokinin, secretin and insulin,[4,64] may also be important, but

their physiological role in switching the gut from a fasting to a fed motor pattern requires further study.

GASTRIC EMPTYING

As indicated earlier, intragastric contents after a physiological meal separate into three phases – aqueous, solid and oil – which are emptied by the stomach at different rates. Plain water or isotonic aqueous solutions with low nutrient content leave the stomach most rapidly and are continuously replaced by gastric secretion.[48] Fluids of high osmolality or soluble nutrient content, or both, have slower emptying rates than water, allowing for gradual adjustment of the chyme osmolality to isotonicity in the upper intestine (*Figure 3.18*). Fats which are liquid at body temperature (the oil phase) and solids leave the stomach much more slowly than the aqueous phase.

There is evidence that different mechanisms and regions of the stomach are involved in the emptying of the solid and liquid components of gastric contents. Experimental studies suggest that tonic fundal activity is primarily responsible for the emptying of fluids, whereas the antrum is mostly concerned with the emptying of solids.[33] This concept represents a departure from the earlier view that an 'antral pump' was the main determinant of gastric emptying of all kinds of contents. In the case of digestible solids, the antrum plays an important role in reducing the size of the ingested solids to find particulate matter and suspending them in fluid. This grinding–mixing process is accomplished by rhythmic and powerful antral contractions described earlier. Solid

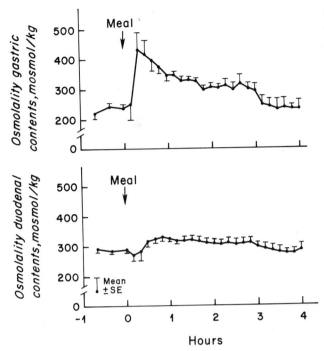

Figure 3.18 Osmolality of gastric and duodenal contents after a meal in health. (a) Osmolality of gastric contents. (b) Osmolality of duodenal contents aspirated at the ligament of Treitz. Note the gradual decrease in gastric osmolality as the meal becomes more diluted with gastric juice and food is emptied from the stomach. In the duodenum, large fluctuations in osmolality are prevented by mechanisms regulating gastric emptying and through dilution of chyme in the duodenum by biliary and pancreatic secretions. (Modified from Malagelada *et al.*[49])

tive migrating motor complexes propels them across the pylorus. This mechanism may explain the development of fibrous bezoars in patients with gastric motility disorders in which gastric interdigestive migrating motor complexes are frequently absent.

Regulation of gastric emptying

Mechanisms regulating gastric emptying have gradually been characterized through several decades of experimental work. They can be divided into central and peripheral mechanisms. Central mechanisms are intimately related with the emetic centre in the medulla oblongata and, indeed, inhibition of gastric emptying is observed preceding vomiting and in response to a variety of nauseating stimuli. Psychological and emotional factors may affect emptying as well, but the mechanisms involved are not well characterized.

The peripheral mechanisms are located on both sides of the pylorus. The gastric mechanisms are largely stimulatory and are triggered by distension of the stomach. Their regulatory role was probably over-estimated by early experimental work carried out with simple crystalloid solutions. With complex, nutrient-containing meals, the intragastric volume is probably not the primary determinant of gastric emptying. The gut mechanisms, which are inhibitory, are probably more important. The key factors are the pH, osmolality and nutrient content of the material being emptied into the duodenum. If the duodenal load or the characteristics of the emptied material are not adequate, inhibitory mechanisms will reduce gastric emptying, even at the expense of an expanding intragastric volume. It is impossible to dissociate postprandial gastric emptying from gastric secretion in a physiological context because the gut regulatory mechanisms 'see' the whole of the gastric contents, which includes the meal itself and two to three times its volume in gastric juice,[48] pass through the pylorus.

Distal to the pylorus, inhibitory mechanisms appear to be arranged in a 'priority system', which sometimes allows stimulation of one receptor to override the effect on others. Volume and osmolality are probably more important factors than acidity, which exerts a more obvious inhibitory effect on gastric secretion than on emptying. The nutrient composition and load are also important. Protein, carbohydrates and lipids are all inhibitory for gastric secretion and, at least for liquid meals, there appears to be an inverse relationship between the energy content of the duodenal load and the rate of gastric emptying. The osmotic receptors are thought to reside in the duodenum, whereas the main acid-sensitive mechanisms are located in the first 5 cm of

particles and some liquid are propulsed forwards, and then backwards by the terminal antropyloric contraction, which allows some liquid to pass through but retains most solid particles in the stomach until they have been finely broken down. Meyer *et al.*,[60] for instance, have shown in the dog that only liver particles of less than 1 mm are allowed to pass into the duodenum. In summary, in this process of emptying of digestible solids, three interacting functions are important: the grinding pressure waves of the distal antrum; the discriminatory mechanism that allows small suspended particles to leave with the liquids and retains large particles for further grinding in the stomach; and the propulsive forces, mostly fundal, that push the fluids (and the small suspended solid particles) into the duodenum.

Non-digestible solids, such as the fibrous, cell wall structures of plants, are rather impervious to mechanical grinding by antral contractions. As a result, the larger non-digestible solid particles in a meal probably remain in the stomach until the rest of the food has left. However, the return of the interdiges-

the duodenum.[11] The nutrient-sensitive areas extend much more distally into the jejunum. Therefore, nutrient load may be more important than initial concentration since a larger load means the nutrients are spread over a longer portion of the intestine where inhibitory mechanisms are located.

The mechanisms of intestinal feedback inhibition of motility are reminiscent of those we have discussed with respect to intestinal inhibition of gastric acid secretion. Vagal and probably other peptidergic influences have some effect but most attention has focused on the potential roles of secretin, cholecystokinin, peptide YY, gastric inhibitory polypeptide etc. The imaginative term 'the ileal brake' has been coined to describe a number of events – delayed gastric emptying, decreased pancreatic secretion and decreased intestinal transit – that occur if unabsorbed nutrients, particularly fat, reach the ileum, all of which will tend to increase digestion and absorption. Neurotensin, peptide YY and enteroglucagon may mediate this.[71]

PANCREATIC SECRETION AFTER MEALS

PHYSIOLOGICAL CONCEPTS

It is estimated that each day the exocrine pancreas secretes about 1 litre of isotonic, alkaline juice containing 5–8 g of protein, most of which is digestive enzymes. Phospholipases and proteases are secreted as inactive precursors; other enzymes are secreted in active form. The functional reserve of the pancreas is enormous. Eighty to ninety per cent of the functional acinar mass must be absent before clinical evidence of malabsorption appears;[17] therefore, normal digestion of a meal occurs in a comfortable abundance of pancreatic enzymes. Most of the acinar mass of the pancreas is located in the head of the gland and drains into the proximal 40% of the main pancreatic duct, and accessory duct if one is present.[18]

The exocrine pancreas also secretes water and electrolytes, which have an important digestive function. The isotonic pancreatic juice increases duodenal flow and helps to solubilize nutrients at a concentration optimal for digestion and absorption. Its high bicarbonate content neutralizes acidic gastric chyme emptied into the duodenum and helps maintain luminal pH in the optimal range for most pancreatic enzymes to act. Small amounts of calcium, magnesium and zinc are also secreted by the pancreas, but their significance in relation to digestive function is unknown.

FASTING AND POSTPRANDIAL PATTERNS OF EXOCRINE PANCREATIC SECRETION

The secretory activity of the pancreas varies a great deal, as does gastric secretion, at different times of the day. During fasting, interdigestive motor complexes are synchronously associated with increased pancreatic secretion of enzymes, bicarbonate and water.[37,98] Ingestion of an ordinary meal breaks the interdigestive motor–secretory cycles and produces a rapid increase in pancreatic secretion. As assessed by measuring duodenal enzyme output,[49] the pancreatic response to a meal begins as soon as the individual starts eating, reaches its peak within the first hour, plateaus and then gradually declines as the input of nutrients into the duodenum declines. This profile is quite monotonous and varies little for a wide range of meals and individuals (*Figure 3.19*). 'Maximal' pancreatic enzyme secretion is consistently caused by a wide range of meals (e.g. liquid formula meals, homogenized mixed meals, ordinary meals), as long as they contain protein and lipid, which are the main dietary stimuli to pancreatic enzyme secretion.[49,61,77] The main difference in enzyme response among these meals is in the duration rather than the magnitude of the response. On the other hand, responses to crystalloid test meals not containing nutrients have not exceeded 50% of the maximal pancreatic response.[41,58]

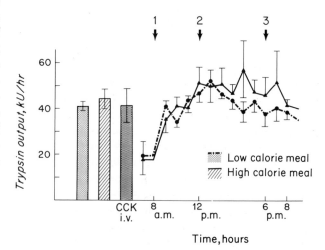

Figure 3.19 Hourly output of trypsin during three liquid meals in healthy individuals. Ingestion of relatively low calorie meals (each 20 cal/kg body weight) and high calorie meals (each 40 cal/kg body weight) resulted in similar pancreatic enzyme responses. (Modified from Brunner, H. *et al.* (1974) *Mayo Clinic Proceedings*, **49**, 851–860.)

CONTROL OF THE PANCREATIC EXOCRINE RESPONSE TO A MEAL

The physiological control of pancreatic secretion is predominantly stimulatory, appears to lack a fine-tuning system, and seems primarily directed to assuring an excess of enzymes whenever food reaches the duodenum. The pancreatic response to a meal is controlled by interacting neurohormonal mechanisms. The most important is the release of regulatory peptides from neuroendocrine cells of the upper small intestines. Of these the stimulating effects of secretin and cholecystokinin are the most powerful. Secretin is released in response to a lowering of duodenal pH,[59] and probably also in response to intraduodenal fat.[101]

Secretin seems to have its primary effect on the ductal systems of the pancreas in stimulating bicarbonate secretion. This is important to generate the proper intraluminal pH for the activity of pancreatic enzymes, as well as for enteric enzymes. The importance of this action is illustrated in gastric hypersecretion, such as that which occurs in the Zollinger–Ellison syndrome, when intraduodenal pH may be reduced to a very low level; maldigestion and malabsorption can become so severe that they constitute the presenting complaint of the patient.

Cholecystokinin is released in response to intraduodenal amino acids, fatty acids and oligopeptides, as well as calcium. It is a very powerful stimulator alone and also synergizes with secretin. Its effectiveness as a pancreatic stimulator and its liberation in response to upper intestinal nutrients, from the upper gastrointestinal tract, all indicate its major significance in regulating pancreatic secretion; recently, the use of cholecystokinin antagonists in animals and humans has confirmed the major role of this neurotransmitter.[5]

Sight, smell, taste and chewing of food generate a 'cephalic phase' of some importance in humans,[79] possibly accounting for a quarter to a third of the maximal response. It is mediated by the vagus nerve, in part through the release of antral gastrin. When food reaches the stomach, further stimulation of pancreatic secretion occurs. Gastropancreatic reflexes, such as those described in the dog,[95] and gastrin release may participate in this gastric phase of pancreatic response to a meal, but their relative contributions to postprandial secretion remains unknown.

When chyme reaches the upper small bowel, an intestinal phase of pancreatic secretion takes place. The role of cholecystokinin and secretin at this stage has already been discussed. Whereas hormonal stimulation has long been thought to be the primary stimulatory mechanism, enteropancreatic vago-vagal reflexes are now being recognized as being of major importance. Interruption of these reflexes may explain the diminished pancreatic response to intraluminal stimuli observed after vagotomy.[84,85] Enteropancreatic reflexes may be critical in obtaining a rapid pancreatic response as chyme begins to flow into the duodenum with hormonal mechanisms providing a sustained subsequent stimulus.

Inhibitory neural and hormonal mechanisms may also come into play in the regulation of postprandial pancreatic secretion. Glucagon, whose serum concentration rises in the postprandial period, and other hormones and active peptides (vasoactive intestinal peptide, pancreatic polypeptide and somatostatin) have been shown to influence pancreatic secretion. The ileal brake mechanism has already been mentioned, and colonic nutrients can do the same.[67] Intraluminal pancreatic enzymes themselves may initiate inhibition of pancreatic secretion, possibly by mechanisms involving inhibition of naturally occurring luminal cholecystokinin-releasing factors.[46] It is impossible at this time to determine which of these mechanisms plays a physiological role in humans. Even less is known about the significance of neural inhibitory mechanisms.

INTERRELATIONSHIPS BETWEEN GASTRIC EMPTYING, NUTRIENT COMPOSITION OF CHYME AND THE PANCREATIC RESPONSE TO A MEAL

Duodenal acid load is an important determinant of the volume and bicarbonate content of pancreatic secretion after a meal. The acid load is mostly gastric hydrochloric acid but weak acids, such as fatty acids, may play a part.[59] Pancreatic enzyme secretion after meals depends largely on stimulation by protein, fat and, possibly, calcium. Human perfusion studies have established the relative potency of luminal digestive products in stimulating pancreatic enzyme output (*Figure 3.20*). Fat appears to be the most potent stimulus, fatty acids and monoglycerides being the active components.[50,51] With long-chain (C_{18}) to medium-chain (C_8) fatty acids there is an inverse relationship between carbon chain length and potency to stimulate pancreatic secretion.[50] In humans, protein is another potent stimulus[21,27,51] because of the essential amino acids it contains (phenylalanine, valine, methionine and tryptophan). In the author's experience, luminal protein can achieve only about 60% of maximal pancreatic enzyme output.[51]

Calcium is also a potent stimulus to human enzyme secretion; magnesium has a weaker but significant effect. Both minerals exert significant stimulatory effects at duodenal concentrations

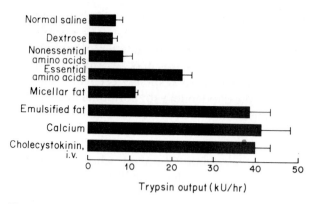

Figure 3.20 Trypsin output during intraduodenal perfusion of digestive products in health. The stimulatory effect of emulsified fat and calcium is comparable to that of 'maximal' intravenous cholecystokinin. In contrast, non-essential amino acids and dextrose lack significant stimulatory effects. Micellar fat and essential amino acids lead to intermediate responses.

above 6 mmol/l.[34,52] It is questionable whether such luminal concentrations of ionic minerals are reached postprandially. Both distension of the duodenum and the presence of hyperosmolar solutions can induce pancreatic secretion.[19] Dextrose is ineffective as a stimulus; it is unlikely that the carbohydrate content influences the pancreatic response to a meal. The effects of alcohol ingestion on pancreatic secretion are confusing. Depending on the amount of alcohol administered and the experimental conditions, either net stimulation[45,93] or net inhibition[55,63] may be observed. The stimulatory effect of alcohol may be mediated through release of antral gastrin and stimulation of gastric acid output.[45,93]

Accepting the premise that intestinal mechanisms are important in the control of postprandial pancreatic secretion, it is appropriate to investigate what segment and length of intestine are required to stimulate and sustain a normal response. Studies[61] suggest that stimulation of the stomach and duodenum is sufficient to elicit a normal pancreatic enzyme response to a meal. It also corroborates the clinical observation that patients with malabsorption secondary to short bowel syndrome do not generally benefit from enzyme therapy, since their malabsorption is not usually compounded by secondary pancreatic insufficiency unless malnourishment has led to pancreatic hypofunction.

BILIARY SECRETION AFTER MEALS

PHYSIOLOGICAL CONCEPTS

The complex structure of the biliary tract seems intended to obtain efficient utilization of a relatively small pool of bile acids. The enterohepatic circulation of bile acids is a conserving mechanism whose integrity is required for bile acids to reach physiological concentrations in the upper gut during digestion. The gallbladder exerts both reservoir and concentrating functions. A fraction of the bile flow is diverted into the gallbladder during fasting and is stored there until required. The biliary excretory system also has a distal sphincter (the sphincter of Oddi) whose function is poorly understood, but it is probably important in the regulation of bile flow into the intestine. The biliary system unlike the excretory systems of other digestive glands, such as the pancreas, depends on motor mechanisms as well as secretory mechanisms for the fulfilment of the physiological role.

FASTING AND POSTPRANDIAL PATTERNS OF BILIARY SECRETION

During fasting, the cyclic changes seen in both the interdigestive motor activity and its secretory counterpart also involve the biliary system. In experimental animals and in humans, duodenal outputs of bile acids and bilirubin increase during phase II of the interdigestive motor cycle, reach peak values just prior to or during phase III activity, and decrease again to low levels during phase I.[37,96,66] The storage capacity of the gallbladder is about 30 ml; up to 10 ml of gallbladder bile may be discharged into the duodenum with each interdigestive motor–secretory cycle, which occurs every 1–2 hours. Phase III probably propels fasting intestinal contents in the aboral direction;[97] therefore, interdigestive motor–secretory cycles probably coincide with an acceleration of the enterohepatic circulation of bile acids. Delivery of bile during fasting probably reflects a combination of partial gallbladder emptying,[88] changes in hepatic secretion of bile and relaxation of the sphincter of Oddi.[68]

Ingestion of a meal disrupts the fasting cyclical pattern of motor and secretory activity and replaces it with the more continuous, although irregular, fed motor pattern. Secretory activity by the digestive glands also markedly increases postprandially. Both motor and secretory responses contribute to a rapid discharge of bile into the duodenum after meals. Contraction of the gallbladder begins within a few minutes of the ingestion of food and reduces its volume by about two-thirds. After reaching a peak within the first postprandial hour, bile acid output usually remains at a high plateau, or declines slightly, until gastric emptying of the meal has been completed, at which time it returns to its basal level. If the profile of duodenal bilirubin output is analysed rather than bile acid output, the early postprandial peak tends to be somewhat sharper; otherwise, it is similar to that of bile acid output.

CONTROL OF THE BILIARY RESPONSE TO A MEAL

Much of what is known about biliary discharge into the duodenum in response to intraluminal stimuli in humans has been gathered from perfusion studies, supplemented by study of gallbladder volume by isotopic techniques and ultrasonography. In response to single intraluminal nutrients, such as fatty acids or essential amino acids, duodenal outputs of bilirubin and bile acids rise sharply within a few minutes as the gallbladder contracts and discharges its contents, but then output drops quickly to a low plateau (*Figure 3.21*).[28,50,51] In contrast, after meals, biliary output of bile acids is more sustained, reflecting the accelerating effect of feeding on the enterohepatic circulation of bile acids.[42,43]

The similarity observed between luminal stimulation of pancreatic enzyme and biliary outputs is due to the fact that both systems share a number of neurohormonal stimulatory mechanisms, chiefly cholecystokinin; this causes gallbladder contraction,[47] produces relaxation of the sphincter of Oddi[26] and, as mentioned earlier, plays an important role in the stimulation of pancreatic enzyme secretion. Cholecystokinin inhibition effectively prevents gallbladder contraction, demonstrating the prime importance of this hormone.[44,65] The contraction of the gallbladder after a meal occurs a few minutes after peak cholecystokinin levels are reached.[104] Secretin increases biliary flow by stimulating secretion of water and electrolytes (mainly bicarbonate) from both the pancreas and the biliary system. Secretin and pancreatic polypeptide may inhibit gallbladder contraction, although it is not known whether these are physiological effects. Neural mechanisms may also be shared but they have not been as well characterized. Cholinergic agonists contract gallbladder smooth muscle and it seems likely that vagal influences control the sham-feeding gallbladder responses that can be elicited.[24] Gastric distensions can also induce gallbladder contraction by a vagally mediated reflex.[15] Vasoactive intestinal peptide immunoreactivity has been demonstrated in close association with gallbladder nerve fibres and may point to neuropeptide mediation of relaxation impulses.[78]

Among the inhibitory mechanisms, the luminal bile acid concentration appears to be an important modulator of biliary response to digestive products, fatty acids and amino acids.[50,51] This effect of bile acids, which is also observed for pancreatic enzyme secretion, is exerted in part through changes in the rate of absorption of nutrients, chiefly fatty acids, which determine the length of proximal small bowel exposed to luminal stimuli, as well as probably by inhibition of the cholecystokinin release.[29] Again, the parallel effect of bile acids on pancreatic enzyme and biliary responses to nutrients suggests that the pancreas and biliary system share common regulatory mechanisms.

Control of biliary flow into the duodenum depends not only on gallbladder contraction but also on changes in tone of the sphincter of Oddi. Phasic contractile activity occurs in the sphincter during the interdigestive period and relaxation of the sphincter occurs during gallbladder contraction in dogs.[9,82] In this field, however, differences in different animals present a complex picture and study in humans is difficult. It seems likely that the mechanisms involved are similar to those controlling gallbladder function.

THE RELATIONSHIP BETWEEN PHYSICAL STATE, NUTRIENT COMPOSITION OF MEALS AND POSTPRANDIAL BILIARY SECRETION

There is a greater variation in the biliary response to meals than that manifested by the exocrine pancreas, although the range of meals tested so far is small. When comparing the effect of meals ingested either in ordinary solid and liquid form or after thorough homogenization,[49] the ordinary meal caused a lower early peak bile acid output into the duodenum, but a more prolonged response, than the homogenized meal. It seems likely that initial

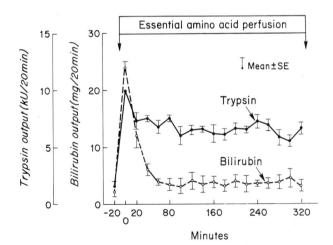

Figure 3.21 Gallbladder and pancreatic response to essential amino acid perfusion in the duodenum in health. Gallbladder contraction at the onset of perfusion causes a sharp peak in bilirubin output followed by a low plateau. The pancreatic enzyme response is more stable since it depends largely on new synthesis and release of enzymes.

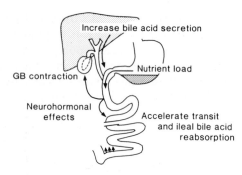

Figure 3.22 Interrelationships between nutrient load, neurohormonal stimulation of gallbladder contraction and small bowel transit, and biliary secretions of bile acids. Postprandial nutrient loads in the upper intestine cause gallbladder contraction and increase duodenal bile acid output. They also shorten transit along the small bowel with a corresponding increase in ileal bile acid reabsorption and acceleration of enterohepatic cycling. These effects are neurohormonally controlled.

emptying of the liquid phase of the ordinary meal (predominantly water and soluble carbohydrates) may have provided insufficient luminal stimulus to fully contract the gallbladder. However, the response would last longer after the ordinary meal because of the more gradual emptying of protein (meat) and fat (butter), which maintain a high level of stimulation.[12,48]

The sustained plateau of duodenal bile acid output which follows the early rise is due to continuing recirculation of the bile acid pool after initial gallbladder contraction. Under constant stimulation by chyme flowing through the duodenum, the gallbladder is largely bypassed, and the sphincter of Oddi remains relaxed, allowing bile acids returning to the liver from the intestine to re-enter the gut.[22] Studies in healthy volunteers ingesting three liquid meals per day suggest that the entire bile acid pool recirculates up to two times per meal.[16] However, the number of times that the pool circulates will vary depending on the size and composition of the meal and its rate of emptying from the stomach (*Figure 3.22*). In turn, enterohepatic bile acid recycling has significant effects on biliary lipid composition. Acceleration of the enterohepatic circulation of bile acids increases total biliary lipid secretion but, since the relationship between bile acid and cholesterol secretion is curvilinear, the mole per cent of cholesterol in the bile, and hence its potential lithogenicity, decreases.

REFERENCES

1. Abrahamson, H. (1973) The inhibitory nervous control of gastric motility. *Acta Physiologica Scandinavica (Supplement)*, **390**, 1–38.

2. Andersson, S., Nilsson, G., Sjodin, L. and Uvnas, B. (1973) Mechanism of duodenal inhibition of gastric acid secretion. In: *Nobel Symposium 16: Frontiers in Gastrointestinal Hormone Research*, pp. 223–238 (Ed.) Andersson, S. Stockholm: Almqvist and Wiksell.

3. Baron, J.H. (1979) *Clinical Tests of Gastric Secretion*. New York: Oxford University Press.

4. Bueno, L. and Ruckebusch, Y. (1976) Evidence for a role of endogenous insulin on intestinal motility. In: *Proceedings of the Fifth International Symposium on Gastrointestinal Motility*, pp. 64–69 (Ed.) Vantrappen, G. Herentals, Belgium: Typoff-Press.

5. Cantos, P., Mortensen, P.E., Gjorup, I. *et al.* (1989) Effect of the cholecystokinin antagonist MK329 on meal-stimulated pancreatic secretion in man. *Digestion*, **43**, 134.

6. Carlson, H.C., Code, C.F. and Nelson, R.A. (1966) Motor action of the canine gastroduodenal function: a cineradiographic, pressure, and electric study. *American Journal of Digestive Diseases*, **11**, 155–172.

7. Chey, W.Y., Kim, M.S., Lee, K.Y. and Chang, T. (1979) Effect of rabbit antisecretin serum on postprandial pancreatic secretion in dogs. *Gastroenterology*, **77**, 1268–1275.

8. Code, C.F. and Schlegel, J.R. (1973) The gastrointestinal interdigestive housekeeper: motor correlates of the interdigestive myoelectric complex of the dog. In: *Proceedings of the Fourth International Symposium on Gastrointestinal Motility*, pp. 631–634 (Eds) Daniel, E.E. *et al.* Vancouver: Mitchell Press.

9. Coelno, J.C.U. and Moody, G.F. (1987) Certain aspects of normal and abnormal motility of sphincter of Oddi. *Digestive Diseases and Sciences*, **32**, 86–94.

10. Cooke, A.R. (1970) Potentiation of acid output in man by a distention stimulus. *Gastroenterology*, **58**, 633–637.

11. Cooke, A.R. (1974) Duodenal acidification: role of first part of duodenum in gastric emptying and secretion in dogs. *Gastroenterology*, **67**, 85–92.

12. Cortot, A., Phillips, S.F. and Malagelada, J.-R. (1981) Gastric emptying of lipids after ingestion of solid–liquid meal in humans. *Gastroenterology*, **80**, 922–927.

13. Csendes, A., Walsh, J.H. and Grossman, M.I. (1972) Effects of atropine and antral acidification on gastrin release and acid secretion in response to insulin and feeding in dogs. *Gastroenterology*, **63**, 257–263.

14. Debas, H.T. and Grossman, M.I. (1975) Chemicals bathing the oxyntic gland area stimulate acid secretion in dog. *Gastroenterology*, **69**, 654–659.

15. Debas, H.T. and Yamagushi, T. (1979) Evidence for a pyloro-cholecystic reflux for gallbladder contraction. *Annals of Surgery*, **190**, 170–175

16. DiMagno, E.P., Go, V.L.W. and Summerskill, W.H.J. (1972) Impaired cholecystokinin-

pancreozymin secretion, intraluminal dilution, and maldigestion of fat in sprue. *Gastroenterology*, **63**, 25–32.

17. DiMagno, E.P., Go, V.L.W. and Summerskill, W.H.J. (1973) Relations between pancreatic enzyme outputs and malabsorption in severe pancreatic insufficiency. *New England Journal of Medicine*, **288**, 813–815.

18. DiMagno, E.P., Go, V.L.W. and Summerskill, W.H.J. (1973) Intraluminal and postabsorptive effects of amino acids on pancreatic enzyme secretion. *Journal of Laboratory and Clinical Medicine*, **82**, 241–248.

19. Dooley, C.P. and Valenzuela, J.E. (1984) Duodenal volume and osmoreceptors in the stimulation of human pancreatic secretion. *Gastroenterology*, **86**, 23–27.

20. Dyck, W.P., Texter, E.C., Lasater, J.M. and Hightower, N.C. (1970) Influence of glucagon on pancreatic exocrine secretion in man. *Gastroenterology*, **58**, 532–539.

21. Ertan, A., Brooks, F.P., Ostrow, J.D. *et al.* (1971) Effect of jejunal amino acid perfusion and exogenous cholecystokinin on the exocrine pancreatic and biliary secretions in man. *Gastroenterology*, **61**, 686–692.

22. Everson, G.T., Lawson, M.J., McKinley, C. *et al.* (1983) Gallbladder and small intestinal regulation of biliary lipid secretion during intraduodenal infusion of standard stimuli. *Journal of Clinical Investigation*, **71**, 596–603.

23. Feldman, M. and Richardson, C.T. (1986) Role of thought, site, smell and taste in the cephalic phase of gastric secretion in humans. *Gastroenterology*, **90**, 428–432.

24. Fisher, R.S., Rock, E. and Malmud, L.S. (1986) Gallbladder emptying in response to sham feeding in humans. *Gastroenterology*, **90**, 1854–1857.

25. Fordtran, J.S. and Walsh, J.H. (1973) Gastric acid secretion rate and buffer content of the stomach after eating: results in normal subjects and in patients with duodenal ulcer. *Journal of Clinical Investigation*, **52**, 645–657.

26. Geenan, J.E., Hogan, W.J., Dodds, W.I. *et al.* (1980) Intraluminal pressure recording from the human sphincter of Oddi. *Gastroenterology*, **78**, 317–324.

27. Go, V.L.W., Hofmann, A.F. and Summerskill, W.H.J. (1980) Pancreozymin bioassay in man based on pancreatic enzyme secretion. *Journal of Clinical Investigation*, **49**, 1558–1564.

28. Go, V.L.W., Hofmann, A.F. and Summerskill, W.H.J. (1970) Simultaneous measurements of total pancreatic, biliary, and gastric outputs in man using a perfusion technique. *Gastroenterology*, **58**, 321–328.

29. Gomez, G., Upp, J.R., Lluis, F. *et al.* (1988) Regulation of the release of cholecystokinin by bile salts in dogs and humans. *Gastroenterology*, **94**, 1036–1046.

30. Grantz, I., Mormwehr, S.R., Lucey, M.R. *et al.* (1989) Gastrotropin, not an entero-oxyntin but a member of a family of cytoplasmic hydrophobic ligand binding proteins. *Journal of Biological Chemistry*, **264**, 20248–20254.

31. Grotzinger, U., Bergegarth, S. and Olbe, L. (1977) The effect of fundic distension on gastric acid secretion in man. *Gut*, **18**, 105–110.

32. Hellemans, J., Vantrappen, G., Janssens, J. and Peeters, T. (1978) Effect of feeding and of gastrin on the interdigestive myoelectric complex in man. In: *Proceedings of the 6th International Gastrointestinal Motility Symposium*, pp. 29–30 (Ed.) Duthie, H.L. Lancaster: MTP Press.

33. Hinder, R.A. and Kelly, K.A. (1977) Canine gastric emptying of solids and liquids. *American Journal of Physiology*, **233**, E335–E340.

34. Holtermuller, K.H., Malagelada, J.R., McCall, J.T. and Go, V.L.W. (1976) Pancreatic gallbladder, and gastric responses to intraduodenal calcium perfusion in man. *Gastroenterology*, **70**, 693–696.

35. Hunt, J.N. and MacDonald, I. (1952) The relation between the volume of a test meal and the gastric secretory response. *Journal of Physiology*, **117**, 289–302.

36. Jahnberg, T., Abrahamsson, H., Jansson, G. and Martinson, J. (1977) Gastric relaxatory response to feeding before and after vagotomy. *Scandinavian Journal of Gastroenterology*, **12**, 225–228.

37. Keane, F.B., DiMagno, E.P. and Malagelada, J.-R. (1980) Role of the migrating motor complex and its secretory counterpart on duodenogastric reflux in man. *Gastroenterology*, **78**, 1192 (abstract).

38. Kelly, K.A. (1970) Effect of gastrin on gastrin myoelectric activity. *American Journal of Digestive Diseases*, **15**, 399–405.

39. Knutson, U. and Olbe, L. (1973) Gastric acid response to sham feeding in the duodenal ulcer patient. *Scandinavian Journal of Gastroenterology*, **8**, 513–522.

40. Kotler, D.P. and Levine, G.M. (1979) Reversible gastric and pancreatic hyposecretion after long-term parenteral nutrition. *New England Journal of Medicine*, **300**, 241–242.

41. Krawisz, B.R., Miller, L.J., DiMagno, E.P. and Go, V.L.W. (1980) In the absence of nutrients, pancreatic-biliary secretions do not exert feedback control of human pancreatic or gastric function. *Journal of Laboratory and Clinical Medicine*, **95**, 13–18.

42. LaRusso, N.F., Korman, M.G., Hoffman, N.E. and Hofmann, A.F. (1974) Dynamics of the enterohepatic circulation of bile acids. *New England Journal of Medicine*, **291**, 689–692.

43. LaRusso, N.F., Hoffman, N.E., Korman, M.G. *et al.* (1978) Determinants of fasting and postprandial serum bile acid levels in healthy man. *American Journal of Digestive Diseases*, **23**, 385–391.

44. Liddle, R.A., Gertz, B.J., Kanayama, S. *et al.* Effects of a CCK receptor antagonist MK-329 on gallbladder contraction and gastric emptying in

humans. *Journal of Clinical Investigation*, **84**, 1220–1225

45. Llanos, O.L., Swierczek, J.S., Teichmann, R.K. *et al.* (1977) Effect of alcohol on the release of secretin and pancreatic secretion. *Surgery*, **81**, 661–667.

46. Lovie, D.S., May, D. and Miller, P. (1986) Cholecystokinin mediates feedback regulation of pancreatic enzyme secretion in rats. *American Journal of Physiology*, **250**, G252–259.

47. Makhlouf, G.M. (1979) Transport and motor function of the gallbladder. *Viewpoints on Digestive Diseases*, **11**, 1–4.

48. Malagelada, J.-R. (1977) Quantification of gastric solid–liquid discrimination during digestion of ordinary meals. *Gastroenterology*, **72**, 1264–1267.

49. Malagelada, J.-R., Go, V.L.W. and Summerskill, W.H.J. (1979) Different gastric, pancreatic and biliary responses to solid–liquid or homogenized meals. *Digestive Diseases and Sciences*, **24**, 101–110.

50. Malagelada, J.-R., DiMagno, E.P., Summerskill, W.H.J. and Go, V.L.W. (1978) Regulation of pancreatic and gallbladder functions by intraluminal fatty acids and bile acids in man. *Journal of Clinical Investigation*, **58**, 493–499.

51. Malagelada, J.-R., Go, V.L.W., DiMagno, E.P. and Summerskill, W.H.J. (1973) Interactions between intraluminal bile acids and digestive products on pancreatic and gallbladder function. *Journal of Clinical Investigation*, **52**, 2160–2165.

52. Malagelada, J.-R., Holtermuller, K.H., McCall, J.T. and Go, V.L.W. (1978) Pancreatic, gallbladder and intestinal responses to interluminal magnesium salts in man. *American Journal of Digestive Diseases*, **23**, 481–485.

53. Malagelada, J.-R., Longstreth, G.F., Summerskill, W.H.J. and Go, V.L.W. (1976) Measurement of gastric functions during digestion of ordinary solid meals in man. *Gastroenterology*, **70**, 203–210.

54. Marik, F. and Code, C.F. (1975) Control of the interdigestive myoelectric activity in dogs by the vagus nerves and pentagastrin. *Gastroenterology*, **69**, 387–395.

55. Marin, G.A., Ward, N.L. and Fisher, R. (1973) Effect of ethanol on pancreatic and biliary secretions in humans. *American Journal of Digestive Diseases*, **18**, 825–833.

56. Marks, I.N. and Shay, H. (1960) Augmented histamine test, Ewald test meal and Diagnex test. *American Journal of Digestive Diseases*, **5**, 1–23.

57. Mayer, G., Arnold, R., Feurle, K. *et al.* (1974) Influence of feeding and sham feeding upon serum gastrin and gastric acid secretion in control subjects and duodenal ulcer patients. *Scandinavian Journal of Gastroenterology*, **9**, 703–710.

58. Meeroff, J.C., Go, V.L.W. and Phillips, S.F. (1975) Control of gastric emptying by osmolality of duodenal contents. *Gastroenterology*, **68**, 1144–1151.

59. Meyer, J.H. (1975) Release of secretin and cholecystokinin. In: *Gastrointestinal Hormones*, pp. 475–490 (Ed.) Thompson, J.C. Austin: University of Texas Press.

60. Meyer, J.H., Thomson, J.B., Cohen, M.B. *et al.* (1979) Sieving of solid food by the canine stomach and sieving after gastric surgery. *Gastroenterology*, **76**, 804–813.

61. Miller, L.J., Clain, J.E., Malagelada, J.-R. and Go, V.L.W. (1979) Control of human postprandial pancreatic exocrine secretion: a function of the gastroduodenal region. *Digestive Diseases and Sciences*, **24**, 150–154.

62. Miller, L.J., Malagelada, J.-R., Taylor, W.F. and Go, V.L.W. (1981) Intestinal control of human postprandial gastric function: the role of components of jejuno-ileal, chyme in regulating gastric secretion and gastric emptying. *Gastroenterology*, **80**, 763–769.

63. Mott, C.B., Sarles, H., Tiscornia, O. and Gullo, L. (1972) Inhibitory action of alcohol on human exocrine pancreatic secretion. *American Journal of Digestive Diseases*, **17**, 902–910.

64. Mukhopadhyay, A.K., Thor, P.J., Copeland, E.M. *et al.* (1977) Effect of cholecystokinin on myoelectric activity of small bowel of the dog. *American Journal of Physiology*, **232**, E44–E47.

65. Niederam, C., Heindinges, T., Rovati, I. and Strohmeyer, G. (1989) Effect of oxiglumide on gallbladder emptying in healthy subjects. *Gastroenterology*, **97**, 1331–1336.

66. Ovist, N., Oster-Jorgensen, E., Rasmussen, I. *et al.* (1988) The relationship between gallbladder dynamics and the migrating motor complex in fasting healthy subjects. *Scandinavian Journal of Gastroenterology*, **23**, 562–566.

67. Owyang, C., Green, L. and Reader, L.J. (1983) Colonic phase of pancreatic and biliary secretion in man. *Gastroenterology*, **84**, 470–475.

68. Peeters, T.L., Vantrappen, G. and Janssens, J. (1980) Bile acid output and the interdigestive migrating complex in normals and in cholecystectomy patients. *Gastroenterology*, **79**, 678–681.

69. Pike, R.L. and Brown, M.L. (1975) *Nutrition: An Integrated Approach*, 2nd edn. New York: Wiley.

70. Preshaw, R.M. (1970) Gastric acid output after sham feeding and during release or infusion of gastrin. *American Journal of Physiology*, **219**, 1409–1416.

71. Read, N.W., McFarlane, A., Kinsman, R.I. *et al.* (1983) Effect of infusion of nutrient solutions into the ileum on gastrointestinal transit and plasma levels of neurotensin and enteroglucagon. *Gastroenterology*, **86**, 224–230.

72. Rees, W.D.W., Go, V.L.W. and Malagelada, J.-R. (1979) Antroduodenal motor response to solid-liquid and homogenized meals. *Gastroenterology*, **76**, 1438–1442.

73. Rees, W.D.W., Go, V.L.W. and Malagelada, J.-R. (1979) Simultaneous measurement of antroduodenal motility, gastric emptying and duodenogastric reflux in man. *Gut*, **20**, 963–970.

74. Rees, W.D.W., Malagelada, J.-R., Miller, L.J. and Go, V.L.W. (1982) Human interdigestive and postprandial gastrointestinal motor and gastrointestinal hormone patterns. *Digestive Diseases and Sciences*, **27**, 321–329.

75. Richardson, C.T., Walsh, J.H., Cooper, K.A. *et al.* (1977) Studies on the role of cephalic-vagal stimulation in the acid secretory response to eating in normal human subjects. *Journal of Clinical Investigation*, **60**, 435–441.

76. Robinson, C.H. (1968) *Normal and Therapeutic Nutrition*. New York: Macmillan.

77. Ruppin, H., Bar-Meir, S., Soergel, K.H. and Wood, C.M. (1979) Effects of liquid diets on proximal gastrointestinal function. *Gastroenterology*, **77**, 1231 (abstract).

78. Ryan, J. and Cohen, S. (1977) Effect of vasoactive intestinal peptide on basal and cholecystokinin-induced gallbladder pressure. *Gastroenterology*, **73**, 870–872.

79. Sarles, H., Dani, R., Preselin, G., Souville, C. and Figarella, C. (1968) Cephalic phase of pancreatic secretion in man. *Gut*, **9**, 214–221.

80. Schaffalitzky de Muckadell, O.B. and Fahrenkrug, J. (1978) Secretion pattern of secretin in man: regulation by gastric acid. *Gut*, 19, 812–818.

81. Schiller, L.R., Walsh, J.H. and Feldman, M. (1980) Distension induced gastrin-release and gastric acid secretion. *Gastroenterology*, **78**, 912–917.

82. Scott, R.B. and Diamont, S.C. (1988) Biliary motility associated with gallbladder storage and duodenal delivery of canine hepatic biliary output. *Gastroenterology*, **95**, 1069–1080.

83. Solcia, E., Capella, C. and Buffa, R. (1987) Endocrine cells of the digestive system. In: *Physiology of the Gastrointestinal Tract*, pp. 111–130 (Ed.) Johnson, L.R. New York: Raven Press.

84. Solomon, T.E. and Grossman, M.I. (1977) Cholecystokinin and secretin release are not affected by vagotomy or atropine. *Gastroenterology*, **72**, 1134(abstract).

85. Solomon, T.E. and Grossman, M.E. (1979) Effect of atropine and vagotomy on response of transplanted pancreas. *American Journal of Physiology*, **236**, E186–E190.

86. Stadaas, J. and Aune, S. (1970) Intragastric pressure–volume relationship before and after vagotomy. *Acta Chirurgica Scandinavica*, **136**, 611–615.

87. Stenquist, B. (1979) Studies on vagal activation of gastric acid secretion in man. *Acta Physiologica Scandinavica Supplementum*, **465**, 7–31.

88. Svenberg, T., Christofides, N.D., Fitzpatrick, M.L. *et al.* (1982) Interdigestive biliary output in man. Relationship to fluctuations in plasma motilin and the effects of atropine. *Gut*, **23**, 1024–1028.

89. Szurszewski, J.H. (1969) A migrating electric complex of the canine small intestine. *American Journal of Physiology*, **217**, 1757–1763.

90. Tache, Y. (1987) Central nervous system regulation of gastric acid secretion. In: *Physiology of the Gastrointestinal Tract*, 2nd edn, pp. 911–927 (Ed.) Johnson, L.R. New York: Raven Press.

91. Thomas, P.A. and Kelly, K.A. (1979) Hormonal control of the interdigestive motor cycle of the canine proximal stomach. *American Journal of Physiology*, **237**, E192–E197.

92. Thomas, P.A., Schang, J.C., Kelly, K.A. and Go, V.L.W. (1980) Can endogenous gastrin inhibit canine interdigestive gastric motility? *Gastroenterology*, **78**, 716–721.

93. Tiscornia, O.M., Gullo, L., Mott, C.B. *et al.* (1973) The effects of intragastric ethanol administration upon canine exocrine pancreatic secretion. *Digestion*, **9**, 490–501.

94. Uvnas-Wallensten, K., Efendic, S. and Luft, R. (1977) Vagal release of somatostatin into the antral lumen of cats. *Acta Physiologica Scandinavica*, **99**, 126–128.

95. Vagne, M. and Grossman, M.I. (1969) Gastric and pancreatic secretion in response to gastric distension in dogs. *Gastroenterology*, **57**, 300–310.

96. Vantrappen, G.R., Peeters, T.L. and Janssens, J. (1979) The secretory component of the interdigestive migrating motor complex in man. *Scandinavian Journal of Gastroenterology*, **14**, 663–667.

97. Vantrappen, G., Janssens, J., Hellemans, J. and Ghoos, Y. (1977) The interdigestive motor complex of normal subjects and patients with bacterial overgrowth of the small intestine. *Journal of Clinical Investigation*, **59**, 1158–1166.

98. Vidon, N., Hecketsweiler, P., Butel, J. and Bernier, J.J. (1978) Effect of continuous jejunal perfusion of elemental and complex nutritional solutions on pancreatic enzyme secretion in human subjects. *Gut*, **19**, 194–198.

99. Walsh, J.H., Richardson, C.T. and Fordtran, J.S. (1975) pH dependence of acid secretion and gastrin release in normal and ulcer subjects. *Journal of Clinical Investigation*, **55**, 462–468.

100. Walz, D.A., Wider, M.D., Snow, J.W. *et al.* (1988) The complete amino acid sequence of porcine gastrotropin, an ileal protein which stimulates gastric acid and pepsinogen secretion. *Journal of Biological Chemistry*, **263**, 14189–14195.

101. Watanabe, S., Chey, W.Y., Lee, K.Y. and Chang, T.M. (1986) Secretin is released by digestive products of fat in dogs. *Gastroenterology*, **90**, 1008–1017.

102. Weisbrodt, N.W., Copeland, E.M., Kearley, R.W. *et al.* (1974) Effects of pentagastrin on electrical activity of small intestine of the dog. *American Journal of Physiology*, **227**, 425–429.

103. Wilen, T., Gustavasson, S. and Jung, B. (1983) Effects of a fatty meal on small bowel propulsion in intact and vagotomised dogs. *European Surgical Research*, **13**, 114–118.

104. Wilner, I., Inove, K., Fagan, C.J. *et al.* (1981) Release of CCK in man. Correlation of blood levels with gallbladder contraction. *Annals of Surgery*, **194**, 321–325.

DIGESTION AND MALABSORPTION OF NUTRIENTS

DIGESTION AND MALABSORPTION OF CARBOHYDRATE *(R.C. Spiller)*

DIETARY SOURCES

Worldwide, carbohydrate is the major energy source of humans, accounting for 40–60% of dietary calories in a Western diet and up to 80% in poorer countries. Dietary carbohydrate is nearly all plant derived, mainly in the form of storage polysaccharides such as starch, which accounts for 64% of UK dietary carbohydrate. The disaccharides sucrose and lactose account for a further 26 and 6%, while the monosaccharides fructose and glucose provide 3 and 1%, respectively.

As all carbohydrates must be reduced to the monosaccharides glucose, galactose or fructose prior to absorption, considerable effort is expended in food processing to aid their extraction from food. These processes include grinding and cooking, which disrupt indigestible structural components allowing access of human digestive enzymes to the digestible parts. This is particularly important for potato starch, which unlike cereal starch is very poorly digested unless it is first cooked.[12] Non-starch polysaccharides such as cellulose, pectin and hemicelluloses are polymers of both hexose and pentose sugars which form the cell walls and other structural components of plants. Although these pass virtually unaltered through the small intestine[9] they are not unimportant since they form gels which trap water and, by increasing the viscosity of the luminal contents, reduce the initial rate of monosaccharide absorption and, by virtue of their indigestibility, increase flow into the colon.[11] A small proportion of starch (1–5%) is 'resistant starch' which cannot be hydrolysed by amylase and therefore passes undigested into the colon where it acts as a nutrient for colonic bacteria. The overall digestibility of starch is improved substantially by grinding and cooking, which increases the surface area/volume ratio, facilitating enzymic attack. Cooking also helps by destroying naturally occurring amylase inhibitors found in whole wheat.[54]

PHYSIOLOGY OF DIGESTION AND CARBOHYDRATE

Digestion begins in the mouth with the action of salivary amylase, which is however inactive at the low pH found in the stomach.[53] Digestion continues in the less acidic media of the small intestine where pancreatic amylase cleaves polysaccharides to oligosaccharides (less than six monomers) which are then acted on by brush border hydrolases to yield monosaccharides which are then transported across the mucosa.

Starch hydrolysis

Starch is a glucose polymer (molecular weight $> 10^6$) composed mostly of amylopectin, α-$(1\rightarrow4)$-linked chains of glucose cross-linked every 20–30 glucose units by an α-$(1\rightarrow6)$ link. About 10–20% of starch is pure α-$(1\rightarrow4)$-linked glucose chains known as amylose. These details are significant because salivary and pancreatic amylase act selectively to cleave α-$(1\rightarrow4)$ bonds in the middle of polymer chains, but not α-$(1\rightarrow6)$ or α-$(1\rightarrow4)$ bonds adjacent to the end of a polymer. It follows therefore (*Figure 3.23*) that the luminal products of starch hydrolysis are maltose, maltotriose and a range of glucose polymers (chain length 5–6) known as α-limit dextrins. Very little free glucose is released by amylase, the process of digestion being completed by brush border hydrolysis. About 10% of the protein of the brush border membrane is formed by high molecular weight glycoprotein (200 kDa) hydrolytic enzymes which are actively synthesized in the cytosol, glycosylated in the Golgi apparatus and then inserted into the microvillous membrane. The active enzyme site protrudes from the membrane and, under the influence of pancreatic proteases, is shed into the lumen to be replaced by newly synthesized enzyme.[2] The enzymes sucrase–isomaltase, maltase, glucoamylase, lactase and trehalase have similar structures, but differ in specificity for cleaving various bonds, as shown in *Table 3.2*. Glucoamylase cleaves α-$(1\rightarrow4)$ bonds at the non-reducing end of linear α-$(1\rightarrow4)$-linked glucose chains, yielding free

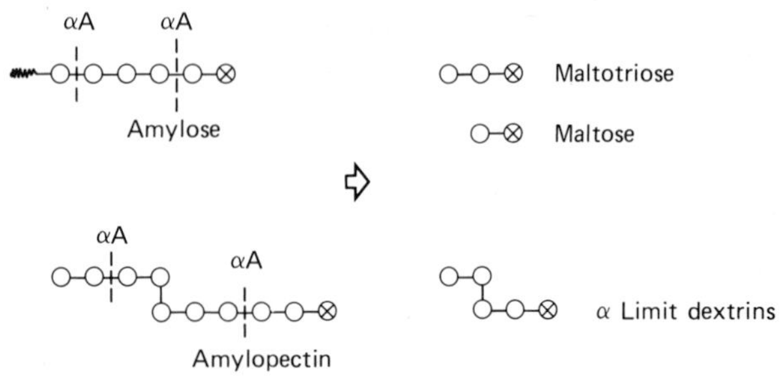

Figure 3.23 Luminal digestion of starch by pancreatic α-amylase (αA). O, glucose units; $\otimes$, reducing glucose unit. Horizontal links indicate α-$(1\rightarrow4)$ bonds, vertical links indicate α-$(1\rightarrow6)$ bonds.

Table 3.2 Brush border hydrolysis of carbohydrates

Carbohydrate	Enzyme	Action	Product
Sucrose	Sucrase	Hydrolysis of α-(1→4) link	Glucose, fructose
Maltose and maltotriose	Glucoamylase or sucrase	Sequential removal of glucosyl residues from non-reducing end	Glucose
α-limit dextrins	Glucoamylase or isomaltase	Initial removal of α-(1→4) linked glucosyl residues from non-reducing end	Glucose and oligosaccharide with terminal α-(1→6) linked glucose
	Isomaltase	Cleavage of α-(1→6) linked glucose residue	Glucose and malto-oligosaccharide
	Sucrase or glucoamylase	Hydrolysis of released malto-oligosaccharides	Glucose
Lactose	Lactase	Hydrolysis of β-(1→4) linkage	Glucose and galactose

Modified from Gray, G.M. (1981) In: *Physiology of the Gastrointestinal Tract*, pp. 1063–1072 (Ed.) Johnson, L.R. New York: Raven Press.

glucose from maltose, maltotriose and α-limit dextrins, whose further digestion requires the cleaving of α-(1→6) bonds by isomaltase. Trehalase catalyses the hydrolysis of trehalose, a disaccharide found mainly in young mushrooms and hence of little clinical significance. Sucrase and isomaltase are linked, being derived from a single precursor polypeptide chain, sequencing of which suggests that this arose because of partial duplication of the gene coding for isomaltase leading to a double isomaltase polypeptide. One end of this polypeptide appears to have undergone mutation to produce an active site capable of splitting sucrose.[22]

Hydrolysis is rapid, so that monosaccharide transport is usually the rate-limiting step in absorption, the only exception being lactose, whose hydrolysis is slower than other disaccharides.[17] Excessive accumulation of monosaccharide would set up an osmotic gradient which would impair water absorption, a situation which does not in fact happen owing to a feedback inhibition whereby the products of hydrolysis inhibit the relevant enzymes.[1]

Monosaccharide transport

Small intestinal enterocytes in humans and animals show active energy-dependent uptake of glucose and galactose. The absorption of fructose is apparently passive and substantially less rapid.[15,20,24]

The absorptive capacity of the small intestine for glucose and galactose is enormous and well in excess of any quantity likely to be ingested, provided motility is normal. The same is not true of fructose, malabsorption being noted in a number of otherwise normal subjects after as little as 37.5 g orally,[48] an amount easily ingested in the form of a few glasses of concentrated fruit juice, or confectionery for diabetics sweetened with fructose.

Glucose–galactose transport

Postprandial luminal concentrations of glucose are often much higher than cellular levels so that much glucose absorption could be passive. However, experimental studies demonstrate active, energy-dependent, saturable glucose–galactose transport linked to Na^+ absorption.

In vitro studies on vesicles created from brush border membranes show that the whole human small intestine contains a high-affinity, low-flux transport system suitable for transporting glucose against a concentration gradient, while in the proximal small intestine there is in addition a low-affinity, high-flux system better suited to rapid absorption from the relatively high glucose concentrations likely to be found postprandially in the region.[18] Similar low- and high-affinity systems for glucose transport exist proximally and distally in the nephron, no doubt evolved to deal with a similar problem of high proximal but low distal glucose concentrations.[4]

Recently, there have been major advances in our understanding of these transport processes. The Na^+/glucose co-transporter had been identified and

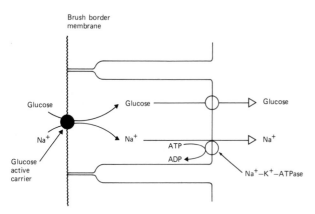

Figure 3.24 Model of active transport of glucose across intestinal epithelial cells. Glucose enters the cell by an Na^+-dependent carrier molecule in the brush border, and leaves via a separate Na^+-independent carrier in the basolateral membrane. The energy needed to operate the brush border carrier is derived from the gradient of Na^+ across the cell membrane which is maintained by Na^+/K^+-dependent ATPase.

its DNA code sequenced.[19] The molecule contains 662 amino acid residues and from its sequence a likely tertiary structure has been devised and the binding sites of Na^+ and glucose separately identified. Two Na^+ ions bind to the carrier protein, increasing its affinity for glucose.[45] The charged Na^+/glucose carrier protein (*Figure 3.24*) then moves down the electrochemical gradient created by the active pumping of Na^+ out of the cell at the basal lateral membrane. On entering the low-Na^+ cytosol, Na^+ leaves the carrier protein, causing its affinity for glucose to fall, leading to the release of glucose as well. The now negatively charged protein is then propelled back to the membrane via electrostatic forces.[26] Fructose is transported by an independent stereospecific carrier[50] which facilitates passive diffusion down the concentration gradients.

CLINICAL FEATURES OF DISORDERED CARBOHYDRATE DIGESTION

The consequences of maldigestion vary with the type of carbohydrate. Osmotically active small molecules like lactose, if not hydrolysed and absorbed, result in large fluid fluxes into the small intestine as water and sodium move down osmotic and concentration gradients. Malabsorption of 50 g of lactose results in about 1 litre of extra fluid entering the colon[7] with symptoms of abdominal colic, flatulence and diarrhoea. Malabsorption of fructose and sucrose have similar effects[48] while malabsorption of the osmotically less active 'resistant starches' leads to much less disturbance.

Colonic bacteria are quite able to metabolize substantial amounts of carbohydrate to short-chain fatty acids which can then be absorbed.[30] This 'colonic salvage' can be overwhelmed if large amounts of fluid also enter the colon, as is seen with lactulose treatment.[56] At standard therapeutic doses of 30 g/day there is a marked reduction in right colonic residence time from approximately 12 to 7 hours. This prevents completion of the degradation and bacterial fermentation processes which are much slower than normal digestion. The result is appearance of unabsorbed starch or sugar in the stool, which becomes frothy and offensive. Children have a relatively shorter and less effective colon than adults and are much more likely to suffer severe symptoms. Most inherited disorders of carbohydrate absorption therefore present in early childhood with failure to thrive, abdominal pain, distension and diarrhoea. Reducing sugar may be detected in the stool using 'Clinitest' tablets.[25] Adults often minimize symptoms by avoiding the relevant foods such as milk, which they have learnt to associate with symptoms. The usual threshold for developing symptoms varies from as little as 10 to as much 50 g. However, it should be noted that total exclusion is not required and that modest amounts of milk are unlikely to cause symptoms, while a whole glass of milk containing approximately 10 g of lactose may well do so.

Specific disorders

Pancreatic insufficiency

Pancreatic enzymes appear to be superabundant because, when α-amylase inhibitors are used, more than 90% inhibition is required before starch malabsorption is noted with increased ileal flow and delivery of carbohydrate to the colon.[29] Under these circumstances, about 1 hour after the meal gastric emptying slows up, probably due to feedback inhibition caused by the presence of excess carbohydrate in the ileum. This is probably analogous to the 'ileal brake' previously described in response to fat infusion into the ileum.[55] This moderates the otherwise excessively rapid gastric emptying characteristic of pancreatic disease in which the normal feedback from the duodenum from gastric emptying is lost, owing to the lack of luminal hydrolysis of starch. These studies have been done with the aid of naturally occurring amylase inhibitors, which have been proposed as a means of improving glucose tolerance in diabetics or reducing weight in obesity. Unfortunately the symptoms of starch malabsorption are unpleasant, including flatulence, abdominal pain and diarrhoea, and one doubts that these treatments will prove acceptable to patients.

Specific enzyme deficiencies

Lactase deficiency is the commonest specific enzyme deficiency encountered, being found in nearly all adults in some races, the incidence in Europeans (1 in 10) being the lowest of any race. Other enzyme disorders are great rarities but nevertheless important because symptoms are often severe. Hyposucrasia may occur in 0.2% of North Americans while glucose–galactose malabsorption has only been described in a few individuals. Trehalase deficiency is rare, interesting but clinically irrelevant since symptoms only occur if one takes very substantial amounts of young mushrooms.[34]

LACTASE DEFICIENCY

Until recently it was traditional to distinguish congenital hypolactasia from adult or acquired hypolactasia, the congenital form being clinically much more severe than the adult form. However, as the molecular basis of the defect is probed it appears likely that in both cases the defect lies in the regulatory genes controlling synthesis of the enzyme rather than a mutant or defective enzyme.[13,52] Furthermore, traces of normal enzyme are present even in the congenital form, suggesting that apart from the variable age of onset the conditions have a similar underlying pathology. Of course, since neonates take upwards of 2 g/kg in body weight of milk for feed, lactose intolerance has a much more marked effect than in an adult who ingests less than 0.1 g/kg body weight per day.

The decline in lactase levels after birth is a normal phenomena in most mammals and, world-wide, lactase persistence is anomalous, being much commoner in populations who have traditionally had access to milk (see *Table 3.3*), presumably because it conferred survival advantages during reproductive life. This fall in lactase levels after weaning appears

to be genetically determined, inherited as an autosomal recessive characteristic.[49]

Although some studies have suggested that, in the laboratory rat, lactase levels are influenced by lactose intake, the effect is small compared to the 10-fold fall in lactase after weaning. Most human studies suggest that lactose ingestion does not prevent the development of hypolactasia nor does it appear to alter mucosal enzyme levels.[14]

As already mentioned, in neonates, hypolactasia is severe in its consequences since lactose is their major energy source. Severe diarrhoea, dehydration and failure to thrive occurs, with frothy stools testing positive for sugars. A lactose-free diet cures the diarrhoea and allows normal weight gain. Since lactose intolerance is very common in a host of other intestinal diseases including viral gastroenteritis, small bowel contamination and drug-induced mucosal injury as well as gluten sensitivity it is important to exclude these underlying diseases. In the 1960s there were a number of reports of lactose intolerance in which lactose tolerance tests showed the absorptions of intact lactose and, as a consequence, lactosuria. These children were all severely malnourished, with diarrhoea and failure to thrive. No new reports have been made and it is now recognized that lactosuria is a non-specific finding in neonates. It seems likely that these patients had some temporary disorder of small intestinal permeability since some years later they appeared to tolerate milk normally.[21]

Symptoms of lactose intolerance become less obvious as the age of onset increases, probably because adults with hypolactasia generally learn to avoid foods containing lactose. When intake is not voluntarily controlled, as for example during enteral feeding via a nasogastric tube, then hypolactasia is associated not only with increased stool but also malabsorption of fat, owing to acceleration of small bowel transit and dilution of digestive enzymes.[27,28,43]

Table 3.3 Incidence of hypolactasia in various ethnic groups[51]

Ethnic group	Incidence of hypolactasia (%)
Southern Nigerians	100
Chinese	100
Japanese	65
Danes	2–3
Finns	6–17
Southern Italians	100
Cypriots	100
American whites	10–15
American blacks	45–77
Eskimos	4
Asians	27–33

Investigation

The diagnosis of mucosal hypolactasia rests most firmly on enzymic assay of a mucosal biopsy. This is tedious, invasive and time-consuming, and many methods have been evolved to make the diagnosis more simple. After an oral dose of lactose, blood glucose and galactose levels rise. Lack of a rise may reflect hypolactasia but can also unfortunately be due to other causes such as delayed gastric emptying or accelerated glucose metabolism. Fortunately, the test which correlates best with the symptoms of lactose malabsorption, the lactose breath hydrogen test, proves also to be the least invasive.[42] This assesses the amount of lactose malabsorbed from the rise in breath hydrogen which occurs as colonic bacteria ferment the lactose which passes into the colon.

Clinical significance of hypolactasia
Most patients with hypolactasia will have few symptoms either because they take little lactose or because when taken with food which delays gastric emptying, the rate of delivery to the small intestine fails to overwhelm its absorptive capacity.[35] However, patients with mucosal disease such as coeliac disease,[6] short bowel syndrome, or with otherwise limited absorptive reserves, who also suffer from hypolactasia are much more likely to have symptoms which will respond to lactose restriction. This is especially true if they are mistakenly ingesting milk under the belief that the abdominal pain they are suffering from is due to a peptic ulcer. Nearly two-thirds of newborn infants develop evening colic in the first few months of life which have many features of lactose intolerance. Colicky infants appear to malabsorb significantly more lactose than those who do not have colic when assessed by breath hydrogen production after a standard dose of lactose.[40] Fortunately, this is usually a transitory phase which disappears on weaning to solid food which does of course have a much lower lactose content.

Treatment
Strict lactose exclusion is not usually necessary since there is usually a threshold below which no symptoms are experienced.[33] Patients can either avoid excessive amounts of milk or take milk in the form of fresh yoghurt, which contains abundant bacterial lactase. This reaches the duodenum in an active state[47] and reduces lactose malabsorption and associated symptoms.[44] Unfortunately, in practice few patients tolerate fresh yoghurt owing to its unfamiliar and bitter taste. Bacterial lactase can be taken in tablet form but this is much less effective than yoghurt.

SUCRASE–ISOMALTASE DEFICIENCY (HYPOSUCRASIA)
Modern Western diets include a substantial quantity of sucrose, a disaccharide which can only be absorbed after hydrolysis to its constituent monomers, glucose and fructose. Patients with sucrase–isomaltase deficiency appear to have no enzyme rather than an inactive variant.[3,16] This deficiency is inherited as an autosomal recessive trait, with asymptomatic heterozygous family members having a reduction in enzyme activity. Although rare in North America (0.2%)[46], it occurs in 10% of Eskimos in western Greenland[36] where, until recently, it had no significance as sucrose was not part of the diet.

Clinical features
Watery explosive diarrhoea with abdominal colic and failure to thrive begins as soon as the child is weaned on to sucrose-containing foods, especially sucrose-sweetened fruit juices.

Investigations
The stool is often acidic, frothy and, after heating to accelerate the hydrolysis of sucrose, will test positive with 'Clinitest' tablets or glucose indicator strips. Sucrose exclusion cures the diarrhoea while sucrose tolerance tests (dose 2 g/kg) result in a flat blood glucose curve and diarrhoea. As with lactose tolerance testing, one can avoid the trauma of blood sampling in a small child by performing a sucrose breath hydrogen test, giving 25 g of sucrose and measuring the breath hydrogen for 30-minute intervals for 3 hours. Sucrose malabsorption results in a rise in breath hydrogen greater than 20 ppm while in normal subjects even 100 g of sucrose gives no rise.[39] Symptoms usually decline with age as colonic salvage improves and the patients learn to avoid the relevant food. However, the diagnosis may sometimes be delayed until adult life and should always be borne in mind when investigating obscure watery diarrhoea.[41]

GLUCOSE–GALACTOSE MALABSORPTION
Patients with this rare, autosomal recessive trait absorb glucose–galactose at a rate only 10% of normal.[32,38] Only a small number of cases of this condition, which presumably reflects absence of the glucose–galactose carrier, have been described.[37] All presented with diarrhoea from birth which could only be controlled by the use of milk-free feeds, usually based on sucrose or fructose. Untreated, dehydration, acidosis and nephrocalcinosis lead to an early death although the occasional patient appears to have survived undiagnosed until adult life.[23] Intestinal perfusion and biopsy studies have shown that, while jejunal morphology and disaccharidase levels are normal, glucose absorption is depressed.[10] Defective monosaccharide absorption cannot be compensated for by uptake of intact disaccharide but, fortunately for these patients, fructose absorption appears to be normal. As with hypolactasia, sugar load is important in determining symptoms, so that while milk leads to violent diarrhoea, slowly digested starches, such as from potatoes, may be tolerated with only minor symptoms. Infants must therefore be maintained on a glucose-galactose-free diet, but once they are weaned to solid food the diet can be liberalized.[37]

FRUCTOSE MALABSORPTION
As already mentioned, fructose is less well absorbed than glucose and otherwise normal subjects may

develop diarrhoea and symptoms of sugar malabsorption after as little as 37.5 g of fructose taken in a liquid form.[48] Indeed, excessive fructose intake in the form of fruit juice can be the often overlooked cause of chronic diarrhoea in otherwise healthy children.[24] This should be clearly distinguished from hereditary fructose intolerance, a disorder of fructose metabolism due to the absence of the hepatic enzyme fructose-1-phosphate aldolase. Oral or intravenous fructose loading produces marked hypoglycaemia with associated sweating and faintness, but fructose absorption is quite normal.[5,8]

Sugar malabsorption secondary to mucosal diseases

Mucosal diseases, especially coeliac disease,[6] tropical sprue, giardiasis and small bowel contamination, can lead to sugar intolerance. Lactase levels are often borderline in adults and the added mucosal insult often leads to symptomatic lactose intolerance. The much greater reserve absorptive capacity for glucose and sucrose means that symptomatic intolerance of these sugars is much less common. However, small bowel contamination with generalized monosaccharide intolerance has been described in malnourished children from the tropics. This appeared to respond to antibiotic therapy and, 2 months later, monosaccharide absorption was quite normal.[31]

Drug-induced sugar malabsorption

Drugs toxic to the mucosa may inhibit disaccharidase levels, e.g. neomycin, as an unintended side-effect. In addition, disaccharidases can be deliberately inhibited by molecules designed to bind to the active site of the enzyme. The best known of these inhibitors, acarbose, binds to sucrase–isomaltase and substantially reduces sucrose and glucose oligosaccharide digestion and absorption, leading to colic, diarrhoea and flatulence. By titrating the dose it is possible to reduce the glycaemic response to a meal without inducing symptoms, raising the possibility of its use in improving glycaemic control in diabetes.[57]

References

1. Alpers, D.H. and Cote, M.N. (1971) Inhibition of lactose hydrolysis by dietary sugars. *American Journal of Physiology*, **221**, 865–868.
2. Alpers, D.H. and Tedesco, F.J. (1975) The possible role of pancreatic proteases in the turnover of intestinal brush border proteins. *Biochimica et Biophysica Acta*, **401**, 28–40.
3. Ament, M.E., Perera, D.R. and Esther, E.J. (1973) Sucrase–isomaltase deficiency – a frequently misdiagnosed disease. *Journal of Paediatrics*, **83**, 721–727.
4. Baly, D.L. and Horuk, R. (1988) The biology and biochemistry of the glucose transporter. *Biochemica Biophysica Acta*, **947**, 571–590.
5. Black, J.A. and Simpson, K. (1967) Fructose intolerance. *British Medical Journal*, **iv**, 138–141.
6. Bode, S. and Gudmand-Hoyer, E. (1988) Incidence and clinical significance of lactose malabsorption in adult coeliac disease. *Scandinavian Journal of Gastroenterology*, **23**, 484–488.
7. Christopher, N.L. and Bayless, T.M. (1971) Role of the small bowel and colon in lactose induced diarrhoea. *Gastroenterology*, **60**, 845–852.
8. Cox, T.M., Camilleri, M., O'Donnell, M.W. *et al.* (1982) Pseudo dominant transmission of fructose intolerance in an adult and three offspring – heterozygote detection by intestinal biopsy. *New England Journal of Medicine*, **307**, 537–540.
9. Englyst, H.N. and Cummings, J.H. (1985) Digestion of the polysaccharides of some cereal foods in the human small intestine. *American Journal of Clinical Nutrition*, **42**, 778–787.
10. Fairclough, P.O., Clark, M.L., Dawson, A.M., Silk, D.B.A., Milla, P.J. and Harries, J.T. (1978) Absorption of glucose and maltose in congenital glucose–galactose malabsorption. *Pediatric Research*, **12**, 1112–1114.
11. Flourie, B., Vidon, N., Florent, C.H. and Bernier, J.J. (1984) Effect of pectin on jejunal glucose absorption and unstirred layer thickness in normal man. *Gut*, **25**, 936–941.
12. Fleming, S.E. and Vose, J.R. (1979) Digestibility of raw and cooked starches from legume seeds using the laboratory rat. *Journal of Nutrition*, **109**, 2067–2075.
13. Freiburghaus, A.M., Schmitz, J., Schindler, M. *et al.* (1976) Protein patterns of brush border fragments in congenital lactose malabsorption and in specific hypolactasia of the adult. *New England Journal of Medicine*, **294**, 1030–1032.
14. Gilat, T., Russo, S., Gelman-Malachi, E. and Aldor, T.A.M. (1972) Lactase in man: a non adaptable enzyme. *Gastroenterology*, **62**, 1125–1127.
15. Gracey, M., Burke, V. and Oshiri, A. (1972) Active intestinal transport of D-fructose. *Biochemica Biophysica Acta*, **266**, 397–406.
16. Gray, G.M., Conklin, K.A. and Townley, R.R.W. (1976) Sucrase–isomaltase deficiency. Absence of an inactive enzyme variant. *New England Journal of Medicine*, **294**, 750–753.
17. Gray, G.M. and Santiago, N.A. (1969) Disaccharide absorption in normal and diseased intestine. *Gastroenterology*, **51**, 489–498.
18. Harig, J.M., Barry, J.A., Rajendram, V.M., Soergel, K.H. and Ramaswamy, K. (1989) D-Glucose and L-leucine transport by human intestinal brush-border membrane residues. *American Journal of Physiology*, **256**, G618–G623.
19. Hediger, M.A., Coady, M.J., Ikeda, T.J. and

Wright, E.M. (1987) Expression cloning and cDNA sequencing of the Na$^+$/glucose co-transporter. *Nature*, **330**, 379–381.

20. Holdsworth, C.D. and Dawson, A.M. (1964) The absorption of monosaccharides in man. *Clinical Science*, **27**, 371–379.

21. Hotzel, A., Mereu, T. and Thompson, M.L. (1962) Severe lactose intolerance in infancy. *The Lancet*, **ii**, 1346–1348.

22. Hu, C.-B., Spiess, M. and Semenza, C. (1987) The mode of anchoring and precursor forms of sucrase–isomaltase and maltase–glucoamylase in chicken intestinal brush-border membrane. Phylogenetic implications. *Biochemica et Biophysica Acta*, **896**, 275–286.

23. Hughes, W.S. and Senior, J.R. (1975) The glucose–galactose malabsorption syndrome in a 21 year old woman. *Gastroenterology*, **68**, 142–145.

24. Hyams, J.S. and Leichtner, A.M. Apple juice: an unappreciated cause of chronic diarrhoea. *American Journal of Diseases in Childhood*, **139**, 503–505.

25. Kerry, K.R. and Anderson, C.M. (1964) A ward test for sugar in faeces. *The Lancet*, **i**, 1981.

26. Kimmick, G.A. and Carter-Su, C. (1978) Membrane potentials and the energetics of intestinal Na$^+$-dependent transport systems. *American Journal of Physiology*, **235**, C73–C81.

27. Launiala, K. (1968a) The mechanism of diarrhoea in congenital disaccharide malabsorption. *Acta Paediatrica Scandinavica*, **57**, 425–432.

28. Launiala, K. (1968b) The effect of unabsorbed sucrose and mannitol on the small intestinal flow rate and mean transit time. *Scandinavian Journal of Gastroenterology*, **39**, 665–671.

29. Layer, P., Zinsmeister, A.R. and DiMagno, E.P. (1986) Effects of decreasing intraluminal amylase activity on starch digestion and postprandial gastrointestinal function in humans. *Gastroenterology*, **91**, 41–48.

30. Levitt, M.D. (1983) Malabsorption of starch: a normal phenomenon. *Gastroenterology*, **85**, 769–770.

31. Lifshitz, F., Coello-Ramirez, P., Gutierrez-Topet, G. *et al.* (1971) Carbohydrate intolerance in infants with diarrhoea. *Journal of Pediatrics*, **79**, 760–767.

32 Lindquist, B., Meeuwisse, G.W. and Melin, K. (1962) Glucose–galactose malabsorption. *The Lancet*, **ii**, 666.

33. Lisker, R., Aguilar, L. and Zavala, C. (1978) Intestinal lactase deficiency and milk drinking capacity in the adult. *American Journal of Clinical Nutrition*, **31**, 1499–1503.

34. Madzarovova-Nohejlova, J. (1973) Trehalase deficiency in a family. *Gastroenterology*, **65**, 130–133.

35. Martini, M.C. and Saraiano, D.A. (1988) Reduced intolerance symptoms from lactose consumed during a meal. *American Journal of Clinical Nutrition*, **47**, 57–60.

36. McNair, A., Gudmand-Hoyer, E., Jarnum, S. and

Orrild, L. (1972) Sucrose malabsorption in Greenland. *British Medical Journal*, **ii**, 19–21.

37. Meeuwisse, G.W. and Melin, K. (1969) Studies in glucose–galactose malabsorption a classical study of 6 cases and a genetic study. *Acta Paediatrica Scandinavica Supplementum*, **188**, 1–24.

38. Meeuwisse, G.W. and Dahlquist, A. (1968) Glucose-galactose malabsorption: a study with biopsy of the small intestinal mucosa. *Acta Paediatrica Scandinavica*, **57**, 273–280.

39. Metz, G., Jenkins, O.J.A., Newman, A. and Blendis, L.M. (1976) Breath hydrogen in hyposucrasia. *The Lancet*, **i**, 119–120.

40. Moore, D.J., Robb, T.A., Davidson, G.P. (1988) Breath hydrogen response to milk containing lactose in colicky and non colicky infants. *Journal of Pediatrics*, **113**, 979–984.

41. Neale, G., Clark, M. and Levin, B. (1965) Intestinal sucrase deficiency presenting as sucrose intolerance in adult life. *British Medical Journal*, **ii**, 1223–1225.

42. Newcomer, A.D., McGill, D.B., Thomas, P.J. and Hofmann, A.F. (1975) Prospective comparison of indirect methods for detecting lactase deficiency. *New England Journal of Medicine*, **293**, 1232–1236.

43. O'Keefe, S.J.D., Adam, J.K., Cakata, E. and Epstein, S. (1984) Nutritional support of malnourished lactose intolerant African patients. *Gut*, **25**, 942–947.

44. Onwulata, C.I., Rao, D.R. and Vankineri, P. (1989) Relative efficiency of yogurt, sweet acidophilus milk, hydrolysed-lactose milk, and a commercial lactase tablet in alleviating lactose maldigestion. *American Journal of Clinical Nutrition*, **49**, 1233–1237.

45. Peerce, B.E. and Wright, E. M. (1984) Sodium-induced conformational changes in the glucose transporter of intestinal brush borders. *Journal of Biology and Chemistry*, **259**, 14105–14112.

46. Peterson, M.L. and Herber, R. (1967) Intestinal sucrase deficiency. *Transactions of the American Association of Physicians*, **80**, 275–283.

47. Pochart, P., Dewitt, O., Desjeux, J.-F. and Bourlioux, P. (1989) Viable starter culture, β-galactosidase activity, and lactose in duodenum after yoghurt ingestion in lactase-deficient humans. *American Journal of Clinical Nutrition*, **49**, 828–831.

48. Ravich, W.J., Bayless, T.M. and Thomas, M. (1983) Fructose: incomplete intestinal absorption in humans. *Gastroenterology*, **84**, 26–29.

49. Sahi, T., Isokoski, M., Jussila, J. *et al.* (1973) Recessive inheritance of adult-type lactose malabsorption. *The Lancet*, **ii**, 823–826.

50. Sigrist-Nelson, K. and Hopfer, U. (1974) A distinct D-fructose transport system in isolated brush border membrane. *Biochimica et Biophysica Acta*, **367**, 247–254.

51. Simoons, F.J. (1978) Geographic hypothesis and lactose malabsorption: a weighing of the evidence. *American Journal of Digestive Diseases*, **23**, 963–980.

52. Skovberg, H., Gudmand-Hoyer, E. and Fenger, H. (1980) Immunoelectrophoretic studies on human small intestinal brush border proteins: amount of lactase protein in adult-type hypolactasia. *Gut*, **21**, 360–364.

53. Skude, G. and Ihse, I. (1976) Salivary amylase in duodenal aspirates. *Scandinavian Journal of Gastroenterology*, **11**, 17–20.

54. Snow, P. and O'Dea, K. (1981) Factors affecting the rate of hydrolysis of starch in food. *American Journal of Clinical Nutrition*, **34**, 2721–2727.

55. Spiller, R.C., Trottman, I.F., Higgins, B.E. *et al.* (1984) The ileal brake – inhibition of jejunal motility after ileal gut perfusion in man. *Gut*, **25**, 365–374.

56. Steed, K.P., Watts, P.J., Blackshaw, P.E. *et al.* (1990) Reservoir function of the ascending colon demonstrated scintigraphically: effect of lactulose. *Gastroenterology*, **98**, A394.

57. Taylor, R.H., Barber, H.M., Bowey, E.A. and Canfield, J.E. (1986) Regulation of the absorption of dietary carbohydrate in man by two new glycosidase inhibitors. *Gut*, **27**, 1471–1478.

DIGESTION AND MALABSORPTION OF FAT *(P.L. Zentler-Munro and T.C. Northfield)*

The assimilation of fat into a largely aqueous organism poses particular problems, as fat is not miscible with water. The process by which humans digest and absorb dietary fat is more complex than that for protein and carbohydrate; it involves several organs in a coordinated series of events, and is therefore more subject to disturbance by disease.

The malassimilation (the term is used to indicate both maldigestion and true malabsorption) of fat is often obvious in the form of steatorrhoea, an unpleasant symptom for the patient and sometimes a threat to his or her nutrition. The clinician looks for steatorrhoea because it is more obvious than creatorrhoea or amylorrhoea, and because it is a more sensitive and specific indicator of alimentary disease.

A physicochemical process

Our understanding of the physiology of fat assimilation[5,6,36] has moved from the elucidation of the chemical processes involved, culminating in the seminal work of Hofmann and Borgström,[21] to the more recent investigation of the physical processes culminating in the recent contributions by Carey and co-workers.[18,35] The chemical work has been largely analytic and reductionist – involving the examin-

ation of biological samples – whilst the physical work has been both analytic and synthetic – involving also the examination of model mixtures of lipids. Classical teaching had it that the first steps were 'chemical' – the digestion of dietary fat into more polar compounds – and were followed by primarily 'physical' processes – the solubilization of these lipids into aqueous solution. This distinction is helpful but false: both chemical and physical forces act simultaneously and in complex coordination.

Dietary lipids

Most people normally eat between 70 and 150 g of fat daily, in the form principally of triglycerides, phospholipids and cholesterol. Triglycerides of animal origin contain largely saturated long-chain fatty acids, important as a source of energy; those of vegetable origin also contain unsaturated fatty acids which, with those of the phospholipids (principally lecithin), are essential in the synthesis of eicosanoids and in the structure of all cell membranes.[36] The influence of the chain length, saturation and configuration of triglyceride and phospholipid fatty acids on their aqueous solubility and mucosal uptake, and the relevance of this to nutrition, has only recently begun to be explored.[6,11,36]

NORMAL PHYSIOLOGY

Intragastric events

The role of the stomach in fat digestion has long been thought only a physical one: the creation of a coarse emulsion in the gastric antrum by the shearing force of the corpus contracting against the closed pylorus.[6] The emulsifiers are at first dietary protein, phospholipids and polysaccharides.

It is now clear, however, that a chemical process occurs in the stomach. The chief cells in the fundus secrete a true lipase[26] (capable of hydrolysing long-chain triglycerides). This gastric lipase was thought to originate in the tongue, and was therefore termed lingual lipase, but is now known to be of gastric origin in humans. The enzyme is peculiar in acting only in an acid environment (pH 3–5), as in the stomach. Its action is independent of colipase, and is not promoted by bile acids at the low concentrations in the stomach caused by bile reflux from the duodenum. It hydrolyses triglycerides incompletely to produce diglycerides and fatty acids at water interfaces at the surface of and within the oil droplet. The released fatty acid, when eventually ionized in the duodenum, contributes to further emulsification of the triglyceride. Released medium- and short-chain fatty acids can be absorbed in the stomach. The potential of this acid-stable lipase for therapeutic use is clear: the enzyme has been sequenced, cloned and prepared by biosynthesis.

The final contribution of the stomach is again a physical one – the sphincter action of the pylorus in releasing gastric contents at an appropriate rate into the duodenum, under the control of peptidergic reflexes originating in duodenal receptors. The emulsified lipid phase of gastric contents empties more slowly than the aqueous protein/carbohydrate phase, depending on the dietary presentation of the fat.[25] How this happens is not clear; it is not simply a result of density and gravity. The relevance of this delay in the gastroduodenal – and more distal – transit of fat to nutritional therapy is now being appreciated.

Intraduodenal events

The entry of chyme into the duodenum sets in motion a train of coordinated and interdependent chemical and physical events. The release of the two major digestive hormones secretin and cholecystokinin is mediated by the entry into the duodenum of acid and larger peptic digest peptides, respectively, and to a lesser extent by fatty acid released in the stomach. These hormones stimulate the pancreas to secrete bicarbonate and several digestive hydrolytic enzymes or proenzymes, including most relevantly here pancreatic lipase, phospholipase and colipase. They also stimulate the simultaneous contraction of the gallbladder to deliver a high concentration of the major digestive detergent – the amphipathic bile acids – into the duodenum. The lipase catalyses a chemical process: the hydrolysis of the substrate (emulsified triglycerides and diglycerides) to produce the *solute* (the more polar lipids – monoglycerides and fatty acids). The biliary amphipaths then act as *solvents* for a physical process: the solubilization of these solutes into aqueous *solution* mainly as micelles.

The first step is the neutralization of gastric effluent (pH 3–5) to near neutral (around pH 6) by bicarbonate secreted mainly by the pancreas. This process is largely completed by the duodenojejunal flexure. It is crucial to all the chemical and physical processes which achieve the necessary phase change (lipid to aqueous) which must precede absorption. The digestors – pancreatic lipase and phospholipase – are most active about pH 6, and are irreversibly inactivated below pH 5. The predominant solvents – glycine (but not taurine) conjugated bile salts – become protonated below pH 5 and precipitate out of solution. The major products of digestion and the ultimate solute – the fatty acids – become protonated below pH 6 and then return to the oil phase; the monoglycerides, being non-ionic, are not influenced by pH. Gastric lipase, on the other hand, is almost inactive at normal duodenal pH and its role is probably confined to the stomach in health.

Lipase is a surface-active enzyme. The emulsified lipids in the gastric effluent become coated with bile acid on entry into the duodenum, preventing access of the active site of the enzyme to its substrate. The function of the pancreatic coenzyme colipase is to penetrate the bile acids coating the emulsion and anchor the lipase to its substrate.[20] Fatty acids probably also contribute to this 'clearing' action: the addition of fatty acids overcomes the delay in the onset of triglyceride hydrolysis seen in the presence of lipase, colipase and bile acid *in vitro*.[3] The fatty acids produced by the rapid action of phospholipase on the more accessible biliary and dietary phospholipids serve this role *in vivo*; it now seems likely that fatty acids produced by intragastric lipolysis also contribute. The other product of phospholipolysis – lysolecithin – is more important in determining the capacity of the micelles to which it later contributes to solubilize, and ultimately release, neutral lipids and cholesterol.[6] A fourth enzyme, carboxyl-ester lipase, hitherto thought important in hydrolysis only of cholesterol and fat-soluble vitamin esters, may also contribute to the initial hydrolysis of triglyceride as it is not inhibited by bile acid.[23] We thus see four enzymes and one coenzyme coordinating in the process of fat digestion.

Pancreatic lipase hydrolyses long-chain dietary triglycerides, and diglycerides produced by lingual lipase, to their constituent monoglycerides and fatty acids; very little glycerol is produced. These more polar lipids are insoluble in water but can be solubilized in the lipid interior of the bile acid/phospholipid micelles secreted in bile (*Figure 3.25*). Micelles are spherical molecular complexes, termed micelles, about 6 nm across, composed of amphipathic bile salts and phospholipids arranged with their hydrophilic poles outwards and their hydrophobic poles inwards, thus creating a lipid interior. Those rather larger mixed-lipid micelles can in turn solubilize a little weakly polar cholesterol, diglyceride and possibly triglyceride. The solubilization of a normal dietary lipid load requires a bile salt concentration of at least 4 mmol/l, the 'critical physiological concentration'. Such a process of micellar solubilization converts an opalescent emulsion into an optically clear aqueous solution, as identified in Hofmann and Borgström's classic study of ultracentrifuged duodenal chyme.[21]

These authors separated chyme into three physical phases by ultracentrifugation: an oil phase (tri-

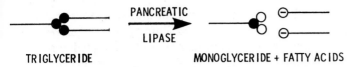

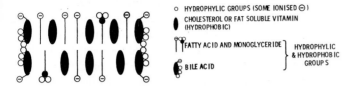

Figure 3.25 Molecular models of triglyceride hydrolysis and micellar solubilization of lipids.

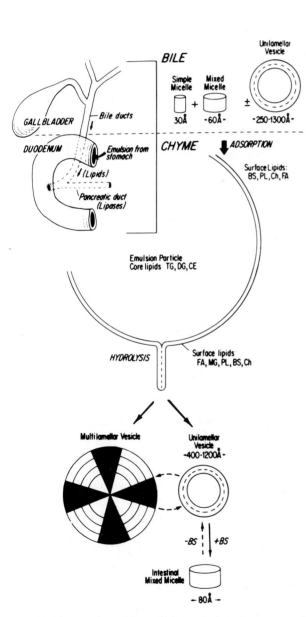

Figure 3.26 Schematic representation of intraluminal processes in fat digestion and solubilization. BS, bile salt; Ch, cholesterol; FA, fatty acid; PL phospholipid. (Reproduced, with permission, from Hernell et al.[18])

glycerides, diglycerides and protonated fatty acids), a micellar phase and a precipitate (protein debris containing protonated bile acid).

More recently, it has been realized that this model is an oversimplification.[4] The chemical composition of the micellar phase does not conform with the phase limits of mixed-lipid micelles created in vitro.[35] Other 'intermediate' phases are present in ultracentrifuged chyme; their constituents have been identified by a variety of microscopic and other imaging techniques and include liquid crystalline structures such as unilamellar vesicles and larger multilamellar liposomes.[18] Patton and Carey's fascinating observation of the process of digestion identified these phases in the process of formation.[28] Their phase limits have been determined and correspond to the chemical composition of the intermediate phases observed ex vivo. Carey's current model (Figure 3.26), based both on the study of the behaviour of model systems in vitro[35] and on the observation and analysis of chyme samples ex vivo,[18] is that the lipolytic products form on the surface of the emulsified oil droplet, bud off as large multilamellar liquid crystal bilayers, and ultimately become free liposomes. These large structures form smaller unilamellar vesicles which, on enrichment with bile salt in solution above the critical physiological concentration, equilibrate with mixed micelles in a two-phase aqueous solution. The whole of this process is probably extremely rapid.

Mucosal events

The unstirred aqueous layer and the small intestinal mucosal cell membrane form, in essence, barriers to the movement of lipid from the lipid-rich aqueous phase within the intestinal lumen down a concentration gradient to the interior of the mucosal cell. This movement is probably the rate-limiting step in fat assimilation. The function of the micelle has always been considered to be to increase the gradient by concentrating lipid in the aqueous phase, thus

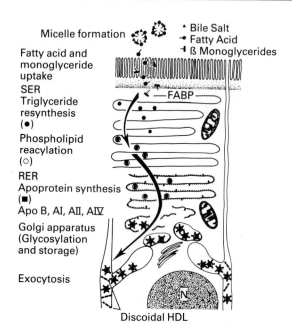

Micelle formation
Fatty acid and monoglyceride uptake
SER Triglyceride resynthesis (●)
Phospholipid reacylation (○)
RER Apoprotein synthesis (■)
Apo B, AI, AII, AIV
Golgi apparatus (Glycosylation and storage)
Exocytosis

▲ Bile Salt
◄ Fatty Acid
◄ ß Monoglycerides

FABP

N

Discoidal HDL

Figure 3.27 Schematic representation of cellular processes in fat absorption. FABP, fatty acid-binding protein; SER, smooth endoplasmic reticulum; RER, rough endoplasmic reticulum. (Reproduced, with permission, from Glickman, R. and Ley, J.R. (1979) *American Journal of Medicine*, **67**, 984.)

facilitating its passage through the unstirred water layer and ultimately presenting it to the lipid exterior of the mucosal microvilli.[41] At this point, it is considered that the micelle disrupts in the acid microclimate under the unstirred water layer,[33] and the released lipid dissolves into and through the lipid of the cell membrane, the 'empty' micelles returning to the lumen. Whether lipid can also be absorbed from the larger lipid-rich vesicles and liposomes remains conjectural. Cholesterol, fat-soluble vitamins and monoglycerides are probably absorbed from micelles alone.

Within the cell cytosol (*Figure 3.27*), fatty acids and, probably, monoglycerides are transported by binding proteins to the smooth endoplasmic reticulum, where they are re-esterified to recreate triglycerides; this process maintains a concentration gradient away from the microvillus cell membrane. The triglyceride is then transported to the Golgi apparatus, where intestinal lipoproteins are synthesized and chylomicrons formed. The chylomicrons are transported by a microtubular system to the lateral cell membrane and pass into the lymphatic system by a process of reverse pinocytosis. This transport process is dependent, at various stages, on an adequate supply of luminal phospholipid, which comes largely from biliary lecithin rather than dietary phospholipid.[6]

This model applies primarily to the digestion,

solubilization, absorption and resynthesis of long-chain triglycerides. Medium-chain triglycerides are present in vegetable oils and artificial feeds; their constituent fatty acids are more water-soluble and may be absorbed without micellar solubilization, although whether they are absorbed as liquid crystals is not known. Their fate after absorption is also different, as they diffuse through the cytosol and pass directly into the portal venous system. The intraluminal and intramucosal processes involved are little understood, but the major difference in aqueous solubility is exploited in nutritional therapy.

PATHOPHYSIOLOGY

Our understanding of the physiology of fat assimilation comes from the study not only of the normal process in health, but also of how these processes are upset in diseases affecting each of the organs involved.[45]

Gastric disorders

Deficiency of gastric lipase has not been reported, and the specific contribution of this enzyme to fat assimilation in adults cannot therefore be quantified. Some, but not all, studies have shown that secretion of the enzyme is increased in chronic alcoholic pancreatitis,[27] perhaps to compensate for deficiency of pancreatic lipase.

Partial gastrectomy involving removal of the antrum and gastrojejunostomy (Bilroth II) almost always leads to mild steatorrhoea. This may be attributable to loss of 'antral mill' emulsification, and to rapid gastric emptying depositing lipid-rich chyme in the jejunum well before the arrival of pancreatobiliary fluid, and perhaps to a reduction in gastric lipase activity. These disturbances have not been explored in sufficient detail to contribute to the physicochemical model.

The Zollinger–Ellison syndrome is, however, the most important gastric disorder of fat assimilation and its pathophysiology has been carefully documented.[17] Massive gastric acid hypersecretion in this condition leads to severe steatorrhoea; the disturbance of digestion and absorption occurs in the duodenum and will be considered later.

Pancreatic disorders (*Figure 3.28*)

The exocrine pancreas has enormous reserves, and exocrine insufficiency is not manifest as steatorrhoea until about 95% of the pancreatic acini are destroyed, or secretion of enzyme into the duo-

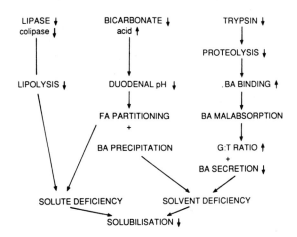

Figure 3.28 Summary of intraluminal disturbances in pancreatic insufficiency. (Reproduced, with permission, from Zentler-Munro *et al.*[45])

denum is reduced by over 90%. The secretion of lipase and colipase can be selectively reduced in rare individuals with pure lipase[12] or colipase[19] deficiency, and both of these disorders result in steatorrhoea. Non-selective exocrine insufficiency much more commonly results from cystic fibrosis, alcoholic and other forms of chronic pancreatitis, infiltrative disorders of the pancreas such as haemochromatosis, and obstructive disorders of the main pancreatic duct.

These conditions lead to the almost complete absence of lipase from duodenal chyme, greatly diminished lipolysis and thus, in theory, steatorrhoea due to solute (monoglyceride and fatty acid) deficiency. The administration of large quantities of pancreatin, however, despite protection against acidic inactivation in the stomach, fails to abolish steatorrhoea in many patients, suggesting that enzyme deficiency cannot be the sole mechanism.[43] Studies in both cystic fibrosis[44] and chronic alcoholic pancreatitis[31] have shown that damage of the ductular epithelium also contributes: decreased secretion of bicarbonate leads to impaired neutralization of gastric effluent, and intraduodenal pH falls to well below 5. This is the pH below which glycine-conjugated bile salts and fatty acids are protonated and leave the aqueous phase, resulting in solvent as well as solute deficiency. Duodenal hyperacidity and its sequelae are particularly marked in cystic fibrosis, because pancreatic ductular function is more gravely affected,[14] and the steatorrhoea in this disease is more severe and difficult to treat.

Diminished secretion of pancreatic protease may also contribute to the problem. Trypsin converts procolipase and prophospholipase into active forms, and an adequate concentration of colipase is particularly important when the lipase concentration is

marginal.[16] More importantly, bile salts bind to various dietary and faecal proteins *in vitro* and *in vivo*, and diminished proteolysis increases the extent of such binding[22] and further decreases the availability of bile salts for solubilization. Both protein binding and pH-dependent precipitation of bile salt, if persistent all down the small intestine, would lead to a functional interruption of the enterohepatic circulation of bile salt. This could in turn decrease the secretion of bile salt by the liver and further limit its availability in the duodenum. Increased bile salt turnover is, in general, accompanied by enrichment with glycine conjugates due to the limited dietary supply of taurine, further predisposing to the pH-dependent precipitation of glycine conjugates.

This model of pancreatic steatorrhoea as a deficiency of solvent as well as solute has been assembled from a series of studies conducted largely in cystic fibrosis.[42] These have shown increased faecal bile salt excretion (to levels similar to those seen in ileectomy steatorrhoea), decreased bile acid pool size, increased glycine:taurine ratio, and decreased intraduodenal bile salt concentration. The last is the most contentious; it is probable that the amount of bile salt is decreased, but the concentration is not, due to the diminished water secretion which characterizes cystic fibrosis.[39] It is also likely that a proportion of the micellar bile salt is 'occupied' by solubilizing protonated bile acid, and is therefore unavailable for lipid solubilization. Despite a similar increase in faecal bile acid excretion in alcoholic pancreatitis,[9] analogous disturbances in the bile acid pool size have not been found.[10]

This model is further supported by interventional studies in cystic fibrosis[42] showing reduction in faecal bile acid excretion and restoration of the bile acid pool size on treatment with pancreatin, particularly in combination with a histamine H_2 antagonist, and on substitution of dietary protein with an oligopeptide feed. Treatment with taurine reduces steatorrhoea, which is also consistent with this model.[8]

Mucosal dysfunction may also contribute to fat malabsorption in cystic fibrosis. Villous architecture is not greatly disturbed, but the villi are thickly coated with an abnormal mucus characteristic of the disease[15] which may increase the functional thickness of the unstirred aqueous layer. Mucosal malfunction has been demonstrated in several respects,[42] but absorption of bile acid is probably normal,[37] and that of fat has not yet been reported.

Hepatobiliary disorders *(Figure 3.29)*

Bile salts are synthesized in and secreted by hepatocytes into the intrahepatic biliary system and then,

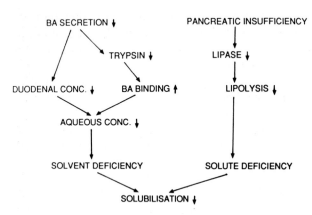

Figure 3.29 Summary of intraluminal disturbances in hepatic cirrhosis. (Reproduced, with permission, from Zentler-Munro et al.[45])

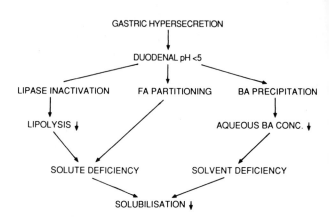

Figure 3.30 Summary of intraluminal disturbances in the Zollinger–Ellison syndrome. (Reproduced, with permission, from Zentler-Munro et al.[45])

after interprandial concentration in the gallbladder, are propelled into the duodenum. Both hepatocellular and cholestatic disorders might therefore be expected to decrease the availability of solvent. Cirrhosis alone leads to only mild steatorrhoea, and only when intraduodenal bile salt concentrations fall below the critical physiological concentration.[2] Cholestasis alone also disrupts fat solubilization only mildly, and appreciable fat absorption can occur even with an external biliary fistula.[30] It is only when cirrhosis and cholestasis are combined, as in primary biliary cirrhosis,[32] that clinically overt steatorrhoea is common. Even in this condition, pancreatic insufficiency may well contribute both as the primary effect of the disease, and because bile salt is a cofactor in the activation of trypsinogen by enterokinase. Similarly, the combination of cirrhosis and pancreatic insufficiency (in alcoholics and haemochromatosis) is a more potent cause of steatorrhoea. Cholecystectomy, although diminishing the postprandial surge of bile salt secretion into the duodenum, does not cause steatorrhoea.

Luminal disorders

The Zollinger–Ellison syndrome is, in the current context, a luminal disorder (*Figure 3.30*). Massive gastric acid hypersecretion leads to severe duodenal hyperacidity (pH < 3), and all the pH-dependent processes already described – irreversible enzyme activation and potentially reversible bile acid and fatty acid protonation – act together to cause a very severe disturbance of fat assimilation.[17] The importance of acid is well documented by the therapeutic response to antisecretory treatment.

Bacterial colonization of the small intestine, whether caused by stagnation in diverticula or in multiple strictures due to Crohn's disease, systemic

sclerosis, ischaemia or irradiation, or by direct contamination through enteric fistulae, promotes deconjugation and dehydroxylation of bile salts. The resultant free secondary bile salts are less effective solvents, and are more susceptible both to premature passive absorption in the jejunum and to pH-dependent precipitation. It is to this that the often severe steatorrhoea of bacterial overgrowth syndrome has been attributed, but this is probably an oversimplification.

Mucosal disorders

Fat digestion is normally completed in the jejunum. Like the pancreas, the small intestine has an enormous reserve capacity and the process is easily displaced downwards when the jejunum is removed or when discrete lengths of small intestine are diseased. The diffuse villous damage which characterizes coeliac disease, Whipple's disease and tropical sprue causes a much more marked loss of absorptive area, for which the intestine cannot compensate, and steatorrhoea results. Duodenal mucosal damage leads to decreased postprandial secretion of cholecystokinin, and resultant pancreatic hyposecretion and gallbladder hypomotility may contribute in some patients.[7]

The distal ileum is the active site of bile salt reabsorption. Resection or disease of a major length of distal ileum (generally over 100 cm) can interrupt the enterohepatic circulation to such an extent as to decrease the bile acid pool size, enrich the pool with glycine conjugates, and reduce intraluminal bile salt concentration.[24,29] In addition, gastric acid secretion increases, probably by a hormonal reflex, and both disturbances combine – as in cystic fibrosis – to aggravate ileectomy steatorrhoea.

In massive intestinal resection, the effect of rapid

transit over a decreased absorptive area, bile salt deficiency and intestinal acidification combine to cause the most severe disturbance of fat assimilation. The relationship between impaired bile acid and fatty acid absorption and water secretion will be discussed in this chapter (p. 460).

Other rare and predictable causes of fat malabsorption include abetalipoproteinaemia, intestinal lymphangiectasia and intestinal amyloidosis.

Compensatory mechanisms

Steatorrhoea is seldom complete in most of these diseases. It is likely that compensatory mechanisms exist, and these further illuminate pathophysiological principles.

In pancreatic exocrine insufficiency, dietary fat is hydrolysed to some extent despite the complete absence of pancreatic lipase, and this has been attributed to the action of the acid-stable gastric lipase persisting in the hyperacid duodenum.[1] Intragastric lipase concentrations are increased in alcoholic pancreatitis,[27] perhaps as a compensatory mechanism. Carey's model describes the formation of liquid crystalline vesicles particularly in conditions of bile salt deficiency, and a preponderance of such forms has indeed been observed in cystic fibrosis. Whether liquid crystals can cross the unstirred water layer and yield their solute to the mucosa is as yet unknown. It is interesting that a few cystic fibrosis patients are able to abandon pancreatin treatment as they get older. These patients have not been studied, unfortunately, but they demonstrate perhaps an extreme degree of compensation – fat digestion and solubilization by the non-pancreatic/bile salt mediated routes, as discussed earlier.

The robustness of fat assimilation to cholestatic or ileectomy bile salt deficiency emphasizes the fact that micellar solubilization is not essential,[24,30] and is again perhaps explained by the Carey model, where liquid crystalline structures may replace micelles as the vehicles for fat solubilization. Cholestasis is likely to lead also to deficiency of the phospholipid later required for transport of lipid across the mucosal cell and into the lymphatic system. There is indirect evidence that neutral long-chain triglycerides are then transported into the portal system, the route normally used by medium-chain length fats.[38]

A well-described change in gastrointestinal motility may also help compensate for disordered digestion, solubilization or absorption. The infusion of nutrients, particularly triglycerides, into the terminal ileum – as if unabsorbed – slows small bowel transit[34] and gastric emptying of meal[13] by a hormonal reflex (the 'ileal brake'). It also induces satiety,[40] and this may contribute to the impaired appetite and food intake seen in most patients with malabsorptive disease.

CONCLUSION

The stomach, pancreas, biliary system and intestine all have a distinct but coordinated part to play in the complex process of fat assimilation. The robustness of this system to disorders of these organs has been explained by recent developments in our knowledge of the chemical and physical processes involved, and it is only generally when more than one organ is involved that clinically significant steatorrhoea occurs.

References

1. Abrams, C.K., Hamosh, M., Dutta, S.K., Hubbard, V.S. and Hamosh, P. (1987) Role of nonpancreatic lipolytic activity in exocrine pancreatic insufficiency. *Gastroenterology*, **92**, 125–129.
2. Badley, B.W., Murphy, G.M., Bouchier, I.A. and Sherlock, S. (1970) Diminished micellar phase lipid in patients with chronic nonalcoholic liver disease and steatorrhoea. *Gastroenterology*, **58**, 781–789.
3. Borgström, B. (1980) Importance of phospholipids, pancreatic phospholipase A_2 and fatty acid for the digestion of dietary fat: *in vitro* experiments with the porcine enzymes. *Gastroenterology*, **78**, 954–962.
4. Borgström, B. (1985) The micellar hypothesis of fat absorption: must it be revisited? *Scandinavian Journal of Gastroenterology*, **20**, 389–394.
5. Borgström, B. (1988) Fat digestion and solubilisation. In: *Bile Acids in Health and Disease*, pp. 217–228 (Eds) Northfield, T.C., Jazrawi, R. and Zentler-Munro, P.L. London: Kluwer Academic.
6. Carey, M.C. (1983) Role of lecithin in the absorption of dietary fat. In: *Phospholipids and Atherosclerosis*, pp. 33–63 (Eds) Avogaro, P., Mancini, M., Ricci, G. and Paoletti, R. New York: Raven Press.
7. Collins, B.J., Bell, P.M., Boyd, S. *et al.* (1986) Endocrine and exocrine pancreatic functions in treated coeliac disease. *Pancreas*, **1**, 143–147.
8. Columbo, C., Arlati, S., Curcio, L. *et al.* (1988) Effect of taurine supplementation on fat and bile acid absorption in patients with cystic fibrosis. *Scandinavian Journal of Gastroenterology*, **23**(suppl. 143), 151–156.
9. Dutta, S.K., Anand, K. & Gadacz, T.R. (1986) Bile salt malabsorption in pancreatic insufficiency secondary to alcoholic pancreatitis. *Gastroenterology*, **91**, 1243–1249.
10. Einarrson, K., Angelin, B. & Johansson, C. (1987) Biliary lipid metabolism in chronic pancreatitis: influence of steatorrhoea. *Gut*, **28**, 1495–1499.

11. Färkkilä, M. and Miettinen, T.A. (1990) Lipid metabolism in bile acid malabsorption. *Annals of Medicine*, **22**, 5–13.

12. Figarella, C., De-Caro, A., Leupold, D. & Poley, J.R. (1980) Congenital pancreatic lipase deficiency. *Journal of Pediatrics*, **96**, 412–416.

13. Fone, D.R., Horowitz, M., Read, N.W., Dent, J. and Maddox, A. (1990) The effect of terminal ileal triglyceride infusion on gastroduodenal motility and the intragastric distribution of a solid meal. *Gastroenterology*, **98**, 568–575.

14. Forstner, G.G., Kopelman, H.R., Durie, P.R. and Corey, M.L. (1987) Pancreatic and intestinal dysfunction in cystic fibrosis. *Progress in Clinical Research*, **254**, 7–17.

15. Forstner, J., Wesley, A., Mantle, M., Kopelman, H., Man, D. and Forstner, G. (1984) Abnormal mucus: nominated but not yet elected. *Journal of Pediatric Gastroenterology and Nutrition*, **3**(suppl. 1), 67–73.

16. Gaskin, K.J., Durie, P.R., Lee, L., Hill, R., Forstner, G.G. (1984) Colipase and lipase secretion in childhood-onset pancreatic insufficiency: delineation of patients with steatorrhoea secondary to relative colipase deficiency. *Gastroenterology*, **86**, 1–7.

17. Go, V.L., Poley, J.R., Hofmann, A.F. and Summerskill, W.H. (1970) Disturbances in fat digestion induced by acidic jejunal pH due to gastric hypersecretion in man. *Gastroenterology*, **58**, 638–646.

18. Hernell, O., Staggers, J.E. and Carey, M.C. (1990) Physical-chemical behaviour of dietary and biliary lipids during intestinal digestion and absorption. 2. Phase analysis and aggregation states of luminal lipids during duodenal fat digestion in healthy adult human beings. *Biochemistry*, **29**, 2041–2056.

19. Hildebrand, H., Borgström, B., Bekassy, A., Erlanson-Albertsson, C. and Helin, I. (1982) Isolated co-lipase deficiency in two brothers. *Gut*, **23**, 243–246.

20. Hofmann, A.F. (1978) Lipase, colipase, amphipathic dietary proteins, and bile acids: new interactions at an old interface. *Gastroenterology*, **75**, 530–532.

21. Hofmann, A.F. and Borgström, B. (1964) The intraluminal phase of fat digestion in man: the lipid content of micellar and oil phases of intestinal content obtained during fat digestion and absorption. *Journal of Clinical Investigation*, **43**, 247–257.

22. Jonas, A. and Diver-Haber, A. (1988) Bile acid sequestration by the solid phase of stools in cystic fibrosis patients: role of pancreatic enzymes. *Digestive Diseases and Sciences*, **33**, 724–731.

23. Lindström, M.B., Sternby, B. and Borgström, B. (1988) Concerted action of human carboxyl ester lipase and pancreatic lipase during lipid digestion *in vitro*: importance of the physicochemical state of the substrate. *Biochimica et Biophysica Acta*, **959**, 179–184.

24. Mansbach, C.M., Newton, D. and Stephens, R.D. (1980) Fat digestion in patients with bile acid malabsorption but minimal steatorrhoea. *Digestive Diseases and Sciences*, **25**, 353–362.

25. Meyer, J.H., Mayer, E.A., Jehn, D., Gu, Y., Fink, A.S. and Fried, M. (1986) Gastric processing and emptying of fat. *Gastroenterology*, **90**, 1176–1187.

26. Moreau, H., Laugier, R., Gargouri, Y., Ferrato, F. and Verger, R. (1988) Human preduodenal lipase is entirely of gastric fundic origin. *Gastroenterology*, **95**, 1221–1226.

27. Moreau, J., Bouisson, M., Balas, B., *et al.* (1990) Gastric lipase in alcoholic pancreatitis. Comparison of secretive profiles following pentagastrin stimulation in normal adults and patients with pancreatic insufficiency. *Gastroenterology*, **99**, 175–180.

28. Patton, J.S. and Carey, M.C. (1979) Watching fat digestion. The formation of visible product phases by pancreatic lipase is described. *Science*, **204**, 145–148.

29. Poley, J.R. and Hofmann, A.F. (1976) Role of fat digestion in pathogenesis of steatorrhoea in ileal resection. *Gastroenterology*, **71**, 38–44.

30. Porter, H.P., Saunders, D.R., Tytgat, G., Brunser, O. and Rubin, C.E. (1971) Fat absorption in bile fistula man. A morphological and biochemical study. *Gastroenterology*, **60**, 1008–1019.

31. Regan, P.T., Malegelada, J.R., Di Magno, E.P. and Go, V.L. (1979) Reduced intraluminal bile acid concentration and fat maldigestion in pancreatic insufficiency: correction by treatment. *Gastroenterology*, **77**, 285–289.

32. Ros, E., García-Pegés, A., Reixach, M., Cusó, E. and Rodés, J. (1984) Fat digestion and exocrine pancreatic function in primary biliary cirrhosis. *Gastroenterology*, **87**, 180–187.

33. Shiall, Y.-F. and Levine, G.M. (1980) pH dependence of micellar diffusion and dissociation. *American Journal of Physiology*, **239**, G177–G182.

34. Spiller, R.C., Trotman, I.F., Adrian, T.E., Bloom, S.R., Misiewicz, J.J. and Silk, D.B.A. (1988) Further characterisation of the "ileal brake" reflex in man – effect of ileal infusion of partial digests of fat, protein, and starch on jejunal motility and the release of neurotensin, enteroglucagon, and peptide YY. *Gut*, **29**, 1042–1051.

35. Staggers, J.E., Hernell, O., Stafford, R.J. and Carey, M.C. (1990) Physical–chemical behavior of dietary and biliary lipids during intestinal digestion and absorption. 1. Phase behavior and aggregation states of model lipid systems patterned after aqueous duodenal contents of healthy adult human beings. *Biochemistry*, **29**, 2028–2040.

36. Thomson, A.B.R., Keelan, M., Garg, M.L. and Clandinin, M.T. (1989) Intestinal aspects of lipid absorption: in review. *Canadian Journal of Physiology and Pharmacology*, **67**, 179–191.

37. Thomson, G.N. and Davidson, G.P. (1988) *In vivo* bile acid uptake from terminal ileum in cystic fibrosis. *Pediatric Research*, **23**, 323–328.

38. Tso, P., Kendrick, H., Balint, J.A. and Simmonds, W.J. (1981) Role of biliary phosphatidylcholine in the absorption and transport of dietary triolein in the rat. *Gastroenterology*, **80**, 60–65.

39. Weizman, Z., Durie, P.R., Kopelman, H.R. Vesely, M. and Forstner, G.G. (1986) Bile acid secretion in cystic fibrosis – evidence for a defect unrelated to fat malabsorption. *Gut*, **27**, 1043–1048.

40. Welch, I., Saunders, K. and Read, N.W. (1985) Effect of ileal and intravenous infusions of fat emulsions on feeding and satiety in human volunteers. *Gastroenterology*, **89**, 1293–1297.

41. Westergaard, H. and Dietschy, J.M. (1976) The mechanism whereby bile acid micelles increase the rate of fatty acid and cholesterol uptake into the intestinal mucosal cell. *Journal of Clinical Investigation*, **58**, 97–108.

42. Zentler-Munro, P.L. (1987) Cystic fibrosis – a gastroenterological cornucopia. *Gut*, **28**, 1531–1547.

43. Zentler-Munro, P.L. and Northfield, T.C. (1987) Pancreatic enzyme replacement – applied physiology and pharmacology (review). *Alimentary Pharmacology and Therapeutics*, **1**, 575–591.

44. Zentler-Munro, P.L., Fine, D.R., Batten, J.C. and Northfield, T.C. (1985) Effect of cimetidine on enzyme inactivation, bile acid precipitation, and lipid solubilisation in pancreatic steatorrhoea due to cystic fibrosis. *Gut*, **26**, 892–901.

45. Zentler-Munro, P.L., Fine, D. and Northfield, T.C. (1988) Fat digestion and solubilisation in disease. In: *Bile Acids in Health and Disease*, pp. 239–252 (Eds) Northfield, T.C., Jazrawi, R. and Zentler-Munro, P.L. London: Kluwer Academic.

DIGESTION AND MALABSORPTION OF PROTEIN *(R.C. Spiller)*

DIETARY INTAKE

Adequate intake of protein is essential for health, but intake is often marginal in many poor countries. Safe levels of protein intake vary with age, being high at 1.85 g/kg body weight per day in the neonatal period, falling with age to 0.75 g/kg body weight per day in adult life, rising again in females during pregnancy and lactation. Gastrointestinal diseases such as malabsorption raise needs in adults to 1 g/kg body weight per day, whilst severe trauma and burns increase needs to double or four times that amount.[54]

The quality of protein varies with source, the highest quality being derived from meat because the balance of amino acids in this food is optimum for digestion and resynthesis within the body. Poor sources are those which lack essential amino acids (e.g. gelatin lacks tryptophan) or those in which the protein is hard to extract because it is surrounded by indigestible coatings as are found in some plant products. Cooking generally improves digestibility by disrupting such coatings, allowing access of digestive enzymes. Essential amino acids are those which must be taken in the diet because they cannot be synthesized in humans, and include valine, leucine, isoleucine, lysine, tryptophan, phenylalanine, methionine and threonine; for children, arginine is also thought to be essential.

ENDOGENOUS PROTEIN SOURCES

Large quantities of endogenous protein enter the gut lumen daily in the form of digestive enzymes and mucus (20–30 g), most of which is reabsorbed.[12] Further substantial amounts of protein (30 g) come from desquamated cells, and small amounts of plasma proteins (1–2 g) are also lost daily into the lumen. These losses can be increased markedly in various disease states known as 'protein-losing enteropathies' characterized by inflammation, ulceration or exudation secondary to lymphatic obstruction[51] (see below). Thus, in addition to 70 g of dietary protein, an average 70 kg adult will receive a further 60 g of endogenous protein. Since only 1–2 g of nitrogen, equivalent to 6–12 g of protein, are excreted in the stool each day, protein absorption must be greater than 90% efficient. This conclusion is supported by direct observation of the flow of protein through the terminal ileum after a 50 g protein load in which it was shown in normal volunteers that only 1% of ingested protein entered the colon.[11]

PHYSIOLOGY OF PROTEIN DIGESTION AND ABSORPTION

Gastric phase

After mastication, digestion starts in the stomach, which secretes pepsin, derived from its precursor zymogen (pepsinogen) by removal of a small basic peptide. Pepsin is most active on peptide bonds involving leucine and the aromatic amino acids phenylalanine and tyrosine. The end-products of pepsin digestion are oligopeptides and small amounts of free amino acids. This prior digestion of food in the stomach enhances the secretion of pancreatic and mucosal secretions, probably by allowing faster liberation of mucosal regulatory peptides such as secretin and cholecystokinin. This is especially important where digestion is impaired, as for example in pancreatic insufficiency.[12] Free amino acids are potent stimulants of pancreatic secretion,[21] probably via the release of cholecystokinin.

Intestinal phase

A mixture of polypeptides and oligopeptides is rapidly hydrolysed by pancreatic and intestinal secretions to free amino acids and di- and tripeptides, which are then absorbed. The main pancreatic enzymes are trypsin, chymotrypsin, elastase and carboxypeptidase, which are secreted as inactive precursors. Activation is initiated by the action of an enzyme, enterokinase,[20] an endopeptidase localized to the villous tip and presumed to be released into the lumen, where it converts the proenzyme trypsinogen to trypsin. Trypsin then activates more trypsinogen as well as the precursors of chymotrypsin, elastase and carboxypeptidase. Chymotrypsin and elastase act as endopeptidases, cleaving internal peptide bonds, while carboxypeptidase attacks the carboxyl end of the peptide chain, the end result being a mixture of free amino acids and a range of oligopeptides. Luminal sampling after a protein meal shows that most amino acids are in peptide form (118 mmol in the jejunum and 65 mmol in the ileum) while free amino acids account for only 16 and 20 mmol, respectively.[5]

Mucosal phase of absorption

Postprandially, virtually all of the absorbed amino nitrogen in the portal blood is present as free amino acids, so it follows that virtually complete hydrolysis occurs at some stage during absorption and assimilation. For the most part this hydrolysis takes place in the gut lumen but further hydrolysis does occur both at the brush border and in the enterocyte cytosol. Whereas virtually all carbohydrates must be reduced to monosaccharides prior to absorption, amino nitrogen can be absorbed both as free amino acids as well as di-, tri- and even tetrapeptides. Absorption of certain dipeptides is actually faster than the free amino acids, improving the efficiency of absorption considerably.

Oligopeptide hydrolysis

The distribution of peptide hydrolases has been extensively researched,[32,38,50] from which it is clear that brush border hydrolases differ significantly from cytosolic ones, with the tendency for hydrolytic activity against the longer oligopeptide chains to be located in the brush border while dipeptidase activity is largely confined to the cytosol.[38] The

brush border aminopeptidases which have been isolated are high molecular weight proteins (200–300 kDa) with active binding sites that show highest affinity for tri- and tetrapeptides.[24,31] These enzymes cleave peptide bonds to liberate the amino-terminal amino acid but generally do not cleave peptides containing proline or diamino acids. The active peptide-binding site and the carbohydrate-rich hydrophilic portion of the enzyme protrudes into the lumen, being anchored into the membrane by a small hydrophobic peptide sequence rather similar to that found in the disaccharidases. Like other cell surface glycoproteins, aminopeptidases are synthesized in the rough endoplasmic reticulum, glycosylated in the Golgi apparatus and are incorporated from there into the plasma membrane.[39]

Other enzymes capable of cleaving peptides from oligopeptides have been described in the brush border as well as cytosolic enzymes capable of splitting proline-containing dipeptides. In addition, as a back-up for situations in which pancreatic secretion is defective, there are brush border neutral endopeptidases, capable of reducing the milk protein casein to oligopeptides and free amino acids.[25] This may well be important in the neonatal period in which control of pancreatic secretion may still be immature and ineffective. Equally, it may also be important in adults with exocrine pancreatic insufficiency. In the rat, at least, these mucosal proteases, when combined with the action of gastric pepsin, allow 37% of orally administered protein to be absorbed in spite of exclusion of all pancreatic enzymes.[12] How important they are in humans is as yet uncertain.

Absorption

Whole protein

Absorption of whole protein in the adult is quantitatively insignificant but may be qualitatively very important, especially in food allergies. In the immediate neonatal period there appear to be specialized transport mechanisms allowing immunoglobulin from the colostrum of the mother to be absorbed intact.[52] This physiological mechanism ceases within about 48 hours of birth. However, intact macromolecules can be absorbed in adults in conditions characterized by increased intestinal permeability such as coeliac disease. One recent study[29] showed the presence of intact egg albumin and β-galactoglobulin from milk after test meals in normal children. They also showed an increase in absorption of these substances in children with coeliac disease who were challenged with gluten, which is known to increase small intestinal permeability.

The nutritional significance of such absorption is of course minimal and most amino acids are absorbed either free or as part of di-, tri- or tetrapeptides. The molecular basis of amino acid transport has been extensively investigated, initially by means of perfusion experiments.[1] and *in vivo* studies using isolated jejunal rings,[34] and more recently using isolated brush border membranes in the form of vesicles.[42] These sophisticated laboratory techniques have allowed much more rapid progress in the last few years, because in isolated brush border vesicles one can exclude other complicating factors such as the cytosolic metabolism of peptides which made interpretation of perfusion studies so difficult.

Amino acid absorption

Amino acids are transported across the brush border by three main mechanisms: (1) non-saturable simple diffusion; (2) Na^+-independent carriers; and (3) Na^+-dependent carriers. The relative importance of these various mechanisms depends on the concentration gradients from lumen to serosa with passive diffusion predominating at high concentrations, Na^+-independent transport predominating at intermediate concentrations and Na^+-linked transport being the most important in the range of concentrations (2–5 mmol) most commonly found for individual amino acid species in the gut lumen postprandially.[49] Two Na^+-independent transport mechanisms have been defined, the L system transporting neutral amino acids at very low concentrations while the y^+ system transports cationic amino acids such as lysine and arginine. There are, in addition, four Na^+-dependent transport systems which derive the energy needed to actively transport amino acids against a concentration gradient from the Na^+-inward concentration gradient generated by sodium pumping at the basolateral membrane. The NBB (neutral brush border) system transports most neutral amino acids, the PHE system transports phenylalanine and methionine while the IMINO system transports proline and hydroxyproline. Acidic amino acids are absorbed by a further unique system.[43] These conclusions are based mainly on work done with brush border vesicles in the last few years but largely confirm earlier studies done in humans and animals using the much more laborious *in vivo* perfusion techniques.[4,34] Amino acids within each group show competitive inhibition but generally do not influence the absorption via other systems.[34] These transport processes are generally common between the renal tubules and enterocytes so that defects in amino acid absorption are usually associated with aminoaciduria. In keeping with the greater concentrations of amino acids found proximally, amino acid transport is faster in the distal jejunum than in the ileum.[1] Recent work has shown that this is due to changes in brush border transport activity.[27]

Peptide absorption

It has been known for some two decades that, in humans, amino acid absorption from certain dipeptides, e.g. glycylglycine[2] and glycylalanine,[46] is more rapid than from the equivalent free amino acid solution. Furthermore, animal studies using non-hydrolysable dipeptides have shown that dipeptides can be absorbed intact, probably by a single carrier[3] because free amino acids do not inhibit peptide absorption but peptides do show competitive inhibition. These findings have been confirmed recently using the purified brush border membrane vesicle, a model which has the advantage that dipeptides are not hydrolysed once they are absorbed.[42] Of course, in the whole enterocyte, transported dipeptides are rapidly hydrolysed by cytosolic peptidase, thereby maintaining a lumen-to-cell concentration gradient which facilitates further dipeptide transport. Although the dipeptide transporter has not been purified, experimental evidence suggests that transport is Na^+-independent and probably linked to the inward H^+ gradient generated by Na^+/H^+ exchange at the brush border, itself energized by Na^+/K^+ exchange at the basolateral membrane.[19]

Significance of peptide transport

The more rapid transport of amino nitrogen by the dipeptide transporter, the so-called 'kinetic advantage of dipeptides', varies with the amino acid type and the overall concentration.[28] Hegarty *et al.*[28] found that the absorption of amino acids from a protein hydrolysate was faster than from a free amino acid solution for some amino acids (serine, phenylalanine, histidine, threonine and glutamic and aspartic acids) but absorption was equal for the remaining amino acids. The peptide transporter appears to have a greater capacity than the free amino acid transport systems,[3] a difference especially noticeable at high luminal concentrations. Another possible advantage of peptides as a nutritional source of amino acids is the way insoluble amino acids can be made much more soluble by being linked to water-soluble amino acids such as glycine. Glyceryl dipeptides can readily be made and have many of the favourable properties discussed above. Mixtures of glycyl peptides show considerable enhancement of absorption of the amino acids, especially those which are otherwise poorly absorbed such as histidine, tryptophan and threonine (*Figure 3.31*)[28,48]

Dipeptide transport is of even greater significance in the rare individuals who have inherited defects of

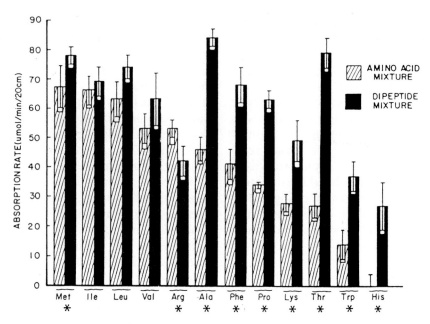

Figure 3.31 Jejunal amino acid absorption rates (mean ± SEM) from a mixture of 12 glyceryl dipeptides and a corresponding mixture of amino acids in five normal volunteers. Except for glycine, the concentration of each dipeptide and amino acid in the test solutions was 6 mmol/l. Because glycine served as the amino terminus of each dipeptide the concentration of glycine in the amino acid mixture was 72 mmol/l, to make the two mixtures similar in glycine content. *, Statistically significant difference. (From Adibi[3].)

amino acid transport, e.g. cystinuria. Subjects cannot absorb cystine, cysteine, arginine or lysine from a free amino acid solution but can absorb them from dipeptides.

DEFECTS OF ABSORPTION

Gastric defects

Surprisingly, loss of gastric proteolysis has little impact unless pancreatic enzymes are also deficient and patients with total gastrectomy absorb protein well.

Exocrine pancreatic insufficiency

Trypsin output has to be reduced to less than 10% of normal values before significant protein malabsorption is detected.[15] Severe pancreatic insufficiency leads, of course, to malabsorption, not only of protein but also of carbohydrate and fat, which in turn leads to flatulence and diarrhoea, largely due to colonic fermentation of malabsorbed carbohydrates and the irritant effect of unabsorbed fat on the colon. Malabsorbed protein causes no very obvious additional symptoms but contributes to the loss of weight and malaise experienced. Gastric surgery, especially a gastroenterostomy, leads to a mismatch between pancreatic secretion and the delivery of

chyme to the small bowel. Thus, in the first few hours of the meal luminal trypsin levels are suboptimal[33] and, if there is in addition rapid small bowel transit owing to dumping, then malabsorption can be expected. Mucosal injury may also lead to defective pancreatic secretion owing to inadequate release of the mucosal peptide cholecystokinin, as is seen in coeliac disease.[10,16] A further cause of inadequate trypsin activity is defective enterokinase action.[26] A congenital deficiency of enterokinase has been described leading to vomiting, diarrhoea, failure to thrive and an associated anaemia and hypoproteinaemia. Diagnosis depends on the demonstration of absent tryptic activity in duodenal juice which rises on the addition of exogenous enterokinase.[20]

Defects in mucosal absorption

Loss of absorptive surface, defective pancreatic secretion, dilution of enzymes and poor appetite all combine to produce defective intake and absorption in coeliac disease. Small bowel overgrowth, resection and damage by cytotoxic drugs or radiation also lead to non-specific malabsorption, which includes malabsorption of protein. Nitrogen balance is particularly impaired in coeliac disease because of its associated accelerated enterocyte turnover leading to an increased loss of endogenous protein. This compounds the malabsorptive problem associated with the reduced surface area and decreased maturity of cells which reduces their digestive and absorptive capacity.[6] A further important factor in causing a negative nitrogen balance in coeliac disease is inadequate protein intake. Coeliac patients, like those with Crohn's disease and other malabsorptive conditions, experience pain and diarrhoea after eating, and patients often eat less because of this. Contamination of the small bowel impairs absorption non-specifically but also increases protein loss in the form of secretions and shed cells.

Specific transport defects

No defects in peptide absorption have been described but there are a number of rare amino acid transport defects which will be described below, most of which are diagnosed in early life.

Cystinuria

Defective intestinal and renal transport of cystine, lysine, ornithine, arginine and cysteine is a rare (1 in 2000–100 000), autosomal recessive, inherited disorder whose sole clinical manifestation relates to the development of renal calculi largely composed of the poorly soluble amino acid cystine.[13]

ABSORPTIVE DEFECT

Oral loading with either cystine,[14] lysine or arginine[36] shows poor absorption, with an increase in faecal excretion. Since the intestinal enterocyte and renal tubular cells share many transport systems, the defect also results in aminoaciduria, free amino acids filtered in the glomeruli being incompletely reabsorbed. Intestinal perfusion experiments in patients confirm a defective absorption of free arginine though, when presented as a dipeptide, arginyl-lysine absorption is normal,[47] explaining why no symptoms of essential amino acid deficiency can be detected in these patients.

INVESTIGATIONS

The diagnosis is usually made after presentation in teenage and early adult life with renal calculi, analysis of which shows the presence of cystine. Alternatively, the screening of urine with the sodium nitroprusside test gives a red colour in dilute ammonia if cystine is present in excess. Quantification is usually necessary to separate heterozygotes from homozygotes.

TREATMENT

Cystine's low solubility (1.3 mmol/l at pH 7.0) results in renal calculus formation, a tendency which can be prevented by diluting and alkalinizing the urine.

The first successful treatment regime devised by Dent and colleagues involved the intake of copious amounts of water together with sodium bicarbonate to obtain more than 3 litres of alkaline urine per day. Indeed, to ensure a continual diuresis through the night, patients were advised to set an alarm clock for 2 a.m. to allow them to awake and drink more water. Though successful, this regime is arduous and there have been many attempts to improve the solubility of cystine in the urine by using chelating agents such as penicillamine and mercaptoproprionyl glycine.[45] Unfortunately, drug toxicity (rashes, nephrotic syndrome and granulocytosis) is a serious problem and requires close monitoring. A more attractive recently developed strategem relies on the reduction in cystine secretion induced by a low-sodium diet. Reducing sodium intake from 150 to 50 mmol/day reduced the crystine excretion in one study from 2.3 to 1.5 mmol/day, which with an alkaline urine would make the difference between insolubility and solubility.[30] One other benefit of sodium depletion may be the stimulation of thirst, which ensures large volumes of dilute urine.

Hartnup disease

This rare autosomal, recessively inherited disorder was first described in a family of this name by Baron and colleagues in a mother and sister who had an excess of neutral amino acids in their urine. Other features which in retrospect are probably due to other metabolic defects included a scaly rash, ataxia and mental retardation.[8] Screening programmes subsequently performed have suggested an incidence of 1 in 33 000 births with a low incidence of photosensitivity (1 in 15) and no cases of mental retardation.[53]

TRANSPORT DEFECT

Oral loading with tryptophan demonstrates excess faecal tryptophan with an increased urinary secretion of indoleacetic acid, produced by colonic bacterial metabolism of malabsorbed tryptophan.[35] Further studies from the same group of investigators demonstrated impaired absorption of phenylalanine and histidine when presented as the free amino acid but not when presented as a dipeptide.[7] The normal absorption of peptide-bound amino acids explains why the clinical features of essential amino acid deficiencies are muted in most cases. It appears that an abnormal diet is necessary before the pellagra symptoms found in the first case are observed.[37]

Other rare defects for amino acid transport

Defective absorption of proline, hydroxyproline and glycine has been reported in a number of cases, most of whom had no defined clinical defects. Case reports tend to overemphasize the incidence of associated pathology and no screening has been performed so it is hard to tell whether the associated features are actually caused by the amino transport defect.[45] The *blue diaper syndrome*[17] is rare but, as its name suggests, presents in neonates with failure to thrive, recurrent fever, irritability and a blueish discoloration of the diaper owing to excess tryptophan in the stool. Some of this excess amino acid is metabolized to indoles which are then absorbed and converted to indican and indigo blue in the liver, to be subsequently excreted in the urine. Unlike Hartnup disease, tryptophan is apparently the only amino acid malabsorbed, the defect being limited to the intestine with no aminoaciduria. The high levels of tryptophan and metabolites in the stool suggest a virtually complete block in tryptophan absorption. This suggests that the block lies more centrally than the enterocyte brush border, perhaps at the basolateral membrane where absorption of both free and peptide-bound tryptophan could be interrupted, as it is in lysinuric protein intolerance. This is also a rare, autosomally recessive inherited defect in absorption of dibasic amino acids (lysine, arginine and ornithine) with aminoaciduria and reduced plasma levels of these amino acids.[40] Unlike cystinuria and Hartnup disease, this syndrome is clinically severe with hyperammonaemia and protein aversion which is due to the nausea, vomiting and diarrhoea which follows a protein-rich meal. Severe growth failure follows unless the defective absorption can be overcome. The protein intolerance is due to lack of urea cycle intermediates within hepatocyte mitochondria so that deamination of amino acids results in accumulation of ammonia, as urea synthesis is insufficient to detoxify the amino groups released. Malabsorption of both free and peptide-bound lysine and, presumably, the other dibasic amino acids appears to be due to a block in transport at the enterocyte basolateral membrane.[40] In addition, there appears to be a defect within the mitochondria because uptake into the hepatocyte is normal but subsequent metabolism and incorporation into the urea cycle is impaired.[41] Management is by supplementation using arginine and ornithine; presumably, high doses allow passive absorption to overcome the defect in absorption.

Malabsorption of methionine (*oasthouse urine disease*)[45] leads to bacterial breakdown of methionine in the colon to 2-hydroxybutyric acid, which is absorbed and excreted in the urine with what is said to be a characteristic malodour. A similar fate befalls the neutral amino acids lysine, isoleucine and valine, leading to the excretion of a range of unusual short-chain fatty acids. Methionine appears with phenylalanine and tyrosine in the urine, suggesting a common transport defect in the renal tubule and enterocyte. Only a very few cases have been reported, one of whom was mentally retarded with convulsions. In the same patient, methionine loading led to diarrhoea. Whether peptide-bound methionine would be normally absorbed and how the transport defect relates to other symptoms is unclear. Similar comments could be applied to *aminoglycinuria*. Again initially reported in a mentally retarded child, it was later recognized in asymptomatic adults.[44] Prolinuria, hydroxyprolinuria and glycinuria are associated with apparently defective absorption of proline on oral loading[23] though, surprisingly, glycine absorption appears normal.

Lowe's syndrome is a rare disorder characterized by mental retardation and aminoaciduria. Although defects in lysine and arginine absorption have been reported,[9] their significance is obscure. Defects in mitochondrial metabolism[22] may underlie this disorder, the apparent transport defect and aminoaciduria being secondary epiphenomena rather than the underlying cause.

PROTEIN-LOSING ENTEROPATHY (*see also* p. 609)

Studies using radiolabelled albumin indicate that, in about 1% of normal subjects, plasma proteins are lost into the gut daily (1 g). Inflammation of the gut, as in Crohn's disease, ulcerative colitis or diseases characterized by increased permeability to large molecules, such as coeliac disease or lymphatic obstruction (e.g. lymphangieactasia or lymphatic infiltration by tumour), are associated with a substantial increase in this loss of plasma protein into the gut which can be as high as 30 g/day.[51] These patients may present with manifestations of hypoalbuminaemia, the specific gastrointestinal symptoms often being occult. Quantification of protein loss by using [135]I-labelled albumin is tedious, and is now rarely done as more specific diagnostic tests are available. If quantification of protein loss is desired, then the 24-hour stool clearance of α_1-antitrypsin can be performed much more easily.[18]

REFERENCES

1. Adibi, S.A. (1969) The influence of molecular structure of neutral amino acids on their absorptive kinetics in the jejunum and ileum of human intestine *in vivo*. *Gastroenterology*, **56**, 903–911.
2. Adibi, S.A. (1971) Intestinal transport of dipeptides in man: relative importance of hydrolysis and intact absorption. *Journal of Clinical Investigation*, **50**, 2266–2275.
3. Adibi, S.A. (1989) Glycyl-dipeptides: new

substrates for protein nutrition. *Journal of Laboratory and Clinical Medicine*, **113**, 665–673

4. Adibi, S.A. and Gray, S.J. (1967) Intestinal absorption of essential amino acids in man. *Gastroenterology*, **52**, 837–845.

5. Adibi, S.A. and Mercer, D.W. (1973) Protein digestion in human intestine as reflected in luminal mucosal and plasma amino acid concentrations after meals. *Journal of Clinical Investigation*, **52**, 1586–1594.

6. Adibi, S.A., Fogel, M.R. and Agrawal, R.M. (1974) Comparison of free amino acid and dipeptide absorption in the jejunum of sprue patients. *Gastroenterology*, **67**, 586–591.

7. Asatoor, A.M., Cheng, B., Edwards, K.D.G. *et al.* (1970) Intestinal absorption of two dipeptides in Hartnup disease. *Gut*, **II**, 380–387.

8. Baron, D.N., Dent, C.E., Harris, H. *et al.* (1956) Hereditary pellagra-like skin rash with temporary cerebellar ataxia, constant renal aminoaciduria and other bizarre biochemical features. *The Lancet*, **ii**, 421–428.

9. Bartsocas, C.S., Levy, H.L., Crawford, J.D. and Thier, S.O. (1969) A defect in intestinal amino-acid transport in Lowe's syndrome. *Americam Journal of Diseases in Childhood*, **117**, 93–95.

10. Calam, J., Ellis, A. and Dockray, G.J. (1982) Identification and measurement of molecular variants of cholecystokinin in duodenal mucosa and plasma. Diminished concentration in patients with coeliac disease. *Journal of Clinical Investigation*, **89**, 218–225.

11. Chung, Y.C., Kim, Y.S., Shadchehr, A., Garrido, A., MacGregor, I.L. and Sleisenger, M.H. (1979) Protein digestion and absorption in human small intestine. *Gastroenterology*, **76**, 1415–1421.

12. Curtis, K.J., Gaines, H.D. and Kim, Y.S. (1978) Protein digestion and absorption in rats with pancreatic duct occlusion. *Gastroenterology*, **74**, 1271–1276.

13. Dahlberg, P.J., Van den Berg, C.J., Wilson, D.M. and Smith, H. (1977) Clinical lectures and management of cystinuria. *Mayo Clinic Proceedings*, **52**, 533–542.

14. Dent, C.E., Heathcote, J.G. and Joran, G.E. (1954) The pathogenesis of cystinuria. I. Chromatographic and microbiological studies of the metabolism of sulphur containing amino acids. *Journal of Clinical Investigation*, **33**, 1210–1215.

15. DiMagno, E.P., Go, V.L.W. and Summerskill, W.H.J. (1972) Impaired cholecystokinin–pancreoenzymic secretion, intraluminal dilution and maldigestion of fat in sprue. *Gastroenterology*, **63**, 25–52.

16. DiMagno, E.P., Go, V.L.W. and Summerskill, W.H.J. (1973) Relations between pancreatic enzyme outputs and malabsorption in severe pancreatic insufficiency. *New England Journal of Medicine*, **288**, 813–815.

17. Drummond, K.N., Michael, A.F., Ulstrom, R.A. and Good, R.A. (1964) The blue diaper syndrome: familial hypercalcaemia and nephrocalcinosis and indolanuria. *American Journal of Medicine*, **37**, 928–948.

18. Florent, C., L'Hirondel, C., Desmazures, C., Aymes, C. and Bernier, J.J. (1981) Intestinal clearance of α-antitrypsin. A sensitive method for the detection of protein-losing enteropathy. *Gastroenterology*, **81**, 77–780.

19. Ganapathy, V. and Leibach, F.H. (1985) Is intestinal peptide transport energised by a proton gradient? *American Journal of Physiology*, **249**, G153–G160.

20. Ghishan, F.K., Lee, P.C., Lebenthal, E., Johnson, P., Bradley, C.A. and Green, H.L. (1983) Isolated congenital enterokinase deficiency. Recent findings and review of the literature. *Gastroenterology*, **85**, 727–731.

21. Go, V.L.W., Hofmann, A.F. and Summerskill, W.H.J. (1970) Pancreanzymin bioassay in man based on pancreatic enzyme secretion: potency of specific amino acids and other digestive products. *Journal Clinical Investigation*, **49**, 1558–1564.

22. Gobernado, J.M., Lousa, M., Gimeno, A. and Gonsalvez, M. (1984) Mitochondrial defects in Lowe's oculocerebrorenal syndrome. *Archives of Neurology*, **41**, 208–209.

23. Goodman, S.I., McIntyre, C.A. and O'Brien, D. (1967) Impaired intestinal transport of proline in a patient with familial aminoaciduria. *Journal of Pediatrics*, **71**, 246–248.

24. Gray, G.M. and Santiago, N.A. (1977) Intestinal surface aminopeptidases. 1. Isolation of two weight isomers and their subunits from rat brush border. *Journal of Biological Chemistry*, **252**, 4922–4928.

25. Guan, D., Yoshioka, M., Erickson, R.H., Heizer, W. and Kim, Y.S. (1988) Protein digestion in human and rat small intestine: role of new neutral endopeptidases. *American Journal of Physiology*, **255**, G212–G220.

26. Hadorn, B., Tarlow, M.J., Lloyd, J.D. and Wolff, O.H. (1969) Intestinal enterokinase deficiency. *The Lancet*, **i**, 812–813.

27. Harig, J.M., Barry, J.A., Rajendran, V.M., Soergel, K.H. and Ramaswamy, K. (1989) D-Glucose and L-leucine transport to human intestinal brush-border membrane vesicles. *American Journal of Physiology*, **256**, G618–G623.

28. Hegarty, J.E., Fairclough, P.D., Moriaty, K.J., Kelly, M.J. and Clark, M.L. (1982) Effects of concentration on *in vivo* absorption of a peptide-containing protein hydrolysate. *Gut*, **23**, 304–309.

29. Husby, S., Fogel, N., Host, A., Svehag, S.-E. (1987) Passage of dietary antigens into the blood of children with coeliac disease. Quantification and size distribution of absorbed antigens. *Gut*, **28**, 1062–1072.

30. Jaeger, P., Portman, L., Saunders, A., Rosenbergy, L.E. and Thier, S.O. (1986) Anticystinuric effects of glutamine and of dietary sodium restriction. *New England Journal of Medicine*, **315**, 1120–1123.

31. Kania, R.K., Santiago, N.A. and Gray, G.M. (1977) Intestinal surface aminopeptidases. II. Substrate kinetics and topography of the active site. *Journal of Biological Chemistry*, **252**, 4929–4934.

32. Kim, Y.S., Kim, Y.W., Gaines, H.D. and Sleisenger, M. (1979) Zymogen studies of human intestinal brush border and cytoplasmic peptidases. *Gut*, **20**, 987–991.

33. MacGregor, L., Parent, J. and Meyer, J.H. (1977) Gastric emptying of liquid meals and pancreatic and biliary secretion after subtotal gastrectomy or truncal vagotomy and pyloroplasty in man. *Gastroenterology*, **72**, 195–205.

34. Matthews, D.M. and Laster, L. (1965) Competition for intestinal transport among five neutral amino acids. *American Journal of Physiology*, **208**, 601–606.

35. Milne, M.D., Crawford, M.A., Girao, C.B. and Loughridge, L.W. (1960) The metabolic disorder in Hartnup disease. *Quarterly Journal of Medicine*. **29**, 407–421.

36. Milne, M.D., Asatoor, A.M., Edwards, K.D.G. and Loughridge, L.W. (1961) The intestinal absorption defect in cystinuria. *Gut*, **II**, 323–337.

37. Navab, F. and Asator, A.M. (1970) Studies on intestinal absorption of amino acids in the case of Hartnup disease. *Gut*, **II**, 372–379.

38. Nicholson, J.A. and Peters, T.J. (1979) Subcellular localisation of peptidase activity in human jejunum. *European Journal of Clinical Investigation*, **9**, 349–354.

39. Quaroni, A., Kirsh, K. and Weiser, M.M. (1979) Synthesis of membrane glycoproteins in rat small intestinal cells. Redistribution of L (1,5,6–^{3}H)fucose-labelled membrane glycoproteins among Golgi, lateral, basal and microvillus membrane. *Biochemical Journal*, **182**, 213–221.

40. Ragantie, J., Simell, O. and Perheentupa, J. (1980) Basolateral membrane transport defect for lysine in lysinuric protein intolerance. *The Lancet*, **i**, 1219–1221.

41. Rajantie, J., Simell, O. and Perheentupa, J. (1983) Basolateral and mitochondrial membrane transport defect in the hepatocytes in lysinuric protein intolerance. *Acta Paediatrica Scandinavica*, **72**, 65–70.

42. Rajendran, V.M., Ansari, S.A., Harig, J.M., Adams, M.B., Khan, A.H. and Ramaswamy, K. (1985) Transport of glycyl-L-proline by human intestinal brush-border membrane vesicles. *Gastroenterology*, **89**, 1298–1304.

43. Rajendran, V.M., Harig, J.M., Adams, M.B. and Ramaswamy, K. (1987) Transport of acidic amino acids by human brush-border membrane vesicles. *American Journal of Physiology*, **252**, 533–539.

44. Scriver, C.R. (1967) Membrane transport in disorders of amino acid metabolism. *American Journal of Diseases in Childhood*, **113**, 170–173.

45. Silk, D.B.A. (1982) Disorders of nitrogen absorption. *Clinical Gastroenterology*, **11**, 47–72.

46. Silk, D.B.A., Perrett, D. and Clark, M.L. (1973) Intestinal transport of two dipeptides containing the same two neutral amino acids in man. *Clinical Science and Molecular Medicine*, **45**, 291–299.

47. Silk, D.B.A., Perrett, D. and Clark, M.L. (1975) Jejunal and ileal absorption of dibasic amino acids and an arginine-containing dipeptide in cystinuria. *Gastroenterology*, **68**, 1426–1432.

48. Silk, D.B.A., Fairclough, P.D., Clark, M.L. *et al.*, (1980) Uses of a peptide rather than free amino acid nitrogen source in chemically defined 'elemental' diets. *Journal of Parenteral and Enteral Nutrition*, **4**, 548–553.

49. Stevens, B.R., Kaunitz, J.D. and Wright, E.M. (1984) Intestinal transport of amino acids and sugars: advances using membrane vesicles. *Annual Review of Physiology*, **46**, 417–433.

50. Tobey, N., Heizer, W., Yeh, R., Huang, T.-I. and Hoffner, C. (1985) Human intestinal brush border peptidases. *Gastroenterology*, **88**, 913–926.

51. Waldman, D.A. (1966) Protein losing enteropathy. *Gastroenterology*, **50**, 422–432.

52. Walker, W.A. and Isselbacher, K.J. (1974) Uptake and transport of macromolecules by the intestine: possible role of clinical disorders. *Gastroenterology*, **67**, 531–550.

53. Wilcken, B., Yu, J.S. and Brown, D.A. (1977) Natural history of Hartnup disease. *Archives of Disease in Childhood*, **52**, 38–40.

54. Young, V.R. and Pellett, P.L. (1987) Protein intake and requirements with reference to diet and health. *American Journal of Clinical Nutrition*, **45**, 1323–1343.

DIGESTION AND MALABSORPTION OF MINERALS   *(R.C. Spiller)*

The Oxford Dictionary defines a mineral as 'a substance obtained by mining', a definition which considerably overlaps with the term 'trace elements'. Biologically important minerals include the elements sodium, magnesium, potassium, calcium, sulphur, phosphorus and chlorine as well as the trace elements (*Table 3.4*) which, in addition to being minerals, also have the distinction of being essential to life while being present in the body in only trace amounts. Recent experiments using total parenteral nutrition to maintain life for prolonged periods have provided a great impetus to our understanding of the importance of such elements. Limitations of space will permit only the absorption of the relatively well researched cations magnesium, zinc and copper to be concentrated upon; calcium and iron absorption is discussed elsewhere. Although knowledge of the precise daily requirements is far from complete in humans, deficiency syndromes have been described

Table 3.4 Trace elements considered to be essential in humans

Element	Daily requirements	Deficiency syndromes in humans
Iron	10–18 mg	Anaemia, lethargy
Iodine	10–20 μg	Myxoedema
Zinc	3–15 mg	Eczema, dwarfism, hypogonadism, anorexia, poor wound healing[37]
Selenium	100–200 μg	Cardiomyopathy[12]
Copper	0.3–0.5 mg	Anaemia, leukopenia, bony abnormalities[8]
Chromium	50–200 μg	Neuropathy, impaired glucose tolerance[22]
Molybdenum	150–500 μg	Amino acid intolerance[1]
Manganese	2–3 mg	?
Vanadium	?	Salt and water retention[15]

for most of these elements (*Table 3.4*), mainly in severe malabsorption and patients requiring long-term total parenteral nutrition.

MAGNESIUM

This ubiquitous, largely intracellular cation is required as a vital part of many essential enzymes, including ATPase. The wide distribution of magnesium in many foods, together with a substantial body pool (25 g in a 70 kg individual) means that deficiency is rare except in chronic malabsorption or excessive urinary losses induced by alcohol, diuretics or cytotoxic drugs.

Absorption

Magnesium salts are ionized once exposed to gastric acid, are thus highly water-soluble and readily absorbed. Radioactive isotope studies show that orally ingested magnesium appears rapidly in the blood within about 1 hour of ingestion and that about 40% of the total dose is absorbed.[3,16] Jejunal perfusion studies in humans show evidence of active jejunal and ileal absorption at low luminal levels of magnesium (<5 mmol), with passive diffusion probably via the paracellular route predominating at higher concentration.[7] Absorption is independent of calcium absorption but the mechanisms show certain similarities, both being stimulated by 1,25-dihydroxyvitamin D_3.[23] Active absorption can be demonstrated in the rat and may well occur in humans, being particularly important in patients with the short bowel syndrome.

Malabsorption

Hypomagnesaemia due to malabsorption has been reported in a range of patients with fat malabsorption due to both massive intestinal resection[18] as well as mucosal disease such as coeliac disease.[6]

Malabsorption of magnesium like that of calcium is also depressed in chronic renal failure, a defect that can be corrected by 1,25-dihydroxyvitamin D_3 treatment.[41]

A rare, specific, inherited disorder of magnesium absorption, primary hypomagnesaemia, has been described, presenting in infancy with convulsions and tetany[14] due to low levels of serum calcium and magnesium. Intravenous magnesium is needed to correct both the hypocalcaemia and the convulsions. Perfusion studies[29] have demonstrated that these patients have a defect of active magnesium transport at low luminal magnesium concentrations even though passive absorption at higher concentrations is normal.

Clinical features of magnesium deficiency

A low serum magnesium concentration is a poor guide to overall deficiency because it represents only 1% of total body stores. Measuring these stores is, however, impractical, and in normal clinical practice a low serum magnesium concentration together with low urinary 24-hour magnesium excretion is usually taken to represent magnesium depletion. Tetany, convulsions, lethargy and cardiac arrhythmias are all features of severe magnesium depletion which, in a 70 kg individual, respond rapidly to parenteral therapy with 50 mmol of magnesium sulphate given in 5% dextrose over a 12-hour period. Small bowel resection, as already mentioned, leads to a proportionate reduction in magnesium absorption so that hypomagnesaemia is common in the short bowel syndrome and also in patients suffering from radiation enteritis. Replacement by oral therapy may be difficult since magnesium salts commonly cause diarrhoea, which in such patients may be severe. Parenteral therapy may be necessary in these cases but an alternative may be to administer the magnesium together with glucose polymers which promote magnesium absorption.[5] Malabsorption of fat due to mucosal damage such as that found in coeliac disease is often associated with magnesium depletion both because of defective magnesium absorption but also because malabsorbed fatty acids bind magnesium in an insoluble form in the gut lumen. Removal of excess malabsorbed fat by means of a low-fat diet prevents this occurring and improves magnesium balance.[4,19,20] Urinary losses are increased by a range of substances including cisplatin, which often induces profound hypomagnesaemia. Increased urinary losses are also seen in alcoholics and the resulting hypomagnesaemia predisposes to withdrawal fits. Magnesium replacement is therefore important when these individuals are admitted for 'drying out'.

ZINC

Zinc is an important constituent of many enzymes, especially those involved in DNA synthesis and transcription. It is present in only trace amounts, total body stores amounting to only 2.5 g. Zinc is widely distributed in animal products and grains but at low concentrations so that, even on a normal diet, dietary intake is relatively low. Dietary interactions altering the bioavailability of zinc in food are therefore crucial in determining whether zinc deficiency develops.

Absorption

Dietary zinc is often bound to proteins and other dietary components such as phytate, complexes from which zinc is unavailable for absorption. This means that only about 15% of ingested zinc is actually absorbed. Orally administered ^{69}Zn results in peak blood levels 2–3 hours after ingestion, implying absorption in the upper and mid small intestine.[4] Intubation studies[28] show that, after a meal, zinc levels in the proximal small bowel actually rise compared to the concentration in the meal, reflecting the endogenous secretion of zinc in intestinal and pancreatic secretions. Further distally, net absorption is observed. Perfusion studies in humans show absorption throughout the small intestine, facilitated by glucose and by the presence of the dipeptide glycyl-lysine.[24,42] Once absorbed, zinc is transferred to albumin and α_2-macroglobulin, which account for 66 and 30%, respectively, of circulating zinc. This high degree of protein binding results in a low renal clearance, and urinary excretion is only a small fraction of the daily zinc flux. Most zinc is excreted in the faeces, derived from gastrointestinal secretions themselves together with unabsorbed dietary zinc. In hot countries, appreciable amounts of

zinc can also be lost by sweating. Perhaps because of its low dietary levels and relative lack of toxicity there are no clear pathways for excreting toxic loads of zinc, high intakes usually leading to a positive zinc balance for many months.

Zinc deficiency due to dietary interactions

Populations which subsist on a largely vegetarian diet are at risk from zinc deficiency, not only because they are excluding the best sources of zinc (meat, poultry and seafood) from their diet but also because they ingest large amounts of fibre, phytate and oxalate compounds which bind zinc and reduce bioavailability.[13,39,40] Some dramatic examples of zinc deficiency characterized by dwarfism and hypopituitarism which respond to zinc supplementation have been reported in Iranians, who ingest clay in addition to a high level of phytate. These two substances together bind zinc salts in insoluble complexes and reduce its bioavailability.[36,37]

Zinc deficiency and gastrointestinal diseases

Crohn's disease is commonly associated with a low serum zinc level, which correlates well with the serum albumin level. True zinc deficiency, that is to say, whole-body zinc depletion, is hard to identify but is usually diagnosed when a low serum zinc concentration is associated with low urinary zinc excretion. This combination was found in 15% of 63 patients with Crohn's disease.[11] There is an associated accelerated clearance of zinc,[34] presumably due to excessive losses in gastrointestinal secretions and desquamated cells. Zinc supplementation has been reported to be helpful in healing eczematous skin lesions in such patients. There have been, however, few controlled trials looking at the benefit of zinc supplementation alone in Crohn's disease since zinc supplements are usually given along with many other nutrients.

There have been some controlled trials of zinc supplementation which appears to correct defective taste in patients with uraemia[27] and also night blindness in patients with cirrhosis, another group who often show evidence of zinc depletion, usually due to excessive urinary losses.[32]

Specific defects in zinc absorption

Acrodermatitis enteropathica is a rare inherited (autosomal recessive) disease characterized by severe diarrhoea, dermatitis and alopecia which often presents when infants are transferred from breast milk to cow's milk. The disorder is associated with a subnormal serum zinc level and responds to either human breast milk or a small amount of zinc supplementation.[31,35] Severe eczema has also been reported in premature infants in association with a low serum zinc concentration and this also responds well to zinc supplements.[33] The fact that normal breast milk heals acrodermatitis enteropathica is explained by the recent finding that, in rats at least, neonates showed defective zinc absorption correctable by a low molecular weight zinc-binding protein found in both rat and human, but not bovine, milk.[10]

COPPER

Copper is found in many animal products, especially liver and kidneys, as well as shellfish, legumes and cola-type soft drinks. It forms a part of many vital enzymes, especially cytochrome-*c* oxidase and lysyl oxidase. In plasma, 90% of copper is in the form of caeruloplasmin, which is important because it facilitates the transfer of cellular iron to transferrin by oxidizing ferrous iron to ferric iron. Copper deficiency leads to an apparent iron deficiency owing to a block at this step in iron metabolism. Body stores of copper are large (100–150 mg) compared with daily intake and needs (*Table 3.4*). Furthermore, absorption increases in dietary deficiency so that deficiency in an adult is rarely due to dietary causes.

Absorption

This varies from 15 to 55% of an oral dose of ^{64}Cu, depending on dietary copper levels. Free copper ions are highly toxic, so copper in the body is usually in a bound form. After an oral dose there is an early rise in plasma copper, which is loosely bound to albumin, there is then a rapid clearance of copper by the liver and, after 24–48 hours, ^{64}Cu reappears in the plasma irreversibly bound to caeruloplasmin[43] (molecular mass 150 kDa). This distribution ensures that little copper is filtered by the glomeruli, urinary excretion being less than 10% of dietary intake.[2] The main route of excretion of this potentially toxic element is in the bile.[25,30] Defective excretion appears to be the main cause of Wilson's disease, a rare autosomal recessive trait (prevalence 1 in 200 000) characterized by a lifelong deficiency of caeruloplasmin and an accumulation of copper within the liver.[44] In biliary excretions, copper is firmly bound to a caeruloplasmin-like protein, probably a fragment of the whole molecule which is missing in Wilson's disease.[21] Caeruloplasmin is unusual in being protease-resistant, thus preventing the reabsorption of copper excreted from the body in this way. In the absence of such an excretory pathway, copper accumulates in the liver where it is stored in lysosomes.[17] Their ultimate rupture and release of toxic free copper together with lysosomal enzymes can lead to attacks of haemolysis with associated hepatic and renal damage.

Copper depletion syndromes

Premature neonates appear to have a much increased requirement for copper since a major part of total body copper stores are accumulated in the last 10 weeks of pregnancy. Copper deficiency has been reported in premature neonates who have malabsorption syndrome.[8]

Specific defects of copper transport

Menkes's kinky-hair disease is an X-linked, recessively inherited defect characterized by infantile seizures, psychomotor retardation, hypopigmentation, tortuous arteries, fragile bones and twisted hair.[9] Serum copper in these patients is at very low levels and the condition shares many features of copper deficiency as demonstrated in laboratory animals kept on a copper-deficient diet. Unfortunately, supplementation is rarely effective in reversing the clinical features. The few studies which have been done in this rare condition[26] suggest that absorption is defective, only about 10% of an oral dose being retained in the body in spite of the low serum copper concentration. Surprisingly, the copper content of the duodenum and kidneys is high while the normal site of copper accumulation, the liver, is depleted. Laboratory work has shown that there is a generalized cellular defect, and even fibroblasts show abnormal retention of copper, suggesting that although uptake is normal the process of transporting copper through the various cellular compartments is ineffective.[9] The various defects are associated with deficiencies of a range of copper-dependent enzymes.

Dietary interactions

Unlike zinc, phytate and other types of cellulose do not appear to significantly impair copper absorption.[45] However, zinc supplementation does run the risk of inducing copper depletion.[37] The mechanism is uncertain but interactions between trace elements are common, perhaps because they compete for similar binding sites. Zinc therapy given to patients with sickle cell disease has been reported to be associated with hypocupraemia, which manifests itself as macrocytosis and a relative neutropaenia. Bone marrow studies suggest iron deficiency, though the serum iron level is in fact normal, suggesting a defect in iron transport compatible with the known functions of copper.[38]

REFERENCES

1. Abumrad, N.W. (1981) Amino acid intolerance during prolonged total parenteral nutrition reversed by molybdenum. *Clinical Research*, **27**, 621A.

2. Adelstein, S.J. and Vallee, B.L. (1961) Copper metabolism in man. *New England Journal of Medicine*, **265**, 892–897.

3. Aikawa, J.K., Gordon, G.S. and Rhoades, E.L. (1960) Magnesium metabolism in human beings: studies with Mg^{28}. *Journal of Applied Physiology*, **15**, 503–507.

4. Andersson, K.E., Bratt, L., Dencker, H. and Lanner, E. (1976) Some aspects of the intestinal absorption of zinc in man. *European Journal of Clinical Pharmacology*, **9**, 423–428.

5. Bei, L., Wood, R.J. and Rosenberg, I.H. (1986) Glucose polymer increases jejunal calcium, magnesium and zinc absorption in humans. *American Journal of Clinical Nutrition*, **44**, 244–247.

6. Booth, C.C., Hanna, S., Babouris, N. and MacIntyre, I. (1963) Incidence of hypomagnesaemia in intestinal malabsorption. *British Journal of Medicine*, **iii**, 141–144.

7. Brannan, P.G., Vergne-Marini, P., Pak, C.Y.C., Hull, A.R. and Fordtran, J.S. (1976) Magnesium absorption in the human small intestine results in normal subjects, patients with chronic renal disease and patients with absorptive hypercalciuria. *Journal of Clinical Investigation*, **57**, 1412–1418.

8. Cordano, A. and Graham, G.C. (1966) Copper deficiency complicating severe chronic intestinal malabsorption. *Pediatrics*, **38**, 596–604.

9. Danks, D.M., Campbell, P.E., Walker-Smith, J. *et al.* (1972) Menkes' kinky hair syndrome. *The Lancet*, **i**, 1100–1103.

10. Duncan, J.R. and Hurley, L.S. (1978) Intestinal absorption of zinc: a role for a zinc-binding ligand in milk. *American Journal of Physiology*, **235**(5), E556–E559.

11. Flemming, C.R., Huizenga, K.A., McCall, J.T., Gildea, J. and Dennis, R. (1981) Zinc nutrition in Crohn's disease. *Digestive Diseases Scientific*, **26**, 865–870.

12. Fleming, C.R., McCall, J.T., O'Brien, J.F. *et al.* (1982) Selenium deficiency and fatal cardiomyopathy in a patient on home parenteral nutrition. *Gastroenterology*, **83**, 689–693.

13. Freeland-Graves, J. (1988) Mineral adequacy of vegetarian diets. *American Journal of Clinical Nutrition*, **48**, 859–862.

14. Friedman, H., Hatcher, G. and Watson, L. (1987) Primary hypomagnesia with secondary hypocalcaemia in an infant. *The Lancet*, **i**, 703–705.

15. Golden, M.H. and Golden, B.E. (1981) Trace elements. Potential importance in human nutrition with particular reference to zinc and vanadium. *British Medical Bulletin*, **37**, 31–36.

16. Graham, L.A., Caesar, J.J. and Burgen, A.S.V. (1960) Gastrointestinal absorption and excretion of Mg^{28} in man. *Metabolism*, **9**, 646–659.

17. Gooneratne, S.R., Howell, J.McM. and Cook, R.D. (1980) An ultrastructural and morphometric study of the liver of normal and copper-poisoned sheep. *American Journal Pathology*, **99**, 429–450.

18. Heaton, F.W. and Fourman, P. (1965) Magnesium deficiency and hypocalaemia in intestinal malabsorption. *The Lancet*, **ii**, 50–52.

19. Hessor, I., Hasselblad, C., Fusth, S. and Hulten, L. (1983) Magnesium deficiency after ileal resections for Crohn's disease. *Scandinavian Journal of Gastroenterology*, **18**, 643–649.

20. Hessor, I., Anderson, H. and Isaksson, B. (1983) Effects of a low fat diet on mineral absorption in small-bowel disease. *Scandinavian Journal of Gastroenterology*, **18**, 551–554.

21. Iyengar, V., Brewer, G.J., Dick, R.D. and Owyang, C. (1988) Studies of cholecytokinin-stimulated biliary secretions reveal a high molecular weight copper-binding substance in normal subjects that is absent in patients with Wilson's disease. *Journal of Laboratory Clinical Medicine*, **111**, 267–274.

22. Jeejeebhoy, K.M., Chu, R., Marliss, E.B. *et al.* (1975) Chromium deficiency, diabetes and neuropathy reversed by chromium infusion in a patient on total parenteral nutrition (TPN) for three and half years. *Clinical Research*, **23**, 636A.

23. Krejs, G.J., Nicar, M.J., Zerwekh, J.E., Norman, D.A., Kane, M.G. and Pak, C.Y.C. (1983) Effect of 1,25-dihydroxy vitamin D_3 on calcium and magnesium absorption in the healthy human jejunum and ileum. *American Journal of Medicine*, **75**, 973–976.

24. Lee, H.H., Prasad, A.S., Brewer, G.F. and Owyang, C. (1989) Zinc absorption in human small intestine. *American Journal of Physiology*, **256**, G67–G91.

25. Lewis, K.W. (1973) The nature of the copper complexes in bile and their relationship to the absorption and excretion of copper in normal subjects and in Wilson's disease. *Gut*, **14**, 221–232.

26. Lucky, A.W. and Hsia, Y.E. (1979) Distribution of ingested and injected radiocopper in two patients with Menkes' kinky hair disease. *Pediatric Research*, **13**, 1280–1284.

27. Mahajan, S.K., Prasad, A.S., Lambujon, J., Abbasi, A.A., Briggs, W.A. and McDonald, F.D. (1980) Improvement of uremic hypogeusia by zinc: a double-blind study. *American Journal of Clinical Nutrition*, **33**, 1517–1521.

28. Matseshe, J.W., Phillips, S.F., Malagelada, J.-R. and McCall, J.T. (1980) Recovery of dietary iron and zinc from the proximal intestine of healthy man: studies of different meals and supplements. *American Journal of Clinical Nutrition*, **33**, 1946–1953.

29. Milla, P.J., Aggett, P.J., Wolf, O.H. and Harries, J.J. (1979) Studies in primary hypomagnesaemia: evidence for defective carrier-mediated small intestinal transport of magnesium. *Gut*, **20**, 1028–1033.

30. Mistilis, S.P. and Farrer, P.A. (1968) The absorption of biliary and non-biliary radio-copper in the rat. *Scandinavian Journal of Gastroenterology*, **3**, 586–592.

31. Moynahan, E.J. (1974) Acrodermatitis enteropathica: a lethal inherited human zinc-deficiency disorder. *The Lancet*, **ii**, 399–400.

32. Morrison, S.A., Russell, R.M., Carney, E.A. and Oaks, E.V. (1978) Zinc deficiency: a cause of abnormal dark adaptation in cirrhotics. *American Journal Clinical Nutrition*, **31**, 276–281.

33. Munro, C.S., Lazaro, C. and Lawrence, C.M. (1989) Symptomatic zinc deficiency in breast-fed premature infants. *British Journal of Dermatology*, **121**, 773–778.

34. Nakamura, T., Higashi, A., Takano, S., Akagi, M. and Matsuda, I. (1988) Zinc clearance correlates with clinical severity of Crohn's disease. A kinetic study. *Digestive Diseases & Sciences*, **33**, 1520–1524.

35. Neldner, K.H. and Hambridge, K.M. (1975) Zinc therapy of an acrodermatitis enteropathica. *New England Journal of Medicine*, **292**, 879–882.

36. Prasad, A.S. (1983) The role of zinc in gastrointestinal and liver disease. *Gastroenterology Clinic*, **12**, 713–741.

37. Prasad, A.S., Miale, A., Farid, Z. *et al.* (1963) Biochemical studies on dwarfism, hypogonadism and anaemia. *Archives of Internal Medicine*, **111**, 407–428.

38. Prasad, A.S., Brewer, G.J., Schoomaker, E.B., Rubbani, P. (1978) Hypocupremia induced by zinc therapy in adults. *Journal of the American Medical Association*, **240**, 2166–2168.

39. Reinhold, J.G., Lahimgarzadek, A., Nasr, K. and Hedayrich, H. (1973) Effects of purified phytate and phytate-rich bread upon metabolism of zinc, calcium, phosphorus and nitrogen in man. *The Lancet*, **i**, 283–288.

40. Reinhold, J.G., Pursu, A., Karimian, N. *et al.* (1974) Availability of zinc in leavened and unleavened whole meal wheaten bread as measured by solubility and uptake by rate intestine *in vitro*. *Journal of Nutrition*, **105**, 976–982.

41. Schmulen, A.C., Lerman, M., Pak, C.Y.C., Zerwekn, J., Morawski, S., Fordtran, J.S. and Vergne-Marini, P. (1980) Effect of 1,25-$(OH)_2 D_3$ on jejunal absorption of magnesium in patients with chronic renal disease. *American Journal of Physiology*, **238**, G349–G352.

42. Steinhardt, H.H. and Adibi, S.A. (1984) Interaction between transport of zinc and other solutes in human intestine. *American Journal of Physiology*, **247**, 176–182.

43. Sternlieb, I. (1967) Gastrointestinal copper absorption in man. *Gastroenterology*, **52**, 1038–1041.

44. Sternlieb, I., Morrell, A.G., Bauer, C.D. *et al.* (1961) Detection of the heterozygous carrier of the Wilson's disease gene. *Journal of Clinical Investigations*, **40**, 707–715.

45. Turnlund, J.R., King, J.C., Gong, B., Keyes, W.R. and Michel, M.C. (1985) A stable isotope study of copper absorption in young men: effect of phytate and alpha-cellulose. *American Journal of Clinical Nutrition*, **42**, 18–23.

DIGESTION AND MALABSORPTION OF VITAMINS* *(R.C. Spiller)*

Vitamins are essential dietary substances present in very low concentration (a few milligrams per litre) in normal food. After dilution in intestinal secretions the luminal concentrations lie in the 10^{-8}–10^{-6} mmol/l range. Since vitamins are essential for life it is not surprising that specific transport mechanisms have evolved to ensure adequate absorption at these very low concentrations. Earlier studies using high concentrations of vitamins suggested absorption was largely passive but it is now clear that at physiologically relevant concentrations there are active, usually sodium-dependent, specific transport mechanisms for most of the water-soluble vitamins. Since these mechanisms are widely distributed throughout the small intestine, failure of absorption is rare except after massive intestinal resection or in severe mucosal damage such as is seen in untreated coeliac disease. The usual cause of deficiency of water-soluble vitamins is therefore inadequate intake.

The fat-soluble vitamins A, D, E and K appear to be absorbed by the same transport mechanism as for fatty acids, and bind to the fatty acid-binding proteins which lie within the brush border of the enterocyte;[20] thus, all conditions characterized by fat malabsorption are likely to lead to varying deficiencies in these particular vitamins.

VITAMIN A

Function

The aldehyde of vitamin A (retinaldehyde) when combined with a protein, opsin, forms the light-sensitive pigment rhodopsin, lack of which leads to night blindness. More recently, it has been recognized that vitamin A also acts directly on the nucleus to control cellular differentiation,[15] and lack of vitamin A has been associated with disorders of growth, cellular differentiation, reproduction and immunocompetence.[38]

*Excluding vitamin D and vitamin B_{12}.

Dietary sources

Vitamin A (retinol) is ingested mainly as retinyl esters and a range of carotenoids, the most abundant of which (β-carotene) is cleaved in the enterocyte to retinaldehyde and then reduced to retinol. Carrots and green leafy vegetables such as spinach contain abundant (2000–3000 μg/100 mg) carotenoids, as do some fruits, and these non-animal sources account for about 40% of vitamin A intake in a normal diet.[31] After absorption, vitamin A in animals, as in humans, is largely stored in the liver, which is also the most concentrated dietary source of vitamin A (3000–15 000 μg/100 mg). Meat, eggs and milk are also important sources, containing 30–70 μg/100 ml.

Absorption

Absorption of vitamin A is 70–80% efficient, though carotenoid absorption is much less so, 6 μg of dietary β-carotene needing to be ingested to ensure absorption of 1 μg of retinol. Uptake of retinol by the enterocyte is by carrier-mediated passive absorption showing saturation kinetics. Competitive inhibition is observed with polyunsaturated fatty acids, suggesting a common carrier, perhaps the fatty acid-binding protein found in the enterocyte brush border. Once in the enterocyte, retinol is re-esterified before being transported in the lymph in chylomicrons as retinyl esters. The hepatic uptake is substantial and excess vitamin A is stored in hepatic fat cells. Vitamin A is secreted from the liver bound to retinol-binding protein, which allows its delivery to peripheral tissues.

Since hydrolysis is necessary to liberate retinol before it can be absorbed, pancreatic insufficiency as seen in cystic fibrosis may be associated with clinical vitamin A deficiency leading to xerophthalmia[45] in spite of daily vitamin A supplements. However, in most cases vitamin A deficiency is due to inadequate intake.

Deficiency syndrome

Overt vitamin A deficiency progresses from night blindness to the development of xerophthalmia, which, if untreated, leads to corneal destruction and, ultimately, permanent blindness. More subtle borderline deficiency appears to manifest itself as an impaired ability to repair mucosal surfaces. The measles virus, which attacks mucosal surfaces, results in a prompt fall in vitamin A levels. Vitamin A supplementation in areas of borderline vitamin A intake has been reported to reduce the mortality of measles by 80%[4] and simultaneously to reduce the overall mortality of whole populations. Fortification

of staple foods such as bread and margarine with vitamin A in the Western world means that in these countries vitamin A deficiency is extremely rare and, in fact, toxicity is a more likely hazard. Habitual consumption of >100 g of liver per day or ingestion of large doses of vitamin A in the form of multivitamin preparations may result in a syndrome characterized by headaches, vomiting, desquamation of the skin and hepatotoxicity. Even modest amounts of liver ingested on a daily basis may be undesirable for pregnant women because vitamin A, even at low doses, can be teratogenic.[30]

VITAMIN E

The term 'vitamin E' covers a family of tocopherols and tocotrienols of which α-tocopherol is the most biologically active. The function of vitamin E in humans is unclear but it may act as an antioxidant, protecting membrane-associated polyunsaturated fatty acids from lipid peroxidation by free radicals.

Dietary sources

Requirements are uncertain but 10–30 mg/day is advised. The naturally occurring tocopherols are synthesized by green plants. Rich dietary sources of the vitamin include dairy products, meat, fish, nuts, green vegetables, and vegetable and nut oils.

Absorption

Bile salts are vital to the absorption of vitamin E, being required to activate a specific esterase needed to liberate free α-tocopherol from its esters and allow micelle formation, which is necessary for tocopherol absorption.[26,27] Unlike vitamin A, tocopherol is not re-esterified but transported unchanged in the chylomicrons via the lymphatics to peripheral tissues. Severe prolonged obstructive jaundice, such as is seen in childhood cholestasis and in adults in primary biliary cirrhosis, leads to malabsorption of vitamin E,[36,37] while in coeliac disease absorption is virtually normal. Severe prolonged deficiency may lead to ataxia, peripheral neuropathy and retinal defects similar to those seen in abetalipoproteinaemia.[12,22] Prolonged deficiency may also be associated with the 'brown bowel syndrome', in which brown pigment accumulates in the smooth muscle of the small intestine, perhaps due to lipid peroxidation.[39]

As descriptions of the neurological consequences of vitamin E deficiency are not readily available, they will be described here. As far as liver disease is concerned, neurological dysfunction secondary to vitamin E deficiency has been described most frequently in children with congenital biliary atresia. Neurological symptoms, chiefly unsteadiness of gait and weakness, developed between the ages of 5 and 15 years, although depression or absence of the tendon reflexes may precede symptoms by a number of years. Ptosis, failure of upgaze and limitation of eye adduction have been described in some children, as has dysarthria. Limb and gait ataxia were prominent features. The tendon reflexes were depressed or absent and the plantar responses often extensor. Proprioceptive and vibration sense loss was common and often severe. Some patients had generalized muscle weakness and lordosis.

The neurological syndrome varied somewhat in relation to progression. A few patients were unable to walk 1 year after the onset of gait ataxia but in others the disorder was more slowly progressive. Serum vitamin E levels were extremely low or undetectable in all these cases. Neurologic dysfunction secondary to vitamin E deficiency has not been described in adults with liver disease.

A neurological disorder similar to that described in biliary atresia has been reported in some patients with cystic fibrosis.[11,53] Symptoms did not develop until the latter part of the second decade of life and these were relatively slowly progressive but disabling. Again, vitamin E levels were undetectable or extremely low. A few adult patients with a spinocerebellar syndrome presumed due to vitamin E deficiency have been described in the setting of extensive small bowel resections and chronic steatorrhoea with intermittent bacterial overgrowth in the gut.

The neurological signs of abetalipoproteinaemia are now regarded as entirely explicable on the basis of vitamin E deficiency. Parenteral or massive oral therapy (100 mg/kg per day) can reverse or prevent further deterioration in neurological abnormalities.

VITAMIN K

Function

Vitamin K catalyses the conversion of glutamyl residues in precursors of plasma clotting factors II, VII, IX, X[16] to γ-carboxyglutamyl residues in the mature proteins. The vitamin is therefore essential for normal blood coagulation.

Dietary sources

Vitamin K activity is found in two main forms, phylloquinone (vitamin K_1) from green vegetables and menaquinones (vitamin K_2) synthesized by colonic bacteria. Daily requirements are about 70 μg, a normal diet supplying an average daily intake of 100–200 μg.[41] Body stores are small and blood levels fall rapidly after only 1 week on a diet deficient in vitamin K. Green vetetables, cow's and formula milk are rich in vitamin K while human breast milk is a poor source. Breast-fed neonates should therefore receive vitamin K supplementation to prevent them developing haemorrhagic disease of the newborn characterized by petechial bruising, spontaneous purpura and bleeding from the gums and skin. Malnourished patients and those on total parenteral nutrition are likely to have marginal vitamin K status.

Broad-spectrum antibiotics, especially cephalosporins, induce hypoprothrombinaemia responsive to vitamin K. The mechanism is unclear because other broad-spectrum antibiotics such as tetracycline do not. Some cephalosporins interfere with hepatocyte regeneration of vitamin K_2 and this may be a possible mechanism. The importance of menaquinones synthesized by the colonic flora is probably overrated because they are certainly not sufficient to prevent vitamin K deficiency if the diet is inadequate.[41]

Absorption

This is similar to vitamin A and E, occurring by means of a saturable transport mechanism competing with other fatty acids.[19] Bile is necessary[14] and, like other fat-soluble vitamins, vitamin K is transported via the lymphatics in chylomicrons. Malabsorption is seen in diseases of fat malabsorption such as cystic fibrosis.[9]

WATER-SOLUBLE VITAMINS

Vitamin B₁ (thiamine)

Function

Thiamine pyrophosphate is a coenzyme for the decarboxylation of α-keto acids such as pyruvic and α-ketoglutaric acid, which form vital steps in intermediary metabolism.

Dietary sources

Most thiamine in an average Western diet comes from cereals and enriched grain products. Pork, beef and wheatgerm are, however, the richest sources on a gram per kilogram basis.

Absorption

As illustrated in *Table 3.5*, active, sodium-dependent transport has been demonstrated at low luminal concentrations.[21,28] This is transiently impaired by alcohol but rapidly reverts to normal

Table 3.5 Water-soluble vitamins: recommended intake and transport properties

Vitamin	Recommended intake	Active transport	Na$^+$ dependence	Comments	Reference
Vitamin B$_1$ (thiamine)	3 mg	+	+	Passive absorption at high concentrations, impaired in coeliac disease and alcoholism	21,42,43
Vitamin B$_2$ (riboflavin)	3–4 mg	+	+		11
Pantothenic acid	15 mg	+	+		13
Vitamin B$_6$ (pyridoxine)	2 mg	–	–	Passive absorption only. Impaired in coeliac disease	29,33
Niacin	15 mg	–	–	Probably passive absorption	35
Vitamin C	60 mg	+	+		28,40
Biothin	60 µg	+	+		7

after a few weeks of abstinence.[43] Coeliacs also showed impaired absorption which rapidly corrected on a gluten-free diet.[42] Deficiency is, however, in most cases, as with other water-soluble vitamins, largely due to inadequate intake.

Deficiency syndromes

Communities subsisting on a low-thiamine diet such as is found in South-East Asia are particularly liable to develop florid deficiency syndromes such as 'wet beriberi' because their diets contain certain antithiamine factors (mechanism unknown) found in fish, especially carp. Wet beriberi consists of high-output cardiac failure with sodium and water retention. Dry beriberi is a syndrome of deficiency in which neurological damage predominates, with haemorrhagic brain-stem lesions leading to nystagmus, opthalmoplegia and ataxia (Wernick's encephalopathy), a syndrome which is reversible by acute thiamine administration. Untreated, a later, irreversible syndrome of severe short-term memory loss develops with associated confabulation (Korsakoff's psychosis). These features are rarely seen in Western societies apart from in alcoholics. Alcoholics not only have a diet poor in thiamine but also have impaired thiamine absorption.[42] Susceptibility to developing neurological sequelae may well be due to a genetically determined abnormality of a thiamine-dependent enzyme which fails to bind thiamine normally.[6]

Vitamin B$_2$ (riboflavin)

Function

This ubiquitous yellow enzyme is one of the mitochondrial cytochromes involved in electron transfer during oxidative reactions (*Figure 3.32*).

Dietary sources

Milk, eggs and leafy green vegetables are the chief sources in an average diet, which contains 2–3 mg of riboflavine a day, about 2–3 times the minimum requirement. A significant amount is made by colonic bacteria, but how much of this is available to the host is uncertain.

Absorption

Active, saturatable, sodium-linked transport has been demonstrated at low concentrations (*Table 3.5*), whereas at higher concentrations, which have often been used in experimental studies, absorption is largely passive.[11] Dietary riboflavine is usually present as FMN and FAD, which require hydrolysis by phosphatases in the brush border prior to absorption as free riboflavine.[1]

Deficiency

Experimentally induced riboflavine deficiency leads to cheilosis, a red, fissured, macerated, angular stomatitis with a smooth 'magenta' tongue as well as photophobia, blurred vision and paraesthesia. The

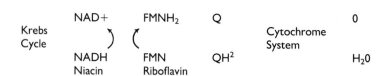

Figure 3.32 The role of NAD in aerobic respiration, resulting in the reduction of molecular oxygen to water.

underlying mechanism in these lesions appears to be capillary dilatation which is most noticeable in the vascular mucosa at mucocutaneous junctions. Response to riboflavine replacement is rapid, with complete resolution after a few weeks.

Diets deficient in riboflavine are also often deficient in pyridoxine and niacin, and in individual cases it is hard to identify which deficiency is responsible. Conversion of pyridoxine to its coenzymes requires riboflavin and conversion of tryptophan to nicotinamide requires pyridoxine, so in many situations there are multiple deficiencies leading to the dermal and connective tissue lesions.[25]

Pantothenic acid

Dietary pantothenic acid occurs primarily in the form of coenzyme A, which is hydrolysed to pantothenic acid in the gut lumen prior to absorption. It is then subsequently converted back to coenzyme A within the cytosol of most cells of the body where, as acetyl coenzyme A, it occupies a central role in the intermediate metabolism of carbohydrate, protein and fats.

Dietary sources
Most animal products including meat, liver, eggs, salt and milk contain abundant pantothenic acid.

Absorption
Active, energy-dependent, sodium-linked transport is observed at low concentrations across the gut mucosa[13] and also from the blood into muscle cells.[23]

Deficiency syndromes
Efficient absorption of pantothenic acid and its very extensive distribution within the body and in the diet mean that deficiency has only been observed in highly artificial settings. After 6–14 weeks on a diet deficient in pantothenic acid, subjects developed muscle soreness, tremor, incoordination and lethargy.[17] In clinical practice it seems unlikely that isolated pantothenic deficiency would occur as such a diet would almost certainly be deficient in many other vitamins.

Niacin

Function
The term 'niacin' includes nicotinic acid and its amide, nicotinamide, as well as derivatives which can be converted *in vivo* to these compounds. Its derivative NAD plays a vital role in many oxidative processes, acting as both a hydrogen acceptor and donor (*Figure 3.32*).

Although referred to as a vitamin, nicotinamide can be synthesized from tryptophan, and dietary deficiency is only seen when the diet is deficient in both niacin and tryptophan.

Dietary sources
Animal products are good sources of niacin. Although grains also contain niacin as nicotinic acid esters, these are not readily hydrolysed by human enzymes and hence not available. Maize diets are commonly associated with deficiency because this cereal is low both in available niacin and tryptophan. A notable exception to this is Mexican tortilla maize flour, which is steeped overnight in a calcium hydroxide solution, which hydrolyses the nicotinic acid esters and liberates free nicotinic acid which is then available for absorption.[8]

Absorption
Normal subjects absorb >90% ingested niacin with nicotinamides being converted within the enterocyte to NAD.[35] Absorption appears to be passive, the only specific defect in absorption is an inherited defect of tryptophan absorption, Hartnup disease.

Deficiency syndromes
Pellagra, a feature of communities in which maize is the staple food, was once common in the Southern USA. It is now rarely seen, except in the poor of Africa and Asia. The three 'Ds' said to characterize pellagra are dermatitis, diarrhoea and dementia. The dermatitis is characterized by dry scaly hyperpigmented skin often associated with soreness of the tongue and mouth. Enterocyte damage leads to diarrhoea and advanced cases are characterized by confusion, delusion, psychosis and epilepsy. The psychiatric changes may relate to 5-hydroxytryptamine depletion because this is usually synthesized from tryptophan.

Isoniazid therapy, by inducing pyridoxine deficiency (see below), interferes with the synthesis of nicotinamide from tryptophan and may lead to pellagra-like features which respond to pyridoxine replacement. Pellagra may also be a feature of advanced carcinoid syndrome, reflecting diversion of tryptophan to serotonin metabolism.

Vitamin B₆ (pyridoxine)

Function
Pyridoxal phosphate is a cofactor for many enzymes, especially those involved in decarboxylation or transamination of amino acids.

Dietary sources

Liver, meat and fish are good sources, as are bananas and avocados, but there is little in other fruits. The grains and legumes also contain some pyridoxine.

Absorption

Unlike other water-soluble vitamins there does not appear to be a specialized transport system.[29] Deficiency is, however, rare, probably because body stores are large and pyridoxine is manufactured by gut bacteria, a source which may be available to the host.

Deficiency syndrome

Pyridoxine-responsive convulsions have been described in neonates fed on milk low in vitamin B_6[10] while a pyridoxine-responsive peripheral neuropathy develops in some patients receiving isoniazid. Isoniazid inactivates pyridoxine by forming an inactive hydrazone. However, symptomatic deficiency can be avoided by the co-prescription of pyridoxine 10 mg daily. Oral contraceptives accelerate the metabolic pathways requiring pyridoxine and may produce a marginal deficiency.[3]

Vitamin C

Function

Vitamin C is a reducing substance with many biological actions. It is important in the hydroxylation of proline and lysine during collagen synthesis and another important function is the facilitation of iron absorption by reducing dietary ferric ions to ferrous ions, which are much better absorbed.

Dietary sources

Citrus fruits and fresh vegetables are good sources of vitamin C. Scurvy was common in 16th century sailors living off biscuits and dried meat and is seen in modern times in elderly patients who live alone and often survive on convenience preprocessed foods containing little vitamin C (bachelor's scurvy).

Absorption

An active, energy-dependent, stereospecific, sodium-linked transport mechanism has been demonstrated in humans (*Table 3.5*) which is distributed throughout the small intestine. Vitamin C is concentrated in the enterocyte, which is capable of converting oxidized vitamin C to its biologically active, reduced form. This may be important in protecting enterocytes from damage from free radicals derived from dietary carcinogens. Malabsorption of vitamin C is rare and most cases of deficiency are due to poor dietary intake. In the UK, intake is often marginal, and low levels of vitamin C are commonly found in the UK in elderly hospitalized patients during the winter months,[34] probably reflecting the decline in intake of vitamin C-rich foods. Body stores (1500 mg) are usually adequate for 4–6 months, so deficiency states are only obvious if defective intake continues for a prolonged period.

Deficiency syndromes

Petechial haemorrhage is followed by spontaneous bruising, swollen gums, hyperkeratosis, coiled hair and follicular congestion, usually most obvious on the buttocks and thighs. Joint pains and effusions are late manifestations occurring when body stores of vitamin C fall below 10% of normal.[18] All these symptoms respond rapidly to modest doses of vitamin C 100 mg daily for a few weeks. Megadose (>500 mg daily) therapy has been advocated for a wide range of conditions without much support from controlled trials.[34] High doses lead to an accelerated catabolism of vitamin C, uricosuria, excessive absorption of food iron and, in a few cases, haemolysis in patients with glucose-6-phosphate dehydrogenase deficiency,[32] features which support a cautious approach to the uncritical and unmonitored use of such therapy.

Biotin

Biotin is the prosthetic group of carboxylases, enzymes which allow the addition of carbon dioxide to elongate short-chain fatty acids, e.g. conversion of pyruvate to oxaloacetate.

Dietary sources

Biotin is found widely in the diet, sources including liver, kidney, chicken, eggs, pulses and cereals.

Absorption

Dietary biotin is usually bound and requires hydrolysis before free biotin is liberated and can be absorbed. Active uptake has been observed, and is greater in the jejunum than in the ileum.[5,7] Absorption can be prevented by the presence of avidin, a protein found in raw egg white. Deficiency states are rare but have been reported during total parenteral nutrition[24] and in an individual who ate 10 raw eggs per day for many years.[46] Experimental biotin deficiency induced by eating raw eggs together with a diet low in biotin induced a macular dermatitis, muscle aches, paraesthesia and anorexia after 4–6 weeks. A genetic defect in biotin metabolism has recently been described in infants in whom 10 mg of biotin corrects a carboxylase deficiency associated with a metabolic acidosis, an erythematous rash, alopecia and keratoconjunctivitis.[44]

REFERENCES

1. Akiyama, T., Selhub, J. and Rosenberg, I.H. (1982) FMN phosphatase and FAD pyrophosphatase in rat intestinal brush border: role in intestinal absorption of dietary riboflavin. *Journal of Nutrition*, **112**, 263–268.

2. Andrassy, K., Bechtold, H. and Ritz, E. (1985) Hypoprothrombinaemia caused by cephalosporins. *Journal of Antimicrobial Chemotherapy*, **15**, 133–135.

3. Barker, B.M. and Bender, P.A. (1980) Vitamin B$_6$. In: *Vitamins in Medicine*, Vol. 1 (Eds.) Barker, B.M. and Bender, D.A. London: Heinemann.

4. Barclay, A.J.G., Foster, A. and Somner, A. (1987) Vitamin A supplements and mortality related to measles: a randomised clinical trial. *British Medical Journal*, **294**, 294–296.

5. Berger, E., Long, E. and Semenza, G. (1972) The sodium activation of biotin absorption in hamster small intestine *in vitro*. *Biochemica et Biophysica Acta*, **255**, 873–887.

6. Blass, J.P. and Gibson, G.E. (1977) Abnormality of a thiamine-requiring enzyme in patients with Wernicke–Korsakoff syndrome. *New England Journal of Medicine*, **297**, 1367–1370.

7. Bowman, B.B., Selhub, J. and Rosenberg, I.H. (1986) Intestinal absorption of biotin in the rat. *Journal of Nutrition*, **116**, 1266–1271.

8. Carter, E.G.A. and Carpenter, K.J. (1982) The bioavailability for humans of bound niacin from wheat bran. *American Journal of Clinical Nutrition*, **36**, 855–861.

9. Congden, P.J., Bruce, G., Rothburn, M.M., Clarke, P.C.N., Littlewood, J.M., Kelleher, J. and Losowsky, M.S. (1981) Vitamin status in treated patients with cystic fibrosis. *Archives of Diseases in Childhood*, **56**, 708–714.

10. Coursin, D.B. (1954) Convulsive seizures in infants with pyridoxine deficient diets. *Journal of the American Medical Association*, **454**, 406–408.

11. Daniel, H., Wille, U. and Rohrer, S. (1983) *In vitro* kinetics of the intestinal transport of riboflavin in rats. *Journal of Nutrition*, **113**, 636–643.

12. Elias, E., Muller, D.P.R. and Scott, J. (1981) Association of spinocerebellar disorder with cystic fibrosis or chronic childhood cholestasis and very low serum vitamin E. *The Lancet*, **ii**, 1319–1321.

13. Fenstermacher, D.K. and Rose, R.C. (1986) Absorption of pantothenic acid in rat and chick intestine. *American Journal of Physiology*, **250**, G155–G160.

14. Forsgren, L. (1969) Studies on the intestinal absorption of labelled fat-soluble vitamins (A, D, E & K) via the thoracic duct lymph in the absorption of bile in man. *Acta Chirurgica Scandinavica Supplementum*, **399**.

15. Goodman, D.S. (1984) Vitamin A and retinoids in health and disease. *New England Journal of Medicine*, **310**, 1023–1031.

16. Hathaway, W.E. (1987) New insights in vitamin K. *Haematology/Oncology Clinics of North America*. **1**(3), 367–377.

17. Hodges, R.E., Olson, M.A. and Bean, W.B. (1958) Pantothenic acid deficiency in man. *Journal of Clinical Investigation*, **37**, 1642–1657.

18. Hodges, R.E., Hood, J., Lonharm, J.E., Sauberlich, H.E. and Baker, E.M. (1971) Clinical manifestations of ascorbic acid deficiency in man. *American Journal of Clinical Nutrition*, **24**, 432–443.

19. Hollander, D. and Muralidhara, K.S. (1977) Vitamin A, intestinal absorption *in vivo*: influence of luminal factors on transport. *American Journal of Physiology*, **232**, E471–E477.

20. Hollander, D., Rim, E. and Muralidhara, K.S. (1977) Vitamin K$_1$ intestinal absorption *in vivo*: influence of luminal contents on transport. *American Journal of Physiology*, **232**, E69–E74.

21. Hoyumpa, A.M., Middleton, H.M., Wilson, F.A. and Schenker, S. (1975) Thiamine transport across the rat intestine. *Gastroenterology*, **68**, 1218–1227.

22. Howard, L., Ovesen, L., Satya-Murti, S. and Chu, R. (1982) Reversible neurological symptoms caused by vitamin E deficiency in a patient with short bowel syndrome. *American Journal of Clinical Nutrition*, **36**, 1243–1249.

23. Lopaschuk, G.D., Michalak, M. and Tsang, H. (1987) Regulation of pantothenic acid transport in the heart. *Journal of Biological Chemistry*, **262**, 3615–3622.

24. McClain, C.J., Baker, H. and Onstad, G.R. (1982) Biotin deficiency in an adult during home parenteral nutrition. *Journal of the American Medical Association*, **247**, 3116–3317.

25. McCormick, D.B. (1989) Two interconnected B vitamins: riboflavin and pyridoxine. *Physiology Review*, **69**, 1170–1198.

26. MacMahon, M.T. and Neale, G. (1970) The absorption of α-tocopherol in control subjects and in patients with intestinal malabsorption. *Clinical Science*, **38**, 197–210.

27. Mathias, P.M., Harries, J.T., Peters, T.J. and Muller, D.P.R. (1981) Studies on the *in vivo* absorption of micellular solutions of tocopherol and tocophenyl acetate in the rat: demonstration and partial characterisation of a mucosal esterase localized to the endoplasmic reticulum of the enterocyte. *Journal of Lipid Research*, **22**, 829–837.

28. Mellors, A.J., Nahrwold, D.L. and Rose, R.C. (1987) Ascorbic acid flux across mucosal border of guinea pig and human ileum. *American Journal of Physiology*, **233**(5), E374–E379.

29. Middleton, H.M. (1977) Uptake of pyridoxine hydrochloride by the rat jejunal mucosa *in vitro*. *Journal of Nutrition*, **107**, 126–131.

30. Nelson, M. (1990) Vitamin A, liver consumption, and risk of birth defects. *British Medical Journal*, **301**, 1176.

31. Olson, J.A. (1987) Recommended dietary intakes (RDI) of vitamin A in humans. *American Journal of Clinical Nutrition*, **45**, 704–716.

32. Omaye, S.T., Skala, J.H. and Jacob, R.A. (1986) Plasma ascorbic acid in adult males: effect of depletion and supplementation. *American Journal of Clinical Nutrition*, **44**, 257–264.

33. Reinken, L. and Zieglauer, H. (1978) Vitamin B_6 absorption in children with acute coeliac disease and in control subjects. *Journal of Nutrition*, **108**, 1562–1565.

34. Schorah, C.J. (1981) The level of vitamin C reserves required in man: towards a solution to the controversy. *Proceedings of the Nutritional Society*, **40**, 147–154.

35. Schuette, S.A. and Rose, R.C. (1983) Nicotinamide uptake and metabolism by chick intestine. *American Journal of Physiology*, **245**, G531–G538.

36. Sokol, R.J., Heubi, J.E., Iannaccone, S., Bove, K.E. and Balistreri, W.F. (1983) Mechanism causing vitamin E deficiency during chronic childhood cholestasis. *Gastroenterology*, **85**, 1172–1182.

37. Sokol, R.J., Kim, Y.S., Hoffnagle, J.H., Heubi, J.E., Jones, A. and Balisteri, W.F. (1989) Intestinal malabsorption of vitamin E in primary biliary cirrhosis. *Gastroenterology*, **96**, 479–486.

38. Somner, A. (1989) New imperatives for an old vitamin (A). *Journal of Nutrition*, **119**, 96–100.

39. Stamp, G.W.H. and Evans, D.J. (1987) Accumulation of ceroid in smooth muscle indicates severe malabsorption and vitamin E deficiency. *Journal of Clinical Pathology*, **40**, 798–802.

40. Stevenson, W. R. (1974) Active transport of L-ascorbic acid in the human. *Gastroenterology*, **67**, 952–956.

41. Suttie, J.W., Mummah-Shendel, L.L., Shah, D.V., Lyle, B.J. and Greger, J.L. (1987) Vitamin K deficiency from dietary vitamin K restriction in humans. *American Journal of Clinical Nutrition*, **47**, 475–480.

42. Thomson, A.D. (1966) The absorption of radioactive sulphur-labelled thiamine hydrochloride in control subjects and in patients with intestinal malabsorption. *Clinical Science*, **31**, 167–179.

43. Thomson, A.D., Baker, H. and Leevy, C.M. (1970) Patterns of ^{35}S-thiamine HCl absorption in the malnourished alcoholic patient. *Journal of Laboratory and Clinical Medicine*, **76**, 34–45.

44. Thoene, J., Baker, H., Yoshino, M. and Sweetman, L. (1981) Biotin-responsive carboxylase deficiency associated with subnormal plasma and urinary biotin. *New England Journal of Medicine*, **304**, 817–823.

45. Vernon, S.A., Neugebauer, M.A.Z., Brimlow, G., Tyrell, J.C. and Hiller, E.J. (1989) Conjunctival xerosis in cystic fibrosis. *Journal of the Royal Society of Medicine*, **82**, 46–47.

46. Williams, R.H. (1943) Clinical biotin deficiency. *New England Journal Medicine*, **228**, 247–252.

DIGESTION AND MALABSORPTION OF HAEMATINICS (INCLUDING GASTROINTESTINAL FEATURES OF PERNICIOUS ANAEMIA) *(A.V. Hoffbrand)*

VITAMIN B_{12}

Dietary sources

Vitamin B_{12} was originally isolated as cyanocobalamin but is now known to consist of a group of compounds, known as cobalamins, each with a nucleotide portion (composed of the base 5,6-benzimdazole attached to the sugar ribose) and a planar corrin ring with a cobalt atom at its centre (*Figure 3.33*). In the four compounds found in human tissues, a methyl (—CH_3), deoxyadenosyl (ado-), hydroxyl (—OH) or cyano (—CH) group is attached to the cobalt atom. Cyanocobalamin has a molecular weight of 1355. The two main naturally occurring compounds are methyl-B_{12} and ado-B_{12} but light rapidly oxidizes them to hydroxocobalamin, which is therefore the main form eaten by humans. Traces of cyanocobalamins and other minor cobalamins are also eaten, as well as non-physiological B_{12} analogues. These B_{12} analogues have an altered or absent nucleotide moiety or different substitutions in the corrin ring compared with cobalamins; like B_{12}, they are made by micro-organisms. Methyl-B_{12} dominates in plasma but forms only about 20% of tissue B_{12}; ado-B_{12} is the

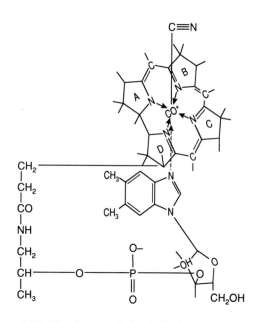

Figure 3.33 The structure of vitamin B_{12} (cyanocobalamin).

main form in tissues. The former is a coenzyme for methylating homocysteine (to methionine) and the latter is a coenzyme in the conversion of methylmalonyl coenzyme A to succinyl coenzyme A.

A normal Western diet contains 5–30 μg of B_{12} daily; it is present in foods of animal origin and absent from cereals, nuts, vegetables and fruits. The foods richest in B_{12} are liver, kidney and red meats. Daily losses, and thus requirements, in adults are 1–2 μg. The Food and Agriculture Organization/World Health Organisation recommends 1 μg daily as a safe level of intake for adults. Body stores are 2–3 mg, i.e. enough for 2–4 years if dietary supplies are completely cut off. The body does not degrade the vitamin and there are no well-documented syndromes of B_{12} deficiency due to increased B_{12} utilization.

Absorption of B_{12}[2,6,21]

All B_{12} in nature is tightly bound to protein. It is released by cooking and by peptic digestion within the stomach. (*Figure 3.34*). B_{12} then binds in the stomach or duodenum, one molecule to one molecule, with one of two glycoproteins, intrinsic factor or the so-called 'R' binding protein. It is now thought that the major binder at the low pH gastric contents is the R binder, derived partly from saliva. 'R' refers to its rapid mobility on electrophoresis. The R binder (molecular weight 56 000) has a higher affinity for B_{12} than intrinsic factor at acid and neutral pH values (intrinsic factor binding constant 10^9–10^{10} M^{-1} at pH 4.5–11.0). The R protein-B_{12} complexes pass into the duodenum, where pancreatic protease degrades both free and B_{12}-bound R protein, freeing B_{12}, which can then transfer to intrinsic factor. The function of gastric and salivary R proteins is probably to bind non-physiological analogues of B_{12} in the gut and to make them unavailable for absorption. Intrinsic factor itself does not bind these analogues.

Intrinsic factor (molecular weight 45 000) consists of 15% carbohydrate. The amino acid structure has regions of homology with both transcobalamin I, an R protein which binds most B_{12} present in plasma and transcobalamin II,[26] the B_{12} transporter to the marrow and other cells. Intrinsic factor is secreted by the rough endoplasmic reticulum of the gastric parietal cells in response to stimulation by food, and its secretion is regulated by histamine and cyclic nucleotides, acid secretion. Membrane-associated vesicular transport is involved. The intrinsic factor–B_{12} complex has a smaller diameter than free intrinsic factor and is more resistant to digestion than free intrinsic factor. It is stable over a pH range of 3–9. The complex subsequently attaches to specific re-

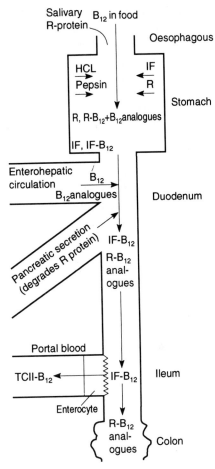

Figure 3.34 Absorption of vitamin B_{12}. R, R-protein; IF, intrinsic factor; TCII, transcobalamin II.

ceptor molecules on the brush border surface of the terminal ileum. This process requires calcium ions and a neutral pH. The receptors are macromolecular (molecular weight >10^6) lipoproteins, which do not bind free intrinsic factor, free B_{12} or R protein–B_{12}. The number of receptors is limited (0.3 $\times$ 10^{12} to 4.9 $\times$ 10^{12} molecules/g mucosa) so that only a few micrograms of B_{12} can be absorbed from a single large dose of intrinsic factor–B_{12} complex. Thus, from 1 μg of B_{12}, 0.3–0.8 μg is normally absorbed, but with smaller doses proportionately more is absorbed and with larger doses proportionately less, to a maximum of 3–4 μg. This is relevant to the interpretation of results from absorption tests using radioactive B_{12}. With the usual 1 μg test done in adults, 30–80% is absorbed. Following a single dose of intrinsic factor–B_{12} complex the ileum is refractory to further B_{12} absorption for 3–4 hours.

The exact fate of the intrinsic factor which attaches to the brush borders is unknown – it is either degraded inside the cell in lysosomes, after uptake by pinocytosis, or digested at the brush border. B_{12} itself appears after a delay of 3–5 hours in the portal blood, largely bound to the transporter transcobalamin II. It becomes attached to transcobalamin II, which is probably synthesized in the ileal cell itself, either within or at the basal surface of the enterocyte. Because of the delay in dietary B_{12} reaching the terminal ileum and the subsequent slow absorptive process, the peak level in systemic blood is only reached 8–12 hours after a single oral dose in humans.

Normally the stomach secretes a vast excess of intrinsic factor. By definition, 1 unit of intrinsic factor binds 1 ng of B_{12} and so only about 1000 units of intrinsic factor are needed for absorption of the normal daily requirements of B_{12}. In response to maximal pentagastrin stimulation, however, the normal adult male stomach secretes 1000–3000 units of intrinsic factor in 1 hour (females secrete about half this, due to a smaller volume of gastric juice). Following histamine or pentagastrin stimulation, there is initially wash-out of preformed intrinsic factor, but after 15 minutes secretion of newly formed intrinsic factor reaches a plateau which may last for several hours with continued maximal stimulation. Although H_2 receptor antagonists block acid secretion by parietal cells, intrinsic factor secretion is not specifically inhibited although the fall in volume of gastric juice results in a proportionate fall in total intrinsic factor secreted. B_{12} absorption is not increased in response to B_{12} deficiency. Indeed, severe B_{12} deficiency may reduce ileal uptake of intrinsic factor–B_{12} complex by damaging the mucosal cells. On the other hand, adaptation of the ileum to an upper intestinal resection may lead to an increased number of ileal receptors and thus increased capacity for B_{12} absorption.

In the absence of intrinsic factor, about 1% of an oral dose of crystalline B_{12} is passively absorbed, mainly through the upper small intestine but also through the buccal and gastric mucosae. This absorption is rapid and occurs by diffusion, in contrast to the active, slow intrinsic factor–mediated normal physiological absorption.

An enterohepatic circulation of B_{12} occurs and is variably estimated to be from 1 to 43 μg of B_{12} daily. This B_{12} is reabsorbed by the intrinsic factor mechanism. The bile may be a route for excretion of unwanted B_{12} analogues which have either been eaten and absorbed or have been produced by degradation of endogenous B_{12} and carried to the liver by transcobalamin I. Since intrinsic factor does not bind these analogues, they are excreted in the stools.

Tests of B_{12} absorption

Since malabsorption is the major cause of B_{12} deficiency, tests of absorption of B_{12} are important.

Cyano-B_{12} labelled with ^{57}Co is usually used since this isotope gives least radiation to the patient. Five techniques are available: whole body, liver uptake, faecal excretion, urinary excretion, or plasma radioactivity measurements. In practice, the urinary excretion (Schilling) test is most widely used. This involves feeding an oral dose of 1 μg of crystalline labelled B_{12} and simultaneously giving an intramuscular flushing injection of 1 mg of unlabelled B_{12} to saturate body B_{12}-binding sites. Cyano-B_{12} was used as flushing dose but hydroxo-B_{12} can be used, although a slightly different normal range is found.[42] The flushing dose allows absorbed labelled B_{12} to remain largely unbound and to be excreted after glomerular filtration in the urine. This is collected for 24 hours or in a more accurate technique with a second flushing dose at 24 hours for 48 hours. The test may be repeated (part II Schilling test), giving intrinsic factor with the oral labelled B_{12} to determine whether malabsorption of B_{12} is due to a gastric or intestinal lesion. If an intestinal lesion is likely, the test may also be repeated after a course of antibiotics to reduce the intestinal bacterial flora (part III test). In the 'Dicopac' test, free and intrinsic factor-bound B_{12}, labelled with ^{57}Co and ^{58}Co, respectively, are given simultaneously and differential counting is performed. Some exchange of labelled B_{12} occurs between free and bound forms, however, and the results do not give such a wide separation of results in pernicious anaemia as when the two tests are carried out separately. The Schilling tests depend on complete urine collection, and give abnormal results in renal failure. Whole-body counting is a more accurate technique which does not require a flushing dose but, in order for unabsorbed labelled B_{12} to be excreted, 7 days must be allowed after ingestion of the test dose before the follow-up whole-body count is performed to estimate amount of labelled B_{12} absorbed.

B_{12} absorption tests using protein (e.g. egg or albumin) bound B_{12} have been developed to provide a better guide to food B_{12} absorption, e.g. in conditions such as atrophic gastritis or following partial gastrectomy where achlorhydria leads to failure of release of food B_{12} from protein binding.[10,20] However these tests are not widely used.

Dietary deficiency of B_{12}

This occurs particularly in vegetarians and especially in vegans, e.g. Hindus whose diet contains less than 2 μg of B_{12} daily.[7] Many remain apparently healthy with subnormal serum B_{12} levels, the enterohepatic circulation helping to maintain body stores, albeit at a suboptimal level. Dietary deficiency may also cause B_{12} deficiency in non-vegetarians, especially in elderly patients and alcoholics living on a poor-quality diet.[24]

Malabsorption of B_{12}

This is due to gastric or intestinal causes (*Table 3.6*).

Gastric causes

By far the commonest in Western countries is acquired (Addisonian) pernicious anaemia in which there is an autoimmune gastritis with achlorhydria and failure of intrinsic factor secretion. Intrinsic factor is usually undetectable or detected in an amount of only a few units per hour. In addition, intrinsic

Table 3.6 Causes of vitamin B_{12} malabsorption

Gastric lesions
  Acquired
    (Addisonian) pernicious anaemia
    Total gastrectomy
    Partial gastrectomy
    Corrosive gastritis
    Gastric bypass
  Congenital
    Absence or abnormality of intrinsic factor

Intestinal lesions
  Acquired
    Abnormal gut flora associated with:
      Jejunal diverticulosis
      Blind loops
      Strictures
      Entero-entero-anastomosis
      Fistulas
      Scleroderma, Whipple's disease
      HIV disease
    Other abnormalities of gut lumen:
      Pancreatic disease
      Giardiasis
      Fish tapeworm
      Zollinger–Ellison syndrome
      Drugs (metformin, phenformin, alcohol, neomycin, anticonvulsants, cholestyramine, slow-release potassium chloride, colchicine)
    Abnormalities of ileal wall:
      Ileal resection or bypass
      Crohn's disease
      Graft versus host disease
      Radiation (e.g. pelvic carcinoma, total body)
      Gluten-induced enteropathy
      Tropical sprue
      Deficiencies of B_{12}, folate, protein, ?iron
      Infiltration, e.g. mastocytosis, lymphoma
  Congenital
    Specific malabsorption with proteinuria (Imerslund–Grasbeck syndrome)
    Transcobalamin II deficiency

factor antibodies in the gastric juice may block the action of any residual intrinsic factor (see below). Total gastrectomy always causes B_{12} malabsorption and B_{12} therapy should be given prophylactically from the time of the operation. Following partial gastrectomy, subsequent intrinsic factor secretion, and thus B_{12} absorption, depends largely on the size of the gastric remnant, but a stagnant loop syndrome may also develop. Malabsorption of B_{12} is present in 32–43% of cases but only about 5% develop megaloblastic anaemia.[6,17] It is more common after surgery for a gastric than a duodenal ulcer. Gastric bypass surgery for obesity may also lead to B_{12} malabsorption.[34]

Congenital intrinsic factor deficiency which is rare, usually presents with megaloblastic anaemia in the first 2 years of life. Neuropathy may occur, especially if folic acid has been given. The inheritance is autosomal recessive. Although the serum B_{12} level is low and B_{12} absorption is similar to that in pernicious anaemia, gastric acid secretion and biopsy are normal. Intrinsic factor and parietal cell antibodies are absent. The disease is heterogenous. Some cases secrete intrinsic factor that does not bind B_{12}, or does not promote its uptake in the ileum, or is unduly sensitive to proteolysis. Others do not secrete intrinsic factor due to failure of its synthesis or a block in its secretion. The parents are haematologically normal and absorb B_{12} normally.

Intestinal causes

A wide variety of intestinal lesions may lead to malabsorption of the vitamin. These usually affect the ileal cell surface or involve bacterial contamination of the upper small intestine. Resection of more than 60 cm of ileum almost always leads to B_{12} malabsorption and B_{12} therapy should be started after this operation. Microorganisms take up free B_{12} (e.g. aerobes such as *Streptococcus faecalis*) or intrinsic factor–B_{12} complex (Gram-negative anaerobes). In a few patients, synthesis of B_{12} analogues by the microorganisms has been demonstrated.[23] B_{12} malabsorption may occur after jejunoileal bypass[18] and B_{12} deficiency due to intestinal malabsorption occurs in chronic tropical sprue and may present with megaloblastic anaemia or B_{12} neuropathy. More recently B_{12} deficiency has been described in a minority of patients with the acquired immune deficiency syndrome (AIDS).[16,29,30] Low serum B_{12} levels are also found in some human immune deficiency virus (HIV)-positive patients before AIDS develops. The lowest levels occur in the patients with the lowest CD4 lymphocyte counts and CD4/CD8 ratios. In a recent study, 10 of 60 HIV-infected patients had subnormal serum B_{12} levels, 9 of the 10 having AIDS. Malabsorption of B_{12} also due to damage to the ileum also occurs after pelvic irradiation,[1] or after bone marrow transplantation, in the latter case either due to total body irradiation, which gradually recovers, or due to chronic graft-versus-host disease.

Causes of intestinal malabsorption of B_{12} also include two rare congenital defects. *Selective malabsorption of B_{12} with proteinuria (Imerslund–Grasbeck syndrome)* is the commonest cause of B_{12} deficiency in early life in Western countries. It is inherited as an autosomal recessive trait. Ninety per cent of cases show proteinuria and usually present in the second year of life. There is a defect of the ileal intrinsic factor–B_{12} receptor. The renal lesion is thought to be in the glomerular podocytes which produce most of the capillary basement membrane. *Congenital deficiency of transcobalamin II* usually presents with severe megaloblastic anaemia at 6–8 weeks of life due to failure of entry of plasma B_{12} into bone marrow cells. The plasma transport defect is associated with intestinal malabsorption of B_{12}, but B_{12} deficiency is not present so early in life since the fetus has acquired B_{12} from maternal transcobalamin II which crosses the placenta. The serum B_{12} is normal, this B_{12} being attached to transcobalamin I, which usually accounts for 80–90% of B_{12} binding in plasma. In some cases, transcobalamin II is undetectable, but in others it is detectable immunologically and partly functional and the disease may present in childhood or even later.

In pancreatic disease, there is failure of release of dietary B_{12} from its binding with the R protein secreted by the stomach. However, this, as with many causes of B_{12} malabsorption shown in *Table 3.7*, rarely, if ever, leads to B_{12} deficiency of sufficient severity to cause megaloblastic anaemia or B_{12} neuropathy.

Pernicious anaemia

Aetiology

Addisonian pernicious anaemia may be defined as severe lack of intrinsic factor due to gastric atrophy.[19] Atrophy of all coats of the body of the stomach is present with relative sparing of the antrum. There is loss of secreting tubules and of parietal and oxyntic cells with replacement by mucous-secreting cells often with intestinal metaplasia. The lamina propria is infiltrated by lymphocytes and plasma cells. A minority of patients show a few remaining parietal cells which produce small amounts of intrinsic factor and acid. These features may occur with severe atrophic gastritis without pernicious anaemia. The essential feature of pernicious anaemia is a humoral and cell-mediated autoimmune reaction to intrinsic factor with consequent malabsorption of B_{12} of sufficient severity to cause B_{12} deficiency with megaloblastic anaemia and/or a neuropathy.[6,13] The frequency of pernicious anaemia is about 1% above the age of 60 years in northern Europe, where the disease is most common, but pernicious anaemia occurs in all races. The female-to-male ratio is 10:7. Only 11% of patients present below the age of 40 years. An incidence of 3.7% over the age of 75 years has been described in north-west England. When there is a positive family history the mean age at diagnosis (51 years) is younger than in patients without such a history (mean 66 years).

In pernicious anaemia there is hyperplasia of endocrine cells in the antrum with very high serum gastrin levels (mean 1000 pg/ml). There is proliferation of gastric enterochromaffin-like cells with secretion of 5-hydroxytryptamine, vasoactive intestinal polypeptide and substance P. Gastric carcinoid is more frequent in pernicious anaemia than controls and may occur in single or multiple microscopic forms.[4] Carcinoma of the stomach is about three times more common in pernicious anaemia than controls and may be present at presentation.

The cause of the autoimmune gastritis may be partly genetic and partly acquired.

Familial incidence

The exact inheritance is unclear but at least 25% of cases of pernicious anaemia have a close relation with the disease and the frequency of the disease among first- and second-degree relatives is about 2.5% compared with 0.13% in controls. Close relatives also show a higher incidence of thyroid diseases

---

Table 3.7 Causes of folate malabsorption

Major causes
    Gluten-induced enteropathy (child or adult)
    Dermatitis herpertiformis
    Tropical sprue
    Congenital specific malabsorption of folate

Minor causes
    Partial gastrectomy
    Jejunal resection
    Intestinal lymphoma
    Systemic infections
    Inflammatory blood disease

Drugs
    Salazopyrine
    Cholestyramine
    Methotrexate
    ?Anticonvulsants
    ?Alcohol

and other diseases associated with pernicious anaemia and of the autoantibodies associated with them than controls. Identical twins are likely to develop pernicious anaemia concordantly. There is a minor association with blood group A and in some, but not all, studies an association with HLA-3. Patients with endocrine disease have a higher incidence of HLA-B8, B12 and B18. There is also an association with HLA-DR2.

Disease associations

Primary myxoedema, Hashimoto's disease and hyperthyroidism are associated in that order of frequency. Antibodies to thyroid antibodies are frequent in the sera of pernicious anaemia patients and their relatives, just as parietal cell antibody occurs with a higher frequency than normal in patients with thyroid diseases. Idiopathic hypoparathyroidism, adrenal failure and premature ovarian failure are also associated with pernicious anaemia, as are vitiligo and alopecia. Up to 35% of patients with acquired hypogammaglobulinaemia develop pernicious anaemia. Pernicious anaemia in association with hypogammaglobulinaemia tends to be present in the third or fourth decade.[43] These patients differ from typical pernicious anaemia patients in having atrophy of the gastric antrum as well as fundus, absence of humoral autoantibodies to intrinsic factor or parietal cells and normal serum gastrin levels. Pernicious anaemia may also be associated with the autoimmune polyglandular syndromes, type I presenting in the second decade and associated with mucocutaneous candidiasis, type II presenting at about 30 years of age, often with diabetes. Humoral antibodies to several endocrine glands are present while impaired supressor T-cell function and cell-mediated immunity may be detected. Pure red cell aplasia is another rare association with pernicious anaemia. It is still uncertain whether there is a real association of pernicious anaemia with diabetes mellitus; if so, it is weak.

Autoantibodies

Of pernicious anaemia patients, 80–90% have serum antibodies against parietal cells. The antigens are α and β subunits of the gastric proton pump (H^+/K^+-dependent ATPase).[14] Type I intrinsic factor antibody directed against the B_{12}-binding site of intrinsic factor occurs in the serum in about 50% of pernicious anaemia patients. Type II antibody directed against the intrinsic factor ileal binding site occurs in about 35% but virtually never in the absence of type I antibody.

Parietal cell and intrinsic factor autoantibodies occur in pernicious anaemia in gastric juice, when they are likely to be IgA (in serum they are IgG).

Cell-mediated immunity against intrinsic factor also occurs in about 86% of pernicious anaemia patients. Decreased numbers of circulating suppressor cells have been found particularly in those with circulating intrinsic factor antibodies. Treatment with corticosteroids reverses some of these abnormalities. There is recovery of acid and intrinsic factor secretion, parietal cells increase in the gastric mucosa, B_{12} absorption returns and there is a fall in the titre of serum intrinsic factor antibody.

Gastric secretion

In pernicious anaemia, the volume of gastric juice is substantially reduced both before and after stimulation. Moreover, the pH of the juice is usually in the range 6–8 with no hydrochloric acid secretion except in a few patients after maximal stimulation. Intrinsic factor secretion is usually undetected but if present it is at low titre, up to 6 units/ml. Normal concentrations after stimulation are 14–114 units/ml. Intrinsic factor antibody in gastric juice may inhibit small amounts of residual intrinsic factor at neutral pH. At low pH (3.0 or less) the intrinsic factor–antibody complex would be dissociated but this pH is not reached in pernicious anaemia gastric juice.

Clinical features

Many patients are now diagnosed on the basis of a 'routine' blood count before symptoms have developed. A rise in the mean corpuscular volume even in the absence of anaemia, and the presence in the peripheral blood film of oval macrocytes and neutrophils with hypersegmented nuclei (more than five nuclear lobes) suggest B_{12} or folate deficiency. If symptoms do occur these are likely to be of anaemia (breathlessness on exertion, tiredness or dyspnoea), due to the neuropathy (paraesthesiae especially of the feet, with difficulty in walking) or due to glossitis (sore tongue). Loss of appetite, diarrhoea, sore mouth and aphthous ulcers are less frequent. Infertility is usual in both males and females. Pernicious anaemia is sometimes diagnosed in patients presenting with symptoms and signs due to gastric carcinoma.

On examination, many show no abnormality. Early greying of the hair and blue eyes are associated clinical features and vitiligo may be present. In the severely anaemic, pallor of the mucous membranes and mild jaundice occur and these patients may be in heart failure. A beefy red tongue or a smooth tongue and angular cheilosis are present in a minority. A mild fever may be due to ineffective haemopoiesis in severe cases but infection such as pneumonia can precipitate presentation to hospital.

Rarely, patients show increased melanin pigmentation of the skin which disappears with therapy.

Mild B_{12} neuropathy causes loss of vibration sense and of superficial sensation in the feet and legs. In more severe cases, the hands are also affected, and if pyramidal tracts are damaged there may be spasticity in the legs with extensor plantar responses. Psychiatric or visual disturbances may occur.

Investigations

In the untreated case, this depends on establishing: (1) megaloblastic haemopoiesis is present, (2) that B_{12} rather than folate deficiency is the cause and (3) that pernicious anaemia is the cause of the B_{12} deficiency.

BLOOD AND BONE MARROW FINDINGS

In early cases the blood count shows only a mild rise in mean corpuscular volume with oval macrocytes and neutrophils with hypersegmented nuclei in the blood film whereas, in severely anaemic patients, pancytopenia is usual. The white cell count rarely falls below 1.5×10^9/l or platelet count below 40×10^9/l however, unless some other cause of inhibition of the marrow is present, such as alcohol. The mean corpuscular volume may be normal if iron deficiency or the thalassaemia trait is also present or in some severe cases with excess fragmentation of red cells.

The bone marrow shows megaloblastic haemopoiesis with delayed nuclear maturation in the erythroid precursors and giant metamyelocytes present. In some laboratories, a deoxyuridine suppression test performed *in vitro* on aspirated bone marrow cells can determine whether B_{12} or folate deficiency is the cause of the megaloblastosis. In other causes of red cell macrocytosis, e.g. liver diseases, aplastic anaemia, myxoedema or myeloma, the marrow is usually normoblastic whereas in other cases, e.g. myelodysplasia, alcoholism and antimitotic drug chemotherapy, the marrow may be normoblastic, or megaloblastic, without B_{12} or folate deficiency. The peripheral blood and marrow appearances are identical in B_{12} or folate. Except when a patient has had a splenectomy or has splenic atrophy (as in adult coeliac disease) morphological abnormalities due to the absence of the spleen (Howel–Jolly bodies and siderotic granules in red cells, target cells) are seen in the peripheral blood.

BIOCHEMICAL TESTS

Raised serum unconjugated bilirubin, lactate dehydrogenase, iron and ferritin levels are found in moderately or severely anaemic patients. Serum haptoglobins are absent and urine haemosiderin may be positive. All these tests are normal in non-anaemic patients and in the anaemic patients return to normal with therapy. Serum homocysteine and methylmalonyl CoA levels are raised and methionine levels are low and urine methyl malonic excretion is raised, but these tests are not performed in routine laboratories.[39]

DIAGNOSIS OF B_{12} DEFICIENCY

The serum B_{12} level is subnormal (less than 160 ng/l) and is particularly low in severely anaemic patients and in patients with B_{12} neuropathy whether or not they are anaemic. The serum folate level is normal or raised in B_{12} deficiency unless folate deficiency is also present but the red cell folate level is frequently subnormal, especially in the more anaemic patients. This is due to failure of formation of folate polyglutamates, the intracellular forms of folate, in B_{12} deficiency.

Diagnosis

This depends on demonstrating B_{12} malabsorption due to a gastric lesion using radioactive B_{12} absorption tests (see above) and in nearly all cases demonstrating autoantibodies to gastric antigens in serum. In addition, it is useful to perform endoscopy and gastric biopsy.

ENDOSCOPY AND GASTRIC BIOPSY

Severe atrophic gastritis or gastric atrophy is present in the fundus with sparing of the antrum unless hypogammaglobulinaemia is present. Parietal cells are absent or very few in the biopsy. Gastric carcinoma, polyps or carcinoid tumours are sought, and biopsied if present. Routine follow-up endoscopy is not performed in most units because of the relative infrequency of gastric carcinoma and the unlikelihood of diagnosing this disease sufficiently early to affect the outcome even with annual endoscopies.

Prognosis

The life expectancy of the female population with treated pernicious anaemia is similar to the rest of the female population. Males have a slightly reduced life expectancy due to gastric carcinoma.

Management

It is usual to treat initially with six intramuscular injections of hydroxocobalamin, each of 1 mg, at approximately 2–3 day intervals. Blood transfusions should be avoided if possible but, in some severely anaemic patients, transfusion of packed cells may be needed, e.g. because of anoxia with angina. Diuretics should be given and an equivalent volume of blood venesected if necessary. If hypokalaemia develops, potassium supplements should be administered. An attack of gout may be precipitated in susceptible individuals in the first 7–10 days of therapy due to increased release of purines from breaking down newly synthesized erythroblasts.

Once the patient has been 'loaded' with B_{12} in this way, 1 mg intramuscularly every 3 months for life is sufficient to maintain body B_{12} stores. Patients who are unable to receive injections (e.g. with severe haemophilia) can be given B_{12} by mouth, but due to lack of intrinsic factor, they will absorb less than 1% of the dose (through the buccal and gastric mucosae) so daily doses will be necessary and it will be impossible to load body stores. About 20% of patients become iron-deficient after starting B_{12} therapy, but if this develops late the possibility of haemorrhage, e.g. from a gastric carcinoma, has to be considered.[3] Careful observation for the development of hypothyroidism is needed in long-term management.

FOLATE

Natural forms

Folate was initially crystallized from spinach as folic (pteroylglutamic) acid (*Figure 3.35*), but most foods contain folates, the richer sources being liver, kidney, yeast, nuts, fruit and green vegetables. An average Western diet contains about 600 μg daily, and adult daily requirements are about 50–200 μg. The recommended daily intake is 3 $\mu g/kg$, and in pregnancy 500 μg daily is recommended.[12] The body stores of 12–15 mg are sufficient for only 4 months if supplies are completely cut off. The body can degrade folates by splitting the C_9—N_{10} bond, and this degradation may be increased in conditions of increased cell turnover such as pregnancy, severe haemolytic anaemia or malignant disease.

Folates occur naturally as a variety of compounds which differ from the parent structure, folic acid, by being reduced to di- or tetrahydro forms, by having additional single-carbon units (e.g. methyl, formyl, methylene, methenyl or fomimino) attached at the N_5 or N_{10} position, and by having additional glutamate residues. In general, folates are not tightly bound to proteins in natural materials and cooking may destroy them by oxidation (particularly if ascorbate has already been destroyed by preheating); folates are also easily extracted by large volumes of water. Human milk contains specific binding proteins which may reduce folate absorption.

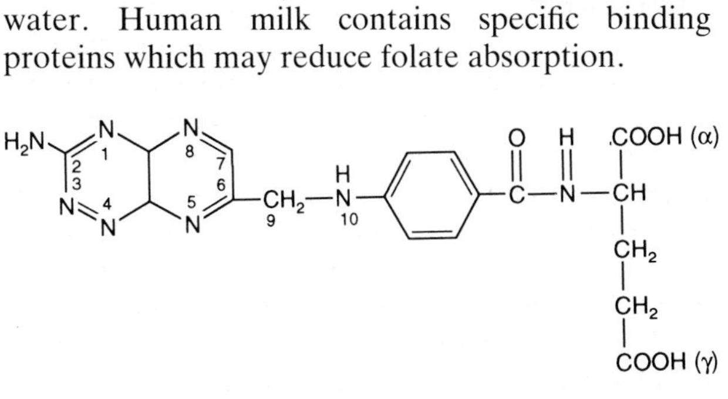

Figure 3.35 The structure of folic (pteroyloglutamic) acid.

Absorption of folate

Absorption takes place largely in the duodenum and jejunum, with conversion of all dietary folates to the single, fully reduced, monoglutamate derivative 5-methyltetrahydrofolate, which enters the portal blood (*Figure 3.36*). Peak levels are reached 1–2 hours after a simple dose. Reduction and methylation occur in the cytoplasm of the enterocyte. The exact site of deconjugation still remains controversal. The enzyme folate conjugase (pteroylpolyglutamate hydrolase or γ-glutamyl carboxypeptidase) is present in pancreatic juice and succus entericus at low concentrations. Higher concentrations are present in the enterocytes, largely in lysosomes. At all these sites, the enzyme has an optimum pH of 4.6 with little activity at neutral pH. An enzyme with a pH optimum of 5.5 and consisting of two polypeptides of molecular masses 145 and 115 kDa, dependent on zinc, is also present in the brush borders of the small intestinal mucosa; it has been proposed that this may be responsible for deconjugation of dietary folates at or near the brush border.[8] Alternatively, a

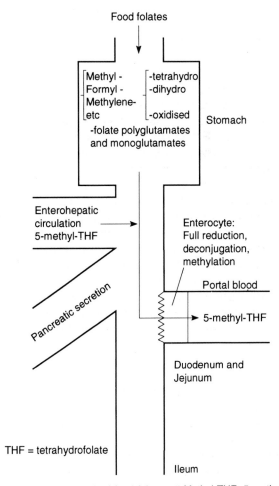

Figure 3.36 Absorption of food folates. 5-Methyl-THF, 5-methyltetrahydrofolate.

microclimate of lower pH than in the lumen has been considered to be present at the small intestinal surface and this may allow deconjugation by the low-pH enzyme.[28,35] A carrier-mediated uptake system in brush border membrane vesicles may also be involved.[33] The brush borders also contain specific folate-binding proteins but their role in folate absorption is unclear. The basolateral membrane of the enterocyte also has a carrier-mediated system which may be involved in transfer of folate into portal blood.[31] Folic acid itself, when used therapeutically in large (5 mg) doses, is largely absorbed passively and unchanged into the portal blood because it is a poor substrate for the reducing enzyme dihydrofolate reductase. It then enters the liver and other tissues, and displaces 5-methyltetrahydrofolate into the plasma. Folate in the plasma is only loosely and non-specifically bound to protein, e.g. albumin, and is easily removed by dialysis. Apart from 5-methyltetrahydrofolate, trace amounts of 10-formyltetrahydrofolate and other minor components have also been identified in plasma, but their physiological significance is unknown. Also, a very small fraction is tightly bound to a specific folate-binding protein, but this is probably not physiologically important.

The proportion of natural folates absorbed depends partly on the length of the polyglutamate chain; monoglutamates are almost completely absorbed whereas only 50–80% of higher polyglutamates is absorbed. The more folate eaten the more is absorbed, with no saturation of the absorptive mechanism. Folate absorbed in excess of the body's needs is largely excreted in the urine, either unchanged or as breakdown products. An enterohepatic circulation exists, the folate concentration in bile ranging from 60 to 90 μg daily.[40] This, and folate from sloughed enterocytes, is largely reabsorbed. Milk contains specific folate-binding proteins which may reduce jejunal folate transport in the neonate and uptake by bacteria but do not affect ileal transport.[32]

Absorption of folates from the lower small intestine is substantially less than from the jejunum, and folates are not absorbed from the large intestine. Bacteria synthesize folates and, if present in the upper small intestine as in the stagnant loop syndrome, produce folate which is absorbed and can lead to excessively high serum, red cell and urine folate levels.

Dietary deficiency

In Western countries, the edentulous, the old and infirm, spirit-drinking alcoholics and psychiatric patients are most at risk.[25] Infants may become deficient because of their relatively high requirements. Their dietary intake is low, especially if superimposed infections and other disease reduces diet intake or absorption. In developing countries, where general malnutrition is frequent, the incidence of nutritional folate deficiency is high. Body stores may be depleted due to inadequate intake in association with general malnutrition and multiple vitamin deficiency. Decreased availability of folate-rich food occurs particularly in the winter season in the poor and is associated with special diets and cooking procedures. Goats milk (folate content 6 μ/l) or milk that has been boiled has less folate than normal human breast milk (50 μg/l).

Folate malabsorption

Gluten-induced enteropathy (coeliac disease, non-tropical sprue)

The commonest cause of folate malabsorption in Western countries is gluten-induced enteropathy. Virtually 100% of untreated cases have low serum folate levels, and the red cell folate level is low (at least 85%). In studies undertaken by the author, 89% of adult untreated cases were anaemic and a raised mean corpuscular volume was present in two-thirds. In some patients, megaloblastic anaemia is the presenting feature with minimal or no diarrhoea or other symptoms of malabsorption. In children, iron deficiency is usually also present but this is so in only 50% of adult cases. Malabsorption of B_{12} occurs in about a third of patients but is not sufficiently severe to cause megaloblastic anaemia due to B_{12} deficiency or neuropathy unless some additional cause of B_{12} deficiency is present.

In dermatitis herpetiformis, malabsorption of folate is frequent but is not usually as severe as in coeliac disease. Similarly, folate deficiency sufficiently severe to cause megaloblastic anaemia is less frequent.

Tropical sprue

In the early stages of tropical sprue, folate deficiency is the predominant cause of megaloblastic anaemia and in about 60% of cases folate therapy produces a cure of the malabsorption syndrome. The additional response to antibiotics implies an infectious aetiology with perhaps folate deficiency of the enterocyte making it susceptible to the infectious agent or its product. Later in the disease, after a chronic phase of 3 years or more B_{12} deficiency due to ileal malabsorption may cause megaloblastic anaemia or neuropathy.

Congenital folate malabsorption

This rare autosomal recessive disease presents in the first few months of life with megaloblastic anaemia. There is failure of transport of all folate analogues through the enterocyte and of 5-methyltetrahydrofolate into the brain, with progressive mental retardation and calcification of the basal ganglia in some cases. Treatment is with parenteral folinic acid or 5-methyltetrahydrofolate in large doses.

Other causes

Malabsorption of folate may also occur after jejunal resection, and has been described in Crohn's disease affecting the upper small intestine, but poor nutrition, excess turnover and sulphasalazine therapy may all contribute to folate deficiency in Crohn's disease, the most ill patients showing the lowest serum and red cell folate levels (present in 38 and 24%, respectively, in one large series of patients).[15]

IRON

Absorption of iron

The human body controls its iron content mainly by regulating iron absorption.[11] With increasing amounts of oral iron, the proportion absorbed falls; there is, nevertheless, some increase in absorption with substantially increased intake so there is no absolute 'mucosal block' to absorption. The amount of iron in the daily diet is generally well in excess of the body's daily needs to make up for iron losses or needs for growth, so normally only a small proportion (5–10%) of the iron in food is absorbed. This may be increased in some situations, e.g. iron deficiency, to a maximum of about 3.5 mg daily, but if, for example, chronic haemorrhage causes loss of more than this, iron deficiency will result.

Dietary iron and daily requirements

The amount of iron in the diet is related to its quality and its caloric value, 6–7 mg of iron per 4000 J (1000 cal) being typical. Iron occurs in non-haem forms as iron oxides or bound to protein (more than 90%) and as haem or porphyrin iron. On average, iron is absorbed better from animal than vegetable foods, although there is a wide variation from food to food, depending on the form of iron and associated compounds in the food.[5]

Iron is needed in both sexes to make up for daily losses from, for example, skin, urine and intestine. In adults this loss is about 1.0 mg daily. In females, menstrual blood loss or pregnancy increases demand for iron and, in children and adolescents, additional iron is needed for growth. In pregnancy, an average of 3.0 mg daily is needed, and in menstruating females 1.5–2.0 mg.

Intraluminal events

Iron in food is largely in the iron(III) state as iron hydroxides, bound to proteins, or in an organic porphyrin or haem complex. Peptic digestion releases inorganic iron which binds to mucoproteins in the gastric and small intestinal juice and subsequently is largely transferred to low molecular weight chelating substances such as sugars, amino acids or vitamin C. Reduction to the more soluble iron(II) state by gastric acid or vitamin C favours absorption whereas alkaline pancreatic secretion has the opposite effect, iron(III) tending to polymerize and form insoluble hydroxides. Inorganic iron is best absorbed in the fasting state, as food generally inhibits absorption by raising the pH and forming insoluble iron complexes, e.g. with phytates, tannates or phosphates. Less than 50% of the iron in most foods is released by peptic digestion and, in general, iron is better absorbed from foods of animal origin such as liver and meat than from vegetables or eggs. Specific inhibitors or activators of iron absorption have been postulated to exist in gastric juice but have not been proven.

In general, haem iron is a better source than inorganic iron. It is less affected than inorganic iron by other substances present in the lumen; some haem enters the intestinal mucosa intact to be digested there by haem oxygenase, some is broken down to release inorganic iron in the lumen. A specific mucosal receptor for haem has been described. The iron released from haem in the mucosa forms a common pool with absorbed inorganic iron for subsequent transfer to portal blood.

Mucosal uptake

Absorption of small amounts of inorganic iron, largely from its low molecular weight chelates, appears to be an active, carrier-mediated process partly related to body needs. The first stage consists of rapid uptake by the brush border and it is uncertain whether this is by passive diffusion or by a specific carrier mechanism.[41] The second stage involves transfer across the cell, possibly by combination with low molecular weight chelates or with a specific transferrin-like carrier protein, and is an active process.[27,38] In vitro, iron-deficient brush borders show increased avidity for iron. Some of the absorbed iron enters cell organelles, particularly mitochondria, or binds with apoferritin to form ferritin. Iron destined to rapidly enter portal plasma, however, remains in the soluble cytoplasmic fraction of the cell.

Iron trapped in the cell, e.g. as ferritin, is shed

into the gut lumen when the cell reaches the tip of the intestinal villous; this is one important control mechanism (or 'block') of the amount of iron absorbed. Iron acts as a stimulus to apoferritin synthesis and, when iron is deficient, ferritin synthesis is reduced.[22] Transferrin receptor synthesis is also modulated by iron levels, so that iron deficiency increases iron uptake, and iron excess reduces iron uptake from transferrin.

Iron leaving the serosal cell surface binds to transferrin in the portal blood, although *in vitro* everted loop experiments have shown that this protein is not essential for this transfer. The overall amount of iron entering the portal plasma increases with the amount of iron presented to the mucosa, but the percentage absorption falls. The amount leaving the serosal surface of the cell is related not only to body stores of iron but also to body iron turnover for erythropoiesis, and it is postulated that plasma iron turnover may partly indicate to the mucosa how much iron to release into portal blood.[9]

Iron deficiency

It has been estimated that it takes up to 8 years for an adult male, starting with normal iron stores, to develop iron deficiency anaemia solely due to absent dietary iron or to impaired iron absorption. This is because iron stores (mainly as haemosiderin and ferritin in the reticuloendothelial cells) of about 1500 mg are large compared to normal daily losses of iron (approximately 1 mg); also, as iron stores are reduced, this small loss becomes even less. Thus, although many factors may reduce iron absorption, iron deficiency anaemia solely due to malabsorption of iron is unusual;[36] excess iron loss as haemorrhage, or increased needs as in growth or pregnancy, are generally more important causes (*Table 3.8*). Tests of iron absorption are thus not used routinely in the investigation of patients with iron deficiency.

In many countries of the world where a low-quality diet is usual, particularly if this is vegetarian and/or malnutrition is frequent, iron stores are low or absent and deficiency due to inadequate intake is common, especially if low intake is combined with growth in children, menstrual blood loss or pregnancy in females.[12]

Malabsorption of iron

Table 3.9 lists causes of iron malabsorption. Reduced absorption of dietary iron occurs with ingestion of foods containing large amounts of phytates or phosphates. Tea has also been shown to reduce absorption of inorganic iron, possibly by

Table 3.8 Causes of iron deficiency

- Dietary (especially in infants, children, adolescents and pregnancy (increased physiological requirements)

- Haemorrhage

  Females
    Uterus
      Menorrhagia
      Antepartum, postpartum
      Postmenopausal

  Males or females
    Gastrointestinal
      Oesophagus:
        Varices
        Carcinoma
      Stomach:
        Ulcer
        Erosions (e.g. aspirin, non-steroidal anti-inflammatory agents)
        Carcinoma
        Gastrectomy
      Small intestine:
        Ulcer
        Hookworm (also schistosomiasis, trichuriasis)
        Crohn's disease
        Meckel's diverticulum
        Tumours
      Large intestine:
        Caecal, colonic or rectal carcinoma
        Colonic polyposis
        Angiodysplasia
        Diverticulosis
        Ulcerative colitis
        Haemorrhoids
        Widespread bleeding disorder (e.g. essential thrombocythaemia, immune thrombocytopenia, scurvy, hereditary haemorrhagic telangiectasia)

    Urinary tract
      Chronic haematuria (e.g. malignancy, schistosomiasis)
      Chronic haemosiderinuria due to intravascular haemolysis (e.g. paroxysmal nocturnal haemoglobinuria, cardiac valves)

    Respiratory tract
      Idiopathic pulmonary haemosiderosis
      Goodpastures syndrome

forming insoluble iron–tannin complexes. In some cases, an unusual craving for substances which impair iron absorption ('pica') such as clay or chalk may be relevant but, in the vast majority of cases, pica is the result of iron deficiency rather than its cause. Gastric atrophy and achlorhydria and ant-

Table 3.9 Causes of iron malabsorption

Dietary factors and drugs
  Phytates
  Phosphates
  Tea (Tannin)
  Chalk
  Desferrioxamine

Gastric lesions
  Achlorhydria
  Atrophic gastritis
  Partial or total gastrectomy
  Gastroenterostomy

Intestinal lesions
  Gluten-induced enteropathy
  Tropical sprue
  Chronic infections

---

acids such as aluminium hydroxide or magnesium trisilicate also reduce iron absorption but it is of interest that the majority of patients with pernicious anaemia do not develop iron deficiency. Iron overload, for example due to multiple transfusions for refractory anaemia, or decreased erythropoiesis as in aplastic anaemia, also reduces iron absorption, as do chronic infections, which may be particularly relevant to deficiency in underdeveloped countries.

Absorption of iron in food is reduced following partial gastrectomy because of reduced acid secretion, chronic gastritis in the remnant with failure of peptic digestion, and because of rapid bypass of duodenal mucosa. Absorption of iron is also reduced in gluten-induced enteropathy of children and adults, but it is difficult to know whether reduced absorption of dietary iron or increased loss of mucosal iron is the main cause of iron deficiency in this condition. Other diseases of the upper small intestine may also impair iron absorption, but haemorrhage is usually present in those patients who develop severe iron deficiency anaemia. In most cases of gastric or intestinal malabsorption of food iron, therapeutic inorganic iron, especially if given in the fasting state, is sufficiently well absorbed to correct the deficiency and replenish body stores.

Iron absorption is increased in iron deficiency and pregnancy, and if there is increased plasma iron turnover owing to increased erythropoiesis, e.g. in some patients with chronic haemolytic anaemias, particularly when erythropoiesis is ineffective such as in thalassaemia intermedia. Iron absorption is particularly increased if patients are carriers of the gene for haemochromatosis.[37] Iron absorption is inappropriately raised in relation to the body stores in the hereditary disorder primary haemochroma-tosis, but the mechanism for this remains controversial.

REFERENCES

1. Anderson, G.C., Walton, K.R. and Chanarin, I. (1981) Megaloblastic anaemia after pelvic radiotherapy for carcinoma of the cervix. *Journal of Clinical Pathology*, **34**, 151–152.
2. Antony, A.C. (1991) Megaloblastic anaemia. In: *Hematology. Basic Principles and Practice* (Eds) Hoffman, R., Benz, E.J., Shattil, S.J., Furie, B. and Cohen, H.J. pp. 392–422. New York: Churchill Livingstone.
3. Atrah, H.I. and Davidson, R.J.L. (1988) Iron deficiency in pernicious anaemia. *Postgraduate Medical Journal*, **64**, 110–111.
4. Borch, K., Renvall, H. and Leidberg, G. (1985) Gastric endocrine cell hyperplasia and carcinoid tumours in pernicious anaemia. *Gastroenterology*, **88**, 638–648.
5. Brittenham, G.M. (1991) Disorders of iron metabolism: iron deficiency and overload. In: *Hematology. Basic Principles and Practice* (Eds) Hoffman, R., Benz, E.J., Shattil, S.J., Furie, B. and Cohen, H.J. pp. 327–349. New York: Churchill Livingstone.
6. Chanarin, I. (1990) *The Megaloblastic Anaemias*, 3rd edn. Oxford: Blackwell.
7. Chanarin, I., Malkowska, V., O'Hea, A.-M., Rinsler, M.G. and Price, A.B. (1985) Megaloblastic anaemia in a vegetarian Hindu community. *The Lancet*, **ii**, 1165–1172.
8. Chandler, C.J., Wang, T.T.Y. and Halsted, C.H. (1986) Pteroylopolyglutamate hydrolase from human jejunal brush borders. Purification and characterisation. *Journal of Biological Chemistry*, **261**, 928–933.
9. Conrad, M.E. Umbreit, J.N., Moore, E.G., Peterson, R.D.A. and Jones, M.B. (1990) A newly identified iron binding protein in duodenal mucosa of rats. *Journal of Biological Chemistry*, **265**, 5273–5279.
10. Dawson, D.W., Sawers, A.H. and Sharma, R.K. (1984) Malabsorption of protein-bound vitamin B_{12}. *British Medical Journal*, **288**, 675–678.
11. Fairbanks, V.F. and Beutler, E. (1990) Iron metabolism. In: *Hematology*, 4th edn (Eds) Williams, W.J., Beutler, E., Erslev, A.J. and Lichtman, M.A. pp. 329–338. New York: McGraw-Hill.
12. FAO (1988) Requirements of vitamin A, iron, folate and vitamin B_{12}. *Food and Nutrition Series*, No. 23. Geneva: Food and Agricultural Organization of the United Nations.
13. Fyfe, J.C., Ramanujam, K.S., Ramaswamy, K., Patterson, D.F. and Seetharam, B. (1991) Defective brush-border expression of intrinsic factor-cobalamin receptor in canine inherited cobalamin malabsorption. *Journal of Biological Chemistry*, **266**, 4489–4494.

14. Gleeson, P.A. and Toh, B.-H. (1991) Molecular targets in pernicious anaemia. *Immunology Today,* **12**, 233–238.

15. Harries, A.D. and Heatley, R.V. (1983) Nutritional disturbances in Crohn's disease. *Postgraduate Medical Journal, 59*, 690–697.

16. Herbert, V. (1988) B_{12} deficiency in AIDS. *Journal of the American Medical Association, 260*, 2837.

17. Hines, J.D., Hoffbrand, A.V. and Mollin, D.L. (1967) The hematologic complications following partial gastrectomy. *American Journal of Medicine*, **32**, 555–569.

18. Hocking, M.P., Duerson, M.C., O'Leary, J.P. and Woodward, E.R. (1983) Jejunoileal bypass for morbid obesity. Late follow-up of 100 cases. *New England Journal of Medicine,* **308**, 995–999.

19. Hoffbrand, A.V. (1983) Pernicious anaemia. *Scottish Medical Journal, 28*, 218–227.

20. Jones, B.P., Broomhead, A.F., Kwan, Y.L. and Grazt, C.S. (1987) Incidence and clinical significance of protein-bound vitamin B_{12}-malabsorption. *European Journal of Haematology,* **38**, 131–136.

21. Kapadia, C.R. and Donaldson, R.M. (1985) Disorders of cebalamin (vitamin B_{12}) absorption and transport. *Annual Review of Medicine, 36*, 93–110.

22. Kuhn, L.C. (1991) mRNA–protein interactions regulate critical pathways in cellular iron metabolism. *British Journal of Haematology,* **79**, 1–5.

23. Murphy, M.F., Sourial, N.A., Burman, J.F., Doyle, D.V., Tabaqchali, S. and Mollin, D.L. (1986) Megaloblastic anaemia due to vitamin B_{12} deficiency caused by small intestinal bacterial overgrowth: possible role of vitamin B_{12} analogues. *British Journal of Haematology, 63*, 7–12.

24. Narayanan, M.N., Dawson, D.W. and Lewis, M.J. (1991) Dietary deficiency of vitamin B_{12} is associated with low serum cobalamin levels in non-vegetarians. *European Journal of Haematology,* **47**, 115–118.

25. Parry, T.E. (1987) Megaloblastic anaemia in the elderly. *Clinical Haematology, 1*, 315–354.

26. Platica, O., Janeczko, R., Quadros, E.V., Regec, A., Romain, R. and Rothenberg, S.P. (1991) The cDNA sequence and the deduced amino acid sequence of human transcobalamin II show homology with rat intrinsic and human transcobalamin I. *Journal of Biological Chemistry,* **266**, 7860–7863.

27. Raja, K.B., Simpson, R.J. and Peters, T.J. (1989) Membrane potential dependence of Fe(III) uptake by mouse duodenum. *Biochimica et Biophysica Acta,* **984**, 262–266.

28. Reisenhauer, A.M., Chandler, C.J. and Halsted, C.H. (1986) Folate binding and hydrolysis by pig intestinal brush border membranes. *American Journal of Physiology, 251*, 481.

29. Remacha, A.F., Riera, A., Cadafalch, J. and

Gimferrer, E. (1991) Vitamin B_{12} abnormalities in HIV-infected patients. *European Journal of Haematology, 47*, 60–64.

30. Rule, S., Hooker, M., Costello, C., Luck, W. and Hoffbrand, A.V. (1992) Vitamin B_{12} deficiency in HIV disease: incidence and significance (in preparation).

31. Said, H.M. and Redha, R. (1987) A carrier-mediated transport of folate in basolateral membranes vesicles of rat small intestine. *Biochemical Journal,* **247**, 141–146.

32. Said, H.M., Horne, D.W. and Wagner, C. (1986) Effect of human milk folate binding protein folate intestinal transport. *Archives Biochemica Biophysica,* **251**, 114–120.

33. Said, H.M., Ghishan, F.K. and Redha, R. (1987) Folate transport by human intestinal brush border membrane vesicles. *American Journal of Physiology, 25*, 229–236.

34. Schilling, R.F., Gondes, P.N. and Hardie, G.H. (1984) Vitamin B_{12} deficiency after gastric bypass surgery for obesity. *Annals of Internal Medicine,* **101**, 501–502.

35. Schron, C.M., Washington, C. and Blitzer, B. (1985) The transmembrane pH gradient drives uphill folate transport in rabbit jejunum. *Journal of Clinical Investigation,* **76**, 2030–2033.

36. Shultz, B.M. and Freeman, M.L. (1987) Iron deficiency in the elderly. *Clinical Haematology, 1*, 291–313.

37. Simon, M., Le Mignon, L., Fauchet, R. *et al.* (1987) A study of 609 HLA haptotypes: (1) mapping of the gene near the HLA-A locus and characters required to define a heterozygous population and (2) lipothesis concerning the underlying cause of HLA–hemochromatosis association. *American Journal of Human Genetics,* **41**, 89.

38. Simpson, R.J. and Peters, T.J. (1987) Transport of Fe^{2+} across lipid bilayers: possible role of free fatty acids. *Biochimica et Biophysica Acta,* **898**, 187–195.

39. Stabler, S.P., Marcell, P.D., Podell, E.R. *et al.* (1988) Elevation of total homocysteine in the serum of patients with cobalamin or folate deficiency detected by capillary gas chromatography–MARS spectrometry. *Journal of Clinical Investigation,* **81**, 466.

40. Steinberg, S.E., Campbell, C.L. and Hillman, R.S. (1979) Kinetics of the normal folate entero-hepatic cycle. *Journal of Clinical Investigation,* **64**, 83–88.

41. Teichmann, R. and Stremmel, W. (1990) Iron uptake by human upper small intestine microvillous membrane vesicles. *Journal of Clinical Investigation,* **86**, 2145–2153.

42. Wallis, J., Clark, D.M. and Bain, B.J. (1986) The use of hydroxocobalamin in the Schilling test. *Scandinavian Journal of Haematology, 37*, 337–340.

43. Wright, P.E. and Sears, D.A. (1987) Hypogammaglobulinaemia and pernicious anaemia. *Southern Medical Journal, 80*, 243–246.

ABSORPTION AND MALABSORPTION OF CALCIUM AND VITAMIN D

(J.R.F. Walters)

Calcium is the most abundant cation in the body; a normal adult has absorbed and retained around 2 kg, 99% of which is in the skeleton. Bone calcium is complexed with phosphate and hydroxyl ions, mostly as hydroxyapatite, and is slowly turned over as bone is remodelled through absorption by osteoclasts and deposition by osteoblasts. Non-skeletal calcium is involved in many physiological regulatory functions. In the extracellular fluid, the total calcium concentration is 2.2–2.6 mmol/l, approximately 50% being ionized, not bound to proteins. In cells, the cytoplasmic calcium concentration is about 0.1 μmol/l, and changes to this have important intracellular messenger functions, such as when calcium is released from stores in the endoplasmic or sarcoplasmic reticulum by a variety of hormones or neurotransmitters.

Bone turnover, and hence calcium metabolism, is influenced by many hormonal agents, including parathyroid hormone, the active vitamin D metabolite, 1α,25-dihydroxycholecalciferol (1,25(OH)$_2$D), calcitonin, prostaglandins, interleukins, oestrogens, corticosteroids, thyroid hormones, parathyroid hormone-related peptide, and other growth factors.[82] Extracellular calcium concentrations are regulated principally by parathyroid hormone acting on bone and kidney. Other hormones interact in many ways with vitamin D metabolism, but it is clear that 1,25(OH)$_2$D is the main physiological regulator of intestinal calcium absorption.[13,77]

MEASUREMENT OF CALCIUM ABSORPTION

The absorption of dietary calcium is inefficient and variable. Depending on diet, intake of calcium varies between 300 and 1300 mg/day. To stay in calcium balance and to compensate for losses from the skin and in urine, about 150 mg/day of calcium must be absorbed from the intestine (*Figure 3.37*). Many normal women need a dietary intake of 1000 mg/day for positive calcium balance and so have net absorption of only 15%. When the reabsorption of calcium in digestive secretions is included, the figure for true net absorption is higher. Calcium absorption can adapt to various physiological demands such as growth, pregnancy, lactation or low-calcium diets. *Table 3.10* gives estimates of net calcium absorption in a variety of states and, calculated from these, the US and UK recommended daily dietary calcium intakes.

The studies which gave these estimates of calcium absorption have used a variety of methods.[13] Balance studies performed over several weeks give the most easily understood values. Radioactive calcium absorption tests are more convenient and correlate well with the results from balance studies.[67] There are several protocols using either ^{45}Ca, a β emitter with a half-life of 165 days, or ^{47}Ca, a γ emitter with a half-life of 4.5 days. Double-isotope methods,[26] where one is given by mouth and the other intravenously, correct for endogenous faecal loss, variable pool sizes and turnover, and should be used for

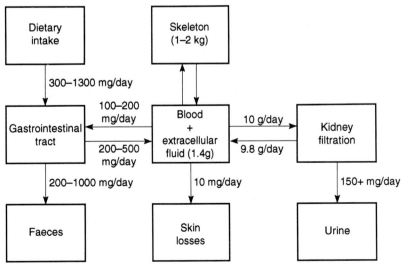

Figure 3.37 Typical daily calcium fluxes in adults. Ca^{2+} intake and estimated fluxes show wide variation.

Table 3.10 Reference values for dietary calcium intake

Period	Estimated net absorption (mg/day)	UK reference nutrient intake (mg/day)	US recommended dietary allowance (mg/day)
0–12 months	160	525	*
1–3 years	70	350	800
4–6 years	110	450	800
7–10 years	150	550	800
11–18 years			
Male	300	1000	1200
Female	250	800	1200
19–24 years			
Male		700	1200
Female		700	1200
24+ years			
Male	160	700	800
Female	160	700	800
Elderly			1200
Pregnancy			+400
Lactation		+550	+400

The figures for estimated net absorption and UK intakes are from Panel on dietary reference values of the committee on medical aspects of food policy (1991) *Dietary Reference Values for food energy and nutrients for the United Kingdom*. London: HMSO. Figures for US intakes are from Food and Nutrition Board, NRC (1989) *Recommended Dietary Allowances*, 10th edn. Washington, DC: National Academy Press.
* US recommended dietary allowance for 0–12 months is 60 mg/kg body weight.

research purposes to estimate dietary or drug effects on absorption. This is unnecessarily complex for most situations.[47,67] A single oral dose of ^{45}Ca, given in a meal with 200 mg of carrier calcium, and blood sampling at 5 hours has been well validated and enables calculation of fractional absorption from a simple equation which includes weight and height.[47,48] Using this method, average fractional absorption was about 30%, but could be as low as 10% or as high as 50% in different individuals.

MECHANISMS OF CALCIUM ABSORPTION

Calcium absorption from food occurs by both an active, transcellular route and a passive paracellular route. These two pathways differ in their distribution in the intestine and in the factors that influence them. From various studies in humans and in animals, it has been established that active absorption is saturable and vitamin D-dependent, whereas passive transport is non-saturable and largely vitamin D-independent.[13]

A careful study was made of the relative importance of these two mechanisms using duodenal intubation and bowel washout techniques in normal subjects and renal dialysis patients with either low or supplemented $1,25(OH)_2D$ levels (*Figure 3.38*).[92] The results indicated that, with a low–normal calcium meal of 120 mg, absorption was entirely by the vitamin D-dependent route. As this pathway was nearly saturated at this intake, when a higher calcium meal of 300 mg was given the increase in absorption was in the passive, vitamin D-independent pathway. Even so, on the higher intake, three times as much calcium was absorbed by the D-dependent as by the D-independent pathway.

Sites of absorption

Passive absorption of Ca^{2+} probably occurs through intercellular tight junctions in both the small intestine and the colon. Active transcellular absorption is largely restricted to the proximal small bowel.[103] In flux chamber studies of rat intestine, in the absence of electrical or chemical gradients, net Ca^{2+} absorption in the duodenum was much greater than in the jejunum or ileum; on a normal calcium diet, net secretion of Ca^{2+} occurred in the distal segments. Adaptation to a low-calcium diet produces a greater proportional change in active absorption in the ileum, however. In rat caecum, absorptive fluxes of Ca^{2+} are also high.[31]

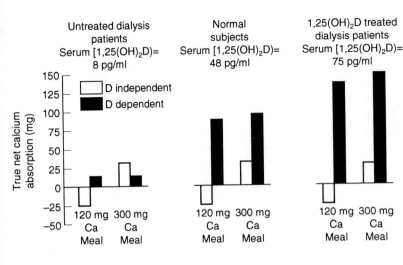

Figure 3.38 Comparison of passive and active Ca^{2+} absorption at different $1,25(OH)_2D$ levels and Ca^{2+} intake. (Reproduced, with permission, from Sheikh *et al.*)[92]

Pathways of transcellular calcium transport

To cross the intestinal epithelial cell, Ca^{2+} has first to enter at the apical membrane, secondly to traverse the cytoplasm and thirdly to exit at the basolateral membrane (*Figure 3.39*).[13,96] As intracellular free Ca^{2+} concentrations are 10 000-fold less than extracellular (approximately 0.1 μmol/l versus 1 mmol/l), entry is down a large concentration gradient. No Ca^{2+} channel or carrier protein has been clearly identified at the brush border membrane although an integral membrane Ca^{2+}-binding protein has been described and changes in membrane lipids and fluidity affect brush border membrane calcium uptake. The microvillus core has large amounts of calmodulin bound to an abundant 110 kDa protein, brush border myosin I protein; binding is affected by $1,25(OH)_2D$.[9] Calmodulin binds calcium and it has been estimated that sufficient is present to buffer Ca^{2+} at millimole per litre concentrations.[41]

The calbindins, previously called vitamin D-dependent Ca^{2+}-binding proteins, chelate Ca^{2+} in the cytoplasm.[102] The mammalian intestinal protein calbindin-D_{9k} is present at high concentrations and binds two Ca^{2+} molecules with sufficient affinity to buffer Ca^{2+} to below micromole per litre levels. Experimental models have shown the overall rate of diffusion of Ca^{2+} to be increased by binding to calbindin.[32] The distribution of calbindin-D_{9k}, higher in duodenum and villus cells, and its response to $1,25(OH)_2D$ are strong evidence of its importance in Ca^{2+} absorption.[14] The structures of calbindin-D_{9k} and the avian equivalent calbindin-D_{28k} (which is also found in mammalian kidney, and certain endocrine and nerve cells) have been determined in several species but human calbindin-D_{9k} has only recently been sequenced.[53] Studies in hu-

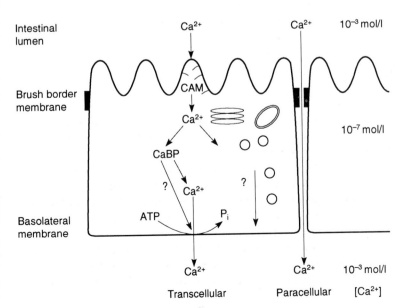

Figure 3.39 Pathways of Ca^{2+} absorption across the enterocyte. The transcellular and paracellular routes are shown. Ca^{2+} may bind first to calmodulin (CAM) in the brush border membrane. Calbindin-D_{9k} (CaBP) binds Ca^{2+} in the cytoplasm, and Ca^{2+} is also taken up by organelles. The ATP-dependent Ca^{2+} pump at the basolateral membrane is depicted.

mans have demonstrated the highest concentrations in duodenojejunal mucosa (6 μg/mg of cytosolic protein or approximately 6 μmol/l) and correlation with circulating 1,25(OH)$_2$D levels but not age.[93]

The ATP-dependent Ca^{2+} pump (Ca^{2+}-transporting ATPase) extrudes Ca^{2+} from the enterocyte into the extracellular fluid at the basolateral membrane and is the energy-requiring step in Ca^{2+} absorption.[96] In animals, the activity of this pump also correlates well with the sites of Ca^{2+} absorption, being higher in duodenum and villus tip cells, and being affected by vitamin D status.[40,100] The transport activity is stimulated by calmodulin[73] and, under certain conditions, by calbindin-D$_{9k}$.[99] Similar activity has been shown in human intestine.[59]

The intracellular organelles in intestinal cells, including the endoplasmic reticulum, mitochondria, lysosomes and Golgi apparatus, take up and sequester Ca^{2+}, as in other cells.[101] It has been suggested that there may be another pathway for Ca^{2+} absorption which follows a transcytotic route. Endocytosis could occur at the brush border, followed by fusion of vesicles with lysosomes and by microtubule involvement in their movement to the basolateral membrane.[74]

FACTORS AFFECTING CALCIUM ABSORPTION

Dietary factors

The bioavailability of calcium varies with different salts and food sources.[1] In the lumen of the gastrointestinal tract, the concentration of ionic Ca^{2+} available for absorption will be affected by solubilization in gastric acid, and reprecipitation by bicarbonate secreted by the pancreas, or by dietary anions.

Dietary components thought to affect Ca^{2+} absorption include lactose, oxalate, phytates, fibre and fatty acids.[1] Milk is the major source of dietary Ca^{2+}; consequently, the effects of lactose on Ca^{2+} absorption have been well studied but with conflicting results. Simultaneous administration of lactose in water increased total fractional Ca^{2+} absorption,[18] though no stimulation was seen in subjects with intestinal lactase deficiency. When milks containing lactose or glucose were compared, both stimulated Ca^{2+} absorption equally in normal subjects and, surprisingly, lactase-deficient were better than normal subjects at absorbing Ca^{2+} from the milk containing lactose.[42] However, milk intake, and hence Ca^{2+} intake, is lower in lactase-deficient subjects and they may be more prevalent in those with osteoporosis.

Various anions complex Ca^{2+} and decrease absorption. Oxalate is present in some vegetable sources of Ca^{2+} such as spinach; fractional Ca^{2+} absorption from spinach was only 5% compared with 28% from milk.[49] Components of fibre, including phytates, cellulose and uronic acids, impair Ca^{2+} absorption as well as that of other cations.[1] Fatty acids are important binders of Ca^{2+} in malabsorption; substitution of medium-chain triglycerides will often improve Ca^{2+} (and fat) absorption. Phosphate intake has little effect on Ca^{2+} absorption, though vitamin D also regulates phosphate metabolism. Diets high in animal protein increase the risk of development of renal stones through hypercalciuria, but do not appear to increase fractional Ca^{2+} absorption.

The action of dietary Ca^{2+} in binding to and precipitating fatty acids, phosphates and bile acids may also be a mechanism whereby high Ca^{2+} intake can help protect against colonic cancer.[63]

Physiological adaptation

Fractional absorption of Ca^{2+} is greater from a low-calcium meal than from a high-calcium meal, as the saturable active transcellular absorptive process predominates at low intakes. Additionally, the body adapts over a period of days to changing to a low calcium intake[57] by increasing fractional absorption. The increase is mediated through changes in parathyroid hormone, increasing 1,25(OH)$_2$D synthesis. The effect on the intestine is most marked distally,[78] where active transport is otherwise minimal.

In pregnancy and lactation, Ca^{2+} absorption is increased to maintain Ca^{2+} balance despite losses to the fetal skeleton and in milk.[45,80] Increases are seen in 1,25(OH)$_2$D concentrations and the vitamin D-binding protein. Studies in rats have indicated that vitamin D may not be the only regulator of this adaptive process;[12] effects of prolactin on the intestine have also been suggested.

Ageing

Fractional absorption of calcium is decreased after the menopause and with advancing age in both sexes, being most marked over the age of 80 years.[4,37] Adaptation to a low-calcium intake is less marked in older subjects.[57] 1,25(OH)$_2$D synthesis is impaired[37] and intestinal resistance to its actions may occur with reduced levels of calbindin-D$_{9k}$ and basolateral membrane Ca^{2+} pump activity being demonstrable in the rat.[2] The decreased efficiency in adapting to low Ca^{2+} intakes is reflected in the higher US dietary allowances recommended for postmenopausal women.

VITAMIN D METABOLISM

Sources of vitamin D

In most people, vitamin D (calciferol) is a physiologically synthesized hormone precursor and not a nutritionally necessary vitamin.[85] Only if exposure to sunlight is inadequate are dietary sources important.[51] Vitamin D_3 (cholecalciferol) is synthesized in the skin from 7-dehydrocholesterol by the action of ultraviolet B radiation (290–320 nm), which opens one of the rings of the steroid nucleus to form the secosteroid ring of previtamin D. This slowly isomerizes to vitamin D_3 (*Figure 3.40*). Vitamin D_3 has a high affinity for the serum vitamin D-binding protein which takes it from the skin for further metabolism. Factors which affect the production of vitamin D in the skin include season of the year, latitude, time of day, use of sunscreens, melanin pigmentation, and age.[52] It has been estimated that sufficient vitamin D_3 will be formed in the elderly by exposure of the face, hands and arms to approximately 15 minutes of midday sunshine (in Boston in the USA; 42° latitude) 2–3 times a week in the summer. By contrast, between November and March, the incident solar radiation is too weak to form any previtamin D.[51]

Vitamin D_2 (ergocalciferol) differs slightly from vitamin D_3 in the side-chain and is made from ergosterol found in some plants and provides a dietary form of vitamin D. Nutritional sources of either form of vitamin D include fish oils and liver, and egg yolks. Many countries fortify milk, margarine and other foods. A daily allowance of 400 IU (10 μg) protects against rickets in children and involves no risk of hypervitaminosis.

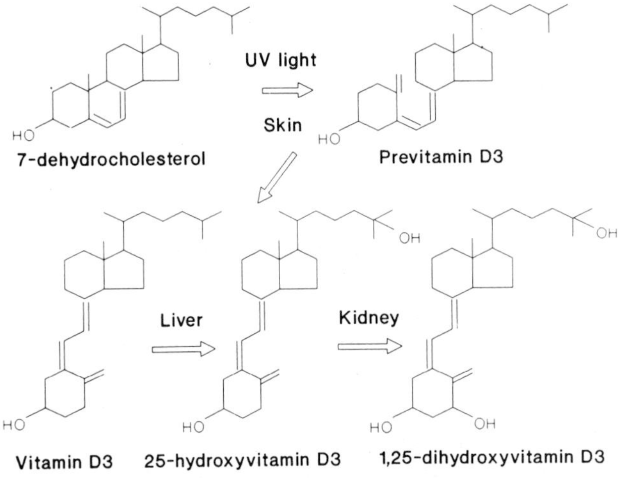

Figure 3.40 Vitamin D metabolism .

Synthesis of vitamin D metabolites

The active hormonal form of vitamin D, $1\alpha,25$-dihydroxycalciferol (calcitriol), was first described in 1970[35] and is produced by successive hydroxylation in the liver and kidney (*Figure 3.36*). 25-hydroxylation of vitamin D by a liver microsomal enzyme produces 25-hydroxyvitamin D (25-OH vitamin D, calcidiol). This circulates with a half-life of several weeks bound to the vitamin D-binding protein and is often used as an estimate of the adequacy of provision of vitamin D in clinical situations. 25-OH vitamin D levels vary with the seasons, reflecting the differing rates of synthesis of vitamin D in the skin.[68] At the circulating concentrations (10–50 μg/l), 25-OH vitamin D is inactive.

25-OH vitamin D is further hydroxylated in the kidney. The enzyme responsible for this, 25-OH vitamin D 1α-hydroxylase, is a mitochondrial mixed-function cytochrome P-450 hydroxylase in the proximal tubule cells and is stimulated by parathyroid hormone.[38] Consequently, hypocalcaemia increases circulating parathyroid hormone, which stimulates synthesis of $1,25(OH)_2D$ and absorption of calcium. $1,25(OH)_2D$ is several hundred-fold more active than 25-OH vitamin D. It is bound in serum at concentrations of 26–65 ng/l and has a circulating half-life of several hours.[51] As the kidney is the major source of production of $1,25(OH)_2D$, this accounts for the severe bone disease found in end-stage renal failure. However, some other sites such as the placenta in pregnancy and macrophages are able to produce small amounts of $1,25(OH)_2D$.[85] Macrophage synthesis gives rise to the hypercalcaemia seen in granulomatous diseases such as sarcoidosis.

Another hydroxylation step which occurs in target tissues including the kidney and intestine is 24-hydroxylation. This is stimulated by $1,25(OH)_2D$ and forms 24,25-dihydroxyvitamin D $(24,25(OH)_2D)$, which circulates at concentrations of 2–4 μg/l. $24,25(OH)_2D$ has been reported to have biological actions, both on its own, or as the further metabolite 1,24,25-trihydroxyvitamin D. These reactions forming more polar metabolites may represent means of deactivating vitamin D. Other hydroxylation steps can occur at carbon-23 and carbon-26, but the consensus view is that $1,25(OH)_2D$ is sufficient to produce all the actions of vitamin D.[11,85]

$1,25(OH)_2D$ inhibits its own production from 25-OH vitamin D in the kidney. Additionally, it acts in the liver to reduce 25-OH vitamin D levels by decreasing synthesis,[6] and by increasing clearance by metabolism to more polar metabolites.[46] Thus, paradoxically, calcium deprivation leads to vitamin

D deficiency by producing secondary hyperpara-thyroidism which increases renal synthesis of the short-lived active metabolite $1,25(OH)_2D$ and also increases metabolic inactivation of 25-OH vitamin D.[17] Primary hyperparathyroidism may also pro-duce the same changes in vitamin D metabolism.

Vitamin D-binding protein

In plasma, vitamin D and its metabolites are bound to a 58 kDa glycoprotein first designated as Gc-globulin and which also binds monomeric actin.[43] This protein is analogous to albumin and α-fetoprotein. Each vitamin D-binding protein mol-ecule has one high-affinity sterol-binding site (K_D 5×10^{-8} mol/l for 25-OH vitamin D) but the concentration of the protein (5 μmol/l) is 50–100 times greater than the vitamin D metabolites.[56] Vitamin D-binding protein is synthesized in the liver and is increased by oestrogens (as in pregnancy) and decreased in liver disease or in protein-losing states.

Intestinal absorption of vitamin D

Absorption of dietary vitamin D is a less important source than synthesis in the skin. Absorption follows the pathway of other fats in being dependent on bile salts and chylomicron formation.[95] The more polar metabolites are absorbed into the portal blood. Vitamin D metabolites are found in bile after intra-venous injection and are subsequently largely reab-sorbed, which has led to the suggestion that there is an enterohepatic circulation resembling that of bile salts. However, as it is now known that these metab-olites result from inactivation of 25-OH vitamin D in the liver by processes which include further hydro-xylation and glucuronidation, it is now considered that a conservative enterohepatic circulation of any form of vitamin D does not occur.[34]

ACTIONS OF $1,25(OH)_2D$

Effects on calcium absorption

The effects of vitamin D metabolites on Ca^{2+} ab-sorption are well known and have been clarified from studies in a variety of experimental situations. For instance, with everted gut sac preparations, active Ca^{2+} transport was shown to be reduced in vitamin D deficiency,[88] and in flux chamber experi-ments to be increased when vitamin D-deficient rats were repleted with $1,25(OH)_2D$.[98] The magnitude of the effects differ along the intestine; injections of $1,25(OH)_2D$ stimulate Ca^{2+} absorption in rat ileum by reversing the normal net secretion to give net

Table 3.11 Actions of $1,25(OH)_2D$ in the intestine

- Increase in transcellular Ca^{2+} transport
- Effects on growth and differentiation of enterocytes

- Receptor-mediated increases in protein expression (alkaline phosphatase, calbindin-D_{9k})
- Stimulation of activity of certain enzymes (ornithine decarboxylase, Ca^{2+} pump etc.)

- Increases in brush border membrane Ca^{2+} uptake and calmodulin binding
- Changes in membrane fluidity and lipid composition
- Activation of second messenger systems (protein kinase C, Ca^{2+} channels etc.)

absorption whereas, in the duodenum, where some active transport remains in the D-deficient state, the stimulation is proportionally less marked.[31] Studies in volunteers have confirmed the relationship in humans between active Ca^{2+} absorption and serum $1,25(OH)_2D$.[37,92]

Many individual steps are implicated in the effects of $1,25(OH)_2D$ on Ca^{2+} absorption (*Table 3.11*) and their relative importance is still controversial.[77] When vitamin D-deficient rats are given a single injection of $1,25(OH)_2D$, the recovery of Ca^{2+} transport is multiphasic, indicating that at least two separate responses occur. Receptor-mediated effects on gene transcription and non-genomic actions are recognized; changes occur at the brush border membrane,[7] basolateral membrane[40,100] and, in particular, to concentrations of the intra-cellular protein calbindin.[14]

Evidence for the relative importance of these effects comes from a recent elegant study,[16] where calcium in transit through the enterocyte was imaged with ion microscopy using a stable isotope, ^{44}Ca. In vitamin D-deficient animals, the rate of transfer from the apical to the basolateral mem-brane was impaired, though initial apical brush border uptake was normal. The decrease in the vitamin D-dependent calcium-binding protein, cal-bindin, seemed to be the predominant reason for this, with other effects less important.

Effects on gene transcription

$1,25(OH)_2D$ is well established as acting as a classic steroid hormone.[77,85] The hormone binds to a specific cytoplasmic receptor which then enters the nucleus. The receptor is a protein of 50 kDa and its nucleotide sequence[5] establishes it as a member of the 'zinc finger' family of transcription activators, which includes glucocorticoid, mineralocorticoid, oestrogen, progesterone, thyroid and retinol receptors. Like other family members, it has steroid-binding and DNA-binding domains. Mutations in the vitamin D receptor have been shown to occur in individuals with hypocalcaemic vitamin D-resistant rickets.[66] The receptor is widely distributed in human tissues, including small intestine, colon, stomach, liver, kidney, thyroid, adrenal, breast and skin.

Expression of the mRNAs coding for many proteins has been shown to be regulated by $1,25(OH)_2D$ and has been reviewed recently.[70,77,85] These include increased expression of specific intestinal proteins (the calbindins and alkaline phosphatase), and bone proteins (including osteocalcin, matrix Gla protein and fibronectin). The levels of a variety of other proteins involved with cellular metabolism (mitochondrial ATP synthetase and cytochrome oxidases), growth and differentiation (c-Ki-*ras* and c-*fos* gene-products, ornithine decarboxylase and others) are also increased. Preproparathyroid hormone, calcitonin, interleukin-2 and γ-interferon, among others, are down-regulated. $1,25(OH)_2D$ also regulates its own receptor.

The regions in the gene that bind the vitamin D receptor have been identified for osteocalcin and both calbindins. These $1,25(OH)_2D$-responsive elements are homologous with those for oestrogen and glucocorticoids. Some of these vitamin D-dependent proteins are also regulated by glucocorticoids and oestrogens acting through separate responsive elements.

Other effects

In addition to the classic steroid hormone effects described above, several groups have reported actions of $1,25(OH)_2D$ which are independent of gene activation yet occur at physiological concentrations.[77] $1,25(OH)_2D$ can increase intestinal Ca^{2+} transport in the presence of inhibitors of RNA and protein synthesis. Changes in the fluidity of enterocyte brush border membranes and in the enzymes regulating membrane phospholipids have been described. A rapid effect on Ca^{2+} absorption occurring within a few minutes of perfusing chick duodenum with $1,25(OH)_2D$ has been termed transcaltachia and may represent effects on calcium channels mediated by activation of second messenger systems. Protein kinase C activation by $1,25(OH)_2D$ has been demonstrated in colonic cells[97] and so has an increase within seconds of inositol trisphosphate and diacylglycerol in rat enterocytes.[62] How these effects interact with the longer-term genomic actions is at present unclear.

The clinical relevance of vitamin D is not only limited to calcium absorption and bone disease. Recent interest has been shown in the association of vitamin D and its metabolites in the prevention of colonic cancer.[39] The effects of $1,25(OH)_2D$ on cellular proliferation and differentiation have led to trials of local therapy in psoriasis and to the development of synthetic metabolites lacking effects on Ca^{2+} absorption.

CALCIUM ABSORPTION AND BONE DISEASES

Osteomalacia

Osteomalacia is a result of defective mineralization of bone and can only be diagnosed with certainty histologically.[79] As bone is diffusely involved, an iliac crest biopsy will be representative. Defective mineralization of the osteoid seam is best demonstrated by double tetracycline labelling, which enables the extent and rate of mineralization to be measured. Clinically, osteomalacia can present with dull bone pain, tenderness, muscle weakness and eventually progresses to pathological fractures and abnormal gait. Radiological findings of pseudofractures (Looser's zones) may only be found in severe cases and biochemical features of hypocalcaemia, hypophosphataemia and raised alkaline phosphatase are not invariable.

Defective mineralization in childhood results in rickets, which has been rarely seen since the discovery of vitamin D and its role in calcium absorption early in this century. Extrinsic deficiency of vitamin D due to inadequate synthesis in the skin and poor dietary intake is now uncommon, but vitamin D deficiency leading to osteomalacia may still be found in migrants from Asia to northern Europe and in the sick and ageing population. The discovery of the role of the kidney in $1,25(OH)_2D$ synthesis and therapy with 1α-hydroxylated metabolites have reduced the incidence of osteomalacia in chronic renal failure. However, bone disease, not necessarily classic osteomalacia, associated with low vitamin D levels, calcium deficiency and hyperparathyroidism is increasingly recognized in gastrointestinal and liver disorders. Hence, more than 75% of all current cases of osteomalacia in US adults, when those with renal failure are excluded, is due to intestinal disease.[79]

Many rare causes of osteomalacia exist, including the hereditary vitamin D-resistant rickets, also called vitamin D-dependent rickets type II. Serum $1,25(OH)_2D$ levels are normal or high but studies have shown abnormal nuclear vitamin D receptors resulting from point mutations.[66] Another inherited disorder, the autosomal recessive vitamin D-dependent rickets type I, has low circulating $1,25(OH)_2D$ levels and an abnormal renal 25-OH vitamin D 1α-hydroxylase.[33] Renal tubule disorders such as the X-linked hypophosphataemic rickets can also lead to bone disease.

Osteoporosis

Osteoporosis is the result of loss of bone where the mineralization of osteoid is normal. Characteristically, when considerable amounts of bone have been lost, it presents with vertebral collapse, wedge fractures and kyphosis, or with forearm or hip fractures. Subclinical osteoporosis can be detected by measurements of trabecular bone density in the vertebrae by quantitative computed tomography (CT) and at other sites such as the femoral neck or forearm by dual-photon absorptiometry or dual-energy X-ray absorption. This osteopenic bone is more than 2 standard deviations from the age- and sex-related mean density and has no evidence of osteomalacia if biopsied. Bone mass gradually decreases with ageing. This is accelerated in women after the menopause. As osteoporotic fractures, particularly of the hip, cause considerable morbidity and mortality, detection of low bone mass and prevention of further bone loss is becoming an important aspect of preventative medicine.[86]

Various risk factors for osteoporosis have been described.[28] A low peak bone mass gives less reserve for subsequent bone loss. Peak bone mass is partly genetically determined and is influenced by nutrition, exercise and menstrual cycle function. A high calcium intake in adolescent females has been suggested to lessen the risk of osteoporosis by ensuring calcium deficiency does not limit peak bone mass. Loss of bone is increased by immobility, oestrogen deficiency, as in an early menopause, cigarette smoking, caffeine and alcohol intake.

Glucocorticoid-induced osteoporosis occurs in at least 50% of patients on long-term therapy and is a problem in many gastrointestinal diseases (see below). Multiple reasons for the osteopenia have been described, including direct effects on bone, increased renal excretion and decreased intestinal calcium absorption. The pathogenesis and management have recently been reviewed in detail.[65]

There is no doubt that hormone replacement therapy will delay the onset of postmenopausal bone loss. Weight-bearing exercise is also beneficial. Calcium absorption and $1,25(OH)_2D$ are reduced in postmenopausal osteoporotic women[37] but whether this is the cause or the effect of the disease, and whether dietary calcium supplementation will pre-

vent bone loss, remains controversial.[58,76] A recent study showed that calcium supplementation slowed bone loss in a group of women more than 6 years after the menopause but was ineffective earlier.[25] As there are wide ranges of calcium intake and fractional absorption, and also rates and sites of bone loss, dietary calcium supplementation may not be universally beneficial but is unlikely to be harmful.

Further bone loss in clinical osteoporosis is prevented by oestrogen, and probably by calcium and vitamin D supplementation.[36] Additionally, calcitonin, bisphosphonates, and fluoride therapy appear to be effective.[30] However, prevention by early detection of reduced bone density is preferable in this largely irreversible condition.

BONE DISORDERS IN GASTROINTESTINAL AND LIVER DISEASE

In view of the central role of the gastrointestinal tract in the absorption of calcium and in the action of vitamin D it is not surprising that bone disorders should be well recognized in a variety of diseases of this system. Vitamin D deficiency, measured by low 25-OH vitamin D levels, has been described in virtually every chronic gastrointestinal and liver disease.[27,89] However, the relative contributions to bone disease of calcium deficiency, vitamin D deficiency, secondary hyperparathyroidism and other factors remain unclear in most cases (*Table 3.12*). Classical osteomalacia may occur, but is usually not seen, and the term 'hypovitaminosis D osteopathy'

Table 3.12 Factors leading to bone disease in gastroenterological patients

---

- Impaired Ca^{2+} absorption:
  Low Ca^{2+} intake (including lactose intolerance)
  Poor solubilization of Ca^{2+} ($\downarrow$ gastric acid, $\uparrow$ fatty acids in lumen)
  Reduction in surface area for absorption
  Decreased contact time

- Vitamin D metabolism:
  Reduced exposure to sunlight impairing vitamin D synthesis
  Inadequate vitamin D intake or absorption
  Increased inactivation of vitamin D metabolites

- Other factors:
  Glucocorticoid therapy
  Amenorrhoea
  Secondary hyperparathyroidism
  Reduced activity levels

---

has been coined to describe the multifactorial bone disease associated with low vitamin D levels and gastrointestinal disorders.[79]

Gastric disease and surgery (p. 290)

Partial gastrectomy, gastroenterostomy and other gastric surgery may all lead to metabolic bone disease which can have the appearances of osteomalacia, osteoporosis or be less specific.[44] Variable prevalance rates are reported but about 10% or more will have bone disease after Billroth I or Polya operations.[29] Multiple factors have been suggested, including inadequate intake of vitamin D or calcium, delayed contact with proximal absorptive sites as a result of altered anatomy or transit times, malabsorption of vitamin D metabolites because of bacterial overgrowth, and impaired solubility of calcium due to hypochlorhydria or soap formation.

Patients with gastroenterostomies may have significantly lower 25-OH vitamin D levels than those without, though very low values are usually associated with additional factors.[27] In a careful study of asymptomatic patients after Billroth II gastrectomy,[60] many had unsuspected vertebral wedge fractures, and although 25-OH vitamin D and parathyroid hormone concentrations were the same as a control group, $24,25(OH)_2D$ levels were significantly lower and $1,25(OH)_2D$ levels were higher. Bone biopsy revealed hyperosteoidosis without osteomalacia, which could be in keeping with the putative actions of the more polar vitamin D metabolites on bone. Another study[75] has also found raised $1,25(OH)_2D$ levels in patients with Billroth I and II gastrectomies, though in that study 25-OH vitamin D levels were low in both groups.

The effects of hypochlorhydria are unclear. In one study, cimetidine did not affect the net absorption of calcium from calcium carbonate and neither did the achlorhydria of pernicious anaemia.[10] Gastric acidity was not needed to solubilize calcium carbonate. Another study showed marked impairment of calcium absorption from calcium carbonate in patients with achlorhydria under fasting conditions, but not from citrate, or when calcium carbonate was taken with a meal.[84]

Coeliac disease (p. 537)

The early descriptions of malabsorption in gluten-sensitive villous atrophy stressed rickets, osteomalacia, tetany and the associated biochemical findings.[22,69,72] Impaired absorption of dietary calcium and high endogenous faecal losses lead to a negative calcium balance. Secondary hyperpara-

thyroidism is common. Steatorrhoea results in excessive calcium soap formation and losses of vitamin D. Circulating levels of vitamin D and its metabolites may be low, and diminished absorption can be demonstrated.[24,94] Treatment with a gluten-free diet reverses these gross changes in calcium and vitamin D metabolism.

Coeliac disease patients may also be at increased risk of developing osteoporosis as many of the demonstrated risk factors are often present. Peak bone mass may be low, reflecting impaired nutrition before diagnosis of gluten-sensitivity, and there may have been delayed menarche or amenorrhoea. Physical exercise may have been less and associated lactose intolerance may have reduced the amount of milk calcium ingested. Although untreated adult coeliac patients were shown to have low forearm bone mineral density, patients treated from childhood have similar bone densities to their controls and a gluten-free diet prevents further significant bone loss.[15,71]

Some evidence suggests that, despite adequate treatment for many years with a gluten-free diet, there may be mild impairment of calcium absorption. In a study of treated patients with coeliac disease, the median value of calbindin-D_{9k} (the cystosolic protein which correlates with calcium absorption) was less than 30% of normal even though other biochemical markers showed no evidence of villous atrophy.[93] Untreated coeliac disease patients had even lower levels of calbindin-D_{9k} though their circulating $1,25(OH)_2D$ concentrations were unaffected. As vitamin D receptors are known to be present in untreated coeliac patients' biopsies, it is possible there is resistance to the action of $1,25(OH)_2D$, leading to failure of adequate calbindin-D_{9k} expression.

Intestinal bypass and resection (p. 666)

Reduced bone mineral content was found in 11% of a group of patients predominantly with Crohn's disease who had had extensive small bowel resection.[54] A weak inverse correlation was shown between calcium absorption and length of resected small bowel. In a further study of 62 Crohn's disease patients, retention of at least half of the colon resulted in higher fractional absorption of dietary calcium.[55]

After ileal bypass for the treatment of obesity, accelerated bone loss was shown to occur, particularly in those with jejunocolostomy.[20] Less than half the patients had osteomalacia, low 25-OH vitamin D levels and secondary hyperparathyroidism, which implied factors other than vitamin D in the bone disease. Patients with partial ileal bypass surgery for familial hypercholesterolaemia had significantly reduced calcium absorption for up to 5 years after operation, but had insignificant bone mineral loss.[83] Patients with resection following intestinal infarction have also been shown to have reduced 25-OH vitamin D.[27]

In addition to loss of small intestinal absorptive area, in bypassed loops, bacterial overgrowth may lead to the development of bone disease. Other causes of bacterial overgrowth can be associated with vitamin D or calcium malabsorption,[23] probably through bacterial deconjugation of bile salts leading to fat malabsorption and brush border damage.

Inflammatory bowel disease (Chapter 7)

In a study of 75 unselected patients with inflammatory bowel disease,[21] 30% were shown to have osteoporosis by single-photon absorptiometry measurements in the forearm, or by spinal quantitative CT scanning. Men were more commonly affected than women. Most patients who had osteoporosis had small intestinal disease with resections. They had significantly higher lifetime steroid doses, weighed less and had lower body mass indices than those without bone disease. Clinical osteoporosis was particularly severe in amenorrhoeic women on steroids. In a subgroup of 13 patients, mostly on steroids, serial measurements showed large losses of spinal and radial bone densities of over 2% a year and larger decreases in total body calcium.[87] These losses were at least double those expected.

Calcium malabsorption was infrequent in a group of patients with Crohn's disease who had not had extensive resection.[61] Low 25-OH vitamin D levels (<8 nmol/l) were found in about 20% of unselected Crohn's patients without previous bowel surgery[27] and all had active disease; a similar incidence was found in patients with resections.

Cholestasis and cirrhosis

Cholestasis interferes with fat absorption and hence that of calcium, vitamin D and its metabolites. Bone disease, calcium malabsorption and low circulating concentrations of 25-OH vitamin D are all well recognized in chronic cholestatic diseases, particularly primary biliary cirrhosis.[3,19,64] Other cholestatic diseases in which low values of 25-OH vitamin D have been reported include sclerosing cholangitis, secondary biliary cirrhosis due to gallstones, benign recurrent intrahepatic cholestasis, and congenital biliary hypoplasia. Calcium malabsorption may not

be important in the development of bone disease in chronic cholestasis in childhood.

Osteopenia is also common in cirrhosis without marked cholestasis, including alcoholic cirrhosis, chronic active hepatitis and cryptogenic cirrhosis.[19] Vitamin D deficiency and osteomalacia have been reported with variable prevalence in these patients and are almost certainly due to factors other than loss of parenchymal liver cells, as several studies have shown that hydroxylation of vitamin D to produce 25-OH vitamin D is not impaired in advanced cirrhosis.[81] However, reduced hepatic synthesis can lead to low values of the vitamin D-binding protein and, consequently, reduced serum total 25-OH vitamin D. Determination of free 25-OH vitamin D shows that this is normal, with a higher than normal free percentage.[9]

Chronic pancreatic disease (p. 1619)

Pancreatic insufficiency resulting in steatorrhoea will also affect calcium and vitamin D absorption. Patients with cystic fibrosis may present with osteomalacia in adult life and respond to vitamin D supplements.[90] Low 25-OH vitamin D levels have been found in patients with chronic pancreatitis and carcinoma of the pancreas but were nearly always associated with other conditions such as severe or prolonged cholestasis.[27]

Alcoholics, even without pancreatic insufficiency or cirrhosis, have been shown to have a high incidence of metabolic bone diseases.[8] Bone turnover was low, usually with normal values of calcium, phosphate, vitamin D metabolites and parathyroid hormone, though magnesium deficiency was frequent. Alcohol may impair calcium absorption and has been suggested to have a direct effect on bone.

PREVENTION AND TREATMENT OF CALCIUM MALABSORPTION

Calcium malabsorption is best treated by reversal of the primary gastrointestinal or endocrine condition. Thus, patients with coeliac disease improve their Ca^{2+} balance on a gluten-free diet, and patients with glucocorticoid-induced problems should have as low and as infrequent courses as possible. Other measures may help Ca^{2+} absorption: medium-chain triglycerides will be better absorbed and so bind less Ca^{2+}, increasing its availability. Hormone replacement therapy in postmenopausal women should be strongly encouraged to prevent osteopenia, particularly in those with gastrointestinal disorders. Provision of adequate vitamin D and ensuring sufficient Ca^{2+} intake are essential.

Calcium supplements

Calcium salts are cheap and well tolerated. It is easy to provide a normal adult intake of 750 mg Ca^{2+}/day and, although the lower limit is debatable, 1.5 g/day is accepted by all workers as sufficient to prevent negative Ca^{2+} balance even in postmenopausal patients with the poorest Ca^{2+} absorption. Debate also exists concerning the relative efficacy of different Ca^{2+} salts which have different solubilities though the variation in absorption between these is much less than that between different subjects. Under experimental fasting conditions, there was little difference in net Ca^{2+} absorption from acetate, lactate, gluconate, citrate or carbonate salts or when compared with milk and milk products.[91] Calcium carbonate preparations are probably adequate, having the highest amount of Ca^{2+} per unit weight, and are some of the cheapest, often being sold as antacid preparations. Co-ingestion of a light meal with Ca^{2+} enhances absorption by 10–30%.[50] Excessive Ca^{2+} intake and absorption increases urinary Ca^{2+} excretion and can result in renal tract stones, and, rarely, in hypercalcaemia and metastatic calcification. Ca^{2+} supplementation may also result in less availability of other minerals such as iron.

Vitamin D supplements

Vitamin D supplementation is less important than ensuring adequate Ca^{2+} intake, particularly as the increase in absorption of Ca^{2+} from high-Ca^{2+} diets is occurring predominantly through the vitamin D-independent passive route. However, sources of adequate vitamin D to prevent deficiency should be provided, particularly as metabolic losses may be increased. Sunlight exposure is the physiological way of providing vitamin D but many ill or aged patients are unable to obtain sufficient exposure. Oral replacement doses of calciferol (10 μg/day) are therefore indicated in those patients at risk for Ca^{2+} malabsorption with documented vitamin D deficiency.

Although in some patients with intestinal disease, malabsorption of vitamin D and 25-OH vitamin D was found and was related to the severity of the steatorrhoea,[94] the extent of the impairment was such that therapy with twice the replacement dose of oral vitamin D (i.e. 20 μg/day) was always sufficient.[24] Absorption of 25-OH vitamin D was shown to be somewhat greater than vitamin D, but use of the more polar metabolites of vitamin D, or parenteral routes, seemed unnecessary. Frequently, larger doses of calciferol (250 μg/day) are prescribed, which run the risk of vitamin D intoxication and necessitate monitoring of serum and urinary calcium values.

More polar metabolites of calciferol (i.e. calcitriol and 1α-hydroxyvitamin D) have the advantage in having a shorter half-life, which lessens accumulation and the risk of toxicity, but, if small replacement doses of calciferol are given, hypercalcaemia should not become a problem in gastrointestinal patients. Treatment with 1α-hydroxylated metabolites of vitamin D is necessary in end-stage renal disease in which the 1α-hydroxylase is lost, or in hypoparathyroidism where the regulation of this enzyme by parathyroid hormone is missing.

REFERENCES

1. Allen, L.H. (1982) Calcium bioavailability and absorption: a review. *American Journal of Clinical Nutrition*, **35**, 783–808.
2. Armbrecht, H.J., Boltz, M., Strong, R., Richardson, A., Bruns, M.E.H. and Christakos, S. (1989) Expression of calbindin-D decreases with age in intestine and kidney. *Endocrinology*, **125**, 2950–2956.
3. Atkinson, M., Nordin, B.E.C. and Sherlock, S. (1956) Malabsorption and bone disease in prolonged obstructive jaundice. *Quarterly Journal of Medicine*, **25**, 299–312.
4. Avioli, L.V., McDonald, J.E. and Lee, S.W. (1965) The influence of age on the intestinal absorption of ^{47}Ca in women and its relation to ^{47}Ca absorption in post-menopausal osteoporosis. *Journal of Clinical Investigation*, **44**, 1960–1967.
5. Baker, A.R., McDonnell, D.P., Hughes, M., Crisp, T.M., Mangelsdorf, D.J., Haussler, M.R. *et al.* (1988) Cloning and expression of full-length cDNA encoding human vitamin D receptor. *Proceedings of the National Academy of Sciences of the USA*, **85**, 3294–3298.
6. Bell, N.H., Shaw, S. and Turner, R.T. (1984) Evidence that 1,25-dihydroxyvitamin D_3 inhibits the hepatic production of 25-hydroxyvitamin D in man. *Journal of Clinical Investigation*, **74**, 1540–1544.
7. Bikle, D.D. and Munson, S. (1985) 1,25-Dihydroxyvitamin D increases calmodulin binding to specific proteins in the chick duodenal brush border membrane. *Journal of Clinical Investigation*, **76**, 2312–2316.
8. Bikle, D.D., Genant, H.K., Cann, C., Recker, R.R., Halloran, B.P. and Strewler, G.J. (1985) Bone disease in alcohol abuse. *Annals of Internal Medicine*, **103**, 42–48.
9. Bikle, D.D., Halloran, B.P., Gee, E., Ryzen, E. and Haddad, J.G. (1986) Free 25-hydroxyvitamin D levels are normal in subjects with liver disease and reduced total 25-hydroxyvitamin D levels. *Journal of Clinical Investigation*, **78**, 748–752.
10. Bo-Linn, G.W., Davis, G.R., Buddrus, D.J.,

Morawski, S.G., Santa Ana, C. and Fordtran, J.S. (1984) An evaluation of the importance of gastric acid secretion in the absorption of dietary calcium. *Journal of Clinical Investigation*, **73**, 640–647.

11. Brommage, R. and DeLuca, H.F. (1985) Evidence that 1,25-dihydroxyvitamin D_3 is the physiologically active metabolite of vitamin D_3. *Endocrinology Reviews*, **6**, 491–511.

12. Brommage, R., Baxter, D.C. and Gierke, L.W. (1990) Vitamin D-independent intestinal calcium and phosphorus absorption during reproduction. *American Journal of Physiology*, **259**, G631–G638.

13. Bronner, F. (1987) Calcium absorption. In: *Physiology of the Gastrointestinal Tract*, pp. 1419–1435, (Ed.) Johnson, L.R. New York: Raven Press.

14. Bronner, F., Pansu, D. and Stein, W.D. (1986) An analysis of calcium transport across the rat intestine. *American Journal of Physiology*, **250**, G561–G569.

15. Caraceni, M.P., Molteni, N., Bardella, M.T., Ortolani, S., Nogara, A. and Bianchi, P.A. (1988) Bone and mineral metabolism in adult celiac disease. *American Journal of Gastroenterology*, **83**, 274–277.

16. Chandra, S., Fullmer, C.S., Smith, C.A., Wasserman, R.H. and Morrison, G.H. (1990) Ion microscopic imaging of calcium transport in the intestinal tissue of vitamin D-deficient and vitamin D-replete chickens: a ^{44}Ca stable isotope study. *Proceedings of the National Academy of Sciences of the USA*, **87**, 5715–5719.

17. Clements, M.R., Johnson, L. and Fraser, D.R. (1987) A new mechanism for induced vitamin D deficiency in calcium deprivation. *Nature*, **325**, 62–65.

18. Cochet, B., Jung, A., Griessen, M., Bartholdi, P., Schaller, P. and Donath, A. (1983) Effects of lactose on intestinal calcium absorption in normal and lactase-deficient subjects. *Gastroenterology*, **84**, 935–940.

19. Compston, J.E. (1986) Hepatic osteodystrophy: vitamin D metabolism in patients with liver disease. *Gut*, **27**, 1073–1090.

20. Compston, J.E., Horton, L.W.L., Laker, M.F. *et al.* (1978) Bone disease after jejuno-ileal bypass for obesity. *The Lancet*, **ii**, 1–4.

21. Compston, J.E., Judd, D., Crawley, E.O. *et al.* (1987) Osteoporosis in patients with inflammatory bowel disease. *Gut*, **28**, 410–415.

22. Cooke, W.T., Peeney, A.L.P. and Hawkins, C.F. (1953) Symptoms, signs and diagnostic features of idiopathic steatorrhoea. *Quarterly Journal of Medicine*, **22**, 59–77.

23. Cooke, W.T., Cox, E.V., Fone, D.J., Meynell, M.J. and Gaddie, R. (1963) The clinical and metabolic significance of jejunal diverticula. *Gut*, **4**, 115–131.

24. Davies, M., Mawer, E.B. and Krawitt, E.L. (1980) Comparative absorption of vitamin D_3 and 25-hydroxyvitamin D_3 in intestinal disease. *Gut*, **21**, 287–292.

25. Dawson-Hughes, B., Dallal, G.E., Krall, E.A., Sadowski, L., Sahyoun, N. and Tannenbaum, S. (1990) A controlled trial of the effect of calcium supplementation on bone density in postmenopausal women. *New England Journal of Medicine*, **323**, 878–883.

26. DeGrazia, J.A., Ivanovich, P., Fellows, H. and Rich, C. (1965) A double isotope method for measurement of calcium absorption in man. *Journal of Laboratory & Clinical Medicine*, **66**, 822–829.

27. Dibble, J.B., Sheridan, P. and Losowsky, M.S. (1984) A survey of vitamin D deficiency in gastrointestinal and liver disorders. *Quarterly Journal of Medicine*, **209**, 119–134.

28. Editorial (1985) Risk factors in postmenopausal osteoporosis. *The Lancet*, **i**, 1370–1372.

29. Editorial (1986) Osteomalacia after gastrectomy. *The Lancet*, **i**, 77–78.

30. Editorial (1990) New treatments for osteoporosis. *The Lancet*, **335**, 1065–1066.

31. Favus, M.J. (1985) Factors that influence absorption and secretion of calcium in the small intestine and colon. *American Journal of Physiology*, **248**, G147–G157.

32. Feher, J.J. (1983) Facilitated calcium diffusion by intestinal calcium-binding protein. *American Journal of Physiology*, **244**, C303–C307.

33. Fraser, D., Kooh, S.W., Kind, H.P., Holick, M.F., Tanaka, Y. and DeLuca, H.F. (1973) Pathogenesis of hereditary vitamin D-dependent rickets: an inborn error of vitamin D metabolism involving defective conversion of 25-hydroxyvitamin D to 1α,25-dihydroxyvitamin D. *New England Journal of Medicine*, **289**, 817–822.

34. Fraser, D.R. (1983) The physiological economy of vitamin D. *The Lancet*, **i**, 969–972.

35. Fraser, D.R. and Kodicek, E. (1970) Unique biosynthesis by kidney of a biologically active vitamin D metabolite. *Nature*, **228**, 764–766.

36. Gallagher, J.C. and Goldgar, D. (1990) Treatment of postmenopausal osteoporosis with high doses of synthetic calcitriol. A randomised controlled study. *Annals of Internal Medicine*, **113**, 649–655.

37. Gallagher, J.C., Riggs, B.L., Eisman, J., Hamstra, A., Arnaud, S.B. and DeLuca, H.F. (1979) Intestinal calcium absorption and serum vitamin D metabolites in normal subjects and osteoporotic patients. *Journal of Clinical Investigation*, **64**, 729–736.

38. Garabedian, M., Holick, M.F., DeLuca, H.F. and Boyle, I.T. (1972) Control of 25-hydroxycholecalciferol metabolism by parathyroid glands. *Proceedings of the National Academy of Sciences of the USA*, **69**, 1973–1976.

39. Garland, C., Shekelle, R.B., Barrett-Connor, E., Criqui, M.H., Rossof, A.H. and Paul, O. (1985) Dietary vitamin D and calcium and risk of

colorectal cancer: a 19-year prospective study in men. *The Lancet*, **i**, 307–309.

40. Ghijsen, W.E.J.M. and van Os, C.H. (1982) 1α,25-dihydroxyvitamin D₃ regulates ATP-dependent calcium transport in basolateral plasma membranes of rat enterocytes. *Biochimica et Biophysica Acta*, **689**, 170–172.

41. Glenney, J.Jr. and Glenney, P. (1985) Comparison of Ca^{2+}-regulated events in the intestinal brush border. *Journal of Cell Biology*, **100**, 754–763.

42. Griessen, M., Crochet, B., Infante, F. *et al.* (1989) Calcium absorption from milk in lactase-deficient subjects. *American Journal of Clinical Nutrition*, **49**, 377–384.

43. Haddad, J.G. and Walgate, J. (1976) 25-Hydroxyvitamin D transport in human plasma. Isolation and partial characterization of calcifidiol binding protein. *Journal of Biological Chemistry*, **251**, 4803–4809.

44. Hall, G.H. and Neale, G. (1963) Bone rarefaction after partial gastrectomy. *Annals of Internal Medicine*, **59**, 455–463.

45. Halloran, B.P. and DeLuca, H.F. (1980) Calcium transport in small intestine during early development: role of vitamin D. *American Journal of Physiology*, **239**, G473–G479.

46. Halloran, B.P., Bikle, D.D., Levens, M.J., Castro, M.E., Globus, R.K. and Holton, E. (1986) Chronic 1,25-dihydroxyvitamin D₃ administration in the rat reduces the serum concentration of 25-hydroxyvitamin D by increasing metabolic clearance rate. *Journal of Clinical Investigation*, **78**, 622–628.

47. Heaney, R.P. and Recker, R.R. (1985) Estimation of true calcium absorption. *Annals of Internal Medicine*, **103**, 516–521.

48. Heaney, R.P. and Recker, R.R. (1988) Estimating true fractional calcium absorption. *Annals of Internal Medicine*, **106**, 905–906.

49. Heaney, R.P., Weaver, C. M. and Recker, R.R. (1988) Calcium absorbability from spinach. *American Journal of Clinical Nutrition*, **47**, 707–709.

50. Heaney, R.P., Smith, K.T., Recker, R.R. and Hinders, S.M. (1989) Meal effects on calcium absorption. *American Journal of Clinical Nutrition*, **49**, 372–376.

51. Holick, M.F. and Adams, J.S. (1990) Vitamin D metabolism and biological function. In: *Metabolic Bone Disease and Clinically Related Disorders*, pp. 155–195. (Eds) Avioli, L.V. and Krane, S.M. Philadelphia: W.B. Saunders.

52. Holick M.F., Maclaughlin, J.A. and Dopplet, S.H. (1981) Factors that influence the cutaneous photosynthesis of previtamin D₃. *Science*, **211**, 590–593.

53. Howard, A., Legon, S., Spurr, N.K. and Walters, J.R.F. (1992) Molecular cloning and chromosomal assignment of human calbindin–D₉ₖ. *Biochemical and Biophysical Research Communications*, **185**, 663–669.

54. Hylander, E., Ladefoged, K. and Madsen, S. (1981) Calcium balance and bone mineral content following small-intestinal resection. *Scandinavian Journal of Gastroenterology*, **16**, 167–176.

55. Hylander, E., Ladefoged, K. and Jarnum, S. (1990) Calcium absorption after intestinal resection. The importance of a preserved colon. *Scandinavian Journal of Gastroenterology*, **25**, 705–710.

56. Imawari, M. and Goodman, D.W.S. (1977) Immunological and immunoassay studies of the binding protein for vitamin D and its metabolites in human serum. *Journal of Clinical Investigation*, **59**, 432–442.

57. Ireland, P. and Fordtran, J.S. (1973) Effect of dietary calcium and age on jejunal calcium absorption in humans studied by intestinal perfusion. *Journal of Clinical Investigation*, **52**, 2672–2681.

58. Kanis, J.A. and Passmore, R. (1989) Calcium supplementation of the diet. Not justified by present evidence. *British Medical Journal*, **298**, 137–140, 205–208.

59. Kikuchi, K., Kikuchi, T. and Ghishan, F.K. (1988) Characterization of calcium transport by basolateral membrane vesicles of human small intestine. *American Journal of Physiology*, **255**, G482–G489.

60. Klein, K.B., Orwoll, E.S., Leiberman, D.A., Meier, D.E., McClung, M.R. and Parfitt, A.M. (1987) Metabolic bone disease in asymptomatic men after partial gastrectomy with Billroth II anastomosis. *Gastroenterology*, **92**, 608–616.

61. Krawitt, E.L., Beeken, W.L. and Janney, C.D. (1976) Calcium absorption in Crohn's disease. *Gastroenterology*, **71**, 251–254.

62. Lieberherr, M., Grosse, B., Duchambon, P. and Drüeke, T. (1989) A functional cell surface type receptor is required for the early action of 1,25-dihydroxyvitamin D₃ on the phosphoinositide metabolism in rat enterocytes. *Journal of Biological Chemistry*, **264**, 20403–20406.

63. Lipkin, M. and Newmark, H. (1985) Effect of added dietary calcium on colonic epithelial-cell proliferation in subjects at high risk for familial colonic cancer. *New England Journal of Medicine*, **313**, 1381–1384.

64. Long, R.G., Skinner, R.K., Wills, M.R. and Sherlock, S. (1976) Serum-25-hydroxy-vitamin-D in untreated parenchymal and cholestatic liver disease. *The Lancet*, **ii**, 650–652.

65. Lukert, B.P. and Raiz, L.G. (1990) Glucocorticoid-induced osteoporosis: pathogenesis and management. *Annals of Internal Medicine*, **112**, 352–364.

66. Malloy, P.J., Hochberg, Z., Tiosano, D., Pike, J.W., Hughes, M.R. and Feldman, D. (1990) The molecular basis of hereditary 1,25-dihydroxyvitamin D₃ resistant rickets in seven related families. *Journal of Clinical Investigation*, **86**, 2071–2079.

67. Marshall, D.H. and Nordin, B.E.C. (1981) A comparison of radioactive calcium absorption tests with net calcium absorption. *Clinical Sciences*, **61**, 477–481.

68. McLaughlin, M., Raggatt, P.R., Fairney, A., Brown, D.J., Lester, E. and Wills, M.R. (1974) Seasonal variations in serum-25-hydroxycholecalciferol in healthy people. *The Lancet*, **i**, 536–538.

69. Melvin, K.E.W., Hepner, G.W., Bordier, P., Neale, G. and Joplin, G.F. (1970) Calcium metabolism and bone pathology in adult coeliac disease. *Quarterly Journal of Medicine*, **39**, 83–113.

70. Minghetti, P.P. and Norman, A.W. (1988) 1,25(OH)$_2$-Vitamin D$_3$ receptors: gene regulation and genetic circuitry. *FASEB Journal*, **2**, 3043–3053.

71. Molteni, N., Caraceni, M.P., Bardella, M.T., Ortolani, S., Gandolini, G.G. and Bianchi, P. (1990) Bone mineral density in adult celiac patients and the effect of gluten-free diet from childhood. *American Journal of Gastroenterology*, **85**, 51–53.

72. Nassim, J.R., Saville, P.D., Cook, P.B. and Mulligan, L. (1959) The effects of vitamin D and gluten-free diet in idiopathic steatorrhoea. *Quarterly Journal of Medicine*, **28**, 141–162.

73. Nellans, N.H. and Popovitch, J.E. (1981) Calmodulin regulated, ATP driven calcium transport by baso-lateral membranes of rat small intestine. *Journal of Biological Chemistry*, **256**, 9932–9936.

74. Nemere, I. and Norman, A.W. (1988) 1,25-Dihydroxyvitamin D$_3$-mediated vesicular transport of calcium in intestine: time-course studies. *Endocrinology*, **122**, 2962–2969.

75. Nilas, L., Christiansen, C. and Christiansen, J. (1985) Regulation of vitamin D and calcium metabolism after gastrectomy. *Gut*, **26**, 252–257.

76. Nordin, B.E.C. and Heaney, R.P. (1990) Calcium supplementation of the diet: justified by present evidence. *British Medical Journal*, **300**, 1056–1060.

77. Norman, A.W. (1990) Intestinal calcium absorption: a vitamin D-hormone-mediated adaptive response. *American Journal of Clinical Nutrition*, **51**, 290–300.

78. Norman, D.A., Fordtran, J.S., Brinkley, L.J. *et al.* (1981) Jejunal and ileal adaptation to alterations in dietary calcium. *Journal of Clinical Investigation*, **67**, 1599–1603.

79. Parfitt, A.M. (1990) Osteomalacia and related disorders. In: *Metabolic Bone Disease and Clinically Related Disorders*, pp. 329–396.(Eds) Avioli, L.V. and Krane, S.M. Philadelphia: W.B. Saunders.

80. Pitkin, R.M. (1985) Calcium metabolism in pregnancy and the perinatal period: a review. *American Journal of Obstetrics and Gynecology*, **151**, 99–109.

81. Posner, D.B., Russell, R.M., Absood, S. *et al.* (1978) Effective 25-hydroxylation of vitamin D$_2$ in alcoholic cirrhosis. *Gastroenterology*, **74**, 866–870.

82. Raisz, L.G. and Rodan, G.A. (1990) Cellular basis for bone turnover. In: *Metabolic Bone Disease and Clinically Related Disorders*, pp. 1–41. (Eds) Avioli, L.V. and Krane, S.M. Philadelphia: W.B. Saunders.

83. Rannem, T., Hylander, E., Jarnum, S. *et al.* (1990) Calcium absorption and bone mineral content in patients subjected to ileal bypass because of familial hypercholesterolaemia. *Scandinavian Journal of Gastroenterology*, **25**, 897–905.

84. Recker, R.R. (1985) Calcium absorption and achlorhydria. *New England Journal of Medicine*, **313**, 70–73.

85. Reichel, H., Keoffler, H.P. and Norman, A.W. (1989) The role of the vitamin D endocrine system in health and disease. *New England Journal of Medicine*, **320**, 980–991.

86. Riggs, B.L. and Melton, L.J. (1986) Involutional osteoporosis. *New England Journal of Medicine*, **314**, 1676–1686.

87. Ryde, S.J.S., Clements, D., Evans, W.D. *et al.* (1991) Total body calcium in patients with inflammatory bowel disease: a longitudinal study. *Clinical Sciences*, **80**, 319–324.

88. Schachter, D. and Rosen, S.M. (1959) Active transport of ^{45}Ca by the small intestine and its dependence on vitamin D. *American Journal of Physiology*, **196**, 357–362.

89. Schoen, M.S., Lindenbaum, J., Roginsky, M.S. and Holt, P.R. (1978) Significance of serum level of 25-hydroxycholecalciferol in gastrointestinal disease. *Digestive Diseases and Sciences*, **23**, 137–142.

90. Scott, J., Elias, E., Moult, P.J.A., Barnes, S. and Will, M.R. (1977) Rickets in adult cystic fibrosis with myopathy, pancreatic insufficiency and proximal renal tubular dysfunction. *American Journal of Medicine*, **63**, 488–492.

91. Sheikh, M.S., Santa Ana, C.A., Nicar, M.J., Schiller, L.R. and Fordtran, J.S. (1987) Gastrointestinal absorption of calcium from milk and calcium salts. *New England Journal of Medicine*, **317**, 532–536.

92. Sheikh, M.S., Ramirez, A., Emmett, M., Santa Ana, C., Schiller, L.R. and Fordtran, J.S. (1988) Role of vitamin D-dependent and vitamin D-independent mechanisms in absorption of food calcium. *Journal of Clinical Investigation*, **81**, 126–132.

93. Staun, M. and Jarnum, S. (1988) Measurement of the 10,000-molecular weight calcium-binding protein in small-intestinal biopsy specimens from patients with malabsorption syndromes. *Scandinavian Journal of Gastroenterology*, **23**, 827–832.

94. Thompson, G.R., Lewis, B. and Booth, C.C. (1966) Absorption of vitamin D$_3$-^{3}H in control

subjects and patients with intestinal malabsorption. *Journal of Clinical Investigation*, **45**, 94–102.

95. Thompson, G.R., Ockner, R.K. and Isselbacher, K.J. (1969) Effect of mixed micellar lipid on the absorption of cholesterol and vitamin D_3 into lymph. *Journal of Clinical Investigation*, **48**, 87–95.

96. Van Os, C.H. (1987) Transcellular calcium transport in intestinal and renal epithelial cells. *Biochimica et Biophysica Acta*, **906**, 195–222.

97. Wali, R.K., Baum, C.L., Sitrin, M.D. and Brasitus, T.A. (1990) $1,25(OH)_2$ vitamin D_3 stimulates membrane phosphoinositide turnover, activates protein kinase C, and increases cytosolic calcium in rat colonic epithelium. *Journal of Clinical Investigation*, **85**, 1296–1303.

98. Walling, M.W. and Kimberg, D.V. (1975) Effects of $1\alpha,25$-dihydroxyvitamin D_3 and *Solanum glaucophyllum* on intestinal calcium and phosphate transport and on plasma Ca, Mg, and P levels in the rat. *Endocrinology*, **97**, 1567–1576.

99. Walters, J.R.F. (1989) Ca[...] the calcium-pump in rat e[...] membranes. *American J[...]* G124–G128.

100. Walters, J.R.F. and W[...] transport by rat duode[...] basolateral membranes. [...] *Physiology*, **252**, G170–G177.

101. Warner, R.R. and Coleman, J.R. (1975) [...] probe analysis of calcium transport by small intestine. *Journal of Cell Biology*, **64**, 54–74.

102. Wasserman, R.H. and Taylor, A.N. (1966) Vitamin D_3-induced calcium-binding protein in chick intestinal mucosa. *Science*, **152**, 791–793.

103. Wensel, R.H., Rich, C., Brown, A.C. and Volwiler, W. (1969) Absorption of calcium measured by intubation and perfusion of the intact human small intestine. *Journal of Clinical Investigation*, **48**, 1768–1775.

INTESTINAL TRANSPORT OF FLUID AND ELECTROLYTES (PHYSIOLOGY AND PATHOPHYSIOLOGY)

N.W. Read

NORMAL INTESTINAL FLUID BALANCE

The turnover of fluid by the gastrointestinal tract can be quite prodigious. It has been estimated that an average of 10 litres of fluid containing about 50 g of sodium enter the gut each day but volumes as high as 20 l/day may be processed without producing diarrhoea. Not all of this fluid is ingested. The average fluid intake with food and drink is usually about 2.5 l/day. To this is added approximately 7.5 litres of digestive secretions. These figures, of course, are subject to considerable variation, depending largely on the quantity and the composition of the diet.

Most of the salt and water that enters the gut is absorbed in the small intestine, the absorptive surface of which is increased many thousand-fold by villous and microvillous projections. Every day, between 1 and 2 litres of liquid effluent from the small intestine enter the colon. In this cavernous and stagnant tube, water and salts are extracted from the solidifying colonic contents against high transepithelial concentration and osmotic gradients.

Although the amount of fluid that passes through the gut is only a fraction of that which passes through the kidney each day (>100 litres), the impaired absorption and excessive secretion that can occur in patients with diarrhoea and vomiting can cause rapid and serious fluid and electrolyte depletion, particularly in children.

MECHANISMS OF ABSORPTION AND SECRETION

Both the small intestine and the large intestine have the capacity to absorb and to secrete fluid, and the balance between the two has been termed the intestinal transport tone.[8,58] It is commonly assumed that intestinal absorption and secretion take place on two separate populations of cells. Absorption occurs on the villi of the small intestine and the surface epithelial cells of the colon while secretion emanates from the small intestinal crypts and the colonic pits.

Under most normal circumstances, and particularly after a meal, the transport tone has a bias in the direction of fluid absorption. The net rate of fluid absorption, however, varies widely from subject to subject and in the same subject on different test days. The transport tone is influenced by many factors. These include the presence of nutrients in nal lumen, the action of various endocrine ...ces and the activity of the enteric and auto- ...c nervous systems. Histological studies have ...onstrated a dense cholinergic innervation of the ...lls in the crypt region of the small intestine. Pharmacological studies suggest that cholinergic agents cause fluid and electrolyte secretion, while adrenergic agents have the opposite effect and cause absorption of salt and water. This implies that sympathetic stimulation induces fluid absorption while vagal stimulation induces fluid secretion, and there is some evidence from experimental animals to support this hypothesis.[20] The transport tone is influenced more directly, however, by local enteric nervous reflexes stimulated by luminal contents. It is reversed, for example, favouring secretion when the intestine is invaded by toxigenic bacteria, irritated by chemicals or stimulated by mechanical factors such as distension.

ABSORPTION FROM THE SMALL INTESTINE

The greatest volumes of fluid are absorbed from the small intestine in the hours immediately following a meal. Much of this fluid travels out of the intestinal lumen in response to osmotic gradients set up by the active cotransport of sodium and non-electrolytes, in particular hexose sugars and amino acids.

SODIUM-LINKED SOLUTE TRANSFER

According to the most widely held hypothesis, both sodium and the organic solute combine with a common carrier protein that is situated on the mucosal membrane of the enterocyte.[25] Separate carrier proteins exist for hexose sugars and for different groups of amino acids. When both loci on the carrier are occupied, the diffusion of sodium from a high concentration in the lumen to a much lower concentration in the cytosol through channels created by the transport protein provides the energy for the transfer of the non-electrolyte into the cell even against a concentration gradient. In order to maintain the inwardly directed sodium gradient, sodium is expelled across the basolateral membrane by active exchange with extracellular potassium using energy derived from the breakdown of ATP (Na^+/K^+-dependent ATPase). Hexose sugars or amino acids diffuse out of the cell across the basolateral membrane on another carrier protein (facilitated diffusion).

OLIGOPEPTIDE TRANSPORT

Much protein is absorbed as small peptides, which are subsequently broken down by intracellular peptidases to amino acids, which escape into the lateral space by facilitated diffusion. Transport of small peptides also stimulates fluid absorption across the epithelium, but the carriers that mediate the active transport of the oligopeptide across the brush border membrane differ from those that transport amino acids.[18] Recent data has shown that they cotransport hydrogen ions. Thus, uptake of oligopeptides is dependent on an inwardly directed gradient of hydrogen ions, which is in turn generated by another transport mechanism that uses the inwardly directed sodium gradient to expel hydrogen ions from the cell across the brush border membrane. Thus, oligopeptide transport also relies on the sodium gradient, but the relationship is less direct than it is with amino acids and hexose sugars.

Not all transport of sodium across the mucosal membrane of the small intestine occurs in combination with non-electrolytes. As indicated above, sodium ions can be absorbed in exchange for hydrogen ions across the brush border membrane,[27,54] acidifying the contents of the upper small intestine. In the ileum, sodium–hydrogen exchange is coupled on a 1:1 basis with a parallel chloride–bicarbonate exchanger.[27,55] In addition, the ileal enterocyte has the capacity to secrete bicarbonate by itself and some chloride absorption can occur independently of bicarbonate.

MECHANISM OF FLUID ABSORPTION

The active absorption of solute across the enterocyte establishes a hypertonic zone in the extracellular fluid space around the enterocytes. This encourages water and low molecular weight solutes to flow from the intestinal lumen into these spaces through the tight junctions, porous connections that join adjacent enterocytes at their mucosal poles. Although active transcellular transport of sodium provides the energy for this process, most sodium is absorbed passively across the epithelium of the upper small intestine dissolved in the water that flows through the tight junctions. This process is known as 'solvent drag'.[12] Recent evidence suggests that the carrier-linked glucose transport across the mucosal membrane facilitates solvent drag by relaxing contractile proteins in the tight junction, so increasing its permeability.[31,32,40]

Several litres of fluid can be absorbed from the upper small intestine in the hours following a meal. This rapid transport of fluid relies on the high permeability of the so-called tight junctions between adjacent enterocytes. In the classic 'standing gradient' hypothesis that is often used to explain small intestinal fluid transport, fluid is 'sucked' into the lateral spaces in response to an osmotic gradient set up by active transcellular transport of sodium and organic solutes. The ensuing hydrostatic pressure gradient then propels fluid towards and into the capillaries.

The requirement for high permeability seems incompatible with the generation of osmotic and hydrostatic pressure gradients within the lateral intercellular space powerful enough to cause rapid absorption. Such gradients would be rapidly dissipated and any increase in intercellular hydrostatic pressure would be just as likely to propel fluid back through the permeable junctions between the cells as to encourage flow onwards towards the capillaries. A more workable hypothesis[21] proposes that the zone of hypertonicity responsible for fluid absorption is normally maintained in the interstitial fluid at the tip of the villus by the operation of a countercurrent multiplier, formed by the hairpin vascular loop configuration of the central capillary supplying the villus with arterial blood and the subepithelial capillary network draining the villus (*Figure 3.41*). This hypothesis proposes that the osmotic gradient set up by the active transport of sodium by the cells on the sides of the villus is quickly dispersed across the

villus to the central capillary and carried towards the villus tip. As in the loop of Henle, this means that water entering the villous via the central capillary can be short-circuited across the base of the villus while sodium is trapped at the villous tip. The osmotic attraction of water from the intestinal lumen into the tip of the villus expands the villous interstitium. This not only increases the interstitial pressure, it also opens up the leaflets on the central lymphatic vessel, which are anchored by fibrous connections to the muscularis mucosae. In this way fluid can be forced into and down the lymphatic vessels. The countercurrent hypothesis could explain why 50% of fluid absorption from the intestine takes place via the lymphatics in spite of the fact that villus blood flow is some 500 times larger than lymphatic flow.[3] It has been suggested that much of the sodium that plays such a crucial role in this model may be secreted from the crypts, and reabsorbed from the lateral surface of the villus.[32] The observation that glucose absorption can increase fluid and electrolyte secretion from the crypt epithelium favours this mechanism.

COLONIC ABSORPTION

THE COLON AS AN ORGAN OF SALVAGE

The capacity of the colon for the absorption of fluid and electrolytes is far less than that of the small intestine, but the colon has the ability to adapt to meet the demands of increased delivery of fluid from the small intestine. Under 'normal circumstances' between 1 and 1.5 litres of fluid enter the colon each day. Water and electrolytes are extracted from the ileal effluent, leaving a residual mass of bacteria of unabsorbable result of about 100 g. Intraluminal perfusion studies have indicated that the human colon is capable of accommodating up to 6 litres of ileal effluent per day without resulting in diarrhoea.[13] Colonic extraction or salvage does not just apply to fluid and electrolytes; the colon can salvage unabsorbed carbohydrate and protein by bacterial conversion to short-chain fatty acids which can be used as a source of energy. Failure of colonic salvage, either because of excessive ileal delivery or impaired colonic absorption, results in diarrhoea.[44]

The ability of the colon to extract salt and water against high transepithelial gradients is arguably the most distinctive feature of colonic transport. By this means, the colon plays an important role in the conservation of salt and water and facilitates the control of defaecation by the production of solid stool.

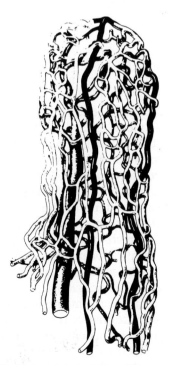

Figure 3.41 The vascular anatomy of a human villus. The dark vessels are the arteries and veins; the light vessels are the capillaries.

TRANSPORT OF SHORT-CHAIN FATTY ACIDS

As in the small intestine, fluid is absorbed in response to osmotic gradients created by the absorption of sodium and non-electrolytes. The human colon, however, does not possess carriers for mucosal transport of hexose sugars and amino acids. Any unabsorbed carbohydrate and protein that enters from the small intestine is broken down by anaerobic bacteria to short-chain fatty acids (carbohydrate is degraded to acetic acid with smaller concentrations of propionic acid and butyric acid), the nitrogen being mainly used for bacterial protein synthesis. Short-chain fatty acids are absorbed rapidly across the colonic epithelium and their transport stimulates the absorption of salt and water.[34,48] The transport of short-chain fatty acids can occur by two mechanisms. At the low colonic pH values generated by rapid bacterial fermentation of carbohydrate, short-chain fatty acids are associated and absorption occurs by non-ionic diffusion. At pH values of 6 and above, however, the anion dissociates and may be absorbed across the epithelium in exchange for bicarbonate.[11,34]

ION TRANSPORT MECHANISMS

While the generation of short-chain fatty acids is a powerful stimulus for the absorption of salt and water in the colon, appreciable quantities can be absorbed by other mechanisms.[6,23] Like the small intestine, the colon possesses a sodium–hydrogen exchange mechanism that is coupled 1:1 with a chloride–bicarbonate exchange mechanism. Independent secretion of bicarbonate can also occur in the colon. Sodium can also be transported independently across the brush border membrane. This important mechanism responds to body requirements and is under the control of the mineralocorticoid aldosterone, which increases the permeability of the mucosal membrane to sodium by insertion of sodium transport proteins.

The colon also differs from the small intestine in its ability to transport potassium.[42] The luminal membrane contains channels for the efflux of potassium. Passive secretion of potassium, particularly in the proximal colon, can be stimulated by transmitters that operate via either cyclic nucleotides or calcium. This efflux of potassium can be enhanced by corticosteroids, which increase the electrochemical gradient for efflux by stimulating sodium absorption across the mucosal membrane and active potassium entry in exchange for sodium across the basolateral membrane. In the distal colon, potassium secretion is partially offset by active absorption of potassium in exchange for hydrogen (K^+ H^+-dependent ATPase).

The surface of the colon is flat and hence the requirements for a countercurrent multiplier do not exist. The osmotic force for colonic transport of water is generated within the lateral intercellular space, which is longer and more tortuous than in the small intestine. The key feature is the configuration of the tight junctions,[12,28] which are much less permeable than in the small intestine. This has three consequences: (1) transport of water is much slower than it is in the small intestine; (2) most sodium is absorbed actively through the colonic enterocyte; (3) backflow of sodium through the tight junctions is virtually impossible. This means that concentrations can be established in the convoluted lateral intercellular spaces that are much higher than those in the colonic lumen, encouraging water to enter via the tight junctions. The resistance to back flow means that a buildup of hydrostatic pressure is more likely to propel salt and water towards the subepithelial capillaries.

ACTIVE INTESTINAL SECRETION

The crucial event that causes the intestinal epithelium to secrete fluid and electrolytes is an increase in the permeability of the luminal membrane of the cells in the small intestinal crypts or colonic pits to the chloride ion.[23,24] This is probably brought about by the opening up of chloride channels in the cell membrane as well as by the fusion of vesicles containing chloride channels with the cell membrane. Chloride leaks into the lumen down its electrochemical gradient, building up a local electronegative charge just adjacent to the mucous membrane. This zone of electronegativity then encourages sodium to leak through the cation-selective tight junctions accompanied by water. It is likely that chloride-driven secretion is facilitated by a local increase in the permeability of the tight junctions[31,39] and by associated vasodilatation and increases in capillary permeability and filtration pressure.[7] The change in mucosal permeability to chloride is subserved by a complicated series of transport mechanisms which are coordinated and triggered by intracellular mediators.[14,15]

If no other changes in membrane transport occurred, the depolarization of the cell membrane induced by the increase in chloride permeability would reduce the electrochemical driving force for chloride exit from the cell and chloride secretion would become self-limiting. The concomitant increase in potassium conductance at the basolateral

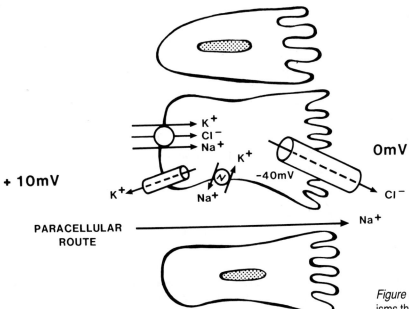

Figure 3.42 A diagram of the ion transport mechanisms that subserve active intestinal secretion.

membrane prevents this happening, hyperpolarizing the cell contents and maintaining the electrical gradient for chloride secretion. Depletion of intracellular chloride and potassium is countered by the entry of chloride across the basolateral membrane by combination with a carrier mechanism that also transports sodium and potassium into the cell.[38] Sodium is actively extruded into the lateral intercellular space by the sodium–potassium exchange mechanism. This not only maintains the electrochemical gradient for cotransport of chloride, it also charges the lateral intercellular space with sodium for passive secretion via the tight junctions, and it helps to replete intracellular potassium concentrations. Secretion can be inhibited by pharmacological agents that act at any of these sites, yielding several possibilities for development of new therapies for diarrhoea (*Figure 3.42*).

INTRACELLULAR CONTROL OF SECRETION[14,15]

The combination of an extracellular secretogogue with the cell membrane causes the changes in ion permeability associated with secretion through the activation of intracellular mediators (*Figure 3.43*). They include the cyclic nucleotides cAMP and cGMP, calcium, calmodulin, the metabolites of phosphotidylinositol, and guanosine triphosphate-dependent regulator proteins (G proteins). These intracellular mediators then alter membrane transport partly by activating specific protein kinases which phosphorylate either the ion channels themselves or the regulator proteins associated with ion channels. Calcium and cAMP do not only mediate secretion in the crypt cell; they also inhibit salt and water absorption across the villus cell by inhibiting sodium–hydrogen exchange. Sodium-coupled non-electrolyte transport is unaffected.

Different secretory transmitters do not necessarily use the same intracellular mediators, although there is considerable interaction between different mediators and mechanisms. Vasoactive intestinal polypeptide, for example, combines with a receptor on the basolateral membrane to release a stimulatory G protein that activates adenylate cyclase, resulting in the formation of cAMP.[10] Prostaglandins can also have the same action. cAMP then induces secretion by binding to the regulatory component of a cAMP-dependent protein kinase. This separates the catalytic subunit which then modifies membrane transport. In contrast, noradrenaline can interact with the epithelial adrenoceptors to release an inhibitory G protein that suppresses adenylate cyclase and interferes with calcium-mediated events.

The heat-stable toxins of *Escherichia coli*, *Yersinia* and *Klebsiella* stimulate secretion by activating guanylate cyclase to cause the release of cGMP.[43] Unlike cAMP, the cGMP-dependent protein kinase does not dissociate upon combination with the nucleotide.

Other transmitters act by increasing the intracellular concentration of calcium. This can occur in several ways. The interaction of substance P with a membrane-bound receptor, for example, causes an increase in membrane permeability to calcium. By

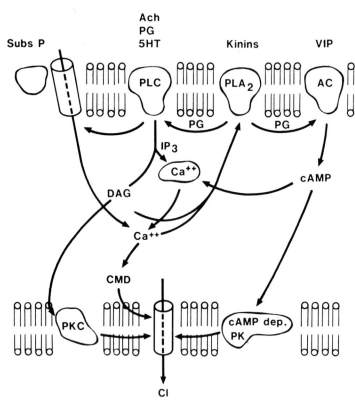

Figure 3.43 A diagram to show the intracellular mediators and their interactions in the production of active intestinal secretion. Ach, acetylcholine; PG, prostaglandin; 5HT, serotonin; VIP, vasoactive intestinal polypeptide; PLC, phospholipase C; PLA₂, phospholipase A₂; AC, adenylate cyclase; IP₃, inositol triphosphate; DAG, diacylglycerol; CMD, calmodulin; PK, protein kinase; PKC, protein kinase C.

contrast, acetylcholine, serotonin and prostaglandin E_2 activate phospholipase C in the basolateral membrane, resulting in the formation of diacylglycerol and inositol triphosphate from membrane components.[4] Inositol triphosphate then releases calcium from organelles within the cytoplasm. Calcium can also be released by cAMP. An increase in cytosolic calcium modifies transport proteins and related enzymes including protein kinases and calmodulin. The calcium-dependent regulator protein calmodulin was thought to play a key role in mediating active chloride secretion but recent studies suggest that it is only responsible for a brief burst of secretion.[14] The activation of protein kinase C by diacylglycerol, causing the enzyme to become bound to the membrane, induces a more sustained secretion which does not depend on increased cytosolic concentrations of calcium.[36] Finally, both diacylglycerol and increases in cytosolic calcium can induce secretion by stimulating the breakdown of arachidonic acid to prostaglandins.

Further information about the way in which chloride channels are regulated has come from studies of cystic fibrosis. In this inherited disease, chloride secretion in epithelia, including the intestine, fails to occur in response to stimulation, although normal chloride channels appear to be present. Recently the gene responsible for cystic fibrosis was identified,

and its gene product, cystic fibrosis transmembrane conductance regulator (CFTR),[47] could therefore be predicted. It is likely that CFTR plays an important role in the control of chloride channels, although its mode of operation and its interaction with intracellular second messengers remain to be elucidated.

The increased understanding of the biochemical transduction of intestinal secretion yields opportunities for the development of novel antisecretory drugs (*Figure 3.43*). The problem is that many organs use the same intracellular machinery to mediate other processes. Thus the probability of unwanted effects from such agents would be high.

EXTRACELLULAR MEDIATORS AND MODULATORS OF INTESTINAL TRANSPORT

A wide variety of chemical substances can modify intestinal transport.[8,15,16] They include neurotransmitters, hormones and normal constituents of intestinal contents as well as bacterial toxins and mediators of the inflammatory process and are listed in *Table 3.13*.

Table 3.13 Some of the factors that influence intestinal salt and water transport

Agents that increase intestinal absorption and inhibit secretion	Agents that decrease intestinal absorption and stimulate secretion

Nutrients
  Glucose
  Amino acids
  Peptides
  Volatile fatty acids (colon)
 	
Neurotransmitters or neuromodulators
  Neuropeptide Y
  Noradrenaline
  Dopamine
  Somatostatin
  Enkephalins
  Angiotensin
  Glucocorticoids
	Bacterial toxins
	  Cholera toxin
	  E. coli toxins
	
	Luminal contents
	  Bile acids
	  Long-chain fatty acids (colon)
	
	Neurotransmitters or neuromodulators
	  Acetylcholine
	  Prostaglandins
	  Leukotrienes
	  Serotonin
	  Histamine
	  Vasoactive intestinal polypeptide
	  Neurotensin
	  Cholecystokinin
	  Secretin
	  Glucagon
	  Bradykinin
	  Substance P
	  Free oxygen radicals
	  Platelet-activating factor
	  Bombesin
	  ATP

FACTORS THAT ENHANCE ABSORPTION AND INHIBIT SECRETION

The range of substances that stimulate absorption is far fewer than those which induce secretion. Luminal nutrients are the most important factors; they include hexose sugars, amino acids and oligopeptides in the small intestine and short-chain fatty acids in the colon.

Neuropeptide Y is said to be the major proabsorptive or antisecretory agent liberated by enteric nerve endings, but noradrenaline also acts on α_2 receptors on the cell membrane, reducing secretion from the crypts and unmasking sodium–hydrogen exchange in the villus. It is uncertain as to whether the action of noradrenaline on the enterocyte is mediated by a decrease in cAMP or a decrease in cell calcium or both. Noradrenaline also acts on receptors in the enteric nervous system to inhibit the release of acetylcholine (and possibly vasoactive intestinal polypeptide) from secretomotor nerve fibres. Enkephalins have a similar action on the enteric nervous system. Somatostatin is released from paracrine cells in the mucosa and inhibits secretion by a direct action on the enterocyte as well as by an indirect effect on the enteric nerves.

Hormones also have an important proabsorptive or antisecretory action. Angiotensin, formed in response to the release of renin from the kidney, promotes absorption of fluid and electrolytes in the gastrointestinal tract, but it probably acts by releasing catecholamines from the adrenal gland and sympathetic nerves. Aldosterone enhances salt and water absorption in the colon by increasing the sodium conductance of the mucosal membrane.[6,23] Glucocorticoids stimulate salt and water absorption in both small intestine and colon by increasing the activity of NA^+/K^+-dependent ATPase at the basolateral membrane.[6,23] Glucocorticoids are also antisecretory; they induce the synthesis of lipomodulin, an intracellular protein that inhibits the action of phospholipase A_2, suppressing the release of the eicosanoid precursor, arachidonic acid, from the cell membrane.[30] Eicosanoids are a large family of local transmitter substances that include prostaglandins and leukotrienes, both of which are potent secretagogues.

FACTORS THAT REDUCE ABSORPTION AND STIMULATE SECRETION

Intestinal secretion can be regarded as a defence mechanism. Fluid is secreted into the intestine

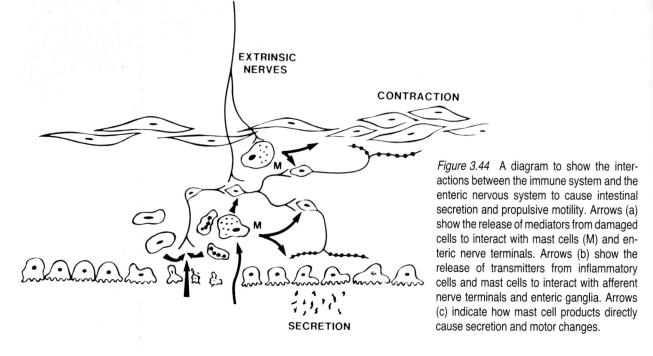

Figure 3.44 A diagram to show the interactions between the immune system and the enteric nervous system to cause intestinal secretion and propulsive motility. Arrows (a) show the release of mediators from damaged cells to interact with mast cells (M) and enteric nerve terminals. Arrows (b) show the release of transmitters from inflammatory cells and mast cells to interact with afferent nerve terminals and enteric ganglia. Arrows (c) indicate how mast cell products directly cause secretion and motor changes.

whenever the epithelium is damaged, irritated or invaded by foreign organisms or chemicals. An enormous range of substances can stimulate the intestine to secrete fluid.[8,15,16] They include bacterial toxins, neurotransmitters and paracrine substances released from leukocytes, lymphocytes, macrophages, mast cells, enteroendocrine cells and damaged enterocytes. Comparatively few of these act directly on enterocytes, most act via the enteric nervous system or inflammatory or immunoreactive cells (*Figure 3.44*).

Bacterial enterotoxins

Bacterial enterotoxins are perhaps the most widely studied cause of intestinal secretion. Cholera toxin combines with a glycoprotein on the cell membrane and induces a watery secretion after a few hours. A subunit of the toxin splits the membrane-bound G protein to release a fragment that is able to traverse the cell and activate adenylate cyclase.[19] Enterotoxic strains of *E. coli* liberate two main toxins. The heat-labile toxin of *E. coli* is thought to act in the same way as cholera toxin, while the heat-stable toxins of *E. coli* and *Klebsiella pneumoniae*, *Yersinia enterocolitica* and enterobacteriaceae induce secretion by activating guanylate cyclase.[43]

A major component of the secretion induced by enterotoxins may be mediated via a local nervous reflex since fluid output can be reduced substantially by treatment with tetrodotoxin, a neurotoxin produced by the puffer fish, or by ganglion blockers.

Furthermore, the observation that the hypersecretion induced by cholera toxin can also be blocked or severely inhibited by serotonin antagonists or tachyphylaxis[29] suggests that the toxins may act by binding to enteroendocrine cells in the epithelium. Enteroendocrine cells release a variety of substances, including neurotensin and serotonin.[8,15,16] Serotonin can induce secretion in several ways, by a direct action on the enterocyte, by interacting with specific receptors on afferent nerves to induce reflex secretion mediated by the release of acetylcholine and/or vasoactive intestinal polypeptide and by stimulating phagocytes to produce prostaglandins. Neurotensin interacts with receptors on the enteric nerves to release substance P, which functions as a secretory neurotransmitter and also causes degranulation of mast cells.

Damage to intestinal epithelium

Other microorganisms, such as viruses and shigella, may invade and damage the intestinal epithelium directly or indirectly via the release of cytotoxic agents. Diarrhoea is a consequence of many inflammatory disorders, and it seems likely that hypersecretion is an important component of the inflammatory reaction of the intestinal epithelium.[42] Most inflammatory mediators are intestinal secretogogues. Damage to the epithelial cells stimulate the metabolism of arachidonic acid, which is metabolized in this cell type by the cycloxygenase pathway to release prostaglandin E_2, which can induce copious intestinal secretion.

Secretagogues can also be released from inflammatory cells and immunocytes, and include histamine, serotonin, prostaglandins, leukotrienes, free oxygen radicals, platelet-activating factor, and kinins.[8,15,16] These substances act in a variety of ways.

Kinins[2,17] stimulate phospholipase A in cell membranes, releasing arachidonic acid to release eicosanoids. The route of arachidonic acid metabolism depends upon the cell type. Epithelial cells and cells in the lamina propria release cyclo-oxygenase products (prostacyclines, prostaglandins and thromboxanes), whereas white cells and mast cells release leukotrienes, the products of the lipoxygenase pathway. Prostaglandins can induce secretion via a direct action on the enterocyte or via an enteric nervous reflex.[29] Leukotrienes can also cause secretion but probably via the release of mast cell products.

The activity of white cells also releases reactive oxygen species (free radicals) which also cause secretion and degranulating mast cells by releasing prostaglandins from enterocytes.

Histamine acts via receptors on the enteric nervous system and on phagocytes. The observation that secretion induced by several of these mediators can be partially inhibited by neurotoxins or anticholinergic agents indicates that many may exert their effects via the enteric nervous system.[29] As a corollary to this, receptors to neuropeptides exist on the membranes of inflammatory cells, so the capacity for interaction between the nervous and immune systems is very large.

Immunological sensitization

Intestinal sensitization of the gut to specific antigens can result in intestinal hypersecretion when the gut is again exposed to that antigen. Sensitization can be induced in experimental animals by replacing drinking water with milk,[1] parasitic infestation,[49] by intraperitoneal injections[50] and by damaging the epithelium with bile acids, detergents and ultraviolet light.[1,50] The mediators of this effect differ in different species, but experiments using specific inhibitors have implicated histamine, serotonin, prostaglandins and tachykinins,[49] suggesting involvement of mast cells. Mast cells can be stimulated by substance P and adenosine as well as by specific combination of the antigen with immunoglobulin E antibodies. Proliferation of submucosal mast cells is a feature of food allergy,[33] coeliac disease,[52] parasitic infestations,[57] inflammatory bowel disease and, possibly, irritable bowel syndrome.[35] Degranulation liberates a cocktail of secretogogues. Mast cells tend to accumulate around enteric nerves[51] and form quite intimate connections with them. This suggests not only the possibility of degranulation of mast cells by activity in nerves, but also activation of enteric nervous system elements by degranulation of mast cells. It is possible that sensitization may occur in humans following an attack of gastroenteritis. This would offer one explanation for postgastroenteritis or food-related diarrhoea. Recent data suggests that responses to food antigens may be conditioned. Bienenstock[5] has shown that if a bell is rung every time food containing the antigen is administered then, after a time, the bell itself can induce degranulation of mast cells.

Nutrient malabsorption

The diarrhoea associated with impaired absorption of nutrients can have an important secretory component. This may be manifested in several ways. First, the atrophy of the villous epithelium in coeliac disease unmasks the background secretion. Second, secretion may be stimulated by the inflammatory or allergic process. Third, the entry of unabsorbed fat or bile acids into the colon stimulates colonic secretion, possibly due to the action of bacterially degraded derivative on enteroendocrine cells.[44] The secretion induced by bile acids and fatty acids has also been partially inhibited by neurotoxins, suggesting involvement of the enteric nervous system.[29]

Starvation-induced hypersecretion

Diarrhoea is a severe and often terminal complication of starvation or malnutrition. It is commonly thought to be related to vitamin deficiency or opportunist infection with enteric pathogens. However, there is new evidence to suggest that starvation may sensitize the epithelium to secretagogues. After rats have been starved for 3 days, the intestine secretes much more fluid and generates a much higher short-circuit current in response to a variety of secretagogues.[58-61] The observations that (1) the intestinal secretory mechanism may be sensitized by factors that act directly on the enterocyte and (2) hypersecretion occurs only in response to those transmitters that act by gating calcium and not in response to agents that act by increasing cyclic nucleotides suggest that this phenomenon is related to a change in cellular response to transmitters rather than an activation of enteric reflexes. Chronic food deprivation, caused by giving rats only 33% of their normal energy supplies, causes a much more prolonged hypersecretion than complete starvation.[58] Discovery of the factors that mediate this important adaptive response could help to prevent a major cause of morbidity and mortality in the developing world.

Neuroendocrine tumours

Copious amounts of secretion, resulting in severe watery diarrhoea, can result from the release of excessive amounts of transmitters from neuroendocrine tumours. Although such neuroendocrine tumours are all extremely rare, those secreting serotonin, vasoactive intestinal polypeptide and gastrin have been described in detail. Vasoactive intestinal peptide can be secreted by some islet cell tumours, by ganglioneuromas, phaeochromocytomas and bronchial carcinomas.[26] Calcitonin released in large amounts by medullary carcinoma of the thyroid is also an intestinal secretogogue. Malignant carcinoids can cause massive diarrhoea through the secretion of serotonin, bradykinin, substance P and prostaglandins.[9] The diarrhoea associated with gastrinomas is not due to the direct action of gastrin on the enterocyte; instead, it is probably explained by the effect of the low pH in the small intestine damaging the intestinal epithelium and inhibiting the digestion of fat.[56]

Irritable bowel syndrome

Patients with the irritable bowel syndrome often present with diarrhoea. Most of these have an increase in rectal sensitivity and motor reactivity of the gut in response to stimuli such as distension, food, stress and injections of cholecystokinin.[46] Most attention has been paid to motor phenomena in irritable bowel syndrome but it seems likely there is also a change in transport tone in the direction of secretion. Abundant secretion of colonic mucus is a classic feature of some patients with irritable bowel syndrome. Also, the secretory response of the ileum to the bile acid glycochenodeoxycholic acid has been shown to be enhanced in some patients with this syndrome.[37] This increased response might be related to release of prostaglandins.

Laxative agents

Copious secretion of fluid and electrolytes resulting in a severe watery diarrhoea can occur after administration of certain drugs, notably laxatives, but also some diuretics, caffeine, theophylline, gold salts and mefanamic acid. Laxative agents probably act on the intestinal epithelium to cause reflex secretion.[29] The other secretogogues are thought to activate the secretory mechanism directly.

ROLE OF MOTILITY

SMALL INTESTINAL MOTOR ACTIVITY

To write about intestinal transport without mentioning motility is to ignore one of the most important modulating factors. After ingestion of a meal, the motor activity of the small intestine is adapted to optimize the exposure of the meal to the small intestinal epithelium and digestive secretions so that maximal absorption can occur before the next meal is ingested.

Postprandial motor activity of the small intestine consists of repetitive and irregular contractions which propagate for very short distances downstream. Such contractions aid the digestive process by breaking up the solids and mixing complex food molecules with digestive juices. They also increase the contact between the products of digestion and the epithelial surface, while at the same time slowly propelling the chyme downstream to the terminal ileum.

At night and in between meals, the motor activity of the small intestine adopts a different motor pattern. This consists of recurrent phases of activity. A period of motor quiescence (phase I) is succeeded by a phase-intermittent contractile activity which may contain bursts of contractions propagated for quite long distances downstream (phase II) and finally by a brief phase of regular contractions (phase III), which only lasts for about 10 minutes and migrates slowly from duodenum to ileum. The whole cycle takes about 90 minutes and the recurrent phases of motor activity are probably associated with corresponding changes in transport tone. Phase III, for example, is associated with an increase in the potential difference across the epithelium that is most likely caused by a burst of intestinal secretion.

COLONIC MOTOR PATTERNS[45]

A quite different pattern of motor activity occurs in the colon. For most of the time this consists of ring-like contractions that divide the colon into compartments or haustra. These haustral contractions form and disappear to re-form in a different position. Occasionally they migrate slowly in an oral or aboral direction. The haustral pattern of colonic motility creates the stagnant conditions that are necessary for the growth of the vast populations of fermentative bacteria, and prolongs the residence of food residue so that there is sufficient time for the extraction of salt and water. Several studies have demonstrated an inverse relationship between colonic transit time and stool weight.

Haustral contractions are not the only motor pattern that the colon exhibits. After getting up from sleep in the morning, and occasionally after meals, the haustral contractions disappear as the colon narrows and a prolonged and powerful contraction propagates slowly from the region of the descending colon towards the rectum. Colonic giant migrating contractions are usually associated with defaecation.

Many of the factors that induce reflex secretion, such as laxatives, enterotoxins, sensitization and infection, are associated with patterns of motor activity than can be propagated over quite long distances and propel intestinal contents downstream at rapid rates.[45] In the small intestine, two manometric patterns have been described though it is possible that they may merge into each other. Discrete clusters of contractions are bursts of usually three or four contractions that occur at intervals of about a minute and appear to be propagated downstream. Giant migrating contractions (otherwise known as prolonged propagated contractions) are high-amplitude contractions of abnormally long duration that are propagated down the intestine at extremely rapid rates. Both of these phenomena are associated with increases in transepithelial potential difference, indicating the possibility of bursts of intestinal secretion.

Laxatives, bile acids and fatty acids increase the frequency of giant migrating contractions in the colon.[45] Inflammation of the colon, as in ulcerative colitis, is also associated with an increase in giant migrating contractions.

DIARRHOEA: AN ENTERIC NERVOUS DISORDER?

The observation that many of the factors that induce active intestinal secretion also cause propagated intestinal contractions suggest that both are components of a programme for clearing the intestine of its contents by promoting diarrhoea. Clearance would be more efficient if the intestinal contents were diluted in a large volume of fluid which is propelled through the intestine by powerful propagated contractions. Many of the factors known to produce propagation and hypersecretion are irritants or toxins, mediators of inflammatory or allergic responses. The motor as well as the secretory responses can be blocked by neurotoxins and ganglion blockers. Others are neurotransmitters. The concept of diarrhoea as an enteric nervous adaptation or disorder may even apply to diarrhoeas that are initiated by impaired absorption. Impaired absorption of bile acids and fatty acids and distension of the caecum caused, for example, by the entry of large volumes of secretions induce reflex colonic secretion and propulsion.

REFERENCES

1. Baird, A.W. and Cuthbert, A.W. (1987) Neuronal involvement in type 1 hypersensitivity reactions in gut epithelium. *British Journal of Pharmacology*, **92**, 647.
2. Baron, D.A., Miller, D.H. and Margolius, H.S. Kinins induce rat structural change in colon concomitant with chloride secretion. *Cell Tissue Research*, **246**, 589–594.
3. Barrowman, J. and Roberts, K.B. (1967) The role of the lymphatic system in the absorption of water from the small intestine of the rat. *Quarterly Journal of Experimental Physiology*, **52**, 19–30.
4. Berridge, M.J. (1984) Inositol triphosphate and diacylglycerol as second messenger. *Biochemical Journal*, **220**, 345–60.
5. Bienenstock, J. (1988) An update on mast cell heterogeneity including comments on mast cell nerve relationships. *Journal of Allergy and Clinical Immunology*, **81**, 763–769.
6. Binder, H.J. and Sandle, G.I. (1987) Electrolyte absorption and secretion in the mammalian colon. In: *Physiology of the Gastrointestinal Tract*, 2nd edn, Vol. 2, pp. 1389–1418 (Ed.) Johnson, L.R. New York: Raven Press.
7. Cedgard, S., Hallback, D.A., Jodal, M., Lundgren, O. and Redfors, S. (1978) The effects of cholera toxin in intramural blood flow distribution and capillary hydraulic conductivity in the cat small intestine. *Acta Physiologica Scandinavica*, **102**, 148–158.
8. Cooke, H.J. (1987) Neural and humoral regulation of small intestinal electrolyte transport. In: *Physiology of the Gastrointestinal Tract*, 2nd edn, pp. 1307–1350 (Ed.) Johnson, L.R. New York: Raven Press.
9. Creutzfeldt, W. and Stockmann, F. (1987) Carcinoids and carcinoid syndrome. *American Journal of Medicine*, **82**, 4–16.
10. Cristophe, J., Svoboda, M., Lambert, M. *et al.* (1986) Effector mechanisms of peptides of the VIP family. *Peptides*, **7** (suppl. 1), 101–107.
11. Cummings, J.H. (1981) Short chain fatty acids in the human colon. *Gut*, **22**, 763–799.
12. Davis, G.R., Santa Ana, C.A., Morawski, S.G. and Fordtran, J.S. (1982) Permeability characteristics of human jejunum, ileum proximal colon and distal colon: results of potential difference measurements and unidirectional fluxes. *Gastroenterology*, **83**, 844–850.
13. Debongnie, J.C. and Phillips, S.F. (1978) Capacity of the human colon to absorb fluid. *Gastroenterology*, **74**, 698–703.

14. Donowitz, M. and Welsh, M.J. (1987) Regulation of mammalian electrolyte secretion. In: *Physiology of the Gastrointestinal Tract*, 2nd edn, pp. 1351–1388 (Ed) Johnson, L.R. New York: Raven Press.

15. Field, M., Rao, M.C. and Chang, E.B. (1989) Intestinal electrolyte transport and diarrhoeal disease. *New England Journal of Medicine*, **321**, 800–806.

16. Field, M., Rao, M.C. and Chang, E.B. (1989) Intestinal electrolyte transport and diarrhoeal disease. *New England Journal of Medicine*, **321**, 879–882.

17. Gaginella, T.S. and Kachur, J.F. (1989) Kinins as mediators of intestinal secretion. *American Journal of Physiology*, **256**, G1–G15.

18. Ganapathy, V. and Leibach, F.E. (1985) Is intestinal peptide transport energised by a proton gradient? *American Journal of Physiology*, **249**, G153–G160.

19. Gill, D.M. and Woolkalis, M. (1985) Toxins which activate adenylate cyclase. *Ciba Foundation Symposium*, **112**, 57–73.

20. Greenwood, B. and Read, N.W. (1986) The effect of vagal stimulation of jejunal fluid transport, transmural potential difference and intraluminal pressure in the anaesthetised ferret. *American Journal of Physiology*, **12**, G651–654.

21. Hallback, D-A., Hulten, L., Jodal, M. *et al.* (1978) Evidence for the existence of a countercurrent exchanger in the small intestine of man. *Gastroenterology*, **74**, 683–690.

22. Hallback, D-A., Jodal, M., Sjoquist, A. and Lundgren, O. (1982) Evidence for cholera secretion eminating from the crypts. *Gastroenterology*, **83**, 1051–1056.

23. Halm, D.R. and Frizzell, R.A. (1992) Ion transport across the large intestine. In: *Handbook of Physiology – The gastrointestinal System* IV. *Absorptive and Secretory Processes of the Intestine*. (Eds) Field, M. and Frizzell, R.R. Bethesda: American Physiological Society.

24. Halm, D.R., Rechkemmer, G.R., Schoumacher, R.A. and Frizzell, R.A. (1988) Apical membrane chloride channels in a colonic cell line activated by secretory agonists. *American Journal of Physiology*, **254**, C505–C511.

25. Hopfer, U. (1987) Membrane transport mechanisms for hexoses and amino acids in the small intestine. In: *Physiology of the Gastrointestinal Tract*, 2nd edn, pp. 499–526 (Ed.) Johnson, L.R. New York: Raven Press.

26. Krejs, C.J. (1987) VIPoma syndrome. *American Journal of Medicine*, **82**, 37–48.

27. Liedtke, C.M. and Hopfer, U. (1982) Mechanism of Cl translocation across the intestinal brush border membrane. I. Absence of NaCl co-transport. *American Journal of Physiology*, **242**, G263–G271.

28. Loeschke, K., Bentzel, C.S. and Csaky, T.Z. (1970) Asymmetry of osmotic flow in the frog intestine, functional and structural correlation. *American Journal of Physiology*, **218**, 1723–1731.

29. Lundgren, O. (1988) Nervous control of intestinal transport. *Bailliéres Clinical Gastroenterology*, **2**, 85–106.

30. Lundgren, J.D., Hirata, F., Marom, Z. *et al.* (1988) Dexamethasone inhibits respiratory glycoconjugate secretion from feline airways in vitro by the induction of lipocortin (lipomodulin) synthesis. *American Review of Respiratory Diseases*, **137**, 353–7.

31. Madara, J.L. (1988) Loosening tight junctions: lessons from the intestine. *Journal of Clinical Function*, **83**, 1089–1099.

32. Madara, J.L. and Pappenheimer, J.R. (1987) Structural basis for physiological regulation of paracellular pathways in intestinal epithelia. *Journal of Membrane Biology*, **100**, 149–164.

33. Marshall, J., Prout, S.G., Jeffery, G. and Bell, E.B. (1987) Induction of an auto-IgE response in rats. Effects on mast cell population. *European Journal of Immunology*, 445–45.

34. McNeil, N.I., Cummings, J.H. and James, W.P.T. (1978) Short chain fatty acid absorption by the human large intestine. *Gut*, **19**, 819–822.

35. Miner, P.B. (1991) Systemic mastocytosis and regional gastrointestinal mast cell disease. In: *Irritable Bowel Syndrome* (Ed.) Read, N.W. Oxford: Blackwell, Oxford.

36. Nishizuka, Y. (1986) Studies and perspectives of protein kinase C. *Science*, **233**, 305–12.

37. Oddson, E., Rash-Madsen, J. and Krag, E. (1978) A secretory epithelium of the small intestine with increased sensitivity to bile acid in irritable bowel syndrome associated with diarrhoea. *Scandinavian Journal of Gastroenterology*, **13**, 409–416.

38. O'Grady, S.M., Palfrey, H.C. and Field, M. (1987) Characteristics and functions of Na–K–Cl co-transport in epithelial tissues. *American Journal of Physiology*, **253**, C177–C192.

39. Pappenheimer, J.S. (1987) Physiological regulation of transepithelial impedance in the intestinal mucosa of rats and hamsters. *Journal of Membrane Biology*, **100**, 128–148.

40. Pappenheimer, J.R. and Reizz, K.Z. (1987) Contribution of solvent drag through intracellular junctions to absorption of nutrients by small intestine of the rat. *Journal of Membrane Biology*, **100**, 123–127.

41. Powell, D.W. (1992) The immunophysiology of intestinal electrolyte transport. In: *Handbook of Physiology – The Gastrointestinal System. IV. Absorptive and Secretory Processes of the Intestine* (Eds) Field, M. and Frizzell, R.A. Bethesda: American Physiological Society.

42. Powell, D.W. (1987) Intestinal water and electrolyte transport in the small intestine. In: *Physiology of the Gastrointestinal Tract*, 2nd edn, Vol. 2, pp. 1267–1305 (Ed.) Johnson, L.R. New York: Raven Press.

43. Rao, M.C. (1985) Toxins which activate guanylate

cyclase: heat-stable enterotoxins. *Ciba Foun[...] Symposium*, **112**, 74–93.

44. Read, N.W. (1982) Diarrhoea: the failure o[...] salvage. *The Lancet*, **ii**, 481–483.

45. Read N.W. (1986) Diarrhee motrice. *Clinic[...] Gastroenterology*, **15**, 657–686.

46. Read, N.W. (1991) The neurotic bowel: a [...] for the irritable bowel. In: *The Irritable Bo[...] Syndrome* (Ed.) Read, N.W. Oxford: Blac[...]

47. Ringe, D. and Petsko, G.A. (1990) Cystic [...] A transport problem. *Nature*, **346**, 312–313[...]

48. Roediger, W.E.W. and Moore, A. (1981) [...] SCFA on sodium absorption in isolated hu[...] colon perfused through the vascular bed. *[...] Diseases and Sciences*, **26**, 100–106.

49. Russell, D.A. and Castro, G.A. (1987) Ph[...] of the Gastrointestinal Tract in the Parasit[...] In: *Physiology of the Gastrointestinal Trac[...] edn, Vol. 2, pp. 1749–1780 (Ed.) Johnson [...] New York: Raven Press.

50. Scott, R.B., Diamant, S.C. and Gall, D.[...] Motility effects of anaphylaxis in the rat. [...] *Journal of Physiology*, **13**, 255.

51. Stead, R.H., Tomioko, M., Quinonez, G[...] G.T., Melten, S.Y. and Bienenstock, J. (1987) Intestinal mucosal mast cells in normal and nematode infected rat intestines are in intimate contact with peptidergic nerves. *Proceedings of the National Academy of Sciences of the USA*, 2975–2979.

52. Strobel, S., Busuttil, A. and Ferguson, A. (1983) Human intestinal mucosal mast cells: expanded population in untreated coeliac disease. *Gut*, **24**, 222–227.

53. Tapper, E.J. (1983) Local modulation of intestinal ion transport by enteric neurones. *American Journal of Physiology*, **244**, G457–468.

model. Jejunal hypersecretion induced by starvation. *Gut*, **31**(1), 43–53.

60. Young, A. and Levin, R.J. (1990) Diarrhoea of famine and malnutrition: Investigations using a rat model 2. Ileal hypersecretion induced by starvation. *Gut*, **31**(2), 162–169.

61. Young, A., Pereira, M.M.C., Warren, M.A. and Levin, R.J. (1988) Hypersecretion associated with the action of *Escherichia coli* STC enterotoxin on jejunum and ileum from starved and chronically undernourished rats. *Medical Science Research*, **16**, 573–576.

MECHANISMS OF MALABSORPTION AND DIARRHOEA

V.S. Chadwick

DEFINITIONS

Malabsorption denotes a failure to absorb exogenous nutrients or substances such as drugs, or to reabsorb endogenous substances such as bile acids.

Diarrhoea may be defined as an increased frequency, fluidity or volume of bowel movements. In many instances, but not all, there is an increase in faecal water and electrolyte excretion with consequent increase in faecal weight. In other instances there is frequent passage of stools of normal consistency and weight, or of blood and pus (exudative diarrhoea).

Malabsorption frequently results in diarrhoea but not necessarily so. When malabsorption of nutrients occurs, nutritional deficiencies usually develop eventually.

PHYSIOLOGICAL CONSIDERATIONS

The normal handling of individual nutrients, fluid and electrolytes, and drugs by the intestinal tract is dealt with elsewhere in this chapter. The gut as a whole exhibits a homeostatic response to fluid and electrolyte depletion mediated by hormonal influ-

...ved
...trast,
...ption of
...omeostati-
...ce of obesity.
...ttle or no part
...n is regulated by
...the kidneys.
...he gut in homeostasis is
...acity to absorb exogenous
...nd to retrieve endogenously
...c acid, bicarbonate, bile salts,
...d water. For absorption or reab-
...s, electrolytes, fat, protein, carbo-
...bile salts the gut operates with about
...ciency. A fall in the efficiency or absorp-
...ne of these substances may or may not have
...diate clinical consequences in the form of diar-
...ea or longer-term consequences in the form of a
nutritional deficiency.

Under certain circumstances the gastrointestinal tract is stimulated to secrete greater than normal volumes of digestive secretions or fluids and electro-

lytes, and when inflamed secretes a protein-rich exudate.

Thus, in simple terms, malabsorption results from a failure to absorb intestinal luminal solute, whereas diarrhoea may result either from failure to absorb solute, from increased secretion of fluids and electrolytes, or from production of an inflammatory exudate (*Table 3.14*).

This section will discuss the clinical physiology of diarrhoea and malabsorption in these terms.

PATHOPHYSIOLOGY OF MALABSORPTION AND DIARRHOEA

Malabsorption may occur as a result of excess ingestion of poorly absorbed solute, or when there is a defect of an essential step in digestion, mucosal uptake, processing or export from enterocyte to blood or lymph of a substance normally well absorbed. In addition, malabsorption may occur in the absence of a specific defect when the exposure time to such mechanisms is markedly reduced by rapid transit (e.g. postvagotomy or diabetic autonomic neuropathy), inadequate mixing (e.g. gut resection), or as a consequence of the metabolic activity of bacteria when bacterial overgrowth occurs in the small bowel lumen. In any clinical malabsorptive state, a disorder at one or more of these stages can be defined.

In this section the clinical pathophysiology of malabsorption and diarrhoea will be discussed, using the loose classification referred to above. Although largely concerned with small intestinal mechanisms, the colon will be considered where relevant.

EXCESS INGESTION OF POORLY ABSORBED SOLUTE

Water absorption from the gut is passive and occurs in response to osmotic gradients. An increase in the luminal osmolality will therefore result in net fluid accumulation in the lumen and may cause diarrhoea.

Polyvalent ions such as magnesium, phosphate and sulphate are only slowly absorbed from normal intestine, as are certain disaccharides such as lactulose or sugar alcohols such as mannitol. Ingestion of substantial amounts of these results in osmotic retention of fluid within the gut lumen, manifest as increased faecal fluid output. Unlike the inorganic ions, poorly absorbed carbohydrates may be susceptible to bacterial degradation with generation of

---

Table 3.14 Mechanisms of diarrhoea in gastrointestinal disorders

Reduced fluid absorption
  Osmotic effects:
    Laxative ingestion
    Monosaccharide or disaccharide intolerance
    Congenital chloridorrhoea
  Mucosal defects:
    Intestinal resections and bypass
    Intestinal mucosal diseases
    Enteropathogenic microorganisms
  Motility effects:
    Irritable bowel syndrome
    Vagotomy and gastrectomy
    Autonomic neuropathy
    Drugs and hormones

Increase fluid secretion
  Bacterial toxins
  Hormones
  Prostaglandins
  Neurotransmitters
  Bile acids and fatty acids in the colon
  Laxatives
  Viral enteritis
  Coeliac disease
  Intestinal obstruction
  Immunosensitization

Exudative diarrhoea
  Rectal carcinoma
  Villous adenoma
  Colitis

osmotically active low molecular weight fatty acids such as acetate, butyrate, propionate and lactate. Colonic mechanisms for reabsorption of small fatty acids exist,[40] so that diarrhoea will occur only if these mechanisms are stressed. The metabolic activity of gut bacteria may adapt to constant ingestion of organic anions such as tartrate (metabolized to bicarbonate),[7] so that initial purgation following ingestion may be replaced by entirely normal stool outputs. Similar mechanisms operate when defects in digestion and absorption of 'absorbable' carbohydrates such as lactose and sucrose occur (see later).

FAILURE OF DIGESTION

Fat

Conditions associated with defective lipolysis are shown in *Table 3.15*. Pancreatic lipase outputs must be below 10% of normal before steatorrhoea results[12] and complete failure of pancreatic secretion results in massive fat malabsorption, with faecal fat levels of 50–100 g/day. This is only seen with end-stage chronic pancreatitis, pancreatic atrophy, fibrocystic disease, complete duct obstruction by carcinoma, or after total pancreatectomy.

Functional pancreatic exocrine deficiency due to failure of cholecystokinin release (e.g. in coeliac disease) is probably not clinically significant because cephalic stimulation via vagal efferents may produce up to 50% of maximal pancreatic secretory responses. After vagotomy, cholecystokinin-mediated pancreatic secretion may be more important, and this may account for the occasional presentation of coeliac disease following vagotomy, when failure of cholecystokinin secretion results in functional pancreatic insufficiency and fat malabsorption.

Steatorrhoea in bile acid deficiency (e.g. total obstructive jaundice) is modest (10–15 g/day) although there is no micellar phase, suggesting that non-micellar lipid is reasonably well absorbed when the small intestine is healthy and complete. After substantial ileal resection (more than 100 cm) the combination of intraluminal bile salt deficiency and loss of the intestinal surface area results in steatorrhoea, which increases with the length of resected gut.[22] Loss of the gut surface area alone (e.g. after jejunal resection) does not result in steatorrhoea, so that, although pancreatic lipase, bile salts and healthy gut mucosa are all requirements for efficient fat absorption, substantial reserve capacity exists for partial failure of any of these components. Failure of two of these components, such as in severe coeliac disease where there is an extensive mucosal abnormality and a failure of gallbladder contraction after meals with poor bile salt delivery to the duodenum, frequently results in fat malabsorption. Luminal precipitation or destruction of bile acids by acid hypersecretion in the Zollinger–Ellison syndrome[20] or by bacterial deconjugation in bacterial overgrowth syndrome[24] is usually accompanied by deleterious effects of acid and bacterial toxins on gut mucosal function, again explaining the frequency and severity of steatorrhoea in these conditions. The absorption of fat-soluble vitamins may be more critically dependent on micellar solubilization than is absorption of triglycerides themselves, which may explain the frequency of vitamin D deficiency after gastric surgery and in cholestatic liver disease.

Protein and carbohydrate

Large polypeptides and polysaccharides are not absorbed well when pancreatic exocrine outputs are below 10% of normal. However, in contrast to fat, their independence from other intraluminal phases of digestion means that in many conditions malabsorption is less evident than for fat. However, the final stage of peptide and disaccharide digestion is at the mucosal brush border, so that either congenital or acquired deficiencies of the brush border enzymes may result in malabsorption. In practice, peptidase deficiency is never clinically important.

Monosaccharide or disaccharide malabsorption due to transport or digestive defects is usually associated with diarrhoea. Fifty grams of unabsorbed disaccharide results in osmotic retention of some 500 ml of water in the small intestine in order to preserve

Table 3.15 Conditions causing defective lipolysis

Failure of emulsification and mixing problems
    Gastric surgery
    Duodenal bypass

Reduced duodenal pH
    Gastrinoma

Impaired cholecystokinin response
    Coeliac disease

Pancreatic lipase deficiency
    Chronic pancreatitis
    Pancreatic cancer
    Congenital lipase deficiency

Luminal bile salt deficiency
    Cholestasis
    Acid hypersecretion
    Drug (neomycin and cholestyramine)
    Ileal resection and disease

isotonicity, and osmotic activity is further increased by the bacterial metabolism of the malabsorbed carbohydrate to short-chain fatty acids, with production of gas (carbon dioxide and hydrogen) in the colon.

Since the normal intestine has a finite capacity to digest and absorb carbohydrate, large loads of hypertonic sugars in the form of proprietary mixtures or elemental diets may provoke nausea, due to fluid distension of the small bowel, and osmotic diarrhoea. The non-fattening sweetener sorbitol may often explain severe symptoms. Any condition which speeds up gastric emptying, shortens the gut transit time or reduces the functional surface area of intestine will impair tolerance to such mixtures.

FAILURE OF MUCOSAL UPTAKE AND INTRACELLULAR PROCESSING

Enterocyte damage

Prior to uptake across the microvillous membrane of the enterocyte, hydrophobic lipid molecules must cross the unstirred water layer. This process is greatly facilitated by incorporation of the lipid products of digestion in the micellar complex.[45] Thereafter, uptake of lipid is passive and depends on its solubility in the lipid components of the cell membrane. A sequence of intracellular events occurs, involving binding to a fatty acid-binding protein, resynthesis to triglyceride on the smooth endoplasmic reticulum, and the addition of apoproteins to form chylomicrons on the rough endoplasmic reticulum; these processes require normal structure and function of the enterocytes.[38] In coeliac disease and tropical sprue, enterocytes are obviously abnormal but their capacity for triglyceride resynthesis and apoprotein synthesis has not been evaluated. In these conditions and others (e.g. viral enteritis), there is an increased crypt cell production rate in response to increased villous cell loss or damage, and the enterocytes populating the villous are relatively immature. It seems likely, as has been demonstrated for salt and water transport,[19] that these cells will not have acquired the full biochemical apparatus for processing lipid. In abetalipoproteinaemia, defective apoprotein B synthesis results in accumulation of lipid within the enterocytes.[29] In coeliac disease this is not seen; it may be that mucosal uptake is more defective than intracellular processing in this and similar conditions. In contrast, where enterocyte morphology is well preserved as in bacterial overgrowth syndromes, a specific defect of triglyceride resynthesis in enterocytes has been postulated.

Enterocyte damage may have marked effects on the uptake and processing of minerals and vitamins, some of which in turn may further reduce enterocyte function.[30] For example, folic acid absorption is diminished by alkalinization of the gut lumen, and it is believed that loss of the acid microclimate adjacent to the brush border reported in coeliac disease and Crohn's disease may have marked effects on folate uptake by the enterocytes.[31] Folate deficiency itself may secondarily impair mucosal structure and function, and many patients with tropical sprue show improvement in jejunal morphology and function following folate administration.[26]

Enterocyte deficits

Congenital absence of specific transport mechanisms for glucose–galactose, various amino acids, folate and vitamin B_{12} have been reported.

Primary defects of electrolyte transport are rare; in congenital chloridorrhoea[44] the ileal and colonic chloride/bicarbonate exchange process is absent and the failure of chloride reabsorption results in osmotic diarrhoea and hypochloraemic alkalosis.

Bowel resection

Bowel resection is one of the more obvious causes of deficient mucosal uptake, and the consequences depend on the extent and region of resection, the state of the residual gut, the presence of adaptive changes in the residual gut and the diet presented to the intestine.[16] Jejunal resection does not result in diarrhoea because the ileum shows marked adaptive hyperplasia and the preservation of the ileal bile salt reabsorptive site maintains the enterohepatic circulation of bile salts. The ability to cope with normal intakes of fat, protein and carbohydrate is preserved. In contrast, ileal resection is frequently complicated by diarrhoea as a result of bile salt malabsorption (see later) and, when more than 100 cm has been removed, by fat malabsorption (see earlier). After total colonic resection, ileostomy outputs reach 800–1000 ml but malabsorption of nutrients is not evident. Smaller colonic resections lead to diarrhoea which is related to the extent of resection and usually diminishes with time due to adaptive mechanisms. In the so-called 'short bowel syndrome' diarrhoea is multifactorial in causation, but the main factors are a reduced capacity to digest and absorb dietary nutrients and a marked sensitivity to luminal osmotic loads.[21]

Enteropathogens

Mucosal abnormalities are important in diarrhoea produced by invasive enteropathogenic microorganisms. Gastroenteritis due to *Salmonella typhimurium* and other species is associated with inflammatory ileitis and colitis and *Shigella dysenteriae* and other species invade the colonic epithelium. Both organisms produce a variety of enterotoxins[23,27] which may be released intraluminally or intracellularly. *Campylobacter jejuni*,[39] *Yersinia enterocolitica*[35] and enteroinvasive *Escherichia coli* also induce mucosal inflammation and release enterotoxins. *Clostridium difficile* produces a cytotoxin which leads to colonic injury with typical inflammatory pseudomembranous characteristics of antibiotic-associated colitis.[28]

Enteropathogenic viruses (e.g. coronavirus and rotavirus) invade small intestinal epithelial cells,[11] resulting in loss of villous height and impairment of absorptive function normally mediated by healthy villous enterocytes. Surviving crypt cells lack a glucose-stimulated sodium transport mechanism and the intestine is in a net secretory state.

FAILURE OF EXPORTATION TO LYMPH OR PORTAL BLOOD

Lymphatic abnormalities

The major effects of congenital or acquired abnormalities of lymphatic drainage from the intestine is in impairing absorption of long-chain fats. In these conditions[13] (primary and secondary lymphangiectasia), chylomicrons accumulate in dilated lymph channels clearly visible in the villous core. Rupture of dilated lymphatics into the bowel lumen results in loss of absorbed lipid and apoproteins, and the other constituents of intestinal lymph (i.e. plasma proteins, immunoglobulins and lymphocytes). The magnitude of fat malabsorption and secondary protein and cell loss is dependent on the amount of ingested long-chain triglycerides and the extent of the lymphatic abnormality.

Infiltrations in the laminia propria

Dense cellular infiltration in the lamina propria occurs in α-chain disease,[3] other types of intestinal lymphoma, and Whipple's disease.[25] In each case the villi may be effaced or grossly distended and misshapen by the accumulation of plasma cells, lymphocytes or periodic acid–Schiff-positive macrophages. While the enterocytes are often morphologically normal, gross fat malabsorption is often seen in these conditions. Secondary lymphatic blockage is likely because gut losses of protein are also great in these conditions.

Table 3.16 Enterotoxin-producing bacteria which lead to intestinal secretion

Vibrio cholerae
Escherichia coli
Shigella dysenteriae, Shigella flexneri
Salmonella enteritidis
Staphylococcus aureus
Clostridium perfringens (welchii)
Clostridium difficile
Pseudomonas aeruginosa
Yersinia enterocolitica
Bacillus cereus
Klebsiella pneumoniae
Aeromonas hydrophila

DIARRHOEA DUE TO INCREASED SECRETION

Table 3.15 summarizes the causes of enhanced intestinal secretion. The individual items are discussed elsewhere. Often, secretion is only one part of the abnormal process leading to diarrhoea. Thus, amongst the bacterial species causing diarrhoea by elaboration of an enterotoxin which is a secretagogue (*Table 3.16*) are a number of bacteria which also cause invasive damage.

Other examples of complex mechanisms of diarrhoea including a component of enhanced secretion are discussed below.

Bile salts and fatty acids

Dihydroxy bile acids and hydroxylated fatty acids[18] are potent stimuli for fluid and electrolyte secretion in the colon. Bile acid malabsorption, or steatorrhoea, will lead to their presence in the colon in unphysiologically high amounts. Both these agents cause mucosal damage and stimulate mucus secretion at concentrations or exposure times less than those required to stimulate fluid secretion.[5] Since the detergent damage markedly increases mucosal permeability to ions,[6] it has been suggested that secretion occurs as a consequence of this altered permeability under the driving force of capillary hydrostatic pressure. Others have demonstrated increased mucosal cAMP levels.[9] The relative importance of these proposed mechanisms is controversial.

Detergent laxatives

Ricinoleic acid (castor oil), a hydroxy fatty acid, and dioctyl sodium sulphosuccinate, a non-ionic detergent, have similar effects to bile acids and fatty acids on colonic morphology and function, and are believed to stimulate secretion by similar pathways.[4]

Immature enterocytes and secretion

A substantial amount of evidence suggests that immature crypt cells differ functionally from mature villous cells, particularly in relation to sodium transport.[19] These observations suggest that intestinal fluid and electrolyte secretion predominates in crypt cells, while absorption predominates in villous cells. In conditions such as coeliac disease, tropical sprue, viral enteritis and a variety of other disorders, villous cells are lost or damaged and the crypts show hyperplasia. The mucosa is thus populated by relatively immature cells with a propensity to secrete fluid and electrolytes. Perfusion studies in conditions associated with villous damage and crypt hyperplasia have shown a net secretion and an absence of glucose stimulation of sodium and water absorption, which is consistent with this hypothesis.

Hormones and neurotransmitters

A variety of hormones and neurotransmitters stimulate intestinal secretion.

Vasoactive intestinal polypeptide is a powerful secretogogue in animal and human small intestine. Pancreatic apudomas or ganglioneuromas which secrete vasoactive intestinal polypeptide cause severe watery diarrhoea and hypokalaemia. The secretory effect is predominantly on the small intestine, and fasting ileal flow rates exceeding the colonic reabsorptive capacity have been recorded.[32] *Calcitonin* is secreted by medullary thyroid carcinomas and promotes small intestinal secretion and decreases intestinal transit time.[10,34] Diarrhoea evident during fasting is markedly increased during feeding, possibly due to fat, carbohydrate and bile acid malabsorption. A similar pattern of secretory and motor responses is seen in the carcinoid syndrome, where *5-hydroxytryptamine (serotonin)* is the most important secretagogue.[15]

Prostaglandins

Prostaglandins are a family of fatty acids which are generated by the cyclo-oxygenase pathway from arachidonic acid, a constituent of mucosal phospholipids. Some of them (E_2, $F_{2\alpha}$) are potent activators of adenylate cyclase in the gut, leading to cAMP production. These prostaglandins are powerful secretagogues at all levels in the gut. Based on findings of elevated prostaglandins in gut luminal fluid in a variety of conditions[36] such as inflammatory bowel disease, small bowel obstruction, coeliac disease, carcinoid syndrome, and irritable bowel syndrome,[1] and reports of the beneficial effects of prostaglandin synthesis inhibitors in some of these conditions, a role for prostaglandins in some of these diarrhoeal disorders has been proposed.

EXUDATIVE DIARRHOEA

Exudation of proteins, mucus or pus from inflammatory sites, ulcers or villous tumours may cause diarrhoea. Prostaglandins have been implicated in diarrhoea associated with ulcerative colitis[41] and villous adenomas.[42]

SMALL BOWEL BACTERIAL OVERGROWTH (an example of composite mechanisms)

The presence of bacterial overgrowth in the small intestine is usually suspected on the basis of a defined anatomical abnormality such as stricture, fistula, diverticulosis or a blind loop. Malabsorption of fat, protein, carbohydrate and vitamins may be profound, and yet the mucosal architecture of the small intestine shows little abnormality, with nearly normal brush borders and enterocytes and minimal cellular infiltration of the lamina propria.[2] However, the enterocytes may be functionally abnormal with swollen mitochondria and lipid accumulation suggesting defective intracellular processing.[14] Deconjugation of luminal bile salts reduces micellar solubilization of lipid, and 'free' bile salts may damage the enterocytes or reduce the function of the brush border disaccharidases and peptidases.

Luminal metabolism of proteins and carbohydrates by bacteria reduces the availability of these substrates. Bacterial generation of low molecular weight fatty acids, hydroxylated long-chain fatty acids and deconjugated bile acids are thought to account for defective salt and water absorption in the small intestine and secretion of fluid and electrolytes into the colon; these effects probably account for the diarrhoea seen in the condition.

Thus, the malabsorption and diarrhoea seen in small bowel bacterial overgrowth is due to a complex combination of enterocyte abnormality and the presence of osmotically active solutes and secretogogues in the lumen.

THE ROLE OF MOTILITY

For intestinal absorption to occur with the maximal possible efficiency, the intestinal contents must be exposed to the absorptive surface area for a critical time period; exposure time is obviously dependent on the small gut transit time.[37] Furthermore, the contents must be adequately mixed with the digestive secretions. Transit time and mixing are dependent on coordinated small gut motility, an area of intestinal physiology which is still in its infancy. Various causes of disordered small bowel motility and transit time have been described and include thyrotoxicosis, medullary carcinoma of the thyroid, carcinoid syndrome, autonomic neuropathy (e.g. diabetic), postvagotomy diarrhoea, and systemic sclerosis. Malabsorption of nutrients, such as fat and carbohydrate, and of bile salts has been described in these disorders but other diarrhoeagenic factors such as bacterial overgrowth (in diabetes and systemic sclerosis) and intestinal fluid and electrolyte secretion (in medullary carcinoma of the thyroid and carcinoid syndrome) may be as important as the altered exposure time for digestion and absorption.

In the colon the role of altered motility is also not well defined. The irritable bowel syndrome in some patients is associated with abnormal motility patterns which appear to be especially sensitive to luminal deoxycholate (a secondary bile acid).[17] Other factors such as ileal secretion in response to bile acids,[33] prostaglandin generation, and food intolerance[1] have also been implicated in the genesis of diarrhoea in this heterogeneous condition. Laxative drugs such as bisacodyl and ricinoleic acid produce marked changes in colonic motility,[43] but are also secretagogues.[18] Evidence is emerging that motility and secretion are to some extent coupled processes in the normal intestine and defining the primary mechanisms for diarrhoea in pathological states may be difficult.

CONCLUSIONS

Mechanisms of malabsorption and diarrhoea are very diverse. In recent years, the major advances have been in our understanding of the intracellular mediators and pathways involved in intestinal secretion. It seems likely that specific pharmacological blockade of these processes will soon be possible.

REFERENCES

1. Alun Jones, V., Shorthouse, M., McLaughlan, P. *et al.* (1982) Food intolerance: a major factor in the pathogenesis of irritable bowel syndrome. *The Lancet*, **ii**, 1115–1117.
2. Ament, M.F., Shimoda, S.S. and Sanders, D.P. (1972) Pathogenesis of steatorrhoea in three cases of small intestinal stasis syndrome. *Gastroenterology*, **63**, 728–747.
3. Asselah, C.H. and Asselah, F. (1982) Alpha chain disease and intestinal lymphoma. In: *Gastroenterology 2: Small Intestine*, pp. 174–202 (Eds) Chadwick V.S. and Phillips, S. London: Butterworth.
4. Binder, H.J. (1977) Pharmacology of laxatives. *Annual Review of Pharmacology and Toxicology*, **17**, 355–367.
5. Camilleri, M., Murphy, R. and Chadwick, V.S. (1981) Dose-related effects of chenodeoxycholic acid in the rabbit colon. *Digestive Diseases and Science*, **25**, 433–438.
6. Chadwick, V.S., Phillips, S.F. and Hoffman, A.F. (1977) Measurement of intestinal permeability using low molecular weight polyethylene glycols (PEG 400). II. Application to normal and abnormal permeability states in man and animals. *Gastroenterology*, **73**, 247–251.
7. Chadwick, V.S., Vince, A., Killingley, M. and Wrong, O.M. (1978) The metabolism of tartrate in man and the rat. *Clinical Science and Molecular Medicine*, **54**, 273–281.
8. Charney, A.N., Kinsey, M.D., Myers, L. *et al.* (1975) Na^+/K^+ activated adenosine triphosphatase and intestinal electrolyte transport. Effect of adrenal steroids. *Journal of Clinical Investigation*, **56**, 653–660.
9. Conley, D.R., Coyne, M.J. and Bonorris, G.G. (1976) Bile acid stimulation of colonic adenylate cyclase and secretion in the rabbit. *American Journal of Digestive Diseases*, **21**, 453–458.
10. Cox, T.M., Fagan, E.A., Hillyard, C.J. *et al.* (1979) Role of calcitonin in diarrhoea associated with medullary carcinoma of the thyroid. *Gut*, **20**, 629–633.
11. Davidson, G.P., Gall, D.G., Petric, M., Butler, D.G. and Hamilton, J.R. (1977) Human rotavirus enteritis induced in conventional piglets. *Journal of Clinical Investigation*, **60**, 1402–1409.
12. Di Magno, E.P., Go, V.L.W. and Summerskill, W.H.J. (1973) Relations between pancreatic enzyme outputs and malabsorption in severe pancreatic insufficiency. *New England Journal of Medicine*, **228**, 813–815.
13. Dobbins, W.O. (1976) Electron microscopic study of the intestinal mucosa in intestinal lymphangiectasia. *Gastroenterology*, **51**, 1004–1017.
14. Donaldson, R.M. (1965) Studies on the pathogenesis of steatorrhoea in the blind loop syndrome. *Journal of Clinical Investigation*, **44**, 1815–1825.
15. Donowitz, M. and Binder, H.J. (1975) Jejunal fluid and electrolyte secretion in carcinoid syndrome. *American Journal of Digestive Diseases*, **20**, 1115–1122.
16. Dowling, R.H. (1982) Intestinal adaptation and its mechanisms. In: *Topics in Gastroenterology*, Vol. 10, pp. 135–156 (Eds) Jewell, D.P. and Selby, W.S. Oxford: Blackwell.
17. Flynn, M., Hammond, P., Darby, C. *et al.* (1979) Faecal bile acids and the irritable colon syndrome. *Gut*, **20**, A946.
18. Gaginella, T.S., Chadwick, V.S., Debongnie, J.C.

et al. (1977) Perfusion of rabbit colon with ricinoleic acid: dose-related mucosal injury, fluid secretion, and increased permeability. *Gastroenterology*, **73**, 95–101.

19. Gall, G. D., Chapman, D., Kelly, M. and Hamilton, J.R. (1977) Na^+ transport in jejunal crypt cells. *Gastroenterology*, **72**, 452–456.

20. Go, V.L.W., Poley, J.R., Hoffmann, A.F. and Summerskill, W.H.J. (1970) Disturbance in fat digestion induced by acidic jejunal pH due to gastric hypersecretion in man. *Gastroenterology*, **58**, 638–646.

21. Griffin, G.E., Fagan, E.A., Hodgson, H.J.F. and Chadwick, V.S. (1982) Enteral therapy in the management of massive gut resection complicated by chronic fluid and electrolyte depletion. *Digestive Diseases and Sciences*, **27**, 202–208.

22. Hofmann, A.F. and Poley, J.R. (1972) Role of bile acid malabsorption in pathogenesis of diarrhoea and steatorrhoea in patients with ileal resection. *Gastroenterology*, **62**, 918–934.

23. Keusch, G.T, Grady, G.F., Mata, L.J. and McIver, J. (1972) The pathogenesis of shigella diarrhoea I. Enterotoxin production by *Shigella dysenteriae* I. *Journal of Clinical Investigation*, **51**, 1212–1218.

24. Kim, Y.S., Spritz, N. and Blum, M. (1966) The role of altered bile acid metabolism in the steatorrhoea of experimental blind loop syndrome. *Journal of Clinical Investigation*, **45**, 956–962.

25. Kirkpatrick, P.M. Jr, Kent, S.P., Mihas, A. and Pritchett, P. (1978) Whipple's disease: a case report with immunological studies. *Gastroenterology*, **75**, 297–301.

26. Klipstein, F.lA. and Falaiye, J.M. (1969) Tropical sprue in expatriates from the tropics living in the continental United States. *Medicine*, **48**, 475–491.

27. Koupal, L.R. and Deibel, R.H. (1975) Assay, characterization and localization of an enterotoxin produced by *Salmonella*. *Infection and Immunity*, **11**, 14–22.

28. Larson, H.E., Price, A.B., Honour, P. and Borriello, S.P. (1978) *Clostridium difficile* and the aetiology of pseudomembranous colitis. *The Lancet*, **i**, 1063–1066.

29. Levy, R.I., Fredrickson, D.S. and Laster, L. (1966) The lipoproteins and lipid transport in abetalipoproteinaemia. *Journal of Clinical Investigation* **45**, 531–541.

30. Lindenbaum, J., Pezzimenti, J.F. and Shea, N. (1974) Small intestinal function in vitamin B_{12} deficiency. *Annals of Internal Medicine*, **80**, 326–331.

31. Lucas, M.L., Cooper, B.T. and Lei, F.H. (1978) Acid microclimate in coeliac and Crohn's disease: a model for folate malabsorption. *Gut*, **19**, 735–742.

32. Modigliani, R., Rambaud, J.C., Matuchansky, C. and Bernier, J.J. (1979) Hormones, intestinal secretion and diarrhoea: human studies. In: *Frontiers of Knowledge in the Diarrhoeal Diseases*, pp. 289–302 (Eds) Janowitz H.J. and Sachar, D.B. Raritan: Ortho Pharmaceutical Co.

33. Oddson, E., Rask-Madsen, J. and Rask-Madsen, J. (1978) A secretory epithelium of the small intestine with increased sensitivity to bile acids in irritable bowel syndrome associated with diarrhoea. *Scandinavian Journal of Gastroenterology*, **13**, 408–416.

34. Rambaud, J.C., Modigliani, R. and Matuchansky, C. (1981) Hormones and diarrhoea. *Clinical Research Reviews*, **1**(suppl. 1), 23–32.

35. Rao, M.C., Guandalini, S., Laird, W.J. and Field, M. (1979) Effects of heat-stable enterotoxin of *Yersinia enterocolitica* on ion-transport and cyclic guanosine-monophosphate metabolism in rabbit ileum. *Infection and Immunity*, **26**, 875–878.

36. Rask-Madsen, J. and Bukhave, K. (1981) The role of prostaglandins in diarrhoea. *Clinical Research Reviews*, **1**(suppl. 1), 33–48.

37. Read, N.W. (1981) The relationship between intestinal motility and intestinal transport. *Clinical Research Reviews*, **1**(suppl. 1), 73–81.

38. Riley, J.W. and Glickman, R.M. (1979) Fat malabsorption: advances in our understanding. *American Journal of Medicine*, **67**, 980–987.

39. Ruiz-Palacios, G.M., Torres, J., Torres, N.I., Escamilla, E., Ruiz-Palacios, B.R. and Tamayo, J. (1983) Cholera-like enterotoxin produced by *Campylobacter jejuni*. Characterisation and clinical significance. *The Lancet*, **ii**, 250–253.

40. Ruppin, H., Bar-Meir, S., Soergel, K.H. et al. (1980) Absorption of short-chain fatty acids by the colon. *Gastroenterology*, **78**, 1500–1507.

41. Sharon, P., Ligumsky, M., Rachmilewitz, D. and Zor, U. (1978) Role of prostaglandins in ulcerative colitis: enhanced production during active disease and inhibition by sulfasalazine. *Gastroenterology*, **75**, 638–640.

42. Steven, K., Lange, P., Bukhave, K. and Rask-Madsen, J. (1981) Diarrhoea in villous adenoma of rectum: effect of treatment with indomethacin. *Gastroenterology*, **80**, 1562–1566.

43. Steward, J.J., Gaginella, T.S. and Bass, P. (1975) Actions of ricinoleic acid and structurally related fatty acids on the gastrointestinal tract. I. Effects on smooth muscle contractility *in vitro*. *Journal of Pharmacology and Experimental Therapeutics*, **195**, 347–354.

44. Turnberg, L.A. (1978) Intestinal transport of salt and water. *Clinical Science and Molecular Medicine*, **54**, 337–348.

45. Wilson, F.A., Sallee, V.L. and Dietschy, J.M. (1971) Unstirred water layers in the intestine: rate determinant of fatty acid absorption from micellar solutions. *Science*, **174**, 1031–1033.

CLINICAL INVESTIGATION OF PATIENTS WITH MALABSORPTION AND DIARRHOEA

V.S. Chadwick

There are many different causes of diarrhoea and malabsorption (*Table 3.17*) and an even larger number of diagnostic tests and procedures available to the clinician. If the full spectrum of investigations were applied to every patient the cost would be enormous. Several investigators have attempted to devise algorithms based on a logical sequence of investigations with appropriate branch points so that, by following the diagnostic route map, successful diagnosis is assured. Others, including the author, have little faith in such systems and prefer a much more selective approach in which the primary aim is to define the anatomical location of the disease, its histological features and the agent or process responsible for the lesion.

A number of disorders producing diarrhoea are associated with normal intestinal anatomy, and a variety of tests are available to sort these problems out. The selection of appropriate radiological, endoscopic and biopsy procedures is based on the results of clinical history, physical examination, and stool, urine and blood tests. There is much debate about the role of intestinal function tests. They are rarely diagnostic and are usually not first-line investi-

Table 3.17   Causes of diarrhoea and malabsorption

Gastric causes	**Small intestinal causes** (*cont.*)
Resection	Amyloidosis
Gastroenterostomy	Visceral myopathy
Vagotomy	Autonomic neuropathy
Gastrinoma	Ulcerative ileojejunitis
Gastroenteric fistula	Immunodeficiency (including AIDS)
	Graft versus host disease
Pancreatic causes	Fistula
Resection	
Chronic pancreatitis	**Colonic causes**
Carcinoma	Resection or bypass
Cystic fibrosis	Infectious agents
Hypoplasia (Schwachman's syndrome)	Ulcerative colitis
Congenital enzyme defects	Microscopic colitis
	Collagenous colitis
Hepatic causes	Crohn's disease
Cholestatic liver disease	Radiation enteritis
Cholecystocolonic fistula	Immunodeficiency (including AIDS)
	Purgative ingestion
Small intestinal causes	Irritable bowel syndrome
Resection or bypass	Diverticular disease
Infections and infestations	Carcinoma
Bacterial overgrowth	Villous adenoma
Tropical sprue	Bile acid malabsorption
Coeliac disease	Unabsorbed fat in colon
Crohn's disease	Graft versus host disease
Eosinophilic enteritis	Fistula
Radiation enteritis	
Whipple's disease	**Extraintestinal causes**
Vasculitis	Hormones
Vascular insufficiency	Prostaglandins
Lymphoma	Serotonin
Lymphangiectasia	Histamine
Abetalipoproteinaemia	Diabetes
Drugs, alcohol	Addisons disease
Systemic sclerosis	Mastocytosis

AIDS, acquired immune deficiency syndrome.

gations in patients with diarrhoea, although tests for fat, vitamin B_{12} malabsorption, lactose intolerance and pancreatic insufficiency are helpful in certain circumstances. A wider spectrum of function tests may be useful in the assessment of patients with gut resections and in monitoring the effects of therapeutic manoeuvres in more complicated cases.

ACUTE DIARRHOEA

The symptom complex of anorexia, nausea, vomiting, abdominal pain, and diarrhoea of sudden onset, often occurring within families or other groups, is loosely termed gastroenteritis. A variety of viruses, bacteria, protozoa or their toxic products may be implicated.[6] These disorders are commonly (though not always) short lived and self-limiting, and the only problem is guarding against significant dehydration.

A specific diagnosis should be sought when there is a 'point' source for the outbreak, when it occurs in a nursery or geriatric unit, or when there is a marked fever and rectal bleeding. Faecal microscopy and culture, sigmoidoscopy and biopsy, and the taking of blood for serological tests is then advisable. Suspect food, milk or water supplies may need to be investigated. Diarrhoea due to preformed enterotoxins in foods (such as those produced by *Staphylococcus aureus*, *Clostridium perfringens* (type A) and *Bacillus cereus*) is usually short lived (less than 48 hours) while that due to enterotoxins formed in the gut lumen (by *Escherichia coli*, *Vibrio cholerae*, *Enterobacter*, *Citrobacter serratia* and *Pseudomonas* spp.) is rarely of prolonged duration though it may be very severe; none of these types produces inflammatory changes in the gut mucosa or cause significant fever. *Clostridium perfringens* and *Clostridium difficile* produce both enterotoxins, causing intestinal secretion and cytotoxins which damage gut mucosa, the former species causing severe, sometimes fatal, necrotizing enterocolitis[24] and the latter causing a severe colitis, often pseudomembranous.[3] Fever and a more prolonged course characterize these infections. Invasive organisms include viruses[8] such as rotaviruses, coronaviruses and adenoviruses, which damage small intestine enterocytes (with sometimes severe fluid losses, but running a short-lived, self-limiting course); bacteria such as *Salmonella*, *Campylobacter* and *Yersinia enterocolitica*[26] are also invasive and predominantly affect the ileum and colon, often causing high fever, severe abdominal pain and diarrhoea with blood and pus. Ideally, electron microscopy of jejunal mucosa and immune electron microscopy of stools should be

used to detect viruses, but routine identification of viruses is impractical. In all but the most short-lived diarrhoeal illnesses, appropriate *in vitro* tests to detect faecal cytotoxins and the usual cultures for pathogens should be performed. It is important that the bacteriologist is provided with fresh faecal specimens so that microscopy for inflammatory exudate, protozoa (*Giardia* and amoebae) and parasites is optimal.

CHRONIC DIARRHOEA AND MALABSORPTION

When diarrhoea persists for more than a week or two it should be fully investigated. It is convenient to divide the investigation into two stages as illustrated in *Table 3.18*. Stage 1 includes the history, physical examination, and blood, stool and urine tests, and takes place in the outpatient clinic or consulting room. Stage 2 procedures are selected on the basis of findings in stage 1, and the emphasis is on 'anatomical' studies, supported where necessary by tests of gut or pancreatic function. There should also be access to the special blood and urine tests which are necessary in some disorders.

STAGE 1

History

Time–frequency relationships
The duration of symptoms of diarrhoea should be determined. Marked physical deterioration with weight loss and a short history of a few weeks or months suggests malignancy, severe inflammatory disease or severe malabsorption, and will rarely be a diagnostic problem. Intermittent symptoms extending over years with periods of normality may occur in organic disorders such as coeliac disease or Crohn's disease, but the irritable bowel syndrome

Table 3.18 Stages in investigation of chronic diarrhoea

Stage 1
    History
    Physical examination
    Stool test
    Screening blood tests

Stage 2
    Anatomical investigations
    Gastrointestinal function tests
    Special blood and urine tests

may also present in this way. Diarrhoea occurring in the night almost always indicates organic disease. Normal bowel frequency is variable, but in the irritable bowel syndrome frequency rarely exceeds 3–4/day, commonly occurring in clusters in the early part of the day; a frequency of 5–10/day, especially if spread throughout the day, usually indicates organic disease.

Nature of the stools

The nature of the stools may be diagnostic in that passing oil per rectum indicates pancreatic insufficiency, whereas the very pale voluminous 'floating' stools of steatorrhoea indicate a gross disorder proximal to the ileocaecal valve such as extensive jejunoileal disease (coeliac disease, tropical sprue, diverticulosis, Crohn's disease, lymphoma) or pancreatic insufficiency. It is important to differentiate between bleeding associated with diarrhoea and blood loss accompanying otherwise normal stools. Colitis and carcinoma may cause the former, whereas bleeding from a polyp, carcinoma, benign vascular malformation or haemorrhoids may give the latter pattern. Watery diarrhoea may occur with a wide variety of conditions affecting all levels of the gut and is the main problem in diagnosis. The presence of undigested food in the stools is a manifestation of rapid transit and is not of diagnostic importance. Sour-smelling stools suggest carbohydrate malabsorption.

Abdominal pain

Colicky abdominal pain preceding bowel movements is common in most diarrhoeas. Small bowel colic is peri-umbilical and large bowel colic usually suprapubic in location. Severe colic following meals or associated with vomiting, temporary cessation of diarrhoea and flatus production suggests partial intestinal obstruction. Prolonged episodes of continuous abdominal pain occur in both organic and non-organic disorders. The typical dull, continuous upper abdominal pain or back pain of chronic pancreatitis or pancreatic cancer, with frequent superimposed paroxysms of burning or boring discomfort forcing the patient to adopt a characteristic 'leaning forward' or crucifix position, clearly focus attention on the pancreas. Postprandial pain, remorseless in nature, which varies in severity in proportion to meal size, and is accompanied by freedom of pain on starvation (fear of eating) suggests mesenteric ischaemia. In general, in organic disease the site and nature of the pain are consistent on repeated history taking, in contrast to the variable location, bizarre radiation and dramatic associations of psychogenic pain. The pain associated with the irritable bowel syndrome most commonly has the features of gut spasm, with an abrupt onset and often lasting several hours with a slow decline but with occasional pronounced exacerbations after bowel movements. Continuous pain in patients with inflammatory bowel disease suggests severe bowel ulceration, or complications such as abscess or perforation with peritonitis; in those with malignancy, continuous pain suggests involvement of adjacent structures with neural infiltration or pressure.

Drugs

A wide variety of drugs produce diarrhoea (*Table 3.19*) and the relationship between starting the drug and onset of diarrhoea is crucial in diagnosis. Stopping the drug for a trial period under these circumstances is wise. Alcohol is a common cause of diarrhoea but usually patients are obviously heavy imbibers with other clinical, haematological and biochemical features of alcoholism. Occasionally, diarrhoeal illnesses are empirically treated with neomycin-containing preparations which can themselves provoke diarrhoea.

Dietary factors

Patients often report that specific foods provoke diarrhoea but an allergic mechanism, though poss-

Table 3.19 Drugs causing diarrhoea and proposed mechanisms

Drug	Proposed mechanism
Laxatives	
Senna	Intestinal secretion
Phenolphthalein	Increased motility
Cascara	
Castor oil	
Magnesium salts	Osmotic
Lactulose	
Antibiotics	
Ampicillin	?Altered gut flora
	Occasionally haemorrhagic colitis
Tetracycline	?Altered gut flora
Lincomycin	
Clindamycin	} Colitis (*C. difficile* toxin)
Neomycin	Steatorrhoea and mucosal damage
Antimetabolites	
Methotrexate	
6-Mercaptopurine	Mucosal damage
Colchicine	
Sympathetic blockers	
Guanethidine	Increased motility
Ethanol	?Mucosal damage

ible, is rarely defined. Initially, these patients should be investigated for common organic disorders. Ingestion of milk leading to gaseous distension and diarrhoea suggests lactose intolerance and this is worth checking for in those individuals who might otherwise be classified as having irritable bowel syndrome. In the author's experience, exclusion diets for conditions other than coeliac disease and lactose intolerance often produce temporary benefit but, within a few weeks or months, the patient returns with recurrence of symptoms, claiming intolerance to more and more dietary factors. Nevertheless, there are now several reports implicating food intolerance in the irritable bowel syndrome, especially in those with a history of disorders such as atopic dermatitis and asthma.[5] One or more of the foods wheat, corn, dairy products, coffee, tea and citrus fruits have been identified as provoking diarrhoea in patients, rectal prostaglandin E_2 levels rising after ingestion of the offending dietary component.[2] Intolerance to the polyhydric alcohol sorbitol used as an artificial sweetener and present in several fruits and plants has been identified in both children[21] and adults,[22] resulting in abdominal pain, distension and diarrhoea. Fructose, the major sugar in fruits, and particularly fructose–sorbitol mixtures may produce malabsorption and abdominal disorders.[31] A detailed dietary history may help to identify patients with lactose, sorbitol or fructose intolerance and exclusion diets can be tried. The role of other dietary components in the pathogenesis of irritable bowel syndrome remains controversial.

Other important historical facts

The presence of weight loss suggests organic disease. Diarrhoea dating from a surgical operation may be due to resection of bowel (terminal ileum resection leading to bile salt malabsorption, left hemicolon resection leading to loose stools for a period of time); in the absence of substantial gut resection, postoperative diarrhoea points to the possibility of a stricture, fistula or surgically created stagnant loop with bacterial overgrowth. Failure to thrive following weaning suggests coeliac disease; delayed growth and development or a history of unexplained anaemia suggest coeliac disease or inflammatory bowel disease. A history of foreign travel alerts one to the possibility of intestinal parasites or tropical sprue. A number of patients have diarrhoea lasting several months following an acute diarrhoeal illness on holiday (not always abroad). While a few of these will have Crohn's disease or even coeliac disease, many have minor abnormalities of blood tests and jejunal histology, and slowly recover to normality. This condition is conveniently classified as 'temperate sprue' though its pathophysiology is poorly understood. The time-course of this condition is the main factor in making the diagnosis and a gradually improving symptomatology is reassuring.

Other points

A history of long-standing confirmed steatorrhoea with no diagnosis after hospital investigation suggests either small intestinal lymphangiectasia[35] or pancreatic hypoplasia (Schwachman's syndrome).[34] A history of severe watery diarrhoea previously investigated with no diagnosis suggest either an endocrine tumour-associated diarrhoea (e.g. medullary carcinoma of the thyroid or vipoma),[27] or chronic purgative abuse. A history of 'pernicious anaemia' in a young adult with diarrhoea suggests immunoglobulin deficiency of the common variable type.[14] During the 1980s, sexually transmitted diseases and AIDS have been recognized as major causes of intestinal disease, diarrhoea being one of the major consequences (*Table 3.20*). An assessment of risk and exposure should be an integral part of the clinical history.

Physical examination

Obvious weight loss and anaemia suggest a chronic infective, inflammatory or neoplastic disorder. These symptoms also occur in severe malabsorption syndromes, when they are usually accompanied by abdominal distension and obvious steatorrhoea on rectal examination. Vascular insufficiency[15] or a systemic vasculitis[11] may be suspected if the history is typical and there is a prominent abdominal bruit or a cutaneous vasculitic rash.

Skin lesions are frequently associated with gastrointestinal disorders: dermatitis herpetiformis with coeliac disease, erythema nodosum with inflammatory bowel disease (*Yersinia* enteritis, Crohn's disease and ulcerative colitis), flushing and telangiectasia with carcinoid syndrome, pigmentation with chronic malabsorption and Whipple's disease, and pyoderma with colitis. Common

Table 3.20 Causes of diarrhoea in sexually transmitted diseases and AIDS

Neisseria gonorrhoeae	*Cryptosporidium*[a]
Chlamydia trachomatis	*Isospora belli*[a]
Herpes simplex virus	Cytomegalovirus[a]
Entamoeba histolytica	*Mycobacterium*
Giardia lamblia	*avium-intracellulare*[a]
Shigella spp.	AIDS enteropathy[a]

[a]Only associated with immunodeficiency.

disorders like lichen planus and psoriasis appear to be more common in patients with inflammatory bowel disease. Skin features of systemic sclerosis (scleroderma) are sometimes quite subtle, even though gut involvement may be severe.

Lymphadenopathy with splenomegaly suggest lymphoma, while hepatomegaly must raise the suspicion of malignancy. A careful search for abdominal and pelvic masses is mandatory. Perianal lesions such as fistulas suggest Crohn's disease. Anorectal disease is common in patients with sexually transmitted diseases and AIDS. Typical herpetic lesions of herpes simplex virus or anorectal warts due to human papilloma virus should alert the physician to these possibilities, and appropriate viral cultures arranged.

Sigmoidoscopy and rectal biopsy

Rectal examination and sigmoidoscopy should enable up to 40% of large bowel cancers to be diagnosed in the clinic or consulting room. The macroscopic appearances of severe inflammation and mucosal friability indicate a colitis, whereas discrete ulcers with patchy inflammation are found in Crohn's disease and amoebiasis. It is now accepted that, when an obvious colitis is present, histological examination of rectal biopsies can help to distinguish an acute self-limited colitis from an initial presentation of chronic inflammatory bowel disease (ulcerative colitis or Crohn's disease).[1,36] Frank 'pus' in the lumen should alert one to the possibility of venereal proctitis (gonococcal) and appropriate swabs for microscopy and culture should be taken. Lymphogranuloma venereum serovars of C. trachomatis can cause a severe proctitis; culture of biopsies and serological tests are essential for diagnosis to distinguish this from Crohn's disease.

Very mild reddening of the mucosa without friability should not be labelled 'colitis' in a patient with severe diarrhoea because this is not an uncommon finding in non-inflammatory disorders. Rectal biopsies should be taken routinely and processed for histology. Despite a normal mucosal appearance, microscopic inflammation may be seen in microscopic colitis, subepithelial collagen in collagenous colitis, pigmented macrophages in chronic purgative abuse and granulomas in Crohn's disease: amyloid or schistosoma ova may also be seen.

The stool test

Visual inspection of the faeces at sigmoidoscopy or of a collected sample is vital. A simple classification into 'oily', 'steatorrhoeic', 'exudative' (pus with or without blood), 'watery' or 'within normal limits' will suffice. The presence of blood should be recorded and an occult blood test performed. A fresh stool sample should be looked at microscopically by a skilled person; the presence of large numbers of neutrophil leukocytes indicates inflammatory disease, eosinophils and Charcot–Leyden crystals suggest eosinophilic gastroenteritis, and a relative absence of cells is good evidence against either pathology. Mobile parasites (amoebae, *Giardia*), cysts (protozoa or nematodes) and ova (nematodes and trematodes) should be carefully searched for and if there is a high suspicion (e.g. a history of foreign travel or blood eosinophilia) several samples should be examined. Culture for specific organisms and, if suspected, assays for cytotoxins should be performed. Ideally as a routine procedure, but particularly in all patients with diarrhoea previously investigated without a diagnosis, a fresh watery stool sample should be centrifuged and the supernatant pH determined; a pH below 6 indicates fermentation of unabsorbed carbohydrate to volatile fatty acids and prompts investigation of carbohydrate intolerance (lactose or sucrose–isomaltose). Stool supernatant osmolality is usually 280–340 mosmol/kg but is often much higher in carbohydrate malabsorption and during ingestion of osmotic purgatives. Stool water electrolytes measured in the supernatant or by the *in vivo* dialysis technique[38] permit calculation of the osmotic gap (osmolality $- [(Na^+ + K^+) \times 2]$), which if more than 15 mosmol/kg suggests the presence of an additional cation such as magnesium (in magnesium salt purgative abuse). The sodium/potassium ratio, which is high in colonic disorders and low in small bowel disorders, can also be calculated. Perfection in routine stool analysis is only achieved by attention to detail, and discussion and cooperation with the bacteriology department. In practice, this relatively cheap investigation is badly performed on inadequate samples and therefore too often leads to multiple inappropriate investigations. As an example of this, a patient with the rare condition of asucrasia comes to mind. He complained of passing 'sour, stinking stools' and of gross abdominal distension and flatulence. After multiple investigations he underwent exploratory laparotomy which revealed nothing abnormal. After many referrals, a registrar finally made a careful examination of the stools and recorded a pH of 5.1 and a growth in culture of pure lactobacilli, which led to a series of disaccharide tolerance tests (which were positive for sucrose and starch) and finally a deficiency of sucrose–isomaltase was demonstrated in a peroral jejunal biopsy.[13]

Screening blood tests

Table 3.21 lists the blood tests which are helpful in early evaluation of patients with diarrhoea and should be performed in all cases. These tests may provide positive clues which, taken together with the history, physical examination and stool test, point to the most direct diagnostic approach. In those individuals who have no worrying features in the history and who have a normal physical examination and stool test, a set of completely normal blood tests excludes all but a modest number of organic pathologies.

Iron deficiency anaemia always demands explanation in patients with diarrhoea. Bleeding from the gut is likely if the anaemia is associated with elevated reticulocyte and platelet counts and should lead to faecal occult blood tests. Malabsorption or dietary deficiency of iron produces a hypochromic microcytic anaemia with a low or normal reticulocyte count. The changes of hyposplenism (target cells and Howell–Jolly bodies) suggest coeliac disease. A macrocytic anaemia suggests folate or vitamin B_{12} malabsorption. A low serum or red blood cell folate level suggests proximal small intestinal disease and may be the only abnormality in coeliac disease. A low serum vitamin B_{12} level points to a gastric lesion like pernicious anaemia, to ileal disease, or to bacterial overgrowth at any point in the small intestine. A low serum albumin level may reflect protein-losing enteropathy from a lesion in the stomach, small bowel or large bowel.

Viewed as a whole, the pattern of results should point to the correct diagnostic pathway if this is not already clinically obvious. Thus, for example, a barium follow through or small bowel enema and jejunal biopsy is indicated for diarrhoea in association with folic acid deficiency, for iron deficiency

Table 3.21 Screening blood tests in chronic diarrhoea and malabsorption

Nutritional
Haemoglobin, red blood cell indices
Serum and red cell folate
Serum vitamin B_{12}
Serum iron and transferrin
Serum calcium, phosphorus and alkaline
phosphatase
Serum albumin

General
Erythrocyte sedimentation rate
C-reactive protein
Serum potassium
Thyroid function tests

with negative faecal occult blood and stool test, and for a low serum albumin with normal liver function and negative urine test for protein. Steatorrhoea without abnormalities of the nutritional blood tests is usually pancreatic, prompting a careful look for calcification on plain abdominal radiography, and ultrasound or, preferably, computed tomography (CT) scan to image the pancreas. Abnormalities of liver function prompt delineation of hepatic and pancreatic anatomy by CT scanning and ultrasound. A very low serum potassium level with otherwise normal blood tests in a patient with severe watery diarrhoea and a normal stool test would prompt assays for peptide hormones and a search for a pancreatic neuroendocrine tumour or thyroid medullary carcinoma. Pattern recognition of this type requires careful attention to each aspect of investigation.

Abnormal blood tests must never be ignored; a diagnosis of irritable bowel syndrome or nervous diarrhoea must never be made unless the blood tests are normal and there is no suspicion of organic pathology in the history, physical examination or stool test.

If no abnormalities are found in stage 1 investigations, the physician must ask him- or herself 'Should I do a barium enema or colonoscopy now, or see the patient after 4–6 weeks and re-evaluate then?' It is the author's policy to order a barium enema directly in all those over 30 years of age on the pretext that an early carcinoma might be discovered or, in more elderly subjects, diverticular disease. Occasionally in patients with rather severe diarrhoea and in those who have already had barium studies elsewhere, it is wise to proceed directly to colonoscopy, taking serial biopsies to look for microscopic inflammation (see later). In younger subjects in the same category the author reviews and, if necessary, repeats the screening tests. As a matter of policy, the author is never happy with a diagnosis of irritable bowel syndrome appearing for the first time in middle-aged men because it is usually incorrect – as in many branches of medicine, clinical instincts should lower one's threshold for definitive investigation.

STAGE 2

Investigations of intestinal anatomy

Table 3.22 illustrates the value of different diagnostic techniques.

Barium enema

Double-contrast enemas are performed first in those patients with watery or exudative (pus with or with-

Table 3.22 Investigations of intestinal anatomy and their diagnostic value in chronic diarrhoea and malabsorption

Anatomical investigation	*Diagnosis*
Barium enema	Carcinoma Ulcerative colitis Crohn's disease Diverticular disease Polyposis Fistulas Ischaemic colitis Tuberculosis Megacolon
Barium follow through or small bowel enema	Non-specific malabsorption pattern (e.g. coeliac disease) Crohn's disease Diverticulosis Stricture Stagnant loop Fistulas Lymphoma Tuberculosis Whipple's disease Lymphangiectasia Nodular lymphoid hyperplasia
Sigmoidoscopy and rectal biopsy or colonoscopy and serial biopsy	Carcinoma Ulcerative colitis Crohn's disease Amoebiasis Melanosis coli Amyloid Lymphoma Microscopic colitis
Endoscopic duodenal biopsy or Crosby capsule jejunal biopsy	Coeliac disease Tropical sprue Lymphoma Whipple's disease α-chain disease Giardiasis Lymphangiectasia Immunodeficiency syndromes Disaccharide deficiency (after enzyme analysis)
Endoscopic pancreatography	Carcinoma of the pancreas Chronic pancreatitis
Liver/spleen ultrasound (or CT) scan and liver bopsy	Carcinoma Carcinoid Lymphoma

out blood) diarrhoea and in those with 'change of bowel habit' or rectal bleeding. The diagnostic accuracy depends on adequate bowel preparation, radiological technical expertise and experienced reporting. These three criteria are not always optimal. Even under the best circumstances, caecal carcinomas, polyps and low-grade colitis are occasionally missed. Re-reporting of films in the light of further clinical information, repeat studies, or colonoscopy increases the diagnostic yield where there is any doubt. Studies from other hospitals may be acceptable, but if more than 1–2 months old may need to be repeated.

Colonoscopy

In the author's view, colonoscopy is still not a routine investigation for diarrhoea. It is clearly helpful for defining the nature or extent of a lesion seen on barium enema. For example, a stricture in the transverse colon in a patient with Crohn's colitis could be inflammatory or neoplastic, or a caecal lesion could be carcinoma, amoeboma, Crohn's disease or tuberculosis; similarly, bleeding could be coming from a small polyp, carcinoma or a vascular malformation. It is now recognized that there are a group of patients presenting with diarrhoea who have normal macroscopic appearances at colonoscopy but in whom serial biopsies show extensive microscopic inflammation. This microscopic colitis appears to have two forms, lymphocytic and collagenous.[25] Performing colonoscopy and serial biopsies as an early investigation in patients with substantial diarrhoea may help to define these disorders. Colonoscopy is also essential for surveillance of the colon in individuals with long-standing colitis to detect dysplasia[9] and other stigmata of incipient malignancy.

Small intestine radiology

This should be the first investigation in patients with steatorrhoea or watery diarrhoea with blood tests suggesting small intestinal pathology. Otherwise, it usually follows the barium enema. The interpretation of small bowel radiographs requires considerable experience, and, in many instances, discussion with the radiologist who performed the study is essential to aid interpretation. An intubated follow through enables double-contrast images of high quality to be obtained and is especially useful in detecting areas of narrowing and mucosal lesions which may be missed with conventional studies. Adequate visualization of the terminal ileum requires spot views and careful positioning of the patient and, where ileal loops are low in the pelvis, a lateral view may be helpful. To obtain better views of the terminal ileum, air can be insufflated per rectum or, as an alternative, a tube can be inserted into the terminal ileum at colonoscopy and contrast medium instilled.

It is important to realize that disease of the small intestine (e.g. coeliac disease, Crohn's disease) may be found even when small bowel radiographs appear normal. Abnormalities of the mucosal pattern may be characteristic of, for example, Crohn's disease but the possible differential diagnosis of lymphoma, vasculitis (e.g. Henoch–Schönlein purpura) with submucosal haemorrhage, or tuberculosis must be carefully considered. Whenever possible, histological confirmation of the diagnosis should be obtained, and, if reasonable doubt exists, a laparotomy

may be necessary. A decision to repeat a follow-through examination should be taken whenever symptoms suggestive of intermittent small bowel obstruction occur or after an interval if the diarrhoea persists and no clear diagnosis has been made.

Radiolabelled-leukocyte scans

This technique[29] involves taking a sample of venous blood, separating the polymorphonuclear leukocytes using centrifugation with percol or metrizamide plasma gradients, and labelling the cells with ^{111}In using tropolonate as the chelating agent. Labelled cells are reinjected intravenously and, after 40 minutes, abdominal scans are performed. A normal (negative) scan shows maximal activity in the spleen, lesser activity in the liver and least activity in the bone marrow (*Figure 3.45*), while the bowel is not visualized. Abnormal activity in bowel loops is readily seen in early scans (*Figure 3.46*). In the colon, the extent of acute inflammation and the presence of skip lesions is usually obvious[32] whereas, in the small bowel, clearly defined inflamed bowel loops or more diffuse activity representing overlapping loops may be seen. Labelled cells rapidly migrate from diseased bowel wall to bowel lumen and later scans show a column of cells

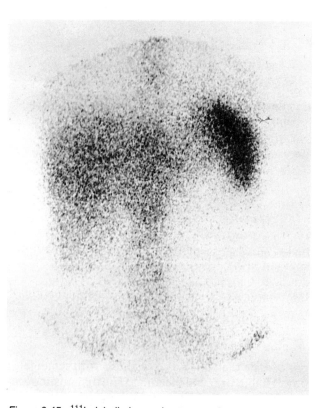

Figure 3.45 ^{111}In-labelled granulocyte scan in a normal subject obtained by external imaging at 40 minutes after reinjection of labelled cells. Note the normal appearance with uptake in liver, spleen, vascular pool, and the bone marrow of the spine and pelvis.

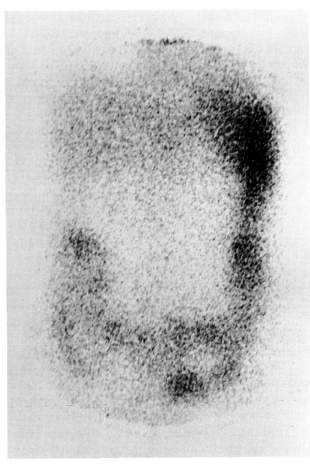

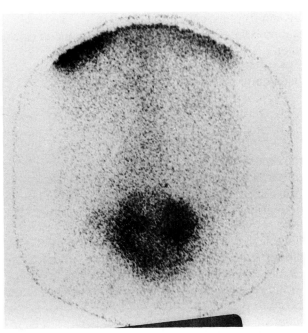

Figure 3.47 ^{111}In-labelled scan at 24 hours after reinjection of labelled cells. Note the dense persistent accumulation of activity in the central part of the lower abdomen and pelvis, indicating an abscess at this site.

Figure 3.46 ^{111}In-labelled granulocyte scan at 40 minutes after reinjection of labelled cells. Note the accumulation of activity throughout the large intestine, indicating pancolitis.

in transit through the bowel with clearance of activity at the diseased segment. Sequential scans thus distinguish bowel inflammation from an abscess, where activity persists at the original site of localization for up to 48 hours (*Figure 3.47*). In patients with inflammatory disease, faecal collections and γ counting of the stool permit calculation of the percentage excretion of labelled cells, which is a measure of disease severity.

The sensitivity of ^{111}In scanning in detecting inflammation in bowel is substantially greater than radiology and in the colon is equivalent to colonoscopy and biopsy; in detecting abscesses it is superior to ultrasound. Although the technique is not widely available, it offers the potential for rapid diagnosis of inflammatory disease and assessment of activity and extent of disease in patients presenting with diarrhoea. No bowel preparation is required and it is therefore a suitable early investigation in the sick and elderly. The finding of normal faecal indium excretion (less than 2%) virtually excludes inflammatory disease as a cause of diarrhoea; gut carcinoma, coeliac disease, endocrine diarrhoea,

diverticular disease and irritable bowel syndrome are usually associated with negative scans and normal faecal indium excretion. Positive scans and an elevated faecal indium level confirm inflammation but are not specific to any particular inflammatory process, so that Crohn's disease, ulcerative colitis, tuberculosis, pseudomembranous colitis and colitis due to other toxigenic or infective causes would all give a positive scan. Nevertheless, the combination of these techniques with selective use of colonoscopy, biopsy techniques and bacteriological studies represents a major advance in the assessment of patients with diarrhoea.

Other scanning techniques

[99m]Tc-labelled hexamethyl propylene amine oxime (^{99m}Tc-HMPAO) leukocyte scanning is also of value in demonstrating bowel inflammation,[30] showing good correlations with the disease extent as assessed by radiology, endoscopy and surgery in patients with Crohn's disease,[33] though does not have the same potential for quantifying disease activity as ^{111}In techniques. Nevertheless, images with ^{99m}Tc are of high quality and there are advantages in terms of expense, convenience and radiation dose with this technique. The main disadvantages are that the technetium label accumulates in the normal colon on late scans unlike the situation with indium and there is substantial renal excretion with bladder activity. Techniques based on *in vitro* phagocytosis

by neutrophils and monocytes of ^{99m}Tc-labelled stannous colloid particles (0.5–2 mm diameter) have been successfully used by some groups.[4,20]

Duodenal or jejunal biopsy

Duodenal or jejunal biopsy should be performed in all patients with steatorrhoea, in those with watery diarrhoea and blood tests suggesting small bowel disease, in those with a radiological abnormality of the small intestine, and in those in whom a suspicion of parasitic disease of the small intestine is raised because of country of origin, foreign travel or immunodeficiency. It is wise to perform barium studies first because the presence of single or multiple diverticula represent a risk of perforation should the biopsy capsule enter a diverticulum. Under these circumstances, duodenal biopsies via an endoscope would be safer. In any case, many groups have now opted to perform small bowel biopsies (four endoscopic biopsies from the distal duodenum) at endoscopy because of the convenience and speed of this procedure. Examination of the biopsy under the dissecting microscope, and of the duodenal juice under dark-ground illumination for motile parasites, is very valuable because a flat or convoluted appearance of the tissue may provisionally confirm suspicions of coeliac disease or tropical sprue, and a positive finding of *Giardia* or *Strongyloides* permits rapid institution of therapy. Histological confirmation of the diagnosis is, of course, essential. The problem of patchy mucosal abnormalities in Crohn's disease or dermatitis herpetiformis has led several authorities to stress the need for multiple biopsies. This is essential for duodenal biopsies (endoscopic) because of their small size. In any case, careful orientation of biopsies prior to fixation and embedding is essential if an adequate assessment of villous morphology is to be assured.

Attempts to biopsy more distal regions of the small intestine are problematic and the author is unable to recall a single example where this has provided a definite diagnosis. This means that a clear pathological diagnosis of a lesion in the lower small intestine demonstrated radiologically is not possible except at laparotomy. In practice, for Crohn's disease, classic radiological appearances together with abnormalities in biopsies from more accessible sites (e.g. rectum, colon, or terminal ileum at colonoscopy) may suffice or, for an ileitis, the finding of positive serological tests for *Yersinia* may confirm the diagnosis. In other instances, laparotomy may be necessary.

Gastroscopy and endoscopic pancreatography

Gastroscopy is advisable in all patients with diarrhoea who have upper gastrointestinal symptoms or abnormalities of the oesophagus, stomach or duodenum on barium radiography. In several units it is now performed in all patients with diarrhoea and malabsorption. The frequency of gastric abnormalities in patients with Crohn's disease has recently been emphasized, though the biopsy appearances are rarely diagnostic.

Typical appearances of effacement of circular folds and absence of villi under magnification are recognized in coeliac disease, and stippling and club-shaped villous enlargement due to lymphatic distension are seen in Whipple's disease. Visible enlargement of lymph vessels may also be seen in intestinal lymphangiectasia. Aspiration of duodenal fluid for microbiological studies is also useful. Duodenal biopsies for culture and histology (see above) should always be obtained.

Endoscopic pancreatography may define the characteristic duct abnormalities of chronic pancreatitis. In patients with steatorrhoea with or without diabetes, in whom blood tests, radiography and jejunal biopsy have excluded small bowel disease, pancreatic insufficiency is likely. If such patients have obvious pancreatic calcification on plain radiography or CT then endoscopic pancreatography is unnecessary. A pancreatic function test in these circumstances is convenient, useful and safe. In the absence of calcification or suggestive abnormalities on ultrasound or CT, it is wise to examine the duct anatomy using endoscopic pancreatography and to obtain cytology for malignant cells.

Intestinal and pancreatic function tests

Small gut function tests

Table 3.23 illustrates the pattern of abnormal function tests to be expected with disease in different anatomical locations. It has already been stressed that these are usually not first-line investigations for diarrhoea.

The jejunum, pancreas and colon are accessible to the anatomical diagnostic approach previously outlined, but the ileum is relatively inaccessible and, in the absence of obvious radiological abnormality, a sensitive function test may exclude or suggest significant ileal disease. Furthermore, to confirm bacterial overgrowth in those patients with an anatomical basis (e.g. stricture, fistula, diverticulosis or dilated gut) or in those with immunodeficiency, function tests before and after antibiotics are useful. Although of limited value in diagnosis, function tests may be repeated at intervals as a parameter of treatment response or to assess functional reserve after gut resection (e.g. Schilling test after ileal resection). Finally, carbohydrate tolerance tests are

Table 3.23 Intestinal function tests in chronic diarrhoea and malabsorption

Disease location or type	*Intestinal function tests*
Jejunal disease	Reduced xylose and glucose absorption Normal or increased faecal fat
Ileal disease	Normal xylose and glucose absorption Increased faecal fat (with greater than 100 cm of disease or resection) Schilling test abnormal Increased faecal bile salt excretion [14C] Bile acid breath test positive
Pancreatic insufficiency	Normal xylose absorption Diabetic glucose tolerance Increased faecal fat and nitrogen Abnormal pancreatic function test
Small bowel bacterial overgrowth[a]	Normal glucose absorption Reduced xylose absorption Increased faecal fat Schilling test abnormal Normal faecal bile salt excretion [14C] Bile acid breath test positive Hydrogen breath test with glucose positive Bacterial counts greater than 10^5 in jejunal fluid
Colonic disease	Normal faecal fat, absorption and breath tests High sodium/potassium ratio in stool

[a]Normalized after antibiotics.

convenient methods of demonstrating lactose and sucrose intolerance, which should have been suspected on the basis of history and a low faecal pH.

The *measurement of faecal fat* is extremely unpopular among biochemists for obvious reasons, though it is an established and sensitive test. Reliable results depend on adequate fat intake so that, on an outpatient basis, supplements in the form of cream must be given to ensure a fat intake of more than 70 g/day. Since the normal coefficient of fat absorption is 5%, a young male adult who may eat up to 200 g of fat in a day will have a normal faecal fat excretion of about 10 g. For inpatients, dietary supervision excludes these obvious pitfalls. A 2-day run-in period is usually followed by a 3-day collection period. Faecal markers to estimate recovery are useful but not essential. Attempts have been made to replace the faecal fat test with radioisotopic breath tests. The [14C] triolein test, for example, detects all patients with steatorrhoea but gives no assessment of the severity of fat malabsorption.[28] It is obvious that a decrease in efficiency of fat absorption from 95 to 90% will increase faecal fat excretion by 100% but change fat absorption by only 5%, so that any test based on events reflecting variable

absorption and subsequent metabolism is intrinsically less sensitive than measurement of the fraction appearing in faeces. Several reports confirm the anticipated insensitivity of this test but others[37] have reported a sensitivity of 85% and a specificity of 93%. Metabolic disorders such as diabetes, hyperlipidaemia and thyroid disease can give erroneous results as can significant lung or liver disease. The test also takes up to 8 hours to perform. In the author's view this test is not likely to replace the standard faecal fat measurement.

Of the other 'tubeless' isotopic function tests, the *Schilling test* remains popular and is useful providing it is correctly carried out and there is a complete urine collection. Modifications of the Schilling test to detect pancreatic insufficiency[10] mean that it is possible to use this test to detect pernicious anaemia, ileal disease, bacterial overgrowth and pancreatic disease.

The [14C] *cholylglycine breath test*[18] is usually positive in patients with bacterial overgrowth of the small intestine, but quantitative faecal [14C] excretion is essential to differentiate between bacterial overgrowth (faecal excretion less than 10% of the dose) and ileal disease or resection with bile acid malabsorption (faecal excretion greater than 10% with or without increased breath[14]CO_2 output). Faecal[14]C counting is difficult and requires expensive combustion apparatus. As a test of ileal function, total body counting at 7 days after administration of SeHCAT (tauro-23 (^{75}Se) selena-25 homocolic acid, a selenium-labelled bile acid) may be more useful in those institutions with whole-body γ counters.[17]

Non-radioisotopic breath tests based on hydrogen excretion[12] after administration of glucose (for bacterial overgrowth), lactose (for lactose malabsorption) or lactulose (for small intestinal transit time or bacterial overgrowth) are simple to perform and the newer hydrogen gas analysers are useful additions to the gastrointestinal function laboratories. It should be remembered that lactose intolerance may be due to organic disease of the small intestine and tests to exclude such disorders are mandatory before a diagnosis of primary hypolactasia is made.

Pancreatic function tests

Tubeless pancreatic function tests are increasingly popular (e.g. PABA (para-amino benzoic acid) test, fluorescein dilaurate test and modified Schilling test). They are useful in assessing pancreatic function in patients with steatorrhoea but not sensitive enough for detection of pancreatic disease in the absence of severe exocrine deficiency.[16] Of the intubation tests, the Lundh test is widely used in clinical gastroenterology, but the secretin or secretin–cholecystokinin test using a continuous intravenous infusion of hormones and a duodenal perfusion system to measure outputs of bicarbonate and enzymes is probably the only test which offers the potential for measurement of lesser degrees of pancreatic insufficiency. The main value of pancreatic function tests in investigation of diarrhoea is that they can define exocrine deficiency as the cause of steatorrhoea. In some instances this will obviate the need for endoscopic retrograde pancreatography, which is not always available, may fail to visualize the ducts, may provoke acute pancreatitis and may introduce infection. In units with appropriate expertise and low complication rates, however, visualization of pancreatic duct anatomy by endoscopic pancreatography is the most definitive procedure. Since duct anatomy and functional reserve do not correlate well, it is quite useful to assess pancreatic function in addition to demonstrating anatomical abnormalities.

Other function tests

Recently, several groups have suggested that the measurement of intestinal permeability is clinically useful in screening for, or monitoring the response to therapy in, small gut disorders such as coeliac disease and Crohn's disease. These tests depend on the administration of molecules of different sizes by mouth and assess gut permeability by the ratio of concentrations excreted in urine. For example, in coeliac disease the mannitol-to-cellobiose ratio is markedly reduced compared to normal, reflecting the decreased absorption of mannitol (due to loss of surface area) and the increased absorption of cellobiose (due to increased permeability). Ratios return towards normal with treatment.[19] The use of single probes such as ^{51}Cr ethylenediaminetetra-acetate has demonstrated increased absorption in coeliac disease and small bowel Crohn's disease.[7] The cellobiose/mannitol test has been prospectively evaluated in a large number of patients presenting with symptoms suggesting a possible diagnosis of coeliac disease.[23] The sensitivity of the test for diagnosis of coeliac disease was 96% and the specificity 70% (positive and negative predictive values 36 and 99%, respectively). False positive tests often indicated other diagnoses explaining abnormal permeability. These results suggest that this test could be useful in selecting patients for early duodenal/jejunal biopsy.

Tests of small and large bowel transit time, while of research interest, have no obvious role to play in the diagnosis or management of patients with diarrhoea.

Special blood, stool and urine tests

Endocrine causes of diarrhoea

Table 3.24 illustrates the endocrine causes of diarrhoea and the diagnostic tests most appropriate in each case. Thyrotoxicosis and the Zollinger–Ellison syndrome should be suspected on clinical history or physical examination, while obvious flushing is always, in the author's experience, associated with the diarrhoea of the carcinoid syndrome. The vipoma syndrome (Verner–Morrison or WDHA syndrome) should be suspected when severe watery diarrhoea occurs in any patient who has a negative stool test (normal microscopy, culture and pH), hypokalaemia (usually marked) as the only abnormal blood test (except for minor abnormalities of serum calcium and abnormal liver tests when there are widespread hepatic secondaries), and normal intestinal anatomy. The key investigation is the plasma vasoactive intestinal polypeptide level, which if elevated indicates a pancreatic tumour (children or adults) or a ganglioneuroma (usually children). Pancreatic imaging (ultrasound and CT) may show the tumour, but selective pancreatic angiography is the most sensitive test.

Medullary carcinoma of the thyroid causes a usually persistent, painless diarrhoea, watery in

Table 3.24 Endocrine causes of diarrhoea and diagnostic tests

Endocrine syndromes	Diagnostic tests
Thyrotoxicosis	Plasma T_3 and T_4 Thyroid scan
Medullary carcinoma of thyroid	Plasma calcitonin Thyroid and bone scans CT scan
Zollinger–Ellison syndrome	Plasma gastrin Acid secretion studies Pancreatic angiography CT scan
Vipoma (pancreatic cholera or WDHA syndrome)	Plasma vasoactive intestinal peptide Mesenteric angiography Transhepatic portal venous sampling CT scan
Carcinoid syndrome	Urinary 5-hydroxyindoleacetic acid excretion Liver scan and bopsy

nature, and is the main differential diagnosis of the vipoma syndrome. The mechanism of diarrhoea is not completely understood, but it is clearly different from that in patients with vipomas. Diarrhoea persists during fasting but is much greater when feeding. Stool tests during fasting show normal osmolality and pH but, unlike vipomas, the osmolality increases and the pH falls during feeding, suggesting malabsorption (possibly secondary to fast transit). Hypokalaemia is less marked, though usually present, and again intestinal anatomy is normal. In the absence of an obvious tumour in the neck or elsewhere, diarrhoea usually indicates a substantial tumour mass, and mediastinal lymph nodes, bones and liver are likely sites. If the clinical picture fits, measurement of the plasma calcitonin level is the key investigation and other tests are useful to assess location of the tumour and its metastases.

Endocrine tumour-related diarrhoeas are rare, and in units which act as referral centres occasional patients are seen with a clinical picture resembling the vipoma syndrome but in whom vasoactive intestinal polypeptide levels are normal (including repeat measurements). These patients do not usually have a tumour, but a careful search in the pancreas, lung and liver should be made. There is little point in performing laparotomy on the basis of reports in the literature to date, but careful assessment and surveillance is warranted. The possibility of small tumours secreting uncharacterized secretogogues exists.

Chronic purgative abuse

This condition, which is almost confined to females, may be difficult to diagnose. Patients with diarrhoea who have obvious melanosis coli on sigmoidoscopy or pigment-laden macrophages on rectal histology are almost certainly taking anthraquinone purgatives (e.g. Senokot). Phenolphthalein purgatives may be detected by the development of a red coloration on alkalinization of the stool supernatant and sometimes the urine, and magnesium salt purgatives by the high stool osmolality, high ionic gap and high faecal magnesium concentration. It is important to try and identify any purgatives the patient may have with them; locker searches, although of questionable ethics, may reveal the nature of the purgative. Discharging a patient home for the weekend is usually helpful if stool and urine samples for analysis are obtained immediately on return to hospital. This sometimes overcomes the problem of diminishing diarrhoea and negative tests during hospital confinement, possibly due to the patient not having access to purgatives in the hospital ward. A variety of anatomical, blood test and function test abnormalities may be found in patients with surreptitious laxative ingestion in addition to those already mentioned. The barium enema may show variable dilatation and loss of haustral pattern, there may be an elevated erythrocyte sedimentation rate and a low serum potassium level, and mild abnormalities of xylose, vitamin B_{12} and fat absorption.

CONCLUSION

The diagnostic approach to patients with chronic diarrhoea has been outlined. In order to avoid unnecessary tests and inordinate expense, emphasis is placed on the value of clinical features and screening blood and stool tests. Careful assessment of these permits selection of the further investigations necessary to make a firm diagnosis in almost all patients.

REFERENCES

1. Allison, M.C., Hamilton-Dutoit, S.J., Dhillon, A.P. and Pounder, R.E. (1987) The value of rectal biopsy in distinguishing self-limited colitis from early inflammatory bowel disease. *Quarterly Journal of Medicine*, **65**(248), 985–995.
2. Alun Jones, V., Shorthouse, M., McLaughlan, P. *et al.* (1982) Food intolerance: a major factor in the pathogenesis of irritable bowel syndrome. *The Lancet*, **ii**, 1115–1117.
3. Bartlett, J.G., Change, T.W., Taylor, N.S. and Onderdonk, A.B. (1979) Colitis induced by clostridium difficile. *Reviews of Infectious Diseases*, **1**, 370–378.
4. Bartholomeusz, F.D.L., Durbridge, T.C., Drew, P. *et al.* (1988) The microscopic distribution of ^{99m}Tc-labelled phagocytes in resected bowel in patients with acute Crohn's disease: correlation with histological changes. *Journal of Gastroenterology and Hepatology*, **3**, 93–98.
5. Bentley, S.J., Pearson, D.J. and Rix, K.J.B. (1983) Food hypersensitivity in irritable bowel syndrome. *The Lancet*, **ii**, 295–297.
6. Bishop, F.R. (1982) Spectrum of infectious agents in acute diarrhoea. In: *Gastroenterology 2: Small Intestine*, pp 319–331 (Eds) Chadwick, V.S. and Phillips, S. London: Butterworth.
7. Bjarnason, I., Peters, T.J. and Veall, N. (1983) A persistent defect in intestinal permeability in coeliac disease demonstrated by a ^{51}Cr-labelled EDTA absorption test. *The Lancet*, **i**, 323–325.
8. Blacklow, N.R. and Cukor, G. (1981) Viral gastroenteritis. *New England Journal of Medicine*, **304**, 397–406.
9. Blackstone, M.D., Riddell, R.H., Rogers, B.H.G. and Levin, B. (1981) Dysplasia-associated lesion or mass (DALM) detected by colonoscopy in long standing ulcerative colitis: an indication for colectomy. *Gastroenterology*, **80**, 366–374.
10. Brugge, W.R., Goff, J.S., Allen, N.C. *et al.* (1980) Development of a dual label Schilling test for pancreatic exocrine function on the differential absorption of cobalamin bound to intrinsic factor and R protein. *Gastroenterology*, **78**, 947–949.
11. Camilleri, M., Pusey, C.D., Chadwick, V.S. and Rees, A.J. (1982) Vasculitis and the intestine. In: *Gastroenterology 2: Small Intestine*, pp. 227–248 (Eds) Chadwick, V.S. and Phillips, S. London: Butterworth.
12. Caspary, W.F. (1978) Breath tests. *Clinics in Gastroenterology*, **7**, 351–374.
13. Cooper, B.T., Candy, D.C.A., Harries, J.T. and Peters, T.J. (1979) Subcellular fractionation studies of the intestinal mucosa in congenital sucrose-isomaltase deficiency. *Clinical Science*, **57**, 181–185.
14. Dawson, J., Hodgson, H.J.F., Pepys, M.B. *et al.* (1979) Immunodeficiency malabsorption and secretory diarrhoea. A new syndrome. *American Journal of Medicine*, **67**, 540–545.
15. Dick, A.P. and McC.Gregg, D. (1972) Chronic occlusions of the visceral arteries. In: *Clinics in Gastroenterology*, **1**, 689–706.
16. Di Magno, E.P. (1982) Diagnosis of chronic pancreatitis: are non-invasive tests of exocrine pancreatic function sensitive and specific? *Gastroenterology*, **83**, 143–145.
17. Fagan, E.A., Chadwick, V.S. and McLean Baird, I. (1983) SeHCAT absorption: a simple test of ileal dysfunction. *Digestion*, **26**, 159–165.
18. Fromm, H. and Hofmann, A.F. (1971) Breath test for altered bile acid metabolism. *The Lancet*, **ii**, 621–625.
19. Hamilton, I., Cobden, I., Rothwell, J. and Axon, A.T. (1982) Intestinal permeability in coeliac disease: the response to gluten withdrawal and single-dose gluten challenge. *Gut*, **23**, 202–210.
20. Hanna, R., Braun, T., Levendel, A. and Lomas, F. (1984) Radiochemistry and biostability of autologous leucocytes labelled with ^{99m}Tc stannous colloid in whole blood. *European Journal of Nuclear Medicine*, **9**, 216–219.
21. Hyams, J.L. (1982) Chronic abdominal pain caused by sorbitol malabsorption. *Journal of Pediatrics*, **100**, 772–773.
22. Jain, N.K., Rosenberg, D.B., Ulahannan, M.J. *et al.* (1985) Sorbitol intolerance in adults. *American Journal of Gastroenterology*, **80**, 678–681.
23. Juby, L.D., Rothwell, J. and Axon, A.T.R. (1989) Cellobiose/mannitol sugar test – a sensitive tubeless test for coeliac disease: results on 1010 unselected patients. *Gut*, **30**, 476–480.
24. Lawrence, G. and Walker, P.D. (1976) Pathogenesis of enteritis necroticans in Papua New Guinea. *The Lancet*, **i**, 125–126.
25. Lazenby, A.J., Yardley, J.H., Giardiello, F.M. *et al.* (1989) Lymphocytic ("Microscopic") colitis: A comparative histopathologic study with particular reference to collagenous colitis. *Human Pathology*, **20**, 18–28.
26. Mark, M.I., Pai, C.H., Lafleur, L. *et al.* (1980) *Yersina enterocolitica* gastroenteritis: a prospective study of clinical, bacteriologic and epidemiologic features. *Journal of Paediatrics*, **96**, 26–31.
27. Modigliani, R. and Bernier, J.J. (1982) Pathophysiology of hormonal diarrhoea. In: *Gastroenterology 2: Small Intestine*, pp. 265–279 (Eds) Chadwick, V.S. and Phillips, S. London: Butterworth.

28. Newcomer, A.D., Hofmann, A.F., DiMagno, E.P. et al. (1978) Triolein breath test: a sensitive and specific test for fat malabsorption. *Gastroenterology*, **76**, 6–13.

29. Peters, A.M., Saverymuttu, S.H., Reavy, H.J. et al. (1983) Imaging of inflammation with indium-111 troplolonate labelled leucocytes. *Journal of Nuclear Medicine*, **24**, 39–44.

30. Peters, A.M., Danpure, H.J., Osman, S. et al. (1986) Clinical experience with ^{99m}Tc-hexamethylpropylene-amineoxime for labelling leucocytes and imaging inflammation. *The Lancet*, **ii**, 946–949.

31. Rumessen, J.J., Gudmand-Hoyer, E. (1988) Functional bowel disease: malabsorption and abdominal distress after ingestion of fructose, sorbitol, and fructose-sorbitol mixtures. *Gastroenterology*, **95**, 694–700.

32. Saverymuttu, S.H., Peters, A.M., Hodgson, H.J.F. et al. (1982) [111]Indium autologous leucocyte scanning: comparison with radiology for imaging the colon in inflammatory bowel disease. *British Medical Journal*, **285**, 659–666.

33. Scholmerich, J., Schmidt, E., Schumichen, C. et al. (1988) Scintigraphic assessment of bowel involvement and disease activity in Crohn's disease using Technetium 99m-hexamethyl propylene amine oxine as leukocyte label. *Gastroenterology*, **95**, 1287–1293.

34. Shwachman, H., Diamond, L.K., Oski, F.A. and Khaw, K.T. (1964) The syndrome of pancreatic insufficiency and bone marrow dysfunction. *Journal of Paediatrics*, **65**, 645–663.

35. Strober, W., Wochner, R.D., Carbone, P.P. and Waldmann, T.A. (1967) Lymphangiectasia: a protein losing enteropathy with hypogammaglobulineaemia, lymphocytopenia and impaired homograft rejection. *Journal of Clinical Investigation*, **46**, 1643–1656.

36. Surawicz, C.M. and Belic, L. (1984) Rectal biopsy helps to distinguish acute self-limited colitis from idiopathic inflammatory bowel disease. *Gastroenterology*, **86**, 104–113.

37. Turner, J.M., Lawrence, S., Fellows, I.W. et al. (1987) ^{14}C-triolein absorption: a useful test in the diagnosis of malabsorption. *Gut*, **28**, 694–700.

38. Wrong, O., Morrison, R.B.I. and Hurst, P.E. (1961) A method of obtaining faecal fluid by *in vivo* dialysis. *The Lancet*, **i**, 1208–1209.

THE CONSEQUENCES OF MALABSORPTION

H.J.F. Hodgson

At worst, malabsorption combines the long-term consequences of nutrient deficiency with the more immediate consequences of fluid and electrolyte depletion. The results of malabsorption of individual nutrients and vitamins have been covered previously in the appropriate sections. When all are combined, the patient with advanced malabsorption may be cachectic, pigmented, with peripheral oedema, anaemia, glossitis, angular cheilitis and stomatitis, with a proximal myopathy, nail changes of clubbing or koilonychia, hypotensive and dehydrated. Advanced cases can show peripheral neuropathy and bizarre central nervous manifestations. An extended list of potential physical manifestation of malabsorption is shown in *Table 3.25*. Most of these are reversible with adequate treatment if sufficiently prolonged, although neurological damage may not reverse. None the less, it should be remembered that malabsorptive conditions may be associated with a good general state of health, as studies into the family incidence of coeliac disease emphasize.

Two particular manifestations require comment here as they are not covered in the sections on individual nutrients.

HYPEROXALURIA

Dietary oxalate, in tea, cocoa and vegetables such as spinach and rhubarb is normally poorly absorbed from the intestine. In patients with steatorrhoea, however, paradoxically increased absorption leading to hyperoxaluria may occur, sometimes leading to renal stones and, in extreme cases, interstitial oxalate nephropathy.[1] The presentation of these are with characteristic manifestations of nephrolithiasis (pain, infection, bleeding and diminished renal function).[7] Characteristic oxalate crystals may be identified in the urine.

Although most urinary oxalate is endogenously generated, the hyperoxaluria of malabsorption reflects increased absorption of dietary oxalate due to a combination of small and large intestinal pathophysiology. The basis is increased absorption of oxalate which occurs when malabsorptive states lead to frank steatorrhoea.[6] In the normal state, oxalate ions combine with calcium in the gut lumen to form highly insoluble calcium oxalate, which is not absorbed. In the presence of undigested fat, calcium is diverted to form calcium soaps, and free oxalate

Table 3.25 Manifestations of malabsorption apparent on physical examination[a]

Skin and mucous membranes
  Finger clubbing
  Pigmentations
  Hyperkeratosis
  Eczema
  Purpura
  Folliculitis
  Glossitis
  Cheilosis
  Angular stomatitis
  White nails
  Acrodermatitis

Muscle
  Muscle wasting
  Tetany
  Proximal myopathy

Peripheral nervous system
  Peripheral neuropathy

Central nervous system
  Apathy
  Wernicke–Korsakoff syndrome
  Night blindness
  Ataxia

Blood
  Anaemia
  Coagulopathy

Generalised
  Weight loss
  Dehydration
  Oedema
  Ascites
  Hypotension

Gastrointestinal
  Gut distension

[a] None or all of these may be present.

thus remains which can be absorbed. The diseases in which this occurs therefore tend to be those associated with bile salt malabsorption, and therefore with the passage of excessive quantities of bile salts into the colon, causing damage and enhanced permeability of the colonic epithelium.[5] The overall consequence is enhanced absorption of the still soluble oxalate through the colonic wall. Thus, hyperoxaluria is a common feature in patients with small intestinal Crohn's disease and multiple resections, but does not occur if an ileostomy is present (the ileostomist is prone to uric acid stones due to relative dehydration and loss of bicarbonate-rich faecal fluid leading to a concentrated acid urine).

In addition, the condition is found in patients who have undergone jejunoileal bypass, and is reported in coeliac disease, tropical sprue, bacterial overgrowth syndromes, and chronic pancreatitis.

Treatment is by dietary means, by a combination of dietary restriction to reduce steatorrhoea, and a low-oxalate diet avoiding the foods and drinks already mentioned, and the ubiquitous commercial cola drinks.[2]

HYPOSPLENISM

A variety of chronic intestinal conditions are associated with diminished splenic function, particularly coeliac disease, but also Whipple's disease, tropical sprue, non-ulcerative jejunoileitis, Crohn's disease and ulcerative colitis.[8,9]

The consequence of hyposplenism is most commonly a recognizable blood picture with Howell–Jolly bodies (reflecting aged red cells, which have increased numbers of pits in their surface) and thrombocytosis.[4] This may be an early diagnostic clue to the presence of coeliac disease. Hyposplenism is associated with diminished primary antibody responses, as demonstrated for example following immunization with novel antigens such as ϕX-174, and with a diminished ability to switch from immunoglobulin M to immunoglobulin G production.

In some cases of long-standing inflammatory or malabsorptive disease, the spleen size can be documented to be small, either by ultrasound or by using autologous heat-damaged red cells, which provides an additional means of documenting and quantifying hyposplenism. The functional hyposplenism phenomenon can also be found with a normal-size spleen, and in some cases reversible hyposplenism following the treatment of malabsorption or control of inflammation has been reported.[10,11]

The extent to which hyposplenism is clinically relevant, and whether it contributes to a tendency to overwhelming or severe infections, remains controversial. The condition may contribute to the increase in autoimmune phenomenon noted in patients with coeliac disease.[3]

REFERENCES

1. Anderson, H. and Bosaeus, I. (1981) Hyperoxaluria in malabsorptive states. *Urologia Internationalis*, **36**, 1–19.
2. Anderson, H. and Jagenburg, R. (1974) Fat-

reduced diet in the treatment of hyperoxaluria in patients with ileo-pathology. *Gut*, **15**, 360–366.

3. Bullen, A.W. and Losowsky, M.S. (1979) Consequences of impaired splenic function. *Clinical Science*, **57**, 129–137.

4. Bullen, A.W., Hall, R., Brown, R.C. and Losowsky, M.S. (1977) Mechanisms of thrombocytosis in coeliac disease. *Gut*, **18**, A962.

5. Dobbins, J.W. and Binder, H.J. (1977) Importances of the colonic in enteric hyperoxaluria. *New England Journal of Medicine*, **296**, 298–301.

6. McDonald, G.B., Earnest, D.L. and Admirand, W.H. (1977) Hyperoxaluria correlates with fat malabsorption in patients with sprue. *Gut*, **18**, 561–566.

7. Mandell, I. Krauss, E. and Millan, J.C. (1980) Oxalate induced acute renal failure in Crohn's disease. *American Journal of Medicine*, **69**, 628–632.

8. O'Grady, J.G., Stevens, F.M. and Harding, B. (1984) Hyposplenism and gluten-sensitive enteropathy. Natural history, incidence and relationship to diet and small bowel morphology. *Gastroenterology*, **87**, 1326.

9. Palmer, K.R., Sherrif, S.B., Holdsworth, C.D. and Ryan, F.P. (1981) Further experience of hyposplenism in inflammatory bowel disease. *Quarterly Journal of Medicine*, **50**, 463–471.

10. Robinson, P.J., Bullen, A.W., Hall, R. *et al.* (1980) Splenic size and function in adult coeliac disease. *Clinical Science*, **53**, 532–537.

11. Trewby, P.N., Chipping, P.M., Palmer, S.J. *et al.* (1981) Splenic atrophy in adult coeliac disease: is it reversible? *Gut*, **22**, 628–632.

MOTILITY DISORDERS OF THE INTESTINE

M. Camilleri

INTRODUCTION

Motility disorders of the small intestine and colon are increasingly recognized as clinical syndromes characterized by acute, recurrent or chronic episodes suggestive of mechanical obstruction of the small bowel or colon. However, such episodes are unassociated with any intrinsic or extrinsic occlusion of the gut lumen. These disorders result from impairment of gut motility; they may be intrinsic to the neuromuscular apparatus of the gut, associated with disturbances of extrinsic neural control, accompany systemic diseases, or may result from the effects of medications. The manifestations in any patient are determined by the regions of the gastrointestinal tract affected, by the time-course of the disease, and by extraintestinal effects, such as bladder and ureteric dysfunction. Acute pseudo-obstruction syndromes tend to be associated with severe or catastrophic extraintestinal conditions, and the mechanisms resulting in disturbed gut motility are still largely unexplained. In contrast, chronic disturbances of the neuromuscular apparatus of the gut, whether familial or sporadic, are somewhat better understood and usually result in recurrent or chronic pseudo-obstruction.

In this section, the pathophysiology of disorders primarily affecting both small intestinal and colonic motility and the underlying diseases are discussed. *Table 3.26* summarizes disorders of gastrointestinal motility, and cross-references them to other sections of the book when they lie outside the scope of this chapter.

NORMAL GASTROINTESTINAL MOTOR FUNCTION

Normal gastrointestinal motor function is characterized by the occurrence of cyclical motor activity during the fasting state; postprandially, triturating, mixing and propulsive activity result in the aboral movement of chyme (*Figure 3.48*) The fasting phase is characterized by the interdigestive motor complex, which commences in the gastroduodenal region and propagates for a variable distance down the small bowel.[35] This cyclic activity consists of a period of quiescence (phase I); phase II exhibits intermittent phasic pressure activity (contractile activity that is unassociated with alterations in muscle tone); during the 'activity front', or phase III, there are regular, repetitive contractions at the maximal frequency typical for the locus (three per minute in the human antrum, up to 12 per minute in the human small bowel). The interdigestive motor complex propagates to the distal small bowel; it serves the role of a 'housekeeper', sweeping products of digestion and debris towards the colon. Similar, though less regular, cyclic motor activity occurs in the colon, although it has been well characterized only in the dog.[72] Postprandially, cyclical

Table 3.26   Diseases associated with abnormal small intestinal motility

Type	Comment	Cross-reference
Structural disorders		
Crohn's disease	Identifiable by contrast radiography;	p. 1141
Radiation enteritis	component of secondary	p. 688
Infiltrative disorders	neuromuscular dysfunction (e.g.	p. 591
Postgastric surgery	radiation plexus damage, vagotomy;	p. 290
Small bowel surgery	amyloid neuropathy or myopathy)	p. 666
Jeunal diverticulosis		
Irritable bowel syndrome		
Mucosal disease		
Celiac sprue	Rarely associated with motility disturbance	
Pseudo-obstruction	See *Table 3.27*	
Myopathic, neuropathic		
Acute, chronic		
Neurological disorders	See *Table 3.27*	
Endocrine/metabolic disorders		
Thyrotoxicosis	Direct hormonal effects on	p. 1307
Myxoedema	neuromuscular apparatus; secretory	p. 1308
Carcinoid	effects may alter transit; rarely	p. 643
Hypercalcaemia	associated with neuropathy (e.g.	p. 1303
Zollinger–Ellison syndrome	porphyria)	p. 1656
Vipoma		p. 1660
Somatostatinoma		p. 1662
Porphyrias		

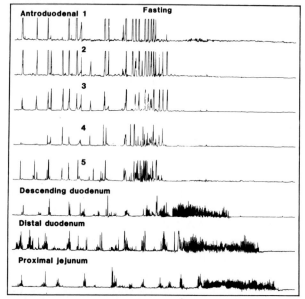
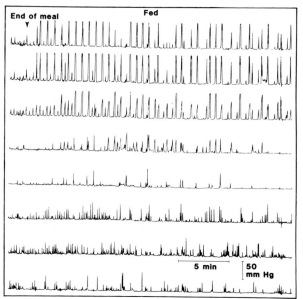

Figure 3.48   Normal manometric profile of the stomach and small bowel (fasting and postprandial). The migrating motor complex characteristic of the fasting state is demonstrated by presence of quiescence (phase I), intermittent activity (phase II), and an activity front (phase III). The postprandial pattern features high-amplitude, irregular, but persistent phasic pressure activity at all levels. (From Malagelada *et al.*[50])

motor activity disappears and gastric and small bowel contractions of variable amplitude occur fairly consistently, although irregularly. These contractions propagate for shorter distances and propel the contents less rapidly than the organized 'activity front' or phase III that occurs during fasting. Postprandial contractions facilitate the trituration (breakdown to a small particle size, on average less than 2 mm in diameter) of solid food in the stomach and the controlled propulsion of solids and liquids from the stomach and through the small bowel. The duration of the 'fed' pattern depends on the size and nutrient content of the meal.

Colonic motility is characterized by cyclical activity during fasting, intermittent irregular contractions, and mass movements. The latter are associated with giant migrating contractions that result in bolus expulsion during defaecation.

SMALL BOWEL MOTILITY: INTEGRATIVE PHYSIOLOGY IN HEALTH AND DISEASE

Some of the effects of deranged small bowel motility can be predicted from a simple understanding of flow dynamics in a hydraulic system. Thus, the motor function of the proximal small intestine is an important determinant of gastric emptying. Inadequate propulsion of chyme from the proximal small bowel (e.g. arising from motor incoordination in diseases such as diabetes mellitus or scleroderma) results in a resistance to flow from the stomach and a delay in gastric emptying.[18] Other characteristics of normal and/or abnormal motility reflect specific functions of certain regions. The propulsion of chyme from the ileum, through the ileocaecal sphincter, and into the right colon is facilitated by the generation of high-amplitude, prolonged and rapidly propagated contractions (*Figure 3.49*) or high-frequency peristaltic rushes that sweep through the region.[41] Such contractile events are rarely observed in the jejunum, presumably because some of the major roles of the jejunum are the mixing of digestive biliopancreatic juices with incoming, partially digested chyme, the transfer of chyme between relatively low-pressure systems, and aboral movement that is slow enough to allow for maximal absorption of nutrients.

The ileocolonic sphincter[64,67] serves as a watershed between the high bacterial counts of the colon and the ileum, with its specialized regional functions for absorption of vitamin B_{12} and bile acids, and its role in the salvage of nutrients not absorbed more proximally. Reflux of colonic contents, such as short-chain fatty acids, into the ileum likely results in the generation of powerful contractions[33] that effectively clear the small bowel of digestive residues and of any colonic contents that had refluxed into the small bowel.

CONTROL OF GASTROINTESTINAL MOTOR FUNCTION

Figure 3.50 summarizes the factors that control gastrointestinal motor function. Motility of the gut is dependent upon the contraction of smooth muscle cells, as mediated by the ion fluxes which alter the cell membrane potential and the contractile state of the cell. Contractions at the level of tissues are integrated and modulated by intrinsic (in the gut wall) or extrinsic nerves. The enteric or intrinsic

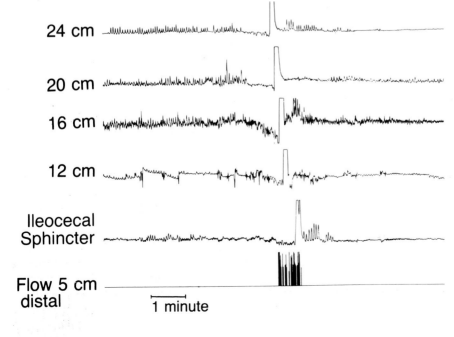

Figure 3.49 Ileal motility patterns in the dog showing a prolonged, propagated contraction and flow of fluid measured by a drop counter. (From Kruis *et al.*[41])

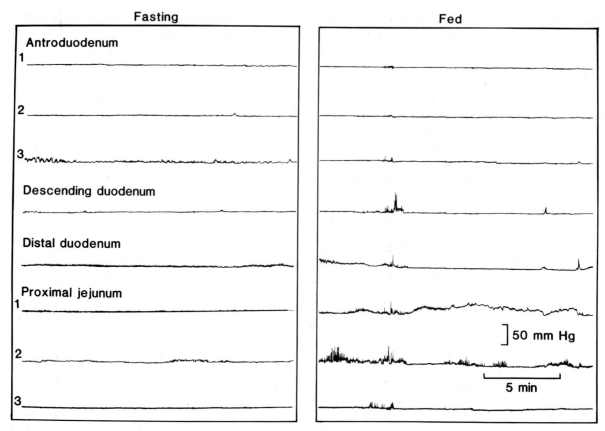

Figure 3.50 Manometric profile (fasting and postprandial) showing pronounced hypomotility in a 30-year-old man with hollow visceral myopathy. Eating causes no change in the featureless record. (From Colemont and Camilleri.[23])

nervous system is vast, and is estimated to contain 10^8 neurones, thus approximating the number of neurones in the spinal cord. It provides an intricate network of excitatory and inhibitory stimuli for the muscle. These stimuli are mediated by specific neurotransmitters (chiefly peptides). The enteric nervous system possesses considerable autonomy and plasticity in its responses to altered conditions (e.g. disease states), but it is also under presynaptic control by extrinsic neural elements. The key extrinsic inputs to the enteric neuromuscular apparatus are cranial (vagal) and sacral (S_2–S_4) parasympathetic nerves, and the thoracolumbar sympathetic outflow. Prevertebral sympathetic ganglia are important in the integration of afferent impulses from the periphery and in central control.[91] Derangements at any of these levels of control may result in abnormal small bowel or colonic motility.

ACUTE INTESTINAL PSEUDO-OBSTRUCTION

Acute intestinal pseudo-obstruction is most frequently encountered as an isolated colonic disturb-ance, usually arising in hospitalized patients as a complication of another, often major, illness, such as cardiac ischaemia, major surgery or trauma.[5] The condition was first described by Ogilvie[62] in 1948 in association with retroperitoneal diseases. In a litera-ture survey of 400 cases reported between 1970 and 1988,[92] the peak age incidence was shown to be in the sixth decade, and the condition was found to be more common in men. It is widely considered to be due to an unexplained disturbance of autonomic innervation of the distal colon. The clinical features are those of mechanical obstruction. The predomi-nant radiological features are evident on a plain abdominal radiograph:[92] gross colonic dilatation, scant air–fluid levels, a gradual transition to col-lapsed bowel, and a normal gas and faecal pattern in the rectum.[26] Barium enema is often recommended in doubtful cases to exclude distal obstruction; the advent of colonoscopic techniques for decompres-sion (see below) also provides the opportunity to prove the diagnosis.

Thus, diagnosis of acute colonic pseudo-obstruction is relatively easy, if suspected. The suc-cess of treatment is critically dependent on early recognition. If the caecal diameter is 12 cm or greater, or if conservative management (with nasogastric decompression, bowel rest, intravenous fluids and antibiotics) is unsuccessful, colonoscopic or operative decompression is indicated.[92] The mode of treatment, age of the patient, diameter of the caecum at the time of intervention, delay in decompression, and status of the bowel significantly influence the mortality rates. With early and appropriate management, the mortality rate is approximately 15%, compared to 36–44% in the presence of perforated or ischaemic bowel.[92]

In the treatment of acute colonic pseudo-obstruction, emphasis has shifted from the use of pharmacological agents (e.g. anticholinesterases such as neostigmine or the cholinergic agonist bethanechol) to the use of mechanical measures for decompression. The first therapeutic colonoscopic decompression was performed by Kukora and Dent,[42] and several series have since confirmed the general efficacy of such treatment. Thus, a 76–90% success rate was reported for acute decompression in those patients non-responsive to conservative treatment.[52,61] In some series, repeated colonoscopic decompression was necessary to allow restoration of normal colonic function.[52] Placement of a colonic decompression tube, which, on average, adds less than 10 minutes to the procedure of colonoscopy, reduces the need for repeated decompressions via colonoscopy;[29] patients with recurrent acute pseudo-obstruction have been successfully treated with a fenestrated colonoscopic overtube introduced transanally.[13] Colonoscopy may also facilitate the fashioning of a caecal fistula by means of percutaneous puncture of the colon and pull-through of a Pezzer catheter.[71] Intravenously administered cisapride has been reported to relieve acute colonic pseudo-obstruction without the need for colonoscopic decompression.[49]

The reversibility of Ogilvie's syndrome suggests that this motility disturbance is not associated with any permanent impairment of the control mechanisms. Indeed, there are other examples of transient disorders of the control of motility. Acute symptoms of nausea and vomiting, which commonly accompany viral gastroenteritis, may be related to gastroparesis, as manifested by delayed gastric emptying of liquids.[56] Idiopathic gastroparesis has been attributed to viral infections,[63] and a recurrent syndrome of cyclic nausea and vomiting, with gastroparesis, has been described.[2]

CHRONIC MOTILITY DISORDERS OF THE SMALL BOWEL

Gastrointestinal complaints of variable severity accompany a number of the diseases of muscle and nerve that are known to affect the gut; however, the spectrum of clinical syndromes is broad. There may be only a few symptoms in patients with dilatation of limited sections of the gut (e.g. megaduodenum) or uncomplicated postsurgical states. On the other hand, extensive involvement by pseudo-obstruction syndromes may result in life-threatening gut failure necessitating nutritional support, decompression or even surgery. Acute gastroenteritis and irritable bowel syndrome are associated with transient and/or subtle disturbances of small bowel motility; at this time, the consequences and responsible mechanisms are unclear. In general, the pathophysiology of abnormal bowel motility can be attributed to myopathic or neuropathic disorders, as the pathogenetic process affects either the smooth muscle directly or its (intrinsic or extrinsic) neural control.

STRUCTURAL DISEASES AND THEIR EFFECT ON SMALL BOWEL MOTILITY

Disturbances of proximal small bowel mobility are frequently observed in symptomatic patients following gastric surgery. Mathias et al.[54] demonstrated incoordinated phasic pressure waves in the Roux-limb after Roux-en-Y gastrectomy, and postulated that these were responsible for the nausea, vomiting and gastric stasis suffered by these patients. Dysfunction in the gastric remnant, which is usually extrinsically denervated, may also play a role in the symptomatology, for tonic contractile activity of the gastric remnant is deranged after vagotomy and partial gastric resection[8] and, in practice, further resection of the gastric remnant sometimes relieves the symptoms of upper gut stasis.[34]

Subacute mechanical obstruction often shows one of two contractile patterns of small bowel motility. Rhythmic, clustered contractions occur as a feature of partial obstruction postprandially, with each cluster lasting approximately 1 minute and each separated from the next cluster by an interval of 1–2 minutes.[14,89] However, these findings are non-specific, being also observed in patients with chronic intestinal pseudo-obstruction[89] and after ileal pouch–anal anastomosis.[87] In a series of patients with distal mechanical obstruction,[14] proximal small bowel manometry was characterized by simultaneous prolonged contractions (Figure 3.51) separated by periods of quiescence. The recognition of such contractile patterns during the evaluation of patients with chronic nausea, vomiting or abdominal pain necessitates the exclusion of mechanical obstruction by careful enteroclysis or even laparotomy.

Small bowel fistulae, diverticula and postsurgical blind loops are all associated with bacterial over-

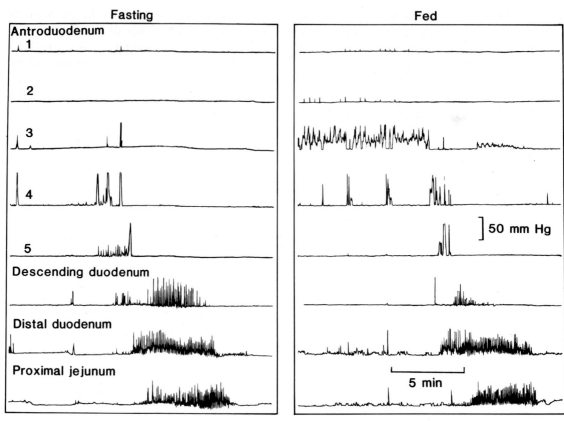

Figure 3.51 Neuropathic intestinal pseudo-obstruction due to diabetic autonomic neuropathy. Note the lack of distal antral contractions (fasting and postprandial), abnormal propagation of the phase III of the interdigestive migrating motor complex (left panel) and the failure of the solid–liquid meal to induce a fed pattern. (From Colemont and Camilleri.[23])

growth, but the pathogenic sequence is not always clear. Experimentally, bacterial toxins induce migrating action potential complexes in the rabbit ileum,[53] abnormal motility, rapid transit through the small bowel, diarrhoea and steatorrhoea. On the other hand, it has also been suggested that multiple jejunal diverticulosis may complicate abnormal neuromuscular function,[39] i.e. anatomical abnormalities of the small bowel may result from the effects of dysmotility. Thus, the more obvious sequence of bacterial overgrowth stemming directly from dysmotility[93] may not always be the case.

'SUPERIOR MESENTERIC ARTERY SYNDROME'

This symptom complex is characterized by nausea, vomiting, early satiety, postprandial bloating and epigastric discomfort, in association with dilatation of the C loop of the duodenum, and radiological evidence of an apparent narrowing of the lumen of the third portion of the duodenum by the superior mesenteric artery.

It occurs in two clinical settings. First, in the patient whose spine is immobilized and in whom

weight loss has been prominent. Such patients are thought to have true mechanical obstruction by the superior mesenteric artery. Second, the condition is considered in ambulant young women with recurrent vomiting and abdominal pain associated with dilatation of the proximal duodenum; the superior mesenteric artery appears to be responsible for partial mechanical obstruction, but it is presently thought that the latter condition is more likely a disorder of small bowel motility. The radiological 'obstruction' of the duodenum is due to dilatation that results from hypomotility or uncoordinated, ineffective contractions of the duodenal loop.

CHRONIC INTESTINAL PSEUDO-OBSTRUCTION

Chronic intestinal pseudo-obstruction is a rare heterogeneous clinical syndrome that is characterized by recurrent episodes of symptoms and signs of intestinal obstruction.[24,75,77,85] As implied in the definition, these symptoms occur in the absence of any mechanical obstruction in any of the organs affected. As with acute pseudo-obstruction, this condition is thought to result from impaired gut motility. The characteristic symptoms in this syndrome[84] are nausea, vomiting, abdominal distention, bloating, abdominal pain and an alteration in bowel movements (most typically, constipation). Weight loss and malnutrition may become prominent features in the more advances stages of the disorder.[84]

This syndrome may be associated with features that reflect the involvement of extraintestinal smooth muscle organs, such as the ureter and urinary bladder. The evolution of the disease and the regions of the gut affected determine the occurrence and variation of the clinical presentation. As the motility disturbances in chronic intestinal pseudo-obstruction are not restricted to the small intestine, but may affect every part of the gastrointestinal tract, the clinical manifestations may vary. Dysphagia and heartburn result from oesophageal involvement; nausea, vomiting, bloating, distention and abdominal discomfort result from involvement of the stomach or small bowel; and colonic involvement leads to distention and constipation. The heterogeneous character of the syndrome is well illustrated by the fact that 4 of 42 patients with idiopathic chronic intestinal pseudo-obstruction studied at the Mayo Clinic[84] had previously undergone colectomy for constipation. In addition, almost half of the young female patients with severe idiopathic constipation in some series had evidence of oesophageal, gastric or small bowel dysmotility, disturbances noted either at the time of colectomy or subsequently.[45,66] Other localized variants of chronic intestinal pseudo-obstruction include megaduodenum and the 'superior mesenteric artery' syndrome (see above), and selective left colonic pseudo-obstruction, which is discussed below.

Pathophysiological types

Chronic intestinal pseudo-obstruction may be due to a variety of underlying diseases (*Table 3.27*).[17,23] In

Table 3.27 Categories of chronic intestinal pseudo-obstruction

Type	Myopathic	Neuropathic	Comments
I. Familial	Familial visceral myopathies (autosomal dominant or recessive)	Familial visceral neuropathies, von Recklinghausen's disease	Rare disorders, usually present in the neonatal period or childhood; neurofibromata may also cause mechanical obstruction
II. Sporadic Infiltrative	Progressive systemic sclerosis	Early progressive systemic sclerosis	Manometry essential to differentiate pathophysiology
General neurological disease	Amyloidosis Myotonic and other dystrophies	Amyloidosis Diabetes, porphyria, brain-stem tumour, multiple sclerosis, spinal cord transection, dysautonomias	Reviewed by Camilleri[15]
Infectious	—	Chagas' disease, cytomegalovirus	Non-specific 'postviral' causes appear common
Drug induced	—	Tricyclic antidepressants, narcotics, anticholinergics, antihypertensives, vincristine, laxative abuse	Exclusion of drug side-effects essential in all patients
Neoplastic	—	Paraneoplastic (bronchial small cell carcinoma)	May require chest CT scan to exclude bronchial carcinoma if chest radiograph is negative
Idiopathic	Non-familial hollow visceral myopathy	Hirschsprung's disease, chronic idiopathic intestinal pseudo-obstruction	Variable manifestations and severity in chronic idiopathic intestinal pseudo-obstruction

clinical practice, identification of the underlying disease process, such as scleroderma or diabetes mellitus, may be all that is necessary to diagnose its associated gut dysmotility. For those patients in whom the aetiology is not immediately apparent, the most practical approach addresses the pathophysiology of the motility disturbance. The pathophysiological features of these disease processes can be broadly subdivided into: (1) a myopathic variety (e.g. scleroderma, amyloidosis or hollow visceral myopathy); and (2) a neuropathic variety (including the 'idiopathic' variant which is thought to result from a disorder of the myenteric plexus). Patterns of gastric and small bowel motility in health (*Figure 3.48*) are easily identifiable and provide the basis for assessing the pathophysiological type of chronic pseudo-obstruction. The myopathic variant is characterized by low-amplitude pressure activity in the affected segments (*Figure 3.50*), whereas the neuropathic type tends to produce excessive or uncoordinated manometric profiles of the small bowel (*Figure 3.51*).[50] Similar features have also been noted in dysmotilities of the oesophagus; low-amplitude pressure waves in myopathic processes, motor incoordination in neuropathic disorders. Some conditions, such as amyloidosis and, less commonly, scleroderma,[27] seem to evoke a neuropathic pattern initially, followed by a myopathic one.

Elicitation of the pathophysiological nature or the motility disorder leads to a logical approach to the diagnosis of the underlying disease process. In eliciting the history, symptoms suggesting an underlying disease process should be sought: for example, postural dizziness, visual disturbances, and sweating abnormalities are indicative of an autonomic neuropathy, and urinary symptoms suggest genitourinary involvement by a generalized visceral neuromyopathic disorder. The family history is particularly relevant in myopathic pseudo-obstruction and suggests a congenital disorder. Patients should also be questioned about the use of anticholinergic drugs, phenothiazines, antihypertensive agents such as clonidine, and tricyclic antidepressants. Physical examination should include a neurological assessment, including pupillary examination, measurement of blood pressure with the patient both in supine and standing positions, and a search for abdominal distension or a succussion splash.

Identification of the neuropathic variant of pseudo-obstruction necessitates a more detailed search for the underlying cause.[15] The aetiological factor may be a disturbance in the extrinsic neural supply (for example, a brain tumour or autonomic neuropathy) or a disorder of the intrinsic or enteric nervous system (for example, idiopathic or paraneoplastic chronic intestinal pseudo-obstruction). The extrinsic neural supply may be assessed by

structural examinations (such as computed tomography (CT) scanning or magnetic resonance imaging (MRI) of the brain) or non-invasive tests of autonomic function (such as pharmacological tests of the pupils, the thermoregulatory sweat test, screening of autonomic reflexes, the plasma pancreatic polypeptide response to hypoglycaemia or sham feeding, and plasma noradrenaline levels after intravenous edrophonium).[15] Such studies may help to identify the level at which the neural supply is deranged, and application of these tests in the diagnosis of motility disorders is discussed more fully elsewhere.[15] This information may lead to the identification of a potentially treatable lesion, e.g. a tumour of the posterior cranial fossa.[99]

Identification of a myopathic variant of pseudo-obstruction should lead to a more thorough family history, fat or rectal biopsy to look for amyloid and infiltrative disorders such as scleroderma, or search for a generalized muscle disease.[15]

Disorders of the enteric nervous system are suspected when manometrically confirmed neuropathic chronic intestinal pseudo-obstruction is unassociated with a demonstrable lesion in the extrinsic neural supply. The classic example of an enteric or intrinsic nervous system disorder is Hirschsprung's disease,[24] in which a localized aganglionosis results in significant abnormalities in motor function, dilatation of the bowel and impairment of colonic transit proximal to the obstructed segment. This is also the best example of a condition with a clear-cut morphological lesion. To date, histological studies of the myenteric plexus in other patients with gastrointestinal motility disturbances have been predominantly based on light microscopy or silver staining techniques.[40] These methods have demonstrated either neuronal intranuclear inclusions, reductions in the number of ganglion cells and replacement by glial cells, inflammatory cell infiltration of the enteric plexus ganglia, or abnormalities in the neuronal process (dendritic or axonal). Immunohistochemical studies revealed no significant abnormalities in gut neuropeptides in severe idiopathic constipation in one study,[68] and the presence of abnormal vasoactive intestinal polypeptide and substance P in the muscularis layer in another study.[38] Apart from the indirect study of myoelectric activity under baseline conditions and in response to neostigmine,[88] no methods can evaluate adequately the function of the myenteric plexus before resection of a full-thickness segment of the affected bowel.

Diagnosis of chronic intestinal pseudo-obstruction

The diagnosis of chronic intestinal pseudo-obstruction is dependent first on recognition of the clinical syndrome, and exclusion of mechanical obstruction or mucosal disease of the gastro-intestinal tract by radiological or endoscopic assessment. In a referral practice, the patient has often undergone exploratory laparotomy before the diagnosis is considered. The greatest diagnostic difficulties presented by chronic intestinal pseudo-obstruction are: (1) the lack of specificity of the clinical features and the absence of diagnostic radiological tests; and (2) overlap with the symptoms and signs of other so-called functional syndromes, such as non-ulcer dyspepsia, irritable bowel syndrome, and chronic idiopathic constipation. In the last condition, some data suggest that histological abnormalities of the colonic myenteric plexus are uniformly present;[45] other studies show no abnormalities.[68] The clinical features detailed above must be carefully sought in evaluating each patient.

Radiological studies

The most important role of radiology in the diagnosis of chronic intestinal pseudo-obstruction is in the exclusion of mechanical obstruction. The radiological findings in patients with this syndrome depend on the anatomical regions affected, and may suggest whether the disorder is due to a neuropathy or a myopathy. Rohrmann et al.[70] reported that visceral myopathy is typified by pronounced duodenal enlargement, lack of haustration, increased colonic calibre and poor-to-absent contractions. On the other hand, visceral neuropathy is mainly characterized by disordered smooth muscle contractility, which is best appreciated on fluoroscopy. Progressive systemic sclerosis, which results in close approximation of the valvulae conniventes in the small bowel and wide-mouthed sacculations in the colon, is most specific. Dilatation of the small intestine is a non-specific feature of all types of chronic intestinal pseudo-obstruction.

In the group of 42 patients with chronic intestinal pseudo-obstruction studied by Rohrmann et al.,[70] some patients had findings of paralytic ileus on plain abdominal film; whereas many others had radiological findings that mimicked true mechanical obstruction. In a minority of patients, dilatation of other smooth muscle viscera, such as the renal pelvis, ureters or urinary bladder, is identified.[84] Small bowel dilatation is not invariably found, suggesting that this may be a manifestation of more advanced disease.[84]

Other radiological studies may be indicated to discover the aetiology of the syndrome. These include brain CT or MRI in patients with neuropathic chronic intestinal pseudo-obstruction in whom autonomic function tests suggest an extrinsic autonomic neuropathy,[15] or chest radiographs and CT scans in heavy smokers or others with risk factors for lung cancer.[83]

Histological analysis

Currently, investigators generally agree that a full-thickness biopsy specimen of the small bowel obtained during laparotomy should be part of the diagnostic work-up of patients with chronic intestinal pseudo-obstruction. This approach may enable the pathologist to identify the neuropathic (myenteric plexus) or myopathic (smooth muscle) abnormalities that might be of pathogenetic importance. Histological sections should include transversely cut paraffin sections stained with haematoxylin and eosin, as well as thicker and larger sections cut in the plane of the myenteric plexus. To date, most published studies have used Smith's silver staining technique.

Krishnamurthy and Schuffler[40] extensively reviewed the histopathological findings in full-thickness biopsy sections of the small intestine and colon in patients with a large variety of neuromuscular disorders. In other studies, histological evaluation of full-thickness biopsies has not provided a clear-cut diagnosis of the disorder of motor function. For example, cases are described where the histological features cannot distinguish between systemic sclerosis and visceral myopathy,[31,96] and the histological changes in familial visceral myopathy can be quite variable.[25] In a number of series in adults[48] and children,[30] a significant number of tissue specimens show no specific neural or muscular morphological abnormality. Finally, in selected patients, rectal biopsy may be of value when the diagnosis of intestinal neuronal dysplasia is considered.[3] Such an approach would clearly be advantageous. Further characterization of the histopathological features and development of immunohistochemical techniques for the study of peptidergic innervation may provide further insights into the diagnosis and pathogenetic mechanisms in chronic intestinal pseudo-obstruction.

Motility studies

Qualitative analysis of small bowel manometric studies[84] may provide complementary evidence of a motility disorder in the small bowel, which is a region of the gut that seems to be most frequently involved in chronic pseudo-obstruction syndromes. Patterns of gastric and small bowel motility in health are easily identifiable and provide the basis for identification of dysmotility in disease states.[23,50] This information is more specific than the abnormalities of oesophageal motility and anorectal sphincter responses to rectal distention that were previously reported in such patients.[75,77] In fact, patients with pseudo-obstruction in the pediatric age group usually show a normal rectoanal inhibitory reflex. Thus, small bowel motility should be assessed when the predominant clinical features suggest small bowel disturbances.[50] The abnormalities of small bowel motility are similar in pediatric and adult patients and include aberrant configuration or propagation of phase III of the interdigestive migrating motor complex, sustained uncoordinated pressure activity, intense bursts of phasic pressure activity, and the inability of a meal to induce a fed pattern or to interrupt cyclical interdigestive motor activity.[50,84] A study of 42 patients with idiopathic chronic intestinal pseudo-obstruction demonstrated that at least two such manometric abnormalities were found in 36 patients.[84]

Until more specific and less invasive histological or electrophysiological assessments of bowel specimens are developed to provide diagnostic evidence of chronic intestinal pseudo-obstruction, manometry is necessary to confirm the clinical impression of pseudo-obstruction, after excluding the possibility of mechanical obstruction by radiological and/or endoscopic methods. Such a strategy avoids the dilemma frequently facing the clinician during subsequent episodes of pseudo-obstruction; these are often mistaken for postoperative mechanical obstruction and can lead to a further, possibly unnecessary, laparotomy. Tests of autonomic function[15] help to determine whether an associated underlying disease, especially one that might be treatable, could be responsible for the patient's problem, and may also provide insights on the mechanisms causing dysfunction in patients with functional gastrointestinal motility disorders.[10,16,95] Changes in colorectal function[48] in chronic colonic pseudo-obstruction include decreased motility and increased rectal wall elasticity.

Gastrointestinal transit

Mouth-to-caecum transit of solids and liquids, and transit of a solid radiolabel (^{131}I-labelled fibre) through the small bowel, are significantly prolonged. Gastric emptying of solids is also delayed in chronic intestinal pseudo-obstruction. In addition, the ileocolonic transfer of radiolabelled solid 1 mm resin pellets occurs less frequently and less efficiently in patients with myopathic pseudo-obstruction than in those with neuropathic disorders and healthy controls.[28] These and other non-invasive methods may help assess motor dysfunction in the more inaccessible segments of bowel.

Localized forms of pseudo-obstruction

There are numerous reports of localized forms of chronic pseudo-obstruction, usually those affecting the entire colon[45] or the duodenal loop[22] in the 'superior mesenteric artery syndrome'. Surgical treatment is sometimes justifiable and efficacious in localized forms of pseudo-obstruction, particularly when the colon is affected. The report of a selective left colonic pseudo-obstruction is intriguing,[90] particularly since a subgroup of patients with severe idiopathic constipation has selective delays in transit in the left colon.[21,86] Confirmation of these findings may lead to novel approaches to treatment such as more restrictive surgery of the left colon, which has been successful in at least one case.[90] Prolonged follow-up of such patients will be necessary to determine whether or not other regions of the colon become affected later.

Pseudo-obstruction in the pediatric age group

In a survey conducted by members of the North American Society of Pediatric Gastroenterology and Nutrition,[94] 87 pediatric patients were identified; 19 of these had symptoms at birth, and 37 (43%) within the first month of life. This survey excluded Hirschsprung's disease, which should always be considered in the differential diagnosis of abnormal colonic motility or distention in the pediatric age group. Sixty-four per cent of pediatric pseudo-obstruction patients were diagnosed by the first year of life. The predominant clinical features were distention (80%), vomiting and constipation (both 57%), diarrhoea and failure to thrive (23%), and urinary tract abnormalities and failure to void (12%). Diagnosis was established by clinical features, radiology and laparotomy. Oesophageal manometry was abnormal in all 14 patients in whom it was performed. Anorectal manometry was generally unhelpful, being abnormal in only 1 of 16 patients studied. Full-thickness biopsies of the intestine were abnormal in 12 cases (8 with plexus disorders, 4 with muscle degeneration) reported in this series. However, 22 other miscellaneous gut biopsies were non-contributory. Among the group with adequate follow-up, 31.4% died, almost half the deaths being attributed to complications of central parenteral nutrition within the first 6 months of starting treatment.

While this retrospective experience is the most comprehensive information available about pediatric pseudo-obstruction, specific reports highlight other features. Hyman et al.[30] found qualitative abnormalities in the patterns of antroduodenal pressure profiles in all 13 of their patients, and those features were similar to the abnormalities reported in adults.[84] Pathological abnormalities were only detected in 4 of 7 full-thickness intestinal biopsy specimens.[50] The histological features in visceral neuropathy and myopathy were essentially similar to those reported in subtypes of pseudo-obstruction in adults.[79] In the pediatric age group, the underlying disease processes that result in pseudo-obstruction also include conditions that are specifically manifested in that age group, such as Kawasaki disease (or mucocutaneous lymph node syndrome)[59] and Duchenne's dystrophy.[45] The familial forms of pseudo-obstruction are more frequently evident in the pediatric age group than in adults; thus, of 87 cases in the North American pediatric group series,[94] 15 cases were familial (three with dominant inheritance).

Neonatal pseudo-obstruction rarely occurs alone, and is more often found in association with other anomalies requiring surgical correction; these include gastroschisis, duodenal atresia, or megacystis.[9] Uncoordinated intestinal motility can be noted radiographically[9] or by small intestinal manometry.[9] Manometric abnormalities must be differentiated from those 'dysmotilities' observed as part of the normal developmental process.[11,57] Anorectal manometry and histology of intestinal biopsies are generally unhelpful.[9] Prokinetic medications are usually ineffective, and many patients require parenteral nutrition and bowel decompression, including gastrostomies or enterostomies.

Treatment of chronic intestinal pseudo-obstruction

The goals of treatment of chronic intestinal pseudo-obstruction are the restoration of normal intestinal propulsion and adequate nutrition,[75,77] and treatment of complications such as bacterial overgrowth. Similarly, the goal of treatment in severe idiopathic constipation or chronic colonic pseudo-obstruction is the restoration of normal colonic propulsion and bowel movements.

Nutritional support

The physical nature of food can be important in the delivery of oral nutrients for the absorption by the intestine, especially if gastric emptying is impaired; thus, food processed in a blender or liquid food is tolerated better. Other dietary measures include the use of a low-lactose, low-fibre polypeptide or hydrolysed protein diet with multivitamins and specific supplementation with iron, folate, calcium and vitamins D, K and B_{12}. With these manipulations, only a minority of patients will be controlled adequately, usually those with mild to moderate symptoms.[75] Supplementation of oral nutrition with a liquid caloric and protein-rich formula is necessary in more severe cases. Deficiencies of trace elements and vitamins should be sought and corrected in patients with chronic intestinal pseudo-obstruction.

Many patients with chronic intestinal pseudo-obstruction ultimately require home central parenteral nutrition because dietary and medical treatments are generally ineffective and surgical intervention is indicated in only a few selected cases. In the author's experience, supplementation with a liquid formula administered orally or enterally, or central parenteral nutrition, are the mainstays of treatment for patients with myopathic pseudo-obstruction in whom prokinetic agents are unlikely to prove beneficial. Central parenteral nutrition is successful in maintaining the patient's weight and reversing trace element and vitamin deficiencies.[32] However, treatment is associated with significant morbidity and mortality and is costly. During a 10-year period, 4 of 10 infants with neonatal intestinal pseudo-obstruction in one series had died, two of sepsis and two of hepatic failure related to central parenteral nutrition.[98] Among 10 adults receiving home parenteral nutrition with a maximal follow-up of 5 years, four required reinsertion of their lines, three for catheter sepsis and septicaemia; one developed immune complex glomerulonephritis and another thrombosed the superior vena cava preterminally.[98]

Nevertheless, these potentially diastrous complications have to be accepted since the prognosis of patients with severe forms of chronic intestinal pseudo-obstruction, particularly the myopathic variants, is poor. In one study,[7] 5 of 8 young children with chronic intestinal pseudo-obstruction had died at the time of the report, although the duration of the follow-up was unclear. Less severely affected persons often suffer considerable morbidity and require repeated hospitalizations for intravenous administration of fluids, nasogastric decompression and a range of nutritional supplementations.

Bacterial overgrowth

Treatment of bacterial overgrowth and secondary fat malabsorption with broad-spectrum antibiotics has only been successful in a small number of patients.[37] In patients with demonstrated steatorrhoea, antibiotics are given on a rotational basis for 7–10 days each month. Commonly used antibiotics are co-trimoxazole, amoxycillin, ciprofloxacin and metronidazole. Very preliminary data in a small number of patients suggest that the motilin agonist erythromycin may be effective in patients with a neuropathic form of chronic intestinal pseudo-obstruction.[58]

Pharmacological agents

Cholinergic agents, including metoclopramide, have been ineffective in the treatment of patients with chronic intestinal pseudo-obstruction. Investigators at the Mayo Clinic[51] were among the first to use cholinergics in patients with pseudo-

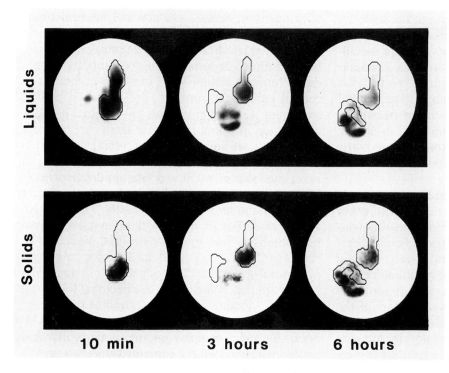

Figure 3.52 Transit of radiolabelled solids and liquids in a patient with chronic (neuropathic) intestinal pseudo-obstruction. Note the prolonged retention of both phases of the meal in the stomach and small bowel. Upper outline depicts stomach, lower outline depicts right side of colon on 3 and 6 hour scans. (From Camilleri *et al.*[19])

obstruction, in five of whom sweating was also abnormal. Intravenous administration of neostigmine had no effect on small bowel motility but, in two patients, the colonic motor response to neostigmine was reported to be normal. A trial of an orally administered cholinergic agonist was unsuccessful in three patients. Sullivan *et al.*[88] reported an increase in colonic spike activity after intravenous administration of neostigmine. Metoclopramide has been used in the treatment of familial visceral myopathy,[24] idiopathic chronic intestinal pseudo-obstruction[46,47] and scleroderma,[77] but its overall efficacy has been disappointing.

Anecdotal reports have suggested that other drugs may be beneficial in restoring the disturbed gastrointestinal motility in patients with chronic intestinal pseudo-obstruction. Subcutaneous naloxone resulted in an increase in gastric emptying of solids and a decrease of small intestinal transit time in a patient with chronic intestinal pseudo-obstruction who had not improved significantly after total colectomy.[74] In two brothers with chronic intestinal pseudo-obstruction, intravenously administered neostigmine or cholecystokinin normalized intestinal activity, as judged by cinematography.[43] Intravenous administration of a trimebutine, a peripheral opiate agonist, induced phase III-like activity (propagated in two cases) in four children with chronic intestinal pseudo-obstruction. Signs of peristalsis were present in one patient.[12] The preliminary experience with erythromycin is mentioned above. Further controlled trials of these agents are necessary to assess their clinical efficacy.

Cisapride, a gastrointestinal non-dopaminergic, non-cholinergic prokinetic drug with serotonin type 4 receptor agonist effects, has been shown to enhance the release of acetylcholine from the myenteric nerve endings in the digestive tract.[80] Because of its selective action on the gut, cisapride is devoid of the systemic side-effects that frequently occur with other cholinergic agonists (such as bethanechol) and inhibitors of acetylcholinesterase (such as neostigmine). In patients with chronic intestinal pseudo-obstruction, cisapride was effective in reducing the delayed intestinal transit time[19] to within the normal range (*Figure 3.52*) Given acutely orally or for up to 6 weeks,[20] cisapride has been shown to correct impaired propulsion in the stomach and small bowel of patients with chronic intestinal pseudo-obstruction. Its long-term beneficial effect on symptoms is less clearly demonstrable;[1] hence, studies of clinical efficacy are awaited.

Surgical treatment

Surgical bypass of affected segments might be beneficial in highly selected patients. Schuffler and Deitch[76] reviewed 73 operations performed on 12 patients with chronic intestinal pseudo-obstruction. Some procedures were not helpful (e.g. gastrojejunostomy and resection of the small bowel); others were beneficial when a short segment of the bowel was involved (e.g. side-to-side duodenojejunostomy for megaduodenum or colectomy for colonic pseudo-obstruction). As already indicated, in planning surgical treatment for these patients it is important to remember that chronic intestinal pseudo-obstruction may be a generalized process.[45,84] In patients with familial visceral myopathy, Anuras *et al.*[6] reported variable results from duodeno-jejunostomy for megaduodenum. They recommended preoperative aerobic and anaerobic cultures of duodenal aspirates and treatment of any bacterial overgrowth. Sometimes, intractable and incapacitating symptoms may necessitate radical resection of the small bowel;[78] even enterectomy has been advocated.[60]

Venting

A venting enterostomy creates an effective means of relieving gaseous distention and bloating, thereby providing symptomatic relief for patients treated with central total parenteral nutrition.[65] Venting can reduce, by a factor of 6, the need for nasogastric intubation and repetitive hospitalization for the 'obstructive' episodes commonly encountered in these patients.[65] The efficacy of a venting enterostomy alone or in combination with a prokinetic agent is currently being investigated. Venting decompresses the small intestine in patients with myopathic pseudo-obstruction, and sometimes restores smooth muscle contractility and the ability to handle enteral nutrition.

Experimental treatments

Electrical pacing and small bowel transplantation[36] are possible future remedies for patients with severe forms of chronic intestinal pseudo-obstruction – particularly the myopathic variant, which is less likely to respond to prokinetic medications. Recent studies have been more successful in achieving capture and entrainment of jejunal pacesetter potentials (K. A. Kelly, personal communication), contrary to earlier studies that suggested that pacing would prove more difficult in humans than in experimental animals.[69] The motor and absorptive behaviour of the transplanted small intestine is also subject to continuing investigations.[73] Whereas the extrinsically denervated autotransplant can assume many normal absorptive, secretory and motor functions, future studies will need to explore such functions when episodes of infection or immunological rejection are superimposed, particularly in view of the increasing evidence of interactions between infection and immunocompetent cells, and the neuromuscular apparatus in the intestine.[4,81,82,97]

REFERENCES

1. Abell, T.L., Camilleri, M., DiMagno, E.P., Hench, V.S. and Malagelada, J.-R. (1987) Cisapride is effective in the long-term treatment of gastric motor disorders. *Gastroenterology*, **92**, 1287.

2. Abell, T.L., Kim, C.H. and Malagelada, J.-R. (1988) Idiopathic cyclic nausea and vomiting: a gastrointestinal motility disorder? *Mayo Clinic Proceedings*, **63**, 1169–1175.

3. Achem, S.R., Owyang, C., Schuffler, M.D. and Dobbins, W.O., III (1987) Neuronal dysplasia and chronic intestinal pseudo-obstruction: rectal biopsy as a possible aid to diagnosis. *Gastroenterology*, **92**, 805–809.

4. Alizadeh, H., Weems, W.A. and Castro, G.A. (1989) Long-term influence of enteric infection on jejunal propulsion in guinea pigs. *Gastroenterology*, **97**, 1461–1468.

5. Anuras, S. and Baker, C.R., Jr (1986) The colon in the pseudoobstruction syndrome. *Clinical Gastroenterology*, **15**, 745–762.

6. Anuras, S., Shirazi, S., Faulk, D.L., Gardner, G.D. and Christensen, J. (1979) Surgical treatment in familial visceral myopathy. *Annals of Surgery*, **189**, 306–310.

7. Anuras, S., Mitros, F.A., Soper, R.T., Pringle, K.C., Maves, B.V., Younoszai, M.K., Franken, E.A., Jr and Whitington, P. (1986) Chronic intestinal pseudo-obstruction in young children. *Gastroenterology*, **91**, 62–70.

8. Azpiroz, F. and Malagelada, J.-R. (1987) Gastric tone measured by an electronic barostat in health and postsurgical gastroparesis. *Gastroenterology*, **92**, 934–943.

9. Bagwell, C.E., Filler, R.M., Cutz, E., Stringer, D., Ein, S.H., Shandling, B., Stephens, C.A. and Wesson, D.E. (1984) Neonatal intestinal pseudoobstruction. *Journal of Pediatric Surgery*, **19**, 732–739.

10. Balm, R., Zinsmeister, A., Greydanus, M., Nelson, D., Walker, D., Low, P. and Camilleri, M. (1990) Visceral dysautonomia in a subset of patients with idiopathic chronic intestinal pseudo-obstruction. *Gastroenterology*, **98**, A324.

11. Bissett, W.M., Watt, J., Rivers, R. and Milla, P.J. (1988) The ontogeny of fasting small intestinal motor activity in the human infant. *Gut*, **29**, 482–488.

12. Boige, N., Cargill, G., Mashako, L., Cezard, J.P. and Navarro, J. (1987) Trimebutine-induced phase III-like activity in infants with intestinal motility disorders. *Journal of Pediatric Gastroenterology and Nutrition*, **6**, 548–553.

13. Burke, G. and Shellito, P.C. (1987) Treatment of recurrent colonic pseudo-obstruction by endoscopic placement of a fenestrated overtube. Report of a case. *Diseases of the Colon and Rectum*, **30**, 615–619.

14. Camilleri, M. (1989) Jejunal manometry in distal subacute mechanical obstruction: significance of prolonged simultaneous contractions. *Gut*, **30**, 468–475.

15. Camilleri, M. (1990) Disorders of gastrointestinal motility in neurologic diseases. *Mayo Clinic Proceedings*, **65**, 825–846.

16. Camilleri, M. and Fealey, R.D. (1990) Idiopathic

autonomic denervation in eight patients presenting with functional gastrointestinal disease: a causal association? *Digestive Diseases and Sciences*, **35**, 609–616.

17. Camilleri, M. and Phillips, S. F. (1989). Disorders of small intestinal motility. *Gastroenterology Clinics of North America*, 405–424.

18. Camilleri, M., Brown, M.L. and Malagelada, J.-R. (1986) Relationship between impaired gastric emptying and abnormal gastrointestinal motility. *Gastroenterology*, **91**, 94–99.

19. Camilleri, M., Brown, M.L. and Malagelada, J.-R. (1986) Impaired transit of chyme in chronic intestinal pseudoobstruction: correction by cisapride. *Gastroenterology*, **91**, 619–626.

20. Camilleri, M., Malagelada, J.-R., Abell, T.L., Brown, M.L., Hench, V. and Zinsmeister, A. R. (1989) Effect of six weeks of treatment with cisapride in gastroparesis and intestinal pseudoobstruction. *Gastroenterology*, **96**, 704–712.

21. Chaussade, S., Khyari, A., Roche, H., Garret, M., Gaudric, M., Couturier, D. and Guerre, J. (1989) Determination of total and segmental colonic transit time in constipated patients. *Digestive Diseases and Sciences*, **34**, 1168–1172.

22. Cohen, L.B., Field, S.P. and Sachar, D.B. (1985) The superior mesenteric artery syndrome. The disease that isn't, or is it? *Journal of Clinical Gastroenterology*, **7**, 113–116.

23. Colemont, L. and Camilleri, M. (1989) Chronic intestinal pseudoobstruction: diagnosis and treatment. *Mayo Clinic Proceedings*, **64**, 60–70.

24. Faulk, D.L., Anuras, S. and Christensen, J. (1978) Chronic intestinal pseudoobstruction. *Gastroenterology*, **74**, 922–931.

25. Fitzgibbons, P.L. and Chandrasoma, P.T. (1987) Familial visceral myopathy. Evidence of diffuse involvement of intestinal smooth muscle. *American Journal of Surgical Pathology*, **11**, 846–854.

26. Gilchrist, A.M., Mills, J.O. and Russell, C.G. (1985) Acute large bowel pseudoobstruction. *Clinical Radiology*, **36**, 401–404.

27. Greydanus, M.P. and Camilleri, M. (1989) Abnormal postcibal antral and small bowel motility due to neuropathy or myopathy in systemic sclerosis. *Gastroenterology*, **96**, 110–115.

28. Greydanus, M.P., Camilleri, M., Colemont, L.J., Phillips, S.F., Brown, M.L. and Thomforde, G.M. (1990) Ileocolonic transfer of solid chyme in small intestinal neuropathies and myopathies. *Gastroenterology*, **99**, 158–164.

29. Harig, J.M., Fumo, D.E., Loo, F.D., Parker, H.J., Soergel, K.H., Helm, J.F. and Hogan, W.J. (1988) Treatment of acute nontoxic megacolon during colonoscopy: tube placement versus simple decompression. *Gastrointestinal Endoscopy*, **34**, 23–27.

30. Hyman, P.E., McDiarmid, S.V., Napolitano, J., Abrams, C.E. and Tomomasa, T. (1988) Antroduodenal motility in children with chronic intestinal pseudo-obstruction. *Journal of Pediatrics*, **112**, 899–905.

31. Jayachandar, J., Frank, J.L. and Jonas, M.M. (1988) Isolated intestinal myopathy resembling progressive systemic sclerosis in a child. *Gastroenterology*, **95**, 1114–1118.

32. Kadowaki, H., Ouchi, M., Kaga, M., Motegi, T., Yanagawa, Y., Hayakawa, H., Hashimoto, G. and Furuya, K. (1987) Problems of trace elements and vitamins during long-term total parenteral nutrition: a case report of idiopathic intestinal pseudo-obstruction. *Journal of Parenteral and Enteral Nutrition*, **11**, 322–325.

33. Kamath, P.K., Hoepfner, M.T. and Phillips, S.F. (1987) Short-chain fatty acids stimulate motility of the canine ileum. *American Journal of Physiology*, **253**, G427–G433.

34. Karlstrom, L. and Kelly, K.A. (1989) Roux-Y gastrectomy for chronic gastric atony. *American Journal of Surgery*, **157**, 44–49.

35. Kellow, J.E., Borody, T.J., Phillips, S.F., Tucker, R.L. and Haddad, A.C. (1986) Human interdigestive motility: variations in patterns from esophagus to colon. *Gastroenterology*, **91**, 386–395.

36. Kelly, K.A. (1984) Pacing the gut: possible clinicial applications. In: *Advances in Gastrointestinal Surgery*, pp. 345–356 (Eds) Najarian, J.S. and Delaney, J.P. Chicago: Year Book.

37. Keshavarzian, A., Isaacs, P., McColl, I. and Sladen, G.E. (1983) Idiopathic intestinal pseudo-obstruction and contaminated small bowel syndrome – treatment with metronidazole, ileostomy, and indomethacin. *American Journal of Gastroenterology*, **78**, 562–565.

38. Koch, T.R., Carney, J.A., Go, L. and Go, V.L.W. (1988) Idiopathic chronic constipation is associated with decreased colonic vasoactive intestinal peptide. *Gastroenterology*, **94**, 300–310.

39. Krishnamurthy, S. and Schuffler, M.D. (1987) Pathology of neuromuscular disorders of the small intestine and colon. *Gastroenterology*, **93**, 610–639.

40. Krishnamurthy, S., Kelly, M.M., Rohrmann, C.A. and Schuffler, M.D. (1983) Jejunal diverticulosis: a heterogeneous disorder caused by a variety of abnormalities of smooth muscle or myenteric plexus. *Gastroenterology*, **85**, 538–547.

41. Kruis, W., Azpiroz, F. and Phillips, S.F. (1985) Contractile patterns and transit of fluid in canine terminal ileum. *American Journal of Physiology*, **249**, G264–G270.

42. Kukora, J.S. and Dent, T.L. (1977) Colonoscopic decompression of massive nonobstructive cecal dilation. *Archives of Surgery*, **112**, 512–517.

43. Laustsen, J., Harling, H. and Fallingborg, J. (1987) Treatment of chronic idiopathic intestinal pseudoobstruction. *Digestive Diseases and Sciences*, **32**, 222–223.

44. Leon, S.H., Schuffler, M.D., Kettler, M. and Rohrmann, C.A. (1986) Chronic intestinal pseudoobstruction as a complication of Duchenne's muscular dystrophy. *Gastroenterology*, **90**, 455–459.

45. Leon, S.H., Krishnamurthy, S. and Schuffler, M.D. (1987) Subtotal colectomy for severe idiopathic constipation: a follow-up study of 13 patients. *Digestive Diseases and Sciences*, **32**, 1249–1254.

46. Lewis, T.D., Daniel, E.E., Sarna, S.K., Waterfall, W.E. and Marzio, L. (1978) Idiopathic intestinal pseudoobstruction: report of a case, with intraluminal studies of mechanical and electrical activity, and response to drugs. *Gastroenterology*, **74**, 107–111.

47. Lipton, A.B. and Knauer, C.M. (1977) Pseudo-obstruction of the bowel: therapeutic trial of metoclopramide. *American Journal of Digestive Diseases*, **22**, 263–265.

48. Loening-Baucke, V.A., Anuras, S. and Mitros, F.A. (1987) Changes in colorectal function in patients with chronic colonic pseudoobstruction. *Digestive Diseases and Sciences*, **32**, 1104–1112.

49. MacColl, C., MacConnell, K.L., Baylis, B. and Lee, S.S. (1990) Treatment of acute colonic pseudoobstruction (Ogilvie's syndrome) with cisapride. *Gastroenterology*, **98**, 773–776.

50. Malagelada, J.-R., Camilleri, M. and Stanghellini, V. (1986) *Manometric Diagnosis of Gastrointestinal Motility Disorders*. New York: Thieme.

51. Maldonado, J.E., Gregg, J.A., Green, P.A. and Brown, A.L., Jr (1970) Chronic idiopathic intestinal pseudo-obstruction. *American Journal of Medicine*, **49**, 203–212.

52. Martin, F.M., Robinson, A.M., Jr and Thompson, W.R. (1988) Therapeutic colonoscopy in the treatment of colonic pseudoobstruction. *American Surgeon*, **54**, 519–522.

53. Mathias, J.R., Carlson, G.M., DiMarino, A.J., Bertiger, G., Morton, H.E. and Cohen, S. (1976) Intestinal myoelectric activity in response to live *Vibrio cholerae* and cholera enterotoxin. *Journal of Clinical Investigation*, **58**, 91–96.

54. Mathias, J.R., Fernandez, A., Sninsky, C.A., Clench, M.H. and Davis, R.H. (1985) Nausea, vomiting and abdominal pain after Roux-en-Y anastomosis: motility of the jejunal limb. *Gastroenterology*, **88**, 101–107.

55. Mayer, E.A., Elashoff, J., Hawkins, R., Berquist, W. and Taylor, I.L. (1988) Gastric emptying of mixed solid–liquid meal in patients with intestinal pseudo-obstruction. *Digestive Diseases and Sciences*, **33**, 10–18.

56. Meeroff, J.C., Schreiber, D.S., Trier, J.S. and Blacklow, N.R. (1980) Abnormal gastric motor function in viral gastroenteritis. *Annals of Internal Medicine*, **92**, 370–373.

57. Milla, P.J. and Fenton, T.R. (1983) Small intestinal motility patterns in the perinatal period. *Journal of Pediatric Gastroenterology and Nutrition*, **2**, S141–S144.

58. Miller, S.M., O'Dorisio, T.M., Thomas, F.B. and Mekhjian, H.S. (1990) Erythromycin exerts a prokinetic effect in patients with chronic idiopathic intestinal pseudo-obstruction. *Gastroenterology*, **98**, A375.

59. Miyake, T., Kawamori, J., Yoshida, T., Nakano, H., Kohno, S. and Ohba, S. (1987) Small bowel pseudo-obstruction in Kawasaki disease. *Pediatric Radiology*, **17**, 383–386.

60. Mughal, M.M. and Irving, M.H. (1988) Treatment of endstage chronic intestinal pseudoobstruction by subtotal enterectomy and home parenteral nutrition. *Gut*, **29**, 1613–1617.

61. Nano, D., Prindiville, T., Paulis, M., Chou, H., Ross, K. and Trudeau, W. (1987) Colonoscopic therapy of acute pseudoobstruction of the colon. *American Journal of Gastroenterology*, **82**, 145–148.

62. Ogilvie, H. (1948) Large intestine colic due to sympathetic deprivation. *British Medical Journal*, **ii**, 671–673.

63. Oh, J.J. and Kim, C.H. (1990) Gastroparesis after a presumed viral illness: clinical and laboratory features and natural history. *Mayo Clinic Proceedings*, **65**, 636–642.

64. Phillips, S.F., Quigley, E.M.M., Kumar, D. and Kamath, P.S. (1988) Motility of the ileo-colonic junction. *Gut*, **29**, 390–406.

65. Pitt, H.A., Mann, L.L., Berquist, W.E., Ament, M.E., Fonkalsrud, E.W. and DenBesten, L. (1985) Chronic intestinal pseudo-obstruction: management with total parenteral nutrition and a venting enterostomy. *Archives of Surgery*, **120**, 614–618.

66. Preston, D.M., Hawley, P.R., Lennard-Jones, J.E. and Todd, I.P. (1984) Results of colectomy for severe idiopathic constipation in women (Arbuthnot Lane's disease). *British Journal of Surgery*, **71**, 547–552.

67. Quigley, E.M.M., Borody, T.J., Phillips, S.F., Wienbeck, M., Tucker, R.L. and Haddad, A. (1984) Motility of the terminal ileum and ileocecal sphincter in healthy humans. *Gastroenterology*, **87**, 857–866.

68. Reynolds, J.C. (1990) Neuron morphology and neuropeptide distribution in colonic inertia determined by immunohistochemical staining of neurofilaments and neuropeptides. *Gastroenterology*, **98**, A384.

69. Richter, H.M., III and Kelly, K.A. (1986) Effect of transection and pacing on human jejunal pacesetter potentials. *Gastroenterology*, **91**, 1380–1385.

70. Rohrmann, C.A., Jr, Ricci, M.T., Krishnamurthy, S. and Schuffler, M.D. (1984) Radiologic and histologic differentiation of neuromuscular disorders of the gastrointestinal tract: visceral myopathies, visceral neuropathies, and progressive systemic sclerosis. *American Journal of Roentgenology*, **143**, 933–941.

71. Salm, R., Ruckauer, K., Waldmann, D. and Faithmann, E.H. (1988) Endoscopic percutaneous cecostomy. *Surgical Endoscopy*, **2**, 92–95.

72. Sarna, S.K. (1985) Cyclic motor activity; migrating motor complex: 1985. *Gastroenterology*, **89**, 894–913.

73. Sarr, M.G., Tanaka, M. and Deunes, J.A. (1987) Jejunoileal autotransplantation: effects on small intestinal motility. *Surgical Forum*, **38**, 160–162.

74. Schang, J.C. and Devroede, G. (1985) Beneficial effects of naloxone in a patient with intestinal pseudoobstruction. *American Journal of Gastroenterology*, **80**, 407–411.

75. Schuffler, M.D. (1981) Chronic intestinal pseudo-obstruction syndromes. *Medical Clinics of North America*, **65**, 1331–1358.

76. Schuffler, M.D. and Deitch, E.A. (1980) Chronic idiopathic intestinal pseudo-obstruction: a surgical approach. *Annals of Surgery*, **192**, 752–761.

77. Schuffler, M.D., Rohrmann, C.A., Chaffee, R.G., Brand, D.L., Delaney, J.H. and Young, J.H. (1981) Chronic intestinal pseudo-obstruction: a report of 27 cases and review of the literature. *Medicine*, **60**, 173–196.

78. Schuffler, M.D., Leon, S.H. and Krishnamurthy, S. (1985) Intestinal pseudoobstruction caused by a new form of visceral neuropathy: palliation by radical small bowel resection. *Gastroenterology*, **89**, 1152–1156.

79. Schuffler, M.D., Pagon, R.A., Schwartz, R. and Bill, A.H. (1988) Visceral myopathy of the gastrointestinal and genitourinary tracts in infants. *Gastroenterology*, **94**, 892–898.

80. Schuurkes, J.A.J., Van Nueten, J.M., Van Daele, P.G.H., Reyntjens, A.J. and Janssen, P.A.J. (1985) Motor-stimulating properties of cisapride on isolated gastrointestinal preparations of the guinea pig. *Journal of Pharmacology and Experimental Therapeutics*, **234**, 775–783.

81. Scott, R.B., Diamant, S.C. and Gall, D.G. (1988) Motility effects of intestinal anaphylaxis in the rat. *American Journal of Physiology*, **255**, G505–G511.

82. Scott, R.B., Gall, D.G. and Maric, M. (1990) Mediation of food protein-induced jejunal smooth muscle contraction in sensitized rats. *American Journal of Physiology*, **259**, G6–G14.

83. Sodhi, N., Camilleri, M., Camoriano, J.K., Low, P.A., Fealey, R.D. and Perry, M.C. (1989) Autonomic function and motility in intestinal pseudoobstruction caused by paraneoplastic syndrome. *Digestive Diseases and Sciences*, **34**, 1937–1942.

84. Stanghellini, V., Camilleri, M. and Malagelada, J.-R. (1987) Chronic idiopathic intestinal pseudo-obstruction: clinical and intestinal manometric findings. *Gut*, **28**, 5–12.

85. Stanghellini, V., Corinaldesi, R. and Barbara, L. (1988) Pseudoobstruction syndromes. *Ballière's Clinical Gastroenterology*, **2**, 225–254.

86. Stivland, T.A., Camilleri, M., Vassallo, M., Proano, M., Rath, D.M., Brown, M.L., Thomforde, G.M., Pemberton, J.H. and Phillips, S.F. (1990) Scintigraphic measurement of regional gut transit in idiopathic constipation. *Gastroenterology*, **101**, 107–115.

87. Stryker, S.J., Borody, T.J., Phillips, S.F., Kelly, K.A., Dozois, R.R. and Beart, R.W., Jr (1985) Motility of the small intestine after proctocolectomy and ileal pouch-anal anastomosis. *Annals of Surgery*, **201**, 351–356.

88. Sullivan, M.A., Snape, W.J., Jr, Matarazzo, S.A., Petrokubi, R.J., Jeffries, G. and Cohen, S. (1977) Gastrointestinal myoelectrical activity in idiopathic intestinal pseudo-obstruction. *New England Journal of Medicine*, **297**, 233–238.

89. Summers, R.W., Anuras, S. and Green, J. (1983) Jejunal manometry patterns in health, partial intestinal obstruction and pseudoobstruction. *Gastroenterology*, **85**, 1290–1300.

90. Suzuki, H., Amano, S., Matsumoto, K., Kitagawa, T. and Masuda, T. (1987) Chronic idiopathic intestinal pseudo-obstruction caused by acquired visceral neuropathy localized in the left colon: report of two cases. *Japanese Journal of Surgery*, **17**, 302–306.

91. Szurszewski, J.H. and Weems, W.A. (1976) Control of gastrointestinal motility by prevertebral ganglia. In: *Physiology of Smooth Muscle*, pp. 313–319 (Eds) Bulbring, E. and Shuba, M.F. New York: Raven Press.

92. Vanek, V.W. and Al-Salti, M. (1986) Acute pseudoobstruction of the colon (Ogilvie's syndrome). An analysis of 400 cases. *Diseases of the Colon and Rectum*, **29**, 203–210.

93. Vantrappen, G., Janssens, J., Hellemans, J. and Ghoos, Y. (1977) The interdigestive motor complex of normal subjects and patients with bacterial overgrowth of the small intestine. *Journal of Clinical Investigation*, **59**, 1158–1166.

94. Vargas, J.H., Sachs, P. and Ament, M.E. (1988) Chronic intestinal pseudo-obstruction syndrome in pediatrics. Results of a national survey by members of the North American Society of Pediatric Gastroenterology and Nutrition. *Journal of Pediatric Gastroenterology and Nutrition*, **7**, 323–332.

95. Vassallo, M., Camilleri, M., Caron, B.L. and Low, P.A. (1991) Gastrointestinal motor dysfunction in acquired selective cholinergic dysautonomia associated with infectious mononucleosis. *Gastroenterology*, **100**, 252–258.

96. Venizelos, I.O., Shousha, S., Bull, T.B. and Parkins, R.A. (1988) Chronic intestinal pseudoobstruction in two patients. Overlap of features of systemic sclerosis and visceral myopathy. *Histopathology*, **12**, 533–540.

97. Vermillion, D.L., Ernst, P.B., Scicchitano, R. and Collins, S.M. (1988) Antigen-induced contraction of jejunal smooth muscle in the sensitized rat. *American Journal of Physiology*, **255**, G701–G708.

98. Warner, E. and Jeejeebhoy, K.N. (1985) Successful management of chronic intestinal pseudo-obstruction with home parenteral nutrition. *Journal of Parenteral and Enteral Nutrition*, **9**, 173–178.

99. Wood, J.R., Camilleri, M., Low, P.A. and Malagelada, J.-R. (1985) Brainstem tumor presenting as an upper gut motility disorder. *Gastroenterology*, **89**, 1411–1414.

BACTERIOLOGY OF THE SMALL GUT AND BACTERIAL OVERGROWTH

P. Ghosh and G. Neale

The normal microbial flora of the lumen of the small intestine in healthy humans has still not been fully characterized and there remains much to be learned about its effect on structure and function. There are many animals, particularly ruminants, which benefit from the bacteria they carry in the upper gastro-intestinal tract, but this does not appear to be so in humans.

THE NORMAL GUT MICROFLORA IN HUMANS

THE GERM-FREE STATE

A germ-free state can be maintained in humans only under the most stringent conditions in a plastic isolator,[71] but even then the condition is relative, depending on the sophistication of the tests used to define microbial sterility.[30] Interesting observations have been made on gut structure and function in the experimental germ-free animal: the epithelium of the small intestine is more regular, the mucosa and lamina propria are thinner, and the crypts of Lieber-kühn are shallower and the enterocytes shorter lived than in controls.[172] Humans are germ-free only *in utero* and the manner in which colonization of the gut occurs immediately after birth is important, particularly to sick, premature infants.

COLONIZATION OF THE INTESTINE AFTER BIRTH

Microbial colonization of the gut of the newborn infant occurs during and after birth and depends on a variety of factors (*Table 3.28*). Differences in gestational age, mode of delivery and type of feeding are associated with significantly different colonization patterns during the first week of life.

Table 3.28 Factors affecting colonization of the small intestine in the newborn

Gestational age
Route of delivery
Degree of exposure to hospital environment
Mode of nutrition

The inoculum of bacteria from the vagina is important. Forty-eight hours after birth, 40% of stools in the normally delivered infant contain anaerobic bacteria and 70% contain aerobic bacteria, compared with 5 and 30% in the infant delivered by Caesarean section.[95] Breast-feeding leads to subsequent predominance of bifidobacteria.[64] *Bacteroides fragilis* is slow to colonize, but at the end of 1 week can be isolated from the faeces of 60% of bottle-fed infants compared with only 20% of those breast-fed. The infrequent finding of *B. fragilis* does not appear to be related to the nature of the aerobic flora as isolation rates for aerobic Gram-negative bacilli and streptococci appear similar in both breast-fed and bottle-fed infants.[95]

The microflora of infant stools at 1 week is already extremely complex – over 100 species of anaerobic bacteria were isolated from a study of 196 neonates and the aerobic organisms were also fully represented, with *Escherichia coli*, *Klebsiella* spp., *Enterobacter* spp., *Proteus* spp., and group D streptococci predominating.[95] These data, of course, tell us nothing about what is occurring in the small intestine, but may be important in our understanding of necrotizing enterocolitis, in many cases of which there appears to be a delay in the normal bacterial colonization of the intestine.[89] It has also been suggested that common bacterial toxins in infants may be a possible cause of the sudden infant death syndrome.[113]

THE ESTABLISHED NORMAL FLORA

The 'normal flora' of the small intestine refers solely to bacteria.[151] Although viruses may be cultured from the gut of otherwise healthy children, a normal viral flora is generally believed not to exist in humans.[129]

There are two groups of bacteria to be considered: firstly, those found in small intestinal fluid which largely reflect the microflora of swallowed saliva and which vary in a phasic manner with the ingestion of meals,[54] and secondly the apparently more stable flora of the mucosal surface.[52]

In the Western world, where most people eat either freshly cooked meals or bacteriologically clean food which has been stored under hygienic conditions, the luminal contents of the upper small intestine contain less than 10^4 (with an average of 10^2) viable organisms per millilitre of fasting aspirate; the organisms are predominantly aerobic and

Table 3.29 Studies on normal flora of human small intestine. Results are expressed as log_{10} (numbers of viable organisms/ml)

Number of control samples studied	Sterile	Aerobic organisms (max.)	Coliform organisms (max.)	Anaerobic organisms (max.)	Bacteroides (max.)	Reference
Upper small intestine						
13	1 (8%)	3.5	—	3.9	—	56
25	17 (68%)	5	2	3	3	40
12	0 (0%)	9.1	2.5	5.0	—	67
13	7 (54%)	5.5	—	6.0	—	26
22	4 (18%)	4.0	1.0	3.0	2.0	35
10^b	2 (20%)	6.9	4.7	2.8	1.6	16
Lower small intestine						
12	—	6.3	6.3	5.5	5.5	56
4	—	6	6	7	7	40
6	—	9.1	8.1	7.8	7.8	67

Gram-positive. Although published reports show considerable differences (*Table 3.29*) and although direct counts of bacteria in aspirates of jejunal fluid suggest that some bacteria are not being grown under standard laboratory conditions (*Figure 3.53*), most workers agree that the jejunum is not sterile but populated by 'transients' originating from the oral cavity. Streptococci, lactobacilli and veillonellae are the principal organisms recovered. After a light meal the concentration of microorganisms in the jejunum increases about 100-fold; although more species may be isolated, enterobacteriaceae and *Bacteriodes* spp. are rarely found.

In contrast, the flora of the small intestine close to the ileocaecal valve is dramatically greater and approximates to that found in the caecum (*Table 3.29*). There is little data to indicate the length of normal ileum carrying such a heavy load of bacteria, but it is probably no more than 50 cm.[56] Removal of the ileocaecal valve may allow an increased growth of bacteria.[63]

Apparently healthy residents of tropical countries carry a richer microflora in the small intestine than their Western counterparts. Studies from India, South-East Asia and South America show that the jejunum often contains 10^4–10^5 coliform organisms per millilitre of fasting fluid. These findings may correlate with a lower normal range for the absorption of xylose and vitamin B_{12} than is accepted in the West.[25]

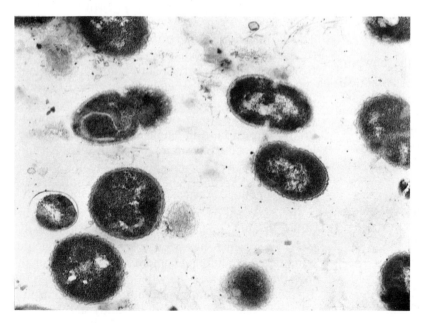

Figure 3.53 Electronmicrograph of bacteria in centrifuged duodenal fluid aspirated from a patient with diverticulosis of the upper small intestine. This sample was one of an unpublished series collected by A. Challen (MRC Dunn Nutrition Unit) and J. Anderson (Department of Pathology, University of Cambridge). In this series, up to 10^9 Gram-positive particles per millilitre of jejunal fluid aspirated were counted under light microscope; by standard methods of aerobic and anaerobic culture the viable bacterial count did not exceed 10^5 organisms/ml.

MAINTENANCE OF THE BACTERIAL FLORA

The bacterial population of fasting jejunal fluid is maintained at a low concentration in part by the peristaltic contractions of the normal gut. Colonization of the mucosal surface appears to depend on the capacity of the bacteria to adhere to epithelial cells. This property of adherence not only prevents the physical expulsion of microorganisms but may also stimulate their growth, since nutrients tend to concentrate at the cell surface.[104] The organisms are also subject to the effects of local immune systems, non-specific host antimicrobial agents, and variations in the biochemical and biophysical environment, and to the shedding of epithelial cells into the lumen of the intestine.

Bacterial properties

Occasionally histologists identify Gram-negative and Gram-positive bacteria in mucus on the mucosal epithelium of the small intestine,[119,125] but the microbial population appears to be extremely sparse. This is quite unlike the situation in many other species. In particular, intimate microbial–epithelial associations throughout the gut are readily demonstrated in rodents.[138] Adherence is mediated by species-specific microbial lectins complementary to host cell surface receptors.[13] These microbial surface antigens are detectable on filamentous projections (pili or fimbriae) of the cell wall and react with proteins (albumin-like or glycoproteins with mannose-containing residues) of the epithelial cell membrane. In addition, dietary lectins may act by promoting bacterial adherence and facilitating colonization leading to bacterial overgrowth.[2] Bacterial properties promoting adherence favour pathogenicity, and secretory antibodies may protect in part by preventing such adherence.

In some species, microorganisms adherent to the surface epithelium may influence the flora of intestinal contents in the fasting state,[98] but in humans this seems unlikely. In South Indian studies, the range of organisms raised from cultures of jejunal aspirates was often very different from those obtained from cultures of jejunal biopsies. Anaerobic organisms were more commonly isolated from the mucosal surface[16] but, as with the luminal flora, there is almost certainly a considerable variation between populations. In a study from Costa Rica the findings were similar to those described above,[73] whereas Plaut[125] in the USA obtained few or no bacteria from the mucosal surface.

One can speculate on the density of bacteria adherent to jejunal mucosa by extrapolating from published data. The culture of 10^5 organisms per millilitre of wet jejunal mucosa[16] sounds impressive, but a milligram of mucosal biopsy may carry 100 villi, each with something like 2000 surface cells. The cell population of the crypts is less than 10% that of the villi. Thus these figures suggest a bacterial concentration of perhaps one organism per villus, or not more than 10 per crypt.

Adherence of bacteria to the epithelium of the small intestine may contribute to damage to brush borders, as for example with E. coli overgrowth in the small intestine of humans and experimental animals.[165]

Epithelial factors

Apart from intestinal motility, important control mechanisms exist at the epithelial surface.[72] Specific secretory immunoglobulin A provides an immunological barrier for unwanted organisms,[173] lysozyme hinders adherence by its steric properties, and blood group-reactive glycoproteins combine with and neutralize bacterial receptors.[174] It is suggested that the growth of bacteria may be influenced by the availability of iron at the epithelial surface,[21] which in turn is controlled by the production of iron-binding proteins. The establishment of a resident normal flora on the epithelial surface might provide a barrier to colonization by other species (Table 3.30).

Luminal factors

Within the lumen of the intestine the antibacterial activity of unconjugated bile acids may play a part by regulating the growth of anaerobic organisms.[17] In addition, physicochemical factors such as pH and the oxidation–reduction potential will favour the growth of some microorganisms but not others.[109]

Table 3.30 Factors which may inhibit bacterial colonization of the epithelial surface

Peristaltic flow of gut contents

Luminal mechanisms
  Variations in pH and oxidation–reduction potential
  Non-specific antimicrobial agents
  Bile acids and volatile fatty acids

Surface mechanisms
  Local immune systems
  Epithelial cell turnover
  Microbial competitors

Exogenous factors

Exogenous influences of importance include age, diet, ingestion of microbes, the debilitation which accompanies serious disease, including severe burns, factors influencing gastrointestinal motility (e.g. pregnancy, drugs, emotional stress) and, probably the most potent of all, antimicrobial agents.

The effects of diet on the normal flora of the small intestine in humans are virtually unknown, although they may explain, at least in part, the differences in the histological appearances of the small intestinal mucosa between normal subjects in the Western world eating a highly purified diet and the people of tropical countries who commonly consume large quantities of unprocessed food. In animals, bacterial flora is altered substantially by the ingestion of, for example, elemental diet rather than laboratory chow.

Serious illness alters the flora of the oropharynx, with an increase in the prevalence of Gram-negative bacilli.[74,75] Similar findings are reported both in diabetics and alcoholics.[18,99,100] One may speculate that this alters bacterial counts in the small intestine.

Viruses may also influence the normal flora. Again there is a paucity of data for the small intestine, but in the respiratory tract there is good evidence that viruses promote colonization of the upper respiratory tract by bacteria which are often pathogenic,[98] possibly by facilitating the adherence of these bacteria to epithelial cells.[46]

Stasis has a critical role in regulating the microbial population of the small intestine. Disruption of normal intestinal peristalsis allows bacteria to proliferate rapidly in the lumen of the intestine,[90] although again there is little data regarding the effect of this on the bacterial population of the epithelial surface. Emotional stress may disrupt the gastrointestinal microbial ecosystem; it has been suggested that this might influence the susceptibility of travellers to diarrhoeal illnesses.[138]

Antimicrobial agents not only kill or inhibit the growth of bacteria, but may also impair their adherence to cell surfaces even when present only in subinhibitory concentrations.[167] The alteration of membrane proteins of bacterial strains developing resistance to antimicrobial agents affects their ability to colonize surfaces.[123]

Finally, inhibition of the growth of sensitive microbes may allow the rapid growth of an otherwise unimportant species of the overall microflora. The development of candidiasis after broad-spectrum antibiotic therapy suggests that the inhibitory mechanisms work against fungi as well as bacterial pathogens. The presence of a normal flora is probably more important than the immune system in warding off overgrowth by *Candida*.[69]

ROLE OF THE NORMAL FLORA

Nutrition

Most bacterial species in the small intestine are capable of synthesizing vitamins in excess of their own metabolic needs, especially vitamin K and constituents of the vitamin B group – riboflavin, pyridoxine, pantothenic acid, biotin, folic acid and vitamin B_{12} – but the balance is often uncertain.[106,134] In disorders of the small intestine allowing bacterial overgrowth, the availability of vitamin B_{12} to the host is usually sharply reduced and nicotinic acid deficiency has also been described.[158] Ascorbic acid (vitamin C) may be broken down by bacteria, although possibly not in significant amounts.

The degradation of urea by the gut flora leads to the release of ammonia which may be absorbed and used for the synthesis of non-essential amino acids,[53,130] but this is estimated to account for no more than 1% of daily amino nitrogen requirements.[166] Moreover, in uraemic patients, the suppression of gut flora with broad-spectrum antibiotics improves the nitrogen balance.

Resistance to infection

There have been several studies of the methods by which the normal flora may act as a barrier to infection by preventing or limiting the colonization of the surface epithelium with pathogenic microorganisms (*Table 3.30*). However, the importance of these mechanisms as barriers to infection remains largely unproven. Some bacteria (e.g. *Streptococcus viridans*) have been shown to be capable of producing protein antibiotics (bacteriocins) which play a role in preventing bacterial overgrowth.[155] The metabolic end-products of anaerobic metabolism such as volatile fatty acids and deconjugated bile acids are toxic to some bacteria; the lowering of the oxidation–reduction potential may also be inhibitory.

In some species, the presence of a normal gastrointestinal flora has been shown to inhibit the passage of bacteria (e.g. indigenous *E. coli*) through the epithelial mucosa into the lymphocytes and mesenteric lymph nodes. In germ-free animals this barrier is reduced.[14] The resident bacteria may even be capable of degrading the toxin of pathogenic bacteria, although this mechanism has so far been demonstrated only in animals with rumina.[3] Bacterial interrelationships may also be important in preventing invasion of epithelial surfaces, as has been demonstrated in mice infected with *Shigella*.[41]

Effect on immune mechanisms

The presence of intestinal bacteria primes the immune system, and this state of readiness may be of marginal benefit to the host. For example, the resistance of germ-free mice to *Vibrio cholerae* after immunization is enhanced by the simultaneous colonization of the gut with intestinal flora obtained from conventional animals.[150] Conversely, the overall decrease in the cellular immune response in germ-free animals appears to decrease the mortality from viruses capable of causing hepatitis and lymphocytic chloriomeningitis.[126,156]

Intestinal bacteria as a cause of systemic infection

The indigenous microflora of the gut can be a major source of disease by translocation. This is most clearly seen in immunosuppressed patients in whom the microorganisms of the intestine are a potent cause of opportunistic infections. The suppression of these bacteria by antibiotics reduces the incidence of complications in susceptible subjects[154] so that prophylactic regimes are generally used in severely neutropenic and other immunocompromised patients. In overwhelming stronglyoidiasis, bacterial invasion of the circulation can result in a serious life-treatening septicaemia.[147]

The role of bacteria in maintaining or promoting the inflammatory process in chronic ulcerative conditions of the small intestine appears to be important in both experimental and clinical situations. Thus, it is possible that the use of a bowel sterilization regimen is beneficial in the short term to patients with Crohn's disease,[79] and experimental and clinical interactions between gut microflora and graft-versus-host disease are described after bacterial colonization. This is supported by experimental evidence showing that the administration of antibiotics inhibits the development of intestinal ulceration in animals given carrageenan.[122]

Conclusion

The role of the normal microflora of the small intestine has not been fully explored. Under experimental conditions it is not a prequisite for life; indeed, if life-span is taken as a marker, germ-free animals often do better than animals reared under conventional conditions.[58] Nevertheless, in a world teeming with microorganisms, it has been suggested that bacteria residing on mucosal surfaces provide a degree of protection against infection by a range of other microorganisms including *Candida albicans*, *V. cholerae* and salmonellae.[98] The effects of the nutritional state of the host appear to be marginal but the role of the intestinal microflora on the health and well-being of poorly nourished people living in unhygienic environments warrants further study.

BACTERIAL OVERGROWTH

From the discussion above it is clear that there cannot be any absolute definition of bacterial overgrowth in the small intestine. For practical purposes the demonstration of viable bacteria in concentrations of more than 10^4–10^5 organisms/ml in the upper small intestine of the fasting subject is adequate evidence of bacterial overgrowth, especially if the flora contains coliform bacteria at a level of more than 10^2–10^3 organisms/ml. These are the sort of results obtained in competent microbiological laboratories using accepted culture techniques, but there are no valid standards against which individual units can check the quality of their work (*Table 3.29*). The problem is compounded by difficulties in obtaining specimens from multiple sites in the small intestine, by the relative paucity of data for normal control subjects, by our incomplete understanding of factors which control bacterial growth, and, in some cases, by the poor correlation between microbiological data and the apparently adverse metabolic effects of bacteria in the small intestine.

For practical purposes the clinician may have to be content with:

1. The demonstration of a lesion known to be associated with bacterial overgrowth.
2. The finding of one or more metabolic disturbances which may occur as a result of bacterial action (classically the malabsorption of vitamin B_{12} and/or steatorrhoea) and a positive breath test to indicate bile salt deconjugation or carbohydrate breakdown in the upper gut.
3. The reversal of such metabolic abnormalities by the oral administration of appropriate antibiotics.

Even this simple scheme may be unsatisfactory, and clinically the impact of antibiotics on diarrhoea may be disappointing, confounded by the emergence of resistant strains and complicated by antibiotic-associated diarrhoea.

HISTORICAL ASPECTS

The combination of bacterial overgrowth and a demonstrable metabolic disturbance reversible by the administration of oral antibiotics has been called the blind loop syndrome,[8] the stagnant loop syndrome,[159] the small intestinal stasis syndrome,[44] and the contaminated small bowel syndrome.[59]

In a review of patients dying with pernicious anaemia at Guy's Hospital, it was suggested a century ago that attention should be paid to the small number of patients with 'changes in the small intestine'.[170] Within the next decade, four separate case reports of intestinal strictures and a 'pernicious anaemia' appeared in the Scandinavian medical literature.[45] Surgical cure of this rare syndrome was attempted successfully in 1924.[148] Shortly afterwards, the use of liver therapy for pernicious anaemia was extended effectively to patients with a megaloblastic anaemia associated with a number of abnormalities of the small intestine, including blind pouches and diverticulae (hence 'blind loop syndrome').[108] Steatorrhoea was demonstrated in many such patients and the major clinical features were summarized in a review by Barker and Hummel.[10] The syndrome was extended to patients with stasis of the contents of the small intestine without self-filling loops, and treatment with appropriate antibiotics was shown to be effective. Gracey[59] used the term 'contaminated small bowel syndrome' to cover patients with conditions in which stasis is not a necessary factor in the maintenance of bacterial overgrowth, such as cholangitis (in which the upper intestine is seeded with bacteria), immune deficiency states, and malnutrition.

Much of our knowledge of the mechanisms of the metabolic disturbances arising from bacterial overgrowth in the small intestine stem from studies of animal models[148,168,169] stimulated by observations on patients.[38,60,118,157] Current attention focuses on interactions between bacteria and the epithelial surfaces with which they are in close association.[137] For example, there is now evidence to show that bacteria in the small intestine can survive on host cell glycoproteins[128] and that they secrete enzymes which damage the enzyme systems of epithelial cell brush borders.[132]

AETIOLOGY AND PATHOGENESIS

The bacterial population in the lumen of the small intestine will depend on the rate of entry of viable organisms into the gut, their rate of reproduction, and the rate of clearance from the gut. Changes in one or more of these mechanisms may lead to bacterial overgrowth in the fluid contents of the fasted small intestine (*Table 3.31*). The normal phasic changes of luminal flora with meals probably become less pronounced, but the effect on the surface flora remains uncertain.[16] With the limited data available one cannot even be certain that the

Table 3.31 Conditions favouring bacterial overgrowth in the small intestine

- *Excess bacteria entering the small intestine*
    Heavily contaminated food (?)
    Impaired gastric barrier
        Achlorhydria[40]
        Gastrojejunostomy[121]
        Partial or total gastrectomy[157]
    Internal bacterial seeding of the small intestine
        Cholangitis[146]
        Fistulas[39]
        Loss of ileocaecal valve[114]

- *Conditions which may allow excess bacterial proliferation in the absence of readily demonstrable stasis*
    With defined mechanisms
        Immune deficiency states[124]
        Bile salt deficiency[48]
    Without clearly defined mechanisms
        Old age,[133] uraemia
        Malnutrition[62]
        Tropical sprue[57,85]
        Monosaccharide malabsorption[61]
    Chronic Pancreatitis[92]

- *Delayed clearance of bacteria from the lumen of the intestine*
    Localized anatomical abnormalities
        Duodenal and jejunal diverticulosis[32]
        Strictures
            Congenital[7]
            Crohn's disease[39,135]
            Tuberculosis[10]
            Caused by ulcers of varying aetiology
    Postoperative problems
        Afferent loop stasis[175]
        Postoperative blind loops[44,91]
        Jejunoileal bypass[11]
        Enteroenterostomy[37]
        Continent ileostomy[143]
    Generalized disorders of the bowel wall
        Coeliac disease (rarely)
        Scleroderma[136]
        Irradiation
        Amyloidosis[161]
        Intestinal pseudo-obstruction[101]
    Neurological disorders affecting motility
        Diabetes mellitus[140]
        Vagotomy
        Degeneration of the myenteric plexus[42]

surface flora is more abundant in subjects with bacterial overgrowth in the lumen. Thus the pathogenetic mechanisms of disorders caused by bacterial overgrowth are discussed principally in relation to concentrations of viable bacteria isolated from aspirates of fluid from the intestine of fasting patients. In patients with bacterial overgrowth, there is characteristically an increase in the concentration of organisms, especially those species normally confined to the lower small intestine and colon (*Table 3.29*).

METABOLIC AND NUTRITIONAL CONSEQUENCES

Caloric undernutrition

It has not been shown that bacterial proliferation in the small intestine *per se* significantly impairs the supply of nutrients for energy production. Indeed, ruminants obtain a major part of their nutrition in the form of volatile fatty acids from the fermentation of complex carbohydrates. However, young experimental animals with surgically created blind loops grow less well than control animals[110] or animals with an equivalent small intestinal resection.[96] Growth impairment seems largely related to diminished food intake and can be reversed by giving antibiotics. This may also be responsible for the failure of growth and infantilism described in children with the blind loop syndrome.[116] Nevertheless, there is also impairment of the absorption of fat and carbohydrate in patients with bacterial overgrowth in the small intestine.

The relationship of malnutrition and diarrhoeal illnesses to the 'normal' flora of the small intestine in malnourished children of Third World countries is incompletely understood, but is of considerable potential importance. The polluted environment is probably the main determinant of bacterial overgrowth, but the role of impaired immune function secondary to malnutrition has not been adequately assessed. The high concentrations of jejunal bacteria, some of which may be enterotoxigenic, almost certainly play a key role in the diarrhoea and malabsorption which may accompany dietary malnutrition in childhood.[60]

Steatorrhoea

Malabsorption of fat is common in patients with bacterial overgrowth and is due primarily to the poor formation of micelles. The structured agglomeration of phospholipids, bile acids, monoglycerides and diglycerides is produced most efficiently by conjugated bile acids. Intestinal bacteria (especially bacteroides, veillonellae, clostridia and bifidobacteria) are capable of deconjugating and dehydroxylating bile salts which then become poorly soluble at the pH of the upper small intestine. As a result, the total concentration of available effective bile acids may fall below the critical level for micelle formation. The importance of this mechanism has been supported by the direct estimation of bile salt concentrations in fluid aspirated from contaminated small intestine of both patients and experimental animals, and by assessing the effect of adding additional conjugated bile salts.[157] As might be expected, however, the clinical situation does not always appear to conform to this elegant mechanism. In some patients with steatorrhoea, the concentration of conjugated bile acids does not appear to fall below the critical micellar concentration.

The adverse effect of bacteria on the ability of the epithelial cell to take up fat has not been adequately assessed, although there is increasing evidence of damage to brush border membranes.[132] In addition, the presence of anaerobic bacteria in the small intestine does not necessarily lead to steatorrhoea. This is particularly true of bacterial overgrowth limited to the ileum and very localized lesions in duodenum (e.g. solitary diverticulum).[55]

Production of hydroxy-fatty acids

Unabsorbed fat may be metabolized by intestinal bacteria to produce long-chain hydroxy-fatty acids, some of which are similar to ricinoleic acid, the major fatty acid in castor oil.[162] Unsaturated hydroxy-fatty acids may also be produced by the bacterially mediated hydration of linoleic acid.[144] These fatty acids stimulate the gastrointestinal mucosa to secrete,[5] and this, together with the increased concentration of intraluminal volatile fatty acids (see below), may contribute to the diarrhoea[4] which is a prominent symptom in many patients with bacterial overgrowth in the small intestine.

Carbohydrate malabsorption

Several groups of workers have documented the malabsorption of carbohydrate in subjects with bacterial overgrowth in the small intestine,[37,60] but some anomalies persist. For example, the transport of glucose by the intestinal mucosa is impaired in the presence of deconjugated bile salts both *in vivo* and *in vitro*, yet the standard glucose tolerance test administered to patients with bacterial overgrowth nearly always gives a normal result. The uptake of glucose from disaccharides may be more consistently depressed, although data regarding this is scanty. In experimental animals the creation of a blind loop depresses the disaccharidase activities of the mucosal brush border.[77] Comparison of the biochemical changes in the jejunal mucosa of dogs suggests that while anaerobes produce brush membrane disruption with alteration of brush border enzymes, aerobes affect the alkaline phosphatase enzyme without affecting either the dissacharidase or aminopeptidase.[12]

The standard test for the absorption of D-xylose is abnormal in the majority of patients with bacterial overgrowth. Bacteria are capable of fermenting many carbohydrates, but the production of bacterial metabolites from xylose is difficult to demonstrate. It seems likely that there is a defect in transport superimposed on the effects of bacterial fermentation.[164]

The relatively small amount of unabsorbed carbohydrate provides an important substrate for the growth of bacteria. In addition, it is readily converted to volatile fatty acids which are then available to the host for energy production.

In children, severe bacterial contamination of the upper small intestine appears to be associated with temporary monosaccharide malabsorption. Bacterial damage to the jejunal mucosa has been postulated as contributing to the malabsorption of all carbohydrates, including the monosaccharides glucose, galactose and fructose. In turn, these may provide an excellent substrate for bacterial growth.[24]

Protein malnutrition

Overt signs of protein–energy malnutrition are not commonly seen in patients with bacterial overgrowth in the small intestine,[127] but mild hypoalbuminaemia is a frequent finding. A number of factors may be responsible, including damage to the intestinal mucosa with protein loss, impaired uptake of peptides and amino acids, and the diversion of protein products into bacterial catabolic pathways.[83] Protein-losing enteropathy is much better documented in the experimental animal with a blind loop than it is in humans. In rats, significant protein loss appears to occur not only from the blind loop but also from the contaminated adjacent small intestine. Reversal of the protein-losing state may require long-term treatment with antibiotics.[80] However, losses of protein into the gut appear to be small compared with the total catabolism of protein.[118]

Impaired uptake of amino acids, especially of the branched-chain group (leucine, isoleucine and valine), correlates with the finding of reduced concentrations of circulating essential amino acids (Figure 3.54). In turn, this may be responsible for the impaired synthesis of proteins.[9,77] Nevertheless, some loose ends remain: the absorption of dipeptides containing branched-chain amino acids is only minimally impaired[9] and, at least in animals with

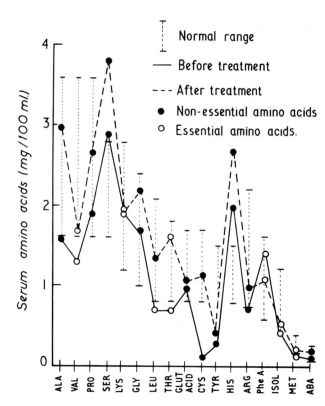

Figure 3.54 Fasting circulating amino acid profile in a patient with protein–calorie malnutrition secondary to malabsorption associated with dual pathology (partial gastrectomy and jejunal diverticulosis). The concentrations of branched-chain essential amino acids are low.

blind loops in the proximal small intestine, overall nitrogen absorption is delayed but not reduced.[34]

The effects of bacterial overgrowth on the metabolism of proteins has been studied in some detail.[78,110] Many of the resulting metabolites are of no value to the host, including indole derivatives from L-tryptophan, volatile phenols from tyrosine, hippuric acid from phenylalanine, piperidine from lysine and pyrollidine from arginine and ornithine. There is some evidence to suggest that the circulating concentrations of L-tryptophan may fall to such low levels that it becomes rate-limiting for protein synthesis.[77] It is estimated that as much as 60% of the dietary intake of L-tryptophan may be diverted into unavailable indolic compounds.

Water and electrolytes

In the Western world, diarrhoea occurs in no more than one-third of patients with anatomical abnormalities of the small intestine leading to bacterial overgrowth. Stool volumes are usually not markedly increased unless there is severe steatorrhoea. In contrast, watery diarrhoea occurs commonly in tropical sprue, especially at the onset of the illness.

Some workers claim that the bacterial flora found in the bowel lumen of patients with tropical sprue is very different from that of patients with the classical blind loop syndrome.[86] In tropical sprue, the coliform organisms (*Klebsiella*, *Enterobacter* and *Escherichia*) are of a limited range of serotypes or biotypes, and enterotoxigenic strains are commonly found. The toxin from these strains will induce water and salt secretion in perfused rat jejunum. In contrast, in the blind loop syndrome, coliform and anaerobic organisms can be cultured and enterotoxigenic bacteria have not been found. This elegant explanation of the symptomatic differences between patients with tropical sprue and those with the blind loop syndrome requires confirmation. Not all reported results are concordant. For example, anaerobic organisms could not be cultured from patients with 'tropical sprue' in the West Indies,[86] but were present in patients with 'sprue' in South India.

Diarrhoea may also be induced by the effect of bacterial metabolites of fatty acids (short-chain fatty acids, hydroxy-fatty acids) on the mucosa of the small and large intestine.[16]

Vitamin deficiencies

Fat-soluble vitamins

In patients with steatorrhoea the absorption of the fat-soluble vitamins will be impaired; however, there are few reported studies. Some data is available for vitamin D and the occasional case of osteomalacia is well documented.[29,141,149] Vitamin E deficiency secondary to malabsorption rarely results in a reversible spinocerebellar degeneration.[20]

Vitamin K deficiency has not been described in the blind loop syndrome perhaps because of the ability of some intestinal bacteria (especialy Gram-positive organisms) to synthesize menaquinones, but it is not uncommon in some patients with severe tropical sprue.

Vitamin B group

Signs of vitamin B deficiency are not uncommon in malnourished patients with bacterial overgrowth in the small intestine, but they rarely progress to dramatic disease. The description of the patient with jejunal diverticulosis responding to an intravenous injection of nicotinic acid remains an isolated case report.[158] There is little good evidence that deficiency of vitamin B may occur as a result of competition by bacteria for a dietary substrate, but it is interesting that nicotinic acid may be the one element of the B Group most required by intestinal bacteria.[50]

VITAMIN B_{12}

Megaloblastic anaemia secondary to vitamin B_{12} deficiency may be regarded as the hallmark of long-term bacterial overgrowth in the small intestine. It dominates the early literature on the subject.[27] This is paradoxical because, although vitamin B_{12} is found in all animal tissues, it is synthesized solely by the bacteria. Unfortunately, vitamin B_{12} synthesized in the colon is not absorbed, thus in both animals and humans a clean vegetarian diet may lead to vitamin B_{12} deficiency, which explains the megaloblastic anaemia sometimes found in vegans.[27] Under natural conditions, bacteria contaminate all foodstuffs and appear to be the natural source of vitamin B_{12} for herbivorous animals which are not coprophagic.

In patients with bacterial overgrowth in the small intestine, tests for the absorption of the vitamin B_{12}–intrinsic factor complex are often abnormal. Intestinal bacteria bind readily with the free vitamin. Furthermore, most species will compete with intrinsic factor and vitamin B_{12}. There appear to be powerful binding sites in the cell walls of some bacteria,[51] especially *Bacteroides* spp., which are capable of taking up most of the vitamin B_{12} from the vitamin B_{12}–intrinsic factor complexes.[169] In clinical experiments it has been shown that more than 50% of orally administered labelled B_{12} is precipitated with the bacterial pellet when aspirates of fluid from the ileum of patients with bacterial overgrowth are centrifuged. In contrast, only 10% of the labelled B_{12} can be precipitated in the ileal fluid of control subjects or of patients shown to have bacterial overgrowth and given appropriate antibiotics.[142]

Bacteria are also capable of metabolizing both intrinsic factor and vitamin B_{12}. It is possible to impair the binding capacity of intrinsic factor by incubating neutralized gastric juice with enteric bacteria. This effect is probably not of great significance. In contrast, the bacterial conversion of vitamin B_{12} to physiologically inactive derivatives (cobamides) is of greater importance. These derivatives block both intrinsic factor and ileal receptors and may even displace vitamin B_{12} from hepatic stores.[19,105]

FOLIC ACID

Folic acid deficiency is uncommon in patients with bacterial overgrowth secondary to intestinal stasis. Indeed, serum values are often abnormally high, which may be due in part to the absorption of folic acid synthesized by the bacteria and in part to the accumulation of folate compounds in the circulation occurring as a result of disordered folate metabolism. The absorption of folic acid is generally normal in the patient with uncomplicated blind loops. Experimentally, elevated levels of serum folic acid can be produced by constructing blind loops in the proximal, but not the distal, small intestine of dogs.[15] Marked folate deficiency is rare, but may occur, and malabsorption of folic acid corrected by treatment with antibiotics has been described.[32]

Once again the situation is different for tropical sprue. In some studies, 90% of patients are folate depleted and, although this is usually ascribed to a poor dietary intake of food folates, malabsorption of folic acid is probably the more important factor.[27]

PRESENTATION

Clinical features

Patients with bacterial overgrowth in the small intestine often present with non-specific symptoms of lassitude and weight loss associated with evidence of disturbed intestinal function such as increased bowel sounds or diarrhoea (Table 3.32).[36] Less frequently, nutritional disturbances are the major presenting feature, with glossitis and stomatitis, anaemia, hypoproteinaemic oedema and, rarely, muscle weakness or bone pain of vitamin D deficiency.

Investigations

Laboratory screening tests often provide pointers, the most significant of which is red cell macrocytosis (usually, but not always, due to vitamin B_{12} deficiency), mild or moderate hypoproteinaemia, and steatorrhoea. One or more standard tests of intestinal absorption (D-xylose absorption, faecal fat excretion, and the Schilling test) will usually be

Table 3.32 Symptomatology of patients with jejunal diverticulosis

Symptom	Percentage presentation
Weight loss	75
Nausea	50
Vomiting	45
Diarrhoea	45
Diarrhoea/constipation	20
Constipation	25
No bowel disturbance	10

Data from a study of 30 patients (mean age 63 years) referred to hospital.[32] More than half of these patients were or had been anaemic (haematocrit less than 12 g/100 ml).

abnormal and provide a baseline for assessing the response to treatment. In themselves they do not provide a diagnosis, but by this stage of the investigation the experienced clinician will have considered the possible aetiology and pathogenesis of the malabsorptive disorder. Often he or she can now arrange the diagnostic test, e.g. radiology of the small intestine, jejunal biopsy, or measurement of pancreatic function.

Radiology

Radiological examination of the small intestine will usually identify sites of potential bacterial overgrowth. It is relatively easy to show anatomical abnormalities such as jejunal diverticulosis (Figure 3.55) and to delineate the extent of intestine involved in a known disorder (Figure 3.56). In addition, the radiologist should be alerted to the possibility of altered transit and motility, although this is difficult to assess with barium. Not all cases will be picked up on a barium examination. In particular, it is easy to miss those cases in which the basic problem is seeding of the small intestine with microorganisms such as may occur from the afferent limb of a Polya gastrectomy, from cholangitis, or from an enteroenteric fistula. Other imaging techniques may be helpful, such as cholangiography and with technetium-labelled iminodiacetic acid (HIDA) scanning (Figure 3.57).

In most cases it is not difficult to detect the presence of a structural disorder which will encourage bacterial overgrowth in the small intestine. In other cases there may be an alternative predisposing condition with the loss of a protective mechanism, such as may occur in the patient with hypogammaglobulinaemia.

Tests for bacterial overgrowth

At this stage of the investigation the clinician needs clear evidence that bacterial overgrowth is present. Three approaches are available: one or more of the indirect tests of bacterial overgrowth may be applied; a sample of the contents may be aspirated and cultured; or the clinical and biochemical response to the administration of antibiotics may be assessed (Table 3.33).

These three approaches may be regarded as complementary. The indirect tests give evidence of the metabolic activities of bacteria and may be used in the long-term monitoring of the effects of therapy; culture of aspirated fluid, although rarely helpful in guiding the choice of antibiotics, provides the background for further clinical research; and monitoring the response to treatment with antibiotics or other forms of therapy is vital to the correct management of such patients.

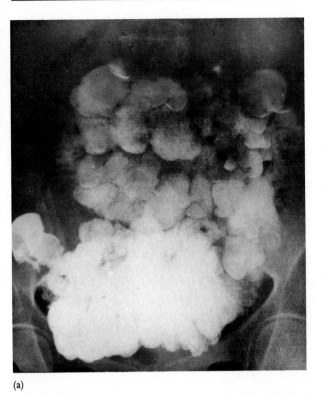
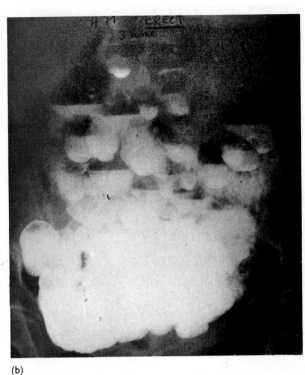

(a) (b)

Figure 3.55 Jejunal diverticulosis. Radiographs taken after the ingestion of barium with the subject (a) supine and (b) erect.

There is a plethora of tests, but they are not always well validated (*Table 3.33*). Their use will depend on the facilities and skills available. It is sensible to limit the range of tests available and ensure good quality control and intelligent use.

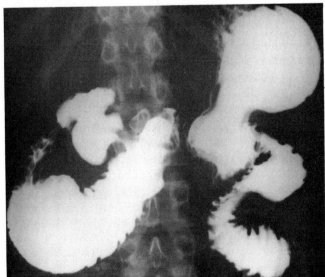

Figure 3.56 Scleroderma. Barium follow through examination showing a dilated duodenum. Culture of fluid aspirated from the upper small intestine yielded 10^6 viable organisms per millilitre.

Table 3.33 Tests for bacterial overgrowth in the small intestine

• *Indirect measures of the effects of bacterial metabolism*
  In the circulation
    Free bile acids
  In urine
    Amino acid derivatives
    Indoles (from tryptophan)
    Phenols (from tyrosine)
    Hippuric acid (from phenylalanine)
    Piperidine (from lysine)
    Pyrrolidine (from arginine and ornithine)
  In expired air
    $^{14}CO_2$ from:
      ^{14}C-labelled bile acids (glycocholic acid)
      ^{14}C-labelled carbohydrate (xylose)
      ^{14}C-labelled amino acid (taurine)
    Hydrogen from:
      Absorbable sugar (glucose)
      Non-absorbable sugar (lactulose)

• *Direct measures of bacteria and their metabolites in aspirates*
    Viable bacterial counts
    Concentration of volatile fatty acids
    Presence of deconjugated bile acids

• *Response to therapy*
    Improvement of clinical measurements of malabsorption (e.g. of fat, vitamin B_{12} and xylose)

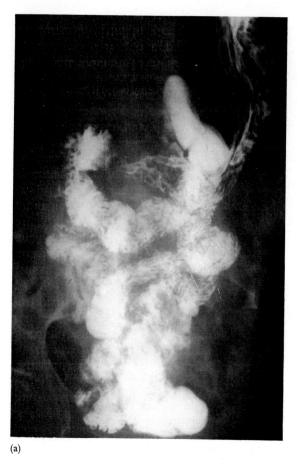

(a)

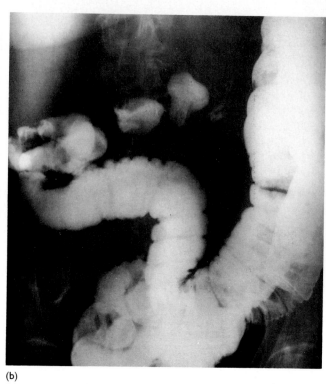

(b)

Figure 3.57 Duodenocolic fistula. Barium studies of a 48-year-old woman who presented with a megaloblastic anaemia (serum vitamin B_{12} 40 pg/ml). (a) A normal barium follow through examination. (b) The fistula is revealed by barium enema. The patient was a seamstress and in the absence of other pathology it was thought that her duodenum was perforated by a swallowed pin. There were no symptoms other than those of anaemia and the diagnosis of fistula was made only after it was shown that the impaired absorption of vitamin B_{12}–intrinsic factor complex could be corrected by the oral administration of tetracycline.

INDIRECT TESTS

Circulating free bile acids

In normal subjects the concentraiton of circulating bile acids in the fasting state is less than 10 μmol/l, whereas in patients with the stagnant loop syndrome levels of 13–52 μmol/l have been described.[93] Another useful test is a 2 hour postprandial rise in unconjugated bile acids. The major drawback is the significant overlap between patients with an interrupted enterohepatic circulation as a result of ileal resection or ileal dysfunction and bacterial overgrowth syndromes.

Bacterial metabolites in the urine

Intestinal bacteria may produce a number of metabolites which, after absorption, are excreted in the urine. The excretion of indican derived from the essential amino acid L-tryptophan has been correlated with bacterial overgrowth, but cannot be used under routine ward conditions because of the many variables involved in the production of indicanuria.

These include the quantity of dietary protein ingested, the efficacy of hydrolysis by proteolytic enzymes, the presence of malabsorption as a result of factors other than bacterial overgrowth, and the composition of intraluminal contents (e.g. the presence or absence of sugars and the hydrogen ion concentration).[118]

In a small series, it has been shown that the measurement of both indican and phenol in urine is a reasonably reliable and specific method of providing support for the diagnosis of bacterial overgrowth in the small intestine.[1] Nevertheless, the measurement of urinary markers is of limited value and, except in a metabolic unit (*Figure 3.58*), is rarely used these days.

Breath tests

The respiratory excretion of gases (carbon dioxide and hydrogen) produced by the metabolism of several substrates provides an elegant way of studying the effect of intestinal bacteria (*Figure 3.59*).[70]

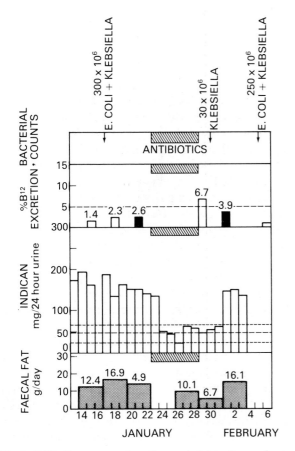

Figure 3.58 Response to the administration of oral tetracycline in a patient with bacterial overgrowth secondary to jejunal diverticulosis. In this case, viable bacterial counts in jejunal fluid can be assessed against measurements of vitamin B_{12} absorption (open columns, B_{12} given alone; closed columns, B_{12} + intrinsic factor), indican excretion (dietary protein 70 g/day) and faecal fat (dietary fat 70 g/day).

These tests are readily accepted by patients because they involve neither intubation nor the collection of urine and faeces. False negative results occur if there is a delay in the ingested substrate reaching the site of bacterial overgrowth or if the bacteria present are incapable of metabolizing that particular substance. Breath tests will not localize the site of bacterial catabolism of the substrate, although this may be overcome to some extent by using a radiopaque or radiolabelled (^{99m}Tc) marker and undertaking serial imaging with the breath test.[70,145] This may be particularly important in patients with rapid transit of material to the colon.

The bile acid breath test. This test, introduced for the diagnosis of altered bile acid metabolism, was the first to be utilized to study bacterial overgrowth.[49] The patient drinks a solution of glycocholic acid labelled with [^{14}C]-glycine, and hourly samples of expired carbon dioxide are collected for 6

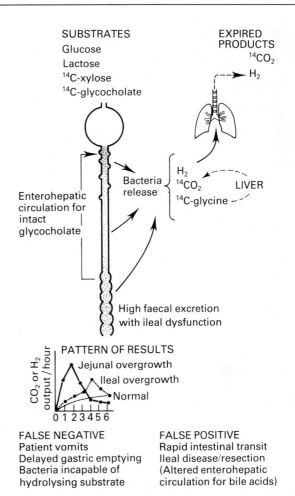

Figure 3.59 The principle of the breath test as used for the detection of bacterial overgrowth in the small intestine.

hours by trapping the gas with a measured quantity of an organic base. The patient must remain in a resting state to ensure a constant rate of carbon dioxide production. Under these circumstances the specific activity of expired $^{14}CO_2$ corrected for body weight gives a measure of the bacterial splitting of the amide bond linking [^{14}C]glycine to cholic acid. The radiolabelled bile acid mixes with the bile acid pool and the rate of excretion of $^{14}CO_2$ reflects its functional catabolic activity. Thus, a high specific activity of expired carbon dioxide may reflect a decreased pool size (e.g. after cholecystectomy or ileal resection) as well as an absolute increase in the breakdown of conjugated bile acids. A high specific activity also occurs in patients with ileal dysfunction sufficiently severe to allow bile acids to spill into the colon. This defect may be detected by the measurement of ^{14}C in the faeces.[139] The value of the bile acid breath test is limited by the fairly high incidence of false positive (10%) and false negative results (30%).[88] Thus, although the test is reasonably specific, it is only moderately sensitive. As a consequence this test is infrequently used nowadays.

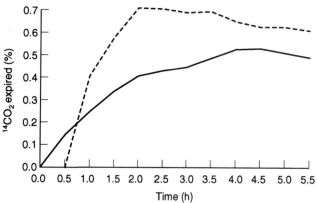

Figure 3.60 Percentage of orally administered [^{14}C]D-xylose expired as $^{14}CO_2$ per millimole of carbon dioxide ($\times 10^{-2}$). - - -, normal control; —, bacterial overgrowth.

[^{14}C]D-Xylose breath test. This test utilizes 1 g of D-xylose as a substrate. Bacterial overgrowth in the small bowel splits D-xylose and the $^{14}CO_2$ produced finds its way out into the breath. The advantages of D-xylose include the near-complete absorption in the proximal small bowel, no colonic dumping (unlike bile acids), very little metabolism of D-xylose by the host and its metabolism by Gram-negative aerobes which are always part of the overgrowth flora. The procedure involves giving 1 g of D-xylose with 5–10 μCI of [^{14}C]D-xylose in 500 ml of water, the breath being analysed at 30 minutes and 1 hour. The concentration of $^{14}CO_2$ can be measured either by liquid scintillation counting of trapped carbon dioxide or as a direct readout of $^{14}CO_2$ concentration from a calibrated $^{14}CO_2$ plastic filament detector system (*Figure 3.60*). The dose received compares favourably with a standard chest or abdominal radiograph and well below that used for contrast radiographs. The sensitivity of this test approaches 95%, which is distinctly superior to the bile acid breath test and probably superior to jejunal fluid culture. The latter is not surprising as the culture fluid is taken from a single location while D-xylose is absorbed over a larger segment of the proximal small bowel. The simplicity of performing the test, its sensitivity and specificity in extensive clinical testing make it an ideal test for detecting bacterial overgrowth.[82,84] The only drawback, perhaps, is the cost.

Hydrogen breath tests. These tests are based on the principle that bacterial metabolism of absorbable (glucose) and non-absorbable (lactulose) sugars produce hydrogen which cannot be utilized by mammalian tissue.[107] This hydrogen is released in the expired air and can be detected by mass spectrometry or commercial electrochemical hydrogen breath meters. A point of some importance is that between 2 and 27%[81] of individuals do not have enteric flora that can produce hydrogen and in this group this test is of little value. The test involves using either 10 ml of lactulose or 80 g of glucose given orally after a 12-hour fast (80 g of glucose is superior in its sensitivity compared to 50 g of glucose). Hydrogen is measured in the breath at half-hourly intervals. A high fasting breath hydrogen level can be found in bacterial overgrowth, in untreated coeliac and in normal individuals after certain diets such as pasta and whole-meal bread. The latter is due to the colonic fermentation of undigested carbohydrate. More specific for bacterial overgrowth is a rise of 18–20 ppm in the expired hydrogen within 2 hours of giving glucose. The lactulose breath test is not only less sensitive than the 80 g glucose breath test (70% compared to 85%) but less specific too.[82] Even in normal individuals, fermentation of lactulose in the caecum produces a rise in the breath hydrogen after a variable period averaging 1.5–2 hours (useful as a test for mouth-to-caecum transit time). Thus, a rise in the breath hydrogen level in the first hour-and-a-half after oral lactulose is suggestive of bacterial overgrowth; any subsequent rise is difficult to interpret. It has been suggested that, by combining a barium meal with the substrate, the site of bacterial proliferation may be identified, but this method is cumbersome and the result is not easy to interpret.

ANALYSIS OF ASPIRATES FROM THE LUMEN OF THE SMALL INTESTINE

Ideally, indirect evidence of bacterial overgrowth in the small intestine should be confirmed by intubating the gut and analysing fluid aspirated from an anatomically abnormal zone.[33] This exercise needs careful attention to detail and the active participation of a microbiologist with an interest in gut bacteria.

The patient should be studied in the fasting state and before treatment with antibiotics. A variety of tubes with devices to prevent contamination from salivary bacteria have been described, but a single-lumen, open-ended sterile tube may provide satisfactory results. In practice, it is easier to use a double-lumen tube. The additional channel should be flushed with carbon dioxide or nitrogen gas to help drive gut fluid up to the aspirating syringe. It is not always easy to pass the tip of the tube to the appropriate segment of the small intestine, and a great deal of patience and encouragement is needed to obtain samples from the ileum. Throughout the period of intubation the patient is asked to spit out saliva and should not be given fluid by mouth unless the study is to include observations on the effects of feeding. It may be possible to recognize salivary contamination of jejunal fluid by comparing the results of cultures of saliva and jejunal fluid taken at the same time.[66]

Aspirated specimens are treated with oxygen-free nitrogen before being passed to the bacteriologist for culture under aerobic and anaerobic conditions. Aliquots should be analysed for bile acids and volatile fatty acid content (if necessary after storage at $-20°C$).

A full bacterial profile in the aspirate could be provided only by a research laboratory, but it should be possible for a good hospital service to quantify viable aerobic and anaerobic organisms and to isolate coliforms and *Bacteroides* spp. Although reports from the literature show a lack of agreement regarding the bacteriology of the upper small intestine of control subjects (*Table 3.29*), most microbiologists agree that total aerobic counts rarely exceed 10^4 organisms/ml and that *E. coli* is never present in more than very small numbers (less than 10^3 organisms/ml). Anaerobic organisms (e.g. *Veillonella*) are usually less plentiful than aerobes, and representatives of the genus *Bacteroides* are only rarely isolated.

Few clinicians will submit their patients to sampling of fluid from the distal ileum except for research purposes and the data on the flora of this segment of the intestine in normal subjects is scanty (*Table 3.29*).

Biochemical study of aspirates

As indicated above, it is not always easy to get reliable results from the bacteriological analysis of fluid aspirated from the small intestine. Not only are there problems in culturing bacteria in the laboratory, but the clinician may not be able to exclude the possibility of contamination of the specimen, especially during a difficult intubation. Thus, biochemical indices of bacterial activity *in situ* are valuable. Bile acids may be measured semiquantitatively using simple thin-layer chromatography. The presence of free cholic, deoxycholic and chenodeoxycholic acids in the jejunum provide good evidence for the presence of bile-splitting organisms.[159] These bile acids may be detected in aspirates from the upper ileum of normal subjects in spite of only apparently small changes in the bacterial flora.[120] It is also useful to measure the concentration of volatile fatty acids in the jejunal contents. The demonstration of acetate (more than 0.5 mmol/l), propionate (more than 0.1 mmol/l) and butyrate (more than 0.01 mmol/l) is reported to occur only in the presence of bacterial overgrowth. Not only is the correlation with bacterial cultures excellent,

but some studies show this to be superior conventional hydrogen breath tests.[28,171]

RESPONSE TO TREATMENT
In some cases the response of metabolic tests to treatment with appropriate antibiotics may be sufficiently brisk to make this a useful method of diagnosis. The Schilling test for the absorption of vitamin B_{12} is particularly useful, and in some studies is as valuable in making a diagnosis as the bile acid breath test.[47] On the other hand, the response to antibiotics may be unpredictable and frequently incomplete.

Selection of tests

Three general problems confront the clinician in testing patients for the possibility of bacterial overgrowth in the small intestine:

1. A lack of absolute bacteriological criteria, especially in the consideration of those with apparently minor abnormalities of structure and function of the small intestine such as the elderly, patients with metabolic diseases such as diabetes and uraemia,[111] and malnourished people living in tropical and subtropical countries.
2. A rather uncertain correlation between bacterial overgrowth and metabolic sequelae, again especially in those with minor abnormalities of structure and function of the small intestine.
3. The variable biochemical potential of intestinal microflora, which means that only a proportion of metabolic tests may give abnormal results.[160]

Thus, members of a specialist gastroenterology unit should know their individual advantages and pitfalls.

TREATMENT

Many patients with bacterial overgrowth in the small intestine appear to suffer little harm. Minor degrees of diverticulosis of the small intestine are common in the elderly population and one suspects that the metabolic consequences are insignificant, although there are few published data to support this.

It is essential to characterize the underlying conditions of patients with suspected bacterial overgrowth and gastrointestinal symptoms or nutritional deficiencies as fully as possible. Obviously ill patients often have more than one disorder and the clinician must be aware of this possibility. Many of the patients are elderly and malnourished and protection against hypothermia may be necessary even under hospital conditions.[117] In such patients, nutritional support is necessary before investigating the

...sorder in detail. The approach to ... depend on the cause of bacterial ... predisposing conditions. Ideally, ...d be removed and the predisposing ...dified. Frequently this is not possible, ho...... ...d then the clinician will consider how best to us... antibiotics to minimize the metabolic consequences of bacterial overgrowth.

Surgical correction of blind loops

Patients with certain anatomical abnormalities (e.g. stricture of the small intestine, enteroenteric fistula, and dilated afferent loop of a Polya partial gastrectomy) can be readily cured by appropriate gastrointestinal surgery.[44,91] These patients must be selected with care because many of those who appear to have a correctable lesion have had previous surgery or have inflammatory disease of the bowel. In such situations, surgery is often difficult and may culminate in the resection of otherwise useful lengths of small intestine. Diverticulosis of the small intestine is rarely an indication for surgery, although the removal of a solitary large duodenal sac may be justifiable. Operations for pseudo-obstruction of the small intestine secondary to neuromuscular abnormalities or to scleroderma (*Figure 3.56*) are usually hazardous and unrewarding. In general, surgery exclusively for bacterial overgrowth is rarely performed and often unhelpful, the majority of patients doing reasonably well on conservative therapy.

Modification of the predisposing causes

Malnutrition is a predisposing cause of bacterial overgrowth in the small intestine.[62] Correction of nutritional deficiencies may play an important part in the recovery of patients with tropical sprue and certain non-specific gastrointestinal disorders such as have been described in elderly subjects.

Patients with immune deficiency frequently have episodes of diarrhoea which may be associated with malabsorption. Bacterial overgrowth and a degree of bile salt deconjugation has been described in such patients. Nevertheless, the cause of the bowel disturbance is not clear cut, as many of the patients have concomitant infection with *Giardia lamblia* or other organisms[124] and a proportion have significant abnormalities of the intestinal mucosa.

Treatment with antibiotics

In most patients with bacterial overgrowth in the small intestine it is not possible to correct the underlying defect and the clinician will wish to use anti-

biotics. Unfortunately, detailed knowledge of the organisms present in the bowel does not help in the selection of the most appropriate drugs. Bacterial overgrowth may be present without causing any problems and the decision to treat must be a matter of clinical judgement. Of bacteria isolated, 60% are resistant to tetracycline and, in particular, this drug has little intrinsic activity against *Bacteroides* yet it is surprisingly effective (*Figure 3.58*), perhaps because it inhibits the growth of many organisms that act synergistically to favour the growth of anaerobes. Control of anaerobic organisms seems to be the must useful step and this can be done using metronidazole or broad-spectrum antibiotics.[76] Treatment for 7–10 days is usually sufficient to get a response which can be monitored clinically and by laboratory tests. Although the numbers and species of the luminal flora may return rapidly to pretreatment levels (*Figure 3.58*), clinical improvement is often sustained for months. There are no set rules regarding the best way of giving antibiotics. Some patients will have remissions but relapse frequently to require intermittent therapy 1 out of 6 weeks while an occasional patient may require several weeks of continuous treatment before beneficial effects are seen. In particular, it often seems necessary to prolong treatment for patients with bacterial overgrowth in association with 'tropical malabsorption'. Tetracycline is given for several months before the functional defects are reversed and even then relapses are not infrequent.[131]

Prolonged clinical remissions despite renewed colonization of the small intestine are well documented,[32,67] but, as mentioned earlier, bacterial overgrowth in the small intestine is often not overtly harmful. Nevertheless, careful follow-up of patients who cannot be cured is desirable because of the risk of development of nutritional deficiency.[60]

Nutritional support

The wide range of nutritional disorders which may occur in patients with bacterial overgrowth in the small intestine have been outlined earlier in this section. It is particularly important to avoid nutritional deficiencies in children because of the danger of irreversible impairment of growth.[60] Regular injections of vitamin B_{12} are desirable not only to prevent the development of B_{12} deficiency but also as a means of keeping a check on the progress of the patient. It may also help to supplement the diet with fat-soluble vitamins, especially in patients with persistent steatorrhoea. Supplements of preparations of medium-chain triglycerides are sometimes prescribed as a means of enhancing the intake of calories without increasing the loss of fat in stools.

SPECIAL PROBLEMS

Diverticular disease of the small intestine

Most of the early reports of the 'blind loop syndrome' concerned patients with intestinal strictures, of which more than a third were ascribed to tuberculosis.[10] Curiously, diverticular disease of the small intestine was rarely mentioned, possibly because it is largely a disorder of the elderly.[8] Certain interesting aspects of this condition are described below.

Duodenal diverticula

Duodenal diverticula are usually benign lesions found by chance, which may cause serious symptoms, including weight loss, bleeding and jaundice.[43] Bacterial proliferation in a diverticulum close to the ampulla of Vater seems to predispose the patient to contamination of bile with the risk of cholangitis and pancreatitis. In patients investigated by endoscopic retrograde cholangiopancreatography, the incidence of common duct stones is distinctly higher in patients with juxtapapillary diverticula.[152] Biliary stasis and cholangitis are thought to be the causes for this observed higher incidence of choledocholithiasis.[153] Precipitated material in the diverticulum may lead to enterolith formation. In patients with recurring symptoms the administration of antibiotics is often not curative and diverticulectomy (not an easy procedure because of its location) may be necessary.

Jejunal diverticula

Diverticulosis of the jejunum may affect up to 5% of the elderly population.[32] The diverticula are usually small in size and number and frequently there are no symptoms. In younger people, diverticulosis may be diffuse and affect the whole of the small and large intestine. There may be an association with congenital disorders of connective tissue.[68] The diverticulae in these patients are not infrequently thin walled and may perforate. Intestinal perforation has occasionally occurred shortly after taking tetracycline tablets. It may be wise to give antibiotics in a liquid suspension to avoid the risk of erosion of the wall of the intestine by the hold up of the tablet in a diverticulum. Spontaneous bleeding from a jejunal diverticulum is also a well-recognized acute complication and it too may be precipitated by tetracycline. Other complications reviewed by Cooke *et al.*[32] include intestinal obstruction, cyst formation by the occlusion of the mouth of the diverticulum, intussusception, diverticulitis, lodgement of foreign bodies and enterolith formation. An enterolith may develop on a nidus of precipitated bile salts and may be seen in strictured intestine as well as in a diverticu-

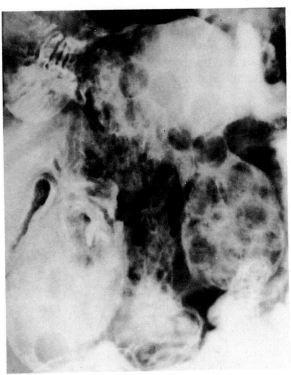

Figure 3.61 Enteroliths in a blind loop. This patient had an operation in infancy for reduplication of the ileum. At 22 years, after a trouble-free childhood, he presented with anaemia secondary to blood loss from the intestine. This view of the ileocaecal region reveals a dilated terminal ileum with a pouch containing enteroliths. The patient felt completely well after correction of the anaemia, and his faeces became free of occult blood. He refused laparotomy and his progress was monitored by his family doctor. Courtesy of A.H. Freeman. (Department of Radiology, Addenbrooke's Hospital, Cambridge.)

lum (*Figure 3.61*). Occasionally, abnormal liver function tests and a liver biopsy simulating alcoholic hepatitis may result from bacterial overgrowth.[115]

Bacterial overgrowth in the elderly

Whilst bacterial overgrowth syndrome may occur in the elderly due to similar causes as in the young, this has been reported in this group of patients in the absence of anatomical intestinal abnormalities. While some patients may have symptoms of diarrhoea, abdominal bloating and pain, many patients are free of gastrointestinal symptoms and present with malnutrition, vitamin B_{12} deficiency or failure to gain weight.[65] The frequency of bacterial overgrowth in the elderly is uncertain as are the consequences of this on overall nutrition. It would, however, seem sensible to treat all symptomatic and malnourished patients with abnormal breath tests. The reasons for bacterial overgrowth are uncertain though gastric achlorhydria, subtle changes in intestinal motility and jejunal diverticulae, not identified radiologically, may all play a part. A course of antibiotics usually improves symptoms and its effect on nutrition is gratifying for both the patient and clinician.[112]

Surgical problems

A further set of special problems are posed by two operations which may predispose to bacterial overgrowth.

Ileal reservoirs (Koch pouches)

The bacterial growth in ileal reservoirs may be close to that of the normal colon. There are occasionally disturbances of small intestinal function with malabsorption of fat and vitamin B_{12}. The morphological changes of the ileal mucosa are very variable. In some cases there is moderate to severe inflammation; in others the changes are minimal.[94] It is probable that malabsorption, when it occurs, is secondary to bacterial proliferation, and this is believed to be the mechanism of the commonly occurring increase in faecal bile acids.[6]

Jejunoileal bypass surgery

Although bypass surgery for obesity involves the creation of a long blind segment of the small intestine, it was originally believed that its self-emptying nature would protect the patient against the dangers of bacterial overgrowth. However, this has not been the case. More than half of all patients develop significant bacterial overgrowth in the jejunum,[127] and the degree of malabsorption is greater than that of an equivalent resection of the small intestine.[96] Appetite appears to be diminished and bacterial metabolites may contribute to life-threatening liver disease and immune complex-mediated arthralgias and skin changes. Bacterial overgrowth has been also implicated in the development of pseudo-obstruction of the colon.[11]

AIDS and AIDS-related complex

Gastrointestinal symptoms are among the most frequent complaints in patients with acquired immune deficiency syndrome (AIDS) and AIDS-related complex (ARC).[102] It is estimated that between 50 and 93% of all AIDS patients will have marked gastrointestinal complaints during their illness.[22,87] These occur secondary to common pathogens, opportunistic infections which are often multiple, and tumours. Infections are often recurrent and in many instances, such as cryptosporidia, no definite treatment exists. Bacterial overgrowth, however, is

an eminently treatable cause of diarrhoea. The incidence of the problem and details of the bacterial interactions are yet to be fully defined. It is believed that the altered immunity, gastric achlorhydria and a motility disorder may all contribute to bacterial overgrowth.[23,87] The diagnosis is by non-invasive breath testing and rarely necessitates jejunal intubation. In fact, once common pathogens have been excluded by culture and examination for parasites, it is reasonable to undertake a 2-week trial of antibiotics prior to undertaking invasive tests, with often gratifying results.

REFERENCES

1. Aarbakke, J. and Schjönsby, H. (1976) Value of urinary simple phenol and indican determination in the diagnosis of stagnant loop syndrome. *Scandinavian Journal of Gastroenterology*, **11**, 409–414.
2. Abud, R.L., Lindquist, B.L. *et al.* (1989) Concanavalin A promotes adherence of *S. typhimurium* to small intestinal mucosa of rats. *Proceedings of the Society for Experimental Biology and Medicine*, **192**(1), 81–86.
3. Allison, M.J., Maloy, S.E. and Mabon, R.R. (1976) Inactivation of *Clostridium botulinum* toxin by ruminal microbes from cattle and sheep. *Applied and Environmental Microbiology*, **32**, 685–688.
4. Ammon, H.V. and Phillips, S.F. (1973) Inhibition of colonic water and electrolyte absorption by fatty acids in men. *Gastroenterology*, **65**, 744–749.
5. Ammon, H.V., Thomas, P.H. and Phillips, S.F. (1974) Effects of oleic and ricinoleic acid on net jejunal water and electrolyte movement. *Journal of Clinical Investigation*, **53**, 374–379.
6. Anderson, H., Fasth, S., Filipsson, S. *et al.* (1979) Faecal excretion of intravenously injected 14C-cholic acid in patients with a conventional ileostomy and in patients with a continent ileostomy reservoir. *Scandinavian Journal of Gastroenterology*, **14**, 551–554.
7. Astley, R. (1975) Radiology of the gastrointestinal tract. In: *Paediatric Gastroenterology*, p. 552 (Eds) Anderson, C.M. and Burke, V. Oxford: Blackwell.
8. Badenoch, J. (1958) The blind loop syndrome. In: *Modern Trends in Gastroenterology*, pp. 231–242. (Ed.) Jones, F.A. London: Butterworth.
9. Bark, S. (1981) Amino acid absorption after intestinal by-pass procedures. *International Journal of Obesity*, **5**, 527–530.
10. Barker, W.H. and Hummel, L.E. (1939) Macrocytic anaemia in association with intestinal strictures and anastomosis. *Bulletin of the Johns Hopkins Hospital*, **46**, 215–254.

11. Barry, R.E., Chow, A.W. and Billesdon, J. (1977) Role of intestinal microflora in colonic pseudo-obstruction complicating jejunoileal bypass. *Gut*, **18**, 356–359.

12. Batt, R.M., Mclean, L. (1987) Comparison of the biochemical changes in the jejunal mucosa of dogs with aerobic and anaerobic bacterial overgrowth. *Gastroenterology*, **93**, 986–993.

13. Beachey, E.H. (1981) Bacterial adherence: adhesion receptor interactions mediating the attachment of bacteria to mucosal surfaces. *Journal of Infectious Diseases*, **143**, 325–345.

14. Berg, R.D. and Owens, W.E. (1979) Inhibition of translocation of viable *Escherichia coli* from the gastrointestinal tract of mice by bacterial antagonism. *Infection and Immunity*, **25**, 820–827.

15. Bernstein, L.H., Gutstein, B., Efron, G. and Wager, G. (1975) Experimental production of elevated serum folate in dogs with intestinal blind loops. II. Nature of bacterially produced folate coenzymes in blind loop fluid. *American Journal of Clinical Nutrition*, **28**, 925–929.

16. Bhat, P., Albert, M.J., Rajan, D. *et al.* (1980) Bacterial flora of the jejunum – comparison of luminal aspirate and mucosal biopsy. *Journal of Medical Microbiology*, **13**, 247–256.

17. Binder, H.J., Filburn, B. and Floch, M. (1975) Bile acid inhibition of intestinal anaerobic organisms. *American Journal of Clinicial Nutrition*, **26**, 119–125.

18. Bode, J.C., Bode, C. *et al.* (1984) Jejunal microflora in patients with chronic alcohol abuse. *Hepatogastroenterology*, **31**, 30–34.

19. Brandt, L.J., Bernstein, L.H. and Wager, A. (1977) Production of Vitamin B_{12} analogues in patients with small bowel bacterial overgrowth. *Annals of Internal Medicine*, **18**, 546–551.

20. Brin, M.F., Fettel, M.R. *et al.* (1985) Blind loop syndrome, vitamin E malabsorption and spinocerebellar degeneration. *Neurology*, **35**, 338–342.

21. Bullen, J.J., Rogers, H.J. and Griffiths, E. (1974) Bacterial iron metabolism in infection and immunity. In: *Microbial Iron Metabolism – A Comprehensive Treatise*, pp. 517–551. (Ed.) Neilands, J.B. New York: Academic Press.

22. Budharaja, M., Levendoglu, H. and Sherer, R. (1985) Spectrum of sigmoidoscopic findings in AIDS patients with diarrhoea. *American Journal of Gastroenterology*, **80**, A828.

23. Budharaja, M., Levendoglu, H. *et al.* (1987) Duodenal mucosal T cell sub-population and bacterial cultures in acquired immunodeficiency syndrome. *American Journal of Gastroenterology*, **82**, 427–430.

24. Burke, V., Houghton, M. and Gracey, M. (1977) Effect of enteric micro-organisms on intestinal sugar and fatty acid absorption. *Australian Journal of Experimental Biology and Medical Sciences*, **55**, 423–430.

25. Cain, J.R., Mayoral, L.G., Lotero, H. *et al.* (1976) Enterobacteriaceae in the jejunal microflora: prevalence and relationship to biochemical and histological evaluation in healthy Columbian men. *American Journal of Clinical Nutrition*, **29**, 1397–1403.

26. Challacombe, D.N., Richardson, J.M. and Anderson, C.M. (1974) Bacterial microflora of the upper gastrointestinal tract in infants without diarrhoea. *Archives of Diseases of Childhood*, **49**, 264–269.

27. Chanarin, I. (1979) Vitamin B_{12} deficiency and abnormal intestinal flora. In: *The Megaloblastic Anaemias*, 2nd edn, pp. 406–419. Oxford: Blackwell.

28. Chernov, A.J., Doe, W.F. and Gompertz, D. (1972) Intrajejunal volatile fatty acids in the stagnant loop syndrome. *Gut*, **13**, 103–106.

29. Clinicopathological conference (1967) A case of osteomalacia, osteoporosis and hypercalcemia. *British Medical Journal*, **i**, 219–223.

30. Coates, M.E. (1975) Gnotobiotic animals in research: their uses and limitations. *Laboratory Animal*, **9**, 275–282.

31. Cook, G.C. (1984) Aetiology and pathogenesis of post-infective tropical malabsorpton. *The Lancet*, **i**, 721–723.

32. Cooke, W.T., Cox, E.V., Fone, D.J. *et al.* (1963) The clinical and metabolic significance of jejunal diverticula. *Gut*, **4**, 115–122.

33. Corazza, G.R., Menozzi, M.G. *et al.* (1990) The diagnosis of bacterial over growth – reliability of jejunal culture and inadequacy of breath hydrogen testing. *Gastroenterology*, **98**, 302–309.

34. Curtis, K.J., Prizont, R. and Kim, Y.S. (1979) Protein digestion and absorption in the blind loop syndrome. *Digestive Diseases and Sciences*, **24**, 929–933.

35. Dickman, M.D., Chappelka, A.R. and Schaedler, R.W. (1976) The microbial ecology of the upper small bowel. *American Journal of Gastroenterology*, **65**, 57–62.

36. Donaldson, R.M., Jr (1964) Normal bacterial population of the intestine and their relation to intestinal function. *New England Journal of Medicine*, **270**, 938–945 and 1050–1056.

37. Donaldson, R.M., Jr (1965) Studies on the pathogenesis of steatorrhoea in the blind loop syndrome. *Journal of Clinical Investigation*, **44**, 1815–1820.

38. Donaldson, R.M., Jr (1965) Malabsorption in the blind loop syndrome. *Gastroenterology*, **48**, 388–395.

39. Donaldson, R.M., Jr (1990) The blind loop syndrome. In: *Gastrointestinal Disease*, p. 928. (Eds) Sleisenger, M.H. and Fordtran, J.S. Philadelphia: W.B. Saunders.

40. Drasar, B.S., Shiner, M. and Mcleod, G.M. (1969) Studies on the intestinal flora. I. The bacterial flora in the gastrointestinal tract in healthy and achlorhydric persons. *Gastroenterology*, **56**, 71–79.

41. Ducluzeau, R., Ladire, M., Callut, C. *et al.* (1977) Antagonistic effect of extremely oxygen sensitive clostridia from the microflora of conventional mice and of *Escherichia coli* against *Shigella flexneri* in the digestive tract of gnotobiotic mice. *Infection and Immunity*, **17**, 415–424.

42. Dyer, N.H., Dawson, A.M., Smith, B.F. and Todd, I.P. (1969) Obstruction of the bowel due to a lesion in the myenteric plexus. *British Medical Journal*, **i**, 686–689.

43. Eggert, A., Teichmann, W. and Wittman, D.H. (1982) The pathological implications of duodenal diverticula. *Surgery, Gynaecology and Obstetrics*, **154**, 62–64.

44. Ellis, H. and Smith, A.D.M. (1967) The blind loop syndrome. *Monographs in Surgical Science*, **4**, 193–215.

45. Faber, K. (1895) Perniciøs Anaemia som Følge afTarmlidelse. *Hospitalstidende*, **4**, 601–615.

46. Fainstein, V. and Musher, D.M. (1979) Bacterial adherence to pharyngeal cells in smokers, non-smokers and chronic bronchitis. *Infection and Immunity*, **26**, 178–182.

47. Farivar, S., Fromm, H. and Schindler, D. (1979) Sensitivity of bile acid breath test in the diagnosis of bacterial overgrowth in the small intestine with and without stagnant (blind loop) syndrome. *Digestive Diseases and Sciences*, **24**, 33–40.

48. Floch, M.H., Gershengoren, W. and Diamond, S. (1970) Cholic acid inhibition of intestinal bacteria. *American Journal of Clinical Nutrition*, **23**, 8–10.

49. Fromm, H. and Hofmann, A.F. (1971) Breath test for altered bile acid metabolism. *The Lancet*, **ii**, 621–625.

50. Gall, L.S. (1970) Normal fecal flora of man. *American Journal of Clinical Nutrition*, **23**, 1457–1465.

51. Gianella, R.A., Broitman, S.A. and Zamcheck, A. (1971) Vitamin B_{12} uptake by intestinal micro-organisms: mechanisms and relevance to syndromes of intestinal bacterial overgrowth. *Journal of Clinical Investigation*, **50**, 1100–1107.

52. Gibbons, R.J. and van Houte, J. (1975) Bacterial adherence in oral microbial ecology. *Annual Review of Microbiology*, **29**, 19–44.

53. Giordano, C. (1963) Use of exogenous and endogenous urea for protein synthesis in normal and uremic subjects. *Journal of Laboratory and Clinical Medicine*, **62**, 231–246.

54. Gorbach, S.L. (1971) Intestinal Microflora. *Gastroenterology*, **60**, 1110–1129.

55. Gorbach, S.L. and Tabaqchali, S. (1969) Bacteria, bile and the small bowel. *Gut*, **10**, 963–972.

56. Gorbach, S.L., Plaut, A.G., Nahas, L. *et al.* (1967) Studies of intestinal microflora. II. Micro-organisms of the small intestine and their relations to oral and faecal flora. *Gastroenterology*, **53**, 856–867.

57. Gorbach, S.L., Banwell, G.J., Jacobs, B. *et al.* (1970) Tropical sprue and malnutrition in West Bengal. Intestinal microflora and absorption. *American Journal of Clinical Nutrition*, **23**, 1545–1558.

58. Gordon, H.A. and Pesti, L. (1971) The gnotobiotic animal as a tool in the study of host microbial relationships. *Bacteriological Reviews*, **35**, 390–429.

59. Gracey, M. (1971) Intestinal absorption in the 'contaminated small bowel syndrome'. *Gut*, **12**, 403–410.

60. Gracey, M. (1979) The contaminated small bowel syndrome: pathogenesis, diagnosis and treatment. *American Journal of Clinical Nutrition*, **32**, 234–243.

61. Gracey, M., Burke, V. and Anderson, C.M. (1969) Association of monosaccharide malabsorption with abnormal small intestinal flora. *The Lancet*, **ii**, 384–385.

62. Gracey, M., Suharjono, S. and Stone, D. E. (1973) Microbial contamination of the gut; another feature of malnutrition. *American Journal of Clinical Nutrition*, **26**, 1170–1174.

63. Griffen, W.O., Jr, Richardson, J.D. and Medley, E.S. (1971) Prevention of small bowel contamination by ileocaecal valve. *Southern Medical Journal*, **64**, 1056–1058.

64. György, P. (1953) Hitherto unrecognised difference between human milk and cow's milk. *Pediatrics*, **11**, 98–107.

65. Haboubi, N.Y., Cowley, P.A. and Lee, G.S. (1988) Small bowel bacterial overgrowth: a cause of malnutrition in the elderly? *European Journal of Clinical Nutrition*, **42**, 999–1005.

66. Hamilton, I., Worsley, B., Shoesmith, J.G. *et al.* (1981) Salivary and jejunal flora in the normal and contaminated small bowel. *Gut*, **22**, A865.

67. Hamilton, J.D., Dyer, N. and Dawson, A.M. (1970) Assessment and significance of bacterial overgrowth in the small bowel. *Quarterly Journal of Medicine*, **39**, 265–285.

68. Hayakawa, A. (1982) Two cases of Ehlers–Danlos syndrome with gastrointestinal complications. *Gastroenterology (Japan)*, **17**, 61–67.

69. Helstrom, P.B. and Balish, E. (1979) Effect of oral tetracycline, the microbial flora and the athymic state on the gastrointestinal colonisation and infection of BALB/c mice with *Candida albicans*. *Infection and Immunity*, **23**, 764–774.

70. Hepner, G.W. (1978) Breath tests in gastroenterology. *Advances in Internal Medicine*, **23**, 25–45.

71. Hutchison, J.C.P., Gray, J., Flewett, T.H. *et al.* (1978) The safety of the Trexler isolator as judged by some physical and biological criteria: a report of experimental work at two centres. *Journal of Hygiene (Cambridge)*, **81**, 311–319.

72. Iacano, V.J., Taubman, M.A., Smith, D.H. *et al.* (1976) In: *Immunological Aspects of Dental Caries* (Eds) Bowen, W.H., Genco, R.J. and O'Brien, T.C. Washington, DC: Information Retrieval Service.

73. Jarumilinita, R., Miranda, M. and Villarejos,

V.M. (1976) A bacteriological study of the intestinal mucosa and luminal fluid of adults with acute diarrhoea. *Annals of Tropical Medicine and Parasitology*, **70**, 165–179.

74. Johanson, W.G., Pierce, A.K. and Samford, J.P. (1969) Changing pharyngeal bacteria flora of hospitalised patients: emergence of Gram-negative bacilli. *New England Journal of Medicine*, **281**, 1137–1140.

75. Johanson, W.G., Pierce, A.K., Sanford, J.P. and Thomas, G.D. (1972) Nosocomial respiratory infections with Gram-negative bacilli: the significance of colonisation of the respiratory tract. *Annals of Internal Medicine*, **77**, 701–706.

76. Joiner, K.A. and Gorbach, S.L. (1979) Antimicrobial therapy of digestive diseases. *Clinics in Gastroenterology*, **8**, 3–35.

77. Jonas, R., Flanagan, P.R. and Forstner, G.C. (1977) Pathogenesis of mucosal injury in the blind loop syndrome. Brush border enzyme activity and glycoprotein degradation. *Journal of Clinical Investigation*, **60**, 1321–1330.

78. Jones, E.A., Craigie, A., Tavill, A.S. *et al.* (1968) Protein metabolism in the intestinal stagnant loop syndrome. *Gut*, **9**, 466–469.

79. Kane, S.P. and Neale, G. (1976) Ileocolitis responding to bowel sterilisation. *Proceedings of the Royal Society of Medicine*, **69**, 266–267.

80. King, C. and Toskes, P.P. (1981) Protein losing enteropathy in human and rat blind loop syndrome. *Gastroenterology*, **84**, 504–509.

81. King, C. and Toskes, P.P. (1983) Use of breath tests in the study of malabsorption. *Clinics in Gastroenterology*, **12**, 591–609.

82. King, C. and Toskes, P.P. (1986) Comparison of the 1 g ^{14}C D-xylose, 10 g lactulose, 80 g glucose H$_2$ breath test in patients with small intestinal bacterial overgrowth. *Gastroenterology*, **91**, 1447–1451.

83. King, C., Lorenz, E. and Toskes, P. (1976) The pathogenesis of decreased serum protein levels in the blind loop syndrome: evaluation including a newly developed ^{14}C-amino acid breath test. *Gastroenterology*, **70**, A43/901.

84. King, C., Toskes, P., Guilarte, T. and Lorenz, E. (1976) Advantages of the xylose breath tests over the bile salt breath test in the diagnosis of blind loop syndrome. *Gastroenterology*, **80**, 504–509.

85. Klipstein, F.A. (1981) Tropical sprue in travellers and expatriates living abroad. *Gastroenterology*, **80**, 590–600.

86. Klipstein, F.A., Engert, R.F. and Short, H.B. (1978) Enterotoxigenicity of colonising coliform bacteria in tropical sprue and blind loop syndrome. *The Lancet*, **ii**, 342–344.

87. Lake-Bakaar, G., Beidas, S. *et al.* (1987) Impaired gastric secretion in AIDS. *Gastroenterology*, **92**, A1488.

88. Lauterburg, B.H., Newcomer, A.D. and Hoffman, A.F. (1978) Clinical value of the bile acid breath test. Evaluation of the Mayo Clinic experience. *Mayo Clinic Proceedings*, **53**, 227–223.

89. Lawrence, G., Bates, G. and Gaul, A. (1982) Pathogenesis of neonatal necrotising enterocolitis. *The Lancet*, **i**, 137–139.

90. Lee, A. (1980) Normal flora of animal intestinal surfaces. In: *Absorption of Micro-organisms to Surfaces*, pp. 145–173. (Eds) Britton, G. and Marshall, K.C. New York: Wiley.

91. Lennert, K.A. (1979) Das Dunndarmstase Syndrom Nachseit-zu-seit-Anastomose. *Chirurg (Berlin)*, **50**, 21–25.

92. Leurbcke, B., Kraus, B. and Lankisch, P.G. (1985) Small intestinal function in chronic relapsing pancreatitis. *Hepatogastroenterology*, **32**(3), 149–151.

93. Lewis, B., Panvelliwala, D., Tabaqchali, S. and Wootton, I.D.P. (1969) Serum bile acids in the stagnant loop syndrome. *The Lancet*, **i**, 219–223.

94. Loesche, K., Bolkert, T., Kiefhaber, P. *et al.* (1980) Bacterial overgrowth in the ileal reservoirs (Koch pouch): extended functional studies. *Hepatogastroenterology*, **27**, 310–316.

95. Long, S.S. and Swenson, R. M. (1977) Development of anaerobic faecal flora in healthy newborn infants. *Journal of Pediatrics*, **91**, 298–301.

96. McGouran, R.C.M., Goldie, A., Ang, L. and Maxwell, J.D. (1979) Weight loss after jejuno-ileal bypass and resection in the rat: food intake, faecal calorie loss and the effect of antibiotics. *Gut*, **20**, A496.

97. Mackowiak, P.A. (1978) Microbial synergism in human infections. *New England Journal of Medicine*, **298**, 21–26, 83–87.

98. Mackowiak, P.A. (1982) The normal bacterial flora. *New England Journal of Medicine*, **307**, 83–93.

99. Mackowiak, P.A., Martin, R.M. and Smith, J.W. (1978) Pharyngeal colonisation by Gram-negative bacilli in aspiration prone persons. *Archives of Internal Medicine*, **138**, 1224–1227.

100. Mackowiak, P.A., Martin, R.M. and Smith, J.W. (1979) The role of bacterial interference in the increased prevalence of oropharyngeal Gram-negative bacilli among alcoholics and diabetics. *American Review of Respiratory Diseases*, **120**, 589–593.

101. Maldonado, J.E., Gregg, J.A., Green, P.S. and Brown, A.L. (1970) Chronic idiopathic intestinal pseudo-obstruction. *American Journal of Medicine*, **49**, 213–222.

102. Malenbranche, R., Guerin, J.M., Laroche, A.C. *et al.* (1983) Acquired immunodeficiency syndrome with severe gastrointestinal manifestations in Haiti. *The Lancet*, **ii**, 873–875.

103. Manny, J., Muga, M. and Eyal, Z. (1981) The continuing clinical enigma of duodenal diverticulum. *American Journal of Surgery*, **142**, 596–600.

104. Marshall, K.C. and Britton, G. (1980) Microbial adhesion in perspective. In: *Adsorption of Micro-organisms to Surfaces*, pp. 1–5. (Eds) Britton, G. and Marshall, K.C. New York: Wiley.

105. Mathan, V.I., Babcor, B.M. and Donaldson, R.M. (1974) Kinetics of the attachment of intrinsic factor bound cobamides to ileal receptors. *Journal of Clinical Investigation*, **54**, 598–608.

106. Metchnikoff, E. (1901) Sur la flore du corps humain. *Manchester Literary and Philosophical Society*, **45**, 1–38.

107. Metz, G., Gassul, M.A., Drasar, B.S. *et al.* (1976) Breath hydrogen test for small intestinal bacterial concentration. *The Lancet*, **i**, 668–669.

108. Meulengracht, E. (1929) Pernicious anaemia in intestinal stricture (with one liver treated case). *Acta Medica Scandinavica*, **72**, 231–240.

109. Meynell, G.G. (1963) Antibacterial mechanisms of the mouse gut. II. The role of volatile fatty acids in the normal gut. *British Journal of Experimental Pathology*, **44**, 209–219.

110. Miller, B., Mitchison, R., Tabaqchali, S. and Neale, G. (1971) The effects of excess bacterial proliferation on protein metabolism in rats with self filling jejunal sacs. *European Journal of Clinical Investigation*, **2**, 23–31.

111. Mitch, W.E. (1978) Effects of intestinal flora on nitrogen metabolism in patients with chronic renal failure. *American Journal of Clinical Nutrition*, **31**, 1594–1600.

112. Montgomery, R.D., Haboubi, N.Y. *et al.* (1986) Causes of malabsorption in the elderly. *Age and Ageing*, **15**, 235–240.

113. Morris, J.A., Havan, D. and Smith, A. (1987) Common bacterial toxins as a possible cause of SIDS. *Medical Hypothesis*, **22**, 211–222.

114. Mutch, W.M., Jr (1977) Stasis syndrome following abdominal colectomy. *Diseases of the Colon and Rectum*, **20**, 340–346.

115. Nazim, M., Stamp, G. and Hodgson, H.J. (1989) Non-alcoholic steatohepatitis associated with small intestinal diverticulae. *Hepatogastroenterology*, **36**, 349–351.

116. Neale, G. (1968) Protein deficiency in the temperate zones. *Proceedings of The Royal Society of Medicine*, **60**, 1069–1073.

117. Neale, G., Antcliff, A.C., Welbourn, R.B. *et al.* (1967) Protein malnutrition after partial gastrectomy. *Quarterly Journal of Medicine*, **36**, 469–481.

118. Neale, G., Gompertz, D., Schonsby, H. *et al.* (1972) The metabolic and nutritional consequences of bacterial overgrowth in the small intestine. *American Journal of Clinical Nutrition*, **25**, 1409–1417.

119. Nelson, D.P. and Mata, L.J. (1970) Bacterial flora associated with the human gastrointestinal mucosa. *Gastroenterology*, **58**, 56–61.

120. Northfield, T.C., Drasar, B.S. and Wright, J.T. (1973) Value of small intestinal bile acid analysis in the diagnosis of stagnant loop syndrome. *Gut*, **14**, 341–347.

121. Nygaard, K. (1967) Changes in the intestinal flora after resections and bypass operations on the small intestine in rats. *Acta Chirurgica Scandinavica*, **133**, 569–583.

122. Onderdonk, A.B. and Bartlett, J.G. (1979) Bacteriological studies of experimental ulcerative colitis. *American Journal of Clinical Nutrition*, **32**, 258–265.

123. Onderdonk, A., Marshall, B., Cioneros, R. and Levy, S.B. (1981) Competition between congenic *Escherichia coli* K-12 strains *in vivo*. *Infection and Immunity*, **32**, 74–79.

124. Parkin, D.M., McCelleland, D.B.L., Moore, R.R.O. *et al.* (1972) Intestinal bacterial flora and bile salt studies in hypogammaglobulinemia. *Gut*, **13**, 182–188.

125. Plaut, A.G., Gorbach, S.L., Nahas, N. *et al.* (1967) Studies of intestinal microflora. III. The microbial flora of human small intestinal mucosa and fluids. *Gastroenterology*, **53**, 868–873.

126. Pollard, M. (1965) The use of germ free animals in virus research. *Progress in Medical Virology*, **i**, 362–376.

127. Powell-Jackson, P.R., Maudgal, D.P., Sharp, D. *et al.* (1979) Intestinal bacterial metabolism of protein and bile acids: role in pathogenesis of hepatic disease after jejunoileal surgery. *British Journal of Surgery*, **66**, 772–775.

128. Prizont, R. (1981) Glycoprotein degradation in the blind loop syndrome. Identification of glycosidases in jejunal contents. *Journal of Clinical Investigation*, **67**, 336–344.

129. Reed, S.E. and Tyrell, D.A.J. (1974) Viruses associated with the healthy individual. In: *The Normal Microbial Flora of Man*, pp. 255–257 (Eds) Skinner, F.A. and Carr, G.J. New York: Academic Press.

130. Richards, P., Metcalfe-Gibson, A., Ward, E.E. *et al.* (1967) Utilisation of ammonia nitrogen for protein synthesis in man and the effect of protein restriction and uraemia. *The Lancet*, **ii**, 845–849.

131. Rickles, F.R., Klipstein, F.W., Tomasini, J. *et al.* (1972) Long term follow up of antibiotic treated tropical sprue. *Annals of Internal Medicine*, **76**, 203–210.

132. Riepe, S., Goldstein, J. and Alpers, D.H. (1980) Effect of secreted Bacteroides proteases on human intestinal brush border hydrolases. *Journal of Clinical Investigation*, **66**, 314–322.

133. Roberts, S.H., James, O. and Jarvis, E.H. (1977) Bacterial overgrowth syndrome without 'blind loop': a cause of malnutrition in the elderly. *The Lancet*, **ii**, 1193–1195.

134. Rosebury, T. (1962) Distribution and development of the microbiota of man. In: *Microorganisms Indigenous to Man*, pp. 310–384. New York: McGraw Hill.

135. Rutgeerts, P., Ghoos, Y., Vantrappen, G. and

Eyssen, H. (1981) Ileal dysfunction and bacterial overgrowth in patients with Crohn's disease. *European Journal of Clinical Investigation*, **11**, 199–206.

136. Salen, G., Goldstein, F. and Wirts, C.W. (1966) Malabsorption in intestinal scleroderma. Relation to bacterial flora and treatment with antibiotics. *Annals of Internal Medicine*, **64**, 834–841.

137. Savage, D.C. (1970) Associations of indigenous microorganisms with gastrointestinal mucosal epithelia. *American Journal of Clinical Nutrition*, **23**, 1495–1501.

138. Savage, D.C. (1980) Colonisation by and survival of pathogenic bacteria on intestinal mucosal surfaces. In: *Adsorption of Microorganisms to Surfaces*, pp. 175–206 (Eds) Britton, G. and Marshall, K.C. New York: Wiley.

139. Scarpello, J.B. & Sladen, G.E. (1977) Appraisal of the ^{14}C-glycocholate acid test with special reference to the measurement of faecal ^{14}C excretion. *Gut*, **18**, 742–748.

140. Scarpello, J.B., Hague, R.V., Cullen, D.R. and Sladen, G.E. (1976) The ^{14}C-glycholate breath test in diabetic diarrhoea. *British Medical Journal*, **ii**, 673–675.

141. Schjönsby, H. (1977) Osteomalacia in the stagnant loop syndrome. *Acta Medica Scandinavica Supplementum*, **603**, 39–41.

142. Schjönsby, H., Drasar, B.S., Tabaqchali, S. and Booth, C.C. (1973) Uptake of vitamin B_{12} by intestinal bacteria in the stagnant loop syndrome. *Scandinavian Journal of Gastroenterology*, **8**, 41–47.

143. Schjönsby, H., Halvorsen, J.F., Hofstad, T. and Hovdenak, N. (1977) Stagnant loop syndrome in patients with continent ileostomy (intra-abdominal ileal reservoir). *Gut*, **18**, 795–799.

144. Schroepfer, J.L., Jr, Niehaus, W.G., Jr and McCloskey, J.A. (1970) Enzymatic conversion of linoleic acid to 10D-hydroxy-Δ12-*cis*-octadenoic acid. *Journal of Biological Chemistry*, **245**, 3798–3801.

145. Sciaretta, G. (1977) Diagnosis of blind loop syndrome by X-ray breath hydrogen test. *The Lancet*, **i**, 310–311.

146. Scott, A.J. and Khan, G.A. (1968) Partial biliary obstruction with cholangitis producing a blind loop syndrome. *Gut*, **9**, 187–192.

147. Scowden, E.B., Schaffner, W. and Stone, W.J. (1978) Overwhelming strongyloidiasis: an unappreciated opportunistic infection. *Medicine (Baltimore)*, **57**, 527–544.

148. Seyderhelm, R., Lehmann, W. and Wichels, P. (1924) Experimentelle Intestinale Perniziose Anamie Biem Hund. *Klinische Wochenschrift*, **3**, 1439–1445.

149. de Seze, S., Bernier, J.-J., Caroit, M. *et al.* (1972) Un cas d'osteomalacie par malabsorption de mechanisme inhabituel au cours d'un syndrome de l'anse borgne. *Revue de Rhumatisme et des Maladies Osteo-Articulares*, **39**, 297–303.

150. Schedlofsky, S. and Freter, R. ( ) between ecologic and immunologic mechanisms of intestinal flora. *Journal Infectious Diseases*, **129**, 296–303.

151. Simon, G.C. and Gorbach, S.L. (1986) Hu intestinal microflora. *Digestive Diseases and Sciences*, **31**(suppl. 9), 1475–1525.

152. Skar, V., Lotveit, T. and Osnes, M. (1989) Juxtapapillary diverticulae predispose to common duct stones. *Scandinavian Journal of Gastroenterology*, **24**, 202–204.

153. Skar, V., Skar, A.J., Bratlie, J. *et al.* (1989) β-glucuronidase activity in the bile of patients both with and without duodenal diverticulae. *Scandinavian Journal of Gastroenterology*, **24**, 205–212.

154. Spiers, A.S.D., Dias, S.F. and Lopez, J.A. (1980) Infection protection in patients with cancer:microbiological evaluation of portable laminar air flow isolation, topical chlorhexidine and oral non-absorbable antibiotics. *Journal of Hygeine* (Cambridge), **84**, 457–465.

155. Sprunt, K., Leidy, G.A. and Redman, W. (1971) Prevention of bacterial overgrowth. *Journal of Infectious diseases*, **123**, 1–10.

156. Szeri, I., Anderlik, P., Banos, Z. and Radnai, B. (1976) Decreased cellular immune response of germ free mice. *Acta Microbiologica Academiae Scientarium Hungaricae (Budapest)*, **23**, 231–234.

157. Tabaqchali, S. (1970) The pathophysiological role of small intestinal bacterial flora. *Scandinavian Journal of Gastroenterology*, **5**(suppl. 6), 139–163.

158. Tabaqchali, S. and Pallis, C. (1970) Reversible nicotinamide deficiency encephalopathy in a patient with jejunal diverticulosis. *Gut*, **11**, 1024–1028.

159. Tabaqchali, S., Hatzioannou, J. and Booth, C.C. (1968) Bile acid deconjugation and steatorrhoea in patients with the stagnant loop syndrome. *The Lancet*, **ii**, 12–16.

160. Taylor, R.H., Argerinos, A., Taylor, A.J. *et al.* (1981) Bacterial colonisation of the jejunum: an evaluation of five diagnostic tests. *Gut*, **22**, A442.

161. Tete, R., Boyer, J.D., Slaoui, H. and Mas, R. (1979) Diarrhée chronique avec malabsorption par amylose intestinale secondairea une polyarthrite rhumatoide au cours d'un diabète. *Lyon Medecin*, **242**, 283–288.

162. Thomas, P.J. (1972) Identification of some enteric bacteria which convert oleic acid to hydroxy-stearic acid *in vitro*. *Gastroenterology*, **62**, 430–435.

163. Tonnis, W. and Brusis, A. (1931) Veranderungen der Morphologischen Blut Bildes Bei Skuter und Chronischer Darminthaltsstaung. *Deutsche Zeitschrift für Chirurgie*, **233**, 133–139.

164. Toskes, P.P., King, C.E., Spivey, J.C. and Lorenz, E. (1978) Xylose catabolism in the experimental rat blind loop syndrome. Studies including the use of a newly developed D-^{14}C-xylose breath test. *Gastroenterology*, **74**, 691–697.

165. Ulshen, M.H. and Rollo, J.L. (1980) Pathogenesis

ritis in man – another
ournal of Medicine,

arson, E.R. *et al.*
on of urea nitrogen for
cally uraemic and
e and Molecular

I., Menge, E.-B. and
abliminal inhibitory
on adhesiveness of
Escherichia coli ....views of Infectious
Diseases; **I**, 845–851.

168. Watson, G.M., Cameron, D.G. and Witts, L.J.
(1948) Experimental macrocytic anaemia in the
rat. *The Lancet*, **ii**, 404–408.

169. Welkos, S.L., Toskes, P.P., Baer, H. (1981)
Importance of anaerobic bacteria in the cobalamin
malabsorption of the experimental rat blind loop
syndrome. *Gastroenterology*, **80**, 313–320.

170. White, W.H. (1890) On the pathology and
prognosis of pernicious anaemia. *Guys Hospital
Reports*, **47**, 149–194.

171. Whitehead, J.S., Kum, Y.S. and Prizont, R.
(1976) A simple quantitative method to determine
short chain fatty acid levels in biological fluids.
Clinica et Chemica Acta, **72**, 315–318.

172. Whitt, D.D. and Savage, D.C. (1980) Kinetics of
changes induced by indigenous microbiota in the
activity levels of alkaline phosphatase and
dissacharidases in small intestinal enterocytes in
mice. *Infection and Immunity*, **29**, 144–151.

173. Williams, R.C. and Gibbons, R.J. (1972)
Inhibition of bacterial adherence by secretory
immunoglobulin A: a mechanism of antigen
disposal. *Science*, **177**, 697–699.

174. Williams, R.C. and Gibbons, R.J. (1975)
Inhibition of streptococcal attachment to receptors
on human buccal epithelial cells by antigenically
similar salivary glycoproteins. *Infection and
Immunity*, **11**, 711–718.

175. Wirt, C.W. and Goldstein, F. (1963) Studies of the
mechanisms of post-gastrectomy steatorrhea.
Annals of Internal Medicine, **58**, 25–36.

POSTINFECTIVE MALABSORPTION (INCLUDING TROPICAL SPRUE)

G.C. Cook

Relatively little is known about the prevalence and severity of malabsorption in acute infective conditions of the small intestine – viral, bacterial and parasitic – and the length of time for which it can continue after the specific organism(s) has been eliminated from the lumen.

In this section, malabsorption following several infective states involving the small intestine – 'postinfective' malabsorption – is described. In some cases, malabsorption persists in the presence of a mixed luminal flora, and a single infective agent cannot be detected. In others the recognizable initiating infective cause (or causes) may continue, culminating in a chronic form; a more precise term is therefore '*postacute* infective' malabsorption. As with all infective diseases the clinical spectrum varies markedly from a subclinical case to one with gross pathology (malabsorption). Postinfective malabsorption is of particular clinical relevance in tropical countries where small (and large) intestinal infections are exceedingly common. The specific infective conditions themselves are considered in more detail in Chapter 9.

There is considerable confusion between postinfective malabsorption and the 'tropical sprue' syndrome; in tropical and subtropical countries the entities now seem certain to be synonymous.

Much of this difficulty is associated with semantics. Sir Patrick Manson first used the term 'tropical sprue' in the English language in 1880.[24] It was afterwards applied to all cases of malabsorption in tropical countries, undoubtedly including some resulting from tuberculosis and parasitoses (both protozoan and helminthic). Historically, chronic diarrhoea accompanied by wasting was, however, known in India prior to 600 BC.[82] Although the Englishman William Hillary is often credited with the first precise description of 'tropical sprue' in Barbados,[8,19,36] it is likely that he described either epidemic *Giardia lamblia* infection or possibly strongyloidiasis. This clinical syndrome was certainly well known to British physicians in India during the 18th and 19th centuries;[24] most descriptions were in the British expatriate population. It was only in the early 1960s that reports of a high prevalence of epidemic postinfective malabsorption in indigenous Indians became available.

Despite suggestions in early descriptions that chronic tropical malabsorption had an insidious onset, it is clear (after careful assessment) that the vast majority of cases have always presented acutely.[24] The confusion is further compounded when acute epidemic cases of small intestinal infection with gross dehydration (in addition to malabsorption of xylose and fat) and acute mortality are labelled 'tropical sprue', as in many reports from southern India.[5,82] It is therefore essential to include a time factor in the definition of the clinical *syndrome* of tropical sprue, e.g. chronic diarrhoea and malabsorption with weight loss, of at least 3–4 months duration. If it is to be used at all, the term 'tropical sprue' would also be better reserved for a condition where the malabsorption of nutrients is quantitatively more important than that of water and electrolytes. Although the pathogenesis of postinfective malabsorption remains in doubt (see below), it now seems clear that most cases follow an acute small intestinal insult from either a bacterial, viral or parasitic (or mixed) infection.

Overall, evidence for postinfective malabsorption following a small intestinal insult is more complete for bacterial and parasitic infections; infections of viral origin might, however, be more important numerically. Lack of precise data may reflect the fact that virology remains a relatively neglected discipline in most developing Third World countries, where infections of all types are far more common than in the West. In a tropical setting it is likely that mixed intestinal infections of viral, bacterial and parasitic origin are responsible for the common small intestinal morphological changes, as demonstrated in preschool Guatemalan village children[80] ('tropical enteropathy', see below). However, many asymptomatic people in tropical countries have at least one pathogenic organism in the small intestinal lumen, which may be viral, bacterial or parasitic. Hence, it is often difficult, or impossible, to incriminate a specific causative agent.

The effect of malabsorption syndromes following the various small intestinal insults on overall nutritional status in the Third World is largely unknown;[118] children are especially at risk. The magnitude of energy loss is unclear;[119] one estimate puts the deficit at 10% of dietary energy, which is substantial in tropical populations subsisting on a marginal diet.[105] The role of anorexia in exacerbating the associated malnutrition is also underexplored.[63]

ACUTE INTESTINAL INFECTIONS PREDISPOSING TO POSTINFECTIVE MALABSORPTION

TRAVELLERS' DIARRHOEA

This disease accounts for vast numbers of cases of transient diarrhoea in travellers to developing Third World countries.[25] Circumstantial evidence[24] indicates that most cases of postinfective malabsorption in a tropical context begin with this disease; small intestinal colonization persists after the acute attack and plays an important role in the pathophysiology of chronic malabsorption.[24,27] Enterotoxigenic serotypes of *Escherichia coli* (see below) account for the majority of cases.[52,99] The enterotoxin attaches to ganglioside receptors on the small intestinal villi, adenylate cyclase is produced, and that in turn raises the luminal cAMP concentration.[46] Other causative organisms are *Shigella* spp., *Campylobacter* spp., the rota and Norwalk viruses, and *G. lamblia*, *Cryptosporidium* spp.[34] and *Isospora belli*. A mixed infection is common. However, 25–30% of cases do not have a recognizable aetiological agent.[52]

Prophylaxis forms the basis of management, but symptomatic treatment is sometimes required. Oral rehydration forms the basis of successful treatment. Diphenoxylate and loperamide, which inhibit peristalsis (and to a lesser extent luminal secretion), promote continuing small intestinal colonization. Antibiotics which are frequently used both prophylactically and therapeutically should be used selectively. Neomycin, doxycycline, co-trimoxazole (trimethoprim and sulphamethoxazole), Streptotriad (streptomycin, sulphadimidine, sulphadiazine), sulphathiazole, and ciprofloxacin are all effective prophylactically.[52] However, they should not be used indiscriminately because the causative organisms are frequently resistant and widespread use encourages the development of further resistant strains. No vaccine is available.

Initiation of chemotherapy early in the disease is the correct management for an established case of moderate to severe magnitude. Many antibiotics have been used; trimethoprim, alone or in combination with sulphamethoxazole (as co-trimoxazole), and ciprofloxacin have given satisfactory results.[43]

VIRAL INFECTIONS

Significant intestinal protein loss (mean 1.7 g daily) and xylose malabsorption have been demonstrated in northern Nigerian children with measles;[42] approximately 25% also had lactose malabsorption. Other infections in children caused by enteroviruses and herpes simplex virus are also associated with diarrhoea and weight loss; malnutrition may follow;[77] the mechanism (involving enterocyte damage) is probably similar to that in measles.

Volunteers infected with enteric viruses develop small intestinal morphological lesions, consisting of broadening and flattening of villi, which are not always associated with symptoms.[2]

Jejunal mucosal changes giving rise to severe

malabsorption have been well documented in viral hepatitis;[23] these may persist for a considerable time after resolution of the hepatic abnormalities. The Norwalk agent, a 27 nm picornavirus, can also produce mucosal damage and malabsorption.[107] Rotavirus infections give rise to morphological abnormalities and, especially in children, malabsorption.[76,106]

These viral infections are invasive, and the resulting diarrhoea and malabsorption are caused by enterocyte destruction. Malabsorption usually occurs after the virus has been shed into the intestinal lumen; the villi contain immature crypt-type enterocytes. In coronavirus infections in piglets, which resemble human rotavirus infections, glucose absorption is significantly impaired.[115] This has practical importance in management since sodium and water secretion cannot be reversed by glucose; oral rehydration fluids, commonly used in small intestinal (including traveller's) diarrhoea, contain high sugar concentrations which overwhelm the limited absorptive capacity.

Baker et al.[6] have suggested that coronavirus infections are responsible for at least some cases of 'tropical sprue' in southern India; this might well be the case, but some asymptomatic individuals also excrete these viruses and this does not necessarily imply a cause–effect relationship. Also in Vellore, a search for evidence of Berne virus infection in 'epidemic tropical sprue' proved negative.[20]

BACTERIAL INFECTIONS

Moderate to severe malabsorption is common during acute intestinal infection of bacterial origin, and subnormal absorptive capacity persists for variable periods after termination of the diarrhoea and apparent clinical recovery. In a study in Bangladesh, approximately 70% of patients still had evidence of xylose malabsorption 1 week after the diarrhoea had ceased; this was less common after cholera than Shigella, Salmonella and Staphylococcal spp. infections; xylose and vitamin B_{12} malabsorption persisted for up to 378 and 196 days, respectively, after the diarrhoea had cleared.[73] This was not the first study to demonstrate persistence of malabsorption after recovery from small intestinal bacterial disease, but it emphasized that it is a relatively common occurrence.

Although many different infective insults to the enterocyte are probably important in postinfective malabsorption, evidence for bacteria being responsible currently has more solid support than that involving other agents.

Escherichia coli

These organisms (with varying modes of pathogenicity) produce diarrhoea and malabsorption by enterotoxin production and mucosal invasion – similar to that caused by Shigella sp. They are frequently food- or water-borne, and may cause outbreaks of gastroenteritis.[15,114] Heat-labile (LT) enterotoxins exert their effect by activating adenylcyclase in the same way as Vibrio cholerae. Both LT and heat-stable (ST) enterotoxins are probably important in traveller's diarrhoea (see above). A large pool of resistant E. coli (often showing resistance to multiple antimicrobials) now exists in the community.[53] Enterotoxin production by E. coli may be transferred simultaneously with antibiotic resistance: 72 and 44% of enterotoxigenic E. coli isolated in South-East Asia were resistant to one or more and four or more antibiotics, respectively.[44] Adhesiveness of E. coli to the enterocyte is also a property of some strains,[17] and that might be important in continuing colonization and subsequent malabsorption.[68] The relationship between adherence and Vero-toxin production remains unclear.[70] Attachment of microorganisms to the enterocyte prevents them being cleared by persistaltic activity; such mucosal receptors may be genetically determined.[101] Ultrastructural studies have shown E. coli adherent to mucosal cells with flattening of the microvilli, loss of the cellular terminal web, and cupping of the plasma membrane around individual bacteria.[98] Intracellular damage was marked in the most heavily colonized cells. Histological improvement was demonstrated following clearing of the E. coli with neomycin backed up by nutritional support. This mechanism can lead to protracted diarrhoea in infants.

In most cases, the resultant malabsorption is short lived. However, some cases of postinfective malabsorption are a long-term result of such infections (see below).

Salmonellosis

Malabsorption occasionally follows infection with Salmonella spp.,[58] but the frequency of this is unknown.

Campylobacter sp.

Although unusual, dysenteric disease (bloody diarrhoea) has for long been known to predispose to tropical postinfective malabsorption;[24,25,27] in additon to shigellosis, it is clear that some cases are caused by enteroinvasive and enterohaemorrhagic E. coli (see above) and others by Campylobacter sp.

Most cases of *Campylobacter* sp. infection presenting with gastroenteritis are acute, and are self-limiting, but the initial symptoms can be prolonged.[16,69] The disease is a zoonosis; poultry are frequently contaminated. Many outbreaks have been traced to infected cow's milk. Dogs are also a source of infection.[57] Although the infection is self-limiting, erythromycin probably hastens recovery when given early in a severe case. The carrier state is common. It is not clear how often the disease progresses to postinfective malabsorption.

Clostridium perfringens *('Pig bel' disease; enteritis necroticans)*

This acute infection, which is more common in children than adults, occurs in several tropical countries, notably Papua New Guinea,[88] Thailand and Uganda,[25] and can cause persisting malabsorption. It is sometimes associated with persisting structural changes in the small intestine.

The disease is caused by the β toxin of *Clostridium perfringens* type C, which is ingested in contaminated pork following pig feasts.[35] Trypsin inhibition is considered important. The acute disease varies from an acute gastroenteritis to a haemorrhagic necrotizing jejunitis with severe dysentery;[88] in the fulminant form, resection of devitalized small intestine may be necessary. The mortality rate is high.

Fluid and electrolyte replacement are essential. Penicillin and type C gas gangrene antisera are of value; laparotomy is often indicated. In Papua New Guinea, immunization against *C. perfringens* type C has given good results;[35] in a controlled trial, a marked reduction in incidence and mortality was demonstrated in the treatment group.

PARASITIC INFECTIONS

Giardiasis

Postinfective malabsorption resulting from infection with this flagellated protozoan has been reviewed.[25,28,32,35,41,47] The reason why some individuals are prone to symptomatic giardiasis is not clear: size of infecting dose, strain variability, genetic predisposition, acquired immunity factors, achlorhydria, a local secretory IgA deficiency, and the presence of blood group A phenotype have all been considered. An increase in IgE and IgD cell numbers has been reported in the jejunal mucosa of 20 affected patients;[50] the former reversed after treatment, when an increase in IgA cell numbers was also recorded. The actual mechanism by which the trophozoites cause an absorptive defect is also not clear. Injury to the mucosa with or without invasion, bacterial overgrowth in association with parasitization, and bile salt deconjugation by bacteria and/or parasites have all been considered. The extent of jejunal morphological abnormality varies widely.[123] Symptoms vary from subclinical cases to those with severe malabsorption and malnutrition.

Clinical features

Clinical presentation is usually between 1 and 3 weeks after infection; contaminated water and, less commonly, food are the usual sources of infection. Infection occurs both endemically and epidemically. The disease can probably be contracted from domestic animals.[47] It is more common in male homosexuals, but is not an 'opportunistic' infection in acquired immune deficiency syndrome (AIDS) sufferers. Diarrhoea of acute onset, flatus, and weight loss may all be present; the stools have the characteristics of malabsorption. The disease is clinically indistinguishable from postinfective malabsorption in the absence of giardiasis; investigations also give similar results. In fact, a 'fully blown' case has all of the clinical and laboratory features of the classical (historical) reports of 'tropical sprue'.[25] Cysts may be found in a faecal specimen; trophozoites can be detected in either a jejunal biopsy or jejunal fluid, or with the string test ('Enterotest'). If mucosal changes and malabsorption exist, circulating antibodies to *G. lamblia* cysts can usually be detected.[87]

Treatment

Treatment is with metronidazole (2 g daily on 3 consecutive days); alcohol should be avoided during the treatment period. A single dose of tinidazole (2 g orally) has been used with success and there are claims that it is equally efficacious. Two 5-nitroimidazoles – ornidazole and tinidazole (in a single dose of 1.5 g) – have been compared;[60] recurrence of the infection during the following 2 months was similar with each agent (about 10%). Nimorazole has also been used. Alternatively, mepacrine (100 mg three times daily for 10 days) – which is less often used – usually gives a satisfactory result.

Cryptosporidium *spp.*

This organism also produces a spectrum of disease – from a travellers' diarrhoea-like syndrome to severe postinfective malabsorption; however, the latter usually, but not always, occurs in the immunosuppressed (including AIDS) sufferer, where the organism is 'opportunistic'.[31,33,110] Diagnosis is similar to that for *G. lamblia* infection; oocysts are usually detectable in a faecal sample. Treatment (which is rarely indicated in the immunointact individual) is with spiramycin,[31] but this is usually ineffective in the immunosuppressed; although at least 70 other compounds have been tested, none is effective.[33]

Other parasites

Several other parasitic infections can give rise to postinfective malabsorption. Although *Ascaris lumbricoides*, *Ancylostoma duodenale* and *Necator americanus* have at various times been implicated,[28] there is no definite evidence except in rare case reports or anecdotal stories.[39] *Diphyllobothrium latum* infections are occasionally associated with a low serum vitamin B_{12} concentration; however, this is caused by uptake of B_{12} by the parasite within the small intestinal lumen, and is not an example of malabsorption.

There is clear evidence that *Strongyloides stercoralis* is causally related to malabsorption.[25,28] This helminth can survive in the human host for several decades; some 10–20% of ex-prisoners of war in South-East Asia during World War II were until recently still infected.[49] Onset of diarrhoea is less acute than with *G. lamblia*. Larvae can be demonstrated by the string test, and less well by jejunal biopsy. Ova and larvae can occasionally be detected in faecal specimens. Eosinophilia may be gross, but is often absent. The immunofluorescent antibody test (IFAT) is positive in approximately 70% of cases; however, cross-reaction with filaria is common. The enzyme-linked immunosorbent assay (ELISA) test, when available, is far more specific. Immunosuppressed patients may have negative serological results. Treatment is with thiabendazole (1.5 g twice daily on 3 successive days); repeated courses may be required. Albendazole (400 mg daily for 3 days) is less effective. In animal experiments, cambendazole has given encouraging results; this has also been the case in limited clinical studies, but the compound has not been released for human use.[33] Other *Strongyloides* species are important, especially in children. *S. fülleborni* has been implicated in the pathogenesis of severe postinfective malabsorption in Zambia and Papua New Guinea, where a significant mortality rate has been recorded.[25,33]

In the northern Philippines and Thailand, *Capillaria philippinensis* has been causally associated with postinfective malabsorption. It can occur in epidemics. An acute onset of diarrhoea is followed by malabsorption and, if untreated, infection carries a substantial mortality rate. Protein-losing enteropathy may also be present. Treatment with mebendazole, and latterly albendazole, has given good results.[33]

The protozoa *I. belli* and *Sarcocystis hominis* (usually conveyed by undercooked pork and beef) are further causes of malabsorption.[21,33] These organisms replicate within the enterocyte. *I. belli*, like *Cryptosporidium* spp., causes a spectrum of disease – from travellers' diarrhoea to postinfective malabsorption – and is more common in the immunosuppressed individual. Pyrimethamine with sulphadiazine, and co-trimoxazole with nitrofurantoin, have been used with some success. Other protozoan parasites, such as *Plasmodium falciparum* (in an acute infection) and visceral leishmaniasis (kala-azar) can also produce significant malabsorption.

CHRONIC INTESTINAL INFECTION PREDISPOSING TO CHRONIC MALABSORPTION

HIV INFECTION

Incontrovertible evidence now exists that human immunodeficiency virus (HIV) infection causes a chronic enteropathy with 'villous blunting';[37] crypt hypoplasia results either from a direct effect of the viruses on cell replication, or by an unknown immunological reaction. This is now a very common cause of persisting malabsorption in Africa.

TUBERCULOSIS

Intestinal tuberculosis is a grossly underdiagnosed cause of malabsorption in a tropical context;[25] in many countries in the tropics and subtropics, including Saudi Arabia,[86] it is the most common cause. The condition should be suspected in immigrants from Africa and Asia in the UK who present with features of malabsorption (even after several years of residence here) as well as in people indigenous to Third World countries.

INTESTINAL TUBERCULOSIS

Clinical features

Presentation is with weight loss, low-grade fever, anorexia, abdominal pain and diarrhoea.[72] Malnutrition may be severe enough to produce adult kwashiorkor. Generalized lymphadenopathy is occasionally present. Miliary spread, dissemination within the peritoneal cavity, and granuloma formation in the ileum and colon may complicate the picture. Clinically, a mass is sometimes palpable (and can be confirmed by ultrasonography) in the right iliac fossa. Transverse ileal ulcers with under-mined edges follow involvement of Peyer's patches; fibrosis and stenosis with stricture formation occur. The resultant malabsorption and steatorrhoea is largely a result of chronic bile salt loss; these are normally reabsorbed in the terminal ileum. The direct effect of unabsorbed bile salts on the colon is an exacerbating factor.

Investigations

Barium meal and follow through, or barium enema, may show multiple ileal strictures; shortening of the ascending colon and caecum with loss of the normal ileocaecal angle are other radiological features. *Mycobacterium tuberculosis* is only rarely detected in a faecal specimen. Protein-losing enteropathy may be present. Anaemia and hypoalbuminaemia are usual. Peritoneoscopy (and peritoneal biopsy) and laparotomy are often required for a positive diagnosis. Crohn's disease is an important differen-tial diagnosis; however, vomiting, fever and men-strual disorders are more common and diarrhoea is less common in tuberculosis. Chest radiography is usually normal.

Treatment

Treatment is with antituberculous agents.[48] Resec-tion of ileal strictures and a right hemicolectomy are often required to deal with stricture formation.

TROPICAL ENTEROPATHY AND SUBCLINICAL MALABSORPTION

The small intestinal mucosa of people living in a developing Third World country possesses minor structural differences compared with that of those who have always lived in a temperate zone.[25,83] These changes, described as *tropical enteropathy*, are not related to the clinical syndrome postinfective malabsorption ('tropical sprue').[62] Although the cause of the changes is not entirely clear, they seem to result from repeated low-grade viral and bacterial infections. Similarly, xylose and glucose malabsorp-tion has been shown to be present in large numbers of people indigenous to tropical countries. The ab-normalities are certainly greater in lower socio-economic groups.[83,116] Subclinical malabsorption exists in many people in Third World developing countries;[25,118] xylose and vitamin B_{12} malabsorp-tion have been demonstrated in 39 and 52%, re-spectively, of Peace Corps workers living under

rural conditions in Pakistan.[74] Apart from repeated small intestinal infections, other factors are prob-ably important.[25,45] Xylose, glucose and folic acid absorption have been shown to be impaired in individuals with systemic bacterial infections such as pulmonary tuberculosis and pneumococcal pneu-monia. There is also good evidence that dietary folate depletion results in xylose malabsorption.[25] Although marginal malnutrition and pellagra have both been suggested as causing subclinical malabsorption, the evidence is contradictory.

The practical importance of subclinical malab-sorption is unclear. It seems likely that it signifi-cantly contributes to malnutrition in people in Third World countries who subsist on a marginally ade-quate dietary intake, consisting largely of carbo-hydrate. Before any rigid conclusions are drawn, however, it should be appreciated that the small intestine has a very substantial functional reserve, and that the role of the colon in absorption of carbohydrates (and other substances) remains unclear (see below).

POSTINFECTIVE MALABSORPTION IN THE TROPICS ('TROPICAL SPRUE')

The clinical entity *postinfective malabsorption related to tropical exposure* has been reviewed by Cook,[25,27,34,36] Tomkins,[118] Baker[4] and Mathan.[82,83]

GEOGRAPHICAL DISTRIBUTION

Figure 3.62 summarizes the geographical localities where postinfective malabsorption has been reported either commonly or less often; it does not include areas where rare sporadic cases have been recorded. Although it is common (and endemic) in Asia and the northern part of South America,[40] it is a very unusual condition in tropical Africa. Until recently it was common in overland travellers from the UK to Asia;[120] the fact that it is now rarely seen is probably largely a result of early antibiotic admin-istration. In the Middle East and Mediterranean littoral, postinfective malabsorption is unusual,[86] but certainly occurs.[85,102]

AETIOLOGY

Taking the available evidence into account, there can be no reasonable doubt that postinfective malabsorption has an infective basis:[22] the disease is more common in geographical areas where enteric

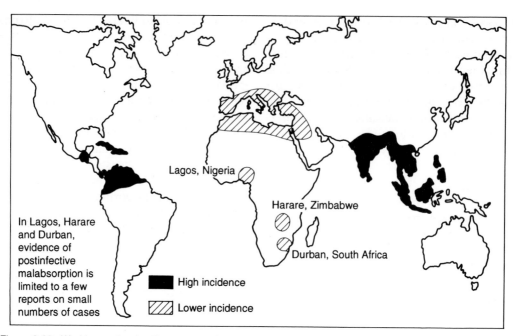

Figure 3.62 World map showing those areas where postinfective malabsorption is a significant medical problem.

infection abounds, it is epidemic in nature in some areas (including southern India),[82] the small intestinal lumen is colonized by aerobic enterobacteria,[109] and recovery usually occurs rapidly (and dramatically) following initiation of broad-spectrum antibiotic treatment.[25,27,34] Despite this, however, Mathan considers that, in southern India, the primary lesion is one of enterocyte damage[83] which results from a 'persistent' lesion of the stem cell compartment, and this occurs on a 'background of tropical enteropathy'.[82] He further considers that 'an immunity conferring agent may be responsible for the initiating damage'. However, as already discussed, the widely used definition for this *clinical syndrome* in southern India, 'intestinal malabsorption of at least 2 nutrients after the exclusion of diseases that give rise to secondary malabsorption (in a tropical environment)',[5] is simply inadequate; it does not exclude acute infections and tropical enteropathy, nor does it introduce a time (chronicity) clause (see above).

Genetic predisposition

It is likely that all infective diseases possess a genetic background. In a limited study in Puerto Rico, 25 out of 27 patients with postinfective malabsorption (which was not very well defined) had at least one antigen of the HLA-Aw19 series;[84] the strongest associated link was with Aw31. In India, a high frequency of HLA-B8 was documented;[89,108] HLA-A1, A28 and Bw35 were significantly decreased in the affected group. It must be emphasized, how-

ever, that more data are required on genetic markers for postinfective malabsorption.

Infection

In severe postinfective malabsorption (in the absence of parasites) bacterial colonization has been demonstrated both within the jejunal lumen and in biopsy specimens.[7,64,121] The importance of adhesive properties of bacteria in the pathogenesis of the disease is unclear; many bacteria, including *E. coli, Salmonella typhimurium* and *V. cholerae*, have adhesive properties which are mediated by a transmissible plasmid. Several groups have demonstrated a higher concentration of aerobic enterobacteriaceae in relation to the enterocyte compared with luminal fluid, in postinfective tropical malabsorption.[121] (In the normal individual, anaerobes outnumber aerobes by about 1000-fold.[109]) It seems likely that a variety of toxins released by these enterobacteria induce net water secretion and malabsorption.[65] (In the blind loop syndrome, the enterobacteria are invariably obligate anaerobes which do *not* produce toxins.[66]) Several months after tropical exposure the intraluminal bacterial flora of the upper small intestine (mucosal biopsy or luminal fluid) may remain abnormal;[121,122] 7 out of 11 patients had enterobacteria in numbers ranging from 10^3 to 10^8/g or ml. The most common organisms are *Klebsiella pneumoniae, Enterobacter cloacae* and *E. coli; Citrobacter feundii, Serratia marcescens* and *Pseudomonas* sp. have also been detected. It seems highly likely therefore, that these organisms had been present since the tropical exposure. The origin of this overgrowth has not been adequately studied in postinfective tropical malabsorption; in patients in the UK with small intestinal bacterial overgrowth, faecal flora account for most of the organisms, but salivary flora seems important in some cases.[56] In southern India, a viral aetiology has been sought for postinfective malabsorption, but there is little convincing evidence for this.

Jejunal morphology

Morphological changes are non-specific and there is a range in severity.[79] Blunting of villi ('partial villous atrophy') with increased lymphocyte and plasma cell infiltration (which is not a feature of tropical enteropathy) are present to a variable degree; a 'flat' mucosa is exceedingly unusual. Although the number of plasma cells is increased, distribution of IgA-, IgM- and IgG-containing cells is normal.[13] T-cell numbers are increased: in untreated gluten-induced enteropathy, T cells expressing T-cell receptor γ/δ heterodimers are disproportionately raised; this is not the case in postinfective malabsorption.[112] The significance of an elevated jejunal surface pH which has been demonstrated in southern India[75] is unclear, but is probably merely an indicator of enterocyte damage. Crypt *hyperplasia* has been demonstrated.[81,83]

Although a predisposing immunological deficit has been postulated in postinfective tropical malabsorption, there is no satisfactory evidence for this; immunological changes (increased IgG, IgE, C4 and orosomucoid, gastric parietal cell antibodies, and lymphopenia with a low peripheral blood T-cell count) seem to be *sequelae* of mucosal damage, and are not causally related.[83,97]

A single case report has documented the occurrence of myeloma in a patient suffering from postinfective tropical malabsorption;[71] chronic immunocyte stimulation with autonomous proliferation of a malignant clone of plasma cells has been suggested.

Small intestinal stasis

In southern India, whole-gut transit time (using a radiopaque marker technique) in tropical postinfective malabsorption has been shown to be unaltered, despite a striking increase in faecal weight.[59] Small intestinal stasis has, however, been documented in postinfective tropical malabsorption and might result from excessive enteroglucagon production in response to ileal (and colonic) mucosal injury (see below).[13,27] However, many patients with postinfec-

tive malabsorption have taken diphenoxylate or loperamide for acute diarrhoea; both of those agents produce relative small intestinal stasis.[67,103] They induce antiperistalsis as well as preventing prostaglandin-induced diarrhoea;[103] inhibition of small intestinal secretion also occurs.[25] This stasis is of particular interest, because peristalsis is usually *increased* in the presence of intraluminal bacteria.

Gut hormones

Gut hormones have been studied in postinfective tropical malabsorption in the fasting state and following a standard meal.[13] Fasting and postprandial concentrations of plasma enteroglucagon (produced by L cells in the distal ileum and colon[61]) and motilin were markedly elevated; furthermore, the high enteroglucagon concentration showed a significant correlation with a reduction in small intestinal transit (using the hydrogen breath test). Both enteroglucagon and motilin concentrations fell after treatment.[27] Recently, the concentration of another gut hormone, plasma peptide YY (also produced by endocrine cells in the ileum and colon) has been shown to be grossly elevated in postinfective malabsorption;[1] it seems possible that this results from a change in peptide YY secretion, resulting from malabsorption, and is a compensatory mechanism in diarrhoea.[91] This hormone is also known to delay gastric emptying and small intestinal transit, and to reduce gastric and pancreatic secretion. Patients with postinfective malabsorption have a reduced postprandial rise in gastric inhibiting polypeptide; gastrin and pancreatic polypeptide are normal.

Role of the colon

The colonic mucosa, in addition to that of the small intestine, is damaged in postinfective tropical malabsorption (tropical colonopathy).[82] Few causes of diarrhoea are strictly confined to one or other of these organs; e.g. shigellosis frequently involves the small intestine, and salmonellosis and *Campylobacter* sp. infection the colon.

Recent recognition of the important role of the colon in absorption is clearly relevant to postinfective malabsorption. The normal colon can absorb 4–7 litres of water every 24 hours,[95] together with 100–160 mmol of carbohydrate as volatile fatty acids.[104] Thus, failure of the diseased colon to 'salvage' the increased ileal effluent increases intensity of diarrhoea.

Colonic abnormalities have been reported in 'tropical sprue';[92] using a colonic perfusion system, impaired water and sodium absorption was demonstrated.[93] These abnormalities might result from impaired fatty acid absorption, and the effect of free fatty acids on the colonocyte.[117] Other suggested mechanisms are colonocyte damage, enterotoxin production by colonic bacteria, and the local action of bile acids (unabsorbed by the small intestine). Bile acids can be converted to deconjugated, dihydroxy bile acids by colonic bacteria, and can impair colonic salvage of water and salt by stimulating colonic secretion and propulsion.[14,111] Colonic bacteria are able to convert long-chain fatty acids to hydroxy-fatty acids, which stimulate colonic secretion,[14] modify colonic motility, and cause diarrhoea. A defect in sodium and water absorption from rectal mucosa has also been demonstrated using an *in vivo* dialysis technique;[94] Na^+K^+-dependent ATPase activity was significantly reduced.

There is still scope for some rigorous clinical and laboratory investigation of colonic function in postinfective malabsorption.[25]

Animal model

A clinical syndrome has been described in the German shepherd dog which bears very close similarities to postinfective malabsorption.[9–12,100] Jejunal biopsy specimens show 'villous atrophy' with a variable infiltration of lymphocytes and plasma cells in the lamina propria.[100] Subcellular biochemical studies are also consistent with the human syndrome.[11] Xylose absorption is impaired and blood folate and serum vitamin B_{12} concentrations reduced. Aerobic bacteria are involved and both clinical and laboratory recovery take place after broad-spectrum antibiotic therapy.[12]

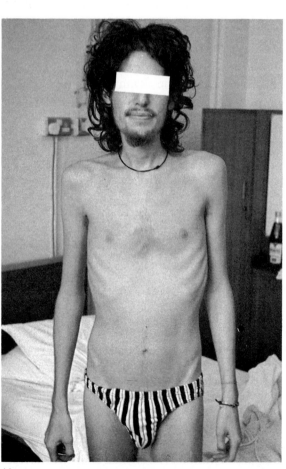
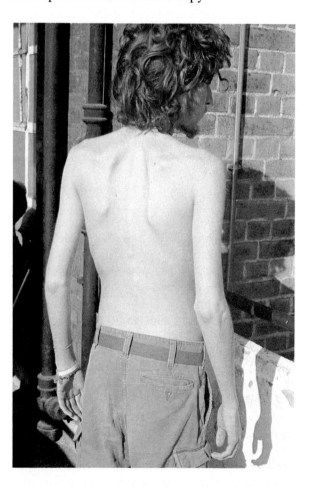

(a)

Figure 3.63 (a) A 19-year-old Englishman presented in London with postinfective tropical malabsorption (tropical sprue). Acute diarrhoea started soon after arriving in Nepal and he lost approximatley 12 kg in weight during the subsequent 2 months. The total urinary xylose excretion after a 25 g oral load was 2.5 mmol/5 hours (normal range 8.0–16.0 mmol/5 hours); the 24 hour faecal fat was 83 mmol (normal range 11–18 mmol); the Schilling test result was 0.16% urinary excretion at 24 hours (normal >10%) and the 8 hour serum concentration was 0% (normal >0.6%) of the loading dose. Jejunal biopsy histology showed marked villous blunting with increased lymphocytes in the lamina propria. Parasites were not found in several faecal samples. Serum albumin 36 g/litre; haemoglobin 13.2 g/dl; mean corpuscular volume 102.9; red blood cell folate 113 ng/l (normal >150 ng/l); serum vitamin B_{12} 322 pg/l (normal >150 ng/l). The patient responded rapidly to treatment with oral tetracycline and folic acid. (*Continued opposite*)

CLINICAL FEATURES

The clinical picture is dominated by chronic diarrhoea with large, pale, fatty stools, and sometimes excessive flatulence, following an acute intestinal infection.[25,120] Weight loss may be gross and is probably related to anorexia as much as to the intestinal disease.[118] *Figure 3.63* shows an affected patient before and after chemotherapy; a brief case history is given. A wide range of clinical presentation has however been recorded, from the very acute onset type, described by Baker and Mathan in Vellore, southern India (which is not in fact *post*infective)[5] often occurring in epidemics (with vomiting and pyrexia in up to 50% of cases), to a far more chronic entity. Most other clinical features, such as glossitis (aphthous ulceration was common in 19th-century reports), megaloblastic anaemia, fluid retention, depression, apathy, amenorrhoea and infertility, occur only after several months duration.

Table 3.34 summarizes the more important causes of chronic malabsorption in relation to tropical exposure. The condition must be differentiated from persisting bacterial overgrowth within the lumen of the small intestine ('blind loop syndrome'), which should be treated early with antibiotics,[96] and giardiasis, which is sometimes difficult to diagnose and for which the correct treatment is one of the 5-nitroimidazoles.[18,33] There are also many non-infective causes of malabsorption in the tropics and subtropics; these should be systematically excluded.[25]

During, and immediately after, an acute small intestinal infection, xylose, glucose, fat, vitamin B_{12} and folate malabsorption frequently occur (see above). After 4 months or so, moderate or severe morphological changes occur in the jejunal mucosa, and serum folate and, later, vitamin B_{12} concentrations decline, often to very low levels. Hypoalbuminaemia and oedema are late signs.

Gastric acid secretion is often depressed, but whether this precedes or is a sequel to the initiating infection is unknown.[5,82] The role of hypochlorhydria in the predisposition to small intestinal infection is unclear.[29] In a small proportion of cases in southern India, vitamin B_{12} absorption either improves or becomes normal with addition of intrinsic factor.[82] Secondary hypolactasia may be present.[25]

There is no indication that postinfective

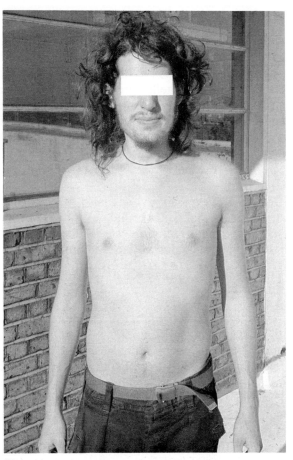
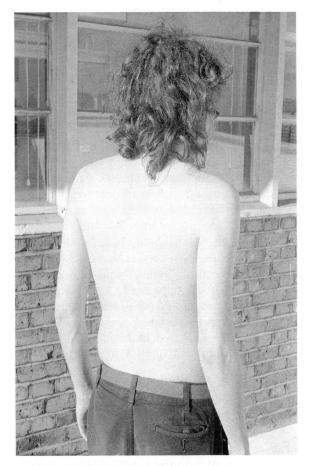

(b)

Figure 3.63 continued   (b) The same man 4 weeks after initiation of treatment.

Table 3.34 Major causes of chronic malabsorption in a tropical environment

Disorder	Cause
Digestive disorders:	
Pancreatic	Chronic calcific pancreatitis (Chapter 11)
Bile salt deficiency	Acute and chronic liver disease
	Ileal tuberculosis (Chapter 9)
	Trauma to ileum
Absorptive disorders:	
Short bowel syndrome	Trauma or surgery
Bacterial colonization of small intestine	Postinfective tropical malabsorption (tropical sprue)
	Severe kwashiorkor
	Blind loop syndrome (Chapter 3)
Viral and bacterial infections	HIV enteropathy
	Viral hepatitis, measles, rotavirus
	Ileocaecal tuberculosis (Chapter 9)
	Pig bel disease
Parasitic infections	*Giardia lamblia*, *Cryptosporidium* spp., *Isospora belli*, *Sarcocystis hominis* (*Plasmodium falciparum*, visceral leishmaniasis)
	Strongyloides stercoralis, *Strongyloides* sp., *Capillaria philippinensis*
Venous and lymphatic obstruction	Right-sided endomyocardial fibrosis, constrictive pericarditis, idiopathic tropical cardiomyopathy, filariasis
Isolated malabsorption.	
Hypolactasia	Primary (genetic) or secondary to absorptive disorders (Chapter 3)

malabsorption predisposes to any gastrointestinal malignancy.

INVESTIGATIONS

Investigations should include urinary D-xylose excretion after a 5 or 25 g loading dose, 72 hour faecal fat estimation, a Schilling test and jejunal biopsy; faecal parasites should be excluded. (The 1 hour blood xylose concentration is in practice probably superior to a 5 hour urinary collection in a tropical environment.[54]) Serum vitamin B_{12} and red blood cell folate concentrations should be estimated; after 4 months of illness, most patients have a low folate concentration. Serum albumin[78] and globulin concentrations are often depressed. Monosaccharide absorption is impaired to a greater extent than that of amino acids.[26] A barium meal and follow-through examination shows dilated loops of jejunum with clumping of barium,[78] in addition to reduced transit rate.

Jejunal mucosal changes are variable, depending on the duration of the disease. By 3 or 4 months, most biopsies are ridged and/or convoluted; a flat mucosa is extremely unusual and, if present, gluten-induced enteropathy should be suspected. Submucosal invasion with lymphocytes (predominantly T cells) and plasma cells is usual.

Ultrastructural changes in jejunal biopsy specimens have been studied;[90] although lyosomes, peroxisomes and mitochondrial enzymes are not depressed, the organelles are more fragile. Endoplasmic reticulum is unchanged. A significant reduction in 5-nucleotidase in the basolateral (plasma) membrane persists after recovery. The latter finding might reflect an underlying abnormality in the enterocyte of individuals susceptible to postinfective malabsorption.

Intestinal permeability has also been investigated;[38] abnormalities in urinary excretion of lactulose and rhamnose after an oral load are similar to results obtained in gluten-induced enteropathy.

TREATMENT

A hypothesis to account fot the aetiology of postinfective tropical malabsorption[27,34] is summarized in *Figure 3.64*. In practice, the vicious cycle can be broken by (1) eliminating the bacterial overgrowth, and (2) aiding mucosal recovery (with folic acid supplements).[55] Whilst this hypothesis has been challenged,[19,51] a satisfactory alternative has not been produced. An adequate diet should be combined with tetracycline (250 mg three times a day for at least 2 weeks) and folic acid (5 mg three times daily for 3 months). Evidence of susceptibility of the

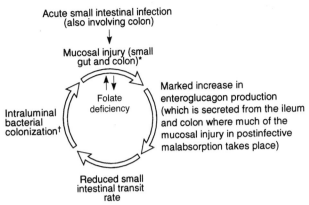

Figure 3.64 Hypothetical scheme to illustrate the pathogenesis of postinfective malabsorption. The open arrows indicate the vicious cycle which, once set in motion, is only broken by elimination of the abnormal luminal flora, and hastening of enterocyte recovery. * Recovery by oral folic acid supplements. †Terminated with antibiotics – tetracycline is most often used.

responsible flora to antibiotics other than tetracycline is very limited.[3] Symptomatic treatment may be necessary in the acute stage of the disease; codeine phosphate (30 mg three times daily), diphenoxylate (2.5–5 mg four times daily), or loperamide (5–10 mg four times daily) are of value if stool frequency is excessive. Mild cases respond without treatment, but this may take several months. Recovery is now usually rapid and straightforward;[25,27,34] in pre-antibiotic days, a mortality rate of 10–20% was usual.

Evidence from south India suggests that the response to antibiotics there is less satisfactory;[4,83] this is used in support of a suggestion that a viral rather than a bacterial aetiology is causative in that locality.

CONCLUSION

The aetiology of postinfective malabsorption – especially that presenting in association with tropical exposure – is slowly becoming clearer.[22,27,30,51] It is probable that several primary insults (of an infective nature) to the enterocyte are involved. Whereas postinfective malabsorption resulting from most viral, bacterial and parasitic causes is usually self-limiting, the 'tropical sprue' syndrome when well established is not usually so. The reason why only a minority of affected individuals who suffer from an acute small intestinal infection are susceptible to postinfective malabsorption is unknown; a genetic (or ethnic) basis for susceptibility now seems likely.

REFERENCES

1. Adrian, T.E., Savage, A[...] A.J., Wolfe, K., Besterm[...] S.R. (1986) Peptide YY a[...] gastrointestinal disease. G[...] 379–384.

2. Agus, S.G., Dolin, R., W[...] Acute infectious non-bacte[...] intestinal histopathology. *Annals of Internal Medicine*, **79**, 18–25.

3. Albert, M.J., Rajan, D.P. and Mathan, V.I. (1984) *In vitro* susceptibility to metronidazole of bacteria from the small intestine of tropical sprue patients. *Indian Journal of Medical Research*, **79**, 333–336.

4. Baker, S.J. (1982) Idiopathic small intestinal disease in the tropics. In: *Critical Reviews in Tropical Medicine*, Vol. 1, pp. 197–245 (Ed.) Chandra, R.K. New York: Plenum Press.

5. Baker, S.J. and Mathan, V.I. (1971) Tropical sprue in southern India. In: *Tropical Sprue and Megloblastic Anaemia. A Wellcome Trust Collaborative Study*, pp. 189–260. London: Churchill Livingstone.

6. Baker, S.J., Mathan, M., Mathan, V.I. *et al.* (1982) Chronic enterocyte infection with coronavirus. One possible cause of the syndrome of tropical sprue? *Digestive Diseases and Sciences*, **27**, 1039–1043.

7. Banwell, J.G. and Gorbach, S.L. (1969) Tropical sprue. *Gut*, **10**, 328–333.

8. Bartholomew, C. (1989) William Hillary and sprue in the Caribbean: 230 years later. *Gut (Festchrift)*, 17–21.

9. Batt, R.M. and Hall, E.J. (1989) Chronic enteropathies in the dog. *Journal of Small Animal Practice*, **30**, 3–12.

10. Batt, R.M. and McLean, L. (1987) Comparison of the biochemical changes in the jejunal mucosa of dogs with aerobic and anaerobic bacterial overgrowth. *Gastroenterology*, **93**, 986–993.

11. Batt, R.M., Bush, B.M. and Peters, T.J. (1983) Subcellular biochemical studies of a naturally occurring enteropathy in the dog resembling chronic tropical sprue in human beings. *American Journal of Veterinary Research*, **44**, 1492–1496.

12. Batt, R.M., McLean, L. and Riley, J.E. (1986) Response of the jejunal mucosa of dogs with aerobic and anaerobic bacterial overgrowth to antibiotic therapy. *Gut*, **29**, 473–482.

13. Besterman, H.S., Cook, G.C., Sarson, D.L. *et al.* (1979) Gut hormones in tropical malabsorption. *British Medical Journal*, **ii**, 1252–1255.

14. Binder, H.J. (1980) Pathophysiology of bile acid and fatty acid induced diarrhoea. In: *Secretory Diarrhoea*, p. 157 (Eds) Field, M., Fordtran, J.S. and Schultz, S.G. Bethesda: American Physiological Society.

15. Black, R.E., Merson, M.H., Rowe, B. *et al.* (1981) Enterotoxigenic *Escherichia coli* diarrhoea:

...d immunity and transmission in an endemic ... *Bulletin of the World Health Organisation*, ..., 263–268.

... Blaser, M.J. and Reller, L.B. (1981) Campylobacter enteritis. *New England Journal of Medicine*, **305**, 1444–1452.

17. Boedeker, E.C. (1982) Enterocyte adherence of *Escherichia coli*: its relation to diarrhoeal disease. *Gastroenterology*, **83**, 489–492.

18. Bolin, T.D., Davis, A.E. and Duncombe, V.M. (1982) A prospective study of persistent diarrhoea. *Australian and New Zealand Journal of Medicine*, **12**, 22–26.

19. Booth, C. (1984) Tropical sprue. *The Lancet*, **i**, 1018.

20. Brown, D.W.G., Selvakumar, R., Daniel, D.J. and Mathan, V.I. (1988) Prevalence of neutralising antibodies to Berne virus in animals and humans in Vellore, South India. *Archives of Virology*, **98**, 267–269.

21. Bunyaratvej, S., Bunyawongwiroj, P. and Nitiyanant, P. (1982) Human intestinal sarcosporidiosis: report of six cases. *American Journal of Tropical Medicine and Hygiene*, **31**, 36–41.

22. Case 15-1990 (1990) Case records of the Massachusetts General Hospital. *New England Journal of Medicine*, **332**, 1067–1075.

23. Conrad, M.E., Schwartz, F.D. and Young, A.A. (1964) Infectious hepatitis – a generalised disease. *American Journal of Medicine*, **37**, 789–801.

24. Cook, G.C. (1978) Tropical sprue: implications of Manson's concept. *Journal of the Royal College of Physicians of London*, **12**, 329–349.

25. Cook, G.C. (1980) *Tropical Gastroenterology*, pp. 228–229, 271–324, 325–339. Oxford: Oxford University Press.

26. Cook, G.C. (1981) Jejunal absorption rates of glucose and glycine in post-infective tropical malabsorption. *Transactions of the Royal Society of Tropical Medicine and Hygiene*, **75**, 378–384.

27. Cook, G.C. (1984) Aetiology and pathogenesis of post-infective tropical malabsorption (tropical sprue). *The Lancet*, **i**, 721–723.

28. Cook, G.C. (1985) Parasitic infection. In: *Disorders of the Small Intestine*, pp. 283–298 (Eds) Booth, C.C. and Neale, G. Oxford: Blackwell.

29. Cook, G.C. (1985) Infective gastroenteritis and its relation to reduced gastric acidity. *Scandinavian Journal of Gastroenterology*, **111**, 17–23.

30. Cook, G.C. (1987) Post-infective malabsorption (including 'tropical sprue'). In: *Oxford Textbook of Medicine*, 2nd edn, pp. 12.115–12.120 (Eds) Weatherall, D.J., Ledingham, J.G.G. and Warrell, D.A. Oxford: Oxford University Press.

31. Cook, G.C. (1988) Small-intestinal coccidiosis: an emergent clinical problem. *Journal of Infection*, **16**, 213–219.

32. Cook, G.C. (1989) Gastrointestinal diseases. In: *Tropical Medicine and parasitology*, pp. 619–631

(Eds) Goldsmith, R. and Heyneman, D. Norwalk: Appleton and Lange.

33. Cook, G.C. (1990) In: *Parasitic Disease in Clinical Practice*, pp. 31–47, 49–75, 91–101. London, Berlin: Springer Verlag.

34. Cook, G.C. (1990) Travellers' diarrhoea and post-infective malabsorption. *Medicine International*, **77**, 3222–3226.

35. Cook, G.C. (1991) Tropical disease and the small-intestine. In: *Diseases of the Gut and Pancreas*, 2nd edn (Eds) Misiewicz, J.J., Pounder, R.E. and Venables, C.W. London: Grant McIntyre.

36. Cook, G.C. (1991) The small intestine and its role in chronic diarrhoeal disease in the tropics. In: *Diarrhea* (Ed.) Gracey, M., pp. 127–162. Boca Raton: CRC Press.

37. Cook, G.C. (1991) Gastroenterological parasitoses in Europe: a growing problem without an obvious solution. *Acta Endoscopica*, **21**, 19–26.

38. Cook, G.C. and Menzies, I.S. (1986) Intestinal absorption and unmediated permeation of sugars in post-infective tropical malabsorption (tropical sprue). *Digestion*, **33**, 109–116.

39. Crosby, W.H. (1987) The deadly hookworm: why did the Puerto-Ricans die? *Archives of Internal Medicine*, **147**, 577–578.

40. Davis, J.S. and Klipstein, F.A. (1985) Tropical sprue in a visitor to Mexico. *The Lancet*, **i**, 454.

41. Desai, H.I. and Chandra, R.K. (1982) Giardiasis. In: *Critical Reviews in Tropical Medicine*, Vol. 1, pp. 109–141 (Ed.) Chandra, R.K. New York: Plenum Press.

42. Dossetor, J.F.B. and White, H.C. (1975) Protein-losing enteropathy and malabsorption in acute measles enteritis. *British Medical Journal*, **ii**, 592–593.

43. Dupont, H.L. (1991) Travelers' diarrhea. In: *Diarrhea* (Ed.) Gracey, M., pp. 115–126. Boca Raton: CRC Press.

44. Echeverria, P., Verhaert, L., Ulyangco, C.V. *et al.* (1978) Antimicrobial resistance and enterotoxin production among isolates of *Escherichia coli* in the Far East. *The Lancet*, **ii**, 589–592.

45. Elia, M., Northrop, C.A., Lunn, P.G. and Goren, A. (1989) Effect of systemic infection on intestinal permeability in man. *Proceedings of the Nutrition Society*, **48**, A80.

46. Evans, N. (1979) Bacterial toxins and diarrhoea. *Tropical Doctor*, **9**, 10–15.

47. Farthing, M.J.G. (1988) Giardia lamblia. In: *Enteric infection: Mechanisms, Manifestations and Management*, pp 397–413 (Eds) Farthing, M.J.G. and Keusch, G.T. London: Chapman and Hall.

48. Findlay, J.M. (1982) Medical management of gastrointestinal tuberculosis. *Journal of the Royal Society of Medicine*, **75**, 583–584.

49. Gill, G.V. and Bell, D.R. (1982) Longstanding tropical infections amongst former war prisoners of the Japanese. *The Lancet*, **i**, 958–959.

50. Gillon, J., Andre, C., Descos, L. *et al.* (1982) Changes in mucosal immunoglobulin-containing cells in patients with giardiasis before and after treatment. *Journal of Infection*, **5**, 67–72.

51. Glynn, J. (1988) Tropical sprue – its aetiology and pathogenesis. *Journal of the Royal Society of Medicine*, **79**, 599–606.

52. Gorbach, S.L. (1992) Travelers' diarrhea. In: *Infectious Diseases* (Eds) Gorbach, S.L., Bartlett, J.G. and Blacklow, N.R. Philadelphia: W.B. Saunders.

53. Gross, R.J., Ward, L.R., Threlfall, E.J. *et al.* (1982) Drug resistance among infantile enteropathogenic *Escherichia coli* strains isolated in the United Kingdom. *British Medical Journal*, **285**, 472–473.

54. Gupta, B., Narru, N. and Dhar, K.L. (1987) Evaluation of surface area corrected peak blood xylose as a screening test of intestinal malabsorption in the tropics. *Indian Journal of Gastroenterology*, **6**, 89–91.

55. Haffejee, I.E. (1988) Effect of oral folate on duration of acute infantile diarrhoea. *The Lancet*, **ii**, 334–335.

56. Hamilton, I., Worsley, B.W., Cobden, I. *et al.* (1982) Simultaneous culture of saliva and jejunal aspirate in the investigation of small bowel bacterial overgrowth. *Gut*, **23**, 847–853.

57. Holt, P.E. (1981) Role of *Campylobacter* spp. in human and animal disease: a review. *Journal of the Royal Society of Medicine*, **74**, 437–440.

58. Iushchuk, N.D. and Abdullaev, Skh. (1981) Sostoianie vsasyvatel'noi funktsii tonkoi kishki pri sal'monelleze u detei. *Pediatriia*, **7**, 23–24.

59. Jayanthi, V., Chacko, A., Gani, I.K. and Mathan, V.I. (1989) Intestinal transit in healthy Southern Indian subjects and in patients with tropical sprue. *Gut*, **30**, 36–38.

60. Jokipii, L. and Jokipii, A.M.M. (1982) Treatment of giardiasis: comparative evaluation of ornidazole and tinidazole as a single oral dose. *Gastroenterology*, **83**, 399–404.

61. Kelly, C.P., Johnston, C.F., Nolan, N., Keeling, P.W.N. and Weir, D.G. (1989) Necrolytic migratory erythema with elevated plasma enteroglucagon in celiac disease. *Gastroenterology*, **96**, 1350–1353.

62. Klipstein, F.A. (1979) Sprue and subclinical malabsorption in the tropics. *The Lancet*, **i**, 277–278.

63. Klipstein, F.A. and Corcino, J.J. (1977) Factors responsible for weight loss in tropical sprue. *American Journal of Clinical Nutrition*, **30**, 1703–1708.

64. Klipstein, F.A., Holdeman, L.V., Corcino, J.J. and Moore, W.E.C. (1973) Enterotoxigenic intestinal bacteria in tropical sprue. *Annals of Internal Medicine*, **79**, 632–641.

65. Klipstein, F.A., Horowitz, I.R., Engert, R.F. and Schenk, E.A. (1975) Effect of *Klebsiella*

66. Klipstein, F.A., Engert, R.F. and Short, H.B. (1978) Enterotoxigenicity of colonising coliform bacteria in tropical sprue and blind-loop syndrome. *The Lancet*, **ii**, 342–344.

67. Lancet Editorial (1981) Loperamide – what does it block? *The Lancet*, **ii**, 1088–1089.

68. Lancet Editorial (1981) Microbial adhesion, colonisation and virulence. *The Lancet*, **ii**, 508–510.

69. Lancet Editorial (1982) Campylobacter enteritis. *The Lancet*, **ii**, 1437–1438.

70. Lancet Editorial (1983) Mechanisms in enteropathogenic *Escherichia coli* diarrhoea. *The Lancet*, **i**, 1254–1256.

71. Levine, D.S., Ree, H.J. and Crowley, J.P. (1986) Tropical sprue and multiple myeloma: chronic immunocyte stimulation may have led to autonomous proliferation of a malignant clone of plasma cells. *Rhode Island Medical Journal*, **69**, 277–279.

72. Lewis, E.A. and Kolawole, T.M. (1972) Tuberculous ileo-colitis in Ibadan: a clinico-radiological review. *Gut*, **13**, 646–653.

73. Lindenbaum, J. (1965) Malabsorption during and after recovery from acute intestinal infection. *British Medical Journal*, **ii**, 326–329.

74. Lindenbaum, J., Kent, T.H. and Sprinz, H. (1966) Malabsorption and jejunitis in American Peace Corps volunteers in Pakistan. *Annals of Internal Medicine*, **65**, 1201–1209.

75. Lucas, M.L. and Mathan, V.I. (1989) Jejunal surface pH measurements in tropical sprue. *Transactions of the Royal Society of Tropical Medicine and Hygiene*, **83**, 138–142.

76. McCormack, J.G. (1982) Clinical features of rotavirus gastroenteritis. *Journal of Infection*, **4**, 167–174.

77. McKenzie, D., Hansen, J.D.L. and Becker, W. (1959) Herpes simplex virus infection: dissemination in association with malnutrition. *Archives of Disease in Childhood*, **34**, 250–256.

78. McLean, A.M., Farthing, M.J.G., Kurian, G. and Mathan, V.I. (1982) The relationship between hypoalbuminaemia and the radiological appearances of the jejunum in tropical sprue. *British Journal of Radiology*, **55**, 725–728.

79. Marsh, M.N. (1985) Functional and structural aspects of the epithelial lymphocyte, with implications for coeliac disease and tropical sprue. *Scandinavian Journal of Gastroenterology*, **114** (suppl.), 55–75.

80. Mata, L.J., Kromal, R.A., Urrutia, J.J. and Garcia, B. (1977) Effect of infection on food intake and the nutritional state: perspectives as viewed from the village. *American Journal of Clinical Nutrition*, **30**, 1215–1227.

81. Mathan, M.M., Ponniah, J. and Mathan, V.I.

(1986) Epithelial cell renewal and turnover and relationship to morphologic abnormalities in jejunal mucosa in tropical sprue. *Digestive Diseases and Sciences*, **31**, 586–592.

82. Mathan, V.I. (1988) Tropical sprue in southern India. *Transactions of the Royal Society of Tropical Medicine and Hygiene*, **82**, 10–14.

83. Mathan, V.I. (1990) Tropical sprue. *Springer Seminars in Immunopathology*, **12**, 231–237.

84. Menendez-Corrada, R., Nettleship, E. and Santiago-Delpin, E.A. (1986) HLA and tropical sprue. *The Lancet*, **ii**, 1183–1185.

85. Montgomery, R.D. and Chesner, I.M. (1985) Post-infective malabsorption in the temperate zone. *Transactions of the Royal Society of Tropical Medicine and Hygiene*, **79**, 322–327.

86. Montgomery, R.D., Atiyeh, M., Scales, W.R. *et al.* (1982) Intestinal absorption in Saudi Arabia: an evaluation of the one-hour blood xylose test. *Transactions of the Royal Society of Tropical Medicine and Hygiene*, **76**, 25–28.

87. Moody, A.H., Ridley, D.S., Tomkins, A.M. and Wright, S.G. (1982) The specificity of serum antibodies to *Giardia lamblia* and to enterobacteria in gastrointestinal disease. *Transactions of the Royal Society of Tropical Medicine and Hygiene*, **76**, 630–632.

88. Murrell, T.G.C. and Walker, P.D. (1991) The pigbel story of Papua New Guinea. *Transactions of the Royal Society of Tropical Medicine and Hygiene*, **85**, 119–122.

89. Naik, S. (1986) HLA and gastrointestinal disorders. *Indian Journal of Gastroenterology*, **5**, 121–124.

90. Peters, T.J., Jones, P.E., Wells, G. and Cook, G.C. (1979) Sequential enzyme and subcellular fractionation studies on jejunal biopsy specimens from patients with post-infective tropical malabsorption. *Clinical Science and Molecular Medicine*, **56**, 479–486.

91. Playford, R.J., Domin, J., Beacham, J., Parmar, K.B., Tatemoto, K., Bloom, S.R. and Calam, J. (1990) Preliminary report: role of peptide YY in defence against diarrhoea. *The Lancet*, **335**, 1555–1557.

92. Ramakrishna, B.S. and Mathan, V.I. (1982) Water and electrolyte absorption by the colon in tropical sprue. *Gut*, **23**, 842–846.

93. Ramakrishna, B.S. and Mathan, V.I. (1987) Role of bacterial toxins, bile acids, and free fatty acids in colonic water malabsorption in tropical sprue. *Digestive Diseases and Sciences*, **32**, 500–505.

94. Ramakrishna, B.S. and Mathan, V.I. (1988) Absorption of water and sodium and activity of adenosine triphosphatases in the rectal mucosa in tropical sprue. *Gut*, **29**, 665–668.

95. Read, N.W. (1982) Diarrhoea: the failure of colonic salvage. *The Lancet*, **ii**, 481–483.

96. Read, N.W., Krejs, G.J., Read, M.G. *et al.* (1980) Chronic diarrhoea of unknown origin. *Gastroenterology*, **78**, 264–271.

97. Ross, I.N. and Mathan, V.I. (1981) Immunological changes in tropical sprue. *Quarterly Journal of Medicine*, **50**, 435–449.

98. Rothbaum, R., McAdams, A.J., Giannella, R. and Partin, J.C. (1982) A clinicopathologic study of enterocyte-adherent *Escherichia coli*: a cause of protracted diarrhoea in infants. *Gastroenterology*, **83**, 441–454.

99. Rowe, B., Taylor, J. and Bettelheim, K.A. (1970) An investigation of travellers' diarrhoea. *The Lancet*, **i**, 1–5.

100. Rutgers, H.C., Batt, R.M. and Kelly, D.F. (1988) Lymphocytic–plasmocytic enteritis associated with bacterial overgrowth in the dog. *Journal of the American Veterinary Medicine Association*, **192**, 1739–1742.

101. Rutter, J.M., Burrows, M.R., Sellwood, R. and Gibbons, R.A. (1975) A genetic basis for resistance to enteric disease caused by *Escherichia coli*. *Nature*, **257**, 135–136.

102. Salem, A.A. and Allam, C.K. (1982) Tropical sprue: a case report from the Middle East. *American Journal of Gastroenterology*, **77**, 51–52.

103. Sandhu, B.R., Tripp, J.H., Candy, D.C.A. and Harries, J.T. (1981) Loperamide: studies on its mechanism of action. *Gut*, **22**, 658–662.

104. Saunders, D.K. and Wiggins, H.S. (1981) Conservation of mannitol, lactulose and raffinose by the human colon. *American Journal of Physiology*, **241**, G397–G402.

105. Schneider, R.E., Shiffman, M. and Faigenblum, J. (1978) The potential effect of water on gastrointestinal infections prevalent in developing countries. *American Journal of Clinical Nutrition*, **31**, 2089–2099.

106. Schoub, B.D. (1981) Enteric adenoviruses and rotaviruses in infantile gastroenteritis in developing countries. *The Lancet*, **ii**, 925.

107. Schreiber, D.S., Blacklow, N.R. and Trier, J.S. (1973) The intestinal lesion of the proximal small intestine in acute infectious nonbacterial gastroenteritis. *New England Journal of Medicine*, **288**, 1318–1323.

108. Sengupta, S., Naik, S. and Naik, S.R. (1983) HLA antigen frequency in endemic tropical sprue. *Indian Journal of Gastroenterology*, **2**, 12–13.

109. Simon, G.L. and Gorbach, S.L. (1986) The human intestinal microflora. *Digestive Diseases and Sciences*, **31**, 147S–162S.

110. Sloper, K.S., Dourmashkin, R.R., Bird, R.B. *et al.* (1982) Chronic malabsorption due to cryptosporidium in a child with immunoglobulin deficiency. *Gut*, **23**, 80–82.

111. Snape, W.J., Shiff, S. and Cohen, S. (1980) Effect of deoxycholic acid on colonic mobility in the rabbit. *American Journal of Physiology*, **238**, G321–G325.

112. Spencer, J., Isaacson, P.G., Diss, T.C. and MacDonald, T.T. (1989) Expression of disulfide-linked and non-disulfide-linked forms of the T cell receptor γ/δ heterodimer in human intestinal

intraepithelial lymphocytes. *European Journal of Immunology*, **14**, 1335–1338.

113. Spreeuwel van, J.P., Meijer, C.J.L.M., Rosekraus, P.C.M. and Lindeman, J. (1986) Immunoglobulin-containing cells in gastrointestinal pathology – diagnostic applications. *Pathology Annuals*, **21**(part 1), 295–310.

114. Taylor, W.R., Schell, W.L., Wells, J.G. *et al.* (1982) A foodborne outbreak of enterotoxigenic *Escherichia coli* diarrhoea. *New England Journal of Medicine*, **306**, 1093–1095.

115. Telch, J., Shephard, R.W., Butler, D.G. *et al.* (1981) Intestinal glucose transport in acute viral enteritis in piglets. *Clinical Science*, **61**, 29–34.

116. Thomas, G., Clain, D.J. and Wicks, A.C.B. (1976) Tropical enteropathy in Rhodesia. *Gut*, **17**, 888–894.

117. Tiruppathi, C., Balasubramanian, K.A., Hill, P.G. and Mathan, V.I. (1983) Faecal free fatty acids in tropical sprue and their possible role in the production of diarrhoea by inhibition of ATPases. *Gut*, **24**, 300–305.

118. Tomkins, A. (1981) Tropical malabsorption: recent concepts in pathogenesis and nutritional significance. *Clinical Science*, **60**, 131–137.

119. Tomkins, A. (1983) Nutritional cost of protracted diarrhoea in young Gambian children. *Gut*, **24**, A495.

120. Tomkins, A.M., James, W.P.T., Walters, J.H. and Cole, A.C.E. (1974) Malabsorption in overland travellers to India. *British Medical Journal*, **iii**, 380–384.

121. Tomkins, A.M., Drasar, B.S. and James, W.P.T. (1975) Bacterial colonisation of jejunal mucosa in acute tropical sprue. *The Lancet*, **i**, 59–62.

122. Tomkins, A.M., Wright, S.G. and Drasar, B.S. (1980) Bacterial colonization of the upper intestine in mild tropical malabsorption. *Transactions of the Royal Society of Tropical Medicine and Hygiene*, **74**, 752–755.

123. Vega-Franco, L., Alvarez, E.L., Romo, G. and Bernal, R.M. (1982) Absorción de proteinas en niños con giardiasis. *Boletin Medico Hospital Infantil de Mexico*, **39**, 19–22.

COELIAC DISEASE AND RELATED DISORDERS

COELIAC DISEASE   *(P.J. Ciclitira)*

DEFINITION

Coeliac disease may be defined as a condition in which there is an abnormal jejunal mucosa, which improves morphologically when treated with a gluten-free diet and relapses when gluten is reintroduced.[23] The condition, commonly called coeliac sprue, or gluten-sensitive enteropathy in the USA, has previously been called non-tropical sprue, coeliac syndrome, idiopathic steatorrhoea or primary malabsorption. Dermatitis herpetiformis is a related condition in which there is an itchy blistering skin eruption, frequently affecting the knees, elbows, buttocks and back, with deposition of granular IgA at the dermoepidermal junction, including uninvolved skin. The majority of patients with dermatitis herpetiformis have a small intestinal enteropathy which improves on gluten withdrawal.

HISTORICAL ASPECTS

The first reported description of coeliac disease was by A retaeus the Cappadocian in the 2nd century AD:[1] 'If diarrhoea does not proceed from a slight cause of only one or two days' duration and if, in addition, the patient's general systems be debilitated by atrophy of the body, the coeliac disease of a chronic nature is formed'. Aretaeus thought that the illness only affected adults.

In 1887, Samuel Jones Gee renewed attention to the condition.[67] He noted that the disease affected all ages. He thought that to 'regulate the food was the main part of treatment'. He wrote that 'a child who was fed upon a quart of the best Dutch mussels daily, throve wonderfully but relapsed when the season for mussels was over. Next season he could not be prevailed upon to take them. This is an experiment I have not yet been able to repeat, but if the patient can be cured at all, it must be by means of the diet'.

Still commented that 'the most striking feature is the surprising inconsistency of the child's size with its age. What appears to be an infant little more than twelve months old, startles one by unexpectedly talking and so reveals the fact that it is at least a year or two older, perhaps three or four years older, than its appearance would suggest'.[149]

In 1924 Haas described his treatment of coeliac disease.[77] Following the successful treatment of anorexia nervosa he thought it logical to try a banana diet in children with coeliac disease and anorexia. Haas's treatment was purely dietary, excluding bread, crackers, potatoes and cereals. Bananas were gradually added to the diet usually from the fourth or eighth day. This treatment was continued for an indefinite period. He believed that, ultimately, all children would tolerate most foods.[78]

This dietary treatment of coeliac disease continued well into the 1950s. During World War II, children with coeliac disease in the UK were treated as a special case, being allowed extra bananas at a time of shortage.

During this same period in The Netherlands there was a scarcity of cereals and bread in particular. Dicke, a Dutch paediatrician, observed that coeliac sprue diminished remarkably during this shortage.[46] Following Swedish planes dropping bread into The Netherlands it was observed that children with coeliac disease quickly relapsed. It was this that helped convince Dicke of the toxicity of wheat to individuals with coeliac disease. Dicke and co-workers went on to prove that wheat flour and not the associated starch was the offending substance and that the toxicity resided in the gluten fraction.[46,156]

Early diagnosis was made on clinical grounds.[137] The relatively late description of the histology was due to the presumption that the abnormal changes seen at autopsy were post-mortem artifacts.[151] In 1954 Paulley reported on the histology of coeliac jejunal mucosa obtained operatively.[122,123]

Shiner and Royer independently developed methods for biopsying the duodenum,[141,142] followed by Crosby, who recognized the need for a more flexible instrument.[45]

EPIDEMIOLOGY

Coeliac disease is essentially a disorder of Europe and those countries to which Europeans have emigrated, including North America and Australasia. The frequency in England is about 1/1500.[7] It was thought that the incidence of coeliac disease in childhood was declining in response to changes in feeding habits, but recent evidence suggests that this reflects presentation at a later stage.

The prevalence in the west of Ireland is as high as 1/300, possibly related to the reliance of the Irish in the past on potatoes rather than wheat.[120] Individuals with coeliac disease on this diet would remain well and survive to have children, unlike those who received wheat in their diet. In mainland Europe the prevalence varies between 1/300 and 1/6000.[74,130,133]

Coeliac disease occurs in non-Caucasians although the prevalence is possibly much lower. It has been reported from wheat-eating areas of Bengal and the Punjab as opposed to the predominantly rice-eating areas of Southern India. The disorder has been reported in Negroes, Arabs, Hispanics, Israeli Jews, Sudanese of mixed Arab Negro stock,

and claims have been made for a rising incidence in Cantonese children.[42]

Sex incidence

A number of papers suggest that the female-to-male ratio is 2:1 but in other series the sexes are more equally affected.[42]

Twin studies

Concordance in identical or apparently identical twins is well documented. Discordance was reported in infancy with normal biopsy findings in an 11-month-old twin who was ahead of his monozygotic twin in developmental age.[159] However, gluten loading was not undertaken. Even in the presence of discordance amongst monozygotic twins, prolonged follow-up is required to determine whether the apparently unaffected twin subsequently develops overt disease.

Mortality

The outlook for individuals with coeliac disease prior to the introduction of the gluten-free diet was poor, with published mortality rates varying between 10 and 30%. Following the introduction of gluten-free diets the mortality in one series fell to 0.4%.[139] Recent statistics suggest that the mortality rate is twice that of a matched control population.[82]

PATHOLOGY

Coeliac disease affects the mucosa of the proximal small intestine with damage gradually decreasing in severity towards the distal small intestine, although in severe cases the lesion extends to the ileum.[131] Abnormalities of the rectal mucosa may also be observed in severe cases.[99]

Examination of the jejunal mucosa with the dissecting microscope is valuable. Most observers can distinguish between normal and flat biopsies with degrees of abnormality falling between these two categories.[131] The normal mucosa exhibits digitate villi, leaf forms and ridges. The villi vary in size, shape and height but are usually three times taller than wide. Convolutions are long ridges, which may be regarded as having fused and buckled. There are differences in appearance of the jejunum in apparently normal subjects, depending on whether they reside in temperate or tropical climates. Fully convoluted appearances occur in more than 5% of normal subjects in tropical areas. Infants exhibit broad leaves and villi, with finger-shaped villi rarely present.[158]

The jejunal mucosa in coeliac disease may be flat and featureless but usually presents a mosaic pattern, caused by intersection of deep depressions leaving elevated mounds. Each mound has 8–40 crypt openings.[126]

Examination of a biopsy by dissecting microscopy is of value in assessing the whole specimen for patchiness of mucosal abnormality. This is particularly important in dermatitis herpetiformis, where a patchy lesion is more common.

The characteristic histological appearance of the jejunal mucosa in normal individuals is shown in *Figure 3.65*. This compares with the appearance of the jejunal mucosa from a patient with untreated coeliac disease in *Figure 3.66*. The classic flat mucosa exhibits no villi, a loss of the normal villous architecture and a reduction in the normal villous height:crypt depth ratio of between 5:1 and 3:1.[143] There is a general flattening of the mucosa which can vary from mild through partial villous atrophy to a total absence of villi. The total thickness of the mucosa may be increased because of crypt hyperplasia and infiltration of the lamina propria by plasma cells and lymphocytes. The surface epithelial cells become pseudostratified compared to their normal tall columnar shape. The surface enterocyte height is reduced. Crypt mitotic activity is normally confined to the lower third of the crypt, but in coeliac disease this activity may be increased and continue to the crypt surface, although the histological appearance of the crypt appears normal.

The time taken for the cells to migrate from the crypt to the surface is reduced from between 3 and 5 to between 1 and 2 days. The number of intraepithelial lymphocytes in relation to the number of surface cell enterocytes is increased in patients with active disease. Crypt abscesses have been described and small ulcers may be encountered. These ulcers may become problematical, developing into the small intestinal T-cell lymphoma that complicates 6–10% of cases of coeliac disease.

Goblet cells are evident throughout the crypts and along the surface of the epithelium. Paneth cells in coeliac disease may more readily discharge their contents into the crypt lumen, making recognition difficult, and resulting in an apparent reduction in their numbers. There have been reports of both increased and decreased numbers of endocrine-secreting cells in the small intestine of patients with untreated coeliac disease. The basement membrane may be thickened, this change often being patchy and having the staining characteristics of collagen rather than reticulin. There was previously controversy regarding the specific diagnosis of collagenous sprue as opposed to coeliac disease. This has now been resolved through the appreciation that this represents a variation of the histological appearance of coeliac disease. The presence of a thickened basement membrane was suggested to imply a slow response to a gluten-free diet.[24]

Chronic inflammatory cells are found infiltrating the jejunal mucosa in untreated coeliac disease. Increased numbers of plasma cells are found in the lamina propria[104] and lymphocytes in the surface epithelium. The majority of the intraepithelial lymphocytes express the common lymphocyte antigen CD3, 70% express the suppressor/cytotoxic phenotypic CD8, 5% express the helper/inducer CD4

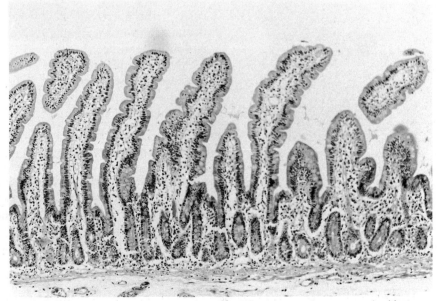

Figure 3.65 Histological appearances of the jejunal mucosa from a normal subject.

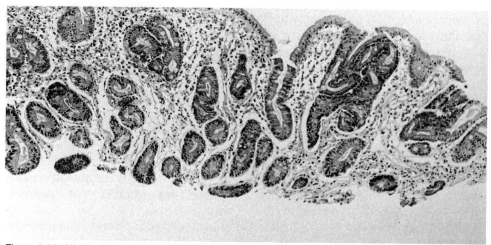

Figure 3.66   Histological appearances of the jejunal mucosa from a patient with untreated coeliac disease.

phenotype and 20% of the cells while they are CD3$^+$ are CD4$^-$ and CD8$^-$.[61,88,147] There is also an increase in the number of intraepithelial lymphocytes expressing the more primitive γ/δ T-cell receptor, in both treated and untreated coeliac disease, compared to controls.[146]

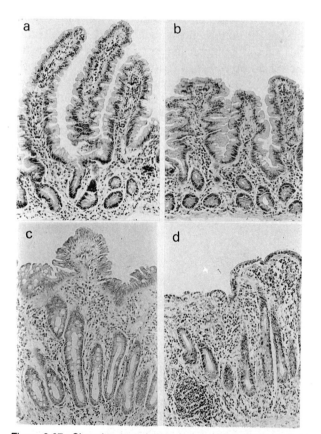

Figure 3.67   Changing morphology of the jejunal mucosa in response to gluten. The light microscopic appearances of the small intestinal mucosa biopsied from a treated coeliac patient before and after gluten challenge, showing the time-course of villous atrophy: (a) time 0; (b) 2½ hours; (c) 4 hours; (d) 6 hours. (From Bailey *et al.*[5])

Gluten challenge in treated coeliac patients, with hourly jejunal biopsy over 6 hours, shows that the earliest morphological appearances in the jejunal biopsy occur 2½ hours after challenge (*Figure 3.67*).[5]

Scanning electron microscopy reveals the surface of villi from normal subjects to be traversed by a series of furrows. In contrast, in untreated coeliac disease shallow depressions on the surface of the mucosa can be seen into which 2–4 crypts open. Higher magnification reveals that the microvilli are thicker than normal and appear to bear rounded projections.

Transmission electron microscopic studies of normal enterocytes show that the brush border is composed of tall, regular microvilli covered by a glycocalyx. Below this is the terminal web where the cells appear tightly bound together by an apparent fusion of the lateral cell membranes. The epithelium in untreated coeliac disease reveals stratified cells;[116] the microvilli show varying degrees of abnormality from shortening to gross disorganization and disappearance.

Abnormalities within the enterocytes include an increase in the number of lysosome-like bodies, swelling of the mitochondria, increased vacuolation and evidence of cellular degeneration.

Dermatitis herpetiformis

Skin disorders in coeliac disease are common, and include psoriasis, eczema and pustular dermatitis.[43] Atopic eczema in coeliac patients may respond to a gluten-free diet. There are a number of rare skin disorders which have been reported in association with coeliac disease, including cutaneous amyloid, cutaneous vasculitis, nodular prurigo, acquired icthyosis, epidermal necrolysis, pityriasis rubra pilaris and mycosis fungoides.

The most important skin disorder associated with coeliac disease, however, is dermatitis herpetiformis. This is because of the enteropathy common to both conditions and the possible mucosal mechanisms linking gluten to the development of the skin lesion.

Dermatitis herpetiformis[54] is characterized by an itchy papular vesicular eruption, usually located symmetrically on the elbows, knees, buttocks, sacrum, face, neck, trunk and, occasionally, within the mouth. The predominant symptoms are itching and burning which may be so severe as to cause pain. Rupture of the blisters leads to rapid relief of symptoms.

The earliest abnormality consists of a small erythematous macule 2–3 mm in diameter which quickly develops into a papule. Small vesicles then appear which coalesce. Scratching causes them to rupture, dry up and possibly leave an area of pigmentation and scarring. The vesicles appear tense and shiny, containing a clear fluid which clouds as the lesion progresses and may be tinged with blood in rapidly growing blisters. Solitary vesicles may occur. The lesions tend to occur in crops, although all stages may be evident at one time. The blisters take 7–10 days to evolve. The tendency to suffer from attacks continues throughout life, although complete remission has been reported. The disorder is common in childhood and usually presents in adults. There tends to be a predominance of males. In 1940 the rash was found to respond to sulphapyridine and subsequently to dapsone.[39]

The common symptoms encountered are the same as those in coeliac disease. They include lassitude, diarrhoea, abdominal pain and distention. The degree of malabsorption found in patients with dermatitis herpetiformis is less than that found in coeliac disease; indeed, only approximately 10% of patients have symptoms attributable to malabsorption, although almost 100% will have a histologically abnormal jejunal mucosa (see below). Dapsone may induce severe but reversible hypoalbuminaemia. The increased risk of gastrointestinal lymphoma and neoplasia that occurs in patients with coeliac disease also affects those with dermatitis herpetiformis.[64]

The serum levels of immunoglobulin in dermatitis herpetiformis tend to parallel those found in coeliac disease, with lowered IgM, raised IgA and variable changes in IgG. Antireticulin antibodies of the IgG class are present in a significant percentage of patients with dermatitis herpetiformis, as in coeliac disease.[104]

The demonstration of IgA in the skin has become the most important investigation to confirm the diagnosis of dermatitis herpetiformis. The deposition, which should be sought in an area of skin not affected by blistering, is granular at the dermoepidermal junction.[66] Confusion should not be made with linear IgA disease, where the deposition is linear, a condition thought not to be associated with coeliac disease.[37] There may be minimal deposition of IgA in the skin in coeliac disease without dermatitis herpetiformis, although this is unusual.

The majority of patients with dermatitis herpetiformis have an abnormal small bowel mucosa, reaching nearly 100% when several biopsies are taken, suggesting that the lesion is patchy.[135] Some patients have apparently normal jejunal biopsies but increased lymphocyte counts in the epithelium, the numbers of which fall towards normal following treatment with a gluten-free diet. The degree of mucosal change may depend on the amount of gluten ingested, as well as individual sensitivity. The exact relationship of the gluten-sensitive enteropathy found in patients with dermatitis herpetiformis to that found in coeliac disease remains unclear.

The pathogenesis of the condition is poorly understood. It has been suggested that antibodies form in the gut as a result of stimulation by gluten, which then circulate to the skin where they fix and create the conditions for the skin lesion to develop.

The treatment of dermatitis herpetiformis is dapsone at a dose of 50–100 mg/day. Patients should also be advised to take a gluten-free diet as this results in a significant improvement after 6–12 months, permitting reduction in the dose of dapsone necessary to control the rash.[66] The diet may eliminate completely the need for dapsone. Months or years are usually necessary for the full benefit to be obtained, which results in many patients being unwilling to continue the diet.

CHARACTERIZATION OF THE TOXIC CEREAL PEPTIDE

Classification of cereal proteins

The precise structure of the part of gluten which causes the damage in coeliac disease remains unclear. Wheat grains have three major constituents which are separated by milling: the outer husk or bran, the germ or semolina and the endosperm or white flour, which constitutes 70–72% of the whole grain by weight (*Figure 3.68*). The storage proteins of cereals fall into two major groups: the ethanol-soluble fraction, termed prolamins, and the glutenins. Prolamins from the different cereals are termed gliadins from wheat, secalins from rye, hordeins from barley, avenins from oats and zeins from coeliac non-toxic maize. The taxononic relationship of the graminae is shown in *Figure 3.69*.

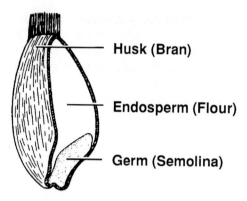

Husk (Bran)

Endosperm (Flour)

Germ (Semolina)

Figure 3.68   The constituents of a wheat grain.

A classification of wheat proteins is shown in *Figure 3.70*. Wheat proteins are subdivided into classes according to their solubility characteristics:[121] gliadins are soluble in 40–90% ethanol; and glutenins are insoluble in neutral aqueous solution, saline and ethanol. The gliadins may be further subdivided according to their relative electrophoretic mobility,[163] α, β, γ and ω in decreasing order of mobility.[29] Their molecular masses rise from 32 to 58 kDa.[96]

Clinical studies

Much of the initial work attempting to characterize the toxic cereal fraction within wheat flour involved Frazer's method for purification and separation of wheat proteins,[60] following physiological digestion of wheat proteins (*Figure 3.71*). All Frazer's six fractions were shown to exacerbate coeliac disease, with the exception of fraction VI, which was only tested in a single patient. Frazer's fraction III is usually used for the investigation of coeliac disease because of its good solubility in physiological solutions. Subfractions from Frazer's fraction III have been prepared using reversed-phase high-pressure liquid chromatography (*Figure 3.72*).[48,63,71]

Hekkens and co-workers purified α-gliadin to 60% purity and investigated its toxicity in a single patient in remission. They concluded that α-gliadin was toxic in the subject, from a deterioration in the small intestinal morphology and a decrease in small intestinal brush border enzyme levels in serial biopsies over 55 hours. However, they did not investigate other wheat protein fractions.[79] Kendall separated gliadin into three groups termed pre-α-, α- and post-α-gliadins. They fed the three fractions to five treated coeliac patients, and concluded that only the α-gliadin fraction was enterotoxic.[98] However, the assessment of toxicity was limited to a xylose absorption test, which has been shown not to reflect accurately the state of the jejunal mucosa.[33]

Jos studied the effects of α, β, γ and ω subfractions of gliadins, by an *in vitro* assay of the effects of the fractions on the normal increase in surface cell height, that occurs when jejunal biopsies of untreated coeliac disease are cultured for 24 hours *in vitro*, in the absence of gliadin. They found that peptic tryptic digests of all four gliadin subfractions had enterotoxic effects.[89,90] They concluded that the

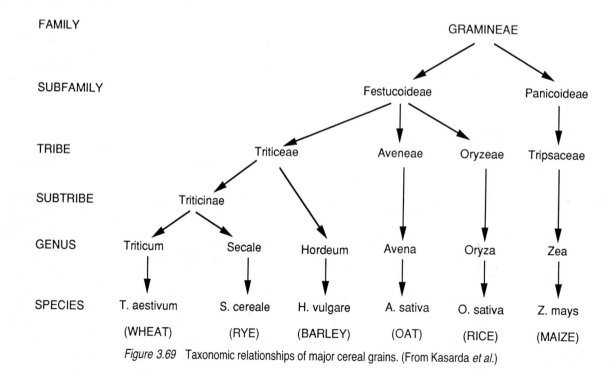

Figure 3.69   Taxonomic relationships of major cereal grains. (From Kasarda *et al.*)

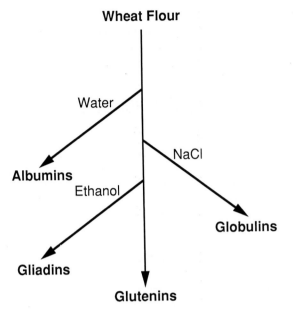

Figure 3.70 The classification of wheat proteins.

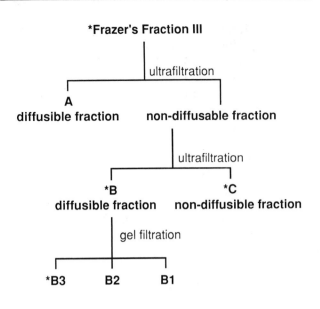

* Toxic fractions

Figure 3.72 Dissanayake's fractionation of Frazer's fraction III. Molecular pore size of Amicon UM10 membrane approximately 1×10^5. Molecular pore size of Amicon XM100a membrane approximately 1×10^4. Fractions C, B and B3 are toxic in feeding trials; 100 g of gluten yielded 15 g of B; 35 g of B yielded 15 g of B2 and B3.

most toxic fraction contained 7–8 kDa peptides rich in proline and glutamine and poor in aromatic amino acids and carbohydrates. Similar results were obtained by Howdle et al.[84]

Kumar suggested that only the α-fraction of wheat gliadin is toxic to coeliac patients but did not provide precise details of their methods of assessment.[102]

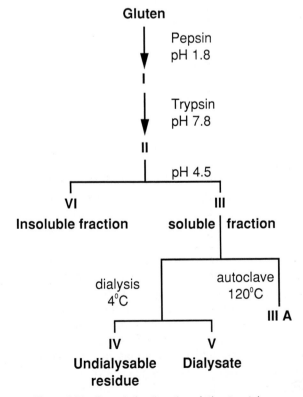

Figure 3.71 Frazer's fractionation of wheat proteins.

The subject remains contentious. Studies by the author indicate that all four gliadin subfractions exacerbated the small intestinal lesions in two treated coeliac patients.[35] The author also assessed the amount of gliadin that would cause damage, using a Quinton multiple jejunal biopsy and infusion technique. Ten milligrams of gliadin produced no light microscopic changes in jejunal biopsies taken over 8 hours. However, there were minimal changes with 100 mg of gliadin, moderate changes with 500 mg of gliadin and marked histological changes commencing 2–3 hours after an infusion of 1 g of gliadin that persisted throughout the 6 hours of this study.

Kagnoff and co-workers suggested that environmental factors may be important in the pathogenesis of coeliac disease. Computer analysis of a bank of protein sequences to look for the proteins that might share amino acid homologies with A-gliadin showed that A-gliadin (an α-gliadin component) shared amino acid residues in a span of 12 amino acids and an identical pentapeptide with the 54 kDa E1b protein of human adenovirus 12, an adenovirus usually isolated from the intestinal tract.[91] Furthermore, they found that an antibody to this adenovirus protein cross-reacted with A-gliadin. They suggested that an encounter of the immune system in susceptible individuals with antigenic determinants produced during intestinal viral infection may be important in the pathogenesis of coeliac disease.[92]

Karagiannis investigated cell-mediated immunity to this same 12 amino acid sequence peptide by an indirect leukocyte migration inhibition assay, and reported that patients with coeliac disease being treated with a gluten-free diet showed a significantly greater response than healthy subjects.[94] However, it is difficult to evaluate their results in the absence of a control peptide.

Other groups have been unable to find a correlation between the presence of coeliac disease and serum antibody titres to the adenovirus 12 protein.[30,47,84] However, further evidence for the coeliac toxicity of the 12 amino acid sequence peptide has recently been found by feeding synthesized peptide to treated coeliac patients and assessing the morphological changes involved.[114] The adenovirus hypothesis is attractive and has analogies to theories regarding the pathogenesis of autoimmune disease.

The fraction of wheat that exacerbates coeliac disease must be protein, as defatted α-gliadin containing less than 0.007 mol of carbohydrate per mole of protein[18] exacerbates the condition. All four gliadin subfractions have common epitopes, and these are also found in rye secalins, as demonstrated by both polyclonal[36] and monoclonal antibody studies.[62,144] Detoxification of wheat gluten proteins by deamidation implies that glutamine, which constitutes more than 35% of the amino acids within gliadin, may be involved, although the method employed may also have altered the structure of the other amino acid residues.[47]

The gliadins constitute a multigene family.[96] Several purified gliadin components have similar amino-terminal amino acid sequences, suggesting that, despite the electrophoretically dissimilar characteristics of the gliadin subfractions, they contain protein groups with shared amino acid sequences.[4,95] At least two such groups occur which Autran termed the α and γ types from their common amino-terminal sequences.[4] α-type sequences were found in some β- and γ-gliadins, and γ-type sequences were present in the gliadin subfractions other than γ-gliadin and in some rye secalins. Shewry reported amino-terminal sequence homology between an ω-gliadin and barley hordeins.[140] Cross-hybridization of storage protein cDNA to barley and rye endosperm poly(A^+) RNA[9,11] confirms these observations, and the deduced amino acid sequences of wheat storage proteins and barley hordeins confirm their close homology.[9,11,97]

Recently, it was shown that wheat storage proteins could be synthesized in *Escherichia coli* using novel expression vectors.[10] This should permit the production of sequenced gliadin proteins, which may be investigated for their coeliac toxicity by the *in vitro* technique described above, and provide the structure of the putative cereal peptide that exacerbates coeliac disease.

HYPOTHESES FOR PATHOGENESIS

There are three main hypotheses for the pathogenesis of coeliac disease: (1) a small intestinal enzyme deficiency; (2) an enterocyte membrane defect, allowing lectin-like binding of gliadin to the small intestine enterocytes; and (3) a primary abnormal immune response to specific cereal peptides.

Enzyme deficiency hypothesis

This postulates that absence of a specific peptidase from the jejunal mucosa of coeliac patients results in an inability to digest gluten which, in turn, damages the small intestinal mucosa. This hypothesis followed the demonstration that gluten, subjected to complete acid hydrolysis, deamidation by acid and treatment with papain,[93] resulted in the loss of its deleterious properties. However, peptic tryptic digestion of gluten does not significantly reduce its toxicity.[60] Batt suggested that the primary abnormality is late development during infancy of the ability to produce small intestinal N-peptidase.[12] This abnormality then permits gluten peptides to be absorbed into the circulation and establish a hypersensitivity to specific cereal peptides.

Lectin-binding hypothesis

This hypothesis suggests there is a defect in the cell surface of small intestinal enterocytes, either an abnormal glycoprotein or glycolipid structured element, or reduced biosynthesis of one of these cell wall components.[132,161] Immunohistochemical studies suggested that gliadin bound only to coeliac and not to normal small intestinal enterocytes, but these findings have not been confirmed, either by similar techniques or by radioimmunoassay binding studies.[31,40] Douglas reported that a carbohydrate-containing component of wheat gluten bound to components of coeliac small intestinal enterocytes but not to those from controls.[53] However, other investigators were unable to repeat these observations. Weiser and Douglas went on to suggest that as a result of this primary abnormality, a sugar residue not normally exposed in coeliac enterocytes interacted with a lectin in wheat gluten, to produce coeliac disease.[161] The lack of confirmation of these observations makes such an aetiology appear unlikely.

Primary immune hypothesis

This hypothesis suggests there is an abnormal primary immune response of the small intestine to gluten that results in allergic phenomena. There is considerable evidence to support this hypothesis. The rare occurrence of 'gluten-shock' (vomiting, diarrhoea, tachycardia and cardiovascular collapse[100]) in a small number of treated coeliac patients after gluten challenge implies an immune aetiology.

There is dense infiltration of the lamina propria of jejunal biopsies from patients with untreated coeliac disease, by lymphocytes and plasma cells. There is a significant increase in the ratio of intraepithelial lymphocytes to surface cell enterocytes,[58] the majority of which express the suppressor/cytotoxic phenotype[147] and which have the appearance of immunoblasts.[115] Freedman recently showed that, in the majority of treated coeliac patients subject to gluten challenge, there is a deterioration in villous morphology concomitant with an increase in the ratio of T lymphocytes to surface small intestinal enterocytes 1–2 hours after the challenge.[61] The reversal of both the symptoms and histological abnormalities of the small intestine in coeliac patients, when treated with a gluten-free diet or systemic steroids, implies an immune-mediated aetiology. Splenic atrophy, which occurs in coeliac patients,[21] and the strong association with the histocompatibility antigens associated with autoimmune disorders, further support this hypothesis.[152]

The presence of circulating antibodies to gluten following gluten ingestion by coeliac patients[34] also points to an immune mechanism, although the presence of antibodies to a variety of food antigens in these patients implies that these antibodies could be secondary to small intestinal damage, allowing non-specific absorption of food antigens. The finding that cultured jejunal biopsies from untreated coeliac patients secrete more total IgM and IgA, but not IgG, than those from controls or treated coeliac patients is evidence of a local immune response.[162] In addition, there is increased secretion of IgG and IgA antibodies to gliadin, but not casein, by cultured jejunal biopsies from untreated coeliac patients compared to those from normal controls.[38]

Further evidence that coeliac disease might be a manifestation of an immune response was the observation that coeliac patients, unlike controls, developed a reaction to intradermal injections of gluten subfractions.[2] However, this was not confirmed with the same batch of fractions.[3,108] Baker and Read obtained positive skin reactions in 52% of coeliac patients, but not in any of their controls (3 hours after the injections), using Frazer's fraction III as the test substance.[6] They suggested this was an immune complex-mediated (Arthus type) reaction. The occasional association of coeliac disease with cryoglobulinaemia, vasculitis and raised circulating immune complexes favours an immune-mediated mechanism.[50]

Holmes demonstrated an *in vitro* response of lymphocytes from coeliac patients, but not controls, to Frazer's fraction III, but only when the coeliac patients were on a gluten-free diet.[81] Leukocyte migration inhibition has been used to suggest that coeliac peripheral blood leucocytes are sensitized to Frazer's fraction III.[28] The finding by Ferguson that coeliac small intestinal lymphocytes are sensitized to gliadin using a leukocyte migration inhibition assay is strong evidence that the condition is mediated by sensitized small intestinal T lymphocytes.[59]

Coeliac patients who possess HLA-B8 were found to show a higher incidence of cell damage when their jejunal mucosa was cultured *in vitro* in the presence of gluten.[55] Gluten challenge in treated coeliac patients was shown to induce abnormal expression of HLA class II gene products in small intestinal enterocytes 1–2 hours after the challenge.[39]

The author has proposed that gliadin is initially presented by small intestinal dendritic cells in the lamina propria to the T-cell receptor of lamina propria helper lymphocytes (afferent limb), which generate immune products to damage the epithelial cells (efferent limb). The lymphocyte products also induce HLA class II gene product expression on the small intestinal enterocytes that may then present further antigen to the sensitized lymphocytes. This is shown schematically in *Figure 3.73*.

GENETICS OF COELIAC DISEASE

The precise inheritance of coeliac disease and dermatitis herpetiformis are unknown, although 10% of first-degree relatives of coeliac patients are affected by the condition. Efforts to understand the mechanisms and genetics of polygenic human disease have focused on the identification of DNA and protein markers that segregate with diseases in populations and families. The most significant observation was the increased frequency of specific serologically defined lymphoid cell surface proteins, encoded in the HLA-D region of the major histocompatability complex and referred to as HLA class II antigens. These consist of α- and β-chain transmembrane glycosylated heterodimers. The genes for these are organized into three related subregions termed DR, DP and DQ,[154] as shown in *Figure 3.74*. The association of HLA-DR3 and DQ2 with coeliac disease and dermatitis herpetiformis has been well

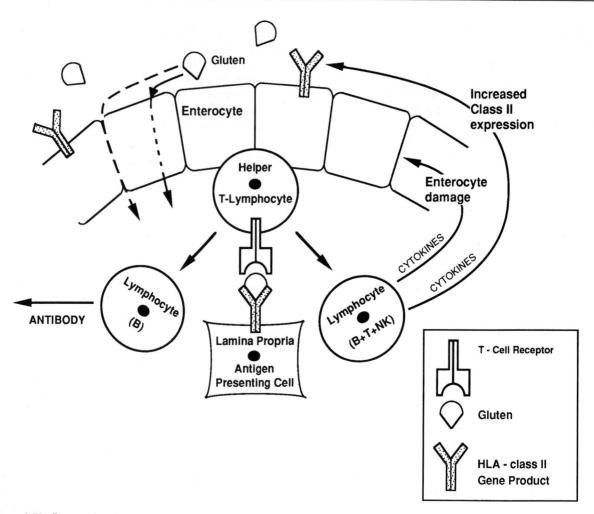

Figure 3.73 Proposed pathogenetic mechanism for coeliac disease. Gluten is absorbed into the lamina propria and presented in conjunction with HLA class II cell surface antigens by dendritic cells to sensitized T lymphocytes via the T-cell receptor (afferent limb). These lymphocytes then activate other lymphocytes to generate immune products which damage the enterocytes (efferent limb). Induction of aberrant HLA class II cell-surface antigens on the enterocytes permits additional antigen presentation by these cells to the sensitized lymphocytes.

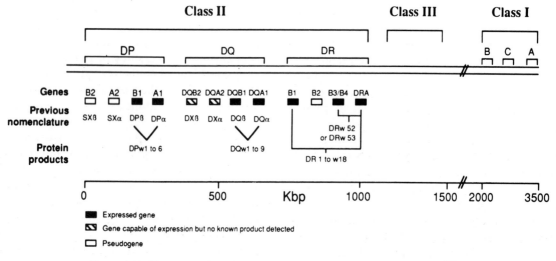

Figure 3.74 The genes of the HLA-D region. (From Trowsdale and Campbell.[153])

established.[72,73,152] Recently a DQ-A gene[27] and an HLA-DP locus association, although weaker, have also been demonstrated.[26,86,127,128]

Restriction fragment length polymorphism (RFLP) analysis of HLA class II genes reveals that 96% of coeliac patients carry the HLA-DR3 marker ($P < 0.001$).[72] Of 50 of the coeliac patients, 47 had the RFLP subtype DR3, which is associated with the serological specificity HLA-B8 ($P < 0.001$).

HLA-DP genotyping by RFLP analysis showed a significant increase in the frequency of DPw1 in the coeliac disease population; of 77 coeliac patients 29 (38%) were typed as DPw1, compared with 7 of 53 controls (13%, $P < 0.005$). DPw1 was only present in those coeliac patients who genotyped DR3a positive. Of DR3a controls, 24% were DPw1 positive compared with 5% of the non-DR3a controls ($P < 0.03$), suggesting that an extended DR3a–DPw1 haplotype occurs in the population that predisposes to coeliac disease.[72]

An independent RFLP analysis in 23 patients with dermatitis herpetiformis has recently revealed that HLA-DQ2 was present in 100% of the dermatitis herpetiformis patients (23/23) versus 40% of the controls (21/53) examined, significant secondary associations were also seen with HLA-DR3 (91% of patients versus 28% of controls) and DPw1 (39% of patients versus 11% of controls). The increase in DPw1 was again thought to be due to linkage disequilibrium between HLA-DR3, DQ2 and DPw1. These findings suggested that dermatitis herpetiformis and coeliac disease share the same HLA class II association.[73] This implies that HLA class II genes directly influence the immune responses to gluten proteins and are involved in generation of the mucosal damage found in the small intestine of individuals with these conditions. The strongest candidate for disease susceptibility to both coeliac disease and dermatitis herpetiformis was found to be DQ2. This suggested the HLA molecule most likely to be involved in gluten-sensitive enteropathy to be a specific DQα–DQβ heterodimer, encoded in a *cis* arrangement in DR3 haplotypes or *trans* in a DR5, 7 genotype.[72,145]

These studies have been extended to investigate 13 families in which several individuals have either coeliac disease or dermatitis herpetiformis. Individuals with coeliac disease in all the families showed the same HLA-B8, DR3, DQ2 haplotype, confirming this association and suggesting that it is due to the presence of these alleles on a disease-associated extended haplotype.[22]

HLA class II analysis by the author and other investigators points to HLA-DQ2 being the major susceptibility molecule in the pathogenesis of gluten-sensitive enteropathy in both coeliac disease

and dermatitis herpetiformis. Studies from Italian and Argentinian coeliac disease populations show an increase in the HLA-DR5, 7 genotype which is not seen in North European coeliac disease patients.[80] However, the common link between these ethnic groups is the potential to express a specific HLA-DQ2–DQα/β heterodimer. The association of DPw1 with the disease is the result of linkage disequilibrium between DPw1 and some B8–DR3 haplotypes, and it is this haplotype that is highly represented in the disease.[22,26,72,128]

CLINICAL FEATURES

The classic description by Gee with its delightfully evocative account was largely concerned with the gross manifestations of the disorder. Clinicians should not neglect the relatively mild symptomatology which represents the common presentation of coeliac disease as it is seen today. Patients may still have a severe illness, although it is now evident that many others have little or no symptoms. Diagnosis may be made by screening relatives of probands and placing a greater awareness of the disorder in the abnormalities encountered in haematological, biochemical and, more recently, HLA class II profiles.

Infancy and childhood

The classical presentation of coeliac disease in infancy occurs after weaning and introduction of cereals into the diet. There is failure to thrive associated with apathy, pallor, anorexia, misery and muscle wasting. There is generalized hypotonia and abdominal distension, with the child passing soft, bulky, clay-coloured, offensive stools. Very young children may present with vomiting, which is often effortless, of large volume, and usually associated with abdominal distension and little or no diarrhoea. Abdominal pain may be so severe that a child undergoes laparotomy under the mistaken diagnosis of intestinal obstruction, which in some cases is brought about by constipation. Retardation of motor activity has been observed. A great variety of symptoms may bring the patient for advice and diagnosis, including rectal prolapse, which is of course more common in cystic fibrosis.

Older children tend to have more varied symptomatology and present with anaemia, rickets or failure to grow normally. Rickets is particularly common in Asian children. Unexplained short stature is an indication for jejunal biopsy, even when gastrointestinal symptoms are mild or absent. A study of 34 such patients revealed that eight had coeliac disease and seven showed significant acceleration in height and weight velocity when given a gluten-free diet.[70]

Gastrointestinal symptoms may date from birth in 25% of children, while more than half become symptomatic in the first 6 months of life. The later presentation and diagnosis of coeliac disease in recent years can be ascribed to the current practice of introducing gluten in the form of cereals later, that is, after the age of 6 months. The exception to this is Sweden, where infant-feeding practices have returned to the early introduction of gluten to infants within the first few weeks of life. This has resulted in an upsurge of cases presenting during infancy. It was suggested that coeliac disease occurs predominantly in infants who had not been breast-fed, but there is little to substantiate this.[52]

Adult life

Adult and adolescent patients with coeliac disease may present with varied symptomatology in almost any hospital department. Diarrhoea is the main presenting feature while those with constitutional disturbances such as lassitude, loss of weight, glossitis and symptoms of anaemia form another group. A much smaller group present because of abnormal neurological or psychiatric symptoms, including schizophrenia. Patients may present with problems related to osteomalacia, including spontaneous fractures and myopathy, skin complaints, bleeding diatheses or infertility.[8,41,44] The age of presentation of coeliac disease in 84 adults is shown in *Figure 3.75*.[57]

Many patients have long-standing ill health for many years and, never having had severe symptoms, come to accept this as normal. Abdominal pain occurs in approximately 5% of cases. Aphthous stomatitis may uncommonly be the sole presenting symptom and therefore coeliac disease should be excluded in cases of severe unexplained recurrent mouth ulceration. The stress of an operation or infection can occasionally induce severe diarrhoea.

Pregnancy may precipitate macrocytic anaemia or the onset of unexplained diarrhoea. Following pregnancy the symptoms may abate and the diagnosis be missed.

The presenting symptoms in many patients with coeliac disease are non-specific and, therefore, a high diagnostic suspicion should be aroused with significant minor abnormalities or haematological or biochemical profiles. In a few patients, investigated for an unrelated problem, the finding of a mild unexplained macrocytic anaemia with a persistent low serum or red cell folate level will suggest further investigation and lead to a diagnosis of coeliac disease. A previous diagnosis of coeliac disease in childhood can be overlooked by both the patient and doctor, only to be a source of symptoms in adult life. Clinicians should therefore explore possible childhood disturbances such as short stature, anaemia or rickets.

There is a high incidence of the condition among the patients' relatives, which may permit the diagnosis of a number of unsuspected individuals.[22]

Certain symptoms warrant particular mention. Lassitude may frequently be attributed to mild psychiatric disturbances. Glossitis of varying severity may be found. Angular stomatitis may occur and, in a few patients, marked chelosis is present. Nausea and vomiting are common, particularly during episodes of diarrhoea, and occur in as much as 50% of coeliac children. The appetite is usually lost, though it may be excessive in some patients. Failure to gain weight despite ingesting 6000–7000 calories/day has been reported.[69] Abdominal distension is common, often associated with flatulence and flatus. Symptoms of cramp and tetany may occur, usually associated with a low serum calcium level. Bowel disturbance is the most frequent problem, usually in the form of loose stools. The motion may be paler than normal, sometimes offensive, occasionally frothy, sometimes difficult to flush away. The frequency of bowel action varies but is commonly 3–4 times a day and rarely more than eight. However, pale stools can occur in other conditions. Normally formed and coloured stools do not preclude the diagnosis; indeed, some patients with steatorrhoea may have stools with a normal appearance. Physicians should not forget to enquire specifically about a subject's stools since patients with long-standing bowel disturbance frequently make no complaint. It

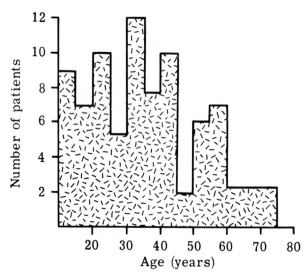

Figure 3.75 Age at time of diagnosis of coeliac disease jejunal biopsy in 84 adults. (From Ferguson.[57])

has been reported that 10% of patients suffer incontinence complicating nocturnal diarrhoea.[69]

Many other factors can disturb bowel habit, including emotional problems. One study revealed that 10% of patients attending a gastroenterology clinic and labelled as suffering from a functional non-organic bowel disorder were subsequently found to be suffering from coeliac disease. Constipation occurs in approximately 10% of subjects with coeliac disease.

Abdominal pain is uncommon and may indicate the need for investigation to exclude intra-abdominal pathology complicating coeliac disease, particularly conditions such as volvulus, intussusception, mesenteric adenitis, cholelithiasis, peptic ulceration and pancreatitis.

Scurvy complicating coeliac disease has been reported. Bleeding into the skin and subcutaneous tissue, though uncommon, may reflect vitamin K deficiency. Prior to the discovery of the value of a gluten-free diet purpura was reported to occur in 10% of patients at some time and be the presenting feature in 2%.

Osteomalacia, rickets or bone pains lead to the diagnosis of coeliac disease in an appreciable number of subjects, reflecting a failure of calcium and vitamin D absorption. Symptoms of rickets and osteomalacia tend to be insidious in onset and may become severe before they are recognized. Negative calcium balances were shown to be associated with excessive endogenous faecal calcium and malabsorption of vitamin D; a gluten-free diet restores these abnormalities to normal.

Physical signs

Personality

Early reports commented on the frequency of mental symptoms. Children with coeliac disease are usually irritable and miserable. Adults may suffer from depression, paranoia, Korsakov's syndrome and neurasthenia.[68,129] The majority of patients do not appear abnormal when judged against their peers, although it is striking to note the significant change in outlook and mood experienced by most patients when they exclude gluten from their diet, however well they had claimed to be before.

Height

Coeliac patients frequently exhibit a short stature, not infrequently dwarfism. Growth retardation in children is well documented and the return to normal growth rate is one of the criteria by which the effect of treatment can be judged. Coeliac patients are on average 8 cm shorter than their peers.[70] Tall patients do, however, exist and a height of over 1.8 m does not preclude the diagnosis.

Weight

Weight loss frequently affects both children and adults when first seen. Sixty per cent of newly diagnosed coeliac children are below the third percentile for weight. The average loss of weight in adults in one series was 12 kg of whom 90% had lost more than 4.5 kg.[69] An increase in weight of the order of 6 kg in adults is usually seen when a gluten-free diet is instituted. None the less, the occasional patient is grossly overweight when first seen.

Teeth

Children exhibit delay in the eruption of teeth, and hypoplasia of the enamel has been described; dental caries is rare.

Fever

A low-grade fever associated with anaemia may be encountered in some individuals, but a recurrent marked pyrexia is usually a manifestation of complications such as septicaemia or lymphoma.

Finger clubbing and koilonychia

Finger clubbing is reported in 5–10% of both children and adults. Koilonychia is usually associated with long-standing severe iron deficiency and anaemia, and responds to iron therapy.

Oedema and ascites

Oedema and ascites may rarely be present in severe cases, reflecting hypoproteinaemia. Abnormal distension and general dilatation of the intestinal tract are, however, common in coeliac disease, and the abdomen feels like dough, making the detection of ascites difficult.

Sexual characteristics

There is some delay in the menarche, typically by 1 year in an untreated group.[138] Amenorrhoea lasting more than 3 months, unrelated to pregnancy, occurs in a third of women of child-bearing age, and menstrual loss is frequently shorter than normal (1–3 days). The average age of the menopause in untreated coeliac patients is 45 compared to 53 years in those on gluten-free diet.

Many coeliac patients appear relatively infertile but eventually conceive. The mean time for coeliac patients to conceive on a normal diet is 19 months, and 12 months on a gluten-free diet. Infertile coeliac patients frequently become pregnant shortly after commencing a gluten-free diet. Spontaneous abortion is more common in untreated coeliac patients (18% of pregnancies) compared to coeliac patients on a gluten-free diet (9%). Recurrent abortions may be a presenting feature.

There is some reduction in the potency of men. Fertility and normal sperm counts are restored by a gluten-free diet after some years of oligospermia. Low levels of plasma testosterone, free testosterone and plasma 5-dihydrososterone are reported; the plasma luteinizing hormone level is frequently raised.[56] This may in part explain the frequently observed marked delay in puberty and development of secondary sexual characteristics in untreated male coeliac patients. These abnormalities usually revert to normal following prolonged treatment.

Lymphadenopathy

Lymphadenopathy is not usually found in coeliac disease. Its presence should suggest the presence of a complicating lymphoma, although very rare cases of lymphadenopathy, that has resolved on treatment with a gluten-free diet, have been reported.

METABOLIC DISTURBANCES

Haematology

Haemoglobin

The characteristic blood picture in adult coeliac disease is a mild hypochromic, macrocytic anaemia. Severe anaemia occurs uncommonly and should raise the suspicion of a superimposed complication such as a malignancy.

The peripheral blood film may show target cells, Howell–Jolly bodies, siderocytes, irregular and crenated cells, Heinz bodies, microspherocytes, acanthocytes and occasional erythroblasts.[65,153,157] An erythroblastic appearance with circulating nucleated red cells, pale ring cells and Howell–Jolly bodies suggests splenic atrophy, which occurs in coeliac disease. Variation in the size and shape of the erythrocytes and the degree of haemoglobinization may give rise to the characteristic appearances of dimorphic anaemia. The mean corpuscular volume varies, but is raised in a third of patients. In children, the predominant picture is that of hypochromic microcytic anaemia, responding slowly to iron therapy. The serum levels of iron and folic acid are usually low. A macrocytic megaloblastic anaemia may occasionally be seen in older children.

Bone marrow

Bone marrow examination in adult patients usually reveals megaloblastic erythropoiesis. Forty-five per cent have pure megaloblastic marrows, 55% have megaloblastosis combined with lack of iron, and a few have pure iron deficiency.

Folic acid

A low serum folate level is present in the majority of patients with untreated coeliac disease. Red cell folate is a better test for total body stores and a reduced level is present in 85% of patients. The levels usually improve with a gluten-free diet, although it is usual to correct this therapeutically.

Vitamin B$_{12}$

The mean serum level of vitamin B$_{12}$ in patients with untreated coeliac disease is lower than in controls, although only 14% have levels below normal. Occasionally, patients will exhibit an anaemia due to a combined deficiency of vitamin B$_{12}$ and folic acid, requiring combined therapeutic replacement. The vitamin B$_{12}$ level will rise to normal in most patients when treated with a gluten-free diet and folic acid.

Iron

Iron deficiency is common in coeliac disease and may occur because of impaired absorption and increased loss into the intestinal tract, either as a result of the rapid epithelial turnover or associated blood loss. Therapy with a gluten-free diet or corticosteroids increases the amount of iron absorbed.

Biochemistry and immunology

Gliadin antibodies

Patients with untreated coeliac disease have elevated titres of IgG, IgM and IgA circulating antibodies to wheat gliadin and other food proteins compared to controls.[17,34] Coeliac patients also have elevated circulating antibody titres to collagen, reticulin[75] and endomysium,[75] the significance of which is unclear. Estimation of gliadin or gluten antibodies can be useful to uncover intentional or inadvertent ingestion of gluten among coeliac patients who are unwell. Raised gliadin antibody titres can also be used to screen for the condition, although raised titres alone should not be used to make a definitive diagnosis because elevated gliadin antibody titres can occur in other disorders, including inflammatory bowel and liver diseases.

Circulating immune complexes

Elevated levels of circulating immune complexes were reported in a group of coeliac patients,[51] but subsequent groups have been unable to confirm this result. Their presence would not be of diagnostic significance.[32]

Malabsorption of fat

Most patients with coeliac disease have steatorrhoea. To assess the amount of fat excreted over a fixed period, it is important that the daily intake is at least 50 g (preferably 100 g) per day (the normal intake of fat in the UK is 60–90 g/day). Patients with steatorrhoea often find that they can moderate their diarrhoea by reducing fat intake; it is therefore advisable to place subjects on a 100 g fat diet, commencing 2 days prior to the study. All the motions should be collected over a 3-day period, eliminating the normal day-to-day variations. The generally accepted upper limit of fat excretion is 5 or 6 g/day.[148] Estimation of faecal fat is a relatively crude test, readily subject to errors of collection and measurement. Thus, while faecal fat determination was considered mandatory at one time for the diagnosis of coeliac disease, the introduction of jejunal biopsy has made quantification of faecal fats superfluous, particularly as 30% of patients with untreated coeliac disease have a normal fat excretion.

Breath tests

Hydrogen and [14C]bile acid breath tests may be mildly abnormal, reflecting a degree of bacterial overgrowth which usually returns to normal when coeliac disease is treated.

Carbohydrate absorption tests

Patients with untreated coeliac disease characteristically have a flat glucose tolerance curve, but this has no diagnostic value since a significant proportion of the normal population also exhibit this. Nearly all patients with untreated coeliac disease have some degree of lactose intolerance. However, a gluten-free diet removes this intolerance, leaving only a small percentage with concomitant constitutional alactasia, necessitating a lactase- and gluten-free diet. More complex sugars are used in gastrointestinal permeability studies (see below).

Pancreatic enzymes

Pancreatic function tests may reveal low intraluminal trypsin and lipase concentrations in resting samples. Following intravenous stimulation by secretin and pancreazymin, the pancreas is able to respond normally in untreated coeliac disease.

Gut hormones

Reduced levels of cholecystokinin following a fatty meal have been recorded in coeliac disease, which may explain the inertia of the gallbladder as well as diminished pancreatic function in response to oral challenge.[110,111] A generalized reduction in many gut hormones found in the condition tends to normalize following introduction of a gluten-free diet, except for the poor rise in plasma gastric inhibitory peptides following an oral stimulus. Grossly elevated levels of enteroglucagon and the abnormal responses to oral glucose are considered unique to the disorder.[19,20]

Sodium and potassium

Individuals who suffer persistent frequent loose stools are at risk of developing sodium and potassium depletion, leading to loss of muscle power and fatigue. Should they become severe, symptoms suggestive of a peripheral neuropathy may appear. Potassium depletion may stimulate a renal disorder with albuminuria, oedema and renal tubular vacuolation, all of which can be reversed with potassium therapy.

Calcium and magnesium

Untreated coeliac patients frequently have hypocalcaemia and hypomagnesaemia. Symptoms do not usually occur until the serum calcium level falls below 1.5 mEq/l.[14] The clinical symptoms include personality changes, tremor of the limbs, uncoordinated movements, convulsions, great variation in the reflexes (either absent or exaggerated), nausea, vomiting, abdominal pain and paralytic ileus. Insensitivity to vitamin D may occur, causing resistant osteomalacia and elevated serum parathormone levels, both of which are corrected by calcium and magnesium therapy.

Serum albumin

Albumin levels in untreated coeliac disease are frequently low, perhaps in a third of subjects. The value usually rises after the introduction of a gluten-free diet. Severe hypoalbuminaemia in a patient under active treatment suggests a complication such as lymphoma, cancer or jejunal ulceration.

Zinc and copper

Zinc deficiency is liable to develop in coeliac disease. Zinc therapy has been reported to be complicated by the development of anaemia, apparently due to induction of copper deficiency.[125]

INVESTIGATIONS

The diagnosis may be suspected on clinical grounds and as a result of various screening tests. However, for confirmation, it is mandatory to proceed to jejunal biopsy.

Biopsy of the small intestine

Indications

A biopsy is indicated in any patient with a history suggestive of coeliac disease. This includes individuals with mild symptoms, particularly relatives of probands. All patients with dermatitis herpetiformis require biopsy. The commonest indications in childhood are diarrhoea, failure to thrive, anaemia and short stature.

Small intestinal biopsy can be undertaken either endoscopically or with a small intestinal biopsy capsule. The haemoglobin concentration, platelet count and prothrombin time should be checked prior to biopsy because of the significant number of untreated coeliac patients who have an increased prothrombin time (correctable by intravenous vitamin K). Anaemia is not a contraindication to small intestinal biopsy unless very marked, for the risk of haemorrhage with a normal prothrombin time is small.

Endoscopic biopsies should be obtained from the second part of the duodenum using the largest forceps available. It is advisable to take at least three biopsies to avoid difficulties in interpretation due to the normal avillous mucosa overlying Brunner's glands. The macroscopic appearance of the duodenum at endoscopy should be noted, as a duodenal ulcer or patchy duodenitis may produce a pattern of inflammation similar to that found in coeliac disease. Occasionally the endoscopist may note a loss of the normal duodenal folds.

Ideally, a biopsy of the proximal jejunum should be obtained with some form of suction–guillotine biopsy capsule, most commonly that of Crosby and Kugler or Watson.[45] An alternative capsule, described by Brandburg and frequently termed a Quinton biopsy capsule, may be used to obtain multiple biopsies from the oesophagus, stomach, small intestine or colon.[25]

Biopsy technique

The patient is fasted overnight. Sedation and local anaesthesia to the throat are not essential but usually help. The patient swallows the capsule attached to a flexible radiopaque tube. A semi-stiff polypropylene outer tube measuring 4 mm diameter with a brass ring at the end facilitates movement of the capsule into the pyloric antrum. Metaclopramide (10 mg intravenously) increases bowel motility. The patient is asked to turn on to their right-hand side and use of the outer tube permits the capsule to be passed into the duodenum. When radiographic screening shows that it is in the proximal jejunum, the capsule is fired, in the case of the Watson or Crosby capsule, by application of rapid suction through the peroral connecting tube with either a 50 or 20 ml syringe. Inexperienced operators may check the position of the capsule prior to firing by injecting 15–20 ml of Gastrograffin through the connecting tube to outline the jejunum. If this is

done, the oral tube should be washed through with 20 ml of tap water followed by 30 ml of air to remove fluid from the capsule and enable it to fire.

With a Quinton multiple jejunal biopsy capsule, the size of the biopsy is dependent on the degree of suction applied. The smallest amount of suction possible (10 lb/in.^{2}) should be used initially, particularly if several biopsies are being taken, to avoid the slight risk of haemorrhage or perforation. In patients with untreated coeliac disease the suction may have to be increased to 20 lb/in.^{2}, as the flat mucosa is more resistant to biopsy. Biopsies should be taken from different areas of the jejunum by repositioning the capsule.

Biopsy orientation

The biopsy should be quickly retrieved from the biopsy capsule and oriented before fixing so that, on sectioning, the villi are cut through a plane parallel to their longitudinal axis and not obliquely, which makes histological interpretation difficult. The cut surface of the biopsy should be placed on to a small square of absorbant paper and the whole immediately placed in fixative. The mucosa should then be viewed under the dissecting microscope for rapid assessment of obvious abnormalities.

Complications

The procedure is usually trouble-free, although complications may rarely arise. These include haemorrhage, perforation (which has been reported to occur in 1:11 000 procedures), retention of the capsule, intramural haematoma and bacteraemia.[137] Retention of the capsule is usually caused by a blunt knife blade. Should this happen, the capsule can be retrieved some hours later when the biopsy will have autolysed (and become uninterpretable). Should the cap of a Crosby or Watson capsule separate from the body, it can be retrieved at no risk to the patient by the patient collecting and inspecting his or her stools, normally passing between 12 and 16 days after the procedure.

Gastrointestinal permeability studies: D-xylose

Monosaccharide and disaccharide small intestinal permeability tests have been used to assess the absorptive capacity of the small intestine. The absorption and excretion of D-xylose, which is absorbed and excreted in the urine within 5 hours, was used for many years as a diagnostic screening test. The 5 g oral loading test was found to be more discriminating than 25 g. A combination of measurements of the plasma level 1 hour after taking an oral load considered in conjunction with the amount excreted in the urine within 5 hours permits discrimination between coeliac disease and a normal small intestine in 95% of cases.[16] Many centres, however, only use the urinary value; since this will not detect a significant number of patients, the test has not achieved wide acceptance.

Screening can be undertaken by simultaneous measurement of excretion of L-rhamnose and lactulose after ingestion of a hypertonic solution containing both of these sugars. One study revealed the lactulose/L-rhamnose urinary excretion ratio to be seven-fold higher in patients with untreated coeliac disease compared to controls; there was no overlap of values for patients and controls.[117,118] These tests can be useful in diagnostic management where a peroral biopsy is contraindicated, for example during pregnancy. They do not, however, replace the diagnostic value of peroral jejunal biopsy, which remains the diagnostic investigation of choice.

Radiology

Dilatation of the colon was an early radiological feature to be noted. Segmentation and dilatation of the bowel and 'moulage' resembling 'a tube into which wax had been poured and allowed to harden' were added later.[93,113] With colloidal preparations of barium, flocculation and segmentation occur in most patients. The most common constant feature in coeliac disease is dilatation. The upper limit for the diameter of the normal proximal small bowel on barium follow through is 30 mm in adults, 24 mm in children at 10 years of age, and 14 mm up to the age of 6 months. The ileum does not show much distension but measures up to 24 mm in the normal adult.

Values for the technique of small bowel enema, in which barium is placed into the duodenum through a peroral or pernasal tube, are higher. The upper limit for the diameter of the small intestine in normal adults, using this technique, is 50 mm.

Barium follow-through examination of the small intestine reveals a loss of the fine feathery mucosal pattern, with thin mucosal folds in 85% of subjects, an example of which is shown in *Figure 3.76*. The normal appearance of the small bowel enema does not, however, include this feathery pattern. There is usually a degree of straightening of the valvulae conniventes, thickening of the mucosal folds and an increase in their separation. Superimposed upon dilatation and thickening of the mucosal folds are varying degrees of flocculation, segmentation and clumping, which are more relevant when they occur early in the examination. These features are not specific to coeliac disease.

Whilst most patients with untreated coeliac disease have radiological findings suggestive of the

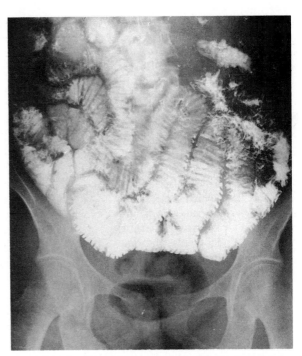

Figure 3.76 Small bowel follow through showing dilated loop of jejunum with the characteristic appearances of untreated coeliac disease.

condition, others have findings resembling Crohn's disease, scleroderma (which should readily be differentiated on screening by decreased motility), tropical sprue and, occasionally, chronic pancreatitis. A quarter of patients with untreated coeliac disease do not have any radiological abnormality. Radiological examination, however, remains important, particularly in the presence of abdominal pain, to exclude complicating lesions such as benign ulceration of the small intestine with strictures, lymphoma or carcinoma.

A dilated and often redundant colon is a feature which renders the untreated patient liable to develop volvulus with associated abdominal pain. Intussusception can complicate coeliac disease and may be diagnosed by its classic radiological appearance.

DISEASE ASSOCIATIONS

Numerous disease associations with coeliac disease have been reported and are shown in *Table 3.35*.[134] There is a high association with a variety of autoimmune disorders which also have a high prevalence of the gene encoding HLA-DR3. The relationship to dermatitis herpetiformis has already been discussed above.

Table 3.35 Factors and diseases associated with coeliac disease

Disease	Approximate reported disease incidence (%)
First-degree relative of coeliac patients	10
Dermatitis herpetiformis	80
IgA deficiency	20
Hyposplenism	100
Aphthous ulceration	5
Cow's milk protein intolerance	10
Small intestinal T-cell lymphoma	6
Thyroid disease	U
Diabetes mellitus	U
Cutaneous vasculitis	U
Fibrosing alveolitis	U
Sjögren's syndrome	U
Polyarteritis	U
Addison's disease	U
Systemic lupus erythematosus	U
Ulcerative colitis	U
Rheumatoid arthritis	U
Idiopathic pulmonary haemosiderosis	U
Glomerulonephritis	U
Schizophrenia	U
Sarcoidosis	U
Histocompatibility antigens HLA-B8 and DR3	U

U, incidence unknown.

Diabetes Mellitus

The coexistence of diabetes and coeliac disease is well recognized in both children and adults. The prevalence of diabetes in coeliac disease has been reported to be between 4 and 6%.[134] Diarrhoea is a symptom of both disorders. However, the control of the diabetes often becomes poor in the months preceding the onset of diarrhoea caused by coeliac disease. Anaemia, finger clubbing, glossitis, mouth ulceration, abdominal discomfort and distention and poor nutritional state in a diabetic may alert one to the diagnosis. Unexpected episodes of hypoglycaemia with exacerbations of diarrhoea are additional pointers. Treatment of coeliac disease aids diabetic control.

Liver disease

A higher than expected incidence of chronic hepatitis, primary biliary cirrhosis and sclerosing cholangitis is found in coeliac disease.[109]

Pulmonary disorders

Chronic fibrosing alveolitis and other interstitial lung diseases, including idiopathic pulmonary haemosiderosis, have been reported in association with coeliac disease.[103]

Inflammatory bowel disease

There is a known association of coeliac disease with inflammatory bowel disease, particularly ulcerative proctocolitis.[99] Patients reporting with proctocolitis complicating coeliac disease improved with a gluten-free diet, and also with therapy with oral salazopyrine and corticosteroid enemas. The demonstration of an inflammatory infiltration of the rectal mucosa in response to local gluten challenge in coeliac disease suggests that the aetiology of the proctocolitis is similar to that of the small intestinal enteropathy.[106,107] The relationship of these conditions to microscopic colitis (which may be associated with small bowel villous atrophy unresponsive to a gluten-free diet) remains obscure.

Jejunal ulceration and lymphoma

Ulcerative jejunitis is characterized by chronic, multiple, apparently benign ulcers which are found most frequently in the jejunum, though occasionally the ileum may be affected.[13] The condition affects those in the fifth and sixth decades of life and presents with fever, lassitude, anorexia, weight loss, abdominal pain and diarrhoea. Anaemia, both microcytic and macrocytic, are common, together with steatorrhoea and a protein-losing enteropathy. The ulcers may be complicated by haemorrhage, perforation or stricture formation, frequently bringing the patients to laparotomy, which represents a common presentation of this complication. A flat jejunal mucosa is found on biopsy similar to that found in coeliac disease. Patients may initially benefit from a gluten-free diet, but response is frequently lost. The nature of this entity is not entirely clear, and is discussed later in this chapter.

The HLA-DR3 genotype in the few reported cases, which is also present in coeliac disease, supports the association of the disorders.[150]

The outlook for this condition is poor, with a third of patients rapidly dying of complications. The prognosis is much improved if the ulcerated or strictured segment is resected.

The clinical features of jejunal ulceration and lymphoma are similar and both tend to occur in coeliac patients during middle life. Some patients with ulceration go on to develop malignancy. Isaacson and Wright have suggested that ulcerative jejunitis, intestinal pseudolymphoma and malignant lymphoma when associated with villous atrophy of adjacent small intestinal mucosa and malabsorption are all one condition, namely malignant lymphoma. They previously designated these cases as malignant histocytosis, but now feel that these tumours are of T-cell origin.[87] The problems of malignancy complicating coeliac disease are discussed in a later section of this chapter.

Intestinal pseudo-obstruction

Intestinal obstruction, without any evidence of an organic lesion obstructing the lumen, is very rarely associated with coeliac disease and when present improves on treatment with a gluten-free diet.[112]

Non-coeliac gluten intolerance

This condition has been described in infants and young children, usually occurring in association with cow's milk intolerance. Ingestion of gluten-containing cereals is associated with diarrhoea, vomiting and, sometimes, dermatitis, rhinitis and bronchitis. Investigations reveal a normal jejunal mucosa, normal intraepithelial lymphocyte count and disacharidase activity. This disorder may also affect adults with abdominal pain and diarrhoea, which may be incapacitating. Others suffer vomiting, headaches or recurrent apthos ulceration. All the patients have dramatic relief with a gluten-free diet and relapse on challenge. Immunological disturbances, including immunoglobulin and gliadin antibody levels, are normal. The cause of the intolerance is unknown. Sodium cromoglycate is not helpful. It is probable that some of the patients have a functional bowel disorder exacerbated by wheat starch. A diet omitting cereals, particularly wheat bran, and replacing dietary fibre with regular ipsaghula husks may prove helpful.

TREATMENT

Coeliac disease is treated with a gluten-free diet, avoiding products containing wheat, rye, barley and oats.[46] Since there is disagreement concerning the toxicity of oats[49] some physicians permit oats to be taken in the diet. Holmes recently showed that a gluten-free diet decreased the incidence of small intestinal T-cell lymphoma in coeliac patients.[83] For this reason, and to protect against dietary deficiency, the author feels that even coeliac patients with relatively few symptoms should be advised to take a strict gluten-free diet. Some patients improve well on a partially gluten-free diet, symptomatic sensitivity to gluten varying widely. It is not customary to discuss this with patients because it might provide a false impression of an easy way out of dealing with their condition. A few patients with untreated coeliac disease may become very ill and require treatment with a short course of oral or parenteral steroids. A gluten-free diet is low in roughage and, therefore, may induce troublesome constipation. This usually responds to the addition of regular dietary rice bran and ispaghula husks. Patients may supplement their diet with commercial gluten-free products, which are available on prescription in many European countries.

Specific dietary deficiences which occur should be corrected. These include iron, folic acid, calcium and, very rarely, vitamin B_{12} deficiency.

Following 3–4 months of treatment with a gluten-free diet, a repeat jejunal biopsy should be undertaken to demonstrate improvement in the appearance of the jejunal biopsy morphology. If this has not occurred, other possible causes of small intestinal villous atrophy, such as giardiasis or cow's milk allergy, should be excluded. Even if improvement in small bowel morphology is not seen, if symptomatic improvement has occurred the diet should be continued and jejunal biopsy should then be repeated after a further 6–9 months.

Should an improvement in jejunal biopsy and morphology and symptoms have occurred, the author advocates further confirmation of the diagnosis by a deterioration of small intestinal morphology in a repeat jejunal biopsy after a gluten challenge. This is particularly important in children, where conditions such as infectious diarrhoea and cow's milk intolerance may produce similar abnormalities in small intestinal morphology. The most convenient way to give a gluten challenge is to ask the patient to ingest at least 10 g of gluten or four slices of normal bread per day for 4–6 weeks. Should this cause severe symptoms then the biopsy date may be brought forward. However, the European Society of Paediatric Gastroenterology and Nutrition (ESPGAN) have suggested recently that it is not mandatory to proceed to a repeat jejunal biopsy following a gluten challenge if a gluten-free diet has produced a good improvement in symptoms and the morphology of a jejunal biopsy.[160] Many physicians do not practise gluten challenge.

The biopsy after the gluten challenge should exhibit relapse in small intestinal morphology, compared to the previous biopsy taken after at least 3 months of treatment with a gluten-free diet. Should the patient's symptoms persist or the jejunal biopsy morphology remain grossly abnormal while continuing a gluten-free diet, commercial gluten-free products based on wheat starch should be discontinued and the initial diagnosis questioned. However, the commonest reason for the lack of response to a gluten-free diet is a lack of patient compliance with dietary therapy.

Failure to respond to a gluten-free diet

Patients who fail to adhere strictly to a gluten-free diet frequently continue with ill-health and recurring symptoms which can usually be traced to dietary lapses, either deliberate or accidental. Difficulty may arise when a food is taken which is thought to be gluten-free but contains gluten. A rare failure to respond to a true gluten-free diet is due to development of small intestinal lymphoma or jejunal ulceration or unmasking of a condition such as chronic pancreatitis. Rarely, a patient on treatment may deteriorate and die unaccountably.

Pink and Creamer reported that 70% of coeliac patients on a gluten-free diet quickly return to normal health, with improvement within 2 weeks. The remaining 30% were divided into three groups. Patients in the first group experienced progressive deterioration which was halted in some cases by corticosteroids but which continued to death in others. Patients in the second group were found to have an associated pancreatic lesion and those in the third group were found not to adhere strictly to the diet but even when this was corrected their minor abdominal symptoms and diarrhoea persisted.[124] It is important not to forget these observations, and it cannot necessarily be assumed that dietary failure is an explanation for poor response.

Steroids and coeliac disease

Coeliac disease can be controlled with systemic corticosteroids, with rapid cessation of diarrhoea, weight gain and improvement of fat absorption. However, within a few days of stopping treatment there is usually deterioration. Steroids are indicated in the treatment of coeliac crises (severe diarrhoea, dehydration, weight loss, acidosis, hypocalcaemia and hypoproteinaemia). They have also been used to treat gliadin shock, an anaphylactic reaction that rarely occurs in treated patients subject to gluten challenge.[100]

The necessity to use steroids in coeliac disease occurs rarely, being given to complement a gluten-free diet when the serum albumin level is markedly depressed, in an attempt to bring the associated protein-losing enteropathy under control. The use of azathiaprine as a steroid-sparing agent has been reported.[76] There is a theoretical potential for the use of more specific immunotherapy in the form of cyclosporin A, in non-responsive life-threatening disease, although the role of these agents in clinical practice remains to be established.

The dose of steroids used depends on each individual case. Should a patient require intravenous fluid replacement because of vomiting, diarrhoea or surgery, hydrocortisone should be given intravenously. A patient who is eating normally but is exhibiting a crisis should be given 40–60 mg of prednisolone daily. The usual dose which would be given for coeliac disease that has not responded adequately to a gluten-free diet is 7.5–20 mg/day. It should be possible within a matter of weeks to reduce the higher dose. Failure to be able to do so should alert clinicians to the possibility of either failure to adhere to the diet or complications such as lymphoma or ulcerative jejunitis.

Treatment of complications

Many patients with coeliac disease have lactose or sucrose intolerance at the time of diagnosis. Only a small percentage of treated coeliac patients continue to be troubled with disaccharidase deficiencies. Such patients develop diarrhoea and abdominal pain with lactose in the case of alactasia, and with sucrose in the case of asucrasia. These conditions may be diagnosed either by enzyme assays of the mucosa from part of a repeat jejunal biopsy or by the appropriate sugar peroral permeability study.[117] Should concomitant disaccharidase deficiency be diagnosed, then the appropriate disaccharide should be excluded from the gluten-free diet.

A small number of treated coeliac patients suffer from small intestinal bacterial overgrowth, diagnosable by abnormal breath hydrogen or bile acid breath tests, an abnormal urinary indican excretion test or an abnormally high small intestinal aspirate bacteriological count. Should small intestinal bacterial overgrowth be a persistent problem, patients may be treated with antibiotics such as oxytetracycline 250 mg four times a day, which may be rotated fortnightly with another agent such as co-trimoxazole one tablet twice a day. A short 10-day course of metronidazole 200 mg three times a day is frequently helpful if small bowel bacterial overgrowth is a problem, although this agent should not be continued in the long term.

The neurological complications of coeliac disease are rare,[121] and are discussed in a later section of this chapter.

CONCLUSION

It has been proposed that coeliac disease is a condition in which susceptible individuals have an abnormal response to the ingestion of certain cereal epitopes. The results of the immunogenetic studies described above suggest that a particular HLA class II antigen is required which presents certain cereal epitopes to a clone of wheat gliadin antigen-sensitive T cells. The increased incidence of gastrointestinal T-cell lymphoma in coeliac disease implies that chronic stimulation of a clone of T cells occasionally proceeds to a neoplastic state, allowing a lymphoma to develop. This is further supported by recent evidence showing a reduction in the incidence of lymphoma complicating coeliac disease in those patients who have been treated with a strict gluten-free diet.[83]

REFERENCES

1. Adams, F. (1856) The extant works of Aretaeus the Cappadocian. London: *London Sydenham Society*, p. 350.
2. Anand, B.S., Truelove, S.C. and Offord, R.F. (1977) Skin test for coeliac disease employing a subfraction of gluten. *The Lancet*, **i**, 118–120.
3. Aurrichio, S., Buffolano, W., Camperi, M. *et al.* (1979) Skin tests for coeliac disease. *The Lancet*, **i**, 611.
4. Autran, J.C., Ellen, J., Law, L., Nimmo, C.C. and Kasarda, D.D. (1979) N-terminal amino acid sequencing of prolamins of wheat and related species. *Nature*, **282**, 527–529.
5. Bailey, A.S., Freedman, A.R., Price, B., Chescoe, D. and Ciclitira, P.J. (1989) Early biochemical responses of coeliac small intestine to wheat gliadin. *Gut*, **30**, 78–85.
6. Baker, P.G. and Read, A.F. (1976) Positive skin reaction to gluten in coeliac disease. *Quarterly Journal of Medicine*, **180**, 603–610.
7. Baker, S.J. (1973) Geographical variation in the morphology of the small intestinal mucosa in apparently healthy individuals. *Pathologia et Microbiologia*, **39**, 222–237.
8. Barry, R.E., Baker, P. and Read, A.E. (1974) The clinical presentation. *Clinics in Gastroenterology*, **3**, 55–69.
9. Bartels, D. and Thompson, R.D. (1983) The characterization of cDNA clones coding for wheat storage proteins. *Nucleic Acids Research*, **11**, 2961–2977.
10. Bartels, D., Thompson, R.D. and Rothstein, S. (1985) Synthesis of a wheat storage protein subunit in E coli using novel expression vectors. *Gene*, **35**, 159–167.
11. Bartels, D., Altosaar, I., Harberd, N.P., Barker, R.F. and Thompson, R.D. (1986) Molecular analysis of γ-gliadin gene families of the complex *gli-1* locus of bread wheat (*T. aestivum* L.). *Theoretical Applied Genetics*, **72**, 845–853.
12. Batt, R.M., Carter, M.W. and McLean, L. (1984) Developmental brush border defect associated with cereal sensitivity in the Irish setter dog. *Clinical Science*, **66**, 38.
13. Bayless, T.M., Kapelowitz, R.F., Shelley, W.M., Ballinger, W.R. and Hendrik, T.R. (1967) Intestinal ulceration, a complication of coeliac disease. *New England Journal of Medicine*, **776**, 996–1002.
14. Bennett, T.I., Hunter, D. and Vaughan, J.M. (1932) Idiopathic steatorrhoea (Gee's disease). A nutritional disturbance associated with tetany, osteomalacia and anaemia. *Quarterly Journal of Medicine*, **i**, 603–677.
15. Benson, G.D., Kowlessar, O.B. and Sleisenger, M.H. (1964) Adult coeliac disease with emphasis upon resistance to the gluten-free diet. *Medicine*, **43**, 1–40.
16. Benson, J.A., Culver, P.J., Ragland, B., Jones, C.M., Drunmey, G.D. and Bougar, E. (1957) The D-xylose absorption test in malabsorption syndromes. *New England Journal of Medicine*, **256**, 335–339.
17. Berger, E. (1958) Zur Allerguchen Pathogenese der Coliakie; mit Versuchenn aber die Spaltung Pathogenes Antigene durch Fermentf. *Bible Paedia*, **67**, 1–55.
18. Bernardin, J.E., Saunders, R.H.M. and Kasarda, D.D. (1976) Absence of carbohydrate in coeliac toxic A-gliadin. *Cereal Chemistry*, **53**(4), 612–614.
19. Besterman, H.S., Bloom, S.R., Sarson, D.L. *et al.*

(1978) Gut-hormone profile in coeliac disease. *The Lancet*, **i**, 785–788.

20. Bloom, S.R., Polak, J.M. and Besterman, H.S. (1978) Gut hormone profile in coeliac disease: a characteristic pattern of pathology. In: *Perspectives in Coeliac Disease*, pp. 399–408 (Eds) McNichol, B., McCarthy, C.F. and Fonredl, P.F. Lancaster: MTP Press.

21. Blumgart, H.L. (1923) Three fatal cases of malabsorption of fat with emaciation and anaemia and in two acidosis and tetany. *Archives of Internal Medicine*, **32**, 113–128.

22. Bolsover, W.J., Hall, M.A., Vaughan, R.W., Welsh, K.I. and Ciclitira, P.J. (1991) A family study confirms that the HLA-DP associations with celiac disease are the result of an extended HLA-DR3 haplotype. *Human Immunology*, **31**, 100–108.

23. Booth, C.C. (1974) Definition of adult coeliac disease. In: *Coeliac Disease. Proceedings of the Second International Symposium*, pp. 17–22 (Eds) Hekkens, W.T.Th.J.M. and Pera, A. Leiden: Steinfert Kroese.

24. Bossart, R., Henry, K., Booth, C.C. and Doe, W.F. (1975) Subepithelial collagen in intestinal malabsorption. *Gut*, **16**, 18–22.

25. Bradburg, L.L., Rubin, C.E. and Quinton, W.E. (1959) A multipurpose instrument for suction biopsy of the oesophagus, stomach, small bowel and colon. *Gastroenterology*, **37**, 1–16.

26. Bugawan, T.L., Horn, G.T., Long, C.M. *et al.* (1988) Analysis of HLA-DP allelic sequence polymorphism using *in vitro* enzymatic DNA amplification of DP-α and DP-β loci. *Journal of Immunology*, **141**, 4024–4030.

27. Bugawan, T.L., Angelini, G., Larrick, J., Aurrichio, S., Ferrara, G.B. and Erlich, H.A. (1989) A combination of a particular HLA-DPβ allele and an HLA-DQ heterodimer confers susceptibility to coeliac disease. *Nature*, **339**, 470–473.

28. Bullen, A.N. and Losowsky, M.S. (1978) Cell mediated immunity to gluten fraction III in adult coeliac disease. *Gut*, **19**, 126–131.

29. Bushuck, W. and Zillman, R.R. (1978) Wheat culture identification by gliadin electropherograms. Apparatus, method and nomenclature. *Journal of Canadian Plant Science*, **58**, 505–515.

30. Carter, M.J., Willcocks, M.M., Mitchison, H.C., Record, C.O. and Madeley, A. (1989) Is a persistent adenovirus infection involved in coeliac disease? *Gut*, **30**, 1563–1567.

31. Ciclitira, P.J. and Nelufer, J.M. (1985) Immunohistochemical investigation of pathogenetic mechanisms in coeliac disease. *Clinical Science*, **68**(11), 64P.

32. Ciclitira, P.J., Harkiss, G.D. and Hunter, J.O. (1979) The incidence of immune complexes by the polyethylene glycol precipitation complement test (PEG-CC) in coeliac disease and inflammatory bowel disease. *Gut*, **20**, A909.

33. Ciclitira, P.J., Hunter, J.O. and Lennox, E.S. (1980) Clinical testing of bread made from nullisomic 6A wheats in coeliac patients. *The Lancet*, **ii**, 234–235.

34. Ciclitira, P.J., Ellis, H.J. and Evans, D.J. (1983) A solid phase radioimmunossay for measurement of circulating antibody titres to wheat gliadin and its subfractions in patients with adult coeliac disease. *Journal of Immunological Methods*, **62**, 231–239.

35. Ciclitira, P.J., Evans, D.J., Fagg, N.L.K., Lennox, E.S. and Dowling, R.H. (1984) Clinical testing of gliadin fractions in coeliac patients. *Clinical Science*, **66**, 357–364.

36. Ciclitira, P.J., Ellis, H.J., Evans, D.J. and Lennox, E.S. (1985) Relationship of antigenic structure of cereal proteins to their toxicity in coeliac patients. *British Journal of Nutrition*, **53**, 39–45.

37. Ciclitira, P.J., Ellis, H.J., Venning, V.A. *et al.* (1986) Circulating antibodies to wheat gliadin in linear IgA dermatosis in children and adults. *Clinical and Experimental Dermatology*, **11**, 502–509.

38. Ciclitira, P.J., Ellis, H.J., Wood, G. M., Howdle, P.D. and Losowsky, M.S. (1986) Secretion of gliadin antibody by jejunal mucosal biopsies cultured *in vitro* from patients with coeliac disease. *Clinical and Experimental Immunology*, **64**, 119–124.

39. Ciclitira, P.J., Nelufer, J.M., Ellis, H.J. and Evans, D.J. (1986) The effect of gluten on HLA-DR in the small intestinal epithelium of patients with coeliac disease. *Clinical and Experimental Immunology*, **63**, 101–104.

40. Colyer, J., Farthing, M.J.G., Kumar, P.J., Clark, M.L., Obannesian, A.D. and Waldron, N.M. (1986) Reappraisal of the lectin hypothesis in the aetiopathogenesis of coeliac disease. *Clinical Science*, **71**, 105–110.

41. Comfort, M.W. (1958) Non-tropical sprue: diagnosis and therapy. *Gastroenterology*, **34**, 476–483.

42. Cooke, W.T. and Holmes, G.K.T. (1983) Coeliac disease definition and epidemiology. In: *Coeliac Disease*, pp. 2–22 (Eds) Cooke, W.T. and Holmes, G.K.T. London: Churchill Livingstone.

43. Cooke, W.T. and Holmes, G.K.T. (1984) Skin manifestations and dermatitis herpetiformis. In: *Coeliac Disease*, pp. 204–224 (Eds) Cooke, W.T. and Homes, G.K.T. London: Churchill Livingstone.

44. Cooke, W.T., Peeney, A.L.P. and Hawkins, C.F. (1953) Symptoms, signs and diagnostic features of idiopathic steatorrhoea. *Quarterly Journal of Medicine*, **22**, 59–77.

45. Crosby, W.H. and Kugler, H.W. (1957) Intraluminal biopsy of the small intestine.

American Journal of Digestive Disease, **2**, 236–241.

46. Dicke, W.K., Weijers, N.A. and van de Kamer, J.H. (1953) Coeliac Disease. The presence in wheat of a factor having a deleterious effect in cases of coeliac disease. *Acta Paediatrica*, **42**, 34–42.

47. Dieleman, L.A., Pena, S., van Doornick, J.H., Mearin, M.L., Duijn, W.V. and Lamers, C.B.H.W. (1991) No humoral response to the E1B-54Kb protein of adenovirus Ad12 in patients with coeliac disease. *European Journal of Gastroenterology and Hepatology*, **3**(3), 255–258.

48. Dissanayake, A.J., Jerome, D.W., Offord, R.E., Truelove, S.C. and Whitehead, R. (1974) Identifying toxic fractions of wheat gluten and their effect on the jejunal mucosa in coeliac disease. *Gut*, **15**, 931–946.

49. Dissanayake, A.J., Truelove, S.C. and Whitehead, R. (1974) Lack of harmful effect of oats on small intestinal mucosa in coeliac disease. *British Medical Journal*, **i**, 189–191.

50. Doe, W.F., Evans, D., Hobbs, J.R. and Booth, C.C. (1972) Coeliac disease, vasculitis and cryoglobulinaemia. *Gut*, **13**, 112–123.

51. Doe, W.F., Booth, C.C. and Brown, D.L. (1973) Evidence for complement-binding immune complexes in adult coeliac disease, Crohn's disease and ulcerative colitis. *The Lancet*, **i**, 402–403.

52. Dosseter, J.F.B., Gibson, A.A.M. and McNeish, A.S. (1981) Childhood coeliac disease is disappearing. *The Lancet*, **i**, 322–323.

53. Douglas, A. (1976) The binding of a glycopeptide component of wheat gluten to intestinal mucosa of normal and coeliac human subjects. *Clinical Chemical Acta*, **73**, 357–361.

54. Duhring, L.A. (1884) Dermatitis herpetiformis. *Journal of the American Medical Association*, **3**, 225–229.

55. Falchuk, Z.M., Nelson, D.L., Katz, A.Z. *et al.* (1980) Gluten sensitive enteropathy: influence of histocompatability type on gluten sensitivity *in vitro*. *Journal of Clinical Investigations*, **66**, 227–233.

56. Farthing, M.J.G., Edwards, C.R.W., Rees, L.H. and Dawson, A.M. (1982) Male gonadal function in coeliac disease. I. Sexual dysfunction, infertility and semen quality. *Gut*, **23**, 608–614.

57. Ferguson, A. (1976) Coeliac disease (gluten hypersensitivity). *Journal of Human Nutrition*, **30**, 193–201.

58. Ferguson, A. and Murray, D. (1971) Quantitation of intraepithelial lymphocytes in human jejunum. *Gut*, **12**, 988–994.

59. Ferguson, A., MacDonald, T.T., McClure, J.P. and Holen, R.J. (1975) Cell-mediated immunity to gliadin within the small intestinal mucosa in coeliac disease. *The Lancet*, **i**, 895–897.

60. Frazer, A.C., Fletcher, R.F., Ross, C.A.S., Shaw, B., Sammons, H.C. and Schneider, R. (1959) Gluten-induced enteropathy. The effect of partially digested gluten. *The Lancet*, **ii**, 252–255.

61. Freedman, A.R., Macartney, J.C., Nelufer, J.M. and Ciclitira, P.J. (1987) Timing of infiltration of T-lymphocytes induced by gluten into the small intestine in coeliac disease. *Journal of Clinical Pathology*, **40**, 741–745.

62. Freedman, A.R., Galfre, G., Gal, E., Ellis, H.J. and Ciclitira, P.J. (1988) Western immunoblotting of cereal proteins with monoclonal antibodies to wheat gliadin to investigate coeliac disease. *International Archives of Allergy and Applied Immunology*, **85**, 346–350.

63. Freedman, A.R., Wieser, H., Ellis, H.J. and Ciclitira, P.J. (1989) Monoclonal antibody immunoblotting for gliadin separated by high performance liquid chromatography. *Journal of Cereal Science*, **8**, 231–238.

64. Freeman, H.J., Weinstein, W.M., Shintka, T.K., Piercy, J.R.A. and Wensel, R.H. (1977) Primary abdominal lymphoma. Presenting manifestation of coeliac sprue and complicating dermatitis herpetiformis. *American Journal of Medicine*, **63**, 585–594.

65. Fry, L., Keir, P., McMinn, R.M.H., Cowan, J.H. and Hoffbrand, A.V. (1967) Small intestinal structure and function and haematological changes in dermatitis herpetiformis. *The Lancet*, **ii**, 729–734.

66. Fry, L., Seah, P.P., Riches, D.J. and Hoffbrand, A.V. (1973) Clearance of skin lesions in dermatitis herpetiformis after gluten withdrawal. *The Lancet*, **i**, 288–291.

67. Gee, S. (1888) On the coeliac affection. *St Bartholomew's Hospital Reports*, **24**, 17–20.

68. Goldberg, D. (1970) A psychiatric study of patients with disease of the small intestine. *Gut*, **11**, 459–465.

69. Green, P.A. and Wallaeger, E.E. (1960) The clinical behaviour of sprue in the United States. *Gastroenterology*, **38**, 399–418.

70. Groll, A., Candy, B.C.A., Preece, M.A., Tanner, J.M. and Harries, J.T. (1980) Short stature as the primary manifestation of coeliac disease. *The Lancet*, **ii**, 1097–1099.

71. Guan, R., Rawcliffe, P.M., Priddle, J.D. and Jewell, D.P. (1987) Cellular hypersensitivity to gluten derived peptides in coeliac disease. *Gut*, **28**, 426–434.

72. Hall, M.A., Lanchbury, J.S.S., Bolsover, W.J., Welsh, K.I., Ciclitira, P.J. (1990) Celiac disease is associated with an extended HLA-DR3 haplotype which includes HLA-DPw1. *Human Immunology*, **27**, 220–228.

73. Hall, M.A., Lanchbury, J.S.S., Bolsover, W.J., Welsh, K.I. and Ciclitira, P.J. (1991) The HLA association with dermatitis herpetiformis is accounted for by a *cis-* or *trans*-associated DQ heterodimer. *Gut*, **32**, 487–490.

74. Hallart, C., Gotthard, R., Norby, K. and Wallace,

A. (1981) On the prevalence of adult coeliac disease in Sweden. *Scandinavian Journal of Gastroenterology*, **16**, 257–261.

75. Hallstrom, O. (1989) Comparison of IgA class reticulin and endomysium antibodies in coeliac disease and dermatitis herpetiformis. *Gut*, **30**, 1225–1232.

76. Hamilton, J.R., Chambers, R.A. and Wynn-Williams, A. (1976) Role of gluten, prednisolone and azathiaprine in non-responsive coeliac disease. *The Lancet*, **i**, 1213–1216.

77. Haas, S.V. (1924) Value of bananas in the treatment of coeliac disease. *American Journal of Diseases of Children*, **38**, 42.

78. Haas, S.V. (1932) Coeliac disease, its specific treatment and care without nutritional relapse. *Journal of the American Medical Association*, **99**, 488.

79. Hekkens, W.Th.J.M., Haex, A.J. and Willihager, R.G.J. (1970) Some aspects of gliadin fractionation and testing by a histochemical method. In: *Coeliac Disease*, pp. 11–19 (Eds) Booth, C.C. and Dowling, R.H. Edinburgh: Churchill Livingstone.

80. Herrera, M., Chertkoff, L., Palavecino, E. (1989) Restriction fragment length polymorphism in HLA-class II genes of Latin American Caucasian Coeliac disease patients. *Human Immunology*, **26**, 272.

81. Holmes, G.K.T., Asquith, P. and Cooke, W.T. (1976) Cell-mediated immunity to gluten fraction III in adult coeliac disease. *Clinical Experimental Immunology*, **24**, 259–265.

82. Holmes, G.K.T., Stokes, P.L., Sorahan, T.M., Prior, P., Waterhouse, J.A.H. and Cooke, W.T. (1976) Coeliac disease, gluten-free diet and malignancy. *Gut*, **17**, 612–619.

83. Holmes, G.K.T., Prior, P., Lane, M.R., Poke, D., Allan, R.N. (1989) Malignancy in coeliac disease – effect of a gluten-free diet. *Gut*, **30**, 333–338.

84. Howdle, P.D., Ciclitira, P.J., Simpson, F.G. and Losowsky, M.S. (1984) Are all gliadins toxic in coeliac disease? An *in vitro* study of α, β, γ and ω gliadins. *Scandinavian Journal of Gastroenterology*, **19**, 41–47.

85. Howdle, P.D., Blair, L. and Zajdel, M.R. (1989) Lack of serological response to an E1B protein of adenovirus 12 in coeliac disease. *Scandinavian Journal of Gastroenterology*, **24**, 282–286.

86. Howell, M.D., Smith, J.R., Austin, R.K. *et al.* (1988) An extended HLA-D region haplotype associated with coeliac disease. *Proceedings of the National Academy of Sciences of the USA*, **85**, 222–226.

87. Isaacson, P.G., O'Connor, N.R.J., Spencer, J.O. *et al.* (1985) Malignant histocytosis of the intestine: a T-cell lymphoma. *The Lancet*, **ii**, 616–621.

88. Jenkins, D., Goodall, A. and Scott, B.B. (1986) T-lymphocyte populations in normal and coeliac small intestinal mucosa defined by monoclonal antibodies. *Gut*, **27**, 1330–1337.

89. Jos, J., Charbonnier, L., Mougenet, J.F., Mosse, J. and Rey, J. (1978) Isolation and characterisation of the toxic fraction of wheat gliadin in coeliac disease. In: *Perspectives in Coeliac Disease*, pp. 75–90 (Eds) McNicholl, B., McCarthy, C.F. and Fotterall, P.F. Lancaster: MTP Press.

90. Jos, J., Charbonnier, L., Mosse, J., Oliver, J.P., De Tand, M.F. and Rey, J. (1982) The toxic fraction of gliadin digests in coeliac disease. Isolation by chromatography in Biogel P10. *Clinica et Chemica Acta*, **119**, 263–274.

91. Kagnoff, M.F., Raleigh, K.A., Hubert, J.J., Bernardin, J.E. and Kasarda, D.D. (1984) Possible role for a human adenovirus in the pathogenesis of coeliac disease. *Journal of Experimental Medicine*, **160**, 1544–1547.

92. Kagnoff, M.F., Paterson, N.Y., Kumar, P.J. *et al.* (1987) Evidence for the role of a human intestinal adenovirus in the pathogenesis of coeliac disease. *Gut*, **28**, 995–1001.

93. Kantor, J.L. (1939) The roentgen diagnosis of idiopathic steatorrhoea and allied conditions. Practical value of the 'moulage' sign. *American Journal of Roentgenology*, **41**, 738–778.

94. Kariagiannis, J.A., Priddle, J.D. and Jewell, D.P. (1987) Cell-mediated immunity to a synthetic gliadin peptide resembling a sequence from adenovirus 12. *The Lancet*, 884–886.

95. Kasarda, D.D. (1981) Structure and properties of α-gliadins. *Annals of Technology and Agriculture*, **29**, 151–173.

96. Kasarda, D.D. (1981) Toxic proteins and peptides in coeliac disease; relations to cereal genetics in food nutrition and evolution: food as an environmental factor in the genesis of human variability. In: *Food as an Environmental Factor in the Genesis of Human Variability*, pp. 201–215 (Eds) Walcher, D. and Kretchmer, H. New York: Masson.

97. Kasarda, D.D., Okita, T.W., Bernardin, J.E. (1984) Nucleic acid (cDNA) and amino acid sequences of alpha-type gliadins from wheat (Triticum Aestivum). *Proceedings of the National Academy of Sciences of the USA*, **87**, 4712–4716.

98. Kendall, R.J., Cox, P.S., Schneider, R. and Hawkins, C.E. (1972) Gluten subfractions in coeliac disease. *The Lancet*, **ii**, 1065–1067.

99. Kiln, G., Holmes, G.K.T., Cooper, B.T., Thompson, H. and Allan, R.N. (1980) Association of coeliac disease and inflammatory bowel disease. *Gut*, **21**, 636–641.

100. von Krainick, H.G., Debatin, F., Gautier, E., Tobler, R. and Velasco, J.A. (1958) Additional research on the injurious effect of wheat flour in coeliac disease. I. Acute gliadin reactions (gliadin shock). *Helvetica et Paediatria Acta*, **13**, 432–454.

101. Kruizing, E.E. and Hamminga, A. (1953) Treatment of dermatitis herpetiformis with

diamino-diphenyl-sulphone (DDS). *Dermatologien*, **106**, 387–394.

102. Kumar, P.J., Sinclair, T.S. and Farthing, M.J.G. (1984) Clinical toxicity testing of pure gliadins in coeliac disease. *Gastroenterology*, **86**, 1147 (abstract).

103. Lancaster-Smith, M.J., Benson, M.K. and Strickland, I.D. (1971) Coeliac disease and diffuse interstitial lung disease. *The Lancet*, i, 473–476.

104. Lancaster-Smith, M.J., Kumar, P.J., Marks, R., Clark, M.L. and Dawson, A.M. (1974) Jejunal mucosa immunoglobulin containing cells and jejunal fluid immunoglobulins in adult coeliac disease and dermatitis herpetiformis. *Gut*, **15**, 371–376.

105. Lancaster-Smith, M.J., Kumar, P.J. and Dawson, A.M. (1975) The cellular infiltrate of the jejunum in adult coeliac disease and dermatitis herpetiformis following the reintroduction of dietary gluten. *Gut*, **16**, 683–688.

106. Loft, D.E., Marsh, M.N., Jandle, G.I. *et al.* (1989) Studies of intestinal lymphoid tissue XII. Epithelial lymphocyte and mucosal responses to rectal gluten challenge in coeliac sprue. *Gastroenterology*, **97**, 29–37.

107. Loft, D.E., Marsh, M.N. and Crowe, P.T. (1990) Rectal gluten challenge and diagnosis of coeliac disease. *The Lancet*, **335**, 1293–1295.

108. Logan, R.F.A. and Ferguson, A. (1978) Skin tests for coeliac disease. *The Lancet*, ii, 1042–1043.

109. Logan, R.F.A., Ferguson, A., Finlayson, N.D.C. and Weir, B.G. (1978) Primary biliary cirrhosis and coeliac disease. An association? *The Lancet*, i, 230–233.

110. Low-Bear, T.S., Heaton, K.W., Heaton, S.T. and Read, A.E. (1971) Gall bladder inertia and sluggish enteropathic circulation of bile-salts in coeliac disease. *The Lancet*, i, 991–994.

111. Low-Bear, T.S., Harvey, R.F., Davies, E.R. and Read, A.E. (1975) Abnormalities of serum cholecystokinin and gall bladder emptying in coeliac disease. *New England Journal of Medicine*, **292**, 961–963.

112. McClelland, H.A., Lewis, M.J. and Naish, J.M. (1962) Idiopathic steatorrhoea with intestinal pseudo-obstruction. *Gut*, **3**, 142–145.

113. Mackie, T.T., Miller, D.K. and Rhoah, C.P. (1935) Sprue. Roentgenologic changes in the small intestine. *American Journal of Tropical Medicine*, **15**, 571–589.

114. Mantzaris, G. and Jewell, D.P. (1991) *In vivo* toxicity of a synthetic dodecapeptide from A-gliadin in patients with coeliac disease. *Scandinavian Journal of Gastroenterology*, **26**, 392–398.

115. Marsh, M.N. (1983) Immunocytes, enterocytes and the lamina propria: an immunopathological framework of coeliac disease. *Journal of the Royal College of Physicians, London*, **17**, 205–212.

116. Marsh, M.N., Brown, A.C. and Swift, J.A. (1979) The surface ultra-structure of the small intestinal mucosa of normal control human subjects and of patients with untreated and treated coeliac disease using the scanning electron microscope. In: *Coeliac Disease*, pp. 26–44 (Eds) Booth, C.C. and Dowling, R.H. Edinburgh: Churchill Livingstone.

117. Menzies, I.S. (1984) Transmucosal passage of inert molecules in health and disease. In: *Intestinal Absorption and Secretion* (Eds) Heintze K. and Sradhauge, E. Lancaster: MTP Press.

118. Menzies, I.S., Laker, M., Pounder, R., Bull, J., Heyer, S., Wheeler, P.G. and Creamer, B. (1979) Abnormal intestinal permeability to sugar in villous atrophy. *The Lancet*, ii, 1107–1109.

119. Missen, G.A.K. (1966) Intestinal malignant lymphoma and cerebellar cortical degeneration complicating idiopathic steatorrhea: report of a case with a review of the literature. *Guy's Hospital Report*, **115**, 359–385.

120. Mylotte, M., Egan, F., Mitchell, B., McCarthy, C.F. and McNicholl, N. (1973) Incidence of coeliac disease in Western Ireland. *British Medical Journal*, i, 703–705.

121. Osborne, T.B. (1907) *The Protein of the Wheat Kernel*. Washington, DC: Carnegie Institute.

122. Paulley, J.W. (1949) Personal communications. *Proceedings of the Royal Society of Medicine*, **42**, 241.

123. Paulley, J.W., Fairweather, F.A. and Leemin, A. (1957) Postgastrectomy steatorrhea and patchy jejunal atrophy. *The Lancet*, i, 406–407.

124. Pink, I.J. and Creamer, B. (1967) Response to a gluten-free diet of patients with the coeliac syndrome. *The Lancet*, i, 300–304.

125. Porter, K.G., McMaster, D., Elmes, M.E. and Love, A.H.G. (1977) Anaemia and low serum copper during zinc therapy. *The Lancet*, ii, 774.

126. Ray-Choudhury, D.C., Cooke, W.T., Tan, D.T., Banwell, J.G. and Smits, B.J. (1966) Jejunal biopsy: criteria and significance. *Scandinavian Journal of Gastroenterology*, **1**, 57–74.

127. Roep, B.O., Bontrop, R.E., Pena, A.S., Van Eggermond, M.C.J.A., Van Rood, J.J. and Giphart, M.J. (1988) An HLA-DQ alpha allele identified at DNA and protein level is strongly associated with coeliac disease. *Human Immunology*, **23**, 271–279.

128. Rosenberg, W.M.C., Wordsworth, B.P., Jewell, D.P., Bell, J.I. (1989) A locus telomeric to HLA-DPB encodes susceptibility to coeliac disease. *Immunogenetics*, **30**, 307–310.2.

129. Ross, J.R. and Garabedian, M. (1970) Systemic manifestations of gluten enteropathies and gluten sensitivity in some other diseases. In: *Progress in Gastroenterology*, vol. 2, pp. 430–449 (Ed.) Glass, G.B.J. New York: Grime & Stratton.

130. Rossipal, E. (1975) Incidence of coeliac disease in children in Austria. *Zeitschrift für Kinderheilkunde*, **119**, 143–149.

131. Rubin, C.F., Brandborg, L.L., Flick, A.L. *et al.* (1962) Biopsy studies on the pathogenesis of coeliac sprue. In: *Intestinal Biopsy*, pp. 67–83

(Eds) Wolstenholme, G.E.W. and Cameron, M.P. London: Ciba Foundation Study Group 14.

132. Rubin, C.F., Cauci, A.S., Sleisenger, M.H., Jeffries, G.H. and Margolis, S. (1965) Immunofluorescent studies in adult coeliac disease. *Journal of Clinical Investigation*, **44**, 475–485.

133. Schmerling, D.H., Leisinger, P. and Prader, A. (1972) On the familial occurrence of coeliac disease. *Acta Paediatria Scandinavica*, **61**, 501.

134. Scott, B.B. and Losowsky, M.S. (1975) Coeliac disease: a cause of various associated diseases. *The Lancet*, **ii**, 956.

135. Scott, B.B. and Losowsky, M.S. (1976) Patchiness and duodenal-jejunal variation of the mucosal abnormalities in coeliac disease and dermatitis herpetiformis. *Gut*, **17**, 984–992.

136. Seah, P.P., Fry, L., Hoffbrand, A.V. and Holborrow, E.J. (1971) Tissue antibodies in dermatitis herpetiformis and adult coeliac disease. *The Lancet*, **i**, 834–936.

137. Sheehy, T.W. (1964) Intestinal biopsy. *The Lancet*, **i**, 959–962.

138. Sheldon, W. (1959) Coeliac disease. *Paediatrica*, **23**, 132–145.

139. Sheldon, W. (1969) Prognosis in early adult life of coeliac children treated with a gluten-free diet. *British Medical Journal*, **ii**, 401–404.

140. Shewry, P.R., Autran, J.C., Nimmo, C.C., Ellen, J., Law, I. and Kasarda, D.D. (1980) N-terminal amino acid sequence homology of storage protein components from barley and a diploid wheat. *Nature*, **286**, 520–522.

141. Shiner, M. (1956) Duodenal biopsy. *The Lancet*, **i**, 17–19.

142. Shiner, M. (1956) Jejunal biopsy tube. *The Lancet*, **i**, 85.

143. Shiner, M. and Doniach, I. (1960) Histopathological studies in steatorrhea. *Gastroenterology*, **38**, 419–440.

144. Skerrit, J.M., Smith, R.A., Wrigley, C.W. and Underwood, P.A. (1984) Monoclonal antibodies to gliadin proteins used to examine cereal grain homologies. *Cereal Science*, **12**, 215–224.

145. Sollid, L.M., Markussen, G., Ek, J., Gjerde, H., Vartdal, F., Thorsby, E. (1989) Evidence for a primary association of coeliac disease to a particular HLA-DQ α/β heterodimer. *Journal of Experimental Medicine*, **169**, 345.

146. Spencer, J., Isaacson, P.G., Diss, T.C. and MacDonald, T.T. (1989) Expression of disulphide-linked and non-disulphide linked forms of the T-cell receptor γ/δ heterodimer in human intestinal intra-epithelial lymphocytes. *European Journal of Immunology*, **19**, 1331–1338.

147. Spencer, J., MacDonald, T.T., Diss, T.C., Walker-Smith, J.A., Ciclitira, P.J. and Isaacson, P.G. (1989) Changes in ultra-epithelial lymphocyte subpopulation in coeliac disease and enteropathy associated T-cell lymphoma (malignant histocytosis of the intestine). *Gut*, **30**, 339–349.

148. Stewart, J.S., Pollock, D.J., Hoffbrand, A.V., Mollin, D.L. and Booth, C.C. (1967) A study of proximal and distal intestinal structure and absorptive function in idiopathic steatorrhoea. *Quarterly Journal of Medicine*, **36**, 425–444.

149. Still, C.F. (1918) Lumleian lectures on coeliac disease. *The Lancet*, **ii**, 163–166, 193–197, 227–229.

150. Swinson, C.M., Storm, G., Coles, F.C. and Booth, C.C. (1983) Coeliac disease and malignancy, *The Lancet*, **i**, 111–115.

151. Thaysen. In: *Non-tropical Sprue*. London: Humphrey Milford.

152. Tosi, R., Vismara, D., Tanigaki, N., Ferrar, G.B., Cicimarra, F., Buffolowd, V.Y., Follo, D. and Aurrichio, S. (1983) Evidence that coeliac disease is intimately associated with a DC locus allelic specificity. *Clinical Immunology and Immunopathology*, **28**, 395–404.

153. Trowell, H.C. (1943) Dimorphic anaemia, deficiency of iron associated with nutritional macrocytic anaemia. *Transactions of the Royal Society of Tropical Medicine and Hygiene*, **37**, 19–40.

154. Trowsdale, J. and Campbell, R.D. (1988) Physical map of the human HLA region. *Immunology Today*, **9**, 2–34.

155. van de Kamer, J.H. and Weijers, H.A. (1955) Coeliac disease with some experiments on the cause of the harmful effect of wheat gliadin. *Acta Paediatrica*, **44**, 465–469.

156. van de Kamer, J.H., Weijers, H.A. and Dicke, W.K. (1953) Coeliac disease. IV. An investigation into the injurious constituents of wheat in connection with their action on patients with coeliac disease. *Acta Paediatrica*, **42**, 223–231.

157. Vaughan, J.J. (1936) *The Anaemias*, 2nd edn. London: Oxford University Press.

158. Walker-Smith, J.A. (1969) Small bowel morphology in childhood. *Medical Journal of Australia*, **1**, 382–387.

159. Walker-Smith, J.A. (1973) Discordance for childhood coeliac disease. *Gut*, **14**, 374–375.

160. Walker-Smith, J.A., Guandalini, S., Schmitz, J., Schmerling, D.M. and Visakorpi, J.K. (1990) Revised criteria for diagnosis of coeliac disease. *Archives of Disease in Childhood*, **65**, 909–911.

161. Weiser, M.M. and Douglas, A.P. (1976) An alternative mechanism for gluten toxicity in coeliac disease. *The Lancet*, **i**, 567–569.

162. Wood, G.M., Shires, S., Howdle, P.D. and Losowsky, M.S. (1986) Immunoglobulin production by coeliac biopsies in organ culture. *Gut*, **27**, 1151–1160.

163. Woychik, J.H., Boundy, J.A. and Dimiter, R.J. (1961) Starch gel electrophoresis of wheat gluten protein with concentrated area. *Archives of Biochemistry and Biophysics*, **194**, 477–482.

CHRONIC NON-SPECIFIC ULCERATIVE ENTERITIS *(R. Modigliani)*

Chronic non-specific ulcerative enteritis, first described by Nyman in 1949,[17] is a rare disease with less than 50 published cases. It is characterized by multiple chronic benign small bowel ulcerations of unknown aetiology, without distinctive pathological findings, resulting in abdominal pain, fever, diarrhoea, malabsorption, and surgical complications. It carries a poor prognosis and no specific treatment is available.

PATHOLOGY

Ulcerations are multiple, and always involve the jejunum, usually the ileum and rarely the duodenum and the colon. Histologically, the ulcers vary in depth, penetrating frequently to the muscularis propria and sometimes to the serosa causing perforation (*Figure 3.77*). Submucosal oedema and fibrosis may be prominent, the latter causing stenosis in many cases. The ulcer base is infiltrated by lymphocytes, plasma cells, histiocytes and polymorphonuclear leukocytes. The mucosa adjacent to the ulcerations may have normal or atrophic villi; pyloric metaplasia is sometimes found. The intervening mucosa may be completely flat or show blunted or normal villi. Most importantly, no specific histological features are found anywhere (no tuberculoid granulomas, no sign of vasculitis or neoplastic disease). Mesenteric lymph node enlargement is often seen, but microscopical examination reveals only reactive hyperplasia.

CLINICAL FEATURES AND DIAGNOSIS

The mean age at onset is 50 years (the range being 18–78 years) with a small majority (58%) of females.[15] Chronic diarrhoea with steatorrhoea, periumbilical or epigastric pain, and marked weight loss are almost constant features of the condition. Vomiting, fever, finger clubbing, wasting, and signs of multiple nutritional deficiencies are frequent. Laboratory findings are non-specific: anaemia, usually due to iron deficiency, is frequent; Howell–Jolly bodies and target cells have been rarely reported; neutrophil leucocytosis is found in one-third of patients. Serum calcium, folate, iron and albumin levels are usually low. Serum immunoglobulins are frequently normal but an increased level of IgA may occur, or a deficiency of IgA[13] or IgG.[6] Malabsorption of xylose and fat is almost always present. Vitamin B_{12} absorption is variable. Small bowel radiographs are constantly, but not specifically, abnormal; the most suggestive appearance is a diffuse narrowing of the intestinal loops with total effacement of the mucosal pattern (moulage sign) (*Figure 3.78*). Mucosal folds may also be coarsened, with spiculation of the intestinal margins. Duodenal or jejunal strictures may be seen,

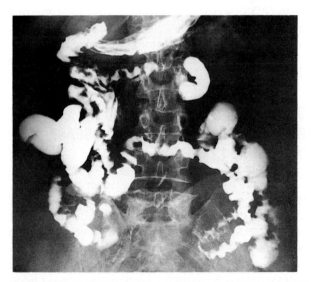

Figure 3.78 Radiograph of upper gastrointestinal tract showing diffusely narrowed jejunum and effacement of the normal mucosal pattern. (Reproduced, with permission, from Modigliani *et al.*[16])

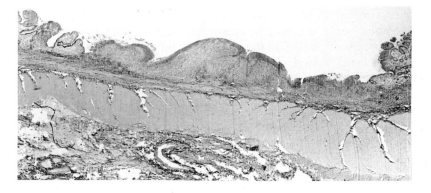

Figure 3.77 Ileal resection specimen. Chronic ulceration surrounded by dystrophic mucosa. (Reproduced, with permission, from Modigliani *et al.*[16] with kind permission of the authors and the editor of *Gut.*)

but radiographic documentation of ulceration is exceptional.[2,19]

Blind peroral small bowel biopsies may show a diffuse or patchy subtotal villous atrophy or a normal mucosa (see below); this procedure, however, is of little use in making the diagnosis of chronic non-specific ulcerative enteritis because it almost never shows ulceration, even when biopsies are taken at multiple levels and from areas ultimately shown to be ulcerated. The only histological clue to the diagnosis might be the discovery of a dystrophic mucosal pattern (variable villous height and shape, irregularity of crypt distribution, and sclerosis of the lamina propria) suggestive of scarred ulceration.[16] Jejunoscopy with biopsies has been rarely performed[4] and is a potentially useful tool to demonstrate the ulcerations, but does not preclude the need for laparotomy to establish their nature. Thus, surgical exploration with biopsy–resection of the small bowel and mesenteric nodes is, at present, the only reliable diagnostic method. The usual findings are of small bowel thickening or oedema, and hyperaemia of the serosa; mesenteric lymph node enlargement has been often described. However, the serosa of the small intestine may look normal at operation. Peroperative enteroscopy is helpful in locating the ulcerations and guiding surgical sampling.[5]

DIFFERENTIAL DIAGNOSIS AND RELATIONSHIP WITH COELIAC DISEASE AND INTESTINAL LYMPHOMA

Due to the absence of any available specific diagnostic criterion, the diagnosis of chronic non-specific ulcerative enteritis can only be made after ruling out all other causes of secondary small bowel ulceration such as Crohn's disease, Zollinger–Ellison syndrome, tuberculosis, fungal infections, ingestion of enteric coated potassium tablets, small bowel malignancy (particularly lymphoma), and vascular diseases. Association of chronic non-specific ulcerative enteritis with systemic disease has been reported.[7] Primary non-specific ulcer of the small intestine is different from chronic non-specific ulcerative enteritis; usually the ulcer presents with a surgical complication, is not associated with diarrhoea or malabsorption, is single, and does not recur after surgical resection.[14]

The relationship between chronic non-specific ulcerative enteritis and coeliac disease has been extensively studied. Patients with chronic non-specific ulcerative enteritis fall into three categories which occur with approximately similar frequency.[16]

1. Chronic non-specific ulcerative enteritis may be clearly associated with coeliac disease, as demonstrated by the presence of the mucosal lesion characteristic of this disease in the intervening non-ulcerated mucosa of the proximal small bowel, and a clear-cut improvement on a gluten-free diet. Both diseases are often diagnosed simultaneously and ulcerations may be found distal to the area of total villous atrophy, at a site where the villous height is normal.[16] Chronic non-specific ulcerative enteritis may also supervene in patients with coeliac disease whose villous height has returned to normal after prolonged treatment with a gluten-free diet.[2,16] Thus, the ulcerative process complicating coeliac disease does not seem to be directly related to villous atrophy nor to be gluten-induced.

2. The second group of patients only differs from the previous one in the failure of a gluten-free diet to improve intestinal villous height.[18,19] The search for a family history of coeliac disease, HLA typing or organ culture of a jejunal biopsy specimen[13] may then be helpful in the diagnosis of coeliac disease.

3. In the third group of patients the histological pattern of the intervening non-ulcerated mucosa, with normal villi, or patchy villous atrophy with flat and strictly normal mucosa adjacent,[11] clearly rules out coeliac disease. A single peroral biopsy may falsely suggest coeliac disease by showing a flat mucosa; multiple small intestinal biopsies are thus necessary.

Relationship of chronic non-specific ulcerative enteritis with intestinal lymphoma and malignant histiocytosis

The diagnosis of chronic non-specific ulcerative enteritis obviously implies that an intensive search for lymphoma had been carried out and is negative. In a few cases, however, lymphomatous cells, especially of the histiocytic type, have been obscured by the inflammatory cells in the base of an ulcer and thus overlooked, leading to a false diagnosis of chronic non-specific ulcerative enteritis.[1,8] Furthermore, intestinal lymphoma may be preceded by, or associated with, truly benign small bowel ulcerations.[1] An intensive search for a lymphomatous process is therefore mandatory before diagnosing chronic non-specific ulcerative enteritis. However, the suggestion that chronic non-specific ulcerative enteritis 'is but a manifestation of malignant histiocytosis of the intestine'[10] is excessive.

TREATMENT

There is no specific treatment for chronic non-specific ulcerative enteritis. Most patients will require surgery either for a complication (obstruction, haemorrhage or perforation) or for diagnostic purposes. When feasible, surgical excision of the worst affected segment of small bowel is the most appropriate therapy. Gluten withdrawal may be beneficial to patients with associated coeliac disease, but only after the ulcerative process has been surgically controlled; it does not influence or prevent the ulcerative process itself. Corticosteroids have been useful in a limited number of patients.[7,9,12] Exclusive parenteral nutrition can overcome severe nutritional deficiencies but our limited experience does not suggest it improves small intestinal function or morphology.[16]

PROGNOSIS

The overall prognosis of chronic non-specific ulcerative enteritis is poor; two-thirds of patients whose follow-up has been reported are dead at the time of publication,[16] with a mean survival period of 37 months (the range being 5–120 months) from the onset of the illness.[15] The cause of death is almost invariably related to a surgical complication of the ulceration, especially perforation. The prognosis seems to be slightly better in the group of patients with associated proven coeliac disease, and worst in those with normal villi or patchy villous atrophy.[16]

References

1. Baer, A.N., Bayless, T.M. and Yardley, J.H. (1980) Intestinal ulceration and malabsorption syndromes. *Gastroenterology*, **79**, 754–765.
2. Bayless, T.M., Kapelowitz, R.F., Shelley, W.M. *et al.* (1967) Intestinal ulceration. A complication of celiac disease. *New England Journal of Medicine*, **276**, 996–1002.
3. Belaiche, J., Modigliani, R., Modigliani, E. *et al.* (1977) Jejuno-iléite ulcéreuse chronique non spécifique. Présentation d'un nouveau cas. *Gastroentérologie Clinique et Biologique*, **1**, 553–560.
4. Cerf, M., Gouerou, H., Marche, E. *et al.* (1977) Jéjunoiléite ulcéreuse diffuse: intérêt diagnostique de la jéjunoscopie. *Gastroentérologie Clinique et Biologique*, **1**, 571–576.
5. Conley, D.R., Feffer, M. and Cove, H. (1975) Duodenal jejunal ulcers and recurrent hemorrhage: diagnostic value of total enteroscopy. *American Journal of Digestive Diseases*, **20**, 876–881.
6. Corlin, R.F. and Pops, M.A. (1972) Nongranulomatous ulcerative jejunoileitis with hypogammaglobulinemia. Clinical remission after treatment with gammaglobulin. *Gastroenterology*, **62**, 473–478.
7. Coupe, M.O., Barnard, M.L., Stamp, G., Hodgson, H.J.F. (1988) Ulcerative ileojenunitis associated with pulmonary fibrosis and polymyositis. *Hepato-gastroentérol*, **35**, 144–146.
8. Freeman, H.J., Weinstein, W.M., Shnitka, T.K. *et al.* (1977) Primary abdominal lymphoma: presenting manifestation of celiac sprue or complicating dermatitis herpetiformis. *American Journal of Medicine*, **63**, 585–594.
9. Goulston, K.J., Skyring, A.P. and McGovern, V.J. (1965) Ulcerative jejunitis associated with malabsorption. *Australasian Annals of Medicine*, **14**, 57–64.
10. Isaacson, P. (1980) Malignant histiocytosis of the intestine: the early histological lesion. *Gut*, **21**, 381–386.
11. Jeffries, G.H., Steinberg, H. and Sleisenger, M.H. (1968) Chronic ulcerative (nongranulomatous) jejunitis. *American Journal of Medicine*, **44**, 47–59.
12. Jones, P.E. and Gleeson, M.H. (1973) Mucosal ulceration and mesenteric lymphadenopathy in coeliac disease. *British Medical Journal*, **3**, 212–213.
13. Klaeveman, H.L., Gebhard, R.L., Sessoms, C. and Strober, W. (1975) In vitro studies of ulcerative ileojejunitis. *Gastroenterology*, **68**, 572–582.
14. Mills, P.R. (1988) Small intestinal ulceration. Current opinion. *Gastroenterology*, **4**, 260–276.
15. Mills, P.R., Brown, I.L. and Watkinson, G. (1980) Idiopathic chronic ulcerative enteritis. Report of five cases and review of the literature. *Quarterly Journal of Medicine*, **194**, 133–149.
16. Modigliani, R., Poitras, P., Galian, A. *et al.* (1979) Chronic non-specific ulcerative duodenojejunoileitis: report of four cases. *Gut*, **20**, 319–328.
17. Nyman, E. (1949) Ulcerous jejuno-ileitis with symptomatic sprue. *Acta Medica Scandinavica*, **134**, 275–283.
18. Shiner, M. (1963) Effect of a gluten-free diet in 17 patients with idiopathic steatorrhea. A follow-up study. *American Journal of Digestive Diseases*, **8**, 969–983.
19. Stuber, J.L., Wiegman, H., Crosby, I. and Gonzalez, G. (1971) Ulcers of the colon and jejunum in celiac disease. *Radiology*, **99**, 339–340.

THE MALIGNANT COMPLICATIONS OF COELIAC DISEASE (*P.J. Ciclitira*)

Adult coeliac disease is associated with an increased incidence of neoplasia. This includes (1) lymphoma of the intestine, predominantly small intestinal,[5] and (2) carcinoma of the gastrointestinal tract, particularly small intestinal and oesophageal.[3,9]

This enhanced predisposition to malignancy extends to patients with dermatitis herpetiformis and associated enteropathy.[1] In contrast, coeliac disease diagnosed and treated in childhood does not appear to be associated with a greater incidence of neoplasia than the greater population.[4,16]

A particular point of concern is whether, when villous atrophy and lymphoma of the small intestine are diagnosed within a few years of each other, or even simultaneously, the malignancy should be viewed as a complication of pre-existing coeliac disease, or whether villous atrophy can be a manifestation of the lymphoproliferative process. It was also argued that carcinoma could itself give rise to villous atrophy.[3] These arguments are of particular relevance, as they affect the possibility of preventing malignant change by adequate treatment of gluten-sensitive enteropathy, as discussed below.

INCIDENCE

Malignancy is not uncommon in the general population, and the recorded incidence in surveys of patients with coeliac disease – between 11 and 15%[4,6,8,14] – is not grossly different from the general population. Furthermore, they reflect cross-sectional surveys from specialist referral centres in whom the malignancy rate is likely to be particularly high. One study suggests that, on long follow-up, the incidence of malignancy is approximately doubled in coeliac disease.[10]

It is, however, clear that two particular types of tumour are substantially more common than in the general population. Adenocarcinoma of the small intestine has an incidence of 50 per 100 000 per year in adult coeliac patients, compared with less than 1 per 100 000 in the general population, giving a relative risk in coeliac disease of over 80.[16] It has been suggested from studies in the 1970s and 1980s that the life-long chances of a patient with adult coeliac disease developing lymphoma are of the order of 1–7%, and a relative risk of 77% is quoted.[10]

CARCINOMA

In a large UK survey of over 200 patients with coeliac disease (with biopsy evidence of villous atrophy) and malignancy, over half had carcinoma and half lymphoma.[16] Amongst the adenocarcinomas, over half were from the gastrointestinal tract. Comparison with Cancer Registry figures demonstrated an increased risk of small intestinal adenocarcinoma as described above, and (particularly in men) oesophageal and pharyngeal squamous carcinoma. Of the small intestinal carcinomas, the majority affected the jejunum, followed by the duodenum, with

fewer in the ileum than would be expected from studies in the general population. Whether enhanced epithelial cell turnover in untreated coeliac disease has predisposed to malignancy is speculative. Apart from associated features of malabsorption, present if coeliac disease was untreated, the clinical features and presentation did not differ from similar tumours in the general population.

LYMPHOMA

Controversy has surrounded the association of lymphoma and coeliac disease, with respect to the nature of the lymphoma, the relationship with the enteropathic process, and the relationship between dietary exposure to gluten and the chances of developing lymphoma.

Clinical features

The incidence is equal in both sexes, and most cases of lymphoma present during the sixth decade.[16] In a large proportion of cases, the presence of diffuse small intestinal villous atrophy had only been detected a year or two before, or at the same time as, the diagnosis of malignancy was made, although there are patients in whom the diagnosis of coeliac disease had been made several decades before.[14]

There are a few cases of predominantly stomach or colonic lymphoma associated with coeliac disease, but in over 80% the lymphoma is small intestinal, and symptoms are either from the small intestine or have spread from the small intestinal site systemically.

A common pattern is the return of symptoms of diarrhoea, associated with both weight loss and particularly pain, in a patient with established coeliac disease. This combination of symptoms strongly suggests the need to seek for the presence of a lymphoma. The standard diagnostic dilemma with such a return of symptoms in a previously well-controlled patient with adult coeliac disease is to distinguish dietary lapses from the development of lymphoma, with the possibility of ulcerative ileojejunitis (whose relation to coeliac disease and lymphoma is problematical, as discussed later in the chapter) a third possibility. Manifestations such as fever, spread with lymphadenopathy, hepatomegaly or splenomegaly, or abdominal masses or ascites may help the diagnostic conundrum but imply more advanced disease. As an alternative to such insidious presentations, acute perforation or obstruction, or less commonly haemorrhage, may lead to emergency presentation.

Early diagnosis usually requires exploratory laparotomy, and a high index of suspicion. An approach based on standard small intestinal diagnostic manoeuvres of biopsy and barium examination is likely to have a low yield, particularly if the condition is suspected when both these studies are abnormal due to associated subtotal villous atrophy. Histology of peripheral lymph nodes, the liver or bone marrow may be diagnostic, and lymphangiography, ultrasound or computed tomography scanning to detect lymphadenopathy may be positive, but these investigations cannot exclude the diagnosis of early intestinal lymphoma. Blood tests are unhelpful, although hypoalbuminaemia, a high erythrocyte sedimentation rate, a high IgA level,[2] and an increase in the serum lysozyme level may all occur,[7] but these are not specific. Thus, laparotomy is an early diagnostic tool, with resection of apparently suspicious areas of intestine, plus full thickness biopsy of normal areas, together with lymph node and liver biopsies. Whether this procedure should include splenectomy is debatable.

Pathological appearance

Lesions may be multiple or single, most commonly in the jejunum, but also in the duodenum or ileum, and may vary from diffuse infiltration to simple ulcers. The appearances are not clearly distinguishable from those outlined for other small intestinal lymphomas later in this chapter. In particular, however, the appearance may be very similar to that reported in diffuse ileojejunitis, and a prolonged histological search may be required to identify the abnormal cells.

Histological appearances and classification

For some years influential opinion described this tumour as a malignant histocytosis of the small intestine.[15] With the advent of molecular biological techniques it has been identified as of T-cell origin,[11] which contrasts with the majority of lymphomas arising *de novo* in the small intestine or in the context of the immunoproliferative small intestinal disease, which are of B-cell origin. The T-cell origin in coeliac disease may imply that chronic T-cell activation associated with the underlying immunopathology of coeliac disease has led to development and proliferation of a malignant T-cell clone.

The histological appearances are variable,[12,13] including cells resembling histocytes with large irregular nuclei and abundant cytoplasm, or monomorphic infiltration with blast cells. Giant cells may be present. An inflammatory infiltrate of lymphocytes, plasma cells, and eosinophils may make recognition of the malignant cells difficult.[15]

Prognosis

The prognosis of lymphoma complicating coeliac disease is poor, with 5-year survival rates of approximately 10% with combined surgical therapy and chemotherapy. One feature contributing to this is that diagnosis is often delayed, as early symptoms of lymphoma may be attributed to dietary indiscretion. Emergency presentation, or a diagnostic laparotomy, may allow resection of macroscopic intestinal disease, but the diffuse nature of the small intestinal pathology and predisposing villous atrophy, as well as the propensity for local and systemic spread, clearly indicate that chemotherapy is required. There are no controlled trials of different regimes, which are therefore likely to be selected on the basis of local advice and expertise.

RELATIONSHIP OF MALIGNANCY TO TREATMENT OF COELIAC DISEASE

The association of malignancy with coeliac disease diagnosed in adulthood rather than childhood car-

Table 3.36 Malignant tumours in 210 patients, all followed for at least 13 years, either on strict gluten-free diet, or normal diet

Tumours	Gluten-free diet (108)	Normal diet (102)
All sites	14	17
Mouth/pharynx/oesophageal carcinomas	1	5
Lymphoma (non-Hodgkins)	2	7
Others	11	5

Data from Holmes *et al.*[10]
Significant excess for mouth/pharynx/oesophageal carcinoma for patients on a normal diet (observed : expected = 22).
Significant excess for lymphoma in patients on a normal diet (observed : expected = 78, $P < 0.001$), and patients on gluten-free diet (observed : expected = 16, $P < 0.01$).

ries with it the implication that early treatment of coeliac disease may prevent the development of malignancy specifically associated with coeliac disease. This has been regarded by some as the main reason for treating coeliac disease with gluten withdrawal rather than, for example, with vitamin supplementation. Recent studies of cohorts of patients, particularly from the Birmingham group who have followed patients with adult coeliac disease over three decades, suggest that the frequency of both gastrointestinal carcinoma and lymphoma falls if patients are treated with gluten withdrawal (*Table 3.36*).

References

1. Anderson, H., Dotevall, G. and Mobacken, H. (1971) Malignant mesenteric lymphoma in a patient with dermatitis herpetiformis. *Scandinavian Journal of Gastroenterology*, **6**, 397–400.
2. Asquith, P. Thompson, A.R. and Cooke, W.T. (1969) Serum immunoglobulins in adult coeliac disease. *The Lancet*, **ii**, 129–131.
3. Brzechwa-Ajdukiewicz, A., McCarthy, C.F., Austad, W. *et al.* (1966) Carcinoma, villous atrophy and steatorrhoea. *Gut*, **7**, 572–577.
4. Cooper, B.T., Holmes, G.K.T. and Cooke, W.T. (1989) Lymphoma risk in coeliac disease of later life. *Digestion*, **23**, 89.
5. Gough, K.R., Read, A.E. and Naish, J.M. (1962) Intestinal reticulosis as a complication of idiopathic steatorrhoea. *Gut*, **3**, 232–239.
6. Harris, O.D., Cooke, W.T., Thompson, H. and Waterhouse, J.A.H. (1967) Malignancy in adult coeliac disease and idiopathic steatorrhoea. *American Journal of Medicine*, **42**, 899–912.
7. Hodges, J.R., Isaacson, P., Eade, O.E. and Wright, R. (1978) Serum lysozyme levels in malignant histocytosis of the intestine. *Gut*, **19**, A933.
8. Holmes, G.K.T., Stokes, P.L., Sorahan, T.M. *et al.* (1976) Coeliac disease, gluten-free diet and malignancy. *Gut*, **17**, 612–619.
9. Holmes, G.K.T., Dunn, G.I., Cockel, R. and Brookes, V.S. (1980) Adenocarcinoma of the upper small bowel complicating coeliac disease. *Gut*, **21**, 1010–1016.
10. Holmes, G.K.T., Prior, P., Lane, M.R. *et al.* (1989) Malignancy in coeliac disease – effect of a gluten-free diet. *Gut*, **30**, 333.
11. Isaacson, P.G., O'Connor, N.T.J., Spencer, J. *et al.* (1985) Malignant histocytosis of the intestine. A T-cell lymphoma. *The Lancet*, **ii**, 688–691.
12. Isaacson, P., Jones, D.B. Sworn, M.J. and Wright, D.H. (1982) Malignant histocytosis of the intestine: report of three cases with immunological and cytochemical analysis. *Journal of Clinical Pathology*, **35**, 510–516.
13. Salter, D.M., Krajewski, A.S. and Dewar, A.E. (1986) Immunophenotype analysis of malignant histocytosis of the intestine. *Journal of Clinical Pathology*, **39**, 8.
14. Selby, W.S. and Gallagher, N.D. (1979) Malignancy in a 19 year experience of adult coeliac disease. *Digestive Diseases and Sciences*, **24**, 684.
15. Spencer, J. and Isaacson, P.G. (1987) Gastrointestinal lymphoma. *Baillières Clinical Gastroenterology*, **1**, 605–623.
16. Swinson, C.M., Slavin, G., Coles, E.D. *et al.* (1983) Coeliac disease and malignancy. *The Lancet*, **i**, 111–115.

THE NEUROLOGICAL COMPLICATIONS OF COELIAC DISEASE *(P.D. Lewis)*

Patients with coeliac disease may rarely show evidence of severe neurological disease. This may take the form of encephalopathy, cerebellar dysfunction, myelopathy, peripheral neuropathy or a combination of these. The available clinical and pathological evidence does not clearly indicate the cause of such neurological complications. However, data implicating dietary vitamin E deficiency will be considered. In a few cases direct involvement of the nervous system by histiocytic lymphoma, itself a complication of coeliac disease, may occur. In contrast to tropical sprue, the development of myopathy in coeliac disease is uncommon,[14] though a number of reports[8,9,12,13] describe a spectrum of features that may be encountered.

The early documentation of neurological manifestations in patients believed to have coeliac disease was either deficient in clinical detail or lacked pathological support. It was only with the important clinicopathological study of Cooke and Smith[4] that the existence of coeliac encephalomyeloradiculoneuropathy became certain.

Earlier reports had described three patients with non-tropical sprue with transient extensor plantar responses[7,10,16] or noted the finding of posterior column changes in autopsy material. In 1957, Sencer[15] described the neurological symptoms and signs in 94 patients with a malabsorption syndrome presumed to be due to coeliac disease. Forty-nine had features suggesting nervous system involvement. Twenty patients had evidence of tetany but no objective reflex or sensory changes. Ten patients had experienced paraesthesiae and were found to be anaemic but had no abnormal neurological signs. A further 12 patients had reflex or sensory abnormalities on examination. There were two cases of severe myeloradiculopathy (referred to by the authors as 'pseudo-tabes'). In a review of 124 patients with 'non-tropical sprue' Green and Wollaeger[6] encountered six patients with neurological signs. Abnormalities included peripheral neuropathy, areflexia and (in one case) 'subacute combined sclerosis'.

The 16 patients described by Cooke and Smith[4] all had a definite jejunal biopsy-proven diagnosis of coeliac disease and all had severe neurological disease. Autopsy was performed in nine cases and data obtained on peripheral nerve or muscle biopsy in the other seven. Two patients were found to have 'neuropathy' at the time of original referral for their gastrointestinal symptoms. Four patients were referred on account of the neuropathy complicating their primary disorder and nine developed neurological complications while under treatment for adult coeliac disease.

The patients usually presented with symptoms affecting the lower limbs and sensory ataxia soon dominated the clinical picture in nearly all cases. Posterior column deficit and distal impairment of pain and tactile sense with absent ankle jerks were frequently encountered. Weakness was often marked but wasting relatively slight. One patient developed an extensor plantar response shortly before death, three had cerebellar signs and five had suffered from unexplained episodes of unconsciousness. One patient presented with neurological signs and symptoms suggestive of motor neurone disease, and probably had that condition.

In 10 patients the 'neuropathy' proved steadily progressive, the rate of progression varying considerably from case to case. Of the nine fatal cases, 'neuropathy' was considered the main cause of death in four. Among the neurological findings reported were demyelination (often of spongiform type) of the posterior and lateral columns of the spinal cord, producing a subacute combined degeneration-like picture, dorsal column degeneration alone, and cerebellar cortical degeneration. Not surprisingly, in view of the rarity of the condition, there has been no comparable case series to substantiate these dramatic findings, though several thorough and convincing case studies with necropsy findings have since been published.

An overview of these cases shows a mainly male preponderance (against a background of a higher incidence of coeliac disease in women) and again, in general, the development of neurological dysfunction years after the onset of coeliac disease. Unsteadiness of gait is a universal feature, with dementia, cranial nerve palsies and myoclonus being among the additional changes encountered. From the neuropathological standpoint, two contrasting patterns of disease predominate. These are dorsal spinal column degeneration, of a type dissimilar to that encountered in subacute combined degeneration, and a diffuse cerebellar degeneration affecting mainly the cortical Purkinje cell population but also involving dentate nuclei. The role of circulating anti-neuronal antibodies in producing cerebellar cortical changes is not yet clear.

Additional unusual pathological changes that may be found include malignant infiltration of spinal nerve roots in the cauda equina secondary to multiple histiocytic lymphomas in small and large bowel,[3] brainstem encephalitis[1] and central pontine myelinolysis, a generally nutrition-related phenomenon.[2] This last point emphasizes the often posited but still unconfirmed role of dietary deficiency in the genesis of the encephalomyeloradiculopathy of coeliac disease. In the majority of affected patients the neurological disease progresses inexorably despite treatment with essential dietary trace constituents. However, the spinal disease may improve in subjects receiving vitamins A, B and E[3] and, obviously, multivitamins and trace element supplementation should always be tried. Response to vitamin E has suggested that the development of neurological changes in coeliac disease may be related to deficiency of this substance, at least in some cases.

References

1. Brucke, T., Kollegger, H., Schmidbauer, M. *et al.* (1988) Adult coeliac disease and brainstem encephalitis. *Journal of Neurology, Neurosurgery and Psychiatry*, **51**, 456–457.
2. Camilleri, M., Krausz, T., Lewis, P.D. *et al.* (1983) Malignant histiocytosis and encephalomyeloradiculopathy complicating coeliac disease. *Gut*, **24**, 441–447.
3. Case Records of the Massachusetts General Hospital (1976) Case 48. *New England Journal of Medicine*, **295**, 1242–1248.
4. Cooke, W.T. and Smith, W.T. (1966) Neurological disorders associated with adult coeliac disease. *Brain*, **89**, 683–722.
5. Finelli, P.F., McEntee, W.I., Ambler, M. and Kestenbaum, D. (1980) Adult coeliac disease presenting as cerebellar syndrome. *Neurology*, **30**, 245–249.
6. Green, P.A. and Wollaeger, E.E. (1960) The clinical behaviour of sprue in the United States. *Gastroenterology*, **28**, 399–418.
7. Hansen, K. and von Staa, H. (1936) *Die Einheimische Sprue*. Leipzig: Thieme.
8. Hardoff, D., Sharf, B. and Berger, A. (1980) Myopathy as a presentation of coeliac disease. *Developmental Medicine and Child Neurology*, **22**, 781–783.

9. Henriksson, K.G., Hallert, C., Norrby, K. and Walan, A. (1982) Polymyositis and adult coeliac disease. *Acta Neurologica Scandinavica*, **65**, 301–319.

10. Hotz, H.W. and Luthy, F. (1939) Funikuläre Spinaler-krankung bei einheimischer Sprue; Mitteilung eines Falles mit pathologisch-anatomischem Befund. *Helvetica Medica Acta*, **6**, 415–426.

11. Kinney, H.C., Burger, P.C., Hurwitz, B.J. *et al.* (1982) Degeneration of the central nervous system associated with coeliac disease. *Journal of Neurological Science*, **53**, 9–22.

12. Lundberg, A., Eriksson, B.O. and Jansson, G. (1979) Muscle abnormalities in coeliac disease: studies on gross motor development and muscle fibre composition, size and metabolic substrates. *European Journal of Pediatrics*, **130**, 93–103.

13. Nanji, A.A., Freeman, H.J. and Anderson, F.H. (1982) Paralysis and rhabdomyolysis: a presenting feature of coeliac disease. *Western Journal of Medicine*, **136**, 273–274.

14. Pallis, C.A. and Lewis, P.D. (1974) *The Neurology of Gastrointestinal Disease*. London. W.B. Saunders.

15. Sencer, W. (1957) Neurological manifestations in malabsorption syndrome. *Journal of the Mount Sinai Hospital*, **24**, 331–345.

16. Thaysen, T.E.H. (1932) *Non-tropical Sprue*. London: Oxford University Press.

WHIPPLE'S DISEASE

H.J.F. Hodgson

DEFINITION

Whipple's disease (intestinal lipodystrophy) is a rare but well-recognized condition affecting the small intestine in which infiltration with characteristic foam-laden macrophages leads to a severe and potentially fatal malabsorption state. The condition may affect virtually any organ of the body, and frank intestinal disease may have been preceded by years of non-specific systemic complaints such as arthralgia or fever.

AETIOLOGY AND PATHOPHYSIOLOGY

The universal finding of rod-shaped bacilli in addition to the characteristic macrophages within the tissues of affected individuals, together with a usually good response to antibiotic therapy, has led to the classification of Whipple's disease as an infective process. Many questions regarding the nature of the infecting agent and the possible role of diminished host immunity remain to be answered.

PATHOLOGY

Small intestine

In virtually every case of untreated Whipple's disease, diffuse small intestinal disease is present.[17]

The jejunum and ileum, and sometimes the duodenum, are thickened and oedematous, and the mucosa shows either total loss of the villous pattern or clubbed, flattened villi (*Figure 3.79*). Ulceration

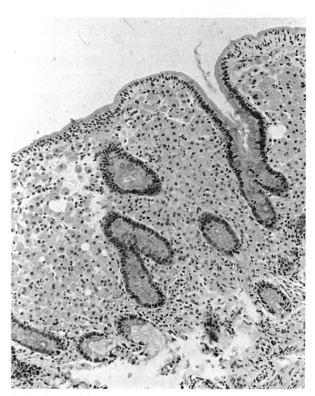

Figure 3.79 Jejunal biopsy appearances of untreated Whipple's disease, showing villous atrophy, a well-preserved epithelial cell layer, and the uniform appearance of the lamina propria due to macrophage infiltration (haematoxylin and eosin).

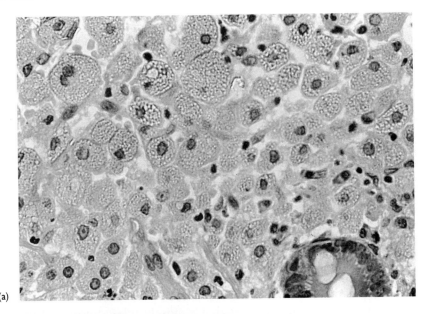

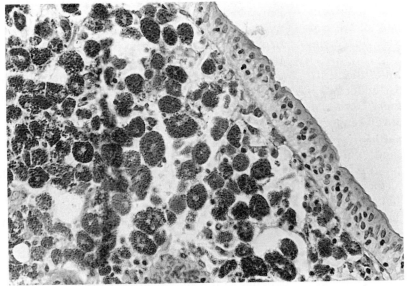

Figure 3.80 (a) High power of the lamina propria of the same tissue as in *Figure 3.79* demonstrating the foam-laden macrophages (haematoxylin and eosin). (b) PAS staining of same tissue, demonstrating the typical glycoprotein material within the macrophages and also scattered within the lamina propria.

is rare. The intestinal lacteals are dilated, and yellow lipid deposits may be seen in all layers of the small intestine beneath the epithelium in untreated cases at autopsy. This latter finding, together with irregular fat-filled cystic spaces in the enlarged mesenteric lymph nodes, led Whipple to coin the name 'intestinal lipodystrophy', for the condition, but these fatty deposits are probably merely the consequence of lymphatic damage and obstruction.[13]

Histologically the villi are distorted by the classic microscopic abnormality of Whipple's disease, the foam-laden macrophages. These are large cells, usually 20–30 μm across, and are often densely packed within the lamina propria, giving it a uniform appearance without any other marked inflammatory cell infiltrate (*Figure 3.80*). The foamy cells stain a dramatic magenta colour with periodic acid–Schiff (PAS) reagent; this stain is diastase-resistant.[4]

Occasional PAS-positive macrophages may be seen in the small intestine of normal individuals, and more commonly in normal colonic tissues, but differentiation from those of Whipple's disease can usually readily be made, based on the number present and the light microscopic appearances of the cells.[36]

Other histological features in the small intestinal mucosa include dilated lymphatics with a virtually normal enterocyte layer and normal numbers of intraepithelial lymphocytes;[2] occasional acute inflammatory cells are occasionally seen. An arteritic process has been noted.[23] Aetiologically, the most interesting finding is the presence of bacilli. With both light and electron microscopy, bacilli are found within and between the foam-laden macrophages, and they also stain brilliant magenta with PAS.[6,47] It seems probable that it is the presence of whole and degenerating bacteria, and of granules of membranous glycoprotein-rich material derived from bacteria, that explains the PAS staining properties of the macrophages. The bacilli are similar in all reported cases. They are rods, 1–1.5 μm long and 0.25 μm across, and may occasionally be seen in division. In the small intestine they are most abundant just beneath the epithelial basement membrane and decrease in number towards the submucosa, perhaps supporting the concept of invasion from the luminal side.

Other pathological findings

In advanced cases, mesenteric lymph nodes may be greatly enlarged, up to 3–4 cm across, with cystic fat-filled spaces and fibrosis apparent macroscopically. Histology confirms the presence of PAS-positive macrophages and bacilli, and granulomas are fairly frequently seen. Other intra-abdominal findings include peritoneal adhesions, thickening of the capsule of the liver and spleen, and ascites, which may be transudate or chylous in nature.[11]

Outside the abdomen, involvement of the heart, lung, brain and skin occurs. Valvular endocarditis occurred in one-third of an autopsy series of patients, with a similar distribution of valve involvement to that seen in rheumatic endocarditis.[13] Fibrinous pericarditis, myocarditis, and coronary arteritis may also occur.[43] The respiratory system may be involved with pleural adhesions, pleural effusions, and nodular pulmonary involvement.[39] Approximately 10% of cases show involvement of the central nervous system at autopsy, with cortical atrophy, spongy demyelination, and areas of infarction.[16] Both macrophages and bacilli have now been identified in all these affected areas.[35] Very rarely, amyloidosis has been reported as a complication of long-standing Whipple's disease.[14]

The presence and distribution of bacteria within the body suggest that Whipple's disease is an infection, entering via the gastrointestinal tract. However, despite clear visualization within the tissues, the bacteria have not been cultured. This, together with the histological evidence of an abnormal response from the macrophage cell line, has led to the concept that pre-existing immunodeficiency in the host is a prerequisite for the development of Whipple's disease.

BACTERIOLOGY

The bacteria appear morphologically similar in all reported cases.[12] Recent electron microscopic studies suggest they are Gram-positive, with an extra surface membrane to explain the characteristic trilaminar appearance.[37] Culture of gut tissues had been disappointing due to a high incidence of contaminated specimens; a wide variety of organisms have been grown from such tissues. These include corynebacteria, *Haemophilus*, *Klebsiella*, streptococci, *Nocardia* and *Brucella*-like organisms. Contamination is less likely in cultures of lymph node tissue; corynebacteria of different strains,[5,20] and cell wall-deficient strains of streptococci and enterococci have been isolated from this site. Some of these corynebacteria would now probably be classified as propionobacteria.

Grouping antisera to streptococci of group A, B and G, and *Shigella* B have reacted strongly with material in Whipple's macrophages, and fluorescence has also been observed with antisera and other groups of streptococci and propionobacteria. The findings of various workers have been similar, and suggest that a closely related group of organisms, whose surface carbohydrate includes rhamnose, occurs in Whipple's tissue.[20,26,27] Analysis of bacterial ribosomal RNA by two groups[33,46] has recently suggested that a bacteria closely related to actinomycetes, named *Trophyrema whippelli* by one group,[33] is indeed the elusive Whipple's bacterium.

IMMUNOLOGY

Even if the organism found in Whipple's tissue has been identified, the ability of this bacteria to survive over years despite the host immune response requires explanation. Many authors have suggested that this is evidence of an immune deficiency in the host, and have provided evidence of this by describing a variety of immunological abnormalities in patients with active Whipple's disease.[8] These abnormalities have mainly affected cell-mediated immunity, and include decreased *in vitro* proliferative response of lymphocytes, decreased numbers of circulating lymphocytes, and abnormal delayed hypersensitivity. Whilst such observations have been fairly frequently made in untreated patients with active disease, investigations in treated patients, who should show a persistent defect if a primary immune deficiency is of importance, have been less dramatic. Some studies have suggested diminished monocyte phagocytic function, persisting after treatment.[3]

An interesting finding in patients with acquired immune deficiency syndrome (AIDS) has been occasional endoscopic and histological findings mimicking Whipple's disease, including PAS-positive macrophages, explained by infection with *Mycobacterium avium-intracellulare*.[18,42] This may act as a paradigm indicating that these histological appearances can arise from inadequate elimination of bacteria in an immunocompromised host.

The involvement of immune factors is also supported by the higher than expected incidence of HLA-B27 (28%) in patients with Whipple's disease compared to the general population (8%).[10]

CLINICAL FEATURES

The majority of patients are middle-aged males, presenting between the ages of 30 and 70 years.[9,29] However, affected women and infants have been reported. Most patients are Caucasian, but affected Negroes and Indians have also been reported. Two sets of affected brothers have been recorded, but most of the cases are sporadic, and there is no obvious aetiological clue from geographical or occupational factors.

The disease is systemic and, as the pathological findings would suggest, symptoms and signs of involvement of almost any organ system may occur. Most patients, however, are not diagnosed until frank symptoms of gastrointestinal disease have developed, at which time routine investigation of a malabsorption state should lead to the diagnosis. Retrospectively, a set of early symptoms, present for many years (anything from 1 to well over 10 years) before the development of symptoms of intestinal disease, can usually be recognized. These commonly include arthritis, fever, malaise, and pulmonary complaints; the challenge for the clinician is to make the diagnosis in this early stage.

INTESTINAL SYMPTOMS

Despite the historical concept of Whipple's disease as a disease of the small intestine, the clinical features of small gut involvement are non-specific. However, they are of great importance, as it is usually investigation of this organ that leads to the diagnosis. In advanced cases, diarrhoea, weight loss, abdominal pain and distension may occur. Investigation may show steatorrhoea, often of the order of 20–30 g/day, and a protein-losing enteropathy. Abdominal distension may be due to gas, ascites, or mesenteric node enlargement. Bleeding from ulcerations of the gastrointestinal tract rarely occur.[15] In a few patients a diffuse colitis resembling ulcerative colitis has been reported.[22]

SKIN MANIFESTATIONS

Pigmentation is seen, particularly in exposed areas, in about half of the patients. Non-specific cutaneous manifestations, similar to those seen in other malabsorptive states, are also seen, such as petechiae, ecchymoses, and follicular hyperkeratosis. Finger clubbing is unusual but can occur, and skin nodules with characteristic histology have been reported.[19] General examination may also reveal oedema, which may be lymphoedema.

RETICULOENDOTHELIAL SYSTEM

Peripheral lymphadenopathy occurs in about 50% of patients, but hepatomegaly and splenomegaly in less than 5%. Biopsy of lymph nodes may be diagnostic.[30] However, occasionally lymph nodes containing granuloma have not been PAS-positive, though they have revealed characteristic bacilli on electron microscopy.[38]

ARTHRITIS

Most patients have some history of arthritis – up to 90% in some series.[25] The arthritis is non-specific in nature and affects peripheral joints, either with frank swelling or, less commonly, with arthralgia alone. Arthritic symptoms are the commonest early manifestation of Whipple's disease, often for years before diagnosis. The symptoms are episodic, and affect the knees, ankles, wrists, hands and elbows most frequently, but virtually any joint can be involved. The arthritis may be symmetrical or asymmetrical, unilateral or bilateral. It is seronegative in type, does not cause abnormal radiological signs, and rarely leads to deformity. Sacroiliitis and spondylitis are also associated with Whipple's disease but occur much more rarely – probably in less than 10% of cases. Synovial biopsies have only rarely been performed, but both characteristic macrophages and bacteria have been identified in such material.[21]

CARDIAC AND PULMONARY MANIFESTATIONS

Pericarditis is reported at some time in about 10% of cases,[44] and may even lead to cardiac constriction. Myocarditis with conduction defects, and valvular disease, mainly of the aortic and mitral valve, also occur;[20] the combination of these may lead to presentation with cardiac failure. The diseased valves may subsequently be the site of conventional bacterial endocarditis; affected valves have been treated by the insertion of prostheses. Pulmonary manifestations are very common; a recurrent cough, associated either with pleurisy or with pulmonary infiltrates, may be one of the early features of

Whipple's disease and occurs in about 50% of cases.[39]

CENTRAL NERVOUS SYSTEM

Clinical central nervous system involvement is rare, occurring in perhaps 5% of cases. Most commonly it occurs after some years of systemic involvement. The manifestations of central nervous system involvement are non-specific, and include depression, apathy, dementia, fits, myoclonus and dizziness. A rare syndrome of oculomasticatory myorhythmia has been reported. A variety of ocular manifestations occur, including supranuclear ophthalmoplegia, papilloedema, optic atrophy and scotomas, uveitis, and vitreous haemorrhages and opacities.[28] Meningitis, with PAS-positive cells in the cerebrospinal fluid has also been reported.[41] In some patients, central nervous system disease has occurred after apparently adequate antibiotic treatment of intestinal Whipple's disease; presentation under these circumstances with apparent hypothalamic involvement, with insomnia, hyperphagia or polysipsia, has been reported.[16,28] Such recurrences clearly have implications for the treatment and follow-up of patients with Whipple's disease.

INVESTIGATIONS

Apart from the histological findings, there are no specific investigations in Whipple's disease.

The cardinal investigation is a jejunal biopsy which, in virtually every case of untreated Whipple's disease, shows the characteristic histological abnormality. Very occasionally patchy changes occur and multiple biopsies are necessary, but in the majority the changes are diffuse. There are very rare cases in which Whipple's tissue has been found elsewhere in the body at a time when small intestinal disease has not been present. The best documented of such cases are those in which central nervous system relapse has occurred after the treatment of Whipple's disease involving the small intestine.[16]

Routine laboratory tests will show an elevated erythrocyte sedimentation rate, an anaemia which may show the combined effects of folate and iron deficiency, and chronic inflammation; vitamin B_{12} levels and absorption are usually normal. Thrombocytosis and an elevated white blood count may be seen.[31] The serum albumin level may be very low, but globulin levels may be normal or elevated and serum IgA levels may be high.

Radiological investigation of the small gut often shows a characteristic pattern of dilatation and

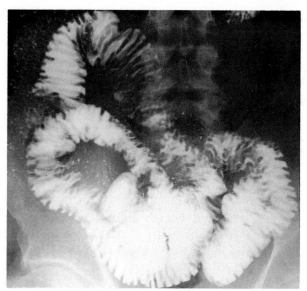

Figure 3.81 Small bowel radiograph showing dilated oedematous intestine in Whipple's disease.

oedema (*Figure 3.81*), but in about 15% of patients the small bowel radiograph will be normal.[29] Endoscopic examination of the duodenum may show thickened folds and yellow-white areas, which on histology prove to be enlarged club-shaped villi; however, the duodenum is not infrequently spared.[45]

Computed tomography scanning[34] and ultrasound[1] may show para-aortic or other lymphadenopathy.

TREATMENT

Early cases of Whipple's disease were fatal. A dramatic and sustained clinical response in a patient with Whipple's disease following chloramphenicol therapy was reported in 1952;[32] since the electron microscope description of bacteria in the tissues, the central role of antimicrobial therapy has been recognized. Corticosteroids, initially advocated during the 1950s for the treatment of this condition, would seem now to have a very restricted role for the short-term support of desperately ill patients.

A variety of antimicrobial treatments have proved successful, although there have been no controlled trials. Penicillin, streptomycin, tetracycline, and sulphonamides have all been used, but there are also well-documented instances in which one or other of these antibiotics have proved unsuccessful.[24] Treatment can be seen to be effective within a few days, with a rapid improvement in general condition, and cessation of fever, diarrhoea or arthritis; weight gain occurs over the ensuing few weeks. Occasionally, an initial febrile Herxheimer-like reaction has been reported. Follow-up biopsies of the small intestine show that the bacteria disappear within a few weeks, followed by restoration of the normal villus architecture, although occasionally PAS-positive macrophages may persist for some years.[40]

Despite the good initial response to a wide variety of antibiotics, there is a high incidence of relapse after stopping treatment.[24] Probably up to one-third of patients will relapse at some time, indicating the need for life-long follow-up. Interestingly, relapse may occur despite, and even during, long-term antibiotic therapy with a drug which was initially responsible for causing remission. Clinical relapse can be foretold by the reappearance of bacteria within serial small intestinal biopsies.[40] Clinical follow-up, including measurement of the sedimentation rate and serum and red cell folate levels, may also be of value.

The appearance of relapses within the ental nervous system, despite apparently successful treatment of intestinal disease some years before, is well recognized; it is therefore appropriate to commence treatment with high doses of parental antibiotics in the hope that this will provide a sufficient concentration within the central nervous system. A regimen of 1.2 g (2 megaunits) of penicillin and 1 g of streptomycin daily for 2 weeks, followed by 1 year of treatment with an oral high-dose tablet of trimethoprim–sulphamethoxazole, has been recommended.

CONCLUSION

To the gastroenterologist, Whipple's disease is a treatable cause of malabsorption, and is particularly important because much systemic disease may be associated with it. To the general physician, the early presentation with arthritis, fever, pericarditis, central nervous system involvement, or ill-defined collagenosis, offers an important diagnostic opportunity.

REFERENCES

1. Alabano, O., Carrieri, V., Vinciguerra, V. *et al.* (1984) Ultrasonic findings in Whipple's disease. *Journal of Clinical Ultrasonography*, **12**, 286–288.
2. Austin, L.L. and Dobbins, W.O. (1982) Intraepithelial leucocytes of the intestinal mucosa in normal man and Whipple's disease. *Digestive Diseases and Sciences*, **27**, 311–320.
3. Bjerknes, R., Laerum, O.D. and Degaards, H. (1985) Whipple's disease. Demonstration of a persisting monocyte and macrophage dysfunction. *Scandinavian Journal of Gastroenterology*, **23**, 611–617.
4. Black-Shaffer, B. (1949) Tinctorial demonstration of glycoproteins in Whipple's disease. *Proceedings of the Society for Experimental Biology and Medicine*, **72**, 225–227.
5. Caroli, J., Julien, C., Eteve, J. *et al.* (1963) Trois cas de maladie de Whipple. *Seminars Hopitaux de Paris*, **31**, 1457–1480.
6. Chears, W.C. and Ashworth, C.T. (1961) Electron microscopic study of the intestinal mucosa in Whipple's disease – demonstration of encapsulated bacilliform bodies in these lesions. *Gastroenterology*, **41**, 129–138.
7. Clancy, R.L., Tomkins, W.A.F., Muckle, T.J. *et al.* (1975) Isolation and characterization of an aetiologic agent in Whipple's disease. *British Medical Journal*, **ii**, 568–570.
8. Dobbins, W.O. (1981) Is there an immune deficit in Whipple's disease? *Digestive Diseases and Sciences*, **26**, 247–252.
9. Dobbins, W.O. (1985) Whipple's disease: an historical perspective. *Quarterly Journal of Medicine*, **56**, 523–531.
10. Dobbins, W.O. (1987) HLA antigens in Whipple's disease. *Arthritis and Rheumatism*, **30**, 102–105.
11. Dobbins, W.O. (1988) Whipple's disease. *Mayo Clinic Proceedings*, **63**, 623–624.
12. Dobbins, W.O. and Kawanishi, H. (1981) Bacillary characteristics in Whipple's disease: an electron microscopic study. *Gastroenterology*, **80**, 1468–1475.
13. Enzinger, F.M. and Helwig, E.B, (1963) Whipple's disease – a review of the literature and report of 15 patients. *Virchows Archiv A Pathologische Anatomie*, **336**, 238–269.
14. Farr, M., Hollywell, C.A., Walton, K.W. *et al.* (1983) Amyloidosis in Whipple's disease. *Journal of the Royal Society of Medicine*, **76**, 963–965.
15. Feldman, M. (1989) Intestinal bleeding in patients with Whipple's disease. *Gastroenterology*, **96**, 1207–1209.
16. Feurle, G.E., Volk, B. and Waldherr, R. (1979) Cerebral Whipple's with negative jejunal histology. *New England Journal of Medicine*, **300**, 907–908.
17. Fleming, J.L. Wiesner, R.H., Shorter, R.G. (1988) Whipple's disease. Clinical, biochemical and histopathological features and assessment of treatment in 29 patients. *Mayo Clinic Proceedings*, **63**, 539–551.
18. Gillin, J.S., Urmacher, C., West, R. and Shike, M. (1983) Disseminated mycobacterium avium intracellulare infection in AIDS mimicking Whipple's disease. *Gastroenterology*, **85**, 1187–1191.
19. Good, A.E., Beals, T.F., Simmons, J.L. and Ibrahim, M.A.H. (1980) A subcutaneous nodule with Whipple's disease – key to early diagnosis. *Arthritis and Rheumatism*, **23**, 856–858.
20. Gupta, S., Pinching, A.J., Onwuabili, A. *et al.*

(1986) Whipple's disease with unusual clinical, bacteriological and immunological findings. *Gastroenterology*, **90**, 1286–1289.

21. Hawkins, C.F., Farr, M. Morris, C.J. *et al.* (1976) Detection by electron microscopy of rod-shaped organisms in synovial membrane from a patient with the arthritis of Whipple's disease. *Annals of Rheumatic Diseases*, **35**, 502–509.

22. Hendrix, J.P., Black-Shaffer, B., Withers, R.W. and Handler, P. (1950) Whipple's intestinal lipodystrophy: report of 4 cases and discussion of possible pathogenic factors. *Archives of Internal Medicine*, **85**, 91–131.

23. James, T.N., Buckley, H.B. and Kent, S.P. (1984) Vascular lesions of the gastrointestinal system in Whipple's disease. *American Journal of Medical Sciences*, **288**, 125–129.

24. Keinan, R.D., Merrell, E.D., Vletstra, R. and Dobbins, W.O. (1985) Antibiotic treatment and relapse in Whipple's disease. Long-term follow-up of 88 patients. *Gastroenterology*, **88**, 1867–1873.

25. Kelly, J.J. and Weisiger, B.B. (1963) The arthritis of Whipple's disease. *Arthritis and Rheumatism*, 615–632.

26. Kent, S.P. and Kirkpatrick, S.M. (1980) Whipple's disease. Immunological and histopathological studies of either cases. *Archives of Pathology and Laboratory Medicine*, **104**, 544–547.

27. Keren, D.F., Weisburger, W.R., Yardley, J.H. *et al.* (1976) Whipple's disease: demonstration by immunofluorescence of similar bacterial antigens in macrophages from three cases. *Johns Hopkins Medical Journal*, **139**, 51–59.

28. Knox, D.L., Bayless, T.M. and Pittman, F.E. (1976) Neurologic disease in patients with treated Whipple's disease. *Medicine (Baltimore)*, **55**, 467–476.

29. Maizel, H., Ruffin, J.M. and Dobbins, W.O. (1970) Whipple's disease. A review of 19 patients from one hospital and a review of the literature since 1950. *Medicine (Baltimore)*, **49**, 175–205.

30. Mansbach, C.M., Shelbourne, J.D., Stevens, R.D. and Dobbins, W.O. (1978) Lymph node bacilliform bodies resembling those of Whipple's disease in a patient without intestinal involvement. *Annals of Internal Medicine*, **89**, 64–66.

31. Nuzum, C.T., Sandler, R.S. and Paulk, H.T. (1981) Thrombocytosis in Whipple's disease. *Gastroenterology*, **80**, 1465–1467.

32. Paulley, J.W. (1952) A case of Whipple's disease (intestinal lipodystrophy). *Gastroenterology*, **22**, 128–133.

33. Relman, D.A., Schmidt, T.M., MacDermott, R.P. and Falkow, S. (1992) Identification of the uncultured Whipple's bacillus. *New England Journal of Medicine*, **327**, 293–300.

34. Rijke, A.M., Falke, R.H. de Vries, R.R. (1983) Computed tomography in Whipple's disease.

Journal of Computer Assisted Tomography, **7**, 1101–1102.

35. Sieracki, J.C. (1958) Whipple's disease – observations on systemic involvement. I. Cytologic observations. *American Medical Associations Archives of Pathology*, **66**, 464–467.

36. Sieracki, J.C. and Fine, G. (1959) Whipple's disease – observations on systemic involvement. II. Gross and histologic observations. *American Medical Associations Archives of Pathology*, **67**, 81–93.

37. Silver, M.T., Macedo, P.M. Moura Nunes, J.F. (1985) Ultrastructure of bacilli and the bacillary origin of the macrophagic inclusions in Whipple's disease. *Journal of General Microbiology*, **131**, 4001–4013.

38. Spapen, H.D., Segers, O., deWit, N. *et al.* (1989) Electron microscopic detection of Whipple's disease bacillus in sarcoid-like PAS negative granulomas. *Digestive Diseases and Sciences*, **34**, 640–643.

39. Symmons, D.P. (1985) Pulmonary manifestations of Whipple's disease. *Quarterly Journal of Medicine*, **56**, 497–504.

40. Trier, J.S., Phelps, J.C., Eidelman, S. and Rubin, C.E. (1965) Whipple's disease. Light and electron microscopic correlation of jejunal mucosal histology with antibiotic treatment and clinical status. *Gastroenterology*, **48**, 384–407.

41. Thompson, D.G., Ledingham, J.M., Howard, A.J. and Brown, C.L. (1978) Meningitis in Whipple's disease. *British Medical Journal*, **ii**, 14–15.

42. Vazquez-Iglesias, J.L., Yanez, Y. and Arnal, F. (1988) Infection by *Mycobacterium avium intracellulare* in AIDS: endoscopic duodenal appearances mimicking Whipple's disease. *Endoscopy*, **20**, 279–282.

43. Vliestra, R.E., Lie, J.T., Kuhn, W.E. *et al.* (1978) Whipple's disease involving the pericardium. Pathological confirmation during life. *Australian and New Zealand Journal of Medicine*, **8**, 649–651.

44. Volpicelli, N.A., Salyer, W.R., Milligan, F.D. *et al.* (1976) The endoscopic appearance of the duodenum in Whipple's disease. *Johns Hopkins Medical Journal*, **138**, 19–23.

45. Whipple, G.H. (1907) A hitherto undescribed disease characterised anatomically by deposits of fat and fatty acids in the intestinal and mesenteric lymphatic tissues. *John Hopkins Hospital Bulletin*, **198**, 382–391.

46. Wilson, K.H., Blitchington, R., Frothingham, R. and Wilson, J.A.P. (1991) Phylogeny of Whipple's disease associated bacterium. *The Lancet*, **338**, 474–475.

47. Yardley, J.H. and Hendrix, T.R. (1961) Combined electron and light microscopy in Whipple's disease – demonstration of bacillary bodies in the intestine. *John Hopkins Hospital Bulletin*, **109**, 76.

IMMUNOLOGICAL DISORDERS AFFECTING THE SMALL INTESTINE

BASIC GASTROINTESTINAL IMMUNOLOGY *(A. Bousvaros and W.A. Walker)*

The gut is the largest immune organ in the body, possessing more than 10^{10} plasma cells. The intestinal mucosal immune system prevents the passage of potentially harmful antigens and pathogens into the systemic circulation of the host. Lymphoid elements in the gut are present as either isolated cells within the lamina propria, or as lymphoid aggregates (Peyer's patches, mesenteric lymph nodes, and appendix) termed *gut-associated lymphoid tissues (GALT)*. Antigens which penetrate the gut epithelium are processed by underlying lymphoid tissues, leading to stimulation of B and T lymphocytes and the generation of IgA-producing plasma cells. Alternatively, a state of systemic tolerance (immune unresponsiveness to antigen) may occur.[26,29]

ANTIGEN UPTAKE

Non-immune defences limit the amount of antigen that comes into contact with the intestinal epithelium. Most antigenic compounds are either large peptides or proteins, and can thus be digested. Salivary amylase, gastric acid, pepsin, and pancreatic proteases hydrolyse macromolecules in the gastric and intestinal lumen. Intestinal peristalsis transports proteins through the digestive tract. Intestinal mucin coats the mucosal surface, and decreases antigen adhesion to the mucosal epithelium. Lastly, the enterocytes themselves are connected by tight junctions, and thus form a physical barrier preventing the penetration of antigen into underlying tissues.[11]

In the adult human intestine, uptake of macromolecules preferentially occurs at specialized sites called follicle-associated epithelium (dome epithelium), which overlie lymphoid aggregates or Peyer's patches (*Figure 3.82*). The dome epithelium is characterized by a decrease in goblet cells and mucin, and by the presence of M cells.[22] Morphologically, M cells are epithelial cells with large numbers of endocytic vesicles, and few microvilli and lysosomes. M cells specialize in the uptake and delivery of intact antigen to lymphoid cells in the Peyer's patches. In animal models, M cells bind and endocytose substances as diverse as horseradish peroxidase, reovirus type 3, and *Escherichia coli* strain RDEC-1.[21,30] In rat intestine, M cells express

proteins of the class II major histocompatibility complex (MHC class II), and thus may be capable of presenting antigens to lymphocytes.[3]

ANTIGEN PROCESSING

Macrophages, dendritic cells, T lymphocytes, and B lymphocytes are all present within the Peyer's patch. *Figure 3.83* illustrates how cellular handling of antigen may result in a mucosal IgA response. B lymphocytes recognize whole antigen directly via immunoglobulin molecules present on the B-cell surface. Cross-linking of immunoglobulin receptors on the B-cell surface provides the initial signal for cellular activation and replication. Further B cell differentiation is promoted by T-cell cytokines (soluble chemical messengers secreted by cells of the immune system).[1]

Antigenic molecules also stimulate helper T cells to produce cytokines, but T cells do not recognize antigen directly. Instead, antigen must be presented to T cells as an antigenic fragment in association with proteins of *antigen-presenting cells* (*Figure 3.83*). The mechanism of antigen processing involves endocytosis of whole antigen, lysosomal degradation, and transport of antigenic fragments to the cell surface, where they may complex with proteins of the major histocompatibility complex (MHC). Macrophages, dendritic cells, and B cells all possess the capability to process antigen in this manner. Thus, all three of these cell types within the Peyer's patch are potential antigen-presenting cells.[9] Intestinal epithelial cells also express MHC proteins on their cell surfaces, and are capable of *in vitro* antigen presentation to T lymphocytes, but their role *in vivo* is yet to be determined.[5]

T cells bind antigen via the T-cell receptor on the T-cell surface (*Figure 3.83*). Accessory molecules (including CD4, CD8, and LFA1), are thought to strengthen the interaction between the antigen-presenting cell and the T cell. The class of MHC protein associated with the antigen determines which T-cell subset recognizes the antigen. T cells of the CD4 phenotype (which includes most helper T cells) recognize antigen in association with MHC class I proteins, while T cells of the CD8 phenotype (which includes most suppressor and cytotoxic T cells) recognize antigen in association with class I proteins.[9] The interaction of antigen with the T-cell receptor triggers a complex series of intracellular events mediated through the molecules CD3 and protein kinase C to generate an 'activated' T cell. An

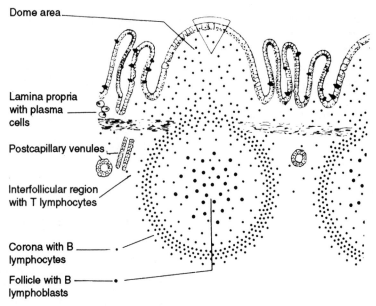

Figure 3.82 Schematic drawing of Peyer's patch and overlying dome epithelium. M cells in the dome area transport antigen to the underlying lymphoid tissue containing B cells, T cells, dendritic cells and macrophages. (Reproduced, with permission, from Pabst.[21])

activated helper T cell is characterized by increased DNA and protein synthesis, increased release of interleukins, and increased responsiveness to both autocrine and exogenous growth factors (e.g. interleukin-2).[10]

B CELL MATURATION AND IgA PRODUCTION

Once stimulated by antigen, Peyer's patch B cells undergo differentiation and maturation into IgA-producing plasma cells. Such differentiation is felt to be under the regulation of Peyer's patch T cells that have also been activated by antigen. For example, human appendiceal T-cell clones have been generated that can promote B-cell isotype 'switching' (i.e. transformation from a B cell producing IgM to one producing IgA); other T-cell clones promote B-cell 'post-switch' differentiation.[13,14]

A stimulated Peyer's patch B cell migrates to the systemic circulation after passing through the

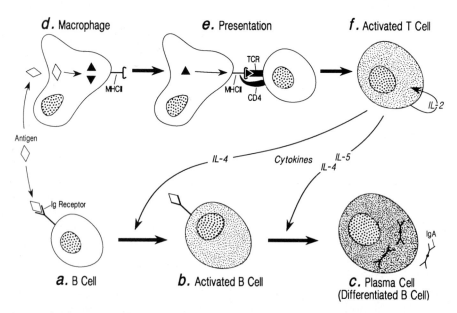

Figure 3.83 Antigen processing by gut-associated lymphoid tissue. Antigen binding to B-cell surface immunoglobulin (a) provides the initial stimulus promoting B-cell activation (b). The B cell may then differentiate into an immunoglobulin producing plasma cell (c). Alternatively, antigen may be degraded by an antigen-presenting cell such as a macrophage (d), and antigen fragments presented to a helper T cell via MHC class II molecules present on the macrophage cell surface (e). The activated helper T cell secretes lymphokines which regulate B-cell maturation, and also autocrine growth factors such as interleukin-2 (IL-2) (f).

afferent lymphatic circulation, mesenteric lymph nodes, and thoracic duct. Once in the systemic circulation, the B cell may be distributed to immune organs throughout the body, including spleen, tonsils, and other mucosal sites (e.g. bronchi). However, intestinal B cells preferentially return to intestinal lamina propria through poorly characterized 'homing' mechanisms, and there mature into plasma cells. The B-cell migration from Peyer's patches to the systemic circulation and return to the intestinal lamina propria is referred to as the IgA cell cycle (*Figure 3.84*).[20,26]

Over 3 g/day of secretory IgA is produced by the greater than 10^{10} plasma cells present in human intestinal lamina propria. In normal adult human intestinal mucosa, IgA-producing plasma cells are six times more prevalent than IgM-producing cells, and 20 times as common as IgG-producing plasma cells.[6] Plasma cells synthesize IgA molecules of both the IgA1 and IgA2 subclasses. Two IgA molecules then combine with a single J-chain molecule within the plasma cell to form an IgA dimer connected by disulphide bonds.[17] The IgA dimer–J chain complex is then transported into the lamina propria, where it combines with secretory component, an 80 kDa glycoprotein present on the basal lamina of the enterocyte.[2] This completed secretory IgA molecule is then transported by the enterocyte into the intestinal lumen, where it may bind to antigens, viruses or bacteria. In rats, secretory IgA is present in high concentrations in bile; however, biliary secretory IgA is minimally present in humans.[15]

OTHER MUCOSAL IMMUNE CELLS

Cytotoxic cells are present in the intestinal lamina propria, and possibly in the epithelial cell layer. CD8 cytotoxic T cells recognize infected cells through T-cell receptor–MHC class I interaction, then kill cells by secretion of cell membrane-destroying enzymes called perforins. In contrast, natural killer cells possess cytotoxic capabilities but do not possess a T-cell receptor that recognizes specific antigens.[23] Lastly, some cytotoxic T cells and natural killer cells require stimulation by cytokines such as interleukin-2 in order to manifest cytotoxic properties, and are termed lymphokine-activated killer cells.[12]

Intraepithelial lymphocytes lie adjacent to the epithelial basement membrane in human intestine, at a concentration of 5–10 intraepithelial lymphocytes per 100 enterocytes. Immunoperoxidase staining has demonstrated that intraepithelial lymphocytes are almost all T lymphocytes, and that 80–90% of human intraepithelial lymphocytes possess the CD8 (suppressor/cytotoxic) phenotype. The role of these lymphocytes in mucosal immunity has not been well defined. However, an increased number of intraepithelial lymphocytes has been seen in various enteropathies, including coeliac disease and autoimmune enteropathy.[7]

Eosinophils are present in intestinal lamina propria, and can be markedly increased in number in pathological conditions such as eosinophilic gastroenteritis, parasitic infestations, and neonatal allergic colitis. In type I (IgE-mediated) hypersensitivity, cross-linking of IgE receptors on eosinophils triggers release of mediators such as leukotrienes and eosinophilic cationic protein.[16]

Mucosal mast cells are also present in intestinal lamina propria, and when stimulated by IgE can degranulate and release mediators such as histamine, heparin and tumour necrosis factor. In animal models, mast cells are important in eradicating infestation with parasites such as *Nippostrongyloides*, but their role in fighting parasitic infections in humans is unclear.[4,16]

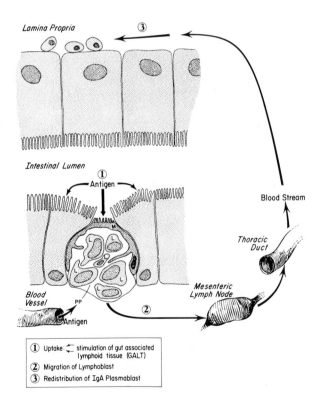

Figure 3.84 The IgA cell cycle. Intestinal B lymphocytes stimulated by antigen leave the Peyer's patch and migrate via mesenteric lymph nodes into the thoracic duct. They subsequently enter the systemic circulation and may enter other lymphoid tissues (e.g. spleen, bronchus or tonsils), but they preferentially return to intestinal lamina propria. (Reproduced, with permission, from Isselbacher, K.J. and Walker, W.A. (1977) *New England Journal of Medicine*, **297**, 768.)

RECENT PROGRESS

Lymphocyte adhesion

Three major classes of adhesion molecules have thus far been identified on lymphocytes: the immunoglobulin, integrin, and selectin superfamilies. The immunoglobulin superfamily includes both isoforms of the T-cell receptor (α/β and γ/δ), as well as the MHC classes I and II, CD2, and LFA-3 molecules. The integrin family includes the molecules LFA1, Mac1, VLA4, and VLA5. The selectin family includes the murine homing antigen MEL14 and its human homologue Leu8.[27]

Lymphocyte adhesion molecules are thought to have three major functions *in vivo*: lymphocyte homing, cell–cell contact, and cell–matrix interactions. B and T lymphocytes both possess the ability to 'home' to tissues from the systemic circulation. In lymph nodes, a specialized blood vessel lined by cuboidal epithelium (the *high endothelial venule*) is the primary site of attachment of circulating lymphocytes, and similar venules exist in gut-associated lymphoid tissues. Recently, homing receptor molecules have been identified on the endothelial cells of these specialized venules that bind adhesion molecules on lymphocyte surfaces. In addition, investigators have demonstrated that antigenic stimulation can alter the adhesion molecules present on lymphocyte cell surfaces. Therefore, an activated lymphocyte may preferentially home to a particular tissue site such as the intestinal mucosa.[24,27]

Cytokines

Cells of the immune system secrete polypeptides that exert both autocrine and paracrine effects on cellular functions such as proliferation, membrane protein expression, and immunoglobulin production. These compounds include interleukins-1–6, tumor necrosis factors α and β, and interferon-γ.[18,28] A summary of the principal actions of some of these compounds is given in *Table 3.37*.

As stated previously, these compounds are probably regulatory signals within the intestinal mucosa. In particular, interleukin-5 has been shown to preferentially enhance IgA production by murine B lymphocytes, and thus may be important in promoting intestinal B-cell differentiation. Altered levels of several interleukins have been demonstrated in inflammatory bowel disease; thus, these compounds are potential mediators of intestinal inflammation.

Table 3.37 Principal Actions of some cytokines

Compound	Chief sources	Stimulates
Interleukin-1	Macrophages, lymphocytes, endothelial cells	Growth and differentiation of lymphocytes Tissue catabolism Prostaglandin synthesis Fever (endogenous pyrogen)
Interleukin-2	Activated T cells	Growth and differentiation of lymphocytes Cytotoxic activity of lymphocyte-activated killer cells
Interleukin-3	Activated T cells	Growth of bone marrow progenitors
Interleukin-4	T cells	Growth and differentiation of B cells Immunoglobulin production
Interleukin-5	Activated T cells	B-cell differentiation
Interleukin-6	T cells	B-cell differentiation Hepatocyte production of acute phase reactants
Tumor necrosis factor α	Macrophages	Fever (pyrogenic) Cachexia Bone resorption
Tumor necrosis factor β	Lymphocytes	Same as tumor necrosis factor α
Interferon γ	T cells, natural killer cells	Activation of macrophages, cytotoxic cells, B cells Immunoglobulin production

Adapted from Strober and James[27] and O'Garra, A. (1989) *Lancet*, **i**, 1003.

In addition, cytokines have important non-immune effects, and may be involved in producing the systemic manifestations of immune-mediated disease. For example, interleukin-1 is a potent pyrogen, and interleukin-6 stimulates production of acute phase reactants by hepatocytes.[18,28]

Chemical mediators produced by other tissues can also modulate intestinal immunity. For example, the neuropeptide substance P and the hormone cholecystokinin can both increase intestinal IgA production in mice.[8,19] In addition, mast cells and eosinophils both release compounds such as histamine and prostaglandins that can modulate immune function, chemotaxis, and gastrointestinal ion transport.[4,25] Thus, mucosal immune cells produce chemical messengers with multiple effects on gastrointestinal physiology, and, conversely, are influenced by mediators produced by non-immune cells of the gastrointestinal tract. The complex network of neuroendocrine–immune interactions is a new area of research termed *immunophysiology*.

In summary, the gastrointestinal immune system processes antigen, resulting in a humoral or cellular immune response. Though stimulated gastrointestinal lymphocytes may migrate to other mucosal sites, they preferentially return to the gastrointestinal mucosa where they mature into differentiated effector cells. The mechanisms controlling the immune response to antigen are poorly understood, but chemical messengers such as cytokines, neuropeptides and gut hormones are important in immunoregulation.

References

1. Abbas, A.K. (1988) A reassessment of the mechanisms of antigen-specific T cell dependent B cell activation. *Immunology Today*, **9**, 89–94.
2. Ahnen, D.J. (1985) Secretory component: the polymeric immunoglobulin receptor. *Gastroenterology*, **89**, 667–682.
3. Allan, C.H., Mendrick, D.L. and Trier, J.S. (1993) Rat intestinal M cells contain endosomal–lysosomal compartments and express class II major histocompatibility compex determinants. *Gastroenterology*, **104**, 698–708.
4. Atkins, F.M. (1987) Intestinal mucosal mast cells. *Annals of Allergy*, **53**, 44–53.
5. Bland, P. (1988) MHC class II expression by the gut epithelium. *Immunology Today*, **9**, 174–177.
6. Brandtzaeg, P. and Baklien, K. (1976) Immunohistochemical studies of the epithelial transport of immunoglobulins. *Scandinavian Journal of Gastroenterology*, **36** (suppl.), 1–15.
7. Dobbins, W.O. (1986) Human intestinal intraepithelial lymphocytes. *Gut*, **27**, 972–985.
8. Freier, S., Eran, M. and Faber, J. (1987) Effect of cholecystokinin on the release of IgA and IgG specific antibodies in the rat intestine. *Gastroenterology*, **93**, 1242–1246.
9. Grey, H.M., Sette, A. and Buus, S. (1989) How T cells see antigen. *Scientific American*, **261**, 56–64.
10. Hadden, J.W. (1988) Transmembrane signals in the activation of T lymphocytes by mitogenic antigens. *Immunology Today*, **9**, 235–239.
11. Israel, E.J. and Walker, W.A. (1988) Host defense development in gut and related disorders. *Pediatric Clinics of North America*, **35**, 1–18.
12. Kanof, M.E. and Strober, W. (1989) Lymphokine-activated killer-cell cytotoxicity in the intestinal immune system. *Gastroenterology*, **97**, 222–224.
13. Kawanishi, H., Saltzman, L. and Strober, W. (1983) Mechanisms regulating IgA class-specific immunoglobulin production in murine gut-associated lymphoid tissue. I. T cells derived from Peyer's patches that switch sIgM cells to sIgA cells *in vitro*. *Journal of Experimental Medicine*, **157**, 433–449.
14. Kawanishi, H., Saltzman, L. and Strober, W. (1983) Mechanisms regulating IgA class-specific immunoglobulin production in murine gut-associated lymphoid tissue II. Terminal differentiation of post-switch secretory IgA Peyer's patch B cells. *Journal of Experimental Medicine*, **158**, 649–669.
15. Kleinman, R.E. and Walker, W.A. (1987) The liver and intestinal immunoglobulin A: up from the "minors"? *Gastroenterology*, **93**, 650–651.
16. Lee, D.G., Swieter, M. and Befus, D. (1988) Mast cells, eosinophils, and gastrointestinal hypersensitivity. *Immunology and Allergy Clinics of North America*, **8**, 469–483.
17. Mestecky, J., McGhee, J.R. and Elson, C.O. (1988) Intestinal IgA system. *Immunology and Allergy Clinics of North America*, **8**, 349–367.
18. Mizel, S.B. (1989) The interleukins. *FASEB Journal*, **3**, 2379–2388.
19. O'Dorisio, M.S. (1988) Neuropeptide modulation of the immune response in gut-associated lymphoid tissue. *International Journal of Neuroscience*, **38**, 189–200.
20. Ogra, P.L. (1979) Ontogeny of the local immune system. *Pediatrics*, **64** (suppl.), 765–773.
21. Owen, R.L. (1977) Sequential uptake of horseradish peroxidase by lymphoid follicle epithelium of Peyer's patches in the normal unobstructed mouse intestine. *Gastroenterology*, **72**, 440–451.
22. Pabst, E. (1987) The anatomical basis for the immune function of the gut. *Anatomy and Embryology*, **176**, 135–143.
23. Peters, P.J., Geuze, H.J., van der Donk, H.A. and Borst, J. (1990) A new model for lethal hit delivery by cytotoxic T lymphocytes. *Immunology Today*, **11**, 28–32.
24. Rosen, S.D. (1989) Lymphocyte homing: progress and prospects. *Current Opinion in Cell Biology*, **1**, 913–919.
25. Russell, D.A. and Castro, G.A. (1989)

Immunological regulation of colonic ion transport. *American Journal of Physiology*, **256**, G396–G403.

26. Schrieber, R.A. and Walker, W.A. (1988) The gastrointestinal barrier: antigen uptake and perinatal immunity. *Annals of Allergy*, **61**, 3–12.
27. Springer, T.A. (1990) Adhesion receptors of the immune system. *Nature*, **346**, 425–434.
28. Strober, W. and James, S.P. (1988) The interleukins. *Pediatric Research*, **24**, 549–557.
29. Walker, W.A. (1986) Antigen handling by the small intestine. *Clinics in Gastroenterology*, **15**, 1–18.
30. Wolf, J.L. and Bye, W.A. (1984) The membranous (M) cell and the mucosal immune system. *Annual Reviews of Medicine*, **35**, 95–112.

IMMUNODEFICIENCY AND THE GUT   *(H.J.F. Hodgson)*

Immunodeficiency and gastrointestinal disease have complex interrelations. A primary defect in antibody-mediated immunity, or less commonly of cell-mediated immunity, can lead to gastrointestinal disease – frequently in the form of infection and infestation, but also of other types.[3,55] Conversely, primary disease of the gut can lead to losses of antibody or lymphocytes into the lumen, thus causing immunodeficiency and predisposing to systemic infections.

A further complexity is introduced by the specialized nature of the gut immune defences. The particular features of this have been outlined in the preceding section, notably the local protective action of secretory IgA, and also its role in inducing tolerance in the systemic immune system when antigens are presented via the gut. Thus, a specific defect in the local immune system may allow ingress of antigens from the lumen, and initiate damaging generalized immune responses.

CLASSIFICATION OF IMMUNODEFICIENCY STATES

Many types of immunodeficiency have now been described, often of considerable rarity, and active research is demonstrating further subgroups in each type. In broad terms, immunodeficiency states may be classified as follows:

1. Primary specific immunodeficiencies – reflecting deficient antibody production, deficient T cell-mediated immunity, or both.
2. Primary non-specific immunodeficiencies – in which immunological memory is intact but there is a deficiency in the function of the mediators of the inflammatory response, such as the complement system or neutrophil polymorphonuclear leukocytes.
3. Secondary immunodeficiency syndromes – the most important of which is the acquired immunodeficiency syndrome (AIDS or SIDA) associated with human immunodeficiency virus (HIV) infection. This topic is dealt with in Chapter 9. Immunodeficiency can also arise secondary to irradiation, neoplasm, or drug therapy. A rare cause of secondary immunodeficiency, relevant to gastroenterology, is the loss of immunoglobulin and lymphocytes into the gut lumen in intestinal lymphangiectasia.

Table 3.38 shows a classification of the major primary immunodeficiency diseases. Most present in childhood. The only diseases commonly encountered by the specialist gastroenterologist in adults

Table 3.38   Primary immune deficiencies

- Antibody deficiency syndromes
  Selective deficiencies of
    IgA
    IgG subclasses
    IgM
  Common variable hypogammaglobulinaemia
  X-linked agammaglobulinaemia
  X-linked lymphoproliferative syndrome

  Selective T-cell deficiency
  Thymic aplasia (DiGeorge syndrome)
  Purine nucleoside phosphorylase deficiency
  Severe combined immunodeficiency
    Primary
      Sporadic
      X-linked
      Bare lymphocyte syndrome (HLA-DR deficiency)
      Adenosine deaminase deficiency
      Reticular dysgenesis
      Biotin-dependent carboxylase deficiency
      Associated with cartilage hair hypoplasia

- Mixed deficiencies
  Wiskott–Aldrich syndrome
  Ataxia telangiectasia
  Bloom's syndrome
  Transcobalamin II deficiency

- Complement deficiencies

- Neutrophil deficiencies
  Congenital neutropenia
  Cyclic neutropenia
  Chronic granulomatous disease
  Complement receptor deficiency

are selective IgA deficiency and, more rarely, common variable hypogammaglobinaemia.

ANTIBODY DEFICIENCY STATES

Common variable hypogammaglobulinaemia

Patients with common variable hypogammaglobulinaemia have abnormally low serum immunoglobulin levels and usually recurrent infections. The serum levels of all three main immunoglobulin classes – IgG, IgA and IgM – are low. The condition has a number of synonyms: common variable immunodeficiency,[20] idiopathic late-onset immunoglobulin deficiency,[24] or primary acquired hypogammaglobulinaemia. These descriptive terms emphasize that the disease is frequently not manifest until adult life, that the serum levels of individual immunoglobulins may vary from time to time in individual patients, and that the condition is heterogeneous.

The condition is rare, reported as 15 per 10^6 of the population in males and 4 in females, with a peak incidence in the third decade.

Aetiology

The aetiology of common variable hypogammaglobulinaemia is unclear. Functionally, there is inadequate production of immunoglobulin by cells of the B-lymphocyte line. In a few rare individuals with strong family histories this may be initiated by an infection with Epstein–Barr virus[41] but this is classified as a disorder separate from common variable hypogammaglobulinaemia, as a sex-linked recessive immunoproliferative disorder. There is no proof of a viral aetiology in most patients with common variable hypogammaglobulinaemia. Some familial cases of common variable hypogammaglobulinaemia are reported, but different pedigrees suggesting autosomal dominant and recessive inheritance exist.

Immune defects

Studies of immunoglobulin production and other immune parameters in patients with common variable hypogammaglobulinaemia indicate that the low serum immunoglobulin levels may have a number of causes. In about 25% of patients, B lymphocytes, the precursors of immunoglobulin-producing plasma cells, are absent from peripheral blood;[28] in others, B cells are present, but in culture they do not synthesize or release normal amounts of immunoglobulin. In some patients, but not all, this decreased production by B cells is attributable to the presence of an overactive regulatory suppressor T cell, removal of which permits normal immunoglobulin production by B cells.[44]

Clinical features

Patients present at any age. The onset is taken as the time at which frequent infections begin: it is usually a supposition that serum immunoglobins become low at that stage, although there are well-documented cases in whom a change from normal serum immunoglobulin levels has been demonstrated.

The majority of patients present with recurrent sinopulmonary infections. There is a small minority in whom these are absent, and gastrointestinal symptoms are the only manifestations. In addition, patients are prone to meningitis, osteomyelitis and other severe systemic bacterial infections; other extraintestinal manifestations may include a sarcoid-like pulmonary infiltration, polyarthritis, haemolysis, neutropenia and thrombocytopenia.

Physical examination may reveal splenomegaly in 20–50% of individuals; lymphadenopathy is much rarer, and should prompt investigation to exclude lymphoma. In patients with severe intestinal disease, the physical signs of a malabsorptive state may be present.

Other immunological studies confirm the heterogeneity of common variable hypogammaglobulinaemia. About one-third of patients have defective cell-mediated immunity demonstrable by *in vivo* or *in vitro* testing, and lymphopenia may be present.[7] Further studies will undoubtedly subdivide common variable hypogammaglobulinaemia. None the less, the similar clinical features and a common susceptibility to infections and a number of gastrointestinal conditions makes the establishment of a diagnosis of common variable hypogammaglobulinaemia useful.

Diagnosis

The diagnosis is suggested by finding hypogammaglobulinaemia (<3 G/L) affecting all main classes. When the albumin level is also low, the possibility of a protein-losing state should be considered as an alternative diagnosis, but when gut inflammatory diseases complicate common variable hypogammaglobulinaemia, the albumin level may also be low.

Gastrointestinal disease

Between 60 and 90% of patients suffer gastrointestinal symptoms; the most common complaints being diarrhoea (intermittent or chronic), weight loss and vomiting. Virtually every part of the gastrointestinal tract may be abnormal in common variable hypogammaglobulinaemia.[5]

GASTRIC DISEASE
Achlorhydria, gastritis and pernicious anaemia are all common. Approximately 50% of patients with

common variable hypogammaglobulinaemia have pentagastrin-fast achlorhydria,[49] often, but not invariably, associated with intrinsic factor deficiency. The histological basis of this is atrophic gastritis with a heavy mononuclear cell infiltrate, absent parietal and chief cells, and intestinal metaplasia. The atrophic inflammatory process tends to involve the whole stomach, without the antral sparing often found in Addisonian pernicious anaemia. This explains why the achlorhydria of common variable hypogammaglobulinaemia is not usually accompanied by a high serum gastrin level;[30] unlike the unaffected antrum of pernicious anaemia, the G cell-bearing area in common variable hypogammaglobulinaemia is atrophic. In addition, there is a lower than expected gastrin response to food and exogeneous bombesin in common variable hypogammaglobulinaemia.[22]

The cause of the gastric atrophy is uncertain; as it occurs in the absence of autoantibodies, it cannot be due to an antibody-mediated autoimmune process. Cell-mediated autoimmunity may play a role, and circulating lymphocytes sensitized to parietal cells and intrinsic factor have been reported.[31]

A frank macrocytic anaemia due to vitamin B_{12} deficiency occurs in many patients with common variable hypogammaglobulinaemia but, as discussed below, it is apparently more frequently due to infestation of the small gut with *Giardia* than a consequence of intrinsic factor deficiency and gastritis.[5] A far more serious consequence of gastric atrophy is the development of gastric carcinoma: in one study, 7 out of 50 patients with common variable hypogammaglobulinaemia were reported to have this complication.[24] This incidence is much higher than the incidence in Addisonian pernicious anaemia: the difference may reflect an additional defect in immunosurveillance against cancer, or differences in the extent and type of bacterial colonization of the stomach, leading to a higher concentration of carcinogenic or co-carcinogenic factors in common variable hypogammaglobulinaemia.[42,55] Whatever the explanation, the risk is high enough in common variable hypogammaglobulinaemia to justify surveillance endoscopy.

SMALL INTESTINE

Between one-third and two-thirds of patients with common variable hypogammaglobulinaemia have chronic or recurrent attacks of diarrhoea. A number of causes have been documented, some occurring with, and others without, abnormal small intestinal morphology. Abnormalities of both small bowel structure and function may occur.

Nodular lymphoid hyperplasia occurs in between 20 and 60% of patients with common variable hypo-

gammaglobulinaemia and diarrhoea. Small nodules of lymphoid cells, 1–3 mm in diameter, appear scattered through the lamina propria of the small intestine.[24] Whether the incidence is as high in patients without diarrhoea in unclear. The nodules are similar to normal lymphoid follicles or intestinal Peyer's patches, and may contain germinal follicles. Immunofluorescence studies have shown IgM to be present in some.[36] The normal villi of the small intestine may be stretched over the nodules. These nodules may be detected either by radiology (*Figure 3.85*), endoscopy,[12] or intestinal biopsy; in one series of patients with diarrhoea in whom biopsies showed nodules in 60%, only half showed the appearances on small bowel radiography.[24] Much less commonly, similar nodules can be detected in the colon and the stomach.[9] Although giardiasis, the common parasitic infection of common variable hypogammaglobulinaemia, may be commoner when nodular lymphoid hyperplasia is present, eradication of the giardiasis does not reverse the nodular lesion.

The differential diagnosis of nodular lymphoid hyperplasia in the context of hypogammaglobulinaemia includes familial polyposis syndromes and other polypoid lesions, and the radiological appearances have been reported in otherwise healthy children investigated for abdominal pain.[52] Nodular lymphoid hyperplasia has been reported in indi-

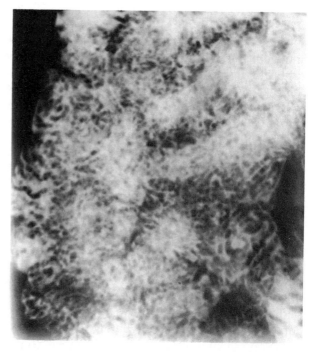

Figure 3.85 Nodular lymphoid hyperplasia shown on a small intestinal radiograph in a patient with common variable hypogammaglobulinaemia

viduals who later developed lymphoma, some with and some without abnormal immunoglobulin levels.

In addition to the nodular lymphoid hyperplasia, a spectrum of small intestinal findings occurs in patients with common variable hypogammaglobulinaemia known as *hypogammaglobulinaemic sprue*. The mucosa may show a normal villous architecture, with the only abnormality being an absence of plasma cells, or there may be varying degrees of lymphocytic infiltration, epithelial atrophy and villous blunting (*Figure 3.86*). Such inflammation or atrophic changes were found on biopsy in one-quarter of a series of patients with diarrhoea.[24] The abnormalities are rarely so severe as to warrant a description of subtotal villous atrophy; they are more commonly patchy, with normal villi present in adjacent areas or when multiple biopsies are taken. Frequently, the changes may be shown to be a consequence of giardial infestation, returning to normal after eradication of the parasite, but in other cases eradication causes no improvement. Other infestations should then be sought, and the possibility of a gluten-sensitive enteropathy be considered, but often no cause other than hypogammaglobulinaemia will emerge.

INFECTIONS

Giardiasis
In some series this is the commonest gut infection in common variable hypogammaglobulinaemia, being found in 60–80% of patients with diarrhoea and occasionally, but much less frequently (approximately 10%), in patients without gastrointestinal symptoms. The importance of using duodenal aspiration, biopsy and imprint techniques rather than simple stool examination to exclude infection has been emphasized.[23] Ament and co-workers have shown that giardiasis may cause not only diarrhoea, but also villous abnormalities, vitamin B_{12} and folate malabsorption, steatorrhoea, lactose intolerance, disaccharidase deficiency and protein-losing enteropathy. In 6 out of 10 patients with common variable hypogammaglobulinaemia, for example, vitamin B_{12} absorption returned to normal after treatment of the infection and, in all infected cases, treatment resulted in improvement of the small intestinal mucosal damage.[6]

Other infections
Many other gut infections occur in common variable hypogammaglobulinaemia. Bacterial overgrowth of the upper small intestine is common with both aerobic and anaerobic organisms. This probably reflects both the achlorhydria and a loss of protective secretory immunoglobulin.[34] However, a high concentration of unconjugated bile acid, as would be expected, were bacterial colonization of the duodenum and jejunum to contribute to malabsorption, is not found.

In patients in the UK, *Campylobacter jejunum*, affecting both the small and large bowel, has been reported as the most common cause of diarrhoea.[50,53,55] This has been associated both with villous atrophy and with granulomata on histology. Infections with *Salmonella* spp. are well reported,[32] and a fastidious Gram-negative organism, dysgomic fermenter-3, not usually a pathogen, has been linked to persistent diarrhoea in common variable hypogammaglobulinaemia.[51]

Chronic viral infections such as with cytomegalovirus also occur.[19] The report of a fatal case of coccidial infection in common variable hypogammaglobulinaemia,[45] and of severe infestations such as cryptosporidiosis in patients with childhood hypogammaglobulinaemia,[15] emphasize that, in patients with immunodeficiency and severe malabsorptive states, parasites and other infective agents should be meticulously sought.

OTHER GASTROINTESTINAL DISEASES
An inflammatory colitis occurs in a minority of patients with common variable hypogammaglobulinaemia and diarrhoea – perhaps in 10%.[11,29] The causes include *Campylobacter*, cytomegalovirus and, rarely, ulcerative colitis or Crohn's disease.

Cholelithiasis is common in common variable hypogammaglobulinaemia, with one series showing a 35% incidence of gallstones, perhaps reflecting either ileal disease or bacterial seeding of stones in the biliary tree.[24] Chronic pancreatitis may be more common but this is poorly documented; some patients with familial pancreatic insufficiency of the Shwachman type also have hypogammaglobulinaemia, and this possibility should be considered.[10]

Mechanisms and management of diarrhoea in common variable hypogammaglobulinaemia

The diarrhoea in common variable hypogammaglobulinaemia is a complex resultant of villous abnormalities, infections and biochemical abnormalities, such as lactase deficiency.[40] Antimicrobial therapy may need to be repeated. In those in whom no definable infection is present, the control of diarrhoea may be a formidable problem.

The relative contributions of lactase deficiency, steatorrhoea, bile salt malabsorption,[7,38] bacterial overgrowth and colitis to the diarrhoea must be assessed; the possibility of a secretory diarrhoea, occasionally reported, must also be considered.[16] Symptomatic treatment of diarrhoea with a low-fat, low-lactose diet, with or without cholestyramine,

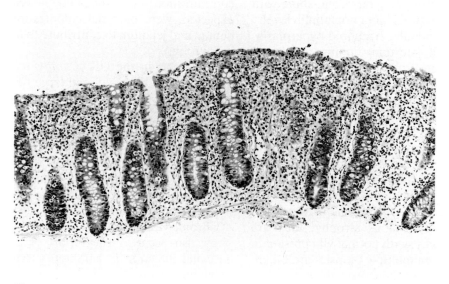

(a)

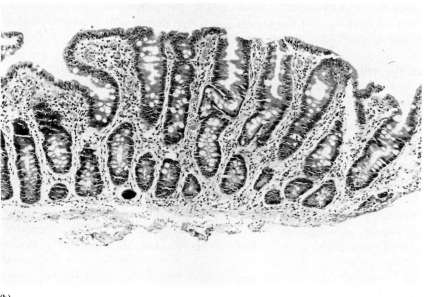

(b)

Figure 3.86 (a) A colonic biopsy illustrating the low grade colitis associated with many cases of hypogammaglobulinaemia (a: H + E, × 115). It produces little crypt architectural distortion but is associated with increased intraepithelial lymphocytes (b: H + E, × 455) and plasma cells are absent or occasional. Subtotal villous atrophy in a jejunal biopsy (c: H+E, × 115) with increased intraepithelial lymphocytes (d: H + E, × 455). There is an absence of plasma cells. (Photomicrographs courtesy of A. Price, Northwick Park Hospital.) (*Continued opposite*)

may be successful. Very occasionally a true gluten-sensitive enteropathy may be present[54] but, in view of the patchy nature of hypogammaglobulinaemic sprue, it is difficult to be certain of the effects of dietary manipulation on villous architecture. There are occasional anecdotal reports of benefit from treatment with fresh frozen plasma infusions, colostral IgA by mouth, or high-dose steroids. In a few unfortunate individuals, persistent diarrhoea and

malabsorption may be resistant to all treatment, and prove fatal.

The general management of common variable hypogammaglobulinaemia will involve parenteral immunoglobulin replacement to prevent systemic infections. Intravenous preparations are now generally well tolerated, given in a dose of about 0.15–0.2 g/kg orally.[17] However, this rarely benefits the gut symptoms.

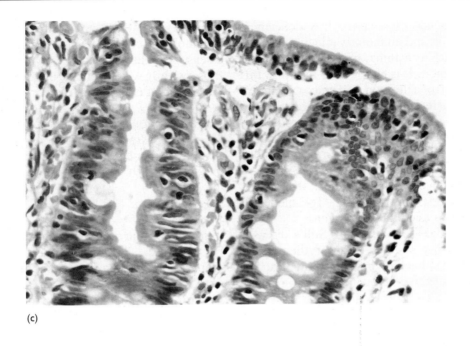

(c)

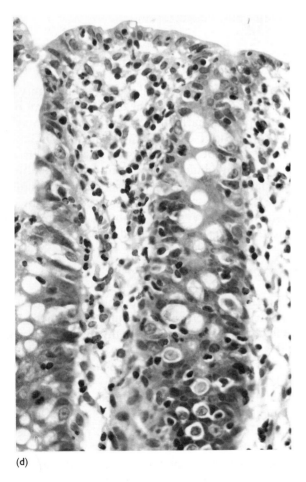

(d)

Other causes of hypogammaglobulinaemia

Childhood, sex-linked (Bruton's) agammaglobuli-naemia presents in male infants with recurrent bacterial infections. Gastrointestinal complications are far less common than in late-onset hypogammaglo-bulinaemia, although minor villous abnormalities, giardiasis and bacterial overgrowth have all been reported. Investigations should follow the lines described for common variable hypogammaglobulin-aemia[7]

Thymomas are associated in about 5% of cases with hypogammaglobulinaemia and in these patients diarrhoea may be a feature.[34] Both *Giardia* and cytomegalovirus infection have been documented.

Selective IgA deficiency

Unlike the immunodeficiencies outlined above, selective IgA deficiency is a common state, often asymptomatic, and frequently not meriting the term 'disease'. The incidence in the general population (estimated on blood donors) is approximately 1 in 500–700.[26] In some individuals, serum IgA is virtually undetectable; in others it is persistently well below the lower limit of normal (approximately 0.7 g/l) but readily detectable. Occasionally IgA deficiency is familial but more often sporadic; in a few patients, IgA deficiency follows therapy with drugs, notably phenytoin. Why one individual with IgA deficiency is symptomatic, but another not, is unclear, but a coexisting deficiency of the IgG2 subclass of IgG has been suggested as a contributing factor.[37]

Clinical presentation

As already mentioned, most affected individuals are asymptomatic. Sinopulmonary disease is the most obvious consequence of selective IgA deficiency, with repeated sinus and pulmonary infections.[6] Atopic disorders, such as asthma, hay fever and atopic eczema are common. It is tempting to interpret this latter fact in terms of a deficiency in mucosal immunity permitting increased ingress of antigens to the body, these antigens then initiating the production of IgE antibodies. It has also been suggested that atopic disorders in patients with normal immunoglobulin levels may be initiated in the same way – a delay in maturation of the IgA system at the mucosa permitting the development of IgE-mediated immune responses to common allergens.[46]

Autoimmune diseases, including Still's disease, rheumatoid arthritis, systemic lupus erythematosus and autoimmune haemolytic anaemia, are all associated with selective IgA deficiency.[6]

Gastrointestinal disease

The gastrointestinal disease associated with IgA deficiency is neither as common nor as dramatic as might be expected in view of the loss of the secretory IgA at the gut surface. Probably in such patients, IgM plays an important protective role, for this immunoglobulin can also combine with secretory component at the mucosal surface and thus function as a secretory immunoglobulin. None the less, food antibodies are relatively common in IgA deficiency, reflecting increased absorption of food protein.[14]

INFECTIONS
Giardiasis, and associated nodular lymphoid hyperplasia, have been reported in selective IgA deficiency, but are far less frequent than in common variable hypogammaglobulinaemia.[21] Candida overgrowth associated with decreased secretory IgA has been reported but the immunoglobulin abnormality was not permanent and may have been secondary to the infection.[47]

COELIAC DISEASE
IgA deficiency is far more common in patients with coeliac disease than the general population – approximately 1 in 50 compared with 1 in 500.[8] The coeliac disease is apparently identical to other cases with normal IgA levels and responds to gluten withdrawal.[43] Again, one may speculate that diminished defences at the mucosa permit increased penetration of gluten or its elements, initiating damaging immune responses.

CROHN'S DISEASE
In virtually every series documenting immunoglobulin levels in patients with Crohn's disease, individuals with IgA deficiency are reported with an overall incidence of approximately 1 in 70. Although this may suggest that individuals with IgA deficiency are more likely to develop or manifest Crohn's disease, the clinical features are indistinguishable in those with IgA deficiency from other patients with normal immunoglobulin levels.[25]

OTHER GASTROINTESTINAL DISORDERS
There is an association between IgA deficiency and severe diarrhoea after gastric surgery, possibly mediated by bacterial overgrowth in the small intestine.[33]

Treatment
Immunoglobulin therapy is usually not required. Furthermore, although purified immunoglobulin preparations contain IgA, this is predominantly the monomer, which lacks the capacity to link with secretory component and thus appear at mucosal surfaces. A few individuals with total deficiency of IgA develop IgG antibodies to IgA, and in these patients administration of IgA or of plasma protein fractions may be dangerous.

DEFECTS IN CELL-MEDIATED IMMUNITY

Primary deficiencies in cell-mediated immunity are rarer than deficiencies of the antibody system; they usually present early in life. The deficiency may be limited to the T-cell system, as in the DiGeorge syndrome, or be associated with B-cell defects and hypogammaglobulinaemia, as in severe combined immunodeficiency. Gastrointestinal disease is often a feature, but poorly documented for obvious reasons in very sick infants. The following conditions are relatively well defined.

DiGeorge syndrome

Afflicted infants present with the consequences of defective development of the third and fourth branchial arch, with absence of the thymus and parathyroid glands, and a selective loss of cell-mediated immune function. Presentation is usually with congenital heart disease or due to hypocalcaemia. Apart from oral Candida infection or occasional associated developmental oesophageal defects, gastrointestinal manifestations are not prominent, but chronic viral infections[56] leading to diarrhoea, and necrotizing enterocolitis,[2] have been reported.

Severe combined immunodeficiency

This is a heterogeneous condition, presenting with recurrent viral, bacterial or fungal infections, failure to thrive, and diarrhoea.[27] Both small intestinal disease, with histological features of villous atrophy and of enlarged macrophages reminiscent of Whipple's disease, and a frank inflammatory colitis may occur. Chronic rotavirus, calicivirus and astrovirus infection may be associated with diarrhoea.[18] Candidiasis is also common. If untreated, the disease may be rapidly fatal without marrow transplantation.

Ataxia telangiectasia

This autosomal recessive condition appears to be due to a primary defect in ability to repair DNA. The clinical manifestations include cerebellar ataxia, telangiectasia, and recurrent infections: defective cell-mediated immunity is combined with IgA deficiency. There is a striking predisposition to malignancy, largely of the lymphoreticular system, and even in heterozygotes there is an increased incidence of gastric carcinoma.[48]

Wiskott–Aldrich syndrome

This sex-linked disorder affects males, and severe cases may present with bloody diarrhoea.[13] Other presentations include bleeding elsewhere, eczema, and recurrent infections; minor small intestinal morphological abnormalities have also been reported. Deficient cell-mediated immunity is associated with a platelet defect and high IgE levels.

Treatment

The treatment of specific complex defects of cellular immunity or mixed immunodeficiencies lies outside the scope of this article. Identification of treatable infection is the prime responsibility of the consulting gastroenterologist. The use of bone marrow transplanation may be life-saving, though bringing with it its own risks of gastrointestinal complications of graft-versus-host disease.

OTHER PRIMARY IMMUNODEFICIENCIES

Chronic granulomatous disease

This condition results from a defect in the non-specific immune function of intracellular killing of phagocytosed material. The defect occurs in the electron transport system of polymorphonuclear leukocytes and monocytes, and may be demonstrated by a failure of these cells to reduce the dye nitroblue tetrazolium. The usual presentation is in infancy with multiple abscesses, lymphadenopathy and recurrent infections. A granulomatous involvement of the small and large intestine may mimic Crohn's disease;[4] appendicitis, hepatic abscesses, cholecystitis, perianal disease, severe mouth ulcers, and gastric outlet obstruction due to inflammatory tissue also occur.[35]

Secondary immunodeficiencies

The growing aggression of medical treatment, with long-term immunosuppressive therapy for collagen–vascular disorders, and particularly with high-dose immunosuppressive or cytotoxic therapy in patients with leukaemia and those undergoing bone marrow transplantation, has demonstrated the importance of the gut as a portal of entry for infection. Oral treatment of such patients with antibiotics reduces the incidence of gut-derived septicaemias or other infective disorders.

Acute neutropenic enterocolitis, or enterotyphlitis, is a dramatic disease mimicking severe complicated appendicitis, presenting with pain, distension, often bloody diarrhoea, and ascites, often complicated by septicaemia. The disease is due to necrosis of the ileocaecal region, with ulceration or perforation, and has a high mortality. Urgent surgery, obviously high-risk, may, however, be beneficial.[2]

Oral and systemic candidiasis develop easily in immunosuppressed patients, and also in those with lymphoma or debilitated by alcohol.

A particular risk applies to the parasite *Strongyloides* which, by autoinfection, may remain resident in the gastrointestinal tract for decades after leaving an endemic area. Hyperinfection leading to dilatation and subacute obstruction of the gut, and systemic strongyloidiasis due to invasion of brain, liver or lung, may be precipitated by immunosuppressive therapy; such patients also develop recurrent bacterial septicaemias, as enteric bacteria are carried into the body by 'piggy-backing' on the invading larvae. Screening of patients from endemic areas is therefore strongly advised before immunosuppression.

The increased risk of tumours in patients undergoing long-term immunosuppression has been highlighted, with non-Hodgkin's lymphoma the major form of neoplasm. Gastrointestinal cancers in general do not seem to be increased, other than an increase in anal carcinoma in renal transplant recipients.

References

1. Alt, B., Glass, N.R., Sollinger, H. (1985) Neutropenic enterocolitis. A review of the literature and assessment of early intervention. *American Journal of Surgery*, **149**, 405–408.

2. Agger, W.A., Glasser, J.E. and Marid-Abakura, R. (1984) Fatal necrotising enterocolitis in a neonate with DiGeorge syndrome. *Wisconsin Medical Journal*, **83**, 16–18.

3. Ament, M.E. (1975) Immunodeficiency syndromes and gastrointestinal disease. *Pediatric Clinics of North America*, **22**, 807–825.

4. Ament, M.E. and Ochs, H.D. (1973) Gastrointestinal manifestations of chronic granulomatous disease. *New England Journal of Medicine*, **288**, 382–387.

5. Ament, M.E., Ochs, H.D. and Davis, S.D. (1973) Structure and function of the gastrointestinal tract in primary immunodeficiency syndromes. *Medicine (Baltimore)*, **52**, 227–248.

6. Ammann, A.J. and Hong, R. (1971) Selective IgA deficiency. *Medicine (Baltimore)*, **50**, 223–236.

7. Asherson, G.L. and Webster, A.D.B. (1980) *Diagnosis and Treatment of Immunodeficiency Disease*. Oxford: Blackwell.

8. Asquith, P., Thompson, R.A. and Cooke, W.T. (1969) Serum immunoglobins in adult coeliac disease. *The Lancet*, **ii**, 129–131.

9. Bird, D.C., Jacobs, J.B., Silbiger, J. and Wolff, S.M. (1969) Hypogammaglobulinaemia with nodular lymphoid hyperplasia of the intestine. *Radiology*, **92**, 1535–1536.

10. Brueton, M.J., Mavromichalis, J., Goodchild, M.C. and Anderson, C.M. (1977) Hepatic dysfunction in association with pancreatic insufficiency and cyclic neutropenia. *Archives of Diseases in Childhood*, **42**, 147–157.

11. Carlos, R., Abramowsky, M.D., Ricardo, U. and Sorensen, M.D. (1988) Regional enteritis-like enteropathy in a patient with agammaglobulinemia: histologic and immunocytologic studies. *Human Pathology*, **19**, 483–486.

12. Christiane Bastlein, R., Burlefinger, E., Hoizberg, A. *et al.* (1988) Common variable immunodeficiency syndrome and nodular lymphoid hyperplasia in the small intestine. *Endoscopy*, **20**, 272–275.

13. Cooper, M.D., Chase, M.P., Lowman, J.T. *et al.* (1968) Wiskott–Aldrich syndrome. An immunologic deficiency syndrome affecting the afferent limb of immunity. *American Journal of Medicine*, **44**, 499–513.

14. Cunningham-Rundles, C., Brandres, W.E., Good, R.A. and Day, N.K. (1970) Bovine antigens and the formation of circulating immune complexes in selective IgA deficiency. *Journal of Clinical Investigations*, **64**, 272.

15. Current, W.S., Reese, N.C., Ernst, J.V. *et al.* (1983) Human cryptosporidiosis in immunocompetent and immunodeficient persons. *New England Journal of Medicine*, **308**, 1252–1253.

16. Dawson, J., Hodgson, H.J.F., Pepys, M.B. *et al.* (1979) Immunodeficiency malabsorption and secretory diarrhoea. *American Journal of Medicine*, **67**, 540–546.

17. EGID report (1986) Intravenous gammaglobulin for immunodeficiency. Report from the European Group for Immunodeficiency. *Clinical and Experimental Immunology*, **65**, 683–690.

18. Eiden, J., Lasonsky, G.A., Johnson, J. *et al.* (1985) Rotavirus RNA variation during chronic infection of immunocompromised children. *Paediatr. Inf. Dis.*, **4**, 632–637.

19. Freeman, H.J., Shnitka, T.K., Percey, J.R. and Weinstein, W.M. (1977) Cytomegalovirus infection of the gastrointestinal tract in a patient with late onset immunodeficiency syndrome. *Gastroenterology*, **73**, 1397–1403.

20. Fudenberg, H.H., Good, R.A., Goodman, H.C. *et al.* (1971) Primary immunodeficiencies. *Bulletin of the World Health Organisation*, **45**, 125–142.

21. Grybowski, J.D., Selft, T.W., Clemett, A. and Herskovic, T. (1968) Selective immunoglobin A deficiency and intestinal nodular hyperplasia. *Paediatrics*, **42**, 833–837.

22. Harteg, G.D., Van der Meer, J., Jansen, J.B.M.J. *et al.* (1988) Decreased gastric secretion in patients with late-onset hypogammaglobulinaemia. *New England Journal of Medicine*, **318**, 1563–1567.

23. Hermans, P.E., Huizenga, K.A., Hoffman, H.N. *et al.* (1966) Dysgammaglobulinaemia associated with nodular lymphoid hyperplasia of small intestine. *American Journal of Medicine*, **40**, 78–89.

24. Hermans, P.E., Diaz-Buxo, J.A. and Stobo, J.D. (1976) Idiopathic late-onset Immunoglobulin deficiency. *American Journal of Medicine*, **61**, 221–237.

25. Hodgson, H.J.F. and Jewell, D.P. (1977) Selective IgA deficiency and Crohn's disease. *Gut*, **18**, 644–648.

26. Holt, P.D.J., Tandy, N.P., and Anstee, D.J. (1977) Screening of blood donors for IgA deficiency. *Journal of Clinical Pathology*, **30**, 1007.

27. Horowitz, S., Lorenzsonn, V.W., Olsen, W.A. *et al.* (1974) Small intestinal disease in T cell deficiency. *Journal of Pediatrics*, **85**, 457–462.

28. Horwitz, D.A., Webster, A.B. and Newton, C. (1977) B and T lymphocytes in primary hypogammaglobulinaemia. *The Lancet*, **ii**, 823–825.

29. Hyder, J.W. and MacKeigan, J.M. (1988) Anorectal and colonic disease and the immunocompromised tract. *Diseases of the Colon and Rectum*, **31**, 971–977.

30. Hughes, W., Brooks, F. and Conn, H. (1972) Serum gastrin levels in primary hypogammaglobulinaemia and pernicious anaemia. *American Journal of Medicine*, **77**, 746–750.

31. James, D., Asherson, G., Chanarin, I. *et al.* (1974) Cell-mediated immunity to intrinsic factor in autoimmune disorders. *British Medical Journal*, **iv**, 494–496.

32. Leen, C.L.S., Birch, A.D.J., Brettle, R.P., Welsby, P.D. and Yap, P.L. (1986) Salmonellosis in patients with primary hypogammaglobulinaemia. *Journal of Infection*, **12**, 241–245.

33. McCoughlin, G.A., Bradley, J., Chapman, D.M. *et al.* (1976) IgA deficiency and severe post-vagotomy diarrhoea. *The Lancet*, **i**, 168–170.

34. Moffatt, R.E. (1976) Radiologic changes in the thymoma–hypogammaglobulinaemia syndrome. *American Journal of Radiology*, **126**, 1219.

35. Mulholland, D.W., Delaney, J.F. and Simmons, R.L. (1983) Gastrointestinal complications of chronic granulomatous disease. Surgical implications. *Surgery*, **94**, 569–575.

36. Nagura, H., Kohler, P.F. and Brown, W.R. (1979) Immunocytochemical characterisation of lymphocytes in nodular lymphoid hyperplasia of the bowel. *Laboratory Investigation*, **40**, 66–70.

37. Oxelius, V.A., Laurell, A.B., Lindquist, B. *et al.* (1981) IgG subclasses in selective IgA deficiency. *New England Journal of Medicine*, **304**, 1476–1477.

38. Parkin, D.M., McClelland, D.B.L., O'Moore, R.R. *et al.* (1972) Intestinal bacterial flora and bile salt studies in hypogammaglobulinaemia. *Gut*, **13**, 182–188.

39. Penn, J. (1986) Cancer of the anogenital region in renal transplant recipients. Analysis of 65 cases. *Cancer*, **58**, 611–616.

40. Perlmutter, D.H., Leicytner, A.M., Goldman, H.S. and Winter, M.D. (1985) Chronic diarrhoea associated with hypogammaglobulinemia and enteropathy in infants and children. *Digestive Diseases and Sciences*, **30**, 1149–1155.

41. Purtilo, D.T. (1976) Pathogenesis and phenotypes of an X-linked recessive lymphoproliferative syndrome. *The Lancet*, **ii**, 882–884.

42. Ruddell, W.S.J., Bone, E.S., Hill, M.J. *et al.* (1976) Gastric juice nitrate, a risk factor for cancer in the hypochlorhydric stomach. *The Lancet*, **ii**, 1037–1039.

43. Savilhati, E. (1973) IgA deficiency in children. *Clinical and Experimental Immunology*, **13**, 395–400.

44. Siegal, F.P., Siegal, M. and Good, R.A. (1978) Role of helper, suppressor and B-cell defects in the pathogenesis of the hypogammaglobulinaemias. *New England Journal of Medicine*, **299**, 172–176.

45. Sloper, K.S., Dourmashti, R.R., Bird, R.B. *et al.* (1982) Chronic malabsorption due to cryptosporidiosis in a child with immunoglobulin deficiency. *Gut*, **23**, 80–82.

46. Soothill, J.F. (1974) Immunodeficiency and allergy. *Clinical Allergy*, **3**, 511–519.

47. Strober, W., Krakauer, R., Klaerman, H.L. *et al.* (1976) Secretory component deficiency. A disorder of the IgA system. *New England Journal of Medicine*, **294**, 351–356.

48. Swift, M., Sholman, C., Perry, M. and Chase, C. (1976) Malignant neoplasms in families of patients with ataxia telangiectasia. *Cancer Research*, **35**, 209–216.

49. Twomey, J.J., Jordan, P.H., Laughter, A.H. *et al.* (1970) The gastric disorder in common variable hypogamma globulinaemia. *American Journal of Internal Medicine*, **72**, 499–504.

50. van der Meer Jos, W.M., Mouton, R., Peter, W., Daha Mohamed, R. and Schuurman Ruud, K.B. (1986) *Campylobacter jejuni* bacteraemia as a cause of recurrent fever in a patient with hypogammaglobulinaemia. *Journal of Infection*, **12**, 235–239.

51. Wagner, D.K., Wright, J.J., Ansher, A.F. and Gill, V.J. (1988) Dysgonic fermenter 3-associated gastrointestinal disease in a patient with common variable hypogammaglobulinemia. *American Journal of Medicine*, **84**, 315–318.

52. Ward, H., Jalan, K.N., Maitra, T.K. *et al.* (1983) Small intestinal nodular lymphoid hyperplasia in patients with giardiasis and normal serum immunoglobins. *Gut*, **24**, 120–126.

53. Ward, T.T., Klein, K., Borthisle, B.K. (1984) Jejunal infection with Campylobacter. *Annals of Internal Medicine*, **144**, 1072–1074.

54. Webster, A.D.B., Slavin, G., Skinner, M. *et al.* (1981) Coeliac disease with severe hypogammaglobulinaemia. *Gut*, **22**, 153–157.

55. Webster, A.D.B. (1987) Immunodeficiency and the gut. *Ballières Clinical Gastroenterology*, **1**, 547–565.

56. Wood, D.J., David, T.J., Chrystie, I.L. and Totterdell, B. (1988) Chronic enteric virus infection in two T-cell immunodeficient children. *Journal of Medical Virology*, **24**, 435–444.

AMYLOIDOSIS   *(H.J.F. Hodgson)*

DEFINITION

The term 'amyloidosis' describes conditions in which amyloid, a waxy substance predominantly consisting of fibrillar proteins, becomes deposited in tissues.

AETIOLOGY AND PATHOGENESIS

A classification of amyloidosis is shown in *Table 3.39*. Common to all is the deposition of amyloid material, which in excess can lead to organ failure or ischaemia. Macroscopically, in organs such as the liver, amyloid deposits give a fatty, waxy or lardy appearance. At the light microscopic level, amyloid is amorphous eosinophilic hyaline material. At the electron microscopic level, amyloid proteins are predominantly fibrillar strands arranged in characteristic β-pleated sheets.

The precise nature of the fibrillary component of the amyloid protein differs in different forms of amyloid.[20] The two major types are:

1. AL amyloid, in which the molecular structure of the fibrils is that of immunoglobulin light chains. This may complicate almost any dyscrasia affecting cells of the B-cell lineage, though it is most commonly seen with multiple myeloma. In a few cases no other evidence of B-cell dyscrasia

Table 3.39 Classification of amyloidosis

Type	Associated conditions	Fibril type and precursor protein
Systemic amyloidosis		
A. Acquired		
AL	Immunocyte dyscrasias	AL, variable portion of immunoglobulin light chain
AA	Chronic inflammation	AA, SAA
B. Hereditary		
Familial		
Mediterranean fever		AA, SAA
Neuropathic types		Prealbumin
C. Senile	Age	Prealbumin
Local amyloidosis		
Dialysis-associated	Renal failure	β_2-Microglobulin
Endocrine amyloid		Insulin, calcitonin
Primary cutaneous		Keratin
Miscellaneous		Various

may be found; in most individuals, however, a monoclonal gammopathy and Bence Jones proteinurea will be present.

2. AA amyloid, in which the fibrillar protein is derived from SAA serum amyloid A protein. This is an acute-phase reactant normally produced from the liver during episodes of inflammation, whose function may be the binding of effete chromatin; in those chronic inflammatory conditions in which a persistent response is mounted, AA amyloid may eventually be deposited systemically (Table 3.40).

In addition to these well-recognized forms of systemic amyloidosis, there are a number of hereditary forms of systemic amyloidosis. Amyloid deposition may also occur in a form in which there are predominantly local deposits, as in senile cardiac amyloid when the fibrils are derived from pre-albumin, or in the joints of patients on long-term haemodialysis when fibrils derived from β-1-microglobulin are deposited.[25] In all types of amyloid, another protein, amyloid P component, is also precipitated in addition to the fibrillary component.

A former classification of amyloid was into primary and secondary, reflecting some tendency of AL and AA amyloid proteins to be deposited in a different spectrum of organs. Now that it is appreciated that similar organ distributions can be found, and that specific reagents are available to classify amyloid protein deposits histologically (Table 3.41), this classification is less used.

Amyloidosis is relevant to gastroenterologists in three main ways – the clinical syndromes reflecting amyloid deposition in the gut (and liver), the occurrence of amyloidosis complicating chronic gastrointestinal disease (largely Crohn's disease), and the involvement of gastroenterologists as technicians to provide biopsy specimens for histological assessment in suspected amyloid.

SYSTEMIC AMYLOiDOSIS

Clinical features

For both AA and AL amyloid, widespread deposits may be present in the organs without clinical symp-

Table 3.40 Conditions predisposing to AA amyloid

Infection	Chronic inflammation	Tumours
Tuberculosis	Rheumatoid arthritis	Hodgkin's disease
Osteomyelitis	Ankylosing spondylitis	Renal carcinoma
Leprosy	Crohn's disease	Carcinoma of lung
Bronchiectasis	Reiter's disease	
Chronic ulceration	Behçet's disease	
Whipple's disease		

Table 3.41 Histological classification of deposits in systemic amyloidosis

Type	Congo red	Birefringence	Permanganate-fast Congo red staining	Histochemistry
AL	+	+	Permanganate-fast	AL positive Amyloid P positive AA negative
AA	+	+	Permanganate-labile	AL negative Amyloid P positive AA positive

toms.[11] Amyloidosis is frequently an unsuspected autopsy finding in conditions such as rheumatoid arthritis.

In AA amyloid, the commonest clinical presentation is proteinurea, often leading to renal failure as the cause of death; Hepatomegaly, or other organomegaly, is another common presentation. Cardiac and gastrointestinal involvement may be prominent. The associated chronic inflammatory conditions have usually been present for 10 years or so.[10,20] In AL amyloid, although the kidney, liver, heart and gut are often involved, typical sites of involvement are the peripheral and autonomic nervous systems, the tongue, and the joints. As a result of this widespread distribution, the clinical features are protean, including nephrotic syndrome, renal failure, cardiac failure, peripheral and autonomic neuropathy, carpal tunnel syndrome, purpura and arthritis. Clinical findings include macroglossia (specific for AL amyloid), cardiac failure, hepatosplenomegaly, and a variety of skin nodules or plaques (*Figure 3.87*).[10,20]

Gastrointestinal manifestations

Any region of the gastrointestinal tract can be involved, and on histopathological survey some deposits are identified in 70–100% of autopsies.[6] It has been suggested that symptomatic involvement is more common in AL amyloid.[12]

The deposition of amyloid begins perivascularly, but subsequently becomes more diffuse, affecting any layer of the gut, leading eventually to macroscopic waxy thickening. Nodular deposits may occur. The classic histological stain is Congo red, staining deposits which turn apple green in polarized light due to birefringence (*Figure 3.88*). The amyloid does not apparently induce any inflammatory response but, when severe, pressure effects lead to distortion, ischaemia and atrophy.

In all areas of the gastrointestinal tract, marked amyloid deposition, if symptomatic, can lead to motility disorders, or may lead to local ischaemia, causing perforation or haemmorhage.

MOUTH

The macroglossia seen in AL amyloid may be severe enough to interfere with eating. Temporomandibular arthritis may also occur.[22]

OESOPHAGUS

The commonest manifestation is dysphagia,[7] with manometric findings similar to scleroderma or diabetic neuropathy, with poorly progressive or aperistaltic segments. Lower sphincter pressures may be low, and relaxation incoordinate.[1]

STOMACH

Failure of the stomach to empty is the most common presentation, reflecting a combination of autonomic neuropathy and muscular involvement or, much less commonly, pyloric obstruction due to an amyloid deposit.[2] Radiology may show a featureless aperistaltic stomach, enhanced gastric rugae or, rarely, local areas mimicking ulcers or tumours.[13]

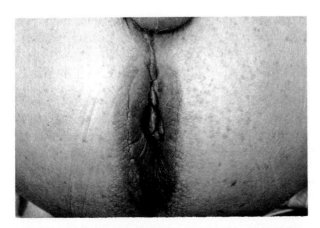

Figure 3.87 Plaque-like perianal amyloid deposit in a patient with long-standing IgA myeloma.

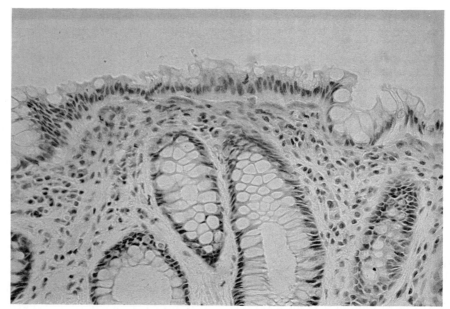

Figure 3.88   Congo red staining of subepithelial deposits of amyloid in rectal biopsy, associated with IgA myeloma.

SMALL INTESTINE

Disordered motility of the small intestine can lead to pseudo-obstruction,[26] or contribute to malabsorption by encouraging bacterial overgrowth. Overall, the clinical picture may therefore be either diarrhoea or constipation. Significant diarrhoea has been reported in up to 40% of individuals in one series, and malabsorption in 6%. Radiological appearances include thickening of the valvulae conniventes, dilatation of small gut loops, slow transit and nodular filling defects.[18,23] Partial villous atrophy may be present, and, in addition, a diffuse subendothelial deposit of amyloid has been thought to contribute to malabsorption. Rarer presentations include intestinal ischaemia and perforation. Substantial enteric protein loss may occur: the mechanism may be either through ulceration of amyloid masses or via lymphatic distortion.[9] It has been suggested that amyloid deposition in the gut may predispose to paralytic ileus in patients with haematological disorders treated with vinca alkaloids.

COLONIC INVOLVEMENT

Amyloid deposits in the colon may present with radiological and clinical features mimicking carcinomas or polyps.[17] Radiological appearances may also resemble inflammatory bowel disease or ischaemic colitis. Other clinical presentations include pseudo-obstruction, diarrhoea or constipation, ischaemic colitis, colonic perforation, and a diffuse colitic form mimicking ulcerative colitis.[21]

GASTROINTESTINAL HAEMORRHAGE

Virtually all patterns of haemorrhage may occur,

from persistent occult blood loss presenting as hypochromic anaemia, to massive haemorrhage from ulcerated deposits or ischaemic areas.[14] Coagulation disorders may contribute, particularly factor X deficiency in AL amyloid.[4]

LIVER INVOLVEMENT[8]

Hepatic involvement may be massive, and is often associated with splenomegaly. Extremely rarely, portal hypertension and oesophageal varices may develop. In most series, hepatic involvement occurs in 50–70%; the characteristic function test abnormality is a mild elevation of alkaline phosphatase. A few patients with hepatic amyloid may develop jaundice due to intrahepatic cholestasis. Liver biopsy is particularly risky in amyloid (see below).

Investigations

Histological assessment remains the investigation of choice for diagnosing and classifying amyloidosis. With multiple biopsies, amyloid deposits can be identified in gastrointestinal tissues of the majority of patients with systemic amyloidosis – in some series nearly 100%.[27] Rectal biopsies are commonly used because, when submucosal tissue is taken, the perivascular area is very likely to be positive; as a single procedure perhaps 80% will be positive. There are sufficient reports of major haemorrhage after liver biopsy to warrant caution; gingival, small intestinal and renal biopsies all have fairly high rates of positivity.

Recently, non-invasive techniques of identifying amyloid deposits utilizing radiolabelled amyloid P component, common to all types of amyloid deposit, have been reported.[5] If available, these may reduce the necessity for multiple biopsies to define sites of involvement.

Treatment

In the absence of effective means of mobilizing amyloid, the treatment strategy is to prevent further deposition by controlling the underlying process. Treatment of the initial process involves either treatment of myelomatosis or similar processes in AL amyloid, or aggressive antibiotic or anti-inflammatory regimes to control the inflammatory conditions precipitating AA amyloid. Attempts to mobilize amyloid deposits with solvents such as dimethyl sulphoxide are experimental. Colchicine diminishes amyloid deposition in familial Mediterranean fever, but not apparently in other conditions.[28]

The gastrointestinal complications of amyloidosis merit individual treatment – nasogastric or parenteral nutrition has been used for severe dysphagia, surgery for acute complications of haemmorhage or perforation, or for obstructing amyloid deposits. Malabsorption requires nutrient replacement, and antibiotic trials for possible bacterial overgrowth. Severe diarrhoea has been reported to respond to a somatostatin analogue.[16]

Prognosis

With a few exceptions, the prognosis of systemic amyloidosis is poor. Fifty per cent of cases of AA amyloid die within 5 years, renal failure being the prime determinant. Prognosis is worse in AL amyloid, reflecting more aggressive amyloidosis and usually associated haematological malignancy. There are some individuals with both types, however, who may survive for a decade or more. Spontaneous regression of amyloidosis, or at least stabilization of the condition, can occur, particularly after removal of the primary inflammatory cause in AA amyloid.[15]

AMYLOIDOSIS SECONDARY TO GASTROINTESTINAL DISEASE

Amyloidosis may complicate long-standing inflammatory disease of the gut. These include generalized conditions such as systemic sclerosis and Behçet's syndrome, but also apparently primarily gastrointestinal disease such as Whipple's disease.[3] The only gastrointestinal condition in which amyloid is other than vanishingly rare is inflammatory bowel

disease. Almost all AA amyloid in the context of inflammatory bowel disease is associated with Crohn's disease, reflecting a more prominent acute-phase protein (including SAA) response in this condition compared with ulcerative colitis.[24] An incidence of 8% in Crohn's disease has been reported.[19] The complication may be recognized early as gut histology is taken to assess the activity of Crohn's disease. Aggressive surgery has been advocated on the basis of occasional case reports of long-term benign clinical courses after removing inflamed bowel, but whether this has any advantage over successful long-term medical control of gut inflammation has not been established.[15] Aggressive surgery when substantial amyloid deposition has occurred may precipitate renal failure.

References

1. Burakoff, R., Rubinow, A. and Cohen, A.S. (1985) Esophageal manometry in familial amyloid polyneuropathy. *American Journal of Medicine*, **79**, 85.
2. Dastur, K.J. and Ward, J.F. (1980) Amyloidosis of the stomach. *Gastrointestinal Radiology*, **5**, 17.
3. Farr, M., Hollwell, C.A., Alton, K.W. *et al.* (1983) Amyloidosis in Whipple's disease. *Journal of the Royal Society of Medicine*, **76**, 963–965.
4. Furie, B., Voo, L., McAdam, K.P.W.J. and Furie, B.C. (1981) Mechanism of factor X deficiency in systemic amyloidosis. *New England Journal of Medicine*, **304**, 827–830.
5. Gilat, T., Revach, M. and Sohnar, E. (1969) Deposition of amyloid in the gastrointestinal tract. *Gut*, **10**, 98–104.
6. Hawkins, P.N., Lavender, P.J. and Pepys, M.B. (1990) Evaluation of systemic amyloidosis by scintigraphy with ^{123}I-labelled serum amyloid P component. *New England Journal of Medicine*, **323**, 508–513.
7. Heitzman, E.J., Heitzman, G.C. and Elliott, C.F. (1962) Primary esophageal amyloidosis. *Archives of Internal Medicine*, **109**, 595–608.
8. Hoffman, M.S., Stein, B.E., Davidian, M.M. and Rosenthal, W.S. (1988) Hepatic amyloidosis presenting as severe intrahepatic cholestasis: a case report and review of the literature. *American Journal of Gastroenterology*, **83**, 783–785.
9. Hunter, A.M., Campbell, I.W., Borsey, D.D.G. and Macaulay, R.A.A. (1979) Protein-losing enteropathy due to gastrointestinal amyloidosis. *Postgraduate Medical Journal*, **55**, 822.
10. Kyle, R.A. (1981) Amyloidosis. *International Journal of Dermatology*, **20**, 20–25, 75–80.
11. Kyle, R.A. and Bayrd, E.D. (1975) Amyloidosis: review of 236 cases. *Medicine* (Baltimore), **54**, 271–299.
12. Kyle, R.A. and Greipp, P.R. (1983) Amyloidosis

(AL) Clinical and laboratory features in 229 cases. *Mayo Clinic Proceedings*, **58**, 665.

13. Legge, D.A., Carlson, H.C. and Wollaeger, E.E. (1970) Roentgenologic appearances of systemic amyloidosis involving the gastrointestinal tract. *American Journal of Roentgenology*, **110**, 406–412.

14. Levy, D.J., Franklin, G.O. and Rosenthal, W.S. (1982) Gastrointestinal bleeding and amyloidosis. *American Journal of Gastroenterology*, **77**, 422–426.

15. Mandelstam, P., Simmons, D.E. and Mitchell, B. (1989) Regression of amyloid in Crohn's disease after bowel resection – a 190 year follow up. *Journal of Clinical Gastroenterology*, **11**, 324–326.

16. O'Connor, C.R. and O'Dorisio, T.M. (1989) Amyloidosis, diarrhoea and a somatostatin analogue. *Annals of Internal Medicine*, **110**, 665.

17. O'Doherty, D.P., Neoptolemos, J.P., Bouch, D.C. and Wood, K.F. (1987) Surgical complications of amyloid disease. *Postgraduate Medical Journal*, **63**, 281–286.

18. Pandannath, G.S., Levine, S.M., Sorokin, J.J. and Jacoby, J.H. (1978) Selective massive amyloidosis of the small intestine mimicking multiple tumours. *Radiology*, **129**, 609.

19. Pepys, M.B. (1982) Goulstonian lecture: C-reactive protein, amyloidosis and the acute phase response. In: *Advanced Medicine*, Vol. 18, pp. 208–229 (Ed.) Sarner, M. London: Pitman.

20. Pepys, M.B. (1987) Amyloidosis. In: *Oxford Textbook of Medicine,* 2nd edn, pp. 145–156 (Eds) Weatherall, D.J., Ledingham, J.G.G. and Warrell, D.A. Oxford: Oxford University Press.

21. Sanchez, G.J.A., Molinero, M.R., Sayans, D.J. and Sanchez, J.F. (1989) Colonic perforation by amyloidosis. Report of a case. *Diseases of the Colon and Rectum*, **32**, 437–440.

22. Schwartz, Y., Tamse, A., Kissin, E. and Shani, M. (1979) An unusual case of temporomandibular joint arthropathy in systemic amyloidosis. *Journal of Oral Medicine*, **34**, 40.

23. Seliger, G., Krassner, R.L., Beranbaum, E.R. and Miller, F. (1971) The spectrum of roentgen appearance in amyloidosis of the small and large bowel. *Radiology*, **100**, 63.

24. Shorvon, P.J. (1977) Amyloidosis and inflammatory bowel disease. *American Journal of Digestive Diseases*, **22**, 209–213.

25. Takahashi, S., Morita, T., Koda, Y., Murayama, H. and Hirasawa, Y. (1988) Gastrointestinal involvement of dialysis-related amyloidosis. *Clinical Nephrology*, **30**, 168–171.

26. Wald, A., Kichler, J. and Mendelow, H. (1981) Amyloidosis and chronic intestinal pseudoobstruction. *Digestive Diseases and Sciences*, **26**, 462–465.

27. Yamada, M., Hatakeyama, S. and Tsukagoshhi, H. (1985) Gastrointestinal amyloid deposition in AL (primary or myeloma-associated) and AA (secondary) amyloidosis: diagnostic value of gastric biopsy. *Human Pathology*, **16**, 1206.

28. Zemer, D., Pras, M., Sohar, E., Modan, M., Cabili, S. and Gafni, J. (1986) Colchicine in the prevention and treatment of amyloidosis of familial Mediterranean fever. *New England Journal of Medicine*, **314**, 1003.

FOOD ALLERGY AND FOOD INTOLERANCE *(P.J. Kumar)*

INTRODUCTION

Ingestion of certain foods can produce severe clinical reactions in some people. However, over recent years, many symptoms such as headaches, palpitations, panic attacks, vomiting and anxiety have been ascribed to being due to a food allergy. 'Food and eating occupy such a prominent position in our phychosocial world that they are only too readily blamed for our most ethereal woes!'[60] Unfortunately, as symptoms are usually subjective, the differentiation of a true food allergy from psychiatric ill health is often difficult. For this reason the clinical section will comprise two headings: acute allergy (probably IgE mediated), which is well established in children and for which there is good evidence, and, secondly, delayed reactions which often occur in adults, but for which firm evidence is still lacking.

DEFINITION

Whether a set of symptoms is due to food allergy, food intolerance or a food fad is often difficult to elucidate.[76] In general, ingested foods can cause clinical symptoms but these are not necessarily due to an allergy and may be idiosyncratic. The term 'allergy' or 'sensitivity' should be reversed for reactions resulting from immunological hypersensitivity, of which the main mediator is IgE. Historically, the first clinical demonstration of the immunological basis of food allergy was in 1921 when Prauznitz transferred food sensitivity from his friend Kustner[72] to his own skin by a subcutaneous injection of serum. Food 'anaphylaxis' is an extremely acute food sensitivity reaction involving IgE antibody and also other chemical mediators. The term 'food intolerance', however, should be reversed for non-immunologically mediated reactions. These adverse reactions may be pharmacological or metabolic (see *Table 3.42*).

Patients may be intolerant of food because the food itself contains substances which have a pharmacological action, e.g. histamine in mackerel or

Table 3.42 Types of food intolerances

| Pharmacological |
| Chemical mediators |
| Toxic substance |
| Irritants |

Idiosyncratic
    Gastrointestinal (e.g. alactasia)
    General (e.g. phenylketonuria)

Allergic
    Gastrointestinal (e.g. cow's milk allergy)
    General (e.g. eczema)

From Soothill.[85]

canned foods, tyramine in certain cheeses, and caffeine.[7] Alternatively, foods may contain substances which release chemical mediators as, for example, histamine released by tomatoes or strawberries. Certain chemicals in food may be toxic and produce clinical disease states, for example hexachlorobenzene, used as a dressing for wheat in Turkey and which produced acquired porphyria,[6,17] and acetanilide in rape-seed oil, which results in respiratory failure.[90]

Metabolic reactions in certain patients may be associated with a deficiency of a particular enzyme involved in the degeneration of certain foods, e.g. milk-induced diarrhoea in patients with alactasia, or fava bean-induced haemolytic anaemia in patients with glucose-6-phosphate dehydrogenease deficiency.

Apart from these difficulties with definition, the subject is further confused by a lack of firmly defined diagnostic criteria and also a paucity of reliable diagnostic tests.

PATHOGENESIS OF TRUE FOOD ALLERGY

The exact mechanisms of the pathogenesis of food allergic disease is still unclear and several factors may be involved. These include the permeability of the gastrointestinal tract, the amount and type of antigen, the development of immune responses to the ingested antigen (both local and systemic), a possible genetic predisposition and, lastly, the effect on the end-organ with the production of clinical symptoms.

Antigenically intact food proteins are known to be absorbed across healthy gastrointestinal mucosa.[96,98] Although the amount absorbed may be nutritionally insignificant, these small amounts are sufficient to immunize and result in the production of antibodies. The presence of these antibodies, however, do not usually cause any clinical symptoms and have no significance.

Permeability

In humans, the gut mucosa is mature by full term of pregnancy and there is evidence that gut 'closure' occurs at about 30 weeks of gestation.[74] The immunological aspects of infant feeding are complex,[85] but when a food is first eaten and appears in the blood, specific antibody (usually IgA) is produced.[56] On subsequent ingestion of the antigen, very little enters the blood due to a protective response (immune exclusion). Ingestion of an antigen also induces partial immunological tolerance to subsequent parenteral contact with the antigen.[18] This tolerance and possibly exclusion may be influenced by nutrition.[89]

Maternal milk (colostrum) contains protective antibodies but may also contain antigens from the food that the mother has eaten.[45] These may trigger symptoms such as atopic dermatitis in the already sensitized infant.[37] It has also been suggested that IgA deficiency predisposes to food allergy by increasing gut permeability,[92] but these patients may also have other defective immunoregulatory processes.[25]

The adult gastrointestinal mucosa has a complex defence mechanism preventing the passage of antigens into the body. The epithelium consists of tightly packed surface cells with overlying mucus and luminal secretory IgA. The mucus contains glycoproteins which inhibit attachment of microorganisms to epithelial cells and interact with allergens. Other factors which minimize epithelial cell penetration are luminal intestinal secretions and gastrointestinal peristalsis, which minimizes the antigenic exposure to the mucosa. Nevertheless, antigens may cross the epithelium through defects in the gut, and the transport of large molecules across intact mucosa has been demonstrated.[97] Even if antigens have crossed the mucosa, the liver and the reticuloendothelial system play a significant part in filtering absorbed substances from the portal venous blood.[88] Other immunological mechanisms are discussed below.

Macromolecules can be absorbed across the intestinal epithelium by passing between the tight junctions of cells (persorption), by pinocytosis, and by uptake through the M or microfold cells which overlie the Peyer's patches. Within the cell, the macromolecules are contained inside membrane bound vesicles (phagosomes) where normal intracellular digestion of macromolecules takes place.

There is evidence to suggest that enhanced jejunal permeability to macromolecules can also occur during acute gastroenteritis both in animals[47] and in infants.[34] This has also been shown after chemotherapy and radiation[36] and other insults causing intestinal surface damage, e.g. alcohol.[103]

Type of antigen

The nature of the allergens in particular foods is still uncertain. Some foods, such as egg, milk, fish and wheat, have a very strong tendency to sensitize[87] whilst others are fairly innocuous. IgE-mediated reactions can be produced by egg white, crab, shrimp, peanuts, tomatoes, soya beans and cow's milk. Milk contains over 20 proteins, but sensitizing reactions are usually observed with casein, α-lactalbumin, β-lactoglobulin and bovine serum albumin. Some substances such as in soya beans can cross-sensitize patients to other related vegetables such as peas, beans and lentils.[30] Contaminating substances in foods, such as penicillin, should also be considered.[5] The response to some foods may be variable. For example, some patients get an enteropathy with gluten whilst others have been reported to have a gluten-sensitive diarrhoea without an enteropathy.[20]

In general, where a reaction is caused by very small amounts of a substance it is likely to have an allergic basis. However, reactions to food additives, e.g. monosodium glutamate,[53] colouring agents such as tartrazine and preservatives such as benzoic acid[57] may well be due to toxicity.

Immunological reactions

Many immunological reactions may be involved in the pathogenesis of food allergies.[81] Hypersensitivity may be antibody or cell mediated, and tissue damage may involve a range of soluble factors, activation products of polymorphonuclear leukocytes, macrophages, eosinophils or direct cell membrane events. The various types of food hypersensitivity are not mutually exclusive and may occur at once or in sequence.

Most common allergic reactions to food are caused by atopic phenomena involving type I IgE-mediated hypersensitivity. These cause immediate-onset reactions. IgE antibodies to foods such as cow's milk protein, eggs or nuts can be detected by the radioallergosorbent test in the serum of some but not all patients.

The tolerance of type III (immune complex mediated) or type IV (delayed cell-mediated hypersensitivity) is uncertain. Secretory IgA antibodies to a variety of foods are found in upper intestinal secretions.[27] Most normal individuals have low

titres of circulating antibody to food proteins.[51] Circulating immune complexes have been demonstrated in both healthy and food allergic subjects after ingestion of food.[66] In healthy subjects these are predominantly IgA-containing[55] whereas in food allergic individuals the complexes may also contain IgG and IgE and may bind complement.[12,13] Their deposition in the gut or elsewhere may lead to local inflammation, as has been demonstrated in the submucosa of the gut in cow's milk allergy.[82] With respect to cell-mediated type IV hypersensitivity, evidence is accumulating that T cells can produce villous atrophy.[28]

Genetic predisposition

A genetic predisposition is suggested by the familial tendency of some food allergies. The best documented is that of the association of coeliac disease with the tissue type of HLA-A1, B8, DR3, DQw2. Atopic patients presenting with eczema have been shown to have an excess of HLA-A1 and B8, whereas atopic patients with hayfever have an excess of HLA-A3 and B8.[86] However, there are many other complex associations, as atopy may be associated with transient IgA deficiency[3] or defects in complement C2 and yeast opsonization.[94]

Other factors such as environment may well play a part, as concordance or atopic allergic disease in monozygotic twins is not 100%.[49] In eczema of childhood, the type of feeding in infancy may be important as there are lower incidences of eczema in offspring of atopic parents fed breast milk when compared to those on artificial feeding.[59]

Miscellaneous factors

It has been suggested that some of the psychiatric changes seen in, for example, coeliac disease or schizophrenia, may be due to the direct toxic action of antigen on brain cells. Klee et al.[48] have shown that some digests of dietary protein have opioid activity. These peptides or exorphins are produced in the gastrointestinal tract, resist digestion by enzymes, cross the blood–brain barrier and eventually act as opioids on central opioid receptors in the brain. However, further studies are required to establish whether there are any direct immunological or endocrine effects of foods on the central nervous system.

Prostaglandins have also been put forward as causing abdominal pain and diarrhoea in acute allergic gastroenteritis. It has been shown that raised stool and blood prostaglandin levels may be associated with gastrointestinal symptoms,[14] but it must be remembered that prostaglandins are generated in many conditions and may not necessarily be responsible for any symptoms.

INCIDENCE AND PREVALENCE

Exact figures for the incidence and prevalence of food allergy are impossible to obtain. In adult life there may be a diagnostic difficulty in differentiating an 'allergy' from a subjective psychological impression. In the USA it has been stated that immediate and delayed hypersensitive reactions to food are present in between 10 and 20% of the population, i.e. 25 million and 50 million people.[11] Food intolerance is a fashionable diagnosis and many of these patients may well not have an allergic reaction to food.

Food allergy presenting in childhood has been more clearly defined. The incidence is probably greatest in the first months and years of life and decreases with age, as most childhood food allergy has a natural tendency to recover.[21,31] Infantile eczema, which is probably largely food allergic, affects 3% of infants[3] and infantile colic is said to be even more common.[41] Estimates of food allergy causing asthma and atopic dermatitis range from 3 to 40%.[38] Bleumink[9] has estimated that foods may cause atopic symptoms in 0.2% of the general population.

CLINICAL FEATURES

Clinically, reactions to food can be divided into 'early' and 'delayed'. The immediate (anaphylactic) reactions to food are easily recognized and can be serious. Reactions occurring within a few hours can also be IgE mediated. However, the delayed reactions (not IgE mediated) are much more difficult to diagnose as they are often non-specific, vague and may be chronic. Here the diagnosis is often confused as it is often difficult for the patient to relate a food to the symptom in a double-blind study and even more difficult to divorce it from a psychiatric origin in adults.

Early or acute reactions to food

The most severe reaction to food is anaphylaxis with urticaria and laryngeal oedema, which can lead to asphyxia and death. Shellfish, eggs and milk have been implicated. Immediate reactions within minutes of eating certain foods, causing swelling of lips and tongue, vomiting, rhinorrhoea, urticaria or asthma, are thought to be IgE mediated. In these cases the total IgE is usually raised, a positive skin

prick test may be elicited or a positive radioallergoabsorbant test obtained. These subjects often have a family history of atophy. In adults, such allergies are not often a clinical problem as patients learn to avoid the offending foods. In infancy, however, features such as vomiting and anaphylactic shock can develop within minutes and may be provoked, for example, with less than 1 ml of milk.[80]

Symptoms related to foods may be widespread or may effect predominantly the gastrointestinal, dermatological, respiratory or any other system. The symptoms described below are some that have been reported frequently in the literature, as single-case reports or uncontrolled studies.

Gastrointestinal symptoms

Gastrointestinal symptoms due to allergic causes have been mainly described in children although they may persist or develop in adult life.

Nausea, vomiting, diarrhoea, abdominal pain, distension, constipation, malabsorption and a protein-losing enteropathy have all been attributed to food intolerance. Vomiting and abdominal pain are common manifestations of food allergy. In children, milk-induced gastrointestinal bleeding in infants with hypochromic microcytic anaemia has been described.[102] Hypoproteinaemia and eosinophilia have been described in an allergic gastroenteropathy.[95]

Allergic gastroenteritis is characterized by eosinophilic infiltration of the mucosa and there may be peripheral eosinophilia and iron deficiency anaemia secondary to gastrointestinal blood loss or a protein-losing enteropathy. The pathological classification is confused[44] and not all reports have a definite food allergic basis. Again in children, Katz et al.[46] have described children between the ages of 6 months and 15 years with eosinophilic infiltration of the gastric mucosa associated with protein and blood loss. There are reports of eosinophilic infiltration of the oesophagus in an infant,[29] and also of the stomach[46] in association with a history of food intolerance, response to food avoidance and laboratory evidence of reaginic allergy.

Much of our knowledge of gastrointestinal allergy comes from work on *cow's milk protein intolerance* in infancy.[23,40] The syndrome results from the sensitization of a child to one or more proteins from cow's milk, which results in damage to the gastrointestinal mucosa. Clinically, patients may present acutely with vomiting and a shock-like state or with a chronic syndrome with colic, diarrhoea or constipation and, possibly, malabsorption.[50] Urticaria and eczema or wheezing and asthma may also be present. Its reported prevalence varies from 3 to 12%,[19,30,32] presumably due to the use of different diagnostic criteria. With the advent of foods containing proteins other than cow's milk, other sensitivities such as those to soya protein have now been described. Soya protein sensitivity can cause various symptoms,[2] and can also produce an enteropathy.[71]

Infantile colic in the first few months of life may be due to cow's milk protein intolerance but studies are not conclusive.[78,100]

Coeliac disease is considered elsewhere (p. 537) and has the pathological lesion of subtotal villous atrophy which reverts to a more normal villous pattern on withdrawal of gluten from the diet. A transient gluten intolerance with intestinal damage has been described in children[99] and possibly in adults.[54]

There is some evidence that certain conditions of the colon and rectum may be due to food sensitivity. An association between ulcerative colitis and cow's milk ingestion was postulated many years ago[91] and Whorwell and Wright[101] favour an association between an early ingestion of cow's milk protein and ulcerative colitis. Most cases of colitis in infants below the age of 1 year are said to be due to food allergy and have a striking eosinophilia apparent histologically,[39,42] and a haemorrhagic proctitis can occur in patients with cow's milk intolerance.[14] Favourable reports of responses to sodium cromoglycate in non-specific proctitis and ulcerative colitis[7] have been documented, but corroborating reports are scanty. Non-specific anal disorders such as pruritus ani have also been associated with food allergies, but there is little supporting evidence.

Recently, cases of the irritable bowel syndrome, which improved on a food exclusion diet, have been reported,[1] and remissions have been obtained in patients with Crohn's disease on elemental diets.[65] There is no evidence to suggest that either of these diseases is related to a food allergy and the temporary improvement may be related to other factors.

Dermatological reactions

Atopic eczema is largely a disease of young children and affects at least 5% of all children at some time. It affects the face and limb flexures as an itchy, red rash with scaling, vesiculation, exudation and crusting. Patients often have asthma, allergic rhinitis, a family history of atopy and a high serum IgE level.[8,59,78] Despite this, the slow evolution and eventual histological appearance are more suggestive of a delayed hypersensitivity reaction possibly due to a cutaneous basophil hypersensitivity. These patients differ from those with asthma and hayfever by having a much higher frequency of positive immediate skin test to foods[6] and much greater levels of circulating food-specific IgE (radioallergosorbent test).[94]

Urticaria consists of oedema and erythema of the skin; the lesions are itchy and last from 30 minutes to 72 hours. Histamine and possibly other mediators are involved in provoking urticarial reactions. Urticaria in children is provoked by food more often than in adults. Halpern[35] found that 44% of children with urticaria had a food intolerance and the foods producing urticaria were similar to those causing other clinical effects.

Some of the more resistant cases of urticaria[4] are thought to be provoked by synthetic food additives such as azo dyes (tartrazine, amaranth, coccine nouvelle, sunset yellow), preservatives (sodium benzoate) and other additives (fat antioxidants, sodium nitrate, sodium metabisulphite, tyramine and drugs such as penicillin, tetracycline, quinine and menthol). Most patients who react to these substances also react to salicylates.[61]

The diagnosis of food-induced urticaria is not difficult if the patient can identify the provoking food eaten within 1 or 2 hours of the development of his symptoms. Recurrent attacks, however, may be difficult to analyse as urticarial rashes can be produced by other non-specific factors, like pressure and exercise. Recurrent challenges with capsules containing tartrazine, yeast, penicillin and placebo may be helpful, but laboratory investigations such as skin prick tests or radioallergosorbent tests are often not helpful.

Respiratory reactions

Food-induced rhinitis in asthma is well recognized and may be associated with other symptoms. Burr *et al.*[15,16] found that 17% of adults believed that a particular food could provoke an attack while this was only true in 3% of children. Asthma may be precipitated by inhalation of the antigen. However, the route of an antigenic stimulation may vary from patient to patient; thus, alcoholic drinks may provoke asthma whereas alcoholic fumes or intravenous alcohol are less likely to do so.[33] In some cases, the congeners in spirits, or histamine in red and white wine may provoke the attacks. Most patients with food-induced asthma have high IgE levels and often positive prick tests or radioallergosorbent tests. However, a subgroup with asthma and low IgE levels and negative tests has also been described.[54]

Symptoms of runny nose, sneezing and nasal obstruction may be caused by certain foods and are often part of a more generalized allergic reaction.

Stimulation is caused not only by inhalation but has also been provoked by nasogastric feeding of milk.[10] Nasal polyps may occur in adults. Other respiratory symptoms include chronic respiratory disease described in children with hypersensitivity to cow's milk; this may be followed by pulmonary haemosiderosis.[5]

Migraine

There are many reports suggesting that food can provoke migraine attacks.[24,62,63] Chocolate, cheese, citrus fruits and alcohol seem to be the major precipitating factors. It has been suggested that foods containing tyramine may provoke headaches but this has not been confirmed. Sandler et al.[79] proposed that migraine is due to reduced phenylethylamine (contained in chocolate) and tyramine oxidation, and that one of the forms of platelet monoamine oxidase is defective. Phenylethylamine is thought to stimulate α receptors and thus produce migraine. A study by Egger and his colleagues[24] reviewed 88 children in a migraine clinic. They put them in a double-blind trial on an oligogenic diet and found that 93% improved. Forty of these children were put into a double-blind, crossover trial and it was found that eight children had no symptoms with any foods, 17 had symptoms with one food item and 24 had symptoms with several foods. In total, 55 food items provoked symptoms. These studies suggest that migraine can be triggered by certain foods.

Arthritis

It has been suggested that joint pains can be due to food sensitivity. Unfortunately, most clinical studies on the relationship between food and arthritis have been performed in an open and uncontrolled fashion. Sköldstam et al.[83] performed a controlled dietary study in patients with rheumatoid arthritis and found reduced symptom scores during the fasting period. Other studies report variable results and trials are in progress.[22]

Another study[67] found that most patients claiming to have food-induced rheumatic symptoms did not show these on blind challenge. The authors suggested that probably not more than 5% of patients with rheumatic disease have an immunological sensitivity to food. In a study in rabbits, Panush and his colleagues[68] looked at food-induced arthritis and found that 53% of rabbits fed on milk produced an inflammatory arthritis. There is no evidence that palindromic rheumatism may be due to food allergies.

Delayed reactions

These reactions develop hours or even days after the ingestion of food and are very difficult to delineate. The course and the relationship between the ingestion of the food and symptoms is difficult to prove. Multiple vague symptoms, e.g. tiredness or malaise, are unlikely to be due to food allergy or an intolerance and probably have a psychiatric basis. Current adult gastroenterological allergy clinics are full of patients with food fads and obsessional neuroses and it is important to distinguish these from patients with true food allergies.[70] Members of the public, clinical ecologists and some health professionals are convinced that reactions to food and environmental agents are common. It has been suggested that vague symptoms such as headaches, insomnia, palpitations, abdominal bloating, fatigue, breathlessness are due to food. In children, where there is good evidence that allergies to certain foods occur, poor school performance and bad behaviour and hyperactivity have been put down to being due to foods. Unfortunately, practitioners may diagnose a food intolerance using unconventional and unscientific techniques such as hair analysis, cytotoxic blood tests, iridology, sublingual and injection provocation tests. Recently, Jewett and his colleagues[43] performed a double-blind study of symptom provocation to food sensitivity. Eighteen patients were selected by clinical ecologists as patients who had reported symptoms on open injection tests with a variety of food extracts. On double-blind testing, patients identified 16 of 60 active injections (27%) as provoking symptoms and 44 of 180 control injections (24%) as active. The symptoms elicited by both the control injections and food extracts were identical. Subsequently, seven patients were given neutralizing injections and these were found to be as effective in relieving symptoms as control injections. This study suggested that the non-blind symptom provocation and relief were based on a placebo reaction and that symptoms were only reproduced if the patients knew the allergen.

The fact that psychiatric problems have a considerable bearing on patients with food allergy was shown in a study of 22 patients who were referred to an allergy clinic and had a full psychiatric evaluation.[73] Only four patients emerged as having clear evidence of food intolerance, three with atopic food allergy and one with salicylate intolerance. The remaining 18 had psychiatric diagnoses of depressive neurosis, neurasthenia, hysterical neurosis etc. These patients were compared to an unselected group of patients referred to a general psychiatric clinic; the two groups of patients had identical patterns of psychiatric symptoms, but the only difference was that the group with unconfirmed food allergies was predominantly composed of professional class people.

Unfortunately, 'self deception affects doctors as well as patients',[26] and in the process of being kind to our patients by seeking a non-psychiatric diagnosis we may in the long run be doing them a great disservice.

The 'total allergy syndrome' has received much publicity. These patients are thought to be very sensitive to contaminants of the environment. Symptoms reported include weakness, lethargy, faintness, convulsions, blackouts, migraine, disorders of bowel and bladder and aching joints. There is at present little evidence to suggest that these patients have an allergic disease and they may well be suffering from anorexia nervosa or hysteria.

The adverse consequences arising from a diagnosis of food allergy was highlighted by Robertson *et al.*[75] They reported four cases where the diagnosis of food allergy and treatment by a practitioner with alternative medicine delayed the diagnosis and treatment of a serious underlying organic disease.

INVESTIGATIONS

A careful history may establish a direct relationship between the ingestion of a particular food and the development of symptoms on repeated occasions; this may be sufficient for diagnosis. Often if a food has already been identified by the patient, he or she avoids eating it and therefore a clinical problem does not arise. A history of atopic disease in childhood and in the family should be taken as the incidence of food allergies is increased in this group of patients.

There are no reliable laboratory tests for food allergy. The main problem is to identify the patient who warrants clinical and laboratory testing. It may be possible to establish, on questioning, whether a patient has a true allergy, a food fad or a personality or psychiatric problem. In general, vague symptoms and those where the reaction is delayed are probably not due to food allergy.

Laboratory tests are usually of more help in diagnosing the immediate type of reaction.

- *Skin prick testing* with a variety of common allergens will help in the diagnosis of atopy. Unfortunately, prick tests to foods may show a high proportion of false positives and have little correlation with the radioallergosorbent test. Bussierett[14] found that only 31% of patients with cow's milk allergy (diagnosed by exclusion and challenge) had a positive skin test. However, tests for eggs, nuts and fish may be slightly more reliable.
- The *serum IgE level* may be high in the immediate type of hypersensitivity reactions.
- *Radioallergosorbant tests (RASTs)* for specific antigen IgE. These may occasionally demonstrate circulating antibodies to specific foods but the correlation with symptoms is poor. Radioallergosorbent tests are affected by the presence of IgG antibodies and the test does not detect cell-bound IgE antibodies. There may also be interlaboratory variations and cross-reactivity problems.
- *Measurements of circulating immune complexes*, leukocyte histamine release test and organ culture test. These have all been performed in various conditions but at the moment are research tools only. Humoral antibodies against foods are also seen in normal individuals, but may be useful in assessing treatment in patients if antibody titres fall.[10,64]
- *Exclusion diets.* If a food has been delineated, the next simple approach is to eliminate it from the diet; most adult patients may already have done so. If the history is vague and the physician is convinced that there is a food-related problem, many would go on to try an elimination diet. These diets, however, are time-consuming and cumbersome and range from being very simple to extremely tedious. With multiple foods involved it is suggested that an elimination diet should not be undertaken unless the patient is atopic, has a high IgE level and, possibly, positive radioallergosorbent tests. A basic exclusion diet usually eliminates colourings, preservatives, milk, eggs, dairy products, fish and nuts, and invariably contains one meat item, one vegetable and spring water initially. Many of these diets have been prescribed by clinical 'ecologists' and workers in fringe medicine.

The effect of dietary challenge is usually easier to evaluate when the patient has been symptom-free on an elimination diet. A 'challenge' can take various forms – it may be by sublingual provocation test, by inhalation, by intragastric or intraduodenal instillation or by using capsules containing the particular food. If possible, these challenges should be performed in a double-blind fashion and the results assessed in terms of symptoms produced. If the symptoms are predominantly respiratory, a peak flow reading may be helpful, and, if gastrointestinal, a jejunal biopsy and the production of clinical symptoms of diarrhoea or pain may be helpful.

TREATMENT

Early and acute reactions

Treatment is dependent where possible, on antigen avoidance. Elimination of a suspect food such as strawberries or shellfish presents no problem as the patient will probably already have learnt to avoid the suspect food. Treatment of asthma, rhinitis, eczema or migraine is again by avoidance of a particular food with symptomatic therapy of the symptom. Desensitization therapy using injections or oral or nasal administration has been used for immediate reactions, but with little success. In cow's milk protein intolerance or coeliac disease, patients are treated with milk-free or gluten-free diets, respectively.

There is no specific drug therapy. Oral sodium cromoglycate has been used prophylactically in patients with IgE-mediated food allergy. Antihistamines, e.g. terfenadine and brompheniramine, have been tried with some success although some have a sedative effect. Prostaglandin synthetase inhibitors, e.g. aspirin and other non-steroidal anti-inflammatory drugs, can be tried although their action is mainly non-specific.

Delayed reactions

As stated earlier, many of these are probably psychiatric in origin. Patients require much reassurance and support and possibly referral to a psychiatrist. However, many are mistaken in their belief that they have a food allergic disorder. They may have been put on very restricted diets which present difficulties in ensuring adequate amounts of protein, calories, vitamins and calcium. A small proportion of patients, however, will not be helped and will probably go from physician to physician to find one who will agree with their preconceived ideas.

References

1. Alun Jones, V., McLaughlan, P., Shorthouse, M. *et al.* (1982) Food intolerance: a major factor in the pathogenesis of irritable bowel syndrome. *The Lancet*, **ii**, 1115–1117.

2. Ament, M.E. and Rubin, C.E. (1972) Soy protein – another cause of the fat intestinal lesion. *Gastroenterology*, **62**, 227–234.

3. Atherton, D.J., Sewell, M., Soothill, J.F. *et al.* (1978) A double-blind cross-over trial of an antigen avoidance diet in atopic eczema. *The Lancet*, **i**, 401–403.

4. August, P.J. (1980) Urticaria. In: *Proceedings of the First Food Allergy Workshop*, pp. 76–81 (Ed.) Coombs, R.R.A. Oxford: Medical Education Services.

5. Bahna, S.L. and Heiner, D.C. (1980) *Allergies to Milk.* New York: Grune and Stratton.

6. Barnetson, R.St.C. (1980) Hyperimmunoglobulinaemia E in atopic eczema is associated with "food allergy". In: *International Symposium on Atopic Dermatitis (Stockholm)* (Ed.) Rajka, G. *Acta Dermatologica Supplementum* **92**, 94–96.

7. Barnetson, R.St.C. and Lessof, M.M. (1983) Challenges to medical orthodoxy. In: *Clinical Reactions to Food,* pp. 15–34 (Ed.) Lessof, M.M. Chichester: Wiley.

8. Barnetson, R.St.C. and Merrett, T.G. (1980) Atopic eczema. In: *Proceedings of the First Food Allergy Workshop*, pp. 69–95 (Ed.) Coombs, R.R.A. Oxford: Medical Education Services.

9. Bleumink, E. (1979) Food allergy and the gastrointestinal tract. In: *Immunology of the Gastrointestinal Tract*, pp. 195–213 (Ed.) Asquith, P. Edinburgh: Churchill Livingstone.

10. Bock, S.A., Buckley, J., Holst, A. and May, C.D. (1977) Proper use of skin tests with food extracts. *Clinical Allergy*, **7**, 375–383.

11. Brenemen, J.C. (1987) Immunology of food allergy. In: *Handbook of Food Allergies*, p. 1 (Ed.) Brenemen, J.C. New York: Marcel Dekker.

12. Brostoff, J., Carini, C., Wraith, D.G. and Johns, P. (1979) Production of IgE complexes by allergen challenge in atopic patients and the effect of sodium cromoglycate. *The Lancet*, **i**, 1268–1270.

13. Brostoff, J., Carini, C., Wraith, D.G. *et al.* (1979) Immune complexes in atophy. In: *The Mast Cell*, pp. 380–383 (Eds) Pepys, J. and Edwards, A.M. London: Pitman.

14. Buisseret, P. (1978) Common manifestations of cow's milk allergy in children. *The Lancet*, **i**, 304–306.

15. Burr, M.L., Eldridge, B.A. and Borysiewicz, L.K. (1974) Peak expiratory flow rates before and after exercise in school children. *Archives of Diseases in Childhood*, **49**, 923–924.

16. Burr, M.L., St Leger, A.S., Bevan, C. and Merrett, T.G. (1975) A community survey of asthmatic characteristics. *Thorax*, **30**, 663–668.

17. Cam, C. and Nigogosyan, G. (1963) Acquired toxic porphyria cutanea tarda due to hexachlorobenzene. *Journal of the American Medical Association*, **183**, 88.

18. Chase, M.W. (1946) Inhibition of experimental drug allergy by prior feeding of the sensitising agent. *Proceedings of the Society of Experimental Biology and Medicine*, **61**, 257.

19. Collins-Williams, C. (1956) The incidence of milk-allergy in paediatric practice. *Journal of Paediatrics*, **48**, 38–59.

20. Cooper, B.T., Holmes, G.K.T., Ferguson, R. *et al.* (1980) Gluten-sensitive diarrhoea without evidence of coeliac disease. *Gastroenterology*, **79**, 801–806.

21. Danneus, A., Inganas, M., Johansson, S.G.O. and Fouchard, T. (1979) Intestinal uptake of ovalbumin in malabsorption and food allergy in relation to serum IgG antibody and orally administered sodium cromoglycate. *Clinical Allergy*, **9**, 263–270.

22. Darlington, G. (1985) Does food intolerance have any role in the aetiology and management of rheumatoid arthritis. *Annuals of Rheumatic Disease*, **44**, 801–804.

23. Eastham, E.J. and Walker, W.A. (1979) Adverse effects of milk formula and ingestion on the gastrointestinal tract. *Gastroenterology*, **76**, 365–374.

24. Egger, J., Carter, C.M., Wilson, J., Turner, M.W. and Soothill, J.F. (1983) Is migraine a food allergy? A double-blind trial of oligo antigenic dietary treatment. *The Lancet*, **ii**, 865–869.

25. Ferguson, A. (1983) Immunology and physiology of digestion. In: *Clinical Reactions to Food*, pp. 59–86 (Ed.) Lessof, M.H. Chichester: Wiley.

26. Ferguson, A. (1990) Food sensitivity or self-deception? *New English Journal of Medicine* **323**, 476–478.

27. Ferguson, A. and Carswell, F. (1972) Precipitins to dietary proteins in the serum and upper intestinal secretions of coeliac children. *British Medical Journal*, **i**, 75–77.

28. Ferguson, A. and Parrott, D.M.V. (1973) Histopathology and time course of rejection of allografts of mouse small intestine. *Transplantation*, **15**, 546–554.

29. Forget, P., Eggermont, E., Marchal, G. *et al.* (1978) Eosinophilic infiltration of the oesophagus in an infant. *Acta Paediatrica Belgica*, **31**, 91–93.

30. Fries, J.H. (1971) Studies on the allergenicity of soy bean. *Annals of Allergy*, **29**, 1–5.

31. Gerrard, J.W., MacKenzie, J.W.A., Goluboff, N. *et al.* (1973) Cow's milk allergy: Prevalence and manifestations in an unselected series of newborns. *Acta Paediatricia Scandinavica Supplementum*, **234**, 2–21.

32. Goldman, A.S., Anderson, D.W., Sellers, W.A. *et al.* (1963) Milk allergy I. Oral challenge with milk and isolated milk proteins in allergic children. *Paediatrics*, **32**, 425–443.

33. Gong, M., Tashkin, D.P. and Calvarese, B.M. (1981) Alcohol-induced bronchospasm in an asthmatic patient. *Chest*, **80**, 167–173.

34. Gruskay, F.L. and Cooke, R.E. (1955) The gastrointestinal absorption of unaltered protein in normal infants and in infants recovering from diarrhoea. *Paediatrics*, **16**, 763–769.

35. Halpern, S.R. (1965) Chronic hives in children: an analysis of 75 cases. *Annals of Allergy*, **23**, 589–593.

36. Hampton, J.C. and Rosario, B. (1968) The distribution of exogenous peroxidase in irradiated mouse intestine. *Radiation Research*, **37**, 209.

37. Hattevig, G., Kjellman, B., Sigurs, N., Björkstén, Kjellman, N.I.M. (1989) Effect of maternal avoidance of eggs, cow's milk and fish during lactation upon allergic manifestations in infants. *Clinical and Experimental Allergy*, **19**, 27–30.

38. Hedström, V. (1958) Food allergy in bronchial asthma. *Acta Allergologica*, **12**, 153–185.

39. Hill, S.M. and Miller, P.J. (1990) Colitis caused by food allergy in infants. *Archives of Disease in Childhood*, **65**(1), 132–133.

40. Hutchins, P. and Walker-Smith, J.A. (1982) The gastrointestinal system. *Clinics in Immunology and Allergy*, **2**(1), 45–48.

41. Jacobsson, I. and Lindberg, T. (1978) Cow's milk as a cause of infantile colic in breast-fed infants. *The Lancet*, **ii**, 437–439.

42. Jenkins, H.R., Milla, P.J., Pincott, J.R., Soothill, J.F. and Harries, J.T. (1982) Food allergy: the major cause of infantile colitis. *Gut*, **23**, A924.

43. Jewett, D.L., Fein, G. and Greenberg, M.H. (1990) A double-blind study of symptom provocation to determine food sensitivity. *New English Journal of Medicine*, **323**, 429–433.

44. Johnstone, J.M. and Morson, B.C. (1978) Eosinophilic gastroenteritis. *Histopathology*, **2**, 335–348.

45. Kaplan, M.S. and Solli, N.J. (1979) Immunoglobulin E in breast-fed atopic children. *Journal of Allergy and Clinical Immunology*, **64**, 122–126.

46. Katz, A.J., Goldman, M. and Grand, R.J. (1977) Gastric mucosa biopsy in eosinophilic (allergic) gastroenteritis. *Gastroenterology*, **73**, 705–709.

47. Keljo, D.J., Butler, D.G. and Hamilton, J.R. (1985) Altered jejunal permeability to macromolecules during viral enteritis in the piglet. *Gastroenterology*, **88**, 998–1004.

48. Klee, W.A. and Iorio, M.A. (1977) Relationships between opiate receptor binding and analgesic properties of prodine-type compounds. *Journal of Medical Chemistry*, **20**(2), 309–310.

49. Konig, P. and Godfreys, S. (1974) Exercise-induced bronchial lability on monozygotic (identical) and dizygotic (non-identical) twins. *Journal of Allergy and Clinical Immunology*, **54**, 280–282.

50. Kuitenen, P., Visakorpi, J.K., Savilhati, E. and Pelkonen, P. (1975) Malabsorption syndrome with cow's milk intolerance. Clinical findings and course in 54 cases. *Archives of Diseases in Childhood*, **50**, 351–356.

51. Kumar, P.J., Ferguson, A., Lancaster-Smith, M.L. and Dawson, A.M. (1973) Relationship between dietary food antigen and jejunal mucosal morphology. *Gut*, **14**, 829–830.

52. Kumar, P.J., O'Donoghue, D.P., Stenson, K. and

Dawson, A.M. (1979) Reintroduction of gluten in adults and children with treated coeliac disease. *Gut*, **20**, 743–749.

53. Kwok, R.H.M. (1968) Chinese restaurant syndrome. *New England Journal of Medicine*, **278**, 796.

54. Lessof, M.H., Wraith, D.G., Merrett, T.G. *et al.* (1980) Food allergy and intolerance in 100 patients – local and systemic effects. *Quarterly Journal of Medicine*, **195**, 259–271.

55. Levinsky, R.J., Paganelli, R., Robertson, D.M. and Atherton, D.J. (1981) Handling of food antigens and their complexes by normal and allergic individuals. In: *The Immunology of Infant Feeding*, pp. 23–30 (Ed.) Wilkinson, A.W. New York: Plenum Press.

56. Lippard, V.M., Schloss, O.M. and Johnson, P.A. (1936) Immune reactions induced in infants by intestinal absorption of incompletely digested cow's milk protein. *American Journal of Diseases of Childhood*, **51**, 562–574.

57. Lockey, S.D. (1972) Sensitizing properties of food additives and other commercial products. *Annals of Allergy*, **30**, 638–642.

58. Maini, V., Lloyd, G., Green, F.H.Y. *et al.* (1976) Treatment of ulcerative colitis with oral disodium cromoglycate. A double-blind controlled trial. *The Lancet*, **i**, 439–441.

59. Matthew, D.J., Taylor, B., Norman, A.P. *et al.* (1977) Prevention of eczema. *The Lancet*, **i**, 321–324.

60. May, C.D. (1980) Food allergy – material and ethereal. *New England Journal of Medicine*, **302**, 1142–1143.

61. Michaëlsson, G. and Juhlin, L. (1973) Urticaria induced by preservatives and dye additives in food and drugs. *British Journal of Dermatology*, **88**, 525–532.

62. Monro, J.A. (1982) Food allergy and migraine. *Clinics in Immunology and Allergy*, **2**(1), 137–163.

63. Monro, J.A., Brostoff, J., Carini, C. and Zilkha, K. (1980) Food allergy in migraine. *The Lancet*, **ii**, 1–4.

64. Nolte, H., Schiotz, P.O., Kruse, A., Stahl-skov, P. (1989) Comparison of intestinal mast cell and basophil histamine release in children with food allergic reaction. *Allergy*, **44**, 554–565.

65. O'Morain, C., Segal, A.W. and Levi, A.J. (1984) Elemental diet as primary treatment of acute Crohn's disease: A controlled trial. *British Medical Journal*, **288**, 1859.

66. Paganelli, R., Levinsky, R.J., Brostoff, J. and Wraith, D.G. (1979) Immune complexes containing food proteins in normal and atopic subjects after oral challenge and effect of sodium cromoglycate on antigen absorption. *The Lancet*, **i**, 1270–1272.

67. Panush, R.S. (1990) Food induced ('allergic') arthritis: clinical and serological studies. *Journal of Rheumatology*, **17**, 291–294.

68. Panush, R.S., Webster, E.M., Endo, L.P., Greer, J.M. and Woodard, J.C. (1990) Food induced ('allergic') arthritis: inflammatory synovitis in rabbits. *Journal of Rheumatology*, **17**, 285–290.

69. Pastorello, E.A., Stocchi, L., Pravettoni, V. *et al.* (1989) Role of the elimination diet in adults with food allergy. *Journal of Allergy and Clinical Immunology*, **84**, 475–483.

70. Pearson, D.J., Rix, K.J.B., Bentley, S.J. (1983) Food allergy: how much in the mind? A clinical and psychiatric study of suspected food allergy. *The Lancet*, **ii**, 1259–1267.

71. Perkkiö, M., Savilahti, E. and Kuitunen, P. (1981) Morphometric and immunochemical study of jejunal biopsies from children with intestinal soy allergy. *European Journal of Paediatrics*, **137**, 63–69.

72. Prauznitz, C. and Kustner, H. (1921) Studien über die verbering Findlichkeit. *Aentralblatt für Bakteriologie, Parasitenkunde, Infektionskrankheiten und Hygiene, Abteilung* I, **86**, 160.

73. Rix, K.J.B., Pearson, D.J. and Bentley, S.J. (1984) A psychiatric study of patients with supposed food allergy. *British Journal of Psychiatry*, **145**, 121–126.

74. Robertson, D., Paganelli, R., Dinwiddie, R. and Levinsky, R.J. (1982) Milk antigen absorption in the premature and term neonate. *Archives of Diseases in Childhood*, **57**, 369–370.

75. Robertson, D.A.F., Ayres, R.C.S., Smith, C.L. and Wright, R. (1988) Adverse consequences arising from misdiagnosis of food allergy. *British Medical Journal*, **297**, 719–720.

76. Royal College of Physicians and the British Nutrition Foundation (1984) Food allergy or food aversion: a joint report of the Royal College of Physicians and the British Nutrition Foundation. *Journal of the Royal College of Physicians, London*, **10**, 83–123.

77. Sampson, M.A. (1989) Infantile colic and food allergy: fact or fiction. *Journal of Paediatrics*, **115**, 583–584 (editorial).

78. Sampson, M.A. and Scanlon, S.M. (1989) Natural history of food hypersensitivity in children with atopic dermatitis. *Journal of Paediatrics*, **115**(1), 23–27.

79. Sandler, M., Youdim, M.B.H. and Hannington, E. (1974) Conjugation defect in tyramine sensitive migraine. *Nature*, **250**, 335–337.

80. Savilhati, E. (1981) Cow's milk allergy. *Allergy*, **36**, 73–88.

81. Scott, H. and Brandtzaeg, P. (1989) Pathogenesis of food protein intolerance. *Acta Paediatrica Scandinavica Supplementum*, **351**, 48–52.

82. Shiner, M., Ballard, J. and Smith, M.E. (1975) The small intestinal mucosa in cow's milk allergy. *The Lancet*, **i**, 136–140.

83. Sköldstam, L., Larsson, L. and Lindström, F.D. (1979) Effects of fasting and a lactovegetarian diet on rheumatoid arthritis. *Scandinavian Journal of Rheumatology*, **8**, 249–255.

84. Soothill, J.F. (1979) Food allergy. In: *The Mast Cell,* pp. 367–376 (Eds) Pepys, J. and Edwards, A.M. London: Pitman.

85. Soothill, J.F. (1983) Immunological aspects of infant feeding. In: *Paediatric Clinical Immunology,* pp. 110–129 (Eds) Soothill, J.F., Haywood, A.R. and Wood, C.B.S. Oxford: Blackwell.

86. Soothill, J.F., Stokes, C.R., Turner, M.W. *et al.* (1976) Predisposing factors and the development of reaginic allergy in infancy. *Clinical Allergy,* **6,** 305–306.

87. Speer, F. (1973) Management of food allergy. In: *Immunology in Children,* pp. 397–402 (Eds) Speer, F. and Dockhorn, R.J. Springfield: Charles. C. Thomas.

88. Stern and Walker, W.A. (1985) Food allergy and intolerance. *Paediatric Clinics in North America,* **32,** 471.

89. Swarbrick, E.T., Stokes, C.R. and Soothill, J.F. (1978) The absorption of antigens after oral immunisation and the simultaneous induction of specific systemic tolerance. *Gut,* **20,** 121–125.

90. Tabuenca, J.M. (1981) Toxic-allergic syndrome caused by ingestion of rape seed oil denatured with aniline. *The Lancet,* **ii,** 567–568.

91. Taylor, K.B. and Truelove, S.C. (1961) Circulating antibodies to milk proteins in ulcerative colitis. *British Medical Journal,* **ii,** 924–929.

92. Taylor, B., Normal, A.P., Orgel, H.A. *et al.* (1973) Transient IgA deficiency and pathogenesis of infantile atropy. *The Lancet,* **ii,** 111–113.

93. Turner, M.W., Mowbray, J.F., Harvey, B.A.M. *et al.* (1978) Defective yeast opsonization and C2 deficiency in atopic patients. *Clinics in Experimental Immunology,* **34,** 253–259.

94. Turner, M.W., Brostoff, J., Mowbray, J.F. and Skelton, A. (1980) The atopic syndrome: *in vitro* immunological characteristics of clinically defined subgroups of atopic subjects. *Clinical Allergy,* **10,** 575–584.

95. Waldmann, T.A., Wochner, R.D., Laster, L. and Gordon, R.S. (1967) Allergic gastroenteropathy: a cause of excessive gastrointestinal protein loss. *New England Journal of Medicine,* **276,** 761–769.

96. Walker, W.A. (1981) Intestinal transport of macromolecules. In: *Physiology of the Gastrointestinal Tract,* p. 1282 (Ed.) Johnson, L.R. New York: Raven Press.

97. Walker, W.A. (1982) Mechanisms of antigen handling by the gut. *Clinics in Immunology and Allergy,* **2**(1), 15–40.

98. Walker, W.A. and Isselbacher, K.J. (1974) Uptake and transport of macromolecules by the intestine: Possible role in clinical disorders. *Gastroenterology,* **67,** 531–550.

99. Walker-Smith, J.A. (1970) Transient gluten intolerance. *Archives of Diseases in Childhood,* **45,** 523–526.

100. Walker-Smith, J.A., Ford, R.P.K. and Phillips, A.D. (1984) The spectrum of gastrointestinal

allergies to food. *Annuals of Allergy,* **53,** 629.

101. Whorwell, P.J. and Wright, R. (1979) Bottle feeding, early gastroenteritis and inflammatory bowel disease. *British Medical Journal,* **i,** 382.

102. Wilson, J.F., Heimo, D.C. and Lahey, M.E. (1964) Milk induced gastrointestinal bleeding in infants with hypochronic microcytic anaemia. *Journal of the American Medical Association,* **189,** 568–572.

103. Worthington, B.S. and Syrotuck, J. (1976) Intestinal permeability to large particles in normal and protein deficient rats. *Journal of Nutrition,* **105,** 21.

EOSINOPHILIC GASTROENTERITIS *(C.J.F. Spry)*

Eosinophilic gastroenteritis has been recognized since 1937 as an uncommon disorder affecting one or more parts of the gut. It is characterized by gastrointestinal thickening with oedema and dense eosinophil infiltrates.[7,22] It usually involves the gastric antrum and proximal small intestine. The disease takes three main forms (*Figure 3.89*). The mucosal form may be associated with protein-losing enteropathy, anaemia and malabsorption and patients may have a history of allergic disorders with high IgE levels. Muscle involvement produces thickening and obstruction which may require surgery, and occasionally bleeding or fistulas occur. Serosal disease gives rise to abdominal pain with peritonitis and ascites.

Eosinophilic gastroenteritis mainly occurs in young adults in their third decade. However, it can occur in children[6,9] and in older people. Males appear to be affected twice as often as females. The

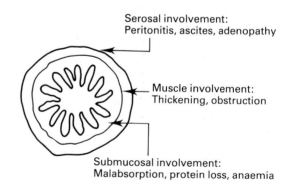

Serosal involvement:
Peritonitis, ascites, adenopathy

Muscle involvement:
Thickening, obstruction

Submucosal involvement:
Malabsorption, protein loss, anaemia

Lesions may be polypoid or diffuse

Figure 3.89 The three main types of eosinophilic gastroenteritis are associated with involvement of different layers of the gut wall.

incidence of the disease is hard to define, but may be as little as 1/10 000 hospital admissions.[6]

The aetiology of eosinophilic gastroenteritis has not been determined. Food antigens are probably not involved, although 20% of patients have a history of allergic diseases. In some patients it may be difficult to distinguish eosinophilic gastroenteritis from allergic gastroenteritis (see p. 596). However, in eosinophilic gastroenteritis the immunoglobulin content of the intestines is normal, in contrast to allergic gastroenteritis, where tissue IgE and IgG levels are usually elevated.[2]

The role of eosinophils in this form of gastroenteritis has not been explained. Eosinophils commonly enter the small intestine, and this may be one of the main sites of eosinophil accumulation in normal individuals. The association of eosinophil infiltrates with a number of tissue lesions, including lesions which progress to fibrosis, has raised the possibility that eosinophils are actively involved in tissue damage in these patients. This has not been tested directly but highly purified eosinophils in ascitic fluid from a patient with eosinophilic gastroenteritis showed many features consistent with an activated and fully functional state.[9,10] Deposits of eosinophil major basic protein, which is toxic to many cells and tissues, have been detected in biopsies from one patient.[23] It is also of interest that some patients with eosinophilic gastroenteritis have associated chronic fibrotic lesions in the lungs, and fibrosis in areas of eosinophil infiltration in the gut has also been noted.

CLINICAL FEATURES

The disease may present as an acute illness with obstruction to the outflow of the stomach or with chronic abdominal pain, distension and ascites, nausea and vomiting. Single episodes may occur, but some patients have a history going back many years.

Involvement of the stomach may be difficult to distinguish from peptic ulcer, adenomas or carcinomas, and helminths in the stomach may produce localized eosinophilic infiltrates. The differential diagnosis of small intestinal involvement includes Crohn's disease, diverticulitis and tropical sprue. Terminal ileal and caecal involvement may mimic Crohn's disease, amoebiasis or intestinal tuberculosis. Localized areas of eosinophilic gastroenteritis are similar in some respects to inflammatory fibroid polyps of the gastrointestinal tract.[8]

Localized forms of eosinophilic gastroenteritis

The stomach alone is involved in about 26% of patients with eosinophilic gastroenteritis (eosino-philic gastritis). Lesions are often circumscribed and similar in appearance to eosinophilic granulomas of the stomach. The antrum is one of the main sites of involvement. A gastric mass may simulate a malignancy,[15] or produce gastric outlet obstruction.[19]

About 50% of patients with eosinophilic gastroenteritis develop symptoms of obstruction even when there is evidence of diffuse involvement.[1] This may require surgery but, wherever possible, a trial of steroids should be given first.

Ileocolitis with narrowing and shortening of the caecum and ascending colon has been described and has led to hemicolectomy for intestinal obstruction,[18] but in the majority of patients eosinophilic gastroenteritis involves the upper small intestine, where the disease is diffuse.

Fourteen patients with the *serosal* form of eosinophilic gastroenteritis have been described.[5,14] These patients have ascites which contain up to 99% eosinophils. Protein in the fluid is usually an exudate. The discovery of eosinophils in ascitic fluid may suggest other diagnoses, including vasculitic disorders, lymphomas, metastatic carcinomas and ruptured hydatid cysts. Peritoneal fluid can contain up to 40% eosinophils in about one-third of patients having peritoneal dialysis, but this is not associated with increased eosinophils in the peripheral blood.

Eosinophilic gastroenteritis may also affect the oesophagus, liver and biliary system,[17] or the large bowel and rectum. Oesophageal involvement can be associated with disorders of motor function,[11] this has also been seen in patients with allergic gastroenteritis. Eosinophilic gastroenteritis is a rare cause of eosinophilic hepatitis[4] and eosinophilic cholangitis and isolated rectal involvement have also been reported.

INVESTIGATIONS

Blood eosinophil counts are raised in only about 20% of patients with eosinophilic gastroenteritis. The counts may fluctuate and follow the course of the disease, but in many patients blood eosinophil counts remain normal throughout their illness. Radiology of the stomach demonstrates gastric antral rigidity with thickened folds and mucosal nodules. In the small intestine the circular folds and walls are thickened, without evidence of ulceration or local abnormality.[12,13] The diagnosis is established by histology; endoscopic biopsies may well be adequate but the lesions may be patchy requiring multiple biopsies. Colonoscopy and fibre-optic sigmoidoscopy have occasionally demonstrated lesions in patients with distal gastrointestinal involvement.[16] Histologically, dense infiltrates of eosinophils are seen in localized or diffuse areas of the gut. There is no necrosis but there may be some fibrosis. Oedema is a constant feature, and where the serosal layer is involved this gives rise to ascites. Further investigations sometimes bring to light malabsorption and/or protein-losing enteropathy, which occurs in about 10% of patients. A full-thickness biopsy is rarely necessary but may be required in the serosal form of the disease, as superficial biopsies can fail to demonstrate the characteristic features of the disease.

TREATMENT

Correct diagnosis of eosinophilic gastroenteritis is rewarding as treatment is extremely effective. Surgery can usually be avoided, and a wide range of more sinister diagnoses can be eliminated. Steroids are the mainstay of treatment. Prednisolone 15–40 mg/day is usually given initially, with doses decreasing to alternate-day therapy when symptoms and clinical signs have resolved. Occasionally, disodium cromoglycate (Intal) has been used with success.[3] Some patients show spontaneous remission of their disease. However, in others, relapses can occur; these usually also respond to treatment, even though it may have to be continued for many months.

Surgery is usually of little benefit and recurrence can occur even after partial gastrectomy in patients who have not received steroids.

The prognosis is usually excellent, providing the disorder is recognized and treated early. Occasional fatal cases have been reported in childhood. Since perforation and bleeding can also occur, some patients may need additional therapeutic measures.

RELATED DISORDERS

A number of vasculitic and granulomatous diseases can also give rise to eosinophil infiltrations into the gastrointestinal tract.[20,21] Patients with these disorders differ from those with eosinophilic gastroenteritis as they are usually older, frequently in their sixth decade. Of these patients 40% have gastric involvement and 26% ileal involvement, but they may also present with epigastric pain, vomiting and obstruction; they may respond to treatment with steroids. The Churg–Strauss syndrome can affect the gut, producing areas of eosinophilic infiltration and focal necrotic lesions. The gut is also involved in some patients with the hypereosinophilic syndrome, which is characterized by high blood eosinophil counts of unknown cause, usually with characteristic

lesions in other sites including the heart (eosinophilic endomyocardial disease), skin and lung. These similarities between different eosinophilic disorders affecting the gastrointestinal tract raise the possibility that they are related, differing only in the sites where eosinophils localize and cause tissue injury. If eosinophilic gastroenteritis is part of a wider spectrum of hypereosinophilic disorders, it appears to be one of the most benign forms, with a good response to treatment with steroids, and an excellent prognosis in most patients.

References

1. Caldwell, J.H., Mekhjian, H.S., Hurtubise, P.E. and Beman, F.M. (1978) Eosinophilic gastroenteritis with obstruction. Immunological studies of seven patients. *Gastroenterology*, **74**, 825–828.
2. Caldwell, J.H., Sharma, H.M., Hurtubise, P.E. and Colwell, D.L. (1979) Eosinophilic gastroenteritis in extreme allergy. Immunopathological comparison with nonallergic gastrointestinal disease. *Gastroenterology*, **77**, 560–564.
3. Di Gioacchino, M., Pizzicannella, G., Fini, N. *et al.* (1990) Sodium cromoglycate in the treatment of eosinophilic gastroenteritis. *Allergy*, **45**, 161–166.
4. Everett, G.D. and Mitros, F.A. (1980) Eosinophilic gastroenteritis with hepatic eosinophilic granulomas. Report of a case with 30-year follow-up. *American Journal of Gastroenterology*, **74**, 519–521.
5. Harmon, W.A. and Helman, C.A. (1981) Eosinophilic gastroenteritis and ascites. *Journal of Clinical Gastroenterology*, **3**, 371–373.
6. Hoefer, R.A., Ziegler, M.M., Koop, C.E. and Schnaufer, L. (1977) Surgical manifestations of eosinophilic gastroenteritis in the pediatric patient. *Journal of Pediatric Surgery*, **12**, 955–962.
7. Johnstone, J.M. and Morson, B.C. (1978) Eosinophilic gastroenteritis. *Histopathology*, **2**, 335–348.
8. Johnstone, J.M. and Morson, B.C. (1978) Inflammatory fibroid polyp of the gastrointestinal tract. *Histopathology*, **2**, 349–361.
9. Keshavarzian, A., Saverymuttu, S.H., Tai, P.C. *et al.* (1985) Activated eosinophils in familial eosinophilic gastroenteritis. *Gastroenterology*, **88**, 1041–1049.
10. Klebanoff, S.J., Durack, D.T., Rosen, H. and Clark, R.A. (1977) Functional studies on human peritoneal eosinophils. *Infection and Immunity*, **17**, 167–173.
11. Landres, R.T., Kuster, G.G. and Strum, W.B. (1978) Eosinophilic esophagitis in a patient with vigorous achalasia. *Gastroenterology*, **74**, 1298–1301.
12. MacCarty, R.L. and Talley, N.J. (1990) Barium

studies in diffuse eosinophilic gastroenteritis. *Gastrointestinal Radiology*, **15**, 183–187.

13. Marshak, R.H., Lindner, A., Maklansky, D. and Gelb, A. (1981) Eosinophilic gastroenteritis. *Journal of the American Medical Association*, **245**, 1677–1680.

14. McNabb, P.C., Fleming, C.R., Higgins, J.A. and Davis, G.L. (1979) Transmural eosinophilic gastroenteritis with ascites. *Mayo Clinic Proceedings*, **54**, 119–122.

15. Milman, P.J. and Sidhu, G.S. (1978) Case report: eosinophilic gastritis simulating a neoplasm. *American Journal of Medical Science*, **276**, 227–230.

16. Partyka, E.K., Sanowski, R.A. and Kozarek, R.A. (1980) Colonoscopic features of eosinophilic gastroenteritis. *Diseases of the Colon and Rectum*, **23**, 353–356.

17. Rumans, M.C. and Lieberman, D.A. (1987) Eosinophilic gastroenteritis presenting with biliary and duodenal obstruction. *American Journal of Gastroenterology*, **82**, 775–778.

18. Schulze, K. and Mitros, F.A. (1979) Eosinophilic gastroenteritis involving the ileocecal area. *Diseases of the Colon and Rectum*, **22**, 47–50.

19. Snyder, J.D., Rosenblum, N., Wershil, B., Goldman, H. and Winter, H.S. (1987) Pyloric stenosis and eosinophilic gastroenteritis in infants. *Journal of Pediatric Gastroenterology and Nutrition*, **6**, 543–547.

20. Spry, C.J. (1982) The hypereosinophilic syndrome: clinical features, laboratory findings and treatment. *Allergy*, **37**, 539–551.

21. Suen, K.C. and Burton, J.D. (1979) The spectrum of eosinophilic infiltration of the gastrointestinal tract and its relationship to other disorders of angiitis and granulomatosis. *Human Pathology*, **10**, 31–43.

22. Talley, N.J., Shorter, R.G., Phillips, S.F. and Zinsmeister, A.R. (1990) Eosinophilic gastroenteritis: a clinicopathological study of patients with disease of the mucosa, muscle layer, and subserosal tissues. *Gut*, **31**, 54–58.

23. Torpier, G., Colombel, J.F., Mathieu Chandelier, C., Capron, M., Dessaint, J.P., Cortot, A., Paris, J.C. and Capron, A. (1988) Eosinophilic gastroenteritis: ultrastructural evidence for a selective release of eosinophil major basic protein. *Clinical Experimental Immunology*, **74**, 404–408.

PROTEIN-LOSING ENTEROPATHY

W. Strober

In 1957 Citrin[11] and his colleagues studied a patient with giant hypertrophy of the gastric rugae (Ménétrier's disease) who had severe hypoalbuminaemia. Using metabolic turnover studies with radioactive iodine-labelled albumin they determined that the patient had an increased rate of albumin catabolism accompanied by an increased rate of loss of albumin into the stomach. At about the same time, Steinfeld et al.[58] made similar observations in patients with inflammatory bowel disease and hypoalbuminaemia. Here again, metabolic studies with radioactive iodine-labelled albumin disclosed an increased rate of albumin catabolism which, in this case, was associated with a normal or even increased rate of albumin synthesis. In addition, an excessive amount of radioactive iodine was found in the stool, suggesting that there was loss of intact protein into the small intestine. These reports were the first to suggest that hypoproteinemia could be due to loss of protein into the gastrointestinal tract. As such, they ushered in a period of intense study of the phenomenon that came to be known as protein-losing enteropathy. Subsequent investigation of this pathological process has involved first the search for better tools for measuring gastrointestinal protein loss, and second the identification of protein-losing enteropathy in a myriad of gastrointestinal conditions, ranging from diseases in which protein-losing enteropathy is a minor and incidental feature of the overall pathological picture to diseases in which protein-losing enteropathy is the dominant abnormality. In the latter regard, the study of protein-losing enteropathy has allowed a better definition of several important gastrointestinal diseases, such as Ménétrier's disease, allergic gastroenteropathy and intestinal lymphangiectasia.

Protein-losing enteropathy is considered here first from a physiological point of view, emphasizing the basic features of serum protein metabolism and the methods used to measure both serum protein turnover and losses to the gastrointestinal tract. Following this, the range of diseases associated with protein-losing enteropathy are discussed, drawing attention to the major mechanisms accounting for this abnormality in these diseases. Finally, the clinical and pathophysiological features of intestinal lymphangiectasia, the prototype protein-losing state, is discussed at some length.

GENERAL FEATURES OF SERUM PROTEIN METABOLISM

Protein-losing enteropathy may be defined as the abnormal loss of serum proteins into the gastro-intestinal tract resulting from a variety of gastro-intestinal abnormalities and leading to reduced serum protein levels, particularly albumin levels. From a pathophysiological point of view, protein-losing enteropathy is a disorder of serum protein metabolism, and for this reason is best described by metabolic turnover studies utilizing radiolabelled proteins.

PROTEIN TURNOVER STUDIES

Metabolically speaking, the body consists of a central intravascular compartment or pool which exchanges material with one or more extravascular compartments (*Figure 3.90*). Synthesis of serum proteins, such as albumin or proteins of similar size and characteristics (here called albumin-like proteins), is followed by their rapid entry into the intravascular compartment, where they circulate or move into one of the extravascular compartments. Catabolism of an albumin-like serum protein is quantitatively defined as the fraction of protein in the intravascular compartment that is irreversibly lost from this compartment per unit time. Such loss may be due to degradation of protein within the body (endogenous catabolism) as well as leakage of protein to the outside via the gastrointestinal tract, kidney, lungs or skin. In the steady-state condition (i.e. the normal condition), the intravascular compartment remains constant in size. This means that the amount of albumin-like protein catabolized per unit time (i.e. the fraction of the intravascular pool catabolized/unit time × pool size) equals the synthetic rate. Thus, during the steady state, the pool size and hence the serum albumin-like protein level is inversely proportional to the fractional catabolic rate. Metabolic turnover studies (such as those described below) have shown that the amount of albumin-like protein that is catabolized or lost is a constant fraction of the total amount of protein in the intravascular compartment, but is not a constant fraction of the amount of protein in the extravascular compartments or the total metabolic system (which includes the extravascular compartments). On this basis, it can be inferred that the catabolism of albumin-like protein occurs in a compartment in rapid equilibrium with the intravascular compartment and that the fraction of the intravascular pool catabolized per day is an accurate reflection of the

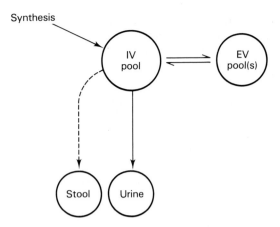

Figure 3.90 Compartmental model of protein metabolism. Synthesis of serum protein is followed by its rapid introduction into the intravascular (IV) compartment or pool. The diagram shows that protein may circulate in this compartment, leave it temporarily by entering one or more extravascular (EV) compartments, or leave the IV pool permanently as a result of endogenous catabolism or loss of intact protein into the bowel (stool). The rate at which protein irreversibly leaves the IV pool can be expressed as a fractional catabolic rate – the fraction of the IV pool catabolized/unit time. In the diagram this is indicated by the vertical arrows leading into the urinary and stool compartments.

total fractional catabolic rate. In addition, for proteins (non-albumin-like proteins) that are catabolized in compartments removed from the intravascular compartment, the fractional catabolic rate is a weighted mean of the fractional catabolic rate relative to each of the compartments in which catabolism occurs.

The quantitative assessment of the metabolism of an albumin-like protein involves measuring various metabolic parameters defined above: the compartment sizes, the intercompartmental transfer rates (which allow calculation of the percentage of the serum protein present in the intravascular compartment), and the fractional catabolic rate. These measurements are generally made by performing metabolic turnover studies using proteins labelled with radioactive tracers which are handled by the body in the same way as endogenously synthesized, unlabelled proteins.[42,68] Radioactive iodine is the label of choice for such metabolic turnover studies because it can be incorporated into proteins in a way that does not alter the metabolic characteristics of the protein and because it is not reincorporated into new protein after the protein to which it is bound is degraded; furthermore, the radioactive iodine label, once separated from degraded protein, is rapidly cleared from the metabolic system as a result of uptake in and excretion by the kidney.

In a typical metabolic turnover study, a purified radiolabelled protein such as ^{125}I-labelled albumin is injected intravenously into the individual under study. Ten minutes after injection, when the radio-labelled protein has had time to be distributed evenly throughout the intravascular compartment, but has not yet undergone significant catabolism and has not yet left the intravascular space, a sample is taken to estimate plasma volume (plasma volume equals counts injected divided by counts/millilitre in the 10-minute sample). The plasma volume can then be used to calculate the size of the intravascular protein compartment: plasma volume multiplied by protein concentration is equal to the intravascular pool size.

The fractional catabolic rate is, in turn, determined from an analysis of the plasma die-away curve (*Figure 3.91*) or from the urinary clearance of radioactive iodine released from degraded protein. In the former, or plasma die-away curve method, one first constructs a die-away curve by plotting the amount

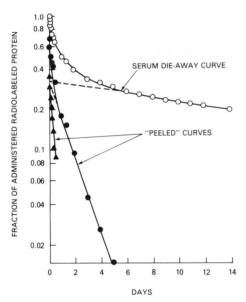

Figure 3.91 Die-away curve of a radiolabelled protein (such as ^{125}I-labelled albumin) following injection into the intravascular (circulating) protein pool. Die-away is initially very rapid because protein is lost from the pool as a result of transfer to extravascular compartments as well as because of endogenous catabolism. Later, when the labelled protein has entered the various compartments, the die-away curve assumes a straight-line (exponential) decline. The reciprocal of the area under the die-away curve is the fractional catabolic rate of the protein (see text for definition); it is obtained by 'curve peeling', i.e. obtaining the slope and intercept of the terminal exponential of the die-away curve, subtracting the latter from the die-away curve to obtain a new curve and repeating the process. The fractional catabolic rate is obtained from the expression

$$\frac{1}{C_1/b_1 + C_2/b_2 + \cdots + C_n/b_n}$$

where C_n and b_n are respectively the slope and intercept of the initial and peeled curves.

of radioactive protein in the plasma at various time points (on semilogarithmic paper) as a percentage of the radioactive protein in the 10-minute plasma.[50] One then performs 'curve peeling' on the plasma die-away curve, i.e. successive subtraction of the terminal exponential curve from the overall exponential curve to obtain a series of slopes and intercepts that can be used to calculate the reciprocal of the area under the die-away curve (see legend to *Figure 3.91*). This latter value is equal to the fractional catabolic rate of the protein under study.[50] In the second, or urinary clearance method, one first determines the clearance of radioactive iodine into the urine per unit time as well as the mean plasma radioactivity value of the intravascular compartment during the period of clearance (from the plasma die-away curve). One then divides the clearance value by the mean plasma radioactivity value. In a well-conducted metabolic study, these two methods will result in fractional catabolic rates that are similar to each other; thus their simultaneous use can serve as a check on the validity of the metabolic study.

To study the metabolism of non-albumin-like proteins which undergo significant extravascular catabolism and/or manifest other metabolic complexities, plasma die-away curves, urinary excretion data and other relevant information are analysed by complex computer programs which allow the metabolic data to be fitted to preselected compartmental models.[7,42] The simplest compartmental model that approximates the data is then assumed to describe the metabolic system under study and is used to generate values for the mean (weighted) catabolic rate and other metabolic parameters.

SERUM PROTEIN METABOLISM IN PROTEIN-LOSING ENTEROPATHY

Metabolic turnover studies performed in individual patients with protein-losing enteropathy reveal several abnormalities. Most importantly, they show that in such patients the fractional catabolic rate is increased, indicating that protein is lost from the intravascular compartment at an increased rate, either because of increased endogenous catabolism or because of excessive loss of intact protein into the gastrointestinal tract.[31,72] Studies with labelled proteins that allow one to determine whether or not the increased catabolic rate is due to loss into the gastrointestinal tract are described below. In addition, the metabolic turnover studies show that the synthesis of albumin is normal or increased, a finding indicative of the fact that the low protein level is due to a defect involving protein catabolism rather than one involving protein synthesis.

In addition to this basic information, metabolic turnover studies provide certain important insights into the nature of gastrointestinal protein loss. First, they show that the effect of protein loss on serum protein concentration depends on the underlying metabolic characteristics of the protein.[72] Thus, if the normal rate of catabolism of a particular serum protein is high, the addition of even a considerable extracatabolic pathway leads to only a small fractional change in the total catabolism of that protein; however, if the normal rate of catabolism is low, a small additional catabolic pathway leads to a large fractional change in total catabolism. For example, if the normal fractional catabolic rate is low, say 10% of the intravascular pool per day (as it is for albumin), a gastrointestinal loss rate of 10% of the intravascular pool per day gives rise to a doubling of the fractional catabolic rate and, provided there is no increase in protein synthesis, a halving of the serum protein level. In contrast, if the normal fractional catabolic rate is high, say 25% of the intravascular pool per day (as it is for IgA), a gastrointestinal loss rate of 10% would lead to only a 25% increase in total catabolism and a corresponding decrease in serum IgA concentration. Thus, any level of protein-losing enteropathy will most affect those proteins with relatively low fractional catabolic rates such as albumin and IgG; in contrast, even severe protein-losing enteropathy will have little impact on these serum proteins with normally rapid rates of catabolism, such as IgE.[29]

A second point that emerges from metabolic turnover data is that the protein loss that occurs in protein-losing enteropathy is a 'bulk loss', i.e. in this condition, proteins are lost regardless of size, charge or any other physical characteristic. This means that the increase in fractional catabolic rate accounted for by gastrointestinal loss, expressed as the fraction of the intravascular pool lost per day, is the same for all serum proteins, regardless of their underlying fractional catabolic rate.[30] In this way protein-losing enteropathy differs from the urinary protein loss process encountered in the nephrotic syndrome, where proteins of intermediate and small size are affected more markedly than larger proteins.

Finally, metabolic turnover studies provide important information on the capacity of the body to increase protein synthesis in the face of protein-losing enteropathy. In general, such studies have disclosed that a low protein level *per se* is not a strong stimulus to protein synthesis and that gastrointestinal tract protein loss is not accompanied by large compensatory increases in the rate at which proteins are added to the system.[75]

MEASUREMENT OF PROTEIN-LOSING ENTEROPATHY

Protein-losing enteropathy can be identified and quantified by measuring the excretion of circulating protein into the gastrointestinal tract. This is best accomplished by using a protein labelled with a radioactive marker which: (1) is not broken down in or reabsorbed from the gastrointestinal tract; (2) is not excreted into the gastrointestinal tract unless it is bound to the protein; and (3) is attached to the protein in a permanent (covalent) and non-denaturing fashion so that the labelled protein can be used both in metabolic turnover studies, such as those described above, as well as in measurements of gastrointestinal protein loss. Alternatively, protein-losing enteropathy can be measured with a circulating protein, such as α_1-antitrypsin, which is not digested in the gastrointestinal tract if and when it is secreted into the latter as a result of a protein-losing state. In this case the immunological specificity of the protein as a whole serves as the 'label' and the protein is quantified both in stool and serum by immunological means rather than by radioactivity measurements.

Over the years a variety of substances have been tested for their ability to measure protein-losing enteropathy. Radioactive iodine-labelled proteins were considered first because they offered the theoretical advantage that they could be used for concomitant studies of protein turnover. However, it rapidly became apparent that radioactive iodine-labelled proteins were, in fact, unsuitable for this purpose because radioactive iodine that is released from protein during digestion within the gastrointestinal tract is readily reabsorbed; in addition, radioactive iodine released from protein during endogenous catabolism can be excreted into the gastrointestinal tract in a non-protein-bound form. Subsequently, a series of other labelled proteins (and non-proteins) were considered for measurement of protein-losing enteropathy including ^{131}I-labelled polyvinylpyrrolidone, ^{59}Fe-labelled dextran, [95]Nb-labelled albumin, [67]Cu-labelled ceruloplasmin and ^{51}Cr-labelled albumin (or [51]CrCl$_3$).[25,31,32,70,72] One such material, ^{131}I-labelled polyvinylpyrrolidone, was used in early studies of protein-losing enteropathy with some success,[25] but was ultimately discarded because it was a non-physiological material that was rapidly cleared from the circulation; in addition, it could be broken down in the gastrointestinal tract and the ^{131}I released could be reabsorbed. Another such material, [67]Cu-labelled ceruloplasmin, seemed at first to be the ideal radiolabelled protein for measurement of protein-losing enteropathy because the labelled moeity, ^{67}Cu, is an integral part of the protein and remains with the protein throughout the latter's biological life; in addition, ^{67}Cu released into the gastrointestinal lumen upon degradation of ceruloplasmin does not undergo significant reabsorption.[70] However, ^{67}Cu-labelled ceruloplasmin proved to be an impractical means of measuring protein-losing enteropathy because ^{67}Cu-labelled ceruloplasmin is difficult to obtain and ^{67}Cu has a short half-life. It should be mentioned, however, that ^{67}Cu-labelled ceruloplasmin was used to advantage in early research studies to show that the gastrointestinal tract accounts for no more than 10% of the total catabolism of ceruloplasmin; this finding put to rest the view that the gastrointestinal tract is normally an important site of degradation of ceruloplasmin and, by extension, other serum proteins.[70]

The radiolabelled materials that ultimately gained the widest use in the measurement of protein-losing enteropathy was ^{51}Cr-labelled albumin or ^{51}CrCl$_3$.[65,72] This resulted from the fact that the radiolabel, ^{51}Cr, is not excreted into the gastrointestinal tract unless it is linked to a serum protein and, once in the gastrointestinal tract, is not absorbed; in addition, ^{51}Cr has a reasonably long half-life and is readily obtained. Initially, the ^{51}Cr label was administered in the form of ^{51}Cr-labelled albumin with the hope that the ^{51}Cr die-away would be a measure of albumin metabolism and ^{51}Cr excretion would be a measure of protein-losing enteropathy. However, it was found that the ^{51}Cr label does not remain associated with the albumin molecule to which it was initially bound and thus it can not be used as a protein tracer. Interestingly, this does not impair the ability of ^{51}Cr-labelled albumin to measure protein-losing enteropathy because the release of ^{51}Cr from the albumin molecule to which it was originally bound is followed by rapid uptake by other serum proteins (notably transferrin) and thus any ^{51}Cr excretion into the gastrointestinal tract is still due to ^{51}Cr attached to a serum protein; furthermore, provided the excreted ^{51}Cr-labelled protein has the same specific activity as the circulating ^{51}Cr-labelled protein, the amount of ^{51}Cr excreted reflects a constant loss rate into the gastrointestinal tract regardless of the protein to which it is attached.

The recognition that the ^{51}Cr label in ^{51}Cr-labelled albumin is dispersed to many proteins *in vivo* without compromise of its ability to measure protein-losing enteropathy led to the use of ^{51}CrCl$_3$,[65] a ^{51}Cr preparation which, following intravenous injection, attaches to many circulating proteins directly rather than residing initially with

albumin. This material provided data equivalent to that obtained with ^{51}Cr-labelled albumin, thereby verifying the fact that a label used to measure protein-losing enteropathy does not have to be attached to only one protein throughout the entire study. While neither ^{51}Cr-labelled albumin or ^{51}CrCl$_3$ could, as mentioned, be used to measure serum protein metabolism, neither material interferred with the simultaneous use of ^{131}I-labelled albumin for the latter purpose. This results from the fact that ^{51}Cr and ^{125}I have widely separated energy peaks and can be independently counted in biological specimens using appropriate radioactivity detection devices. Dual-isotope studies with ^{51}CrCl$_3$ or ^{51}Cr-labelled albumin on the one hand, and ^{125}I-labelled albumin on the other, provided precise data on the extent to which an increase in protein catabolism is accounted for by protein-losing enteropathy.

In recent years, the use of ^{51}Cr-labelled substances for the measurement of protein-losing enteropathy has largely been supplanted by the use α_1-antitrypsin.[22,61] α_1-Antitrypsin is a 54 kDa glycoprotein synthesized in the liver that accounts for some 80% of the circulating human α_1-globulin protein fraction. It is useful for the measurement of protein-losing enteropathy because its antiproteolytic activity renders it resistant to digestion by intestinal proteases and the amount of α_1-antitrypsin in the stool is thus an accurate reflection of the amount excreted into the gastrointestinal tract. The only limitation in the use of α_1-antitrypsin arises from the fact that this protein is broken down by acid in the stomach; hence, it cannot be used to measure protein-losing enteropathy due to protein loss into the stomach, such as that occurring in Ménétrier's disease (see below).

In both the earlier use of ^{51}Cr and the more recent use of α_1-antitrypsin, one quantifies protein-losing enteropathy by one of two methods. In the first method, either injected ^{51}Cr (in the form of ^{51}Cr-labelled albumin or ^{51}CrCl$_3$) or endogenously secreted α_1-antitrypsin is measured only in stool samples. In normal individuals, excretion of ^{51}Cr in the 4 days following injection does not exceed 0.7% of the injected dose. This is a reliable upper bound value that correlates with clearance values of ^{51}Cr determined by methods described below; however, it cannot be quantitatively related to any metabolic parameter, such as the fractional catabolic rate of an albumin-like protein. A similar normal upper bound for α_1-antitrypsin excretion is $<140 \mu g/100$ g dry stool. In this case, however, the faecal α_1-antitrypsin sometimes does not accurately predict clearance values since random stool weights may be low (giving rise to artificially high α_1-antitrypsin excretion values).

In the second or more quantitative method of measuring protein-losing enteropathy, ^{51}Cr clearance or α_1-antitrypsin clearance is measured in manner similar to that in the determination of creatinine clearance. Here, the clearance is calculated from the amount of 'label' (^{51}Cr or α_1-antitrypsin) excreted over a period of time divided by the mean serum concentration of the label during that time (*Figure 3.92*). In practice, the performance of a ^{51}Cr clearance is inherently more difficult than an α_1-antitrypsin clearance because, in the former case, the ^{51}Cr value is changing and one must account for excretion delay (usually 24 hours). This problem does not exist with the use of α_1-antitrypsin, because in this case the serum concentration of the label, the α_1-antitrypsin molecule itself, is constant in any given patient.

The normal clearance value for α_1-antitrypsin is 13–14 ml/day, with an upper limit of normal of 24 ml/day. This value agrees well with the upper limit value of 40 ml/day obtained with ^{51}Cr, if one allows for the fact that α_1-antitrypsin clearance does not include normal protein loss occurring in the stomach. Recent studies have shown that the α_1-antitrypsin may be increased slightly in patients with

diarrhoea induced by laxatives; however, a clearance of >50 ml/day even in such patients is clearly abnormal. Two additional facts concerning the use of α_1-antitrypsin in the measurement of protein-losing enteropathy deserve emphasis. First, the stool concentration of α_1-antitrypsin may be a poor measure of protein-losing enteropathy because it depends on widely varying stool weights and patient-to-patient variation in serum α_1-antitrypsin levels; for this reason, α_1-antitrypsin clearance values are a more reliable index of protein-losing enteropathy than simple stool values; secondly, α_1-antitrypsin values (or indeed ^{51}Cr clearance values) may be erroneously elevated in patients with occult bleeding and the latter should be ruled out before a test for protein-losing enteropathy is performed.

PATHOLOGICAL MECHANISMS RESPONSIBLE FOR PROTEIN-LOSING ENTEROPATHY

The various gastrointestinal diseases associated with protein-losing enteropathy fall into several broad categories (*Table 3.43*). The first such category, dealt with at greater length below, comprises those disorders which lead to obstruction of the intestinal lymphatics. This includes congenital or idiopathic lymphatic abnormalities as well as lymphatic obstruction secondary to a large number of widely different pathological processes. It is in this category that one finds the most severe protein-losing states.

A second category of diseases associated with protein-losing enteropathy are the inflammatory diseases of the gastrointestinal tract. This includes the various ulcerative diseases as well as the diseases in which the bowel wall contains an inflammatory infiltrate such as gluten-sensitive enteropathy (coeliac disease), immunodeficiency states, specific infections of the bowel and gastrointestinal damage caused by radiation or toxins. In addition, anatomical defects such as diverticulosis, stenotic lesions, fistulas, polyps, adenomas, blind loops and neoplasms also lead to protein-losing enteropathy through an inflammatory pathway. The mechanism of protein-losing enteropathy in an inflammation of the bowel is not precisely defined. It seems reasonable to suggest, however, that in the presence of inflammation various substances are released which affect vascular permeability and which thus cause protein-losing enteropathy. Evidence in support of this concept comes from Kondo *et al.*, who have shown that both experimental protein-losing enteropathy induced by irradiation and protein-losing

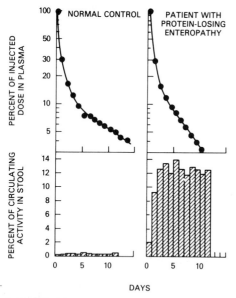

Figure 3.92 ^{51}Cr-labelled albumin study. The serum die-away curve of ^{51}Cr-albumin in a normal individual (left panel) and a patient with protein-losing enteropathy (right panel) is shown. This die-away is more rapid than that of ^{125}I-labelled albumin even in a normal individual because the ^{51}Cr label does not remain with albumin but shifts to other, more rapidly degraded, proteins. Nevertheless, ^{51}Cr-labelled albumin provides accurate data on protein loss into the gastrointestinal tract (see text). Also shown is stool excretion data (expressed as a fractional loss rate); whereas ^{51}Cr excretion is almost non-existent in the normal control, it is quite considerable in the patient.

Table 3.43 Classification of diseases producing protein-losing enteropathy

- *Disorders of intestinal lymphatics*
  - Idiopathic intestinal lymphangiectasia
    - Familial
    - Sporadic
  - Secondary intestinal lymphangiectasia due to:
    - Cardiac disease (see *Table 3.94*)
    - Inflammatory disease resembling lupus erythematosus
    - Non-specific inflammatory disease, Crohn's disease
    - Blockage of lymphatics by lipid filled macrophages, Whipple's disease, abetalipoproteinemia
    - Blockage of lymphatics by neoplastic disease
    - Specific infection involving mensenteric lymphatics, tuberculous peritonitis
    - Non-specific or undefined infection involving mesenteric lymphatics, retroperitoneal fibrosis
- *Inflammatory and/or ulcerative diseases of the gastrointestinal mucosa*
  - Inflammatory bowel disease
  - Specific infections of the gastrointestinal tract
    - Parasitic infections: roundworm, hookworm, amoebae
    - Bacterial infections: Shigella, pseudomembranous colitis
    - Viral infections: gastrointestinal viruses associated with diarrhoea, measles
    - Fungal infections: histoplasmosis
  - Non-specific infections of the gastrointestinal tract associated with:
    - Blind loop syndrome, stenotic and obstructive lesions, diverticula
    - Immunodeficiency states especially common variable hypogammaglobulinaemia
  - Ulcerative diseases
    - Ulcerative gastritis, Zollinger–Ellison syndrome
    - Carcinomas of oesophagus, stomach, small and large bowel
    - Polypoid lesions, villous adenoma, Cronkhite–Canada syndrome
  - Sprue syndromes
    - Gluten-sensitive enteropathy (coeliac disease)
    - Dermatitis herpetiformis
    - Tropical sprue
    - Ulcerative jejunitis (non-granulomatous jejunitis)
    - Kwashiorkor
  - Inflammation or ulceration caused by drugs or physical agents
    - Chronic laxative ingestion
    - Radiation enteritis
    - Retained foreign body (intestinal tube)
  - Vascular diseases of the bowel
    - Vasculo-occlusive diseases, ischaemic bowel disease, diabetes mellitus
    - Haemangiomas, angiomas
    - Malrotation of the bowel
  - Collagen–vascular diseases
    - Henoch–Schönlein purpura
    - Sjogren's syndrome
    - Scleroderma
    - Rheumatoid arthritis
- *Diseases associated with mediator release and changes in vascular permeability*
  - Allergic gastroenteropathy, eosinophilic gastroenteritis
  - Systemic mastocytosis
  - Angioneurotic oedema
  - Ménétrier's disease (giant hypertrophy of the gastric rugae)
  - Carcinoid syndrome

enteropathy due to hypertrophic gastritis and Ménétrier's disease are associated with increased tissue fibrinolytic activity.[39] In addition, these investigators have shown that intraperitoneal administration to rats of streptokinase and urokinase, substances which are activators of plasminogen, lead to protein-losing enteropathy.[40] In general, the extent of protein loss in this category of protein-losing enteropathy is generally mild and for this reason the protein-losing enteropathy in these conditions is usually an incidental finding.

A final group of diseases characterized by protein-losing enteropathy comprises those in which mediator release is a central event, rather than being secondary to inflammation. This category includes the various diseases in which mast cell activation is prominent, such as allergic gastroenteropathy, eosinophilic gastroenteropathy and systemic mastocytosis. In addition, it includes diseases of the complement system, such as Cl esterase inhibitor deficiency (angioneurotic oedema) in which there is an acquired or hereditary lack of a protein which inhibits various complement proteins and elements of the kallikrein system.[23] The mechanism of protein-losing enteropathy in this group of diseases is not intrinsically different from that presumed to occur in inflammation. However, in this case the mediator release may be more massive and, correspondingly, the protein-losing enteropathy more severe.

All three mechanisms of protein-losing enteropathy given above lead to accumulation of fluid (of vascular or lymphatic origin) in the interstitium of the mucosa. Munro has shown, in experimental protein-losing enteropathy induced by reducing agents, that such fluid finds its way into the gastrointestinal lumen by passing between epithelial cells through the tight junctions rather than through the epithelial cells themselves. This fits well with the fact that protein-losing enteropathy can occur when epithelial cells are intact.[47]

GASTROINTESTINAL DISEASES ASSOCIATED WITH PROTEIN-LOSING ENTEROPATHY

Gluten-sensitive enteropathy (coeliac disease)

Mild to moderate hypoalbuminaemia is not an infrequent accompaniment of gluten-sensitive enteropathy, particularly in adult patients with moderate to severe villous atrophy.[12] Studies of albumin metabolism in such patients frequently reveal abnormally low albumin synthesis rates, which is probably secondary to malabsorption of amino acids; this defect in synthesis appears to be mainly responsible for the low albumin level. Patients also have mild to moderate gastrointestinal protein loss as measured with $^{51}CrCl_3$; however, this does not directly correlate with the presence of hypoalbuminaemia, except when the latter is severe. Thus, protein-losing enteropathy probably plays only a minor role in causing the hypoalbuminaemia of gluten-sensitive enteropathy.

Although not proven, the protein-losing enteropathy found in gluten-sensitive enteropathy is probably inflammatory in origin due to infiltration of the lamina propria with inflammatory cells and the consequent release of mediators which change mucosal vascular permeability sufficiently to allow protein-rich fluid to leak into the bowel lumen. Indirect evidence for this comes from recent studies of protein-losing enteropathy in patients with gluten sensitivity in which it was shown that protein-losing enteropathy measured with α_1-antitrypsin correlates with adherence to a gluten-free diet and disease activity.[4]

Malignancy

Hypoalbuminaemia is a frequent finding in all forms of malignancy and is a finding that has a tendency to become more pronounced as the neoplastic disease progresses.[73] In most instances the hypoalbuminaemia is due to a defect in the hepatic synthesis of albumin, even in those cancer patients without obvious liver disease or malabsorption. In a few instances, however, the hypoalbuminaemia of malignancy is due, at least in part, to protein-losing enteropathy. Indeed, the presence of protein-losing enteropathy has been demonstrated in a wide variety of malignancies, including oesophageal, gastric and pancreatic carcinomas, in various polyposis syndromes, in carcinoid syndrome, and in various metastatic carcinomas. In addition, it has been found in lymphomas and in myelomas associated with amyloidosis of the bowel. Protein-losing enteropathy in most patients with malignancy is due to inflammation and ulceration of the bowel accompanied by loss of protein-rich exudate. In addition, disordered lymphatic channels resulting from a malignancy can also cause protein-losing enteropathy, particularly in patients with lymphomas, patients subjected to abdominal irradiation, and in patients with neoplasms associated with right heart failure (carcinoid syndrome).

Inflammatory bowel disease

Inflammatory bowel disease (ulcerative colitis and Crohn's disease), particularly when extensive, is frequently associated with hypoproteinaemia and hypoalbuminaemia. Albumin values in the range 2.5–3.0 g/dl are not uncommon and values below 2.0 g/dl are occasionally seen.[5,58] Steinfeld et al.[58] showed that many patients with inflammatory bowel disease had normal or increased albumin synthesis values but decreased albumin survival (increased albumin fractional catabolic rates) associated with loss of ^{13}I-labelled polyvinylpyrrolidone into the stool. They thus concluded that the hypoalbuminaemia may be largely due to protein-losing enteropathy. Subsequently, it was shown that clearance of ^{51}Cr-labelled albumin (or ^{51}CrCl$_3$) correlated better with the extent of radiological abnormalities than absorptive studies such as fat and D-xylose absorption.[5]

There are probably several causes of protein-losing enteropathy in inflammatory bowel disease. Most importantly, the mucosa is ulcerated and inflamed and this, as discussed above, leads to exudation of protein-rich fluid into the bowel lumen. In addition, lymphatic blockage can occur in Crohn's disease and, therefore, in this disease, leakage of lymphatic fluid may contribute to the protein-losing enteropathy.

Immunodeficiency states

In patients with immunodeficiency and associated gastrointestinal disease (see p. 582), hypoalbuminaemia and protein-losing enteropathy are frequent findings.[67] However, in most cases, the protein-losing enteropathy is not a prominent abnormality and the hypoalbuminaemia observed may be due to a defect in albumin synthesis as well as protein-losing enteropathy. The mechanism of protein-losing enteropathy in patients with immunodeficiency is uncertain, although it seems reasonable to suggest that it is due to a low-grade mucosal inflammatory process attributable to either low-grade bacterial overgrowth, or to concomitant autoimmune-induced inflammation of the gastrointestinal tract.

Ménétrier's disease

Ménétrier's disease (giant hypertrophy of the gastric rugae, giant rugal hypertrophy) is a relatively uncommon abnormality of the gastric mucosa (see p. 345) which has the distinction of being the first disease in which protein-losing enteropathy was clearly demonstrated.[11]

Hypoalbuminaemia occurs in about 70% of patients with Ménétrier's disease and, in all cases studied, this has been shown to be due to an increased fractional catabolic rate of albumin.[34] The protein is lost chiefly, if not exclusively, into the stomach, so that, strictly speaking, Ménétrier's disease is a protein-losing gastropathy, rather than a gastroenteropathy.

Among the factors that may be responsible for this abnormality, release of vasoactive substances in the gastric mucosa is the best substantiated. Thus, protein loss into the stomach was dramatically reduced in one patient with Ménétrier's disease by atropine, and in another patient by hexamethonium bromide.[30] Additionally, one group of investigators has noted reduced protein-losing enteropathy in patients with Ménétrier's disease following administration of trans-4-(aminomethyl)cyclohexane-carboxylic acid, a substance said to act on plasminogen activators and therefore indirectly on substances capable of stimulating kinin release.[39] The fact that protein-losing enteropathy in Ménétrier's disease can be treated in this way places this form of protein-losing enteropathy within the category of protein-losing enteropathy-producing states due to changes in vascular permeability.

Allergic gastroenteropathy

Allergic or eosinophilic gastroenteropathy is characterized by diffuse eosinophilia of the gastric mucosa associated with diarrhoea, abdominal pain and malabsorption (see p. 606). In addition, these gastrointestinal manifestations are associated with allergic symptoms and, at times, peripheral oedema. That allergic mechanisms underlie allergic gastroenteropathy is supported by the fact that patients have high serum IgE levels and an increased number of IgE cells in the lamina propria of the mucosa.[43] In addition, gastrointestinal symptoms are accompanied by frank allergic manifestations and eczema. However, only in occasional cases can a single allergen (most often milk protein) be identified; in most cases, patients seem to be sensitive to most foods and treatment with elimination diets are ineffective. This may be explained by the possibility that oral sensitization with one antigen can lead to sensitization to other antigens because of allergy-induced changes in mucosal permeability.

Patients with allergic gastroenteropathy are generally young individuals who display a somewhat variable clinical picture, ranging from diarrhoea, abdominal pain and malabsorption to peripheral oedema and anaemia. In the latter case, protein-losing enteropathy rather than malabsorption is a major pathological feature. This clinical spectrum is reflected in small intestinal findings which range from a normal villous structure to a mild to moderate villous atrophy reminiscent of gluten-sensitive enteropathy. Whatever the clinical findings, most patients with allergic gastroenteropathy have positive ^{51}Cr-labelled albumin tests and shortened survival of albumin associated with normal albumin synthesis rates.[35,71] The protein-losing enteropathy thus revealed explains the immunoglobulin levels, which are, with the exception of IgE, uniformly low.

The mechanism of protein-losing enteropathy in

allergic gastroenteropathy is not precisely defined. However, it is quite likely to be related to interactions between allergen and IgE bound to mucosal mast cells and subsequent release of mast cell-derived vasoactive substances such as histamine. Davenport has shown that chemically induced histamine release caused by exposure to gastric mucosa to sulphydryl reagents is associated with vascular permeability changes and protein exudation into the lumen.[13] Thus, allergic sensitization of the mucosal surface probably leads to protein-losing enteropathy because of mediator-induced changes in vascular permeability.

INTESTINAL LYMPHANGIECTASIA

Intestinal lymphangiectasia is a distinctive and physiologically informative abnormality whose manifold clinical features have their origin in a central defect in the patency of the intestinal lymphatics. This disease was first recognized by Waldmann et al.,[69] who showed that certain patients with idiopathic hypoalbuminaemia had a protein-losing enteropathy associated with dilated and presumably blocked intestinal mucosal lymphatics. Subsequently, these authors and others showed that intestinal lymphangiectasia is distinguished from other protein-(line missing) signs and symptoms which dominate the clinical picture; secondly, the protein loss of intestinal lymphangiectasia is accompanied by concomitant lymphocyte loss, which leads in turn to lymphocytopenia and immunodeficiency.

Forms of intestinal lymphangiectasia

Intestinal lymphangiectasia is basically divisible into a primary (idiopathic) form in which the disease is due to a congenital defect in lymphatic development and a secondary (acquired) form in which the lymphatics are abnormal due to a more primary disease. Primary intestinal lymphangiectasia is part of a spectrum of abnormalities of lymphatic development. At one end of the spectrum there are the idiopathic lymphoedemas characterized by lymphatic abnormalities which mainly (if not exclusively) affect the extremities of the body.[36,37,41] This includes patients without a family history of disease as well as patients with a variety of autosomal dominant diseases such as Milroy's disease, Noonan's syndrome and Turner's syndrome as well as other autosomal recessive conditions.[26,41,46] Such idiopathic lymphoedemas may be marked by an almost complete lack of development of lymphatics, hypoplastic lymphatics or dilated, tortuous and incompetent lymphatics. In addition, it is occasionally associated with other mesodermal abnormalities such as arteriovenous fistulas, lymphangiomata and neurofibromatosis.[41] Intestinal lymphatic abnormalities may occur in patients with idiopathic lymphoedema,[20,26] but when it does it is generally an inapparent or subclinical aspect of the overall disease. At the other end of the spectrum are patients with primary intestinal lymphangiectasia who have no peripheral lymphatic abnormalities and whose disease is limited to the intestine; such patients are clinically similar to and must be distinguished from patients with secondary (acquired) intestinal lymphangiectasia (see discussion below). Finally, in the middle of the spectrum are patients who have both peripheral abnormalities and intestinal lymphatic abnormalities. In this case the patient is usually considered part of the intestinal lymphangiectasia group, since it is the intestinal lymphatic abnormalities and the result in protein-losing enteropathy which dominates the clinical picture.

The fundamental defect or group of defects leading to the various forms of primary intestinal lymphangiectasia is/are obscure. Thus, while it is clear that lymphatic obstruction is present, either as a central abnormality of a major lymphatic structure or a distal (and more inapparent) abnormality of microscopic tissue lymphatics, the actual origin of the lymphatic lesion is unexplained. Logically, one might postulate the presence of a defect in the lymphatic endothelium or the lymphatic supporting structures which somehow leads to lymphatic hypoplasia and maldevelopment. However, no morphological or biochemical evidence for such a defect has been found.[10,16] In one patient studied at the National Institutes of Health in Bethesda, USA, a defect in fibroblast monolayer formation was observed, suggesting that in this patient an adhesion defect in connective tissue cells are present; however, whether this abnormality can lead to intestinal lymphangiectasia in this or other patients is unknown. In another patient, intestinal lymphangiectasia was successfully treated with anti-plasmin therapy, suggesting that, in some instances of primary intestinal lymphangiectasia, an lymphatic defect may arise from a defect in fibrinolytic activity.[44]

Secondary intestinal lymphangiectasia is due to a variety of diseases which lead to either direct or indirect lymphatic blockage caused by lymphatic fluid overload. Direct blockage can be due to a number of abnormalities including: (1) various forms of cardiovascular disease such as constrictive pericarditis, tricuspid insufficiency or venous thrombosis of a major vein, all of which lead to elevated right-sided venous pressure and impaired emptying of major lymphatics into the subclavian vein; (2) various intestinal conditions marked by an inflammatory cell infiltration caused by infections with known bacteria, fungi or parasites, poorly defined infectious processes such as Whipple's disease[57] and non-specific (autoimmune?) inflammations such as Crohn's disease; (3) intestinal conditions where there is lipophage infiltration such as hypolipoproteinaemia;[17] (4) frank neoplasms of various kinds; (5) inflammatory processes that impinge on major lymphatics such as sclerosing mesenteritis, retroperitonitis and mediastinitis;[6] and (6) post-radiation fibrosis.[53]

Indirect blockage of lymphatics caused by overload of a normal lymphatic system, on the other hand, is probably the mechanism of intestinal lymphangiectasia associated with lupus erythematosus (inflammatory intestinal lymphangiectasia).[21] In this case, it is assumed that intestinal vasculitis leads to gastrointestinal wall tissue fluid production at a rate which exceeds the collecting capacity of the normal lymphatic system. In effect, then, one has functional obstruction of intestinal lymphatics (see further discussion below). This form of intestinal lymphangiectasia may explain the occurrence of occasional cases of transient intestinal lymphangiectasia and/or some cases of idiopathic intestinal lymphangiectasia, since the inflammatory process could be fleeting or could be clinically silent during an early phase and become manifest as lymphatic obstruction during a late phase.[6,51]

Morphological findings in intestinal lymphangiectasia

Gross examination of the small intestine in intestinal lymphangiectasia, either at operation or at autopsy, reveals an oedematous bowel wall with prominent mucosal folds. In addition, the bowel may also have a brownish coloration because of lipofuscin pigment infiltration. Finally, dilated lymphatics may be seen on the serosal surface and these may be associated with yellow nodules representing local accumulations of fat-filled macrophages.

Light microscopic examination of intestinal lymphangiectasia intestinal tissue discloses dilated intestinal lymphatics, the hallmark feature of the disease (*Figure 3.93*). The abnormal lymphatics are most in evidence at the tips of villi, but are often present in the submucosa as well. They are generally intact, i.e. are not in communication with the bowel lumen, and they may contain lymphocytes, foamy macrophages or proteinaceous material representing lymph fluid precipitated during tissue fixation. Failure to observe abnormal lymphatics in intestinal lymphangiectasia may result from the fact that the lymphatic abnormality is patchy in distribution or because the lymphatics are collapsed in the tissue specimen obtained. To some extent, these possibilities can be ruled out by performing a repeat biopsy at the appropriate time after administration of a fatty meal. It is important to recognize, however, that the failure to find dilated intestinal lymphatics in a duodenal or jejunal biopsy specimen does not rule out the diagnosis of intestinal lymphangiectasia.

Intestinal villi in intestinal lymphangiectasia have a normal length, but may appear clubbed because of the dilated lymphatics at their tips. On light microscopic examination, the villous epithelial cells have a normal morphology and there is generally no increase in lamina propria mononuclear cells. (One exception to this is intestinal lymphangiectasia secondary to Whipple's disease, where macrophage

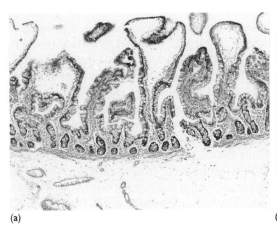
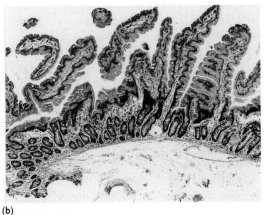

(a)   (b)

Figure 3.93 Jejunal biopsies taken from a patient with intestinal lymphangiectasia due to constrictive pericarditis. (a) The typical lymphatic dilatation can be seen at the villous tips with lymphocytes visible in the dilated channels. (b) The normal histological picture obtained after cardiac surgery which resulted in resolution of the cardiac constriction and the intestinal lymphangiectasia.

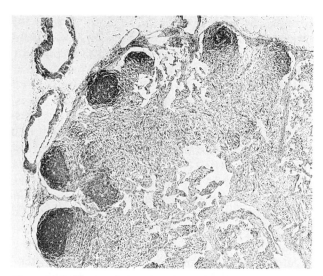

Figure 3.94 Mesenteric lymph node obtained from a patient with intestinal lymphangiectasia. The B-cell areas (germinal centres) have a normal cellularity whereas T-cell areas (paracortical areas) are depleted of lymphocytes. This lymphoid histology indicates that the lymphocyte loss into the gastrointestinal tract drains the lymphoid tissue pool as well as the circulating pool of T cells.

infiltration accompanies the lymphangiectasia.) The lack of epithelial cell abnormalities and mononuclear cell infiltration in intestinal lymphangiectasia generally distinguishes this disease from gluten-sensitive enteropathy (coeliac disease) and other malabsorptive states due to epithelial cell injury. Mesenteric nodes and other lymph nodes in intestinal lymphangiectasia show marked lymphocyte depletion (*Figure 3.94*), correlating well with the chronic and massive lymphocyte loss associated with the disease (see discussion below).

In most cases of intestinal lymphangiectasia abnormality is limited to the small intestine. However, an occasional patient with disease apparently limited to the colon has been described. In these cases one may see (in addition to dilated intestinal lymphatics) giant folds composed of oedematous tissue containing hypoplastic glands and glandular cysts. This picture in not unlike that found in the gastric mucosa of Ménétrier's disease.

On electron microscopic examination of intestinal lymphangiectasia tissue one finds that the endothelial cells forming the wall of the dilated lymphatics have closed intracellular junctions and prominent intracellular filaments.[16] In addition, the lymphatic endothelium has a prominent basal lamina with increased numbers of supporting cells and collagen fibres. This probably represents a secondary response to increased intralymphatic pressure. Another electron microscopic finding is the pres-

ence of lipid droplets (chylomicrons) at the base of absorptive cells, within the lymphatics and in the extracellular areas of the lamina propria. This is attributable to an 'exit-block' of absorbed lipid similar to that seen in abetalipoproteinaemia.

Clinical features

Intestinal lymphangiectasia is generally a disease of early life, with onset of symptoms occurring in the great majority of cases before the age of 30 years; when lymphangiectasia does occur later in life it is likely to be secondary to a cardiac, neoplastic or inflammatory condition.

In early onset disease (i.e. during the neonatal period or during the first few months of life), intestinal lymphangiectasia can manifest as a severe illness characterized by massive oedema, diarrhoea, malabsorption and overwhelming infection; such patients usually die early. Next most devastating is the intestinal lymphangiectasia of childhood which affects growth, sexual development and emotional maturation. Finally, there is the most common pattern of disease, with onset in adolescence or early adulthood, in which chronic difficulties with oedema, various abdominal symptoms and excessive fatigue dominate the clinical picture. Even in primary intestinal lymphangiectasia, most affected individuals are without similarly affected family members. In an occasional case, however, a familial disease is evident, although never in a clearly definable genetic pattern.

The major symptom of intestinal lymphangiectasia is oedema. This may be asymmetrical, indicative of peripheral lymphatic abnormalities (*Figure 3.95*), or may be generalized, in which case it arises from hypoalbuminaemia and reduced tissue oncotic pressure. Fluid in the abdominal (or pleural) cavity is quite common (occurring in about 50% of patients) and is characteristically of a chylous nature, arising from spillage of lymphatic fluid. In long-standing disease, such chylous fluid accumulation can give rise to peritoneal fibrosis and loculation of intestinal loops within fibrotic 'cocoons'. Other manifestations related to fluid accumulation are macular oedema (causing reversible visual difficulties) and chronic stasis dermatitis, which is sometimes associated with peripheral ulcer formation.

Gastrointestinal symptoms are quite frequent in intestinal lymphangiectasia but, particularly in later-onset disease, are usually mild. Diarrhoea is seen in only a minority of intestinal lymphangiectasia patients as a whole, but is both more common and more severe in young children with the disease.[66] In

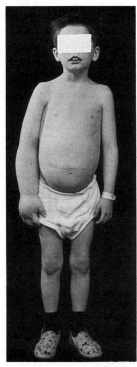

Figure 3.95 An intestinal lymphangiectasia patient with asymmetrical oedema characteristic of fluid accumulation occurring as a result of a lymphatic abnormality. This patient also has abdominal distension due to the presence of chylous ascites.

addition, it is always observed in the occasional patient with intestinal lymphangiectasia of the colon (in which case it is associated with the presence of mucus and blood).[3] Clinically significant steatorrhoea is also relatively uncommon and tends to be more severe in those cases characterized by massive protein-losing enteropathy since both are attributable to blocked intestinal lymphatics. The cause of the steatorrhoea in intestinal lymphangiectasia is probably not not solely to reduced lymphatic uptake of fat, as steatorrhoea may persist even when fat is completely removed from the diet; the latter argues for the presence of a 'fat-losing' enteropathy in some cases.[45] Abdominal pain occurs in perhaps 15% of patients. Its cause is poorly understood, but it may be related to disturbances in intestinal motility. In some cases it may suggest the presence of intestinal obstruction and the latter may in fact be present as a consequence of intestinal fibrosis. Other symptoms attributable to gastrointestinal dysfunction include tetany secondary to hypocalcaemia, growth retardation due to malabsorption and recurrent thrombotic episodes due to intestinal loss of antithrombotic serum factors.[48]

As discussed later, patients with intestinal lym-

phangiectasia frequently, if not always, have an immunodeficiency state and may therefore have manifestations attributable to an inadequate immune response. These include persistent and generalized warts, presumably due to persistent viral infection, infection with atypical mycobacteria, and various signs and symptoms arising from the presence of malignant disease. Finally, patients with intestinal lymphangiectasia frequently complain of chronic fatigue. This symptom is quite important from the patients' point of view and may be severe enough to preclude a normal level of activity. Its cause is probably related to the huge intestinal fluid losses often associated with intestinal lymphangiectasia.

The physical examination in primary intestinal lymphangiectasia is dominated by evidence of lymphatic obstruction. This includes the characteristic physical finding of intestinal lymphangiectasia, an asymmetrical oedema which is usually but not always dependent and which is resistant to diuretics (*Figure 3.93*). Such oedema in severe and chronic cases may be associated with lower limb stasis dermatitis, superficial skin weeping and ulceration, and local skin infection. Lymphatic obstruction may also lead to peritoneal (or pleural fluid) accumulations; these can be quite massive and lead to respiratory difficulties. As alluded to earlier, lymphatic abnormalities in primary intestinal lymphangiectasia may be associated with the occurrence of cutaneous or even intra-abdominal lymphangiomas as well as vascular and nerve tissue tumours. Finally, occasional patients with primary intestinal lymphangiectasia manifest a peculiar dystrophy of the nails of unknown aetiology known as the 'yellow nail syndrome'.[19]

The physical examination in secondary intestinal lymphangiectasia is different from that in the primary disease in that the fluid accumulation, due solely to an intestinal lymphatic dysfunction and protein-losing enteropathy, is symmetric and dependent. In addition, patients may show evidence of a specific underlying abnormality, e.g. jugular venous distension in constrictive pericarditis, skin rash in systemic lupus erythematosus or hyperpigmentation in Whipple's disease.

Investigations

Laboratory abnormalities in intestinal lymphangiectasia are due chiefly to the protein-losing enteropathy or the malabsorption that is present. Patients have markedly decreased total serum protein levels (the mean level in a large group of National Institutes of Health patients was 3.5 g/dl, the normal range being 6.0–8.0 g/dl) which, in turn, is due to low serum albumin levels (mean level of 1.8 g/dl, the normal range being 3.1–4.5 g/dl) and to low serum IgG levels (mean level of 4.5 ± 2.1 mg/ml, mean level in controls being 12.1 ± 2.7 mg/ml). The decrease in both albumin and IgG levels in intestinal lymphangiectasia is attributable to the fact that both of these are long-lived proteins which are most profoundly affected by a bulk loss process such as protein-losing enteropathy (see discussions above). The concentrations of serum proteins with intermediate half-lives, such as IgA, IgM and transferrin, are only moderately decreased in intestinal lymphangiectasia, and the concentrations of proteins with short half-lives, such as IgE and protein hormones, are virtually normal in intestinal lymphangiectasia.

The majority of intestinal lymphangiectasia patients have increased stool fat excretion, but in only a quarter of patients is fat excretion greater than 10% of ingested fat. This is in keeping with the observation, mentioned above, that steatorrhoea is rather uncommon in intestinal lymphangiectasia. Tests of carbohydrate absorption in intestinal lymphangiectasia, such as the D-xylose absorption test, tend to be normal; this is not surprising inasmuch as intestinal epithelial cells in intestinal lymphangiectasia are morphologically intact. Finally, in the majority of intestinal lymphangiectasia patients, although total calcium levels are low (owing to low protein levels), ionized calcium levels are normal except in those patients with significant malabsorption.

Most patients with intestinal lymphangiectasia are not anaemic; on the contrary, many have a high haematocrit due to a reduced intravascular volume (due, in turn, to low oncotic pressure). However, for reasons that are not clear, an occasional patient with hypochromic anaemia associated with low serum iron levels is seen. In addition, patients with severe anaemia due to leakage of blood into the lymphatic system have been observed; this is thought to be due to the presence of abnormal connections between the venous and lymphatic systems.[15]

Radiographic, lymphangiographic and endoscopic findings in intestinal lymphangiectasia

Radiographic studies in intestinal lymphangiectasia show abnormalities that are found in other malabsorption states and are therefore not diagnostic of intestinal lymphangiectasia. In the radiographic study of a large intestinal lymphangiectasia group conducted at the National Institutes of Health, 15 out of 20 patients showed abnormalities of various kinds, whereas 5 out of 20 patients showed no abnormalities.[54] Major abnormal features included increased thickness of intestinal folds, presumably due to oedema of the bowel wall (characteristically this was seen in the ileal region and led to 'jejunization' of the ileum), dilution of the barium column unassociated with significant dilatation of bowel lumen, and mucosal nodularity and punctuate radiolucencies attributable to lymphatic dilatation. In contrast to small bowel radiographs, radiological studies of the oesophagus, stomach, duodenal bulb and colon were generally normal.

Lymphangiographic studies in intestinal lymphangiectasia have revealed a variety of abnormalities rather than one consistent or pathognomonic change.[8,54] In patients with primary intestinal lymphangiectasia and asymmetrical oedema, one commonly finds hypoplastic or varicose peripheral lymphatics which may be accompanied by dermal back-flow. This finding is attributable to lymphatic obstruction and is also observed in idiopathic lymphoedema. In the abdominal area, lymphatic blockage at a particular level (usually at the level of the cisterna chyli), tortuous lymphatic channels, absence of abdominal lymph nodes and obstruction or even absence of the thoracic duct may be seen. In occasional cases one may observe reflux of contrast material into the mesenteric lymphatics and entry of contrast material into the small bowel or into the peritoneal cavity; this finding usually signifies severe leakage of lymph fluid into the bowel lumen or even the presence of a frank lymphatic–duodenal fistula.[24] In patients with intestinal lymphangiectasia secondary to cardiac disease a somewhat different picture is seen; in this case one may observe a dilated, tortuous thoracic duct, probably due to obstruction at the point of entry of the duct into the subclavian vein.

Endoscopic findings in intestinal lymphangiectasia are consistent with the morphological lesion present.[2] Thus, on the jejunal surface one finds scattered white spots (which probably represent dilated lymphatics), white, swollen villi and prominent intestinal folds. In addition, chylous fluid may be present in the bowel lumen.

Ultrasonography and scintigraphy are two newer imaging techniques that can be used to determine the presence of intestinal lymphangiectasia. Ultrasonic findings in intestinal lymphangiectasia include evidence of a diffusely thickened bowel wall, ascites, mesenteric oedema and dilated mesenteric lymphatics.[18] Scintigraphy findings, as performed with ^{99m}Tc/Sb colloid, include massive accumulations of tracer in the intestinal lumen.[56]

Protein-losing enteropathy associated with intestinal lymphangiectasia

Just as obstructed lymphatics are the major anatomical abnormality in intestinal lymphangiectasia, protein-losing enteropathy resulting from this lesion is the main physiological abnormality.

Studies of protein-losing enteropathy in patients with intestinal lymphangiectasia studied at the National Institutes of Health showed that intestinal lymphangiectasia patients excrete into the gastrointestinal tract 5–30% of the administered dose of ^{51}Cr within 4 days of its injection as ^{51}Cr-labelled albumin (normal 4-day excretion is less than 1%) and 'clear' 5–40% of their intravascular compartment into the gastrointestinal tract per day (normal loss by this route is <2%/day). Not surprisingly, study of intestinal lymphangiectasia patients with ^{125}I-labelled serum proteins (such as ^{125}I-labelled albumin) discloses high fractional catabolic rates. These metabolic data indicate that the intestinal loss of protein in intestinal lymphangiectasia is both constant and, in many cases, massive, so that it cannot be treated by plasma infusions of albumin.

Immunological abnormalities associated with intestinal lymphangiectasia

The intestinal loss process in intestinal lymphangiectasia is unique in that it includes lymphocytes present in lymphatic fluid as well as the fluid itself. As a result, intestinal lymphangiectasia is accompanied by an immunodeficiency state marked by abnormalities of T cell-mediated immune function.[59] The main feature of the immunodeficiency in intestinal lymphangiectasia is a lymphocytopenia (mean count in National Institutes of Health patients was 710 ± 34 cells/mm³, the normal mean count being 2500 ± 600 cells/mm³) and a depletion of lymphocytes in lymphoid tissues, particularly of T-cell areas (*Figure 3.94*). This is associated with markedly reduced *in vitro* T-cell responsiveness to mitogens, specific antigens and to allogeneic cells (MHC antigens). In addition, *in vivo* T-cell responses are deficient as manifested by weak or non-existent reactions to standard 'delayed' skin test materials, and reduced ability to reject skin allografts, even when second set grafts are emplaced (*Figure 3.96*).

The cells most at risk for loss in intestinal lymphangiectasia are the long-lived cells which recirculate through the lymphatic and vascular circulations.[74] These cells are, for the most part, T cells, and it is therefore not surprising that it is this lymphocyte population (rather than B cells) which is diminished in intestinal lymphangiectasia. Recent

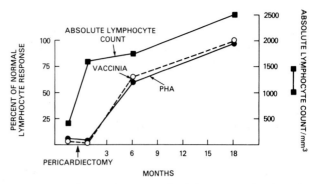

Figure 3.96 Graph of recovery of cellular immune function after pericardiectomy in a patient with secondary intestinal lymphangiectasia due to constrictive pericarditis. It should be noted that lymphocyte levels and immune function return to normal rather slowly. PHA, phytohaemaglutinin.

studies have disclosed that the reduction in T cells involve CD4 T cells in particular, although CD8 T cells are also reduced.[55] The selective reduction in the CD4 T-cell subset probably explains the fact that *in vitro* proliferation responses are reduced in intestinal lymphangiectasia, as the presence of this subset is critical to such responses.

Whereas the intestinal loss of lymph fluid in intestinal lymphangiectasia has a major effect on cellular immunity, its effect on humoral immunity is relatively minor.[59] Thus, in a large group of National Institutes of Health patients, IgG levels were about 30% of normal and IgA and IgM roles were 50% of normal. Such reductions are not usually low enough to result in an increased frequency of infection due to hypogammaglobulinaemia. Measurements of specific antibody responses in intestinal lymphangiectasia indicate that, while patients as a group have tangibly reduced responses, such responses are still substantial.

The question naturally arises as to whether or not patients with intestinal lymphangiectasia are more susceptible to infection as a result of their lymphatic abnormalities. The answer is that, except for perhaps very young intestinal lymphangiectasia patients (who have not had time to develop their immune systems), intestinal lymphangiectasia patients are not subject to excessive infection, although isolated occurrence of chronic infection with low-grade pathogens is encountered from time to time.

Intestinal lymphangiectasia associated with systemic lupus erythematosus – inflammatory intestinal lymphangiectasia

In recent years, a number of cases of intestinal lymphangiectasia due to an underlying inflammatory disease similar to or identical with systemic erythematosus have been observed.[21,38,63] This form of intestinal lymphangiectasia occurs mainly in young women and is marked by oedema, hypoalbuminaemia and protein-losing enteropathy. On intestinal biopsy or endoscopic examination, dilated lymphatics are noted in some, but by no means all, of these patients, and, in those patients that it does occur, the dilatation is usually less marked than in other forms of intestinal lymphangiectasia. Another pathological finding, one not usually found in other forms of intestinal lymphangiectasia, is the presence of a mild inflammatory infiltrate in the lamina propria.

Patients with intestinal lymphangiectasia associated with systemic lupus erythematosus can be distinguished from other patients with intestinal lymphangiectasia by the fact that they have elevated sedimentation rates, normal or elevated immunoglobulin levels and, in many instances, positive serological tests for systemic lupus erythematosus. In addition, patients may have one or more clinical features normally associated with systemic lupus erythematosus, such as carditis, glomerulonephritis, arthritis or skin rash.

The cause of the intestinal lymphangiectasia associated with systemic lupus erythematosus is not known. One possibility suggested by the occurrence of intestinal venulitis in some patients with this condition[38] is that perivascular inflammation leads to changes in vascular permeability, leakage of fluid into the interstitial tissue and lymphangiectasia due to interstitial fluid overload rather than frank obstruction. This mechanism, rather than frank lymphatic obstruction, may explain the fact that patients with intestinal lymphangiectasia associated with systemic lupus erythematosus manifest a relatively small amount of intestinal lymphatic dilatation and are not lymphocytopenic.

Intestinal lymphangiectasia due to cardiac abnormalities

Not long after the initial patients with primary intestinal lymphangiectasia were described, it became apparent the intestinal lymphangiectasia could also occur as a secondary manifestation of certain forms of cardiac disease.[14] Intestinal lymphangiectasia resulting from cardiac disease was first seen in patients with constrictive pericarditis, and indeed this condition remains the most frequent cardiac cause of dilated intestinal lymphatics and protein-losing enteropathy. However, it is now recognized that several different cardiac lesions can lead to intestinal lymphangiectasia (*Table 3.44*).

Table 3.44 Cardiac abnormalities associated with secondary intestinal lymphangiectasia

Constrictive pericarditis
  Idiopathic
  Secondary to lupus erythematosus
  Secondary to radiation

Congenital cardiac abnormalities
  Atrial septal defect (ASD)
  Lutembacher's syndrome (ASD, mitral stenosis)
  Noonan syndrome (ASD, pulmonary stenosis, cleft mitral valve)
  Pulmonary stenosis

Cardiomyopathy
  Familial
  Idiopathic, associated with generalized myopathy

Rheumatic heart disease
  Tricuspid regurgitation
  Mitral regurgitation

Metabolic/toxic cardiac disease
  Myxoedema
  Carcinoid syndrome

Postsurgical cardiac syndromes
  Glenn shunt (vena cava–right pulmonary artery shunt)
  Mustard procedure for transposition of the great vessels

The pathophysiological mechanism which accounts for intestinal lymphangiectasia secondary to cardiac disease undoubtedly involves the fact that lymphatic drainage into the venous system is impeded in the presence of right-sided cardiac disease associated with elevated venous pressures.[60] Increased lymph production may also play some pathogenic role, but cannot be the sole explanation of cardiac intestinal lymphangiectasia since dilated lymphatics and protein-losing enteropathy is slight or non-existent in patients with portal hypertension due to liver disease.[52] This being said, intestinal lymphangiectasia secondary to cardiac disease must also involve certain poorly defined local lymphatic factors, since the vast majority of patients with constrictive pericarditis or right-sided cardiac failure do not develop intestinal lymphangiectasia.[60]

When intestinal lymphangiectasia secondary to a cardiac abnormality occurs, a typical protein-losing enteropathy and lymphocytopenia ensues which leads, in turn, to a secondary immunodeficiency state.[49] The anergy that results may confuse certain diagnostic procedures often performed in the work-up of the cardiac disease such as skin testing with purified protein derivative (PPD) or other antigens. In several National Institutes of Health patients, successful surgical treatment of the constrictive pericarditis led to disappearance of the intestinal lymphangiectasia syndrome as well as the immunodeficiency state[49] (*Figure 3.96*). Such cases provide dramatic evidence that the immunodeficiency of intestinal lymphangiectasia is secondary to the intestinal loss of lymphatic fluid and its cellular contents, since treatment that eliminates the intestinal loss, but which has no direct effect on the lymphoid system, also lead to resolution of the immunological defect.

Cardiac lesions causing intestinal lymphangiectasia can be subtle and inapparent, and patients have been observed in whom cardiac disease was established only by cardiac catheterization. This emphasizes the need for careful cardiac evaluation in each new intestinal lymphangiectasia patient.

Malignant disease and intestinal lymphangiectasia

In common with many other immunodeficiency states, intestinal lymphangiectasia is associated with an increased incidence of lymphoid malignancy. Amongst the National Institutes of Health patients, 3 out of the approximately 60 patients studied have developed malignancy, two with lymphoma and one with the reticulum cell sarcoma. While in 2 of the 3 cases the neoplasm had its origin in the gastrointestinal tract, these malignancies cannot be considered the cause of the intestinal lymphangiectasia since they appeared long after its onset.

The association of intestinal lymphangiectasia with malignancy could stem from defective immunosurveillance and consequent impaired elimination of nascent neoplastic cell colonies. Alternatively, the chronic lymphocyte loss in intestinal lymphangiectasia, consisting mainly of T cells, may lead to defective T-cell regulation of B-cell proliferation and the emergence of neoplastic B cells. This latter possibility is supported by the observation that one patient with intestinal lymphangiectasia seen at the National Institutes of Health developed a monoclonal B-cell malignancy.[9]

Diagnosis and differential diagnosis of intestinal lymphangiectasia

The diagnosis of intestinal lymphangiectasia should be strongly suspected in a patient with oedema who has hypoalbuminaemia (usually less than 3.0 g/dl) associated with lymphocytopenia (usually less than 1500 cells/mm^3); these abnormalities suggest the presence of lymphocytopenic protein-losing gastroenteropathy. In primary intestinal lymphangiectasia one may also see evidence of systemic lymphatic abnormalities (asymmetrical oedema) as well as cutaneous lymphangiomas.

Two studies should be performed in potential intestinal lymphangiectasia patients to establish the diagnosis. The first is a protein leak study to verify the presence of protein-losing enteropathy. In the past, this was performed using ^{51}Cr-labelled proteins but, more recently, α_1-antitrypsin has been used instead. The second is a peroral biopsy of the jejunum to verify the presence of dilated intestinal lymphatics and to rule out other intestinal diseases. As noted above, whilst dilated lymphatics are the hallmark lesion of intestinal lymphangiectasia, their absence does not exclude the diagnosis, because the blocked lymphatics may have a patchy distribution.

Another diagnostic test of potential use in the diagnosis of intestinal lymphangiectasia is the lymphangiogram. However, while this test may provide useful adjunctive data about the lymphatic system in intestinal lymphangiectasia patients, it rarely, if ever, leads to a change in therapy. This, together with the fact that it is not without potential side-effects, has led to its use only in cases where the presence of a neoplasm must be ruled out.

One normally encounters little difficulty in distinguishing intestinal lymphangiectasia from other protein-losing states and/or gastrointestinal disorders. Gluten-sensitive enteropathy with hypoalbuminaemia may be differentiated by the biopsy appearances. Patients with allergic disease of the gastrointestinal tract may have protein-losing enteropathy as severe as in intestinal lymphangiectasia, but lymphocytopenia and immunodeficiency are not present, diffuse oedema of the bowel wall sometimes associated with villous atrophy rather than dilated lymphatics is noted on biopsy, serum IgE levels are usually elevated, and there is a history of relation of symptoms to food ingestion.

Combined immunodeficiency, common variable immunodeficiency and other immunodeficiency states may resemble intestinal lymphangiectasia in that they are sometimes associated with diarrhoea, protein-losing enteropathy and malabsorption; in addition, immunodeficiency patients have low immunoglobulin levels, lymphocytopenia and anergy. Nevertheless, immunodeficiency states are usually distinguishable from intestinal lymphangiectasia in that the immunoglobulin levels are much lower than in intestinal lymphangiectasia, particularly IgA and IgM levels, and the gastrointestinal disease is dominated by malabsorption rather than protein-losing enteropathy, reflecting the fact that villous atrophy, not dilated lymphatics, is the main anatomical lesion present.[1,28]

Finally, dilated intestinal lymphatics also occur in Behçet's syndrome, a disease characterized by neurological abnormalities, aphthous ulcers of the mouth, eye inflammation and arthritis.[64] The cause of this disease is unknown, as is the reason for its association with dilated intestinal lymphatics. It should be noted, however, that the dilated lymphatics in Behçet's syndrome are not associated with the presence of protein-losing enteropathy and Behçet's syndrome is not a form of secondary intestinal lymphangiectasia.

Treatment

The treatment of intestinal lymphangiectasia depends on whether the intestinal lymphangiectasia is primary or secondary. In the former instance, treatment is largely supportive, since no definitive therapy is available to restore the disordered lymphatic channels. Surgical treatment of primary intestinal lymphangiectasia, i.e. surgical excision of severely affected segments of small bowel, has been attempted from time to time,[36] but this form of therapy is rarely, if ever, beneficial and may, in fact, lead to serious complications. The one exception to this rule is in intestinal lymphangiectasia of the colon, where surgical resection of the colon has led to amelioration of protein-losing enteropathy and other disease manifestations.[3] Recently, it has been reported that antiplasmin therapy (i.e. with *trans*-4-(aminomethyl)cyclohexanecarboxylic acid) was dramatically effective in primary intestinal lymphangiectasia associated with an elevated plasma fibrinolytic activity.[44] However, it was ineffective in two other intestinal lymphangiectasia patients with normal plasma fibrinolytic activity.[27]

Supportive therapy in primary intestinal lymphangiectasia consists of diuretics and/or a low-salt diet to control the oedema and ascites. In addition, a diet exceedingly low in fat (<20 g/day) has led to increases in the serum albumin level of 0.5–1.0 g/dl.[33] The low-fat intake probably is beneficial because it reduces the load on the intestinal lymphatics, thereby reducing intralymphatic pressure and protein leakage. The low-fat diet can be supplemented by medium-chain triglycerides because this form of fat is absorbed via the intestinal venous system rather than the lymphatics.[62] Protein repletion of intestinal lymphangiectasia patients by albumin infusion is not generally useful, as the intestinal protein loss in intestinal lymphangiectasia (equivalent at times to a third to a half of the intravascular pool each day) precludes the possibility of meaningful protein replacement. It is nevertheless sometimes useful to augment the serum albumin of intestinal lymphangiectasia patients with parenteral albumin during periods of crisis or prior to surgery.

In secondary intestinal lymphangiectasia, definitive therapy is frequently possible, depending on the underlying disease present. For instance, intestinal lymphangiectasia secondary to constrictive pericarditis can usually be cured by pericardiectomy. Similarly, intestinal lymphangiectasia secondary to systemic lupus erythematous disease may be effectively treated with steroid therapy. The possibility of cure in secondary intestinal lymphangiectasia is so important that every intestinal lymphangiectasia patient should be assumed to have this form of the disease until proven otherwise. In effect, this means that an exhaustive search for cardiac, inflammatory, infectious and neoplastic causes of intestinal lymphangiectasia should be conducted in every new patient.

REFERENCES

1. Ament, M.E., Ochs, H.D. and Davis, S.D. (1973) Structure and function of the gastrointestinal tract in primary immunodeficiency syndromes. A study of 39 patients. *Medicine*, **52**, 227–248.
2. Asakura, H., Miura, S., Morishita, T. *et al.* (1981) Endoscopic and histopathological study on primary and secondary intestinal lymphangiectasia. *Digestive Diseases and Sciences*, **26**, 312–320.
3. Asakura, H., Tsuchiya, M., Katoh, S. *et al.* (1986) Pathological findings of lymphangiectasia of the large intestine in a patient with protein-losing enteropathy. *Gastroenterology*, **91**, 719–724.
4. Bai, J.C., Sambuelli, A., Niveloni, S. *et al.* (1991) Alpha-1-antitrypsin clearance as an aid in the management of patients with coeliac disease. *American Journal of Gastroenterology*, **86**, 986–991.
5. Beeker, W.L., Busch, H.J. and Sylvester, D.L. (1972) Intestinal protein loss in Crohn's disease. *Gastroenterology*, **62**, 207–213.
6. Belaiche, J., Vesin, P., Chaumette, M.T. *et al.* (1980) Intestinal lymphangiectasia associated with fibrosis of the mesenteric nodes. *Gastroenterologie Clinique et Biologique*, **4**, 52–58.
7. Berman, M., Shahn, E. and Weiss, M.F. (1962) The routine fitting of kinetic data to models: a mathematical formalism for digital computers. *Biophysical Journal*, **2**, 275–287.
8. Bookstein, J.J., French, A.B. and Pollard, H.M. (1965) Protein-losing gastroenteropathy: concepts derived from lymphangiography. *American Journal of Digestive Diseases*, **10**, 573–581.
9. Broder, S., Callihan, T.R., Jaffe, E.S. *et al.* (1981) Resolution of longstanding protein-losing enteropathy in a patient with intestinal lymphangiectasia after treatment for malignant lymphoma. *Gastroenterology*, **80**, 166–168.
10. Bujanovir, Y., Liebman, W.M. and Goodman, J.R. (1981) Primary intestinal lymphangiectasia: case

report with radiological and ultrastructural study. *Digestion*, **21**, 101–114.

11. Citrin, Y., Sterling, K. and Halsted, J.A. (1957) The mechanism of hypoproteinemia associated with giant hypertrophy of gastric mucosa. *New England Journal of Medicine*, **257**,906–912.

12. Cluysenaer, O.J.J., Corstens, F.H.M., Hafkenscheid, J.C.M. *et al.* (1974) Mechanisms of hypoalbumenaemia in coeliac sprue. In: *Coeliac Disease, Proceedings of the Second International Coeliac Symposium*, pp. 386–396. (Eds) Hekkens, W.Th.J.M. and Pena, A.S. Leiden: H.E. Stenfort Kroese.

13. Davenport, H.W. (1971) Protein-losing gastropathy produced by sulfhydryl reagents. *Gastroenterology*, **60**, 870–879.

14. Davidson, J.D., Waldmann, T.A., Goodman, O.S. and Gordon, R.S., Jr (1961) Protein-losing gastroenteropathy in congestive heart failure. *The Lancet*, **i**, 899–902.

15. Davidson, J.D., Flynn, E.P. and Kirkpatrick, J.B. (1966) Protein-losing enteropathy and intestinal bleeding. *Annals of Internal Medicine*, **64**, 628–635.

16. Dobbins, W.O. (1966) Electron microscopic study of the intestinal mucosa in intestinal lymphangiectasia. *Gastroenterology*, **51**, 1004–1017.

17. Dobbins, W.O., III (1968) Hypo-beta-lipoproteinemia and intestinal lymphangiectasia. *Archives of Internal Medicine*, **122**, 31–38.

18. Dorne, H.L. and Jequier, S. (1986) Sonography of intestinal lymphangiectasia. *Journal of Ultrasound Medicine*, **5**, 13–16.

19. Duhra, P.M., Quigley, E.M.M. and Marsh, M.N. (1985) Chylous ascites, intestinal lymphangiectasia and the "yellow-nail" syndrome. *Gut*, **26**, 1266–1269.

20. Eustace, P.W., Gaunt, J.I. and Croft, D.N. (1975) Incidence of protein-losing enteropathy in primary lymphoedema using chromium-51 chloride technique. *British Medical Journal*, **iv**, 737.

21. Fleisher, T.A., Strober, W., Muchmore, A.V. *et al.* (1979) Corticosteroid-responsive intestinal lymphangiectasia secondary to an inflammatory process. *New England Journal of Medicine*, **300**, 605–606.

22. Florent, C., L'Hirondel, C., Dezmazures, C. *et al.* (1981) Intestinal clearance of alpha-1-antitrypsin. A sensitive method for the detection of protein-losing enteropathy. *Gastroenterology*, **81**, 777–780.

23. Frank, M.M., Gelfand, J.A. and Atkinson, J.P. (1976) Hereditary angioedema: the clinical syndrome and its management. *Annals of Internal Medicine*, **84**, 580–590.

24. Gold, R.H. and Youker, J.E. (1973) Idiopathic intestinal lymphangiectasia (primary protein-losing enteropathy). Lymphographic verification of enteric and peritoneal leakage of chyle. *Radiology*, **109**, 315–316.

25. Gordon, R.S., Jr (1959) Exudative enteropathy: abnormal permeability of the gastrointestinal tract demonstrable with labelled polyvinylpyrolidone. *The Lancet*, **i**, 325–326.

26. Hennekam, R.C., Geerdink, R.A., Hamel, B.C. *et al.* (1989) Autosomal recessive intestinal lymphangiectasia and lymphedema, with facial anomalies and mental retardation. *American Journal of Medical Genetics*, **34**, 593–600.

27. Herebach, D., Raoul, J.L., Bretagne, J.F. and Gosselin, M. (1991) Intestinal lymphangiectasia: Lack of efficacy of antiplasmin therapy? *Gastroenterology*, **100**, 1152–1153.

28. Hermans, P.E., Diaz-Buxo, J.A. and Stobo, J.D. (1976) Idiopathic late-onset immunoglobulin deficiency. Clinical observations in 50 patients. *American Journal of Medicine*, **61**, 221–237.

29. Iio, A., Strober, W., Broder, S. *et al.* (1977) The metabolism of IgE in patients with immunodeficiency states and neoplastic conditions. *Journal of Clinical Investigation*, **59**, 743–755.

30. Jarnum, S. and Jensen, K.B. (1972) Plasma protein turnover (albumin, transferrin, IgG, IgM) in Ménétrier's disease (giant hypertrophic gastritis): evidence of non-selective protein loss. *Gut*, **13**, 128–137.

31. Jarnum, S., Westergaard, H., Yssing, M. and Jensen, H. (1968) Quantitation of gastrointestinal protein loss by means of Fe[59]-labelled iron dextran. *Gastroenterology*, **55**, 229–241.

32. Jeejeebhoy, K.N., Jarnum, S., Singh, B. *et al.* (1968) [95]Nb-labelled albumin for the study of gastrointestinal albumin loss. *Scandinavian Journal of Gastroenterology*, **3**, 449–457.

33. Jeffries, G.H., Chapman, A. and Sleisenger, M.H. (1964) Low fat diet in intestinal lymphangiectasia. *New England Journal of Medicine*, **270**, 761–766.

34. Jones, E.A., Young, W.B., Morson, B.C. and Dawson, A.M. (1972) A study of six patients with hypertrophy of the gastric mucosa with particular reference to albumin metabolism. *Gut*, **13**, 270–277.

35. Katz, A.J., Goldman, H. and Grand, R.J. (1977) Gastric mucosal biopsy in eosinophilic (allergic) gastroenteritis. *Gastroenterology*, **73**, 705–709.

36. Kinmonth, J.B. and Cox, S.J. (1974) Protein-losing enteropathy in primary lymphoedema: Mesenteric lymphography and gut resection. *British Journal of Surgery*, **61**, 589–593.

37. Kinmonth, J.B., Taylor, G.W., Tracy, G.D. and Marsh, J.D. (1957) Primary lympheodema. Clinical and lymphangiographic studies of series of 107 patients in which the lower limbs were affected. *British Journal of Surgery*, **45**, 1–10.

38. Kobayashi, K., Asakura, H., Ghinozawa, T. *et al.* (1988) Protein-losing enteropathy in systemic lupus erythematosus. Observations by magnifying endoscopy. *Digestive Disease and Science*, **34**, 1924–1928.

39. Kondo, M., Bomba, T., Hosokawa, K. *et al.* (1976) Tissue plasminogen activator in the pathogenesis of protein-losing gastroenteropathy. *Gastroenterology*, **70**, 1045–1047.

40. Kondo, M., Nakanishi, K., Bamba, T., Hosokawa, K. and Masuda, M. (1976) Experimental protein-losing enteropathy. Role of tissue plasminogen activator. *Gastroenterology*, **71**, 631–634.

41. Levine. C. (1989) Primary disorders of lymphatic vessels – a unified concept. *Journal of Pediatric Surgery*, **24**, 233–240.

42. Mariani, G. and Strober, W. (1990) Immunoglobulin metabolism. In: *Fc Receptors and the Action of Antibodies*, pp. 94–177 (Ed.) Metzger, H. Washington, DC: American Society for Microbiology.

43. Min, K.-U. and Metcalfe, D.D. (1991) Eosinophilic gastroenteritis. *Immunology and Allergy Clinics of North America*, **11**, 799–814.

44. Mine, K., Matsubayashi, S., Nakai, Y. and Nakagawa, T. (1989) Intestinal lymphangiectasia markedly improved with antiplasmin therapy. *Gastroenterology*, **96**, 1596–1599.

45. Mistilis, S.P., Skyring, A.P. and Stephen, D.D. (1965) Intestinal lymphangiectasia: mechanism of enteric loss of plasma protein and fat. *The Lancet*, **i**, 77–80.

46. Mucke, J., Hoepffner, W., Scheerschmidt, G., Gornig, H. and Beyreiss, K. (1986) Early onset lymphedema, recessive form – a new form of genetic lymphedema syndrome. *European Journal of Pediatrics*, **145**, 195–198.

47. Munro, D.R. (1974) Route of protein loss during a model protein-losing gastropathy in dogs. *Gastroenterology*, **66**, 960–972.

48. Muntean, W. and Rossepal, E. (1979) Verlust von Inhibitoren des Gerinnungssystems bei der Exudativen Enteropathie. *Klinishi Padiatrie*, **191**, 20–23.

49. Nelson, D.L., Blaese, R.M., Strober, W. *et al.* (1975) Constrictive pericarditis, intestinal lymphangiectasia, and reversible immunologic deficiency. *Journal of Pediatrics*, **86**, 548–554.

50. Nosslin, B. (1973) Analysis of disappearance time-curves after a single injection of labelled proteins. In: *Protein Turnover. CIBA Foundation Symposium 9 (New Series)*, pp. 113–128. Amsterdam: Associated Scientific Publishers.

51. Orbeck, H., Larsen, T.E. and Honig, T. (1978) Transient intestinal lymphangiectasia. *Acta Paediatrica Scandinavica*, **67**, 677–682.

52. Petersen, V.P. and Ottosen, P. (1964) Albumin turnover and thoracic duct lymph in constrictive pericarditis. *Acta Medica Scandinavica*, **176**, 335–344.

53. Rao, S.S., Dundas, S. and Holdsworth, C.D. (1978) Intestinal lymphangiectasia secondary to radiotherapy and chemotherapy. *Digestive Disease and Science*, **32**, 939–942.

54. Shimkin, P.M., Waldmann, T.A. and Krugman, R.L. (1970) Intestinal lymphangiectasia. *American Journal of Roentgenology, Radium Therapy and Nuclear Medicine*, **110**, 827–841.

55. Sorensen, R.U., Halpin, T.C., Abramowsky, C.R. *et al.* (1985) Intestinal lymphangiectasia and thymic hypoplasia. *Clinical Experimental Immunology*, **59**, 217–226.

56. Soucy, J.P., Eybalin, M.C., Taillefer, R., Levasseur, A. and Jobin, G. (1983) Lymphoscintigraphic demonstration of intestinal lymphangiectasia. *Clinical Nuclear Medicine*, **8**, 535–537.

57. Southern, J.F., Moscicki, R.A., Magro, C., Dickersin, G.R., Fallon, J.T. and Block, K.J. (1989) Lymphedema, lymphocytic myocarditis, and sarcoid-like granulomatosis. Manifestations of Whipple's disease. *Journal of American Medical Association*, **261**, 1467–1470.

58. Steinfeld, J.L., Davidson, J.D. and Gordon, R.S., Jr and Green, F.E. (1960) The mechanism of hypoproteinemia in patients with regional enteritis and ulcerative colitis. *American Journal of Medicine*, **29**, 405–415.

59. Strober, W., Wochner, R.D., Carbone, P.P. and Waldmann, T.A. (1967) Intestinal lymphangiectasia: a protein-losing enteropathy with hypogammaglobulinemia, lymphocytopenia and impaired homograft rejection. *Journal of Clinical Investigation*, **46**, 1643–1656.

60. Strober, W., Cohen, L.S., Waldmann, T.A. and Braunwald, E. (1968) Tricuspid regurgitation. A newly recognized cause of protein-losing enteropathy and immunologic deficiency. *American Journal of Medicine*, **44**, 842–850.

61. Strygler, B., Nicar, M.J., Santangelo, W.C., Porter, J.L. and Fordtran, J.S. (1990) α_1-Antitrypsin excretion in stool in normal subjects and in patients with gastrointestinal disorders. *Gastroenterology*, **99**, 1380–1387.

62. Tift, W.L. and Lloyd, J.K. (1957) Intestinal lymphangiectasia. Long-term results with MCT diet. *Archives of Diseases in Childhood*, **50**, 269–275.

63. Tokagi, S., Oshimi, K., Sumiya, M., Gonda, N., Kono, S. and Takaku, F. (1983) Protein-losing enteropathy in systemic lupus erythematosus. *American Journal of Gastroenterology*, **78**, 152–154.

64. Tsuchiya, M., Hibi, T., Mizuno, Y. *et al.* (1976) Comparative, immunological studies on lymphangiectasia of the small intestine revealed in protein-losing gastroenteropathy and Behçet's disease. *Gastroenterologia Japonica*, **11**, 88–99.

65. Van Tongeren, J.H.M. and Reichert, W.J. (1966) Demonstration of protein-losing gastroenteropathy: the quantitative estimation of gastrointestinal protein loss using ^{51}Cr-labelled plasma proteins. *Clinica et Chimica Acta*, **14**, 42–48.

66. Vardy, P.A., Lebenthal, E. and Shevachman, H. (1975) Intestinal lymphangiectasia: a reappraisal. *Pediatrics*, **55**, 842–851.

67. Waldmann, T.A. and Laster, L. (1964) Abnormalities of albumin metabolism in patients with hypogammaglobulinemia. *Journal of Clinical Investigation*, **43**, 1025–1035.

68. Waldmann, T.A. and Strober, W. (1969)

Metabolism of immunoglobulins. *Progress in Allergy*, **13**, 1–110.

69. Waldmann, T.A., Steinfeld, J.L., Dutcher, T.F. *et al.* (1961) The role of the gastrointestinal system in idiopathic hypoproteinemia. *Gastroenterology*, **41**, 197–207.

70. Waldmann, T.A., Morell, A.G., Wochner, R.D. *et al.* (1976) Measurement of gastrointestinal protein loss using ceruloplasmin labeled with [67]copper. *Journal of Clinical Investigation*, **28**, 10–20.

71. Walmann, T.A., Wochner, R.D., Laster, L. and Gordon, R.S., Jr (1967) Allergic gastroenteropathy. A cause of excessive gastrointestinal protein loss. *New England Journal of Medicine*, **276**, 761–769.

72. Waldmann, T.A., Wochner, R.D. and Strober, W. (1969) The role of the gastrointestinal tract in plasma protein metabolism studies with ^{51}Cr-albumin. *American Journal of Medicine*, **46**, 275–285.

73. Waldmann, T.A., Broder, S. and Strober, W. (1974) Protein-losing enteropathies in malignancy. *Annals of the New York Academy of Sciences*, **230**, 306–317.

74. Weiden, P.L., Blaese, R.M., Strober, W. and Waldmann, T.A. (1972) Impaired lymphocyte transformation in intestinal lymphangiectasia. Evidence for at least two functionally distinct lymphocyte populations in man. *Journal of Clinical Investigation*, **51**, 1319–1325.

75. Wochner, R.D., Weissman, S.M., Waldmann, T.A. *et al.* (1968) Direct measurement of the rates of synthesis of plasma proteins in control subjects and patients with gastrointestinal protein loss. *Journal of Clinical Investigation*, **47**, 971–982.

TUMOURS OF THE SMALL INTESTINE

SMALL INTESTINAL LYMPHOMAS

(J.-C. Rambaud and A. Ruskoné-Fourmestraux)

The small intestine is frequently involved late in the course of previously diagnosed nodal malignant lymphomas, but primary localizations in this site are rare. This is true even if the definition of primary digestive tract lymphoma is extended to include not only patients in whom lymphoma apparently arises in the intestine, but all patients with predominant gut lesions without previous peripheral lymphadenopathies, or who presented initially with symptoms caused by digestive tract involvement.[27,32] Primary small intestinal lymphomas of the Western type have to be clearly separated from those of the Mediterranean type.[47,51]

Western-type non-Hodgkin's lymphomas are characterized by focal lesion(s) in the gut with residual non-lymphomatous areas of the small bowel. Mediterranean-type lymphomas are characterized by an extensive infiltration of the whole length or at least a large part of the small intestine without intervening normal mucosa. They include immunoproliferative small intestinal disease, mainly α-chain disease, and extensive parafollicular lymphomas often associated with benign nodular lymphoid hyperplasia.[44,45]

Although this chapter is devoted to primary small intestinal lymphomas, it should be emphasized that these lymphoid proliferations are part of lymphomas arising from gut-associated lymphoid tissue, and thus share many features with lymphomas arising in gastric and colorectal sites. Thus, much data from the literature concerning primary digestive tract lymphoma as a whole will be included in this section.

LYMPHOMAS OF THE WESTERN TYPE

This section will mainly deal with primary small intestinal lymphomas, and secondary lymphomatous involvement of the small bowel will be briefly described afterwards.

Primary small intestinal lymphomas

Epidemiology – premalignant conditions

The reported prevalence of gastrointestinal non-Hodgkin's lymphomas is only 4.5–8.7% of all non-Hodgkin's lymphomas. However, the gastrointestinal tract is the most frequent site (36%) of primary extranodal lymphomas.[47] In western Europe and North America, primary small intestinal lymphomas represent 12.5–20% of all small bowel malignancies and 9–49% (mean 28%) of all primary digestive tract lymphomas.[47] Ileocaecal localizations, not included in the above figures, represent another 5–18%. A histogram of age at diagnosis shows two peak frequencies, one before 15 years of age and one in the fifth or sixth decade.[16,22,27,32] In most series there is a male preponderance which is more marked when children are included.[8,9] In underprivileged countries, primary small intestinal lymphomas of the western type are not more frequent than in the industrialized world but they affect younger patients.

Adult coeliac disease and the similar small intestinal lesions of dermatitis herpetiformis may be complicated by small bowel lymphomas, as discussed elsewhere in this book. Primary small intestinal lymphomas can occur during long-standing ulcerative colitis, Crohn's disease and also in non-specific ulcerative jejunoileitis, which could be malignant from its development.[27,47] Extensive small intestinal follicular lymphoid hyperplasia is frequently associated with, or complicated by, lymphoma in the absence of immunoglobulin deficiency,[35,49] as discussed later with Mediterranean lymphomas,[35] but this association is rare when lymphoid hyperplasia is associated with common variable hypogammaglobulinaemia or selective IgA deficiency.

Other types of immunodeficiency syndromes may be complicated by gut non-Hodgkin's lymphoma: immunodeficiency linked to the X chromosome with increased IgM, or the Wiskott–Aldrich syndrome. Lymphoma occurring during the acquired immune deficiency syndrome is frequently localized to the small bowel (17%) and rectum (3.4%).[68] Such tumours may also be seen in patients who have been previously treated with radiotherapy, chemotherapy or immunosuppressive therapy.[23,47]

Pathology

GROSS FEATURES AND SPREAD

Primary digestive tract lymphomas of Western type are characterized by unifocal or multifocal (10–20%) tumours. They affect several segments of the gastrointestinal tract in 8–20% of cases. In the small bowel the prevalence of the disease increases from the pylorus to the ileocaecal valve.[47]

Various gross patterns of primary small intestinal lymphomas have been described.[66] Large polypoid masses are mostly localized to the distal ileum and are often responsible for intussusception. Aneurysmal tumours are pathognomonic of lymphoma whereas deep ulcerations with raised margins simulate adenocarcinoma: both are frequently complicated by perforation. Annular infiltrations of variable length, sometimes associated with small nodules protruding in the lumen, lead to intestinal obstruction. Composite gross patterns may be observed (Figure 3.97) and multiple lesions in the small bowel are highly suggestive of lymphoma.[14,47,66] Voluminous tumours involving the terminal ileum and caecum are suggestive of Burkitt's and lymphoblastic tumours. In lymphomatous polyposis, small polypoid tumours spread to the whole length of the small intestine, the rectocolon and, sometimes, the stomach.

Lymphatic spread occurs frequently and the abdominal draining lymph node groups are involved consecutively early in the course of the disease. Thoracic and peripheral lymph nodes are rarely and lately involved. Remote spread to the liver (6%), Waldeyer's ring (4%), bone marrow (11%), meningeal tissues (4%) and central nervous system appears to be more frequent in recent series of carefully staged patients with primary digestive tract lymphomas.[53]

The mode of dissemination of primary digestive tract lymphomas may be different from that of primary nodal or spleen non-Hodgkin's lymphomas. Indeed, gut-associated lymphoid cells form a distinct compartment (mucosa-associated lymphoid tissue) with a specific pattern of traffic, and this could explain the frequency of multiple lesions of the gut and of the association of Waldeyer's ring and gastrointestinal deposits.[28,30]

HISTOLOGY

Numerous attempts have been made to subclassify non-Hodgkin's lymphoma in an effort to predict outcome so that comparisons of therapeutic results are very difficult. Until recently, most reports on gut lymphomas have used the Rappaport classification, which is now obsolete. New classifications such as the International Working Formulation for Clinical Usage[65] and the updated Kiel classification[61] are now in use.

However, these classifications are not always well-adapted to primary digestive tract lymphomas. Indeed, as most of (if not all) these tumours arise from mucosa-associated lymphoid tissue, they may include, in various proportions, populations of cells derived from all the normal cellular components of the Peyer's patch.[28] A third tentative classification has therefore been proposed to take into account these peculiar features. Since eventually none of these classifications is satisfactory for correct histological typing of all primary digestive tract lymphomas, they need to be used together (Table 3.45). Furthermore, typing cannot rely only on morphological grounds, and immunohistochemistry on paraffin-embedded and deep-frozen material is essential. Most primary digestive tract lymphomas are B-cell tumours with the exception of the T-cell origin of lymphomas complicating coeliac disease. Of adults with primary small intestinal lymphomas, 50–70% have high-grade malignancy, usually diffuse large cell and immunoblastic lymphomas (Figure 3.98). Children's lymphomas are mainly of the Burkitt or Burkitt-like subtypes and are localized in the ileocaecal area.

Table 3.45 Non-Hodgkin's lymphomas: (a) a Working Formulation for Clinical Usage: the non-Hodgkin's lymphoma pathologic classification project; (b) updated Kiel classification; (c) classification project for primary gut lymphomas

(a)

Low grade
  A. Malignant lymphoma
      Small lymphocytic
          Consistent with CLL†
          Plasmacytoid
  B. Malignant lymphoma, follicular
      Predominantly small cleaved
          cell
      Diffuse areas
      Sclerosis
  C. Malignant lymphoma, follicular
      Mixed, small cleaved and large
          cell
      Diffuse areas
      Sclerosis

Intermediate grade
  D. Malignant lymphoma, follicular
      Predominantly large cell
      Diffuse areas
      Sclerosis
  E. Malignant lymphoma, diffuse
      Small cleaved cell
      Sclerosis
  F. Malignant lymphoma, diffuse
      Mixed, small and large cell
      Sclerosis
      Epithelioid cell component
  G. Malignant lymphoma, diffuse
      Large cell
          Cleaved cell
          Non-cleaved cell
          Sclerosis

High grade
  H. Malignant lymphoma
      Large cell, immunoblastic
          Plasmacytoid
          Clear cell
          Polymorphous
          Epithelioid cell component
  I. Malignant lymphoma
      Lymphoblastic
          Convoluted cell
          Non-convoluted cell

  J. Malignant lymphoma
      Small non-cleaved cell
          Burkitt's
          Follicular area
  Miscellaneous
      Composite
      Mycosis fungoides
      Histiocytic
      Extramedullary plasmacytoma
      Unclassifiable
      Other

†Chronic lymphocytic leukaemia.
Working formulation.[65]

(b)

B	T
Low grade	*Low grade*
*Lymphocytic – chronic lymphocytic and prolymphocytic leukaemia; hairy cell leukaemia	Lymphocytic – chronic lymphocytic and prolymphocytic leukaemia
Lymphoplasmacytic/cytoid (LP immunocytoma)	Small, cerebriform cell mycosis fungoides, Sèzary's syndrome
Plasmacytic	Lymphoepithelioid (Lennert's lymphoma)
*Centroblastic/centrocytic – follicular ± diffuse; diffuse	Angioimmunoblastic
	T zone
	Pleomorphic, small cell
High grade	*High grade*
Centroblastic	Pleomorphic, medium and large cell
*Immunoblastic	Immunoblastic
*Large cell anaplastic (Ki-1+)	Large cell anaplastic
Burkitt lymphoma	Lymphoblastic
*Lymphoblastic	
Rare types	*Rare types*

From Stansfeld *et al.*[61]
*Indicate some degree of correspondence, either in morphology or in functional expression, between categories in two columns.

(c)

B cell
  1. Low-grade B-cell lymphoma of MALT
  2. High-grade B-cell lymphoma of MALT, with or without evidence of a low-grade component
  3. Mediterranean lymphoma (immunoproliferative small intestinal disease), low grade, mixed or high grade
  4. Malignant lymphoma centrocytic (lymphomatous polyposis)
  5. Burkitt-like lymphoma
  6. Other types of low- or high-grade lymphoma corresponding to peripheral lymph node equivalents

T cell
  1. Enteropathy-associated T-cell lymphoma
  2. Other types unassociated with enteropathy

From Isaacson *et al.*[29]
MALT, mucosa-associated lymphoid tissue.

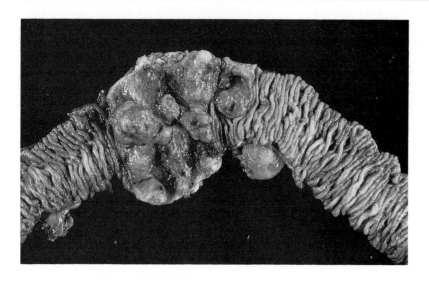

Figure 3.97 Gross appearance of primary small intestinal lymphoma of the Western type. Composite pattern including polypoid masses and an ulcerated tumour. (Courtesy of A. Galian.)

Clinical features

Table 3.46 gives the frequency of presenting symptoms and signs in several large series of primary small intestinal lymphomas. It is often difficult to distinguish in these papers between acute and chronic obstruction and intussusception. However, presentation as a surgical emergency is much more frequent in primary small intestinal lymphomas than with lymphomas in other localizations. A period of malaise, fatigue and vague pains[19,27,32,41] often precedes other symptoms. Weight loss is often said to be mild and the contrast between a short clinical history (mean of 6 months) with minimal emaciation and the finding of an abdominal mass is highly suggestive of abdominal lymphoma.[14] However, many patients are in a poor general condition on presentation.

Investigations

Biochemical, routine haematological and immunological investigations are of little help. Anaemia is frequent but often mild. An increased serum lactate dehydrogenase level indicates rapid growth and/or necrosis of the tumour. A malabsorption syndrome with steatorrhoea and/or protein-losing enteropathy may occur when there is an extensive involvement or partial obstruction (stagnant loop syndrome) of the bowel, massive mesenteric lymph node enlargement or an association with diffuse villous atrophy.[47] Small intestinal radiographs reflect the gross appearance of the lesions.[34] 'Aneurysmal' dilatation with frequent fissure formation, multiple or extensive abnormalities, and extrinsic compression are highly suggestive of lymphoma. However, it is often difficult to distinguish primary small intestinal lym-

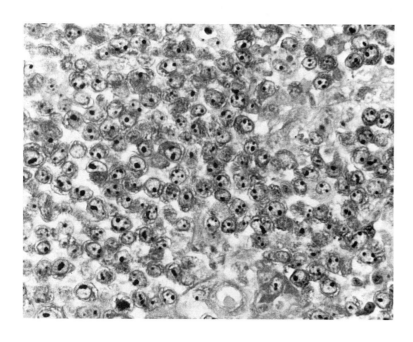

Figure 3.98 Histological pattern of an immunoblastic primary small intestinal lymphoma of the Western type (slow Giemsa). (Courtesy of A. Galian.)

Table 3.46 Clinical presentation in primary small intestinal lymphomas of the Western type

Clinical presentation	References				
			Lewin et al.[32]		
	Loehr et al.[33]	Fu et al.[19]	Small intestinal	Ileocaecal	Rourke et al.[41]
Symptoms and signs					
Abdominal pain	76[a]	81[a]	75[a]	100[a]	67
Nausea/vomiting	48	15	50	38[a]	33
Diarrhoea	20	15	0	38[a]	—
Constipation	—	12	8	7	—
Anorexia	>50		+[b]	+	39
Malaise/fatigue	28	23	37	29	22
Weight loss	52	27	50	31	42
Fever	44[a]	—	—	+	3
Abdominal mass	27	13	29	29	56
Surgical emergency					
Intestinal obstruction	53	44	45	29	25
Intussusception	12	27	0	53	
Peritonitis	16	23	3	0	11
Gross rectal bleeding/melaena	>50	—	16	23	11

[a] Including surgical emergency.
[b] +, frequent.

phomas from other malignant lesions, or even from a benign tumour or from Crohn's disease.[33]

Owing to the usual distal location of the lesions, upper gastrointestinal tract fibre-optic and echo-endoscopy are of little help, whereas colonoscopy usually reaches distal ileum or ileocaecal tumours and allows biopsy. Sonography and computed tomography, with fine-needle aspiration for cytology or microbiopsy, may be of value for the diagnosis of an abdominal mass or of abdominal lymph nodes, but are especially useful for staging and follow-up of the patients.[39,40] However, in most cases of primary small intestinal lymphoma, laparotomy is the only way to confirm the diagnosis.[46]

STAGING

Investigations performed to ascertain the diagnosis of primary small intestinal lymphoma must be complemented by a systematic survey of disease extent for appropriate staging. This staging procedure includes, in addition to careful clinical examination, endoscopy of the upper and lower gastrointestinal tract, abdominal computed tomography, liver and bone marrow biopsies and, in some cases, cerebrospinal fluid study.

PROGNOSTIC FACTORS

Several prognostic factors were shown to influence the outcome in primary digestive tract lymphomas at a time when the treatment was mainly surgery and/or radiotherapy.[17] The influence of the histological

type was clear but often this was merely tautology, if histological grading had been established from survival curves. In all series, the initial extent of the disease was a significant determinant of primary digestive tract lymphoma outcome.[1,2,14,18,31,38] According to the Ann Arbor Staging System modified by Musshoff (*Table 3.47*), localized lymphomas (stages IE, II1E) had a significantly better prognosis than disseminated disease (stages II2E, IIIE, IV). The prognostic value of the size of the primary tumour was unclear. For many of the authors, the large tumours which often invade adjacent tissues, and thus cannot be resected surgically, had a poor survival. The influence of the site of the lymphoma on survival was not well established; it was nil in some series, whereas in others small bowel tumours had a somewhat poorer prognosis than gastric tumours. Multiple sites of tumour seemed to carry a poor prognosis. Old age and severe malnutrition often preclude any curative treatment. Some complications specific to primary digestive tract lymphomas also influenced the outcome, such as digestive tract haemorrhage or perforation.[2]

Modern treatment of primary digestive tract lymphomas, including chemotherapy adapted to the histological grade, to the stage and to the surgical management of the tumour, has markedly modified their outlook. The achievement of a well-documented complete remission at the end of treatment is now the best prognostic factor,[26,53] as it indicates that the therapeutic regimen was well-

Table 3.47 Modified Ann Arbor staging classification for gut non-Hodgkin's lymphomas

Stage	Description
IE	Involvement of one or more localized site of the digestive tract without any lymph node involvement
IIE	Involvement of one or more localized site of the digestive tract and regional lymph nodes without any extra-abdominal lymphomatous localization
	Modification proposed by Musshoff. Stage IIE divided into cases with involvement of regional lymph nodes (II1E) and involvement of regional but non-contiguous lymph nodes (II2E).
IIIE	Involvement of lymph node regions on both sides of the diaphragm with localized tumour of the digestive tract.
IV	Diffuse or disseminated involvement of one or more extralymphatic organs or tissues with or without associated lymph node involvement.

adapted to the characteristics of the particular tumour. It is striking that, by definition, low-grade lymphomas have a spontaneous long survival, whereas patients with high-grade tumours die within a short time untreated; yet a growing percentage of high-grade lymphomas can now be cured, whereas the long-term survival of low-grade lymphomas which respond poorly to chemotherapy has not been markedly improved.

Treatment

There is no current general agreement on therapeutic guidelines in primary digestive tract lymphomas.

Surgery may be performed for several purposes.[46,47] Owing to their frequent localization at sites not reached by endoscopic procedures, diagnosis and histological typing of primary small intestinal lymphomas are often obtained after surgery. Without laparotomy these goals can sometimes be reached by percutaneous aspiration or microbiopsy of lymph nodes. However, high-grade areas may be missed within a low-grade lymphoma when diagnosis is made by perendoscopic or percutaneous procedures.

If no disseminated lesions are disclosed by the usual staging work-up, the evaluation of the local extent of the lymphoma is best achieved by laparotomy. However, surgery should no longer be undertaken for staging purposes alone and can be replaced by echoendoscopy.

It remains unclear whether surgical resection of the whole lesion, or at least of the main focus of tumour, is of value in the treatment of primary digestive tract lymphomas. This certainly avoids local complications of chemotherapy or radiotherapy but the frequency of such complications varies markedly between series.[19,26,63] In localized (stages IE, IIE) low-grade tumours, surgery seems always

advisable since chemotherapy is not effective in the long term and the effectiveness of radiotherapy is not yet well established.[2,26,52] In high-grade primary digestive tract lymphoma many retrospective[2,4,27,33,52,63] and a few prospective[26,53,62] studies seem to show that complete resection of the tumour is an important prognostic feature. It might be argued that tumour resectability merely reflects the fact that a tumour is of limited size and extension. However, even incomplete removal of large tumours allows a better survival than no resection at all.[31,53,63] Nevertheless, extensive resections in order to obtain complete removal of large small bowel lesions should be avoided, at least as the first treatment.

The place of abdominal *radiotherapy* in the treatment of primary digestive tract lymphomas is very ill-defined. It is recommended by some authors instead of surgery.[23,47] The best indications are probably unresectable localized low-grade lymphomas or residual lesions after chemotherapy.[13] Appropriate technique should avoid complications of radiotherapy, the risks of which are greater after surgery and in high-grade lymphomas.

Chemotherapy is now the main therapeutic weapon in the treatment of high-grade primary digestive tract lymphomas as well as of nodal tumours.[2,4,52,54,62] The choice of drug regimen depends on the histological type of the lymphoma, tumour load and tumour dissemination. There is current agreement that adjuvant chemotherapy, probably of short duration, is necessary after apparently complete surgical resection in high-grade primary digestive tract lymphomas, with the possible exception of small tumours removed at stage IE in the absence of serosal infiltration. Some consider that surgery is not indicated in such circumscribed tumours and advocate primary chemotherapy alone. Third-generation chemotherapy regimens are mandatory for the treatment of high-grade large (unresectable) and/or disseminated tumours. In low-grade tumours, current adjuvant chemotherapy regimens do not seem to influence survival; chemotherapy should be limited to patients with residual local tumour or to disseminated (stages IIIE, IVE) tumours.

Treatment of small non-cleaved cell lymphomas, observed in children, relies mainly on intensive chemotherapy regimens. Localized resectable tumours have a very good prognosis but are rare, whereas the common bulky lesions still have a poor prognosis.[42] Extensive resection followed by chemotherapy led to prolonged complete remissions. However, such resections are now avoided because they often delay chemotherapy while tumour growth is very rapid. New drug regimens are currently under evaluation; they all include consolidation and maintenance therapy. Prophylactic treatment of neuromeningeal tissues is systematically performed, consisting of high-dose polychemotherapy, including methotrexate, which may or may not be given intrathecally as well.[42] In other high-grade subtypes this treatment is only undertaken if there is evidence of extension to neuromeningeal tissues.

Prospective series of primary digestive tract lymphomas with accurately histological typing and adequate clinical staging are scarce.[26,53,54] In one series (91 cases, plus 8 multiple polyposis cases),[53] surgical resection of high-grade lymphomas was undertaken whenever possible, followed by combined chemotherapy, including adriamycin. A third-generation chemotherapy protocol was used when there was no or incomplete resection and/or dissemination. The 5-year survival was 91% in the cases with radical surgery and 49% in the others. The 5-year survival for low-grade lymphomas treated by surgical resection when possible and the COP protocol (cyclophosphamide, vincristine, prednisolone) was 78%, but only two-thirds of patients were disease-free. One other series[54] evaluated the effect of a third-generation chemotherapy regime in 71 patients with high-grade lymphomas who had or had not previously undergone radical (31%) or palliative (47%) resection. The overall 4-year survival was 62% and there was no statistically significant difference between the completely resected and non-completely resected cases.

In conclusion, two main guidelines are currently recommended for the treatment of high-grade primary digestive tract lymphomas of whatever site. Both rely on chemotherapy, which may be either preceded by surgery or sometimes followed by radiotherapy. So far, the superiority of one of these alternatives over the other has not been demonstrated. Low-grade primary digestive tract lymphomas are mainly treated by local procedures provided they have not disseminated; most experience in this group has come from gastric tumours.

Plasmacytomas and Waldenström's macroglobulinaemia

Of extramedullary plasmacytomas, 3% are localized in the small intestine, mainly in the ileum.[47] Digestive tract plasmacytomas behave in all respects as other primary digestive tract lymphomas, and evolution to myeloma is infrequent. The finding of a serum monoclonal immunoglobulin is very rare but immunohistochemistry reveals the presence of intracytoplasmic monoclonal immunoglobulin. Radical surgery is considered to be the best treatment but chemotherapy can also achieve complete remission. Thus, extensive resection should be avoided. Small intestinal localizations of Waldenström's macroglobulinaemia are very rare. Localized lymphoplasmacytoid tumours may be found or, in other cases, the small bowel is the site of an extensive infiltration of the lamina propria and of dilated lymphatic vessels by monoclonal IgM and lipids.[43] This form presents with chronic diarrhoea and steatorrhoea and severe protein-losing enteropathy. A variable amount of monoclonal IgM is found in the serum and the bone marrow is usually, but not always, infiltrated by lymphoplasmacytoid cells. The prognosis is very poor.

Secondary small intestinal lymphomas

Digestive tract involvement, often multicentric, was found in 46% of 336 patients dying from malignant lymphoma.[27] Most had widespread systemic and nodal disease and gut involvement was histological only in half of these cases. Indeed, symptomatic secondary involvement of the digestive tract in malignant lymphomas is rare[27] and digestive symptoms occurring during the treatment of a lymphoma are more likely to be due to non-malignant complications, such as moniliasis, acute ulcerations and infection.[47] However, true localization to the digestive tract often remains unnoticed until emergency laparotomy, and postoperative mortality is high; thus, a systemic search for intra-abdominal localization of nodal lymphoma is worthwhile. However, exploratory laparatomy is no longer performed for staging and has been replaced by radiological, endoscopic and computed tomography investigations.

IMMUNOPROLIFERATIVE SMALL INTESTINAL DISEASE, α-CHAIN DISEASE AND MEDITERRANEAN LYMPHOMAS

Much confusion still exists in the literature concerning these entities because of their similar aetiology and clinical presentation, and because of insufficient data on their pathological features and immunological status. As α-chain disease was the first among them to be well described and characterized, a World Health Organisation expert committee proposed the denomination of 'immunoproliferative small intestinal disease' (IPSID)for all those lymphomas whose pathology was identical to that of α-chain disease, whether or not they synthesized the abnormal IgA.[67] In appeared later that the vast majority of immunoproliferative small intestinal disease cases were in fact α-chain disease,[44] but that peculiar extensive lymphomas of the small bowel were a second type of the so-called Mediterranean lymphomas, a denomination which should no longer be used.

α-chain disease

α-chain disease is by far the most frequent of the heavy chain diseases.

Epidemiology and pathogenesis

The digestive form of α-chain disease mostly affects subjects aged 15–30 years, although the disease may be observed in younger children and older patients.[56] The majority of the patients reported originate from the Mediterranean area or from the Middle East but numerous cases have been reported in inhabitants of eastern Europe, the Indian subcontinent, the Far East, Central and South America and sub-Saharan Africa.[44] The only common denominators in these patients, who were of various ethnic origins, were poor socioeconomic status and hygiene.[58] Geophagia since early infancy was almost universal in subjects at risk in Tunisia. It is of great interest that in this country cases of α-chain disease and those of extensive parafollicular small intestinal lymphomas (see later) clustered in distinct geographical areas, with different geological characteristics (M. Ben Jaffar and G. Tufrali, unpublished data).

These peculiar epidemiological features together with the complete remissions achieved by antibiotic treatment alone strongly suggested that microbiological and parasitic factors, operating since early infancy, could play a major role in the pathogenesis of the disease.[57,58] Bacterial counts in the jejunal juice in patients without recent antibiotic treatment revealed moderate bacterial overgrowth with low numbers of strict anaerobes[25] (G. Tufrali, unpublished data).

No specific microorganisms could be found by bacteriological, virological or parasitological studies.[25] However, the putative agent may be present only at the onset of the disease and absent in its usual form at the time of diagnosis. The absence of Fab in α-chain disease protein precludes its use for antigen identification and molecular biology study of nucleic acids of the proliferating cells proved to be disappointing. Even if a specific microorganism is not responsible for the onset of α-chain disease, a non-specific proliferative stimulus, such as bacterial polysaccharide, in the gut lumen could stimulate and perpetuate growth of the abnormal clone growth.[58] Treatment of bacterial overgrowth by suppressing this stimulus could allow the immune defences of the host to eradicate the cellular proliferation. According to this hypothesis, it is remarkable that the putative antigenic stimulation leads in most cases to α-chain disease rather than to myeloma (see later). The α-chain disease clone could have a selective advantage for proliferation because of the lack of idiotypic determinants on the surface of the cells, allowing them to escape from normal immunoregulatory control.[11,45]

The postulated environmental antigenic stimulus might be associated with an underlying immunodeficiency.[58] This could be a defect rendering the host more susceptible to infection with oncogenic organisms or a basic defect of the feedback mechanisms controlling the cellular proliferative response to stimulation. Immunodeficiency could be due to malnutrition, especially in early infancy, or to genetic factors which remain to be identified.

Pathology

The pathological features of α-chain disease are, in general, in accordance with the initial description.[20,21] In the small bowel, lesions extend along the whole length, or at least the major part of the organ, without intervening normal mucosa. Three grades of increasing malignancy can be recognized. In stage A, the cellular infiltrate usually, but not always, remains localized to the mucosal lamina propria and mainly consists of mature plasma cells (*Figure 3.99*). In a few cases, however, small lymphocytes (or centrocytic-like cells?) can be the predominant cell type. Stage C corresponds to an immunoblastic lymphoma with plasmacytic differentiation, forming discrete ulcerated tumours or extensively infiltrating long segments of the small intestine (*Figure 3.100*). Stage B is intermediate between stages A and C. The infiltrate invades at least the submucosa, plasma cells are frankly dys-

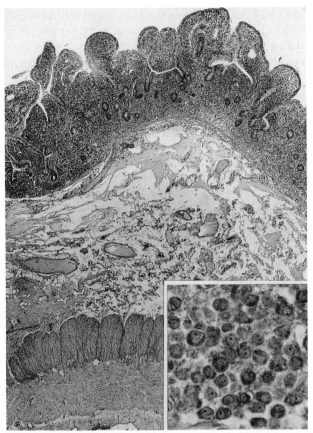

Figure 3.99 α-chain disease: histological pattern of the jejunum at stage A (surgical resection) – short and widened villi; sparse and atrophic crypts; dense cellular infiltrate limited to the lamina propria (HES). *Inset*: the infiltrating cells are mature plasma cells (slow Giemsa). (Reproduced, with permission, from Galian *et al.*[20])

trophic and some large immunoblasts (or centroblasts?) are observed, usually located in the deeper part of the infiltrate and sometimes clustering in small nodules.

Mesenteric lymph nodes are usually involved in the pathological process, although they may be spared in stage A. According to the cellular type(s) of the infiltrate and the degree of architectural disorganization, three histological stages, A, B and C, equivalent to those described in the small intestine, can be identified. Spread to other lymph nodes and organs (liver, spleen, tonsils, retroperitoneal, mediastinal and peripheral lymph nodes) was initially considered to be rare, except when enteromesenteric lesions were at stage C. Histological lesions may progress at a given site from stage A to B and/or from stage B to C, but it must be emphasized that different stages can coexist in different organs or even in different sites of the same organ, especially the small intestine.

This description of α-chain disease pathology requires elaboration and description of nuances.[44] In a few cases, intestinal lesions apparently spare the duodenum and even the jejunum or, in contrast, are limited to a segment of the latter. Spread of the disease outside the enteromesenteric area is not uncommon even when intestinal and mesenteric node lesions are at stage A. Pure gastric, colonic, respiratory tract, thyroid and even systemic localization have been reported.

In his unifying concept of lymphomas arising from mucosa-associated lymphoid tissue, Isaacson[60]

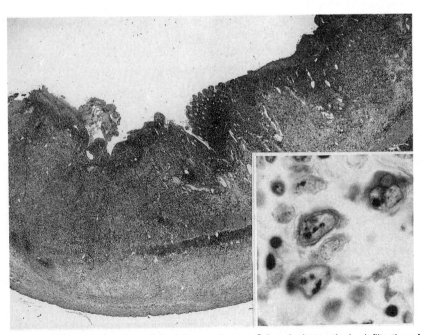

Figure 3.100 α-chain disease: histological pattern of the jejunum at stage C (surgical resection) – infiltration of the whole height of the intestinal wall and ulceration of the mucosa (HES). *Inset*: the infiltrating cells are malignant immunoblasts (slow Giemsa). (Courtesy of A. Galian.)

postulated that in α-chain disease all large cells are neoplastic follicle centre cells, although 'often cytologically bizarre'. Similarly, the invasion, disruption and partial destruction of intestinal crypts, often found even at stage A of α-chain disease, are part of the 'lymphoepithelial lesions', because they are due to centrocytic-like cells, of the same clonal origin as plasma cells.[30] Thus α-chain disease belongs to mucosa-associated lymphoid tissue (MALT) lymphomas. In a few cases, plasma cells synthesizing the α-chain disease protein formed a continuous band in the superficial part of the mucosa, while its middle zone was infiltrated by centrocytic-like cells forming lymphoepithelial lesions,[44] and its deeper part contained hyperplastic follicles penetrated by the centrocytic-like cells.[30]

Clinical features and endoscopic evaluation

The clinical history and presentation of the intestinal form of α-chain disease are well described in several reviews.[44,48,56,58] Briefly, most patients present either with a malabsorption syndrome and a protein-losing enteropathy or with symptoms, signs or complications or intra-abdominal tumours, usually but not always preceded by chronic diarrhoea. Finger clubbing is observed in one-third of cases.

As α-chain disease intestinal lesions nearly always affect the duodenum and the jejunum, endoscopy with biopsies using a colonoscope was suggested as a promising tool for its diagnosis. Thus, the Tunisian–French Digestive Lymphoma Study Group examined in Tunisia its value as the first investigating procedure in patients clinically suspected of the so-called Mediterranean lymphoma.[24] Five primary endoscopic patterns were defined, occurring either alone or in various combinations. The 'infiltrated' pattern was the most sensitive and specific finding with predictive positive and negative values reaching 0.88 and 0.93, respectively; it was followed by the nodular pattern (sensitivity 0.6, specificity 0.84). However, the endoscopic appearance alone of the proximal small intestine could not differentiate α-chain disease from extensive parafollicular small intestinal lymphomas, as defined later, whereas endoscopic biopsies with immunohistochemical study of immunoglobulin chains in the cytoplasm of infiltrative cells could ascertain the diagnosis of α-chain disease in 92% of cases with no false positives.

Immunological diagnosis

In most patients the α-chain disease protein can be found in serum, but its concentration is low or very low in over 50% of cases.[59] Several methods may be used to ascertain the presence in biological fluids of the characteristic incomplete α chains which are unlinked to light chains. Immunoelectrophoresis combined with immunoselection, using for the latter strong anti-$\varkappa$ and anti-λ antisera or anti-Fab-α antiserum to precipitate residual normal IgA proteins, is the most sensitive technique and is 100% specific[15] (*Figure 3.101*). It is noteworthy that in all cases so far studied the α-chain disease protein belonged to the α1 subclass, in spite of the fact that the percentage of IgA2 cells among IgA-synthesizing plasma cells in the intestine is higher than in spleen or peripheral lymph nodes.[3,59]

The concentration of α-chain disease protein in urine is low and Bence Jones proteinuria has never been found. In all cases studied the α-chain disease protein was also found in the jejunal juice when already present in the serum. More interestingly, α-chain disease protein was also found in the intestinal or gastric lumen in two cases although it was undetectable in serum and urine, despite the use of the most sensitive techniques[44] (*Figure 3.101*).

The synthesis of α-chain disease protein by the proliferating cells has been demonstrated by immunohistochemical and/or immunocytochemical methods and by biosynthetic studies *in vitro*.[59] These studies and those of membrane-bound immunoglobulin have shown that immunoblastic cells in stage C of the diseases do synthesize α-chain disease protein.[59] Moreover, these techniques, together with molecular biology studies in one case, allowed the diagnosis of two 'non-secretory' forms

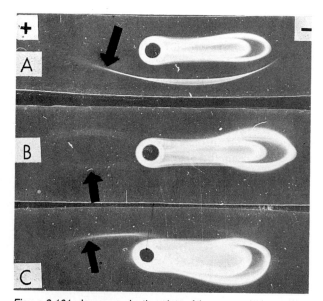

Figure 3.101 Immunoselection plate of the serum of three patients with α-chain disease. The serum samples have been electrophoresed in agar containing anti-$\varkappa$ and anti-λ antibodies. The troughs contain anti-α antiserum. The precipitin lines given by the freely mobile α-chain disease proteins are indicated by arrows. (Reproduced, with permission, from Doe *et al.*[15])

of the disease in which the abnormal protein was absent from serum, urine and jejunal juice.[37,50]

α-CHAIN DISEASE PROTEINS

Most α-chain disease proteins consist largely of multiple polymers. The length of the basic monomeric unit varies between one-half and two-thirds the size of its normal counterpart, the shortening resulting from an internal deletion. Sequence data showed that α-chain disease protein lacked the V_H and the first constant (C_H1) domain.[59] Normal sequence resumed at the beginning of the hinge region with a valine residue corresponding to position 222 of a normal α1-chain.

Recent cytogenetic and molecular biology studies have shown that α-chain disease proliferation is monoclonal from inception. In 3 or 4 cases, cytogenetic studies showed clonal chromosomal abnormalities.[7] In two cases a rearrangement of chromosome 14 was found at band 14q32 where the heavy chain gene cluster locus is located.

Molecular biology studies of the two previous cases with chromosome 14 rearrangement showed three rearranged α bands.[6,64] The α-chain mRNA was short (1.2 kb) compared to that of a normal control (2.0 kb). The cloned α-chain disease protein cDNA contained in the immunoglobulin leader sequence, an insertion variable in length and composition, without any known counterpart, and C_H2 and C_H3 sequences. The leader, the unknown sequence and the second and third (C_H2, C_H3) α exon sequences were in frame.

The α-chain disease productive genes were modified compared to a normal α1 rearranged gene, by the presence of two major deletions in the V_H region and in the switch α C_H1 region. In one case all the C_H1 exon was absent while in the other two-thirds of the 5′ part was lacking, the donor splicing site of the remaining exon being deleted by a mutation.

The high complexity of organization of the 5′ part of the α-chain disease productive gene is without precedent. It includes multiple mutations, insertions and duplications. The presence mainly in the V_H and J_H regions of various inserted sequences of apparently non-immunoglobulin origin within the productive heavy chain gene in the α (and γ) heavy chain is intriguing. Unfortunately, genomic abnormalities in the heavy chain diseases gives no clue to their aetiology.

Finally, it is noticeable that although cellular proliferations do not express light chains, in the two cases mentioned above a short ϰ mRNA (0.9 kb) was found. Interestingly, a short ϰ mRNA has also been observed in three other cases of α-chain disease in which no synthesis of ϰ chains could be detected.[60] Light chain genomic abnormalities are very similar to those of heavy chains.[11] A possible simultaneous defect of heavy and light chain genes in α (and γ) heavy chain diseases would raise the possibility of a coordinated mechanism related to the oncogenic event leading to these diseases.

Course

The natural history of α-chain disease may be unremitting or, more frequently, interrupted by periods of clinical improvement often induced by a blind course of antibiotics. Death may occur at any stage because of complications (infections, hypoglycaemia, surgical emergencies) or cachexia due to malabsorption and tumour growth.[48]

Treatment

Treatment may avoid this fatal outcome, the approach based on a precise knowledge of the extent and histological stage of the disease. Owing to the frequent asynchronism of the histological lesions from one site to another, single sampling at a single site is inadequate and laparotomy must be performed. Complete remission should always be ascertained by multilevel endoscopic gastric, small and large intestinal biopsies studied by immunohistochemical techniques, including double labelling of α and light chains. A second laparotomy may be necessary in a few cases for accurate evaluation.

The authors' present therapeutic guidelines are as follows.[5] Patients with stage A lesions limited to the gut and to mesenteric lymph nodes should be treated first by oral antibiotics and 1 month's treatment with metronidazole, which also eradicates the frequently superimposed Giardia lamblia infestation. Any other parasite should also be treated. Of 28 patients, 39% achieved a complete clinical, histological and immunological remission with antibiotic therapy alone, including one case treated without the classic 2 mg tetracycline regime. Antibiotics usually have a dramatic effect on the malabsorption syndrome, whether or not a true remission of the disease is subsequently obtained. When complete remission is obtained, maintenance antibiotic therapy does not seem necessary.[48]

At stages B and C, antiparasitic and antibiotic treatments are also useful, as they may improve the malabsorption syndrome. At stage C, patients with disseminated immunoblastic lesions of the small intestine require an intensive chemotherapy regimen, as far as is allowed by their nutritional state. When a focal tumour is found, surgical resection followed by combination chemotherapy, including an anthracycline, may induce a complete or prolonged remission. Patients with stage B lesions, or stage A lesions without marked improvement after a 6-month course of antibiotic treatment, or a complete remission within 12 months, should also be given the same combination chemotherapy. Here again, some patients will not improve, even after salvage chemotherapy; some of those patients progress to stage C lesions and die. Others apparently remain at stage A and are asymptomatic for long periods of time on tetracycline treatment. The overall complete remission rate in all Tunisian patients was 52% (64.3% for stages B and C), with a median survival of 67% at 3 years.[5] Relapses, sometimes after a long disease-free interval, may occur after treatment at any stage of the disease. As most patients are young, those with disseminated stage C showing a good response after four cycles of conventional or salvage chemotherapy could be submitted to autologous bone marrow transplantation.

Supportive therapy with intravenous infusion of water, electrolytes, calcium and magnesium salts, blood or albumin and, in some cases, enteral or total parenteral nutrition is often necessary before laparotomy and during the early period of treatment.

Immunoproliferative small intestinal disease distinct from α-chain disease

In three patients with the typical clinical and pathological features of α-chain disease, another monoclonal immunoglobulin was secreted by the cellular proliferation.[44] In a small number of other cases[12,44] the massive small intestinal plasma cells infiltrate was polyclonal. Among these latter patients some had very high plasma levels of polymeric IgA. Evolution to α-chain disease has not been observed thus far.[12] Finally, polyclonal or possibly monoclonal diffuse lymphocytic infiltration can be observed.[36]

Relationships between immunoproliferative small intestinal disease and 'Mediterranean' lymphoma

In 1982, three young patients born in countries where immunoproliferative small intestinal disease is observed, and with a clinical history and presentation identical to this syndrome were reported.[49] However, the pathological lesions, consisting of extensive follicular (or nodular) lymphoid hyperplasia of the small intestine associated in one case with centrocytic-like cell lymphoma were quite different from those of α-chain disease, and immunological studies were unable to show α-chain disease protein synthesis or primary immunoglobulin deficiency.[49]

Review of the literature revealed that the few previously described cases of this entity, which must not be confused with multiple lymphomatous polyposis of the gut, had been mainly observed in the

same epidemiological context as immunoproliferative small intestinal disease. The Tufrali Group in Tunisia therefore evaluated prospectively in this developing Mediterranean country the underlying diseases which would have been previously classified as 'Mediterranean' lymphoma. All consecutive patients referred to the group with the suspicion of intestinal lymphoma from 1981 to 1985 were thoroughly investigated. Among the 55 patients entering the study, 36% had immunoproliferative small intestinal disease and in all of them α-chain disease protein synthesis was demonstrated. In contrast, 46% showed an extensive cellular proliferation infiltrating at least the proximal half of the small intestinal mucosa and submucosa, and consisting of benign-appearing follicular lymphoid structures surrounded, and more or less destroyed, by a malignant lymphoid proliferation of centrocytic or centrocytic-like cells. Gross tumour foci of usually higher malignancy than the diffuse lesions were found in nearly half the cases.[10] No evidence of α-chain disease synthesis immunoglobulin deficiency was observed in any of these patients. A provisional denomination, extensive parafollicular small intestinal lymphoma, can be given to these lymphoid proliferations, which belong to MALT lymphomas. Finally, 15% of patients had a Western-type lymphoma, i.e. localized, small intestinal lymphoma, associated in three cases with coeliac disease.

Thus, it appears that what was called 'Mediterranean' lymphoma is a heterogeneous syndrome, whose common denominators are the young age of the patients, a particular geographical distribution with a marked preponderance of developing countries or populations with low socioeconomic status, and a very similar clinical presentation, including endoscopic pattern. Apart from a few cases of Western-type lymphomas, the syndrome includes in roughly similar proportions immunoproliferative small intestinal disease (α-chain disease in most cases) and extensive small intestinal lymphomas, which are usually associated with extensive follicular lymphoid hyperplasia of the small bowel.

Acknowledgement

The authors would like to thank Professor Annie Galian for allowing them to reproduce the pathological illustrations.

References

1. Aozasa, K., Ueda, T., Kurata, A. *et al.* (1988) Prognostic value of histologic and clinical factors in 56 patients with gastrointestinal lymphomas. *Cancer*, **61**, 309–315.

2. Azab, M., Henry-Amar, M., Rougier, P. *et al.* (1989) Prognostic factors in primary gastrointestinal non Hodgkin's lymphoma. *Cancer*, **64**, 1208–1217.

3. Baklien, K., Fausa, O., Brandtzaeg, P., Froland, S. and Gjone, E. (1977) Malabsorption, villous atrophy and excessive serum IgA in a patient with unusual intestinal immunocyte infiltration. *Scandinavian Journal of Gastroenterology*, **12**, 421–432.

4. Bellesi, G., Alterini, R., Messori, A. *et al.* (1989) Combined surgery and chemotherapy for the treatment of primary gastrointestinal intermediate or high-grade non-Hodgkin's lymphomas. *British Journal of Cancer*, **60**, 244–248.

5. Ben-Ayed, F., Halphen, M., Najjar, T. *et al.* (1989) Treatment of alpha chain disease. Results of a prospective study in 21 Tunisian patients by the Tunisian–French intestinal lymphoma study group. *Cancer*, **63**, 1251–1256.

6. Bentaboulet, M., Mihaesco, E., Gendron, M.-C., Broulit, J.-C. and Tsapis, A. (1989) Genomic alterations in a case of alpha heavy chain disease leading to the generation of composite exons from the J-H region. *European Journal of Immunology*, **19**, 2093–2098.

7. Berger, R., Bernheim, A., Tsapis, A., Brouet, J.-C. and Seligmann, M. (1986) Cytogenetic studies in four cases of α-chain disease. *Cancer Genetic Cytogenetic*, **22**, 219–223.

8. Blackledge, G., Bush, H., Dodge, O.-G. and Crowther, D. (1979) A study of gastro-intestinal lymphoma. *Clinical Oncology*, **5**, 209–219.

9. Blackshaw, A.-J. (1980) Non-Hodgkin's lymphomas of the gut. *Clinical Gastroenterology*, **I**(suppl.), 213–240.

10. Cammoun, C., Jaafoura, H., Tabbane, F., Mourali, N., Halphen, M. and Tufrali, G. (1989) Immunoproliferative small intestinal disease without α-chain disease: pathological study, *Gastroenterology*, **96**, 750–763.

11. Cogné, M., Bakhshi, A., Korsmeyer, S.J. and Guglielmi, P. (1988) Gene mutations and alternate RNA splicing result in truncated Ig L chains in human H chain disease. *Journal of Immunology*, **141**, 1738.

12. Colombel, J.-F., Rambaud, J.-C. Vaerman, J.-P. *et al.* (1988) Massive plasma cell infiltration of the digestive tract. Secretory component as the rate-limiting factor of immunoglobulin secretion in external fluids. *Gastroenterology*, **95**, 1106–1113.

13. Contreary, K., Nance, F.C. and Becker, W.F. (1980) Primary lymphoma of the gastrointestinal tract. *Annals of Surgery*, **191**, 593–598.

14. Dawson, I.M.P., Cornes, J.S. and Morson, B.C. (1961) Primary malignant lymphoid tumours of the intestinal tract. Report of 37 cases with a study of factors influencing prognosis. *British Journal of Surgery*, **49**, 80–89.

15. Doe, W.F., Danon, F. and Seligmann, M. (1979) Immunodiagnosis of alpha-chain disease. *Clinical Experimental Immunology*, **36**, 189–197.

16. Dragosics, B., Bauer, P. and Radaszkiewicz, T. (1985) Primary gastrointestinal non-Hodgkin lymphomas. *Cancer*, **55**, 1060–1073.

17. Fillippa, D.A., De Cosse, J.J., Lieberman, P., Bretsky, S.S. and Weingrad, D.N. (1983) Primary lymphomas of the gastrointestinal tract. Analysis of prognosis factors with emphasis on histological type. *American Journal of Surgical Pathology*, **7**, 363–372.

18. Freeman, C., Berg, J.W. and Cutler, S.J. (1972) Occurence and prognosis of extranodal lymphomas. *Cancer*, **29**, 252–260.

19. Fu, Y.S. and Perkin, K. (1972) Lymphosarcoma of the small intestine. A clinicopathologic study. *Cancer*, **29**, 654–659.

20. Galian, A., Leceste, M.-J., Scotto, J., Bognel, C., Matuchansky, C. and Rambaud, J.-C. (1977) Pathological study of α-chain disease with special emphasis on evolution. *Cancer*, **39**, 2081–2101.

21. Galian, A., Le Charpentier, Y. and Rambaud, J.-C. (1983) La maladie des chaines lourdes alpha. In: *Nouvelles Acquisitions en Pathologie*, pp. 73–112 (Ed.) Nezeloff, C. Paris: Hermann.

22. Green, J.A., Dawson, A.A., Jones, P.F. and Brun, P.W. (1979) The presentation of gastrointestinal lymphoma: a study of a population. *British Journal of Surgery*, **66**, 798–801.

23. Haber, D.A. and Mayer, R.J. (1988) Primary gastrointestinal lymphoma. *Seminars in Oncology*, **15**, 154–169.

24. Halphen, M., Najjar, T., Jaafoura, H., Cammoun, M. and Group Tufrali (1986) Diagnostic value of upper intestinal fiber endoscopy in primary small intestinal lymphoma. *Cancer*, **58**, 2140–2145.

25. Harzic, M., Girard-Pipau, F., Halphen, M., Ferchal, F., Perol, Y. and Rambaud, J.-C. (1985) Etude bactériologique, parasitologique et virologique de la flore digestive dans la maladie des chaines alpha. *Gastroentérologie Clinique et Biologique*, **9**, 472–479.

26. Herrera, A., Solal-Celigny, P., Gaulard, P. *et al.* (1984) Lymphomes primitifs du tube digestif. Résultats thérapeutiques dans une série de 35 cas. *Gastroentérologie Clinique et Biologique*, **8**, 407–413.

27. Herrmann, R., Panahon, A.M., Barcos, M.P., Walsh, D. and Stutzman, L. (1980) Gastrointestinal involvement in non Hodgkin's lymphoma. *Cancer*, **46**, 215–222.

28. Isaacson, P.G. and Wright, D.H. (1987) Extranodal lymphoma. In: *Recent Advances in Histopathology*, pp. 159–184 (Eds) Anthony, P.P. and Macsween, R.N.M. Edinburgh: Churchill Livingstone.

29. Isaacson, P.G., Spencer, J.O., Wright, D.H. *et al.* (1988) Classifying primary gut lymphomas (letter). *The Lancet*, **ii**, 1148–1149.

30. Isaacson, P.G., Dogan, A., Price, S.K. and Spencer, J. (1989) Immunoproliferative small intestinal disease. An immunohistochemical study. *American Journal of Surgical Pathology*, **13**, 1023–1033.

31. List, A.F., Greer, J.P., Cousar, J.C. *et al.* (1988) Non Hodgkin's lymphomas of the gastrointestinal tract: an analysis of clinical and pathologic features affecting outcome. *Journal of Clinical Oncology*, **6**, 1125–1133.

32. Lewin, Kj., Ranchod, H. and Dorfman, R.F. (1978) Lymphomas of the gastrointestinal tract. A study of 117 cases presenting with gastrointestinal disease. *Cancer*, **42**, 693–707.

33. Loehr, J.N., Mujahed, Z., Zahn, F.D., Gray, G.R. and Thorbjarnarson, B. (1969) Primary lymphoma of the gastrointestinal tract: a review of 100 cases. *American Surgery*, **170**, 232–238.

34. Marshak, R.H., Lindner, A.E. and Maklansky, D. (1979) Lymphoreticular disorders of the gastrointestinal tract: roentgenographic features. *Gastrointestinal Radiology*, **4**, 103–120.

35. Matuchansky, C., Morichau-Beauchant, M., Touchard, G. *et al.* (1980) Nodular lymphoid hyperplasia of the small bowel associated with primary jejunal lymphoma. Evidence favoring a cytogenetic relationship. *Gastroenterology*, **78**, 1587–1592.

36. Matuchansky, C., Touchard, G., Babin, P., Lemaire, M., Cogné, M. and Preud'homme, J.-L. (1988) Diffuse small intestinal lymphoid infiltration in nonimmunodeficient adults from western Europe. *Gastroenterology*, **95**, 470–477.

37. Matuchansky, C., Cogné, M., Lemaire, M. *et al.* (1989) Non secretory alpha-chain disease with immunoproliferative small-intestine disease. *New England Journal of Medicine*, **320**, 1534–1539.

38. Mentzer, S.T., Osteen, R.T., Papaas, T.N., Rosenthal, D.S., Canellos, G.P. and Wilson, R.E. (1988) Surgical therapy of localized abdominal non-Hodgkin's lymphomas. *Surgery*, **103**, 609–614.

39. Megiboy, A.J., Balthazare, E.J., Naidich, D.P. and Bosniak, M.A. (1983) Computed tomography of gastrointestinal lymphoma. *American Journal of Roentgenology*, **141**, 541–547.

40. Neumann, C.H., Robet, N.J., Rosenthal, D. and Canellos, G. (1983) Clinical value of ultrasonography for the management of non-Hodgkin lymphoma patients as compared with abdominal computed tomography. *Journal of Computer Assisted Tomography*, **7**, 666–669.

41. O'Rourke, M.G.E., Lancashire, R.P. and Vattoune, J.R. (1986) Lymphoma of the small intestine. *Australian and New Zealand Journal of Surgery*, **56**, 351–355.

42. Patte, C., Philip, Th., Rodary, Ch. *et al.* (1991) High survival rate in advanced-stage B-cell lymphomas and leukemias without CNS involvement with a short intensive polychemo-therapy: results from the French Pediatric Oncology Society of a randomized trial of 216 children. *Journal of Clinical Oncology* **98**, 123–132.

43. Pruzanski, W., Warren, R.E., Goldie, J.H. and Katz, A. (1973) Malabsorption syndrome with infiltration of the intestinal wall by extracellular monoclonal immunoglobulin. *The American Journal of Medicine*, **54**, 811–818.

44. Rambaud, J.-C. and Halphen, M. (1989) Immunoproliferative small intestinal disease (IPSID): relationships with α-chain disease and "Mediterranean" lymphomas. *Gastroenterology International*, **2**, 33–41.

45. Rambaud, J.-C. and Matuchansky, C. (1973) α-chain disease. Pathogenesis and relation to Mediterranean lymphoma. *The Lancet*, **I**, 1431–1432.

46. Rambaud, J.-C. and Najman, A. (1984) Les lymphomes malins primitifs du tube digestif de l'adulte ont des traits particuliers. La laparotomie garde une place pour le diagnostic et le traitement. *Gastroentérologie Clinique et Biologique*, **8**, 432–435.

47. Rambaud, J.-C. and Ruskoné, A. (1985) Small intestinal lymphomas. *Survey of digestive disease*, **3**, 95–113.

48. Rambaud, J.-C. and Seligmann, M. (1976) Alpha chain disease. *Clinical Gastroenterology*, **5**, 341–358.

49. Rambaud, J.-C., De Saint-Louvent, P., Marti, M. *et al.* (1982) Diffuse follicular lymphoid hyperplasia of the small intestine without primary immunoglobulin deficiency. *American Journal of Medicine*, **73**, 125–132.

50. Rambaud, J.-C., Galian, A., Danon, F. *et al.* (1983) α-chain disease without qualitative serum IgA abnormality. Report of two cases, including a "nonsecretory" form. *Cancer*, **51**, 683–686.

51. Rambaud, J.-C., Halphen, M., Galian, A. and Tsapis, A. (1990) Immunoproliferative small intestinal disease (IPSID). Relationships with α-chain disease and Mediterranean lymphomas. *Springer Seminars in Immunopathology*, **12**, 239–250.

52. Richards, M.A., Gregory, W.M., Hall, P.A. *et al.* (1989) Management of localized non-Hodgkin's lymphoma: the experience at St Bartholomew's Hospital 1972–1985. *Hematology and Oncology*, **7**, 1–18.

53. Ruskoné-Fourmestraux, A., Aegerter, Ph., Delmer, A., Galian, A., Brousse, N. and Rambaud, J.C. Groupe d'Etude des Lymphomes Digestifs de l'adulte. (1989) Fondation Française de Cancérologie Digestive. (Primary gastrointestinal non-Hodgkin's lymphoma: prognostic factors and therapeutic results of a prospective multicentric study in 91 patients. *Gastroenterology*, 1992, **102**(4), A393.)

54. Salles, G., Herbrecht, R., Tilly, H. *et al.* (1991) Aggressive primary gastrointestinal lymphomas: review of 91 patients treated with the LNH-84 regimen. A study of the Groupe d'Etude des Lymphomes Agressifs (G.E.L.A.). *American Journal of Medicine*, **90**, 77–84.

55. Seligmann, M. and Rambaud, J.-C. (1969) IgA abnormalities in abdominal lymphoma (α-chain disease). *Israel Journal of Medical Science*, **5**, 151–157.

56. Seligmann, M. and Rambaud, J.-C. (1978) α-chain disease: a possible model for the pathogenesis of human lymphomas. In: *Comprehensive Immunology*, Vol. 4, pp. 425–447 (Eds) Good, R.A. and Day, S.B. New York: Plenum Press.

57. Seligmann, M. and Rambaud, J.-C. (1983) α-chain disease: an immunoproliferative disease of the secretory immune systeme. *Annals of the New York Academy of Sciences*, **409**, 409–478.

58. Seligmann, M., Mihaesco, E. and Frangione, B. (1971) Studies on α-chain disease. *Annals of the New York Academy of Sciences*, **190**, 487–500.

59. Seligmann, M., Mihaesco, E., Preud'homme, J.-L., Danon, F. and Brouet, J.-C. (1979) Heavy chain diseases: current findings and concepts. *Immunology Revue*, **48**, 145–167.

60. Smith, W.J., Price, S.K. and Isaacson, P.G. (1987) Immunoglobulin gene rearrangement in immunoproliferative small intestinal disease (IPSID). *Journal of Clinical Pathology*, **40**, 1291–1297.

61. Stansfeld, A.G., Diebold, J., Noël, H. *et al.* (1988) Updated Kiel classification for lymphomas. *The Lancet*, **i**, 292–293.

62. Steward, W.P., Harris, M., Wasgstaff, J. *et al.* (1985) A prospective study of the treatment of high grade histology non-Hodgkin's lymphoma involving the gastrointestinal tract. *European Journal of Cancer and Clinical Oncology*, **21**, 1195–1200.

63. Talamonti, M.S., Dawes, L.G., Joehl, R.J. and Nahrwold, D.L. (1990) Gastrointestinal lymphoma. A case for primary surgical resection. *Archive of Surgery*, **125**, 972–977.

64. Tsapis, A., Bentaboulet, M., Pellet, P. *et al.* (1989) The productive gene for α-chain disease protein MAL is highly modified by insertion–deletion processes. *Journal of Immunology*, **143**, 3821–3827.

65. The Non-Hodgkin's Lymphoma Pathologic Classification Project (1982) National Cancer Institute sponsored study classification of non-Hodgkin's lymphoma: summary and description of a working formulation for clinical usage. *Cancer*, **49**, 2112–2135.

66. Wood, D.A. (1967) Tumors of the intestine. In: *Atlas of Tumour Pathology*, Section VI, Fasc. 22. Washington, DC: US Armed Forces Institute of Pathology.

67. World Health Organisation Memorandum (1976) α-chain disease and related lymphoma. *Bulletin of the World Health Organisation*, **54**, 615–624.

68. Ziegler, J.L., Beckstead, J.A., Volberding, A.P. *et al.* (1984) Non-Hodgkin's lymphoma in 90 homosexual men. *New England Journal of Medicine*, **311**, 565–570.

CARCINOID TUMOURS AND THE CARCINOID SYNDROME *(H.J.F. Hodgson)*

Carcinoids are solid tumours arising from enterochromaffin cells, usually of the gastrointestinal or respiratory tract. The characteristic histochemical properties of these tumours show them to be related to other tumours of neuroendocrine origin. Carcinoid tumours of the gastrointestinal tract may arise in almost any region of the gut, but the appendix and the small intestine are the commonest sites. Although carcinoids in all sites are potentially malignant, the majority behave as benign tumours and are clinically insignificant. Thus, most clinical attention attaches to the minority of carcinoid tumours that give rise to the carcinoid syndrome – characterized by flushing, diarrhoea and heart disease, and caused by elaboration and release of humoral factors by the tumour.

CARCINOID TUMOURS

Incidence

Carcinoid tumours are not uncommon, occurring as incidental findings in up to 1% of autopsies. In fact, carcinoids are the commonest ileal tumour. By contrast, the carcinoid syndrome is rare – one estimate being that 2 new cases would occur in a population of 250 000 over 10 years.[48]

Pathology

Cell of origin

Enterochromaffin cells, like other cells of the diffuse neuroendocrine system, are scattered throughout the body. Within the gut the cells lie in the lamina propria, mainly near the base of the intestinal crypts; they were originally described as isolated granular cells of the intestine or Kulchitsky cells.[81] Similar cells also occur in the lungs – principally in the submucosal layers of the main bronchi and give rise to bronchial carcinoids and possibly oat cell carcinomas.[6–8] The term 'enterochromaffin' refers to the fact that they stain with potassium chromate, a feature of cells which contain 5-hydroxytryptamine. Thus, other non-Kulchitsky cells which contain 5-hydroxytryptamine, such as mast cells, thyroid C (calcitonin-containing) cells and certain cells in pancreatic islets, the biliary tree, the ovary and the testis, may also give rise to a positive enterochromaffin reaction. Enterochromaffin cells are also stained by other reagents.[28,81] They take up and reduce silver and are thus also termed argentaffin cells. Other closely related cells are stained by silver but do not reduce it spontaneously – argyrophilic cells; these may simply be argentaffin cells which do not store sufficient reducing material to give the appropriate staining reaction, but the precise relationship remains disputed.

The granules of these cells have a particular configuration, being rod-like or biconcave in shape and heterogeneous in density, though granules in enterochromaffin cells from the stomach, duodenum and distal small intestine may differ in morphology. Certain enterochromaffin cells react with antisera to substance P, enkephalins and motilin.[82]

Thus, within the normal enterochromaffin cell population there is a degree of histochemical heterogeneity reflecting different cell products, which may account for the heterogeneity of histochemical reactions in carcinoid tumours and clinical features seen in the carcinoid syndrome (*Table 3.48*).[80,81]

Macroscopic appearance

The majority of carcinoid tumours arise in the appendix, with the small intestine, colon and stomach being the next most common sites[10] (*Table 3.49*). In the small intestine the tumours usually occur in the ileum; 80% of them within 60 cm of the ileocaecal valve. Tumours in this site are multiple in up to 30% of cases. Gastric carcinoids may also be multiple, though single tumours, usually situated in the antrum, are more common. Bronchial carcinoids are usually solitary and occur in the main bronchi, but in 15% of cases they are peripheral and multiple.[21,67]

When discovered, most gastrointestinal carcinoid tumours are less than 1 cm in diameter and only 5% are greater than 2 cm.[30,60] The cut surface is yellow (but may vary from tan to grey) due to the high lipid content; necrosis is rare. Within the gut, tumours usually arise in the submucosa and spread outwards rather than involving the lumen. Ulceration of the mucosa is thus unusual, though it is more common in gastric tumours, which may therefore bleed. Mac-Donald[51] has emphasized that all carcinoids are potentially malignant, but there are marked differences in the likelihood of these tumours producing metastases depending on their site of origin (see below). Local spread from the muscularis mucosa extends to the serosa, by which time the intramural lymphatics are usually involved. A striking feature that may occur at this stage is a dense fibrotic reaction occurring in the region of the primary tumour and sometimes extending into the mesentery. In cases of carcinoid syndrome, such fibrosis may be seen not only around the primary tumour but also in the heart and other sites (see below). Once regional lymph nodes are involved they often become much larger than the primary tumour, so that occasionally massive nodal deposits are found associated with a primary tumour that is only a few millimetres across. Hepatic involvement occurs after nodal involvement late in the disease. Deposits may occur in lung and in bone and rarely other tissues – metastases have been described in nearly every organ.[13] Apparently primary hepatic carcinoids are occasionally reported.

Microscopic appearance

The microscopic appearance of carcinoids is usually

Table 3.48 Characteristics of carcinoid tumours from various sites

| | Site of tumour | | |
	Foregut	*Midgut*	*Hindgut*
Histology	Trabecular	Solid mass of cells	Mixed
Cytoplasmic granules (EM)	Variable density, about 180 μm	Uniformly dense, about 230 μm in size	Variable density, about 190 μm in size
Silver staining	Argyrophil or negative	Argentaffin	Negative
Products			
Blood	5HTP, histamine	5HT	Negative
Urine	5HTP, 5HT, 5HIAA, histamine and others	5HT, 5HIAA	Negative
Metastasis to bone and skin	Common	Unusual	Common

Modified from Williams and Sandler[91] and Soga and Tazawa[80]
EM, electron microscopy; 5HTP, 5-hydroxytryptophan; 5HT, 5-hydroxytryptamine; 5HIAA, 5-hydroxyindoleacetic acid.

Table 3.49 Carcinoid tumours: site of the primary, and the presence of metastases and the carcinoid syndrome[a]

	Number of cases	*Percentage with metastases*	*Number of cases with carcinoid syndrome*
Foregut			
Oesophagus	2	0	—
Stomach	84	23	8
Duodenum	115	20	4
Pancreas	5	20	1
Gallbladder	18	30	1
Bile duct	5	0	—
Ampulla	7	14	—
Larynx	4	50	—
Bronchus	2% of lung tumours	5	66
Thymus	74	25	0
Midgut			
Jejunum	56	35	}91
Ileum	1013	35	
Meckel's diverticulum	44	19	6
Appendix	1687	2	6
Colon	89	60	5
Liver	4	—	—
Ovary	34	6	17
Testis	2	—	0
Cervix	33	25	0
Hindgut			
Rectum	573	18	1

Modified from Cheek and Wilson,[10] with data from Mengel and Shaffer,[55] Hsu *et al.*,[37] Okike *et al.*,[67] Ricci *et al.*,[70] Riddle *et al.*,[72] Wick *et al.*,[77] Matsuyama *et al.*,[53] and Viteaux *et al.*[88]
[a]Other rare primary sites included the middle ear, parotid, breast, kidney, bladder and prostate. None were associated with the carcinoid syndrome.

characteristic, although on occasions metastases initially classified as an adenocarcinoma will be reclassified on review as neuroendocrine in origin. The tumours have no capsule and the cells are uniform in size and polygonal in shape with a centrally situated nucleus containing speckled chromatin and basal granules (*Figure 3.102*). Three major patterns of cellular arrangement have been described[80,91] – alveolar clusters, ribbons or columns of cells; the rare scirrhous pattern may also occur. Correlation of these types with prognosis have been suggested.[40] On electron microscopy, electron-dense granules are seen (*Figure 3.103*) which may differ depending on the site of the primary tumour[80] (*Table 3.50*).

Histochemical reactions

The cells may stain red with eosin (eosinophilic), brown with potassium chromate (chromaffin), black with iron haematoxylin (siderophilic), orange-red with Erlich's diazo reaction, and brownish black with silver nitrate (argentaffin). Echoing the heterogeneity of the normal enterochromaffin cell popu-

lation, different carcinoid tumours may exhibit different staining reactions to these and other agents. For example, tumours arising from embryological foregut (bronchus, oesophagus and stomach) do not usually give positive argentaffin reactions, but do stain with silver when reducing agents are also applied (argyrophilic). As with normal enterochromaffin cells, application of histochemical techniques using the electron microscope may be useful (*Figure 3.104*).[80] Some workers have attempted to correlate the histochemical staining reactions with the embryological origin of the primary tumour and the clinical features of the carcinoid syndrome arising from tumours of different sites (*Table 3.48*).

In addition to these 'classic' histochemical reactions, the use of antisera to a number of peptides has expanded the concept of heterogeneity of substances produced by carcinoid tumours. Particular carcinoids have been shown to contain a wide variety of biologically active products, including insulin, somatostatin, glucagon, cholecystokinin, substance P, enkephalins, gastrin, pancreatic poly-

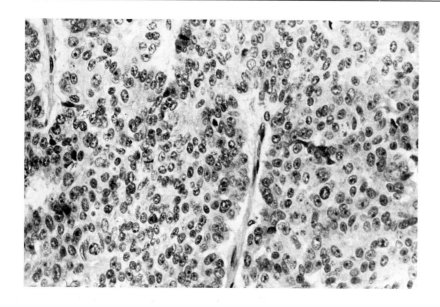

Figure 3.102 Carcinoid of the gastro-intestinal tract (haematoxylin and eosin). (Courtesy of J. Polak, R.P.M.S.)

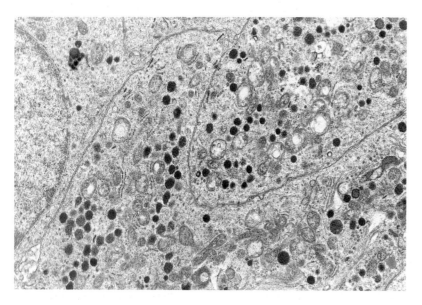

Figure 3.103 Electron micrograph of carcinoid showing electron-dense polymorphic granules with a mean diameter of 280 nm. (Courtesy of J. Polak, R.P.M.S.)

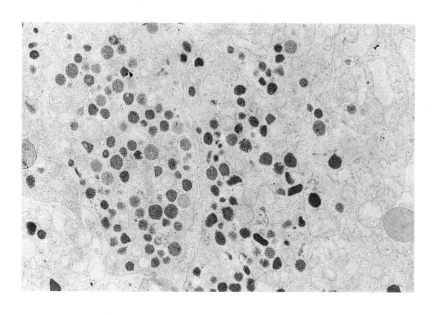

Figure 3.104 Electron micrograph of carcinoid following application of the Masson–Fontana argentaffin reaction. Not counterstained. (Courtesy of J. Polak, R.P.M.S.)

Table 3.50 Prognosis of carcinoid tumours

Site	Number of cases	Percentage with metastases	Age-adjusted 5-year survival rate (%)	
			Local tumour only	Distant metastases present
Appendix	783	5	99	27
Small intestine	147	60	75	19
Stomach	19	55	93	0
Colon	33	71	77	17
Rectum	252	15	92	7
Lung and bronchus	151	21	96	11

Modified from Godwin.[25]

peptide, adrenocorticotrophic hormone, β-melanocyte-stimulating hormone, parathyroid hormone, calcitonin, growth hormone, growth hormone-releasing factor, dopamine or adrenaline and prostaglandins.[26,48,53,83] Carcinoid tumours also give positive reactions with neurone-specific enolase (*Figure 3.105*).

The relationship between the primary tumour and the development of the carcinoid syndrome

The carcinoid syndrome occurs only when the tumour produces vasoactive and other substances which reach the systemic circulation. With gastrointestinal carcinoids, the presence of the syndrome is therefore associated with the presence of hepatic metastases in 95% of cases.[15] Occasionally, however, primary tumours in the gut or tumours with extensive nodal involvement and direct access to the systemic venous circulation will produce the syndrome.[15,19] Carcinoid elements in ovarian teratomas can produce a syndrome in the absence of hepatic metastases, reflecting the direct venous drainage of these tumours into the systemic circulation.[89] Bronchial carcinoids can give rise to the syndrome in the absence of metastases, though in fact metastases are present in most cases.[70] In addition, rarely tumours of thyroid C cells may produce the carcinoid syndrome,[59] as may oat cell carcinomas of the lung.[28] Not all carcinoids produce the carcinoid syndrome when metastases are present. The approximate incidence of primary carcinoid tumours, their propensity to metastasize and their ability to produce the carcinoid syndrome are shown in *Table 3.49*.

Clinical features

Carcinoid tumours are usually unrelated to other disease processes, but there is an apparent association with von Recklinghausen's neurofibromatosis (an autosomal-dominant condition affecting tissues of neural crest origin).[41] Multiple gastric carcinoids have been reported in a few patients with pernicious anaemia and diffuse hyperplasia of enterochromaffin

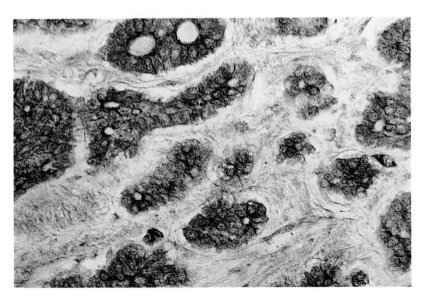

Figure 3.105 Carcinoid of the gastrointestinal tract showing positive immunostaining for neurone-specified enolase (NSE). (Courtesy of J. Polak, R.P.M.S.)

cells.[35] The association in experimental animals of enterochromaffin cell hyperplasia, and multiple gastric carcinoids, with prolonged hypergastrinaemia induced by powerful anti-gastrin acid secretory drugs, offers a potential explanation of this link, and induces a note of caution concerning the long-term use of such drugs in humans. The possibility that multiple gastric carcinoids associated with pernicious anaemia may regress after antrectomy has been reported.[71] Carcinoid tumours of lung, intestine or thymus or the carcinoid syndrome may arise as part of the multiple endocrine neoplasia syndrome type 1.[2,19,90] Carcinoids have been described which not only contain but also secrete other hormones, including insulin,[79] growth hormone, adrenocorticotrophic hormone, gastric, calcitonin, antidiuretic hormone, β-melanocyte-stimulating hormone and vasoactive intestinal polypeptide.[28,47,54] It seems that carcinoids of foregut origin are more likely to produce such peptides than are those from the midgut.

An association of carcinoids with other neoplasms in 17–53% of cases has been claimed.[28] Whether this is a true association, or only an apparent association occurring in a group of patients undergoing extensive investigation, is not clear.

Carcinoid tumours without systemic features

The presentation of carcinoid tumours that have not caused the carcinoid syndrome is diverse and related mainly to the site of origin. In the commonest position – the appendix – the majority of tumours are found at appendicectomy. In about 30% of these cases it is possible that the tumour may have led to the appendicitis by causing luminal obstruction, but usually the carcinoid represents a coincidental finding.[60] Similarly, in the small intestine the majority of carcinoids are asymptomatic, but a minority (possibly 20%) give rise to pain.[28] Usually this is related to subacute small intestinal obstruction by the tumour, although the fibrous reaction, mesenteric vascular occlusion, intussusception or direct tumour spread may also be responsible. Rarely, perforation or haemorrhage occurs. Primary tumours within Meckel's diverticulum behave in a similar fashion to small intestinal rather than appendiceal primaries.[10]

Duodenal carcinoids may present as duodenal or biliary obstruction but may be found during the investigation of pain suggestive of a duodenal ulcer.[10] Gastric carcinoids are often asymptomatic but pain or bleeding following surface ulceration may also occur. The rare oesophageal carcinoids present with dysphagia. Colonic carcinoids present like cancer of the colon with changes in bowel habit, obstruction or bleeding.[10]

Investigation

The radiological features of gut carcinoids are non-specific but tumours impinging on the gut lumen may be seen during barium studies as a smooth swelling or polyp indistinguishable from other intestinal tumours, though multiple ileal polyps are highly suggestive of carcinoids.[3,38] Mucosal irregularity may occur secondary to invasion, lymphatic obstruction or oedema. Mesenteric metastatic deposits may calcify. Bony deposits may be osteoblastic or osteolytic.[28] Angiography may demonstrate distorted stellate vessels in the region of the primary tumour.

Hepatic imaging is particularly relevant, as the liver is the prime site for metastatic spread.[32] Hepatic ultrasound should demonstrate deposits of 1 cm or greater diameter, of variable echogenicity. Computed tomography scans should be more sensitive, but regional low attenuation areas may be more difficult to interpret, representing either diffuse tumour or fatty infiltration due to local compromise of the portal circulation. Using angiography, different patterns of tumour deposit have been defined – diffuse fine or diffuse coarse nodules or single masses.[77] Most deposits are very vascular with dramatic blushing during the capillary phase. Isotopic techniques for imaging carcinoids, relying on uptake of iodinated benzyl guanidine, have been reported.

Bronchial carcinoids may present simply as a coin lesion on routine chest radiographs, or with cough, wheezing or haemoptysis together with symptoms of segmental obstruction and infection with bronchiectasis, pneumonia or anaemia.[46] Bronchoscopy may demonstrate a submucosal mass in one of the larger bronchi (as with the gut, much of the tumour spread may occur away from the lumen – a dumb-bell tumour). The mass may, of course, ulcerate. Lung carcinoids are very vascular: torrential bleeding may occur after a diagnostic biopsy.

Ovarian carcinoids present simply as a pelvic mass. Thymic carcinoids may be asymptomatic or present with the symptoms of an intrathoracic mass, with chest pain, dyspnoea and cough or superior vena caval obstruction. They may also present with Cushing's syndrome.[90]

Treatment of carcinoid tumours without systemic features

Management of carcinoid tumours, whether of the intestine or the bronchus, presenting without the syndrome is surgical – at least for disease which is not advanced.[10,46,70] Debate centres on two points: the management of large appendiceal tumours and the operative approach to apparently benign isolated intestinal carcinoids.

As noted above, appendiceal carcinoids are only infrequently malignant. Furthermore, tumours may not be recognized at operation but only subsequently by the pathologist. The incidence of recurrent or metastatic tumour is very small, even if apparent danger signals are present. In one series, even though there was serosal involvement in some 60% of cases and intramural lymphatics were involved in 90% of cases, there was no evidence of recurrent tumour after a simple appendicectomy.[60] It has been suggested, therefore, that a simple appendicectomy is adequate for most cases,[60] but some authors suggested a right hemicolectomy should be performed if the primary tumour is greater than 2 cm in diameter or if there is evidence of extensive local spread.[10]

Unlike appendiceal tumours, the incidence of metastatic spread with small intestinal and colonic carcinoids is high. It seems appropriate in cases without apparent metastases to undertake more radical surgery involving excision of the tumour with relatively wide margins and removal of adjacent lymph nodes and mesentery.[10,84]

The optimal surgical policy for apparently solitary hepatic secondaries is unclear, but if metastases are surgically amenable then local hepatic resection may be appropriate. Radiotherapy and chemotherapy have been used in carcinoid tumours with widespread metastases but results have been disappointing.[21] This is discussed below with reference to patients with metastatic carcinoid tumours and the carcinoid syndrome. An initial report suggesting benefit from external radiation in carcinoid tumours[24] was not borne out in a subsequent report from the same unit.[42] Hepatic embolization of massive tumour deposits causing severe pain may produce good symptom relief.

THE CARCINOID SYNDROME

Clinical features

General features
The syndrome affects both sexes equally, with the sixth decade being the most common time to present. All forms of temporal relationship to the appearance of the primary tumour have been reported, from an initial presentation with the syndrome in the absence of physical signs of primary or secondary tumour to presentation years after resection of a primary. However, over half the patients have physical signs of advanced metastatic disease at the time of presentation.

The cardinal features of the syndrome are flushing, diarrhoea and heart disease. The differing symptoms of individual patients reflect tumour origin and mass, the length of the history, and qualitative and quantitative differences in the release of tumour products. However, a patient with advanced disease is readily diagnosed at the bedside, being a weak cachectic individual with a continuous flush, plethora, facial and peripheral oedema, and marked knobbly hepatomegaly, often with an hepatic friction rub. As already stated, however, many patients lack one or more of these features.

Cutaneous manifestations
Flushing attacks affecting mainly the upper part of the body are the commonest manifestations of the syndrome, occurring in about 90% of patients. Flushes vary from patient to patient and may last from a few minutes to hours, and may be associated with a violaceous tinge, sweating, lacrimation, itching, facial and conjunctival oedema, palpitations, hypertension or diarrhoea. Whilst some patients are acutely disturbed by their flushes, others may be entirely unaware of them. The episodes may be spontaneous or precipitated by stress, alcohol, exertion, certain foods or abdominal palpation, and may be pharmacologically induced by infusions of noradrenaline.[28] Grahame-Smith[28] has classified flushing into four clinical types but only one of these is clinically distinctive: gastric carcinoids which produce histamine as well as other products may cause a specific pattern of a bright red geographical flush of the face and neck. However, there is a tendency for the flushing due to bronchial carcinoma to also follow a pattern, which is associated with salivation, lacrimation, hypotension, oedema, nausea, vomiting and diarrhoea.

As well as flushing, more permanent changes may occur in the skin, including facial telangiectasia and morphoea-like thickening of the skin, and, more rarely, the syndrome may be complicated by the skin manifestations of pellagra.[88]

Gastrointestinal manifestations
Diarrhoea is common, occurring in about 79–80% of patients,[28,88] but is said to be less evident with gastric carcinoids.[63] In some cases it seems clearly related to circulating products, the diarrhoea being episodic and associated with obvious hypermotility and borborygmi. Such episodes of diarrhoea may or may not be related to episodes of flushing. In some patients a secretory state may occur in the upper small intestine as demonstrated by perfusion studies,[18] whilst in others the diarrhoea may be related to rapid transit. Steatorrhoea may occur, though this is rarer than watery diarrhoea.[44] The abdominal symptoms

and diarrhoea may, however, be due to other causes: subacute intestinal obstruction may occur associated with the primary tumour or fibrosis of the gut wall, whilst intestinal resection for a primary tumour, bile salt spillage, bacterial overgrowth and lymphatic obstruction may all contribute to the symptoms. Abdominal pain may reflect intestinal obstruction, spontaneous necrosis of hepatic metastasis or, rarely, gut ischaemia due to fibrosis causing narrowing of mesenteric vessels.

Cardiac manifestations

Only a minority of patients (up to 40%) with malignant carcinoids and the carcinoid syndrome have heart disease;[28,80] it seems to be less common in those with gastric tumours.[63] Unlike the flushing and diarrhoea which may appear as immediate responses to released tumour products, the cardiac disease is due to a slowly developing, histologically unique form of fibrosis usually involving the endocardium of the right side of the heart.[74] This fibrosis mainly involves the ventricular aspect of the tricuspid valve and the associated chordae. Less commonly the pulmonary valve is also involved and left-sided cardiac fibrosis has also been described, though this seems to be more severe when the primary carcinoid tumour is situated in the lung and therefore drains directly into the left side of the heart. By the time patients develop cardiac manifestations, other symptoms of the syndrome have usually been present for a number of years. The clinical signs of the cardiac disease include a raised venous pressure with obvious evidence of right ventricular hypertrophy, and the presence of right-sided cardiac murmurs indicative of tricuspid regurgitation and stenosis or pulmonary stenosis. Together with these findings there is evidence of cardiac failure. Peripheral oedema develops as the cardiac failure worsens. All cardiac signs may be more striking during episodes of flushing.

Other manifestations

A similar fibrosis to that seen in the heart and around primary ileal tumours may occur on the intima of the great veins, the coronary sinuses or the great arteries, and in the pleura or the pericardium, the latter causing constrictive pericarditis. Retroperitoneal fibrosis may cause ureteric obstruction and Peyronie's disease of the penis may occur.[28]

Wheezing occurs in about 10% of patients and late-onset asthma may occasionally be the presenting feature of the syndrome. As well as true bronchoconstriction, some patients get episodes of hyperventilation during flushing attacks.

Confusional states may occur in the carcinoid syndrome for a number of reasons; during prolonged flushing episodes, particularly in patients with gastric or bronchial carcinoids; as a feature of liver failure in advanced disease; as a side-effect of therapy, particularly if parachlorophenylalanine is used; as part of the pellagra syndrome; or possibly as a specific carcinoid encephalopathy.

Ophthalmic changes may occur in flushing attacks, with fundal changes of 'sludging' within retinal vessels sometimes leading to occlusion.[92]

A minority (about 10%) of patients suffer with arthralgia with stiffness and pain in the hands and minor periarticular changes in the hands may be seen on radiography. Some reports also suggest a myopathy may occur.

Pathogenesis

5-Hydroxytryptamine (serotonin)

Midgut carcinoids secrete large amounts of 5-hydroxytryptamine which is responsible for several of the clinical features. 5-Hydroxytryptamine markedly increases gastrointestinal motility[33] and probably induces a secretory state in the small intestine.[18] In addition it may affect the kidney, reducing blood flow and changing renal handling of salt and water. Together with histamine, 5-hydroxytryptamine may be responsible for producing asthma.[34] Foregut tumours lack the decarboxylase enzyme (*Figure 3.106*) and thus secrete 5-hydroxytryptophan, not 5-hydroxytryptamine, though circulating 5-hydroxytryptophan may be decarboxylated by other tissues to produce 5-hydroxytryptamine. 5-Hydroxytryptamine secretion is therefore characteristic of the midgut carcinoids (*Table 3.48*) but not foregut carcinoids, and may account for the different clinical manifestations of these tumours.

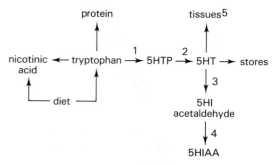

Figure 3.106 Major pathways of tryptophan metabolism and the sites of action of drugs: 1, hydroxylase (blocked by paracholorophenylalanine); 2, aromatic 1-amino-acid decarboxylase present in tissues and midgut carcinoids (partially blocked by methyldopa); 3, monoamine oxidase present in liver and lung and some carcinoid tumours; 4, aldehyde dehydrogenase; 5, site of action of cyproheptadine and methysergide receptor antagonists.

5-Hydroxytryptamine is metabolized principally by monoamine oxidase (*Figure 3.106*). Certain carcinoid tumours contain monoamine oxidase and may thus secrete 5-hydroxytryptamine metabolites into the circulation. Furthermore, the liver contains large amounts of monoamine oxidase and thus 5-hydroxytryptamine secreted by gastrointestinal tumours does not reach the systemic circulation unless hepatic metastases are present – accounting for the lack of symptoms in gastrointestinal carcinoids without metastases.

Histamine

Primary gastric carcinoids produce histamine as well as tryptophan derivatives. Histamine production seems to be associated with a distinctive flush (see above) and responds to combined histamine H_1 and H_2 receptor blockade. Presumably the histamine production may also partially account for the reported increase in incidence of duodenal ulcer in the carcinoid syndrome.

Kallikrein

Carcinoids contain kallikrein, an enzyme which when released into the blood is capable of converting plasma kininogen to lysylbradykinin, which in turn may be converted to bradykinin (*Figure 3.107*). These kinins are vasoactive and may be important in producing flushing in some, but not all, cases of the carcinoid syndrome.[65] Other actions of kinins include effects on intestinal motility and increased vascular permeability. Kallikrein release may be stimulated by sympathomimetic amines and may account for the precipitation of flushing by noradrenaline and alcohol.

Prostaglandins

Prostaglandins E and F (both of which are found within the normal gastrointestinal tract and which increase intestinal motility and induce fluid secretion) and other unidentified prostaglandins have been extracted from carcinoid tumours.[76] In addition, elevated serum concentrations of prostaglandins E and F have been found in patients with the syndrome. However, a review of these reports with an analysis of the response to prostaglandin synthesis inhibitors suggested that prostaglandins are unlikely to be major mediators of flushing and diarrhoea in most patients with the syndrome.[56]

Peptide hormones

During induced flushing or diarrhoea no changes have been reported in plasma concentrations of insulin, gastrin vasoactive intestinal polypeptide, gastric inhibitory peptide, somatostatin or neurotensin. In some patients, flushing episodes have

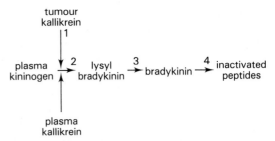

Figure 3.107 Generation of bradykinin and the sites of action of drugs: 1, release of tumour kallikrein promoted by noradrenaline and blocked by α-adrenergic antagonists; 2, kallikrein, which is blocked by aprotinin; 3, plasma amino peptidase; 4, kininases.

been associated with elevated plasma levels of calcitonin gene-related peptide. The short-term action of somatostatin infusions in abolishing flushing and diarrhoea suggests inhibition of either release or action of one or more peptide hormones.

Disturbed tryptophan metabolism

Even though not all patients with the carcinoid syndrome produce large amounts of 5-hydroxytryptamine, all patients have disturbed metabolism of the essential amino acid tryptophan. Tryptophan is used for protein synthesis and as a precursor of the vitamin nicotinic acid, as well as being the precursor for 5-hydroxytryptamine. Normally only 1% of dietary intake of tryptophan is converted to 5-hydroxytryptamine, but in patients with the carcinoid syndrome this may increase to 70% or more.[55] This diversion of tryptophan to 5-hydroxytryptamine synthesis reduces the availability of tryptophan to the rest of the body and may result in reduced protein synthesis with hypoalbuminaemia, and nicotinic acid deficiency with or without the clinical manifestations of pellagra (photosensitive dermatitis, neurological signs of diarrhoea).[85] These deficits of tryptophan and nicotinic acid may well be exacerbated by anorexia or malabsorption.

Other factors

In vitro studies of substances released from a carcinoid tumour cell line have suggested that transforming growth factor β_1 may contribute to the fibrosis induced by carcinoid tumours.[4]

Various cases of the carcinoid syndrome have been shown to produce a number of other biologically active peptides and amines (see above). In view of the rarity of these associations it seems unlikely that any of these substances are important in the pathogenesis of the features of the carcinoid syndrome.

Investigation

In most patients, once the suspicion has been raised, making the diagnosis of the carcinoid syndrome is not difficult. Urinary 5-hydroxyindoleacetic acid may be estimated quantitatively in a 24-hour urine sample. False positives can occur if patients are eating foods containing large amounts of 5-hydroxytryptamine, such as bananas, avocados, pineapples or walnuts, or taking drugs such as reserpine, acetanilide, mephenesin, methocarbamol, or cough medications containing glyceryl guaiacolate. Other drugs such as the phenothiazines interfere with the assay and may produce false negative answers. Mild elevations of urinary 5-hydroxyindoleacetic acid are also seen in the blind loop syndrome, Whipple's disease and coeliac disease; nevertheless, levels of greater than 30 mg (90 μmol)/ 24 hours are otherwise diagnostic.[28,87] As already mentioned, foregut carcinoids tend to produce 5-hydroxytryptophan and not 5-hydroxytryptamine, because they lack the appropriate decarboxylase. This can occasionally give rise to normal urinary 5-hydroxyindoleacetic acid excretion despite the presence of the carcinoid syndrome. If there is a high degree of clinical suspicion, the urine may be screened for earlier metabolites of tryptophan by use of paper chromatography.[14] However, this is not usually necessary as even foregut carcinoids usually produce raised urinary 5-hydroxyindoleacetic acid excretion as the majority of circulating 5-hydroxytryptophan is excreted as 5-hydroxyindoleacetic acid following metabolism by other tissues.[64]

Prognosis

Primary carcinoid tumours grow only slowly and this is often true of the metastases. Patients with raised urinary 5-hydroxyindoleacetic acid levels may have only trivial symptoms of occasional mild flushing or mild diarrhoea for many years which requires no treatment. In one series, the mean survival time in patients with the carcinoid syndrome was 8 years, with some patients surviving for up to 20 years.[68] However, in another series in which all patients had hepatic and/or bony metastases, survival was less than 1 year.[30] In the US National Carcinoid Register containing 2837 cases, the presence of the carcinoid syndrome was not specified, but in patients whose carcinoid tumours had metastasized widely, the relative 5-year survival varied from zero for carcinoids of the stomach to 27% for appendiceal tumours (see Table 3.50).[25]

Treatment

The aims and mode of treatment will differ in different patients and may include removal of the primary tumour, blocking the effects or reducing the amounts of circulating agents by medical or surgical means, or simple palliation of advanced malignant disease.

Supportive and symptomatic therapy

The patients should be advised to avoid any factors known to precipitate carcinoid attacks, such as alcohol, provocative foods or physical activity. Particular attention should be taken to include sufficient nicotinamide in the diet. Heart failure should be treated with diuretics, and asthmatic attacks with aminophylline or salbutamol (this β_2-adrenergic stimulant does not precipitate flushing attacks). Codeine phosphate may be used to control the diarrhoea and potassium supplements may be necessary. If the patient has had an ileal resection for removal of the primary tumour with consequent bile salt spillage into the colon, cholestyramine may be of help.

Drugs

Many drugs have been used to modify or inhibit the attacks of flushing and diarrhoea in the carcinoid syndrome. These act in a variety of ways: by inhibiting synthesis or blocking the peripheral actions of 5-hydroxytryptamine, by inhibiting release of tumour kallikrein, or by inhibiting the generation of vasoactive substances.

INHIBITORS OF 5-HYDROXYTRYPTAMINE SYNTHESIS
Parachlorophenylalanine
This agent has been shown to act by blocking the hydroxylase enzyme that converts tryptophan to 5-hydroxytryptamine (*Figure 3.106*). The major clinical effect is on gastrointestinal symptoms with a reduction in diarrhoea and abdominal pain, though there also seems to be some reduction in the flushing caused by foregut carcinoids. In some patients the drug markedly improves the patient's well-being, possibly due to its effect on gastrointestinal symptoms. The usual dose is up to 1 g four times daily. Side-effects include tiredness, dizziness, anxiety, headache and psychic effects, including depression and hallucinations. Whether these are direct effects of the drug or secondary effects on brain 5-hydroxytryptamine concentrations is not clear.

Methyldopa
This agent partially blocks the conversion of 5-

hydroxytryptophan to serotonin (*Figure 3.106*), but may also reduce catecholamine-stimulated release of flush-producing substances by the tumour. Methyldopa occasionally relieves flushing but has little effect on gastrointestinal symptoms.

Prevention of release of substances by the tumour

Phenoxybenzamine

In some patients the flushes provoked by alcohol or catecholamines may be reduced by the α-adrenergic antagonist phenoxybenzamine in a dose of 10–20 mg four times daily, though patients seem to become refractory to its effects. β-adrenergic antagonists do not seem to reduce flushing.

Phenothiazines

Phenothiazines may on occasion reduce flushing, possibly also through their action as α-adrenergic antagonists.

Inhibitors of kinin production

Aprotinin

In vitro evidence suggests that aprotinin inhibits the action of tumour kallikrein and thus prevents generation of bradykinin. However, it does not seem to be clinically useful in reducing flushing, and suffers from the disadvantage of needing to be administered by intravenous infusion.

5-Hydroxytryptamine antagonists

Serotonin exerts its physiological effects via a number of receptors ($5HT_1$, $5HT_2$, $5HT_3$) present in different tissues, particularly on smooth muscle, and exerts different effects on muscle tone depending on site.[9]

Methysergide

This drug is a $5HT_2$ antagonist with mild vasoconstrictor actions. It frequently alleviates diarrhoea when used in doses of 3–8 g/day, but has little or no effect on flushing. Side-effects include heartburn, nausea, vomiting and abdominal pain, and it may cause diarrhoea as well as producing central effects including unsteadiness, drowsiness, confusion, insomnia, hallucinations and psychosis. Exacerbation of angina has also been reported. The major side-effect is, however, retroperitoneal fibrosis. Although this limits the usefulness of the drug in migraine, in the carcinoid syndrome (which may also lead to ectopic fibrosis) the benefits outweigh the risks.

Cyproheptadine

This agent blocks the actions of 5-hydroxy-tryptamine on smooth muscle and is therefore useful for the treatment of diarrhoea. It also has weak anticholinergic activity, is a histamine H_1 receptor blocker and is also a mild central nervous system depressant. The usual dose is 4 mg four times a day.

Ketanserin

Ketanserin is a $5HT_2$ antagonist, occasionally reducing diarrhoea but of more value in alleviating flushing.[1,29] The usual dose is 20 mg three or four times daily.

Histamine antagonists

In patients with the carcinoid syndrome due to a gastric primary, a combination of histamine H_1 and H_2 receptor antagonists (diphenhydramine hydrochloride 50 mg six-hourly and cimetidine 300 mg six-hourly) may be uniquely effective in reducing the flushing and hypertension.[73]

Somatostatin

After intravenous administration of natural somatostatin had been shown to abolish flushing due to gastric or ileal carcinoids,[23,49] a somatostatin analogue (octreotide) has become established as the single most effective form of treatment for symptoms of the carcinoid syndrome. In 75–80% of cases, symptoms of flushing and diarrhoea are relieved, initially by administration of 50 μg three times daily. Subcutaneously escalating doses are usually required over time with doses of up to 500 μg three times daily being required after some months. The expense of this treatment may be reduced by low-dose continuous infusion of octreotide, which has a half-life of about 2 hours. Eventually, troublesome steatorrhoea may limit its usefulness. The mode of action is a combination of reduced hormone output and peripheral blockade. Most authors do not find a reduction in tumour mass, although this has been reported.[12]

Steroids

Prednisolone in doses of 20 mg/day has been reported as being effective in reducing flushing, facial oedema, diarrhoea and the hyperdynamic state associated with the carcinoid syndrome due to bronchial carcinoids. However, it seems to be ineffective in relieving symptoms due to gastrointestinal carcinoids.

Surgery

Resection of an ovarian or bronchial carcinoid producing the syndrome is potentially curative. In the more common situation with hepatic metastases, surgery may be employed to reduce tumour mass either by partial hepatectomy[22,34] (when deposits are confined to one lobe) or by shelling out metastases.[21,50,62,99] Orthotopic liver transplantation has been performed and, as the results of this procedure improve, may be considered more frequently in the future. Lesser surgical procedures include hepatic artery ligation,[50] now superseded by interventional radiological techniques, or extensive hepatic devascularization except for the main hepatic artery, which can subsequently be intermittently occluded via a percutaneous sling.[5] Surgical procedures in patients with the carcinoid syndrome are potentially hazardous.[16,61] Hyper- or hypotension, bronchial constriction, hyperpnoea, vomiting, diarrhoea, flushing and hyperglycaemia may all be encountered. The patient should be assessed carefully preoperatively and given 5-hydroxytryptamine antagonists or somatostatin prior to the procedure (see earlier). Precipitants of flushing attacks should be avoided when possible and nerve blockers, acetylcholine, curare and morphine should all be used with care. Hypotensive attacks should be treated with transfusion and angiotensin (not catecholamines) and hypertensive episodes with hydrallazine.

Certain carefully selected patients have undergone tricuspid valve replacement when cardiac fibrosis and heart failure has been a major problem in patients who otherwise seemed quite well.[36] Right-sided balloon valvuloplasty is a lesser procedure which has also been reported as being beneficial, depending on the relative contribution of stenosis and incompetence of the valves.

Radiotherapy

Although there is one report of radiotherapy inducing prolonged disease-free remission of carcinoid tumours with metastases,[24] a follow-up report from the same unit showed no benefit in the carcinoid syndrome.[42] Radiotherapy only has a place in producing symptomatic relief from metastases to bone and skin.

Chemotherapy

Several uncontrolled studies have shown a reduction in tumour size with a variety of chemotherapeutic regimens. Streptozotocin, alkylating agents and 5-fluorouracil seem to be the best single agents, with response rates of 30, 23 and 21%[21] (*Table 3.51*). Drug combinations seem to be more effective than single drug regimens and a combination of cyclophosphamide and methotrexate produced a 58% response rate in a small series. However, in many cases 'response' was merely a reduction in liver size

Table 3.51 Chemotherapy in carcinoid syndrome

	Number of patients	Percentage response
Single agents		
Streptozotocin	23	30
Alkylating agents	39	23
5-Fluorouracil	29	21
Methotrexate	6	16
Dactinomycin	9	11
Mitomycin C	3	—
Doxorubicin	1	—
Dacarbazine	2	—
Combination therapy		
Cyclophosphamide and methotrexate	12	58
5-Fluorouracil and streptozotocin	53	38
Cyclophosphamide and streptozotocin	45	27
Doxorubicin and 5-fluorouracil	3	66
Cyclophosphamide and methyl CCNU	4	50
5-Fluorouracil, doxorubicin and methyl BCNU	2	—
5-Fluorouracil and BCNU	2	—

Modified from Mengel and Shaffer.[55]
Single cases described with responses to streptozotocin and BCNU, cyclophosphamide and vincristine, cyclophosphamide, methotrexate and doxorubicin, and cyclophosphamide, vincristine and CCNU.

and in general chemotherapy is not effective in producing symptomatic relief or prolonging life. Furthermore, cytotoxic therapy may exacerbate symptoms,[57] presumably due to release of tumour products from necrotic cells. The most studied regime recently has been a combination of streptozotocin and 5-fluorouracil, producing a partial remission in 30% of patients treated, lasting for a mean of 8 months.[45] There is no evidence to support the suggestion that chemotherapy administered through a cannula into the hepatic artery is more effective than systemic administration.

The use of human recombinant α-interferon appears to offer a better response rate than conventional chemotherapy, with less toxicity. A series of patients treated daily with 3×10^6 to 6×10^6 units intramuscularly were reported to show a 47% partial remission rate, with remissions persisting for up to 3 years.[66] The side-effects were malaise, predominantly when treatment was initiated, and mild pancytopenia.

Table 3.52 Hepatic artery embolization of carcinoid tumours (Hammersmith Hospital regimen)

Pre-embolization	1. Cyproheptadine 4 mg t.d.s. oral – 24 hours prior and afterwards 2. Nicotinamide 250 mg q.d.s. 3. Octreotide (long-acting somatostatin) 200 μg s.c.
Premedication	Omnopon (papveretum) 15 mg IM. Atropine 0.4 mg IM. Prochlorperazine 12.5 mg IM.
Gentamicin 80 mg Flucloxacillin 500 mg Metronidazole 500 mg IV	Give IV at same time as premedication then continue for 10 days. (NB. Facilities for monitoring gentamicin levels should be available)
During embolization	1. Methylprednisolone 1 g IV at start. 2. Trasylol (aprotinin) 50 000 units hourly (1 hour before and 48 hour after) IV infusion. 3. Octreotide 200 μg s.c./h.
To be available if necessary	Hydralazine IV for hypertension (or nitroprusside) or labetalol. Albumin for hypotension (i.e. plasma). Methylprednisolone.
Monitoring	1. Central Venous Pressure line — insert before embolization (or good peripheral line) 2. Peripheral line (left arm easier for radiologist) 3. Blood pressure: measure very frequently during embolization and immediately afterwards (e.g. every 2–3 minutes 'Ultrason' is useful if available) 4. Experienced physician or anaesthetist should always be present during the procedure
Postembolization	1. Usual postangiogram observations 2. Close watch on blood pressure and urine output 3. Daily 5-hydroxyindoleacetic acid, full blood count, daily liver function tests 4. Adequate hydration throughout is very important.

IV, intravenous, IM, intramuscular, t.d.s., three times a day; q.d.s., four times a day.

Hepatic arterial embolization

This technique (*Table 3.52*) reduces arterial blood flow to both tumour deposits and normal liver cells. The latter survive due to their parallel portal venous blood supply, whilst tumour deposits undergo necrosis as they are dependent on arterial inflow. To prevent systemic disturbance from release of vasoactive and other substances from dying tumour cells, and because of the risk of superinfection, blocking agents and antibiotics are used before and after the procedure.[52]

The procedure involves selective cannulation of the hepatic artery and the portal inflow must be demonstrated to be intact. Successful embolization following injection of either absorbable or non-absorbable materials into the hepatic artery is usually followed by fever, leukocytosis, hepatic pain and a rise in serum enzymes.

The results are variable dependent upon patient selection. Local symptoms due to tumour may be reduced, but the main effect is on hormonally-mediated symptoms. In most patients, flushing and abdominal pain can be abolished, with improvement in diarrhoea and a significant fall in 5-hydroxy-indoleacetic acid excretion. Clinical remissions last for 1–18 months, and successful re-embolization has been performed with further remission of symptoms. Multiple repetitions of the procedure tend to produce diminishing returns, however. Whether long-term survival is affected by embolization is not yet clear and would be difficult to prove.[11]

Other approaches

The possibility of delivering local radiotherapy by the radioactive imaging agent *m*-iodobenzyl guanidine is being explored.[43]

Summary of treatment approaches

In patients presenting with the carcinoid syndrome, the possibility of surgical alleviation should be considered, but few patients will have the localized hepatic deposits suitable. For mild symptoms, no active treatment may be required. As symptoms develop, first-line drug therapy, with cyproheptadine and codeine phosphatase for diarrhoea, and ketanserin for flushing, will be adequate for months or years. Subsequently, worsening symptoms will usually respond to a somatostatin analogue, requiring frequent subcutaneous injections, but an alternative approach at this juncture would be a trial of interferon therapy, or hepatic artery embolization. It should be appreciated that so far none of the 'antitumour' therapies – surgery, embolization or chemotherapy – has been shown to prolong survival, and concern for symptomatic improvement without disabling risk or side-effects seems paramount.

REFERENCES

1. Antonsen, S., Hansen, M.G.M., Bukhare, K. and Rask-Madsen, J. (1982) Influence of a new selective 5-HT$_2$ receptor antagonist (ketanserin) on jejunal PGE$_2$ release and non-secretion due to malignant carcinoid syndrome. *Gut*, **23**, A887.
2. Ballard, H., Frame, B. and Hartsock, R.J. (1964) Familial multiple endocrine adenoma–peptic ulcer complex. *Medicine*, **43**, 481–516.
3. Banks, N.H., Goldstein, H.M. and Dodd, G.D. (1975) The roentgenologic spectrum of small intestinal carcinoid tumours. *American Journal of Roentgenology*, **123**, 274–280.
4. Beauchamp, R.D., Lyons, R.M., Coffey, R.J. *et al.* (1989) Carcinoid-associated desmoplasia. A role for type beta transforming growth factors. *Gastroenterology*, **96**, A35.
5. Bengmark, S., Ericsson, M. and Lunderquist, A. (1982) Temporary liver de-arterialization in patients with metastatic carcinoid disease. *World Journal of Surgery*, **6**, 46–53.
6. Bensch, K.G., Cottin, B. and Pariente, R. (1960) Oat cell carcinoma of the lung and its relation to bronchial carcinoid. *Cancer*, **22**, 1163–1172.
7. Bensch, K.G., Gordon, G.B. and Miller, L.R. (1965) Studies on bronchial counterpart of the Kultschitzky (argentaffin) cell and innervation of bronchial glands. *Journal of Ultrastructural Research*, **12**, 668–686.
8. Bensch, K.G., Gordon, G.B. and Miller, L.R. (1965) Electron microscopic and biochemical studies on the bronchial carcinoid. *Cancer*, **18**, 592–602.
9. Bradley, P.B., Engel, G. and Fenick, W. (1986) Proposals for the classification and nomenclature of functional receptors for 5-hydroxytryptamine. *Journal of Neuropharmacology*, **25**, 563–576.
10. Cheek, R.C. and Wilson, H. (1970) Carcinoid tumours. *Current Problems in Surgery*, November, 4–34.
11. Coupe, M., Hodgson, H.J.F., Hemingway, A. and Allison, D.J. (1989) Effect of hepatic artery embolization on survival in the carcinoid syndrome. *Interventional Radiology*, **4**, 179–181.
12. Coupe, M., Levi, S., Ellis, M. *et al.* (1989) Therapy for symptoms in the carcinoid syndrome. *Quarterly Journal of Medicine*, **73**(271), 1021–1036.
13. Davies, A.J. (1960) Carcinoid tumours (argentaffinoma). *Annals of the Royal College of Surgery*, **25**, 277–297.
14. Davis, R.B. and Rosenberg, J.C. (1961) Carcinoid syndrome associated with hyperserotoninaemia and normal 5-hydroxyindoleacetic acid secretion. *American Journal of Medicine*, **30**, 167–174.
15. Davis, Z., Moetel, C.G. and Mellrath, D.C. (1973) The malignant carcinoid syndrome. *Surgery, Gynecology and Obstetrics*, **137**, 637–644.
16. Dery, R. (1971) Theoretical and clinical considerations in anaesthesia for secreting carcinoid tumours. *Canadian Anaesthetists Society Journal*, **18**, 245–263.
17. Dharmsathaphorn, K., Sherwin, R.S., Cataland, S. *et al.* (1980) Somatostatin inhibits diarrhoea in the carcinoid syndrome. *Annals of Internal Medicine*, **92**, 68–69.
18. Donowitz, M. and Binder, H.J. (1975) Jejunal fluid and electrolyte secretion in carcinoid syndrome. *American Journal of Digestive Diseases*, **20**, 1115–1122.
19. Farid, N.R., Beuhler, S., Russell, N.A. *et al.* (1980) Prolactinomas in familial multiple endocrine neoplasia syndrome type 1. Relationship to HLA and carcinoma tumours. *American Journal of Medicine*, **69**, 874–880.
20. Feldman, J.M. and Jones, R.S. (1982) Carcinoid syndrome from gastrointestinal carcinoids without liver metastases. *Annals of Surgery*, **196**, 33–37.
21. Felton, W.L., Liebow, A.A. and Lindskog, G.E. (1983) Peripheral and multiple bronchial adenomas. *Cancer*, **6**, 555–567.
22. Fosier, J. (1970) Survival after liver resection for cancer. *Cancer*, **26**, 493–502.
23. Frohlich, J.C., Bloomgarden, Z.T. and Oates, J.A. (1978) The carcinoid flush: provocation by pentagastrin and inhibition by somatostatin. *New England Journal of Medicine*, **299**, 1055–1057.
24. Gaitan-Gaitan, A., Rider, W.D. and Bush, R.S. (1975) Carcinoid tumour – cure by irradiation. *International Journal of Radiation Biology*, **1**, 9–13.
25. Godwin, J.D. (1975) Carcinoid tumours: an analysis of 2837 cases. *Cancer*, **36**, 560–569.
26. Goedert, M., Otten, U., Suda, K. *et al.* (1980) Dopamine norepinephrine and serotonin production by an intestinal carcinoid tumour. *Cancer*, **45**, 104–107.
27. Goldstein, H.M. and Miller, M. (1975) Angiographic evaluation of carcinoid tumours of

the small intestine; the value of epinephrine. *Radiology*, **115**, 23–28.

28. Grahame-Smith, D.G. (1972) *The Carcinoid Syndrome*. London: Heinemann.
29. Gustafsen, J., Lendord, A., Raskov, H. and Boesby, S. (1986) Ketanserin versus placebo in carcinoid syndrome. A clinical controlled trial. *Scandinavian Journal of Gastroenterology*, **21**, 816–818.
30. Hajdu, S.I., Winawer, S.J. and Laird Myers, W.F. (1974) Carcinoid tumours: a study of 204 cases. *American Journal of Clinical Pathology*, **61**, 521–528.
31. Haskell, C.M. and Tompkins, R.K. (1980) In: *Carcinoid Tumours in Cancer Treatment*, pp. 609–620 (Ed.) Haskell, C.M. Philadelphia: W.B. Saunders.
32. Hemmingson, A., Lindgren, P.G., Lovelius, L.E. and Oberg, K. (1981) Diagnosis of endocrine gastrointestinal tumours. *Acta Radiologica*, **22**, 657.
33. Hendrix, T.R., Atkinson, M., Clifton, J.A. and Ingelfinger, F.J. (1957) The effect of 5-hydroxytryptamine on intestinal motor function in man. *American Journal of Medicine*, **23**, 886–893.
34. Herxheimer, H. (1953) Influence of 5-hydroxytryptamine on bronchial function. *Journal of Physiology*, **122**, 49P–50P.
35. Hodges, J.R., Isaacson, P. and Wright, R. (1981) Diffuse enterochromaffin-like (ECL) cell hyperplasia and multiple gastric carcinoids: a complication of pernicious anaemia. *Gut*, **22**, 237–241.
36. Honey, M. and Paneth, M. (1975) Carcinoid heart disease; successful tricuspid valve replacement. *Thorax*, **30**, 464–469.
37. Hsu, C., Ma, L., Wong, L.C. and Chan, C.W. (1981) Non-endocrine carcinoid tumour of the uterine cervix – aspects of diagnosis and treatment. *British Journal of Obstetrics and Gynaecology*, **88**, 1056–1060.
38. Hudson, H.L. and Margulis, A.R. (1964) The roentgen findings of carcinoid tumours of the gastrointestinal tract: a report of 12 recent cases. *American Journal of Roentgenology*, **91**, 833–839.
39. Jepson, J.B. (1955) Paper chromatograph of urinary indoles. *The Lancet*, **ii**, 1009–1011.
40. Johnson, L.A., Lavin, P. and Moertel, G. (1983) Carcinoid: the association of histologic growth patterns and survival. *Cancer*, **51**, 882–889.
41. Johnson, L. and Weaver, M. (1981) Von Recklinghausen's disease and gastrointestinal carcinoid. *Journal of the American Medical Association*, **245**, 2496.
42. Keane, T.S., Rider, W.D., Harwood, A.R. *et al.* (1981) Whole abdominal radiation in the management of metastatic gastrointestinal carcinoid tumour. *International Journal of Radiation, Oncology, Biology, Physics*, **7**, 1519–1521.
43. Kimming, B.N., Georgi, P. and Adolphi, J.M. (1987) Carcinoid metastases, CT and ^{131}I-metaiodo benzyl guanidine scintigraphy. *Radiology*, **164**, 199–203.
44. Kowlessar, O.D., Law, D.H. and Sleisenger, M.H. (1959) Malabsorption syndrome associated with carcinoid tumour. *American Journal of Medicine*, **27**, 673–677.
45. Kvois, L.K. (1987) Chemotherapy of metastatic carcinoid and islet cell tumours. *American Journal of Medicine*, **82**, 77–83.
46. Lawson, R.M., Ramanathan, L., Hurley, G. *et al.* (1976) Bronchial adenoma: review of 18-year experience of the Brompton Hospital. *Thorax*, **31**, 245–253.
47. Leveston, S.A., McKeel, D.W. Jr., Buckley, P.J. *et al.* (1981) Acromegaly and Cushing's syndrome associated with a foregut carcinoid. *Journal of Clinical Endocrinology and Metabolism*, **53**, 682–689.
48. Linell, F. & Mansson, K. (1966) On the prevalence and incidence of carcinoids in Malmo. *Acta Medica Scandinavica Supplementum*, **179**, 377–382.
49. Long, R.G., Peters, J.R., Grahame-Smith, D.G. *et al.* (1980) Effect of somatostatin on flushing and gastrointestinal peptides in the carcinoid syndrome. *Clinical Science*, **59**, 9P.
50. McDermott, W.V. and Hensie, T.W. (1973) Metastatic carcinoid to the liver treated by hepatic dearterialization. *Annals of Surgery*, **180**, 305–308.
51. MacDonald, R.A. (1956) A study of 356 carcinoids of the gastrointestinal tract. *American Journal of Medicine*, **21**, 867–878.
52. Maton, P.N., Camilleri, M., Griffin, G. *et al.* (1983) The role of hepatic arterial embolization in the carcinoid syndrome. *British Medical Journal*, **287**, 932–935.
53. Matsuyama, M., Inoue, T., Ariyoshi, Y. *et al.* (1979) Argyrophil cell carcinoma of the uterine cervix with ectopic production of ACTH, βMSHm serotonin, histamine and amylase. *Cancer*, **44**, 1813–1823.
54. Melia, W.M., Nunnerly, H.B., Johnson, P.J. and Williams, R. (1982) Use of devascularization and cytotoxic drugs in 30 patients with the carcinoid syndrome. *British Journal of Cancer*, **46**, 331–339.
55. Mengel, C.E. and Shaffer, R.D. (1973) The carcinoid syndrome: In: *Cancer Medicine*, pp. 1584–1594 (Eds) Holland, J.F. and Frei, E. Philadelphia: Lea and Febiger.
56. Metz, S.A., McRae, J.R. and Robertson, P.R. (1981) Prostaglandins as mediators of paraneoplastic syndromes. Review and update. *Metabolism*, **30**, 299–316.
57. Moertel, C.G. (1975) Clinical management of advanced gastrointestinal cancer. *Cancer*, **36**, 675–682.
58. Moertel, C.G., Sauer, G., Dockerty, M.B. and Bagenstoss, A.H. (1961) Life history of the carcinoid tumour of the small intestine. *Cancer*, **14**, 901–912.
59. Moertel, C.G., Beahrs, O., Woolner, L.B. and Tyce, G.M. (1965) Malignant carcinoid syndrome

associated with non-carcinoid tumours. *New England Journal of Medicine*, **273**, 244–248.

60. Moertel, C.G., Dockerty, M.B. and Judd, E.S. (1968) Carcinoid tumours of the vermiform appendix. *Cancer*, **21**, 270–278.

61. Murphy, D.M., Lockhart, C.H. and Burrington, J.D. (1975) Anaesthetic considerations in bronchial adenoma. *Canadian Anaesthetist's Society Journal*, **22**, 710–714.

62. Murray Lyon, I.M., Dawson, J.L., Parsons, V.A. *et al.* (1970) Treatment of secondary hepatic tumours by ligation of the hepatic artery and infusion of cytotoxic drugs. *The Lancet*, **ii**, 172–175.

63. Oates, J.A., Butler, T.C. (1967) Pharmacological and endocrine aspects of carcinoid syndrome. *Advances in Pharmacology*, **5**, 109–128.

64. Oates, J.A. and Sjoerdsma, A. (1962) A unique syndrome associated with secretion of 5-hydroxytryptophan by metastatic gastric carcinoids. *American Journal of Medicine*, **32**, 333–342.

65. Oates, J.A., Pettinger, W.A. and Doctor, R.B. (1966) Evidence for the release of bradykinin in carcinoid syndrome. *Journal of Clinical Investigation*, **45**, 173–178.

66. Oberg, K., Norheim, I. and Lind, E. (1986) Treatment of malignant carcinoid tumours with human leucocyte interferon. *Cancer Treatment Reports*, **70**, 1297–1304.

67. Okike, N., Berratz, P.E. and Woolner, L.B. (1976) Carcinoid tumours of the lung. *Annals of Thoracic Surgery*, **22**, 270–277.

68. Peskin, G.W. and Kaplan, E.L. (1969) The surgery of carcinoid tumours. *Surgical Clinics of North America*, **49**, 137–145.

69. Reuter, S.R. and Boijsen, W. (1966) Angiographic findings in two ileal carcinoid tumours. *Radiology*, **87**, 836–840.

70. Ricci, C., Patrassi, N., Massa, R. *et al.* (1973) Carcinoid syndrome in bronchial adenoma. *American Journal of Surgery*, **126**, 671–677.

71. Richards, A.T., Hinder, R.A. and Harrison, A.C. (1987) Gastric carcinoid tumours associated with hypergastrinaemia and pernicious anaemia – regression of tumours by antrectomy. *South African Medical Journal*, **72**, 51–53.

72. Riddle, P.J., Font, R.L. and Zimmerman, L.E. (1982) Carcinoid tumours of the eye and orbit. *Human Pathology*, **13**, 459–469.

73. Roberts, L.J., Marney, S.R. and Oates, J.A. (1979) Blockade of the flush associated with metastatic gastric carcinoid by combined H_1 and H_2 receptor antagonists. Evidence for an important role of H_2 receptors in human vasculature. *New England Journal of Medicine*, **300**, 236–238.

74. Roberts, W.C. and Sjoerdsma, A. (1964) The cardiac disease associated with the carcinoid syndrome (carcinoid heart disease). *American Journal of Medicine*, **36**, 5–34.

75. Sandler, M. (1968) 5-Hydroxyindoles and the carcinoid syndrome. *Advances in Pharmacology*, **6B**, 127–142.

76. Sandler, M., Karim, S.M.M. and Williams, E.D. (1968) Prostaglandins in amino-peptide-secreting tumours. *The Lancet*, **ii**, 1053–1054.

77. Sata, T., Sakai, Y. and Sonoyama, A. (1984) Radiological spectrum of carcinoid tumours. *Gastrointestinal Radiology*, **9**, 23–26.

78. Seigel, R.S., Kuhna, L.R., Boriaza, G.S. *et al.* (1980) Computed tomography and angiography in ileal carcinoid tumour and refractile mesenteritis. *Radiology*, **134**, 437–440.

79. Skrabanek, P. and Powell, D. (1978) Ectopic insulin and Occams razor: reappraisal of the riddle of tumour hypoglycaemia. *Clinical Endocrinology*, **9**, 141–154.

80. Soga, J. and Tazawa, K. (1971) Pathologic analysis of carcinoids. *Cancer*, **28**, 990–998.

81. Solcia, E., Capella, C., Buffa, R. *et al.* (1981) Endocrine cells of the digestive system. In: *Physiology of the Gastrointestinal Tract*, pp. 39–58 (Ed.) Johnson, L.R. New York: Raven Press.

82. Solcia, C., Polak, J.M., Larsson, L.I. *et al.* (1981) Update on Lausanne classification of endocrine cells. In: *Gut Hormones*, 2nd edn, pp. 96–100 (Eds) Bloom, S.R. and Polak, J.M. Edinburgh: Churchill Livingstone.

83. Sporrong, B., Falkmer, S., Robboy, S.J. *et al.* (1982) Neurohumoral peptides in ovarian carcinoids. *Cancer*, **49**, 68–74.

84. Strodel, W.E., Talpos, G., Eckhauser, F. and Thompson, N. (1983) Surgical therapy for small bowel carcinoid tumours. *Archives of Surgery*, **118**, 391–397.

85. Swain, C.P., Tavill, A.S. and Neale, G. (1976) Studies of tryptophan and albumin metabolism in a patient with carcinoid syndrome, pellagra and hypoproteinaemia. *Gastroenterology*, **74**, 484–489.

86. Thorson, A. (1958) Studies on carcinoid disease. *Acta Medica Scandinavica Supplementum*, **334**, 7–132.

87. Udenfriend, S., Weussbach, H. and Brodie, B.B. (1958) Assay of serotonin and related metabolites, enzymes and drugs. *Methods in Biochemical Analysis*, **6**, 95–130.

88. Viteaux, J., Salmon, R.J., Languille, O. *et al.* (1981) Carcinoid tumour of the common bile duct. *American Journal of Gastroenterology*, **76**, 360–362.

89. Waldenstrom, J. (1958) Clinical picture of carcinoidosis. *Gastroenterology*, **35**, 575–569.

90. Wick, M., Scott, R.E., Li, C.-Y. and Carney, J.A. (1980) Carcinoid tumour of the thymus. A clinical pathologic report of seven cases with a review of the literature. *Mayo Clinic Proceedings*, **55**, 246–254.

91. Williams, E.D. and Sandler, M. (1963) The classification of carcinoid tumours. *The Lancet*, **i**, 238–239.

92. Wong, V.W. and Melmon, K.L. (1967) Ophthalmic manifestations of the carcinoid flush. *New England Journal of Medicine*, **277**, 406.

93. Zeegan, R., Rothwell-Jackson, R. and Sandler, M. (1969) Massive hepatic resection for the carcinoid syndrome. *Gut*, **10**, 617–622.

OTHER TUMOURS OF THE SMALL INTESTINE *(H.J.F. Hodgson)*

Tumours arise in the small intestine much less frequently than in the stomach or colon. For example, the incidence of neoplasms in the small gut is probably only 1/50th of the incidence in the colon.[5] Small intestinal tumours, however, include a very wide variety of histopathological types, both benign and malignant. Most malignant tumours are either adenocarcinomas, leiomyosarcomas, lymphomas or carcinoids; most benign tumours are leiomyomas, adenomas or lipomas. A tabular classification is given in *Table 3.53*, together with their site of predilection (centimetre for centimetre the duodenum is more susceptible to tumours than the rest of the small intestine).[1,5]

To the clinician, the predominant problem is recognizing the presence of a small intestinal tumour. Many series show that symptoms even of malignant tumours have usually been present for 6–9 months before diagnosis, and tumours may escape detection for years. As symptoms are rarely specific for any histological type, the clinical and diagnostic features of small intestinal tumours will be considered in general first.

CLINICAL FEATURES

Small intestinal tumours are commoner in patients in their seventh decade, and slightly more common in men than women.[30,32] Malignant tumours are more often symptomatic than benign tumours, as shown by the higher incidence of malignant tumours in surgical series of small bowel tumours (about 60–70%) compared with autopsy series (25%). There is also some difference in the spectrum of clinical features shown by benign and malignant tumours. Benign tumours present with pain due to intermittent or subacute obstruction (40–70% of cases) or gastrointestinal blood loss (20–50%). Blood loss is more commonly recognized as chronic anaemia, although major haemorrhage with melaena may occur.[32] Weight loss is rare. If complete obstruction occurs it is usually due to intussusception induced by the tumour, and this is the commonest cause of intussusception in adults.[30] Malignant tumours are more likely to present with a combination of pain (30–90%) and weight loss (70%).[16,32] Haemorrhage may occur in 25% of cases. Up to one-third of patients develop obstruction, usually due to tumour infiltration. Another acute surgical presentation is perforation, particularly with lymphomas where it may be the presenting symptom in 35%, and with sarcomas.[31,32]

Physical findings tend to be unremarkable, unless there is evidence of a genetic predisposing condition *(Table 3.54)*, or cachexia or obstruction have supervened. Palpable masses often represent dilated bowel proximal to sites of obstruction. Jaundice may represent periampullary lesions, or metastatic spread.

INVESTIGATIONS

In many patients, the diagnostic manoeuvres in undiagnosed abdominal pain include upper gastrointestinal endoscopy or radiology, and a barium enema or colonoscopy, but the possibility of small bowel pathology tends to be overlooked. Clearly,

Table 3.53 Type, distribution and relative frequency of small intestinal tumours

Tumour	Total (%)	Site (%)		
		Duodenum	Jejunum	Ileum
Benign tumours				
Leiomyoma	31	17	47	34
Adenoma	22	33	33	33
Lipoma	16	28	19	53
Others	31	23	43	34
Malignant tumours				
Carcinoid	35	6	7	87
Adenocarcinoma	32	42	43	15
Lymphoma	21	4	41	55
Sarcoma	11	18	36	46
Others	1	—	0.5	0.5

After Ashley and Wells 1988[1]

Table 3.54 Familial conditions predisposing small intestinal tumours

Condition	Tumour	Cross-reference
Familial adenomatous polyposis (Gardner's syndrome)	Gastric, duodenal and small intestinal adenomas and adenocarcinomas	p. 845
Neurofibromatosis	Neurofibromas ?Carcinoid tumours	
Cowden's syndrome	Hamartomas	p. 846
Peutz–Jeghers syndrome	Hamartomas in the jejunum and ileum	p. 851
Multiple endocrine adenomatosis type II	Ganglioneuromas	
Osler–Rendu–Weber disease	Haemangiomas	p. 1328
Klippel–Trenaunay syndrome	Haemangiomas	

the recent onset of pain suggestive of small intestinal pathology, notably small intestinal colic regularly occurring after meals, above all in the presence of abnormal blood tests such as anaemia or a low serum iron level, requires full investigation.

Whilst flexible endoscopy will survey the upper duodenum, and improvements in instruments are permitting the upper jejunum to be viewed, small bowel radiology remains the most significant investigation. A combination of plain abdominal radiology and small intestinal contrast radiology will be abnormal in 60–70% of such intestinal tumours, but may not be diagnostic in more than 30–40%.[6] Small bowel obstruction will be identified on plain radiographs, and may demonstrate the site of the lesion. When using contrast radiology, the technique of enteroclysis (an intubated small bowel study) has been demonstrated to show lesions when a conventional barium follow-through examination has failed, probably reflecting the use of a more dilute barium solution against which filling defects can be recognized.[15] Ulcerating mucosal lesions or intramucosal masses can be recognized. Malignant lesions which leave the mucosa intact are more likely to be lymphomas, or leiomyosarcomas. Intraluminal lesions are more likely to be adenomas, leiomyomas or inflammatory polyps.[9] 'Apple-core' malignancies diagnosed on barium studies are often adenocarcinomas, but in one study over half the cases were secondary deposits from other tumours.[12] Despite patterns of small intestinal radiology more or less characteristic of various pathological processes, biopsy confirmation and diagnosis is required before a diagnosis can be made and management decided.

Computed tomography (CT) scanning is of little value in the primary diagnosis of small intestine tumours, as fluid and gas in the gut wall may obscure masses, and fluid–gas interfaces in the presence of obstruction introduce artefacts. Primary tumours may produce thickening of the mesentery, particularly if they are carcinoids, and major lymphadenopathy may support the diagnosis of lymphoma. Metastatic disease in the liver may well be demonstrated.[27] Angiography will probably only be resorted to in the context of the investigation of gastrointestinal bleeding. Both benign and malignant leiomyomas may be demonstrated, or missed, at angiography (*see Figures 108–111*).

TREATMENT

The management of small intestinal tumours is predominantly surgical, particularly in view of the necessity of establishing a histological diagnosis. If histology is unavailable at the time of surgery, decisions as to whether to perform local resection or 'cancer surgery' will depend on clinical appearances. In the undiagnosed cases, wide resection with segmental resection of lymph nodes seems advisable.

MALIGNANT TUMOURS

Carcinoid tumours of the intestine have been dealt with earlier in this chapter (p. 643), as have lymphomas (p. 629).

Adenocarcinomas

Most adenocarcinomas arise in the absence of an obvious predisposing condition, but the incidence is higher in patients with Crohn's disease, coeliac disease, Gardner's syndrome and Peutz–Jeghers syndrome. These special cases are discussed below. After carcinoid tumours, adenocarcinomas are the most common malignant tumour of the small intestine. They are more common in the duodenum (approximately 45% of cases), and jejunum (approximately 40%), compared to the ileum.

Perforation is rare but can occur. Histologically the majority are well-differentiated adenocarcinomas, but about one-third are poorly differentiated, mucinous or adenosquamous. Neuroendocrine cells are commonly found within the tumours, and most express carcinoembryonic antigen histochemically.[13] By the time of surgery, nearly all tumours will have penetrated the serosa, with regional lymph node involvement in 50–70% of cases.[26,30] Lymphatic vessel penetration can be distinguished in about two-thirds of cases, and venous penetration in one-third.[13] About one-fifth of patients will already have distant metastases.[1,26]

Histologically good prognostic findings are a differentiated adenocarcinoma with 'pushing' margins, little or no lymph node or lymph vessel involvement, and absent venous permeation. Poor prognostic features are an undifferentiated tumour with infiltrating edges and vascular permeation. Tumour size itself and local invasion have apparently little prognostic significance.[13]

The prognosis of adenocarcinoma overall is poor because of the spread that has usually occurred by the time of surgery. If apparently curative surgery is undertaken, the 5-year survival is about 30%, which with additional histological evaluation can be divided into a 70% 5-year survival if there is no lymph node involvement, or 10% if there is. If cure seems obtainable, the recommended procedure for duodenal lesions is pancreaticoduodenectomy, and for ileal and jejunal lesions wide excision with segmental resection of the mesentery, and hemicolectomy if the terminal ileum is involved. There seems to be no benefit in radical surgery if lymph nodes are involved. Thus, overall survival rates for the condition vary between 5 and 25%.[26,32] If curative surgery is not successful, there is little to be gained either by chemotherapy – 5-fluorouracil having been evaluated and found of little benefit – or by radiotherapy, the effect of which is limited by radioresistance to the tumour and radiosensitivity of the normal small intestine.[26]

Predisposing causes

CROHN'S DISEASE

Small intestine carcinoma is more common in Crohn's disease, and differs from spontaneous carcinoma in the younger age group (average mid-40s), more striking male predominance (3:1), and a greater tendency to involve the terminal ileum.[8] Over three-quarters of cases are ileal in origin. The excluded ileum, if the operation of ileal bypass was performed, is particularly at risk. The prognosis is said to be poorer, as diagnosis may be delayed as symptoms may be attributed to inflammatory activity.[4,10]

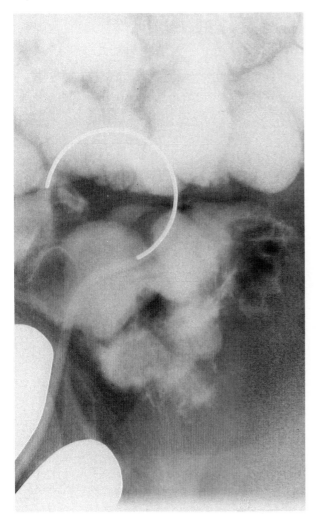

Figure 3.108 Small bowel follow through examination. Shows negative filling defect of intraluminal small intestinal leiomyoma (arrows). (Courtesy of Dr. J. Jackson, RPMS.)

Interestingly, the majority in the duodenum and jejunum are proximal (over three-quarters of duodenal tumours in the bulb, and two-thirds of jejunal cases within the first 80 cm of jejunum), and in the distal ileum (80% within 50 cm of ileocaecal valve).[17,20] They are most frequent between the ages 50 and 80 years, and there is a slight male preponderance. Their aetiology is unknown but, interestingly, adjacent non-malignant adenomatous areas may be found histologically even in the absence of a known genetic predisposition. Macroscopically, adenocarcinomas may be ulcerating areas of mucosa, or less commonly polypoid lesions, and both can cause constriction of the lumen. In the duodenum, proximity to the ampulla may precipitate jaundice, but otherwise the presentation is with pain, obstruction, haemorrhage, weight loss or a combination thereof.

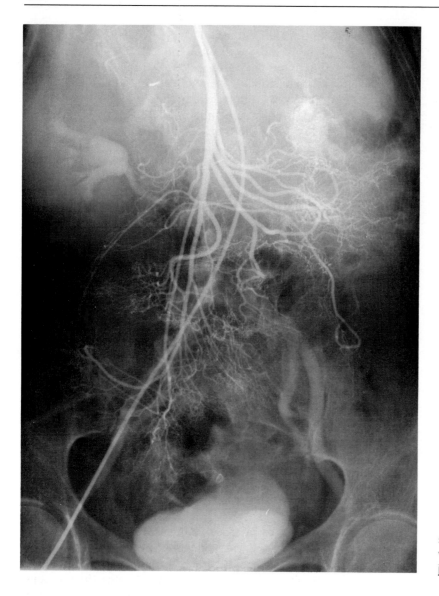

Figure 3.109 Visceral angiogram demonstrating superior mesenteric run with vascular blush from a leiomyoma in upper jejunum. (Courtesy of Dr. J. Jackson, RPMS.)

COELIAC DISEASE

Jejunal adenocarcinoma is in some series the most common carcinoma arising in the context of adult coeliac disease, such patients also being at risk of oesophageal and other cancers, and lymphoma. Evidence now suggests that a strict gluten-free diet may reduce this incidence of the complication. Diagnosis may be delayed, as in Crohn's disease, as symptoms are initially attributed to a relapse of coeliac disease.

PEUTZ–JEGHERS SYNDROME

This genetically determined autosomal-dominant condition gives rise to hamartomous polyps, most commonly small intestinal and biliary, but sometimes affecting the colon, stomach or oesophagus.[28] The characteristic skin lesions are circumoral buccal or lingual pigmentation. Although early studies suggested that fewer than 5% of patients with Peutz–Jeghers syndrome develop neoplastic change, as would be anticipated from the hamartomous nature of the lesions, more recent surveys have reported higher incidences. Spigelman *et al.* reported a 13% incidence of gastrointestinal cancer, and a higher than expected risk of cancer in other sites, resulting in a 48% chance of patients dying of cancer by the age of 57 years.[25] The pathological appearances supported a hamartoma carcinoma sequence, most commonly in the duodenum or jejunum. Histopathological interpretation of specimens in Peutz–Jeghers syndrome can be difficult as epithelium may become displaced submucosally without tumour change. Endoscopic and radiological screening and resection of hamartomas have been advocated to prevent malignant change.[29]

FAMILIAL POLYPOSIS SYNDROME, GARDNER'S SYNDROME

The tendency for small intestinal tumours – particularly periampullary – and gastric adenomas and

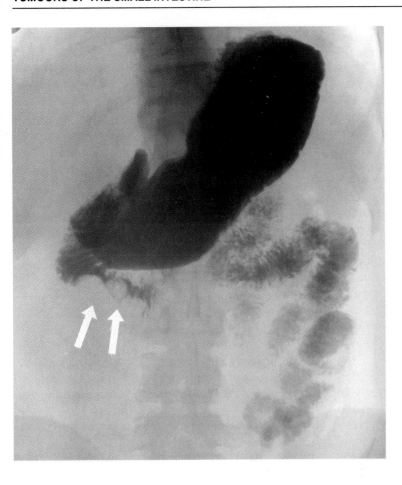

Figure 3.110 Extrinsic compression of third part of duodenum from a leiomyosarcoma demonstrated on barium follow through. (Courtesy of Dr. J. Jackson, RPMS.)

carcinomas to develop in the setting of familial polyposis syndrome predominantly affecting the colon is detailed in Chapter 4.

IMMUNOSUPPRESSION

An increased incidence of small bowel tumours after transplantation has been attributed to the immuno-suppressive drugs.[3,23]

Leiomyosarcomas

Leiomyosarcomas are slow-growing tumours of smooth muscle origin. They are common in men, and typically occur after the age of 40 years. Histologically, differentiation from a benign leiomyoma may be difficult, and depends upon the frequency of mitotic figures. Spindle-shaped cells predominate,

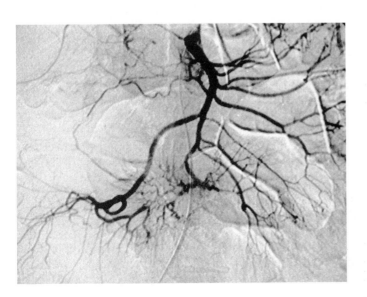

Figure 3.111 Superior mesenteric angiogram showing deformity of vascular supply, stenoid and corkscrewed vessels, typical of a desmoplastic reaction to a carcinoid primary in the ileum. (Courtesy of Dr. J. Jackson, RPMS.)

with variable pleomorphism and hypercellularity. Classically the tumours are intramucosal, within the ileum (45%), jejunum (35%) or duodenum (20%). The characteristic radiological pattern is of an extra-luminal mass, often smooth but with a central or eccentric crater on the luminal surface. The most common presentation is with haemorrhage, either acute or chronic, but rarer presentations include retroperitoneal haemorrhage, protracted fever and peritonitis. At surgery, spread is very commonly present, in 80–90%; this can be local, or to regional lymph nodes, or hepatic, representing a combi-nation of local, lymphatic and haematological spread. The prognosis after surgery is varied, with a 5-year survival rate of 10–50%, but as histological distinction between leiomyomas and leiomyosarco-mas may be difficult, some operative series may have included some benign lesions.

Kaposi's sarcoma

Kaposi's sarcoma, initially recognized as a skin tumour, may arise in the gastrointestinal tract. In Western practice this is almost exclusively in the context of human immunodeficiency virus (HIV) infection. The tumour deposits in the intestine may present with bleeding, perforation, protein loss, obstruction or diarrhoea, particularly in the upper gastrointestinal tract. Radiological appearances are variable, from localized to diffuse nodularity or ulceration.[7]

BENIGN TUMOURS

Whilst histological classification into lipomas and smooth muscle tumours is relatively straight-forward, the classification of adenomas may be com-plex. Non-neoplastic polyps, and hamartomas, can also cause diagnostic difficulties, as discussed below.

Leiomyomas

Leiomyomas arise from smooth muscle, and typi-cally show histologically whorls or sheets of well-differentiated cells without mitotic figures. They may be found at any age, though are commonest in middle age. The most common symptoms are haem-orrhage or anaemia from surface ulceration. Over-all, they appear to be the commonest benign tumour of the small intestine, and are located in the jejunum in about 50% of cases, the ileum in 30–50% and the duodenum in 15–20%. They may project predomi-nantly extraluminally (most commonly), or pre-dominantly intraluminally, or extend in both directions.[18] If symptomatic, local excision is acceptable unless the leiomyoma is more than 5 cm in diameter. Larger lesions may have become malig-nant and, as frozen section is unreliable in excluding a leiomyosarcoma, wide excision is advised in large lesions.

Adenomas

Adenomatous polyps may occur sporadically, or as part of the familial polyposis syndrome (see above).[22] They are evenly distributed between the duodenum, jejunum and ileum, and, if symptoma-tic, present either with obstruction or bleeding. The polypoid nature renders endoscopic removal rela-tively straightforward if they are in the duodenum. They have malignant potential, as judged from the occasional finding of adenomatous tissue at the edge of a carcinoma, but the risk factors and rate of development have not been defined.

Villous adenomas of the small intestine, like ade-nomas occurring in the colon, show a high incidence of malignant change (up to 50%), particularly in large lesions. They are predominantly found in the duodenum, and ideally should be treated by seg-mental resection. The clinical syndrome of hypoka-laemia and watery diarrhoea that occurs with colonic lesions of this histological type does not occur with small intestinal lesions.

Brunner's gland adenomas are discussed in conjunction with Brunner's gland hyperplasia (see below).

Lipomas

Lipomas arise in patients from the age of 50 years onwards, predominantly in males, usually as single (but occasionally multiple), usually smooth, poly-poid masses spreading intraluminally. They may be noted at radiography to conform to the shape of the gut lumen, reflecting their near-liquid consistency, and CT scans can confirm their fatty nature by showing the appropriate attenuation values.[18] They are most commonly found in the ileum, then in the duodenum. They are usually asymptomatic, but may bleed if the surface is ulcerated, or give rise to obstruction. They have no malignant potential, so coincidentally found lesions do not require excision because they rarely if ever cause small bowel obstruction.

Miscellaneous tumours

Neurogenic tumours, from subserosal nerves or cells of Auerbach's and Meissner's plexus, make up about 4% of benign small intestinal tumours. They include neurofibromas, ganglioneuromas, neuro-lemmomas (benign Schwannomas), granular cell tumours, paragangliomas, and gangliocytic para-gangliomas.[14,21] They may be multiple, particularly in the context of neurofibromatosis. All these tend to present as smooth polypoid tumours in any part of the small intestine (except for the gangliocytic para-ganglioma, which is restricted to the duodenum).[18] Haemangiomas are discussed elsewhere in the context of gastrointestinal haemorrhage (Chapter 5).

The Cronkhite–Canada syndrome

In this syndrome, multiple sessile or predunculated polyps occur in the duodenum, less frequently in the jejunum and ileum, as well as in the colon and stomach. They are usually classified as hamartomas of the juvenile type, and the clinical picture is dominated by diarrhoea and malabsorption and electrolyte abnormalities, associated with weight loss, abdominal pain, alopecia, nail atrophy and hyperpigmentation. Corticosteroid therapy and parenteral nutrition may, in combination with local therapy of affected gut, induce remission. In some cases, predisposition to adenocarcinoma of the colon has been noted.

Non-neoplastic tumours

The myoepithelial hamartoma, or 'ectopic pancreas', consists of pancreatic tissue, smooth muscle and epithelial structures. Although predominantly found in the gastric antrum, they can appear in the duodenum or more distally. Radiologically they are smooth polyps 1–5 cm across, and occasionally they are umbilicated. Excision is not normally indicated, and usually they are placed so that endoscopic biopsy can establish the diagnosis.

Brunner's gland hyperplasia/adenoma

About 1% of the population has hyperplasia of Brunner's glands predominantly in the first part of the duodenum, and this may merely produce bosselation of the mucosa recognized at endoscopy. This may be found at any age. Patterns varying from diffuse hyperplasia to localized hyperplasia and apparent adenomas are reported, the last two appearing as sessile smooth submucosal polyps.[18,19] Involvement more distal than the third part of the duodenum is rare. Endoscopic biopsy generally establishes the diagnosis, and therapy is rarely required.

Inflammatory fibroid polyps

Solitary smooth-surfaced polyps in the ileum, in patients aged 50 years and over, may be inflammatory fibroid polyps.[11] They may be up to 12 cm across. A similar polyp is more commonly reported in the stomach, and duodenal examples are also reported.[24]

REFERENCES

1. Ashley, S.W. and Wells, S.A. Jr (1988) Tumours of the small intestine. *Seminars in Oncology*, **15**, 116–128.
2. Bill, K., Belber, J.P. and Carson, J.W. (1982) Adenymoma (pancreatic heterotopia) of the duodenum producing common bile duct obstruction. *Gastrointestinal Endoscopy*, **28**, 182–184.
3. Calne, R.Y., Rolles, K., Thiru, S. *et al.* (1979) Cyclosporin A initially as the only immunosuppressant in 32 recipients of cadaveric organs: 32 kidneys, 2 pancreases and 2 livers. *The Lancet*, **ii**, 1033–1036.
4. Collier, P.E., Turowski, P. and Diamond, D.L. (1985) Small intestine adenocarcinoma complicating regional enteritis. *Cancer*, **55**, 516–521.
5. Darling, R.E. and Welch, E.C. (1959) Tumours of the small intestine. *New England Journal of Medicine*, **260**, 397–408.
6. Ekberg, O. and Ekholm, S. (1980) Radiology in primary small bowel adenocarcinoma. *Gastrointestinal Radiology*, **5**, 49–53.
7. Friedman, S.L., Wright, T.L. and Altman, D.F. (1985) Gastrointestinal Kaposi's sarcoma in patients with AIDS: endoscopic and autopsy findings. *Gastroenterology*, **89**, 102–108.
8. Fresko, D., Lazarus, S.S., Dotan, J. and Reingold, M. (1982) Early presentation of carcinoma of the small bowel in Crohn's disease: case report and review of literature. *Gastroenterology*, **82**, 783–789.
9. Good, C.A. (1963) Tumours of the small intestine: Caldwell lecture. *American Journal of Roentgenology*, **89**, 685–692.
10. Hawker, P.C., Gyde, S.N., Thompson, H. and Allan, R.N. (1982) Adenocarcinoma of the small intestine complicating Crohn's disease. *Gut*, **23**, 188–193.
11. Johnstone, J.M. and Morson, B.C. (1978) Inflammatory fibroid polyp of the gastrointestinal tract. *Histopathology*, **2**, 349–361.
12. Levine, M.S., Drooz, A.T. and Herlinger, H. (1987) Annular malignancies of the small bowel. *Gastrointestinal Radiology*, **12**, 53–58.
13. Lien, G.S., Mori, M. and Enjoji, M. (1988) Primary carcinoma of the small intestine. A clinicopathologic and immunohistochemical study. *Cancer*, **61**, 316–323.
14. Lukash, W.M., Morgan, R.I., Sennett, C.O. and Neilson, O.F. (1966) Gastrointestinal neoplasms in

von Recklinghausen's disease. *Archives of Surgery*, **92**, 905–908.

15. Maglinte, D.D.T., Hall, R., Miller, R.E. *et al.* (1984) Detection of surgical lesions of the small bowel by enteroclysis. *American Journal of Surgery*, **197**, 226–229.

16. Martin, R.G. (1986) Malignant tumours of the small intestine. *Surgical Clinics of North America*, **66**, 779–786.

17. Morgan, D.F. and Busuttil, R.W. (1977) Primary adenocarcinoma of the small intestine. *American Journal of Surgery*, **134**, 331.

18. Olmsted, W.W., Ros, P.R., Hjermstad, B.M., McCarthy, M.J. and Dachman, A.H. (1987) Tumours of the small intestine with little or no malignant predisposition: a review of the literature and report of 56 cases. *Gastrointestinal Radiology*, **12**, 231–239.

19. Osborne, R., Toffler, R. and Lowman, R.M. (1973) Brunner's gland adenoma of the duodenum. *American Journal of Digestive Diseases*, **18**, 689–694.

20. Ouriel, K.K. and Adams, J.T. (1984) Adenocarcinoma of the small bowel. *American Journal of Surgery*, **147**, 56–71.

21. Perrone, T., Sibley, R.K. and Rosai, J. (1985) Duodenal gangliocytic paraganglioma. *American Journal of Surgical Pathology*, **9**, 31–41.

22. Sarre, R.G., Frost, A.G., Jagelman, D.G., Petras, R.E., Sivak, M.V. and McGannon, E. (1987) Gastric and duodenal polyps in familial adenomatous polyposis: a prospective study of the nature and prevalence of upper gastrointestinal polyps. *Gut*, **28**, 306–314.

23. Sheil, A.G.R., Mahoney, J.F., Horvath, J.S. *et al.* (1979) Cancer and survival after cadaveric donor renal transplantation. *Transplantation Proceedings*, **11**, 1052–1054.

24. Shimer, G.R. and Helwig, E.B. (1984) Inflammatory fibroid polyps of the intestine. *American Journal of Clinical Pathology*, **81**, 708–713.

25. Spigelman, A.D., Murday, V. and Phillips, R.K.S. (1989) Cancer and the Peutz–Jeghers syndrome. *Gut*, **30**, 1588–1590.

26. Taggart, D.P., McLatchie, G.R. and Imrie, C.W. (1986) Survival of surgical patients with carcinoma, lymphoma and carcinoid tumours of the small bowel. *British Journal of Surgery*, **73**, 826–828.

27. Thompson, W.M. and Halvorsen, R.A., Jr (1987) Computed Tomographic staging of gastrointestinal malignancies. Part II. The small bowel, colon, and rectum. *Investigative Radiology*, **22**, 96–105.

28. Utsunomiga, J., Gocho, H., Miganaga, T. *et al.* (1975) Peutz–Jeghers syndrome. Its natural course and management. *Johns Hopkins Medical Journal*, **136**, 71–82.

29. Williams, C.B., Goldblatt, M. and Delaney, P.V. (1982) "Top and tail endoscopy" and follow-up in Peutz–Jeghers syndrome. *Endoscopy*, **14**, 82–84.

30. Wilson, J.M., Melvin, D.B., Gray, G.F. *et al.* (1974) Primary malignancies of the small bowel: a report of 96 cases and review of the literature. *Annals of Surgery*, **180**, 175–179.

31. Wilson, J.M., Melvin, D.B., Gray, G. *et al.* (1975) Benign small bowel tumour. *Annals of Surgery*, **181**, 247–250.

32. Zollinger, R.M. Jr, Sternfeld, W.C. and Schreiber, H. (1986) Primary neoplasms of the small intestine. *American Journal of Surgery*, **151**, 654–658.

SURGICAL CAUSES OF MALABSORPTION

JEJUNOILEAL BYPASS *(R.E. Barry)*

Because of the very disappointing results of conservative treatment for gross obesity, many operations were devised to ameliorate the problem by a more radical approach. Until recently, apart from simply excising redundant adipose tissue, the only radical treatment to gain reasonably wide popularity was the operation of jejunoileal bypass, following the publication of their initial results by Payne and De Wind.[13]

The original concept of jejunoileal bypass was to bypass 90% of the small intestine and so produce a state of profound malabsorption which would result in weight loss even in the presence of a large dietary food intake. Once the grossly obese patients reached normal weight, it was intended to restore normal intestinal continuity in the belief that the patient would find the subsequent maintenance of normal weight by dietary means considerably easier than weight reduction. However, the second operation to restore continuity was abandoned as it became apparent that patients soon returned to their preoperative obese state.

The potential incidence of complications is high because the operation produces a state of malabsorption. Consequently, meticulous and conscientious long-term follow-up of the patient is essential after jejunoileal bypass. This burden has proved too great for some centres, with the result that the popularity of this procedure is presently declining.

INDICATION FOR OPERATION

To assess the indications for jejunoileal bypass objectively requires accurate knowledge of the risks of the operation, which can then be compared with the risks of obesity. A large amount of literature is available to assess the operative and postoperative risks, but there is a surprising lack of information on the actual risks of obesity itself. Although the prevalence of diabetes mellitus, hypertension, cholelithiasis etc. is well recorded, the mortality and morbidity from these complications of obesity are not. Even insurance company data are unhelpful because patients with gross obesity tend to be denied life insurance and therefore do not figure prominently in the statistics. Furthermore, the social, economic and emotional morbidity of gross obesity cannot be objectively quantified.

However, some generally agreed principles may be stated although details vary considerably with individual opinion. The patient should be sufficiently obese. This has been defined variably as being over 135 kg, more than 44 kg over the 'ideal' body weight, greater than twice the 'ideal' weight, or having a body mass index (ponderal index) of greater than 30. The body mass index is given by

$$\frac{weight\ (kg)}{height^2\ (m)}$$

The obesity should be long-standing and the patient should have failed in attempts at genuine, concerted and supervised conservative treatment regimes.

Youth (age less than 40 years) is often insisted upon and is clearly advantageous for medical and economic reasons, but a significant complication rate may be anticipated even in otherwise fit adolescents.[15]

Although diabetes mellitus, hypertension or resting hypoventilation may justifiably be considered as an indication for jejunoileal bypass, the presence of diabetic complications, ischaemic heart disease, or respiratory failure must be regarded as relative contraindications. The physical complications of obesity are easily diagnosed but there is an associated psychological morbidity which cannot be ignored. The traumatic effects of isolation, ridicule and low self-esteem cannot be quantified easily but are important considerations in indications for treatment.

Psychiatric illness has been regarded both as an indication and as a contraindication for jejunoileal bypass. Certainly many grossly obese patients are seriously depressed. It can be extremely difficult to decide whether such depression is an effect or a contributory cause of the obesity. If doubt exists then expert help is strongly advised. However, it has been shown that the dramatic alteration of body image following jejunoileal bypass will often improve rather than compound any neurotic traits in properly selected patients.[5]

As in all operative procedures, the patient must give informed consent, which requires an understanding of the inevitable effects and possible complications of jejunoileal bypass. More importantly, the patient should be sufficiently reliable to comply with the requirements of long-term medication and long-term follow-up attendance.

The highest incidence of serious postoperative metabolic complications occurs in those patients with the highest rates of weight loss postoperatively. Because the patients with the highest weight preoperatively are also those who lose weight the fastest postoperatively, some patients are too obese to risk jejunoileal bypass. Unfortunately, the quantification of risks is too difficult to allow this upper limit of weight to be accurately defined.

In practice, these indications mean that relatively small numbers of patients are suitable for this form of radical treatment.

THE OPERATION

The precise details of lengths and regions of small intestine bypassed tend to vary from centre to centre but all aim to achieve a 90% exclusion of the small intestine. In practice this requires 50 cm of functioning small intestine to remain in continuity, and *at least* 10 cm of this must be ileal to prevent the very severe fluid and electrolyte loss which was experienced with the early jejunocolic anastomoses. An anastomosis of 40 cm of jejunum to 10 cm of terminal ileum, or 25 cm of jejunum to 25 cm of terminal ileum, are most commonly used. The jejunoileal anastomosis may be end-to-side (Payne procedure),[13] in which the jejunum is transected 40 cm distal to the ligament of Treitz and the proximal end of the jejunum anastomosed to the side of the ileum 10 cm from the ileocaecal valve (*Figure 3.112a*). The distal end of the transected jejunum is closed and tethered to prevent intussusception. More recently, attempts have been made to minimize postoperative bile salt depletion and catharsis by anastomosing this distal segment to the gallbladder as a cholecystenterostomy. Scott *et al*.[18] believed a more predictable weight loss was achieved by an end-to-end jejunoileal bypass, in which the proximal end of transected jejunum is anastomosed end-to-end to the transected terminal ileum (*Figure 3.112b*). In this procedure, the bypassed jejunum is closed at the proximal end as before and the distal end of

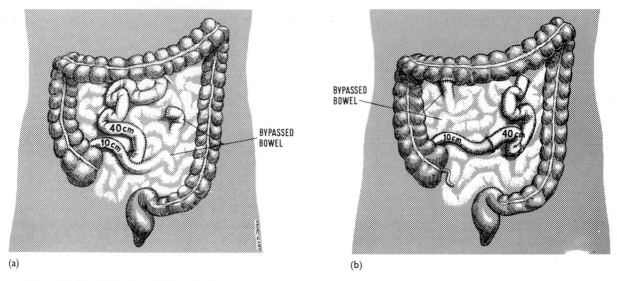

(a)   (b)

Figure 3.112   (a) End-to-side jejunoileal bypass (Payne procedure). (b) End-to-end jejunoileal bypass (Scott procedure).

the bypassed segment is drained by end-to-side anastomosis to the sigmoid or transverse colon.

POSTOPERATIVE MANAGEMENT

Fluid and electrolyte losses due to diarrhoea are considerable in the first few months following surgery, hence prophylactic supplements are essential. Provided patient compliance is good, normal electrolyte status can be maintained with supplements of potassium, magnesium and calcium. Potassium is best tolerated as effervescent potassium chloride. Osmotic catharsis prohibits oral magnesium and supplements must be given intramuscularly if required. Calcium may be taken alone or incorporated in antidiarrhoeal mixtures (such as aromatic chalk with opium mixture) or in combination with vitamin D. Calcium supplements may also be important in preventing renal calculi as discussed later. Early use of vitamin D is desirable to promote calcium absorption and as prophylaxis against metabolic bone disease, which can develop early and subclinically. However, the need for high-potency vitamin D derivatives such as l-hydroxy-cholecalciferol has been questioned.[16]

RESULTS OF JEJUNOILEAL BYPASS

Conservative treatment of gross obesity tends to produce a weight loss which is *small* (rarely 18 kg) and *temporary* without normalization of risk factors. But, provided the patient has been properly selected and the operation accurately performed, the weight loss following jejunoileal bypass is both large and permanent.

Weight loss begins as soon as the immediate postoperative ileus resolves, and is most rapid in the early months after surgery. The total amount of weight which will be lost is difficult to predict; however, in general, the heavier the preoperative weight, the faster the rate of postoperative weight loss will be.

The immediate postoperative consequences of jejunoileal bypass are very similar to those of the short bowel syndrome. *Diarrhoea* is almost invariable but the severity is surprisingly variable. Diarrhoea tends to be most severe in the first few weeks following surgery but is rarely an important problem by 12 months postoperatively provided that the functional segments have been accurately determined. At operation, it is important to measure and mark the proposed functional segments immediately on gaining access to the peritoneum and before much handling of the small intestine has occurred, otherwise the subsequent contraction of the bowel will result in incorrect estimation of the lengths to be used. Similarly, attempts at immediate preoperative weight reduction by starvation are to be avoided as similar errors in measurement may occur in the hypotonic and hypoplastic bowel of the fasting subject.

The rate of *weight loss* usually begins to decline approximately 6 months after jejunoileal bypass but continues at a reduced rate for a further 18 months to 2 years. By 2 years the weight loss is usually maximal and thereafter there is often a slow rise before reaching a plateau. This small rise can usually be controlled by dietary restriction even though preoperative dietary treatment had failed.

The reasons for this cessation of weight loss are

interesting, complex and insufficiently understood. There is no doubt that the malabsorption and steatorrhoea decrease with time. This may be related to the adaptive response of the small intestinal mucosa in the functioning (non-bypassed) segments,[1] a response which is well recorded in the small intestinal mucosa after massive intestinal resections.[8] The importance in quantitative terms of any functional (absorptive) adaptation is uncertain. But there can be no doubt that changes in oral food intake play an important role in weight loss.[15] It was noted early[3] that food intake is considerably decreased following jejunoileal bypass compared with the preoperative state in grossly obese subjects. This decreased intake far outlives any perioperative discomfort associated with eating. This is probably a true alteration in appetite or satiety, particularly since not only does food intake decrease but taste preferences also change towards a more normal pattern. Although this decreased food intake is prolonged, there is an upward trend after about 2 years. However, food intake does not again reach preoperative levels. The timing of the phenomenon tends to suggest that increasing intake may play a part in the arrest and slight reversal of the weight loss described above.

Anorexia is common in the months following jejunoileal bypass and may progress to nausea. In more extreme cases, vomiting may occur which may, when severe or prolonged, be a forerunner of metabolic complications, particularly 'bypass hepatitis'. Such patients tend to be those who are losing weight at the fastest rates. The optimal rate of weight loss in the first year should be less than 4.5 kg/month. If the rate of weight loss is significantly in excess of this, it is desirable to intervene with nutritional support before evidence of hepatic impairment becomes manifest.

Properly selected patients achieving normal weights after bypass may be expected to achieve economic and social rehabilitation. In addition to weight loss, there is a significant and permanent *decrease in serum lipids* and a *decrease in arterial blood pressure*.

COMPLICATIONS

All surgical procedures have an associated morbidity. Perioperative morbidity, even in the grossly obese, can be minimized by the usual precautions, including *pre*operative physiotherapy, early mobilization, the judicious use of prophylactic subcutaneous heparin and good analgesia.

Many metabolic sequelae have been described following jejunoileal bypass. Malabsorption occurs by design, and deficiencies, for example of fat-soluble vitamins, can be anticipated and should never be permitted to develop as a result of an elective procedure.

Although the number of complications described in the literature is large, many of these only occur rarely, e.g. interstitial nephritis. Nevertheless, it can be extremely difficult from the literature to estimate the frequency with which some complications occur. This may reflect regional differences. For example, nephrolithiasis seems common in North America, but relatively rare in Scandinavia. Other complications, such as the varying incidence of thromboembolism or severe electrolyte disturbance, must reflect the quality of postoperative care.

The data presented in *Table 3.55* are a composite of many published series and give an assessment of the lowest and highest rates which may be expected for the commoner or more serious complications listed.

Renal calculi

Deaths from renal failure resulting from obstructive uropathy are well described. Ureteric calculi are usually oxalate in composition. Hyperoxaluria occurs following jejunoileal bypass, as with severe

Table 3.55 Complications of jejunoileal bypass

Complication	Range of incidence (%)
Direct surgical mortality	2–6
Perioperative morbidity (e.g. thromboembolism)	4–13
Renal and ureteric calculi	3–10
Hepatic failure	0–14 (probably approximately 4%)
Arthralgia	7–15
Abdominal distension ± pseudo-obstructive syndromes	13–100
Electrolyte disturbance	Up to 80
Metabolic acidosis	13–80
Metabolic bone disease	Uncertain because of varied diagnostic criteria

steatorrhoea of any cause. Its aetiology is multifactorial but may be related in part to the increased availability of oxalate for absorption as a consequence of steatorrhoea and to increased absorption by the colonic mucosa. An increased calcium intake is desirable following jejunoileal bypass to help prevent this increased oxalate absorption.

Poor hydration in the presence of diarrhoea, and postoperative urinary tract infections related to unnecessary catheterization or poor catheter technique, may be contributory factors to the precipitation of urinary tract calculi. Good hydration is particularly important to minimize crystal-induced renal parenchymal damage.

Liver disease

Although the incidence of liver disease following jejunoileal bypass is relatively small, the mortality from this complication is so high that it is probably the major reason for the decline in the popularity of this procedure. Deaths occur from hepatic failure which may be the end-stage of a cirrhotic process occurring months or years after jejunoileal bypass, or as a consequence of an acute or subacute hepatitic illness. This 'bypass hepatitis' is histologically indistinguishable from alcoholic liver disease but occurs in the absence of alcohol ingestion. The hepatitis tends to occur relatively early after jejunoileal bypass and seems to occur in those patients losing weight at an excessive rate, and is sometimes associated with continued nausea and vomiting. Apart from this, the first sign of serious hepatitic disease may be the appearance of jaundice, by which time restorative surgery is contraindicated. Hepatocellular enzymes are commonly raised in the serum following jejunoileal bypass in the absence of serious liver problems and cannot be used as an indicator of impending hepatic disease.

Although the cause of this hepatitic illness is obscure, there is no doubt it can be ameliorated by nutritional support, if necessary by the intravenous route. A similar syndrome in dogs following jejunoileal bypass can be prevented by antibiotic treatment. However, the similarity to the human counterpart may only be superficial – in humans the incidence of this complication is approximately 4% but in dogs the liver failure is almost universal within a few months of jejunoileal bypass.

The occurrence of liver disease has been regarded as an indication for the restoration of normal intestinal continuity. If a further operation is performed at the time of hepatic insufficiency, as manifested by jaundice, the mortality is unacceptably high. Surgery should be delayed until the hepatic failure has

been controlled by nutritional support. However, cirrhosis may develop insidiously and be detectable only by sequential liver biopsies and hepatic decompensation may occur many years after the surgery.[9]

Arthropathy

Arthralgia is more common than overt arthritis following jejunoileal bypass, but a true reactive arthritis is well described. The larger joints tend to be affected more commonly. The condition is rarely severe but has on occasions necessitated restoration of normal intestinal continuity. The arthritis is transitory and non-destructive, appearing in exacerbations and remissions which tend to peter out. Circulating immune complexes with gut-derived antigens have been suggested as a cause.

Dermatological complications

Some degree of alopecia is almost universal during the period of protein depletion and rapid weight loss. Deficiency states may also be manifested as skin rashes. The incidence of tender red papular or pustular lesions caused by a cutaneous vasculitis may have been underestimated in the literature. Occasionally erythema nodosum occurs. Provided there is no evidence of large vessel vasculitis or haematuria then symptomatic treatment is recommended as usually sufficient. Spontaneous resolution is the rule but treatment with metronidazole or tetracycline is effective.

'Gas/bloat syndrome'

Abdominal distension is caused by gas in the bypassed small intestine and has a wide spectrum of severity. Abdominal bloating, often associated with discomfort or colicky abdominal pain, is common. At the opposite end of the spectrum, distension can be extreme with severe pain, vomiting and obstipation, and is caused by intestinal ileus, apparently due to bacterial colonization of the bypassed intestine.[2] This syndrome of pseudo-obstruction is well described in other conditions associated with small bowel bacterial colonization such as small intestinal diverticulosis and systemic sclerosis.[14] In the acute phase, rapid relief is obtained from oral antibiotics effective against anaerobic organisms such as metronidazole.

Metabolic bone disease

The incidence and severity of metabolic bone disease is controversial, perhaps because of the varying

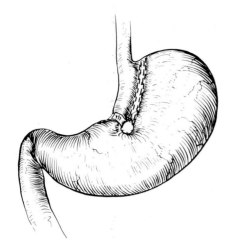

Figure 3.113 Vertical banded gastroplasty. (Reproduced, with permission, from Mason.[11])

diagnostic criteria used in different studies. It would, perhaps, be surprising if some osteopenia did not occur and this may be compounded by the commonly found mild, non-ion gap, metabolic acidosis. Routine supplements of vitamin D are widely employed and monitoring of the serum calcium and alkaline phosphatase levels is recommended.

BYPASS REVISION

The popularity of jejunoileal bypass declined when the prevalence and severity of the metabolic complications became established. Gastric partitioning procedures, particularly Mason's vertical banded gastroplasty (*Figure 3.113*),[11] have largely succeeded jejunoileal bypass – despite the fact that some patients may fail to lose weight and serious *metabolic* complications such as death from liver failure may also occur following gastroplasty.[17] The poor reputation of jejunoileal bypass may merely reflect a poor standard of postoperative follow-up care because, when this is of a high standard, metabolic complication rates as low as 1% can be achieved.[20] Nevertheless, a significant proportion of patients require revision of jejunoileal bypass, despite maintenance of weight loss, because of intolerance or complications. In one careful 13-year follow-up of 180 patients in the UK, the revision rate was 17%.[12] Although most complications tend to occur early after bypass, half of the revisions are required many years following the original surgery. Consequently, although 80% of patients achieve good weight loss and are asymptomatic, constant vigilance is required because such patients remain at a high risk of metabolic decompensation as a consequence of intercurrent illness.[10]

Although longer ileal segments reduce bile salt losses, the complication rate is not influenced by the ratio of functional lengths of jejunum to ileum. Bypass revision for complications usually requires restoration of normal intestinal continuity. This is particularly hazardous in the presence of hepatic decompensation, which must first be adequately corrected by nutritional support and, possibly, antibiotic treatment of the flora in the bypassed loop. Most patients, however, will rapidly regain their pre-bypass weight following restoration of intestinal continuity. Conversion to vertical banded gastroplasty has therefore been suggested to prevent this. Similar operations can be successful, but more usually a mean weight gain of about 20 kg may be anticipated. Twenty per cent of patients may return to pre-bypass weights despite a gastric reduction procedure.[9]

Although the popularity of jejunoileal bypass has undoubtedly declined, many patients remain with a functioning bypass who require continuing supervision, and the operation continues to be performed in a few specialized centres on highly selected patients.

REFERENCES

1. Barry, R.E., Barisch, J., Bray, G.A. *et al.* (1977) Intestinal adaptation after jejunoileal bypass in man. *American Journal of Clinical Nutrition*, **30**, 32–42.
2. Barry, F.E., Chow, A.W. and Billesden, J. (1977) The role of intestinal microflora in colonic pseudoobstruction complicating jejuno-ileal bypass. *Gut*, **18**, 356–359.
3. Bray, G.A., Barry, R.E., Benfield, J.R. *et al.* (1986) Intestinal bypass surgery for obesity decreases food intake and taste preferences. *American Journal of Clinical Nutrition*, **29**, 779–783.
4. Chambers, J.B., Walton, R.T., Coupe, M.O. and Ward, D.E. (1985) QT prolongation after jejunoileal bypass. *The Lancet*, **ii**, 1308.
5. Crisp, A.H., Kalucy, R.S., Pilkington, T.R.E. and Gazet, J.C. (1977) Some psychosocial consequences of ileojejunal bypass surgery. *American Journal of Clinical Nutrition*, **30**, 109–119.
6. Crowley, L.V., Seay, J. and Mullin, G.T. (1986) Long Term Hematopoeitic and Skeletal Effects of Gastric Bypass. *Clinical Nutrition*, **5**(Suppl), 185–187.
7. de Lucia, L.M. and Calabria, R.P. (1986) Gastroplasty for obesity. A Critical Analysis of Techniques, Complications and Results. *Clinical Nutrition*, **5**(Suppl.), 67–72.
8. Dowling, R.H. (1976) Intestinal adaptation. In: *12th Symposium on Advanced Medicine*, pp. 251–261 (Ed.) Peters, D.K. London: Pitman.
9. Hanni, C.L., Pool, L.R., Dean, R.E. and Cronquist, J.F. (1984) Treatment of jejunoileal

bypass failure by reanastomosis and gastroplasty in a single stage procedure: review of 45 cases. *American Surgeon*, **50**, 354–357.

10. Kaminiski, D.L., Herrmann, V.M. and Martin, S. (1985). Late effects of jejunoileal bypass on hepatic inflammation, fibrosis and lipid content. *Hepatogastroenterology*, **32**, 159–162.

11. Mason, E.E. (1982) Evolution of gastric reduction for obesity. *Contemporary Surgery*, **20**, 17–23.

12. McFarland, R.J., Gazet, J-C. and Pilkington, T.R.E. (1985) A 13-year review of jejunoileal bypass. *British Journal of Surgery*, **72**, 81–87.

13. Payne, J.H. and De Wind, L.T. (1969) Surgical treatment of obesity. *American Journal of Surgery*, **118**, 141–147.

14. Phillips, J.H.C. (1953) Jejunal diverticulosis: some clinical aspects. *British Journal of Surgery*, **40**, 350–354.

15. Pilkington, T.R.E., Gazet, J.C., Ang, L. *et al.* (1976) Explanations for weight loss after jejunoileal bypass in gross obesity. *British Medical Journal*, **i**, 1504–1505.

16. Rickers, H., Christiansen, C., Balslev, I. *et al.* (1983) Vitamin D and bone mineral content after intestinal bypass operation for obesity. *Gut*, **24**, 67–72.

17. Bucker, R.D., Chan, E.K., Horstmann, J., Chute, E.P., Varco, R.L. and Buchwald, H. (1984) Searching for the best weight reduction operation. *Surgery*, **96**, 624–631.

18. Scott, H.W., Law, D.H. and Sandstead, H.Y. (1970) Jejunoileal shunt in surgical treatment of morbid obesity. *Annals of Surgery*, **171**, 770–782.

19. Silber, T., Randolph, J. and Robbins, S. (1986). Long term morbidity and mortality in morbidly obese adolescents after jejunoileal bypass. *Journal of Pediatrics*, **108**, 318–322.

20. Zollinger, R.W., Coccia, M.R. and Zollinger, R.W. II. (1983) Critical analysis of jejunoileal bypass. *American Journal of Surgery*, **146**, 626–630.

SHORT GUT SYNDROME

(B.M. Obermayer-Pietsch and G.J. Krejs)

A major loss of intestinal absorptive area due to small bowel resection may be necessitated by such disorders as inflammatory bowel disease, mechanical obstruction with consequent bowel infarction, mesenteric vascular occlusion, trauma, peritonitis, radiation or malignant tumours.

Resection of short segments is usually well tolerated. Specific nutritional disturbances occur if more than 50% of the small bowel is resected. Resection of about 70% can be life-threatening unless parenteral nutrition is provided.

The outcome will depend primarily on the size and type of small bowel resected, the function and adaptation of the remaining bowel, the integrity of the terminal ileum and whether or not the ileocaecal valve is preserved.

Due to the loss of special transport functions, resection of the ileum or ileocaecal area alone may induce severe diarrhoea and malabsorption, even though less than 30% of the small intestine is removed. In addition, the age of the patient and his or her initial physical and nutritional status may be important in determining the severity of the sequelae of small bowel resection.

ANATOMICAL CONSIDERATIONS

Extent of resection

Small intestinal length varies over a wide range between individuals. Also, great differences in length are found with different methods of measurement. A loss in tone of smooth muscle at autopsy elongates the bowel, and telescoping of the intestine occurs during peroral intubation, so the mean length may be measured as 660 or 260 cm, respectively.[53] The length of the removed segment may not be as meaningful as consideration of the length of the remaining bowel expressed as a percentage of the original total length of the small intestine.

In 1935, Haymond[53] was one of the first to review extensive intestinal resection (257 cases), and he concluded that a 33% resection of intestine is well tolerated. To maintain adequate oral nutrition, no more than 50% of the bowel should be resected otherwise problems of malabsorption are common. If less than 25% of the small bowel is left, special management is required. Today, however, survival is possible with as little as 5 cm of bowel remaining or with no small bowel at all if permanent total parenteral nutrition is employed.[50]

Topographical factors

The total surface area of the small bowel is estimated to be about $100 \, m^2$.[150] Since the surface area per unit length decreases markedly from the proximal to the distal region, almost half of the total mucosal surface area is found in the proximal quarter of the small intestine.

The jejunum is particularly important for the absorption of most nutrients, iron, calcium and folic acid.[39,90] However, the ileum acts as a large functional reserve if substances have escaped absorption more proximally. In addition, the transit time in the ileum is longer than in the jejunum, provided that the ileocaecal valve is preserved.

There is no equivalent reserve area to take over specific ileal function after resection of the distal small intestine. Special transport mechanisms for active absorption of bile salts and vitamin B_{12} are localized in the lower ileum. Relatively small resections (60–90 cm) involving the ileum may therefore result in significant malabsorption of vitamin B_{12} and bile acids. Ileal resections interrupt the entero-hepatic circulation of bile salts and may thus result in several disturbances:

1. Bile acids can alter colonic water and electrolyte transport, reducing absorption or even stimulating secretion, and may cause diarrhoea (bile acid diarrhoea, type I).
2. If bile acid loss into the colon exceeds the capacity of accelerated synthesis in the liver, depletion of the bile acid pool will impair micellar formation resulting in fat malabsorption and steatorrhoea. This usually occurs with the loss of 90 cm or more of terminal ileum.[54] In addition, malabsorption of fat-soluble vitamins such as vitamins A, D, E and K may occur.
3. Enhanced oxalate absorption in the colon, due to an increase in oxalate solubility and/or mucosal permeability caused by the abnormal presence of bile acids and long-chain fatty acids in combination with hypomagnesuria and hypocitraturia may result in hyperoxaluria and urolithiasis,[107] and
4. Because of the decreased bile acid pool the lithogenic properties of bile increase and the incidence of gallstones is significantly elevated in such patients.[29,80,124]

Diarrhoea seems to be a minor problem in patients with a preserved ileocaecal valve. The reason for this phenomenon may be protection by the valve from bacterial overgrowth coming from the colon.[127] A dramatic increase in anaerobic bacteria in the distal jejunum after small bowel resection without reconstruction of a nipple valve supports this notion.[89] Bacterial overgrowth may cause diarrhoea by enhancing bile acid loss due to deconjugation and dehydroxylation of bile acids.[54] Bacterial metabolism of vitamin B_{12} may add to the development of vitamin B_{12} deficiency.

A hemicolectomy, as often performed in Crohn's disease, or a total colectomy may significantly influence the outcome after small bowel resection. The normal colon is able to absorb up to 6 litres of fluid per day.[22] Even when there is abnormal delivery of nutrients to the colon, significant absorption of short-chain fatty acids, i.e. metabolic products of unabsorbed carbohydrates, may take place before osmotic diarrhoea occurs.[10] It has in fact been recognized that, following small bowel resection, stool volume and frequency often depend on the length of the remaining colon rather than of the remaining small intestine.[21,85]

In general, the function of the remaining bowel plays a key role in clinical outcome, and disease of the remaining small intestine may lead to severe problems. Examples are the short bowel syndrome in Crohn's disease following multiple resections with recurrence of disease or in scleroderma after surgery for severely dilated segments with subsequent progression of the disease.

Mild lactose intolerance, not noted prior to resection, may contribute to the diarrhoea postoperatively. Any concomitant disease such as chronic liver disease with some degree of portal hypertension or right-sided heart failure may be detrimental for a patient who has lost most of his or her small bowel.

ADAPTATION

Intestinal adaptation is defined as the changes in mucosal morphology and digestive and absorptive functions which allow increased uptake of nutrients over a given length of intestine. Adaptation may develop in response to a variety of stimuli. These changes may be brought about not only by surgical resections, bypass or transposition of segments of intestine, but also by hormonal events such as pregnancy and lactation or changes in oral nutrition, as it is also seen in some diseases of the hypothalamus such as hypothermic hyperphagia.

Morphological adaptation

After extensive small bowel resection, the remnant intestine dilates (*Figure 3.114*),[99,132] and it has been shown by small bowel radiographic studies that there is a several-fold increase in length of the remaining bowel.[69,134] The lengthening goes together with an increase in tissue weight per unit length.[122] Hypertrophy of all segments has been demonstrated by morphometric studies and estimation of nucleic acid content of the mucosa.[28,119]

Resection of the proximal intestine leads to hyperplasia of both villi and crypts,[30] probably because of an increased rate of crypt cell mitoses, cell proliferation and migration.[94] Crypt cell proliferation is proportional to the extent of resection.[111,119] Microscopic morphology is altered, with an increase in the size of villi.[112] Using [³H]thymidine techniques, markedly increased DNA synthesis in the elongated crypts has been shown, along with an increase in the number of dividing cells. This

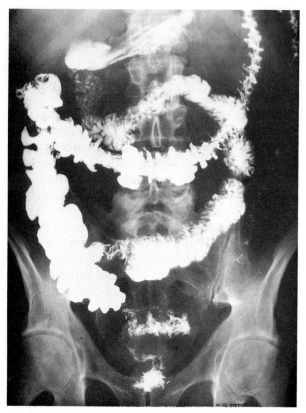

Figure 3.114 Barium meal in a patient 12 months after massive small bowel resection for infarction due to mesenteric vein thrombosis. While barium is still in the stomach, some has already reached the rectum. The remaining loop of small bowel (about 40 cm in length) shows an increase in mucosal folds and dilatation, indicating adaptation with mucosal hyperplasia.

enhanced cell proliferation probably leads to an absolute increase in the number of enterocytes. However, because the life-span of individual cells may be reduced by an increased turnover, it is not clear whether all cells become functionally mature to optimally subserve absorption.

Functional adaptation

Following extensive small bowel resection with less than 25% of the small intestine remaining, patients may often be weaned off intravenous hyperalimentation after prolonged periods of time.[151]

Perfusion techniques showed increased glucose absorption per unit length in the jejunum.[27] *In vitro* passive ileal uptake of fatty acids, cholesterol or L-alanine and L-phenylalanine[119] is increased. Enhanced specific activity of such enzymes as folate conjugase have been found.[103,136]

The transit time of chyme, shortened postoperatively, is prolonged,[120] perhaps due to hormonal influences.[76] A prolongation of gastric emptying is influenced by free fatty acids or fat emulsions in the

distal intestine[143] and by several hyperosmolar nutrients in the upper small bowel.[55]

Adaptive reactions are also found in colonic mucosa, where cell proliferation and increased water and electrolyte transport have been found.[92,137] Patients with an intact colon may benefit from colonic calcium absorption,[57] which may be further increased by 1,25-dihydroxyvitamin D_3.[71]

Luminal nutrients

There is an impressive body of evidence suggesting that luminal nutrients are a major factor in intestinal adaptation after bowel resection. Mucosal mass per unit length decreases from proximal to distal under normal conditions but this difference disappears with starvation. When dogs were fed only intravenously after bowel resection they remained well nourished despite pronounced mucosal hypoplasia.[32] Deficiency of luminal nutrients is also the cause of hypoplasia in bypassed segments of small bowel or self-emptying loops, in transpositioned segments without resection, e.g. in the jejunum, when the ileum is the first to receive nutrients directly from the stomach[28] and in transplanted mucosal autografts.[8] This phenomenon is fully reversible when the segments are put back into the stream of luminal contents. Many nutrients such as triglycerides, especially short-chain triglycerides,[67] several carbohydrates and amino acids are thought to cause intestinal adaptation regardless of whether their absorption is passive or active and whether they are metabolized in the mucosa or not.[144] Mucosal growth seems to be directly dependent on molar concentrations of such nutrients as glucose.[147] Bulk materials have different effects on adaptation. Fermentable fibres produce an adaptive response in the colon and distal small bowel in contrast to nonfermentable fibres or fibre-free diets.[43] Bulk-free chemically defined diets increase cell proliferation in the jejunum, but reduce cell mass in the terminal ileum.[81] Proliferation reaction to inert bulk has been found in the colon together with elevated levels of enteroglucagon and peptide YY.[43]

In addition to a direct topical effect, luminal nutrients may also have an indirect influence far from their site of presence, which suggests the involvement of enterotrophic hormones. An example is jejunal hyperplasia in rats due to intracaecal infusion of hypertonic glucose.[84]

Pancreaticobiliary factors

Jejunal and, particularly, ileal mucosal structure and function are influenced by exocrine pancreatic secretion and, vice versa, pancreatic growth and function are controlled, at least in part, by luminal components in the small bowel.[127] This is supported by the observation that, on total parenteral nutrition, not only the gut but also the pancreas becomes hypoplastic, with a parallel reduction in exocrine function. Whether pancreatic and biliary secretion stimulates mucosal growth in the small bowel and even contributes to the proximal-to-distal decrease in mucosal mass is not clear. Particularly trophic to the ileum are juices from the exocrine pancreas, as shown by isoperistaltic transposition of jejunum and ileum.[105] As the jejunum also showed mucosal growth under these circumstances, mediation of these effects through enterohormones released from the hyperplastic mucosa of the ileum is likely.[26]

Endocrine factors

Local contact with luminal nutrients or pancreaticobiliary secretion alone does not explain many of the trophic effects in the small intestine as mentioned above and there has been evidence for enterotrophic regulatory peptides for a long time.[62] It has remained controversial whether they act as classic hormones.

One of the first 'enterohormones' thought to have a trophic influence was gastrin.[62] However, very high exogenous doses are necessary to obtain these changes. Endogenous plasma levels of gastrin, which are elevated after intestinal resection, may not be high enough to cause such changes. Moreover, in antrectomized rats, adaptation occurs as usual in the shortened bowel with unchanged gastrin levels,[24] and trophic effects on the pancreas are unchanged by any type of resection of the stomach.[127]

Marked hyperplasia of the small intestine, particularly the jejunum, was described in a patient with an enteroglucagonoma in 1971. The morphological changes were reversible after tumour resection.[41] Since then, no definite proof for the enterotrophic properties of enteroglucagon and related peptides has been established.[108] However, in rats with exclusion of 75% of the small bowel, oral feeding resulted in significantly higher plasma enteroglucagon levels and crypt cell production rates in the excluded segment than did intravenous feeding. Mucosal concentration of enteroglucagon is high in the terminal ileum and in the colon, which suggests perhaps an important role of the colon in intestinal adaptation.[84] Enteroglucagon-producing cells have been shown to be in a hyperfunctional state in the remaining short bowel.[15] Nevertheless, studies with immunoneutralization of enteroglucagon and consecutive inhibition of small bowel adaptation have not been carried out.

There is now strong evidence that epidermal growth factor is trophic to the intestine. By using pure synthetic epidermal growth factor a dose-dependent stimulation of crypt cell proliferation rate and mucosal growth has been found.[44] Infusion of the peptide prevented partially, but not completely, hypoplasia of the small bowel mucosa caused by total parenteral nutrition. An interesting observation is that epidermal growth factor is found in saliva, Brunner's gland secretions, pancreatic juice and breast milk, so that this peptide might perhaps act luminally in the intestine of both adults and breast-fed infants.

Ornithine decarboxylase, an enzyme that is stimulated through receptors by epidermal growth factor plays a key role in intestinal adaptation. It stimulates DNA and protein synthesis, crypt cell production and villous hyperplasia. Up to now, receptors for other hormones such as enteroglucagon have not been found on enterocytes.

Other potential enterotrophins are a combination of secretin[146] and cholecystokinin[63] (but not the single peptides), some anterior pituitary hormones such as growth hormone and its analogue, plerocercoid growth factor,[52] adrenocorticotrophic hormone and thyroid-stimulating hormone, human placental lactogen (which enhances vitamin B_{12} absorption), bombesin and insulin. Additional factors may be platelet-derived growth factor and corticosteroids, which seem to stimulate enterocyte transport without changes of morphology or cytokinetics.[47,88] Prostaglandin E_2 has recently been found to stimulate mucosal adaptation after small bowel resection, but suppression of its effects by aspirin was only found in the distal ileum.[140,141] Hormones that do not seem to be responsible for adaptive intestinal growth are gastric inhibitory polypeptide, motilin, neurotensin and peptide YY,[2] even though they are cosecreted in short bowel syndrome[102] or can partly stimulate pancreatic growth.

Hormonal changes are also important for the pathogenesis of gastric acid hypersecretion[17,87,148] and an increase in parietal cell mass.[116,117] First, there is a lack of hormonal clearance of gastrin due to the lost small bowel.[1] Secondly, a putative gastrin-inhibiting hormone may have been lost with the resected bowel. This is supported by the findings that gastrin levels are elevated in some patients after small bowel resection[129] and this is in proportion to the length of resection.[59] Somatostatin and the 'glucose-sensitive insulin-releasing peptide' may suppress gastric secretion[86] and may explain such observations as gastric hyposecretion in dogs after small bowel resection.[115]

Other possible factors

Clinical observations have shown marked increases of arterial and venous vessel size, which may suggest increased mucosal blood flow. It is known that intestinal arteriovenous shunts may sometimes cause tissue hypertrophy. Transient rises in intestinal blood flow and constantly elevated flow in the ileal remnant have been documented. Whether this is the cause or the consequence of intestinal adaptation remains unclear.

The role of the autonomic nervous system, neurotransmitters, some circulating peptides such as neurotensin and enteroglucagon and also the changes in intestinal mesenchymal elements in adaptation have not been extensively evaluated.[2,37,102] The availability of small bowel transplantation has drawn attention to smooth muscle and nerves in the small bowel. In the graft, an extrinsic adrenergic inhibitory innervation is absent, whereas the intrinsic noradrenergic inhibitory nerves and the excitatory innervation are not altered.[130]

CLINICAL FEATURES

Diarrhoea

Patients with short bowel syndrome usually present with watery diarrhoea during the first days and weeks. Daily stool volumes may be as high as 10 litres. Dehydration, electrolyte loss, acid–base disturbances and secondary hyperaldosteronism may pose severe problems. These patients often complain of abdominal pain, perianal discomfort, urgency and faecal incontinence. When the patient is eating, large-volume watery diarrhoea occurs and therefore steatorrhoea may not be clinically appreciated. They usually have bulky, greasy and excessively malodorous stools which float due to their gas content. Causes for these symptoms are multiple. First, due to a significant loss of absorptive surface the approximately 8–9 litres of fluid that enter the jejunum every day overwhelm the transport capacity of the remaining small intestine, and a large fluid load is spilled into the colon. The colon has a high reserve capacity for absorption of up to 6 litres of isotonic solution daily.[22] Unfortunately, many patients cannot benefit from this compensating action of the large intestine because of an additional resection of part or even all of their colon. Secondly, high-calorie nutrients that are usually absorbed in

the upper small bowel are delivered to the colon. Colonic bacteria may then metabolize unabsorbed carbohydrates and cause osmotic diarrhoea by generation of short-chain fatty acids and a low pH as seen in disaccharidase deficiency or lactulose therapy. Bile acid depletion leads to fat malabsorption and the presence of long-chain fatty acids in the colon. They inhibit colonic absorption, particularly if hydroxylated by bacteria.[7,123] Thirdly, bile acids lost into the colon, especially dihydroxy bile acids, can induce colonic secretion by themselves.[82] Bile acid diarrhoea and steatorrhoea may also result from bacterial overgrowth of the remaining bowel due to loss of the ileocaecal valve. Finally, gastric hypersecretion may aggravate the diarrhoea, as is seen in the Zollinger–Ellison syndrome.

Malabsorption

The malabsorption syndrome due to small bowel resection may consist of a wide variety of symptoms such as weight loss, weakness, fatigue, excessive flatus, diffuse abdominal pain, hypotension, bone pain, tetany and paraesthesia. Amenorrhoea, secondary hypopituitarism and peripheral thyroid impairment are caused by protein depletion, i.e. 'calorie starvation'. Other more specific deficiency states are night blindness, coagulopathy with abnormal bruisability, purpura and ecchymosis, peripheral neuropathy, glossitis, stomatitis and cheilosis and macrocytic anaemia due to loss of vitamins A and K and other fat soluble vitamins or vitamin B_{12} or B_6, iron and folic acid. A depletion of trace elements like zinc may cause acrodermatitis and follicular hyperkeratosis due to depletion of essential fatty acids.

Other complications

Frequent vomiting postoperatively accounts for a rapid deterioration of the patient's condition, severe hypochloraemia and hypomagnesaemia may be life-threatening without substitution. Sodium loss leads to severe secondary hyperaldosteronism with very high renin levels.

Gastric acid hypersecretion has been recognized in 17–50% of patients with extensive small bowel resection, particularly during the postoperative period, and is correlated with the extent of bowel resection and the initiation of enteral nutrition. A trial of enteral feeding results in increased basal and maximal output. Exogenous pentagastrin does not further stimulate this basal acid hypersecretion.[4,59]

The formation of gallstones is related to bile acid depletion,[124] stasis, poor oral intake and use of anticholinergic and analgesic drugs. The highest incidence of gallbladder disease is seen in patients with terminal ileal disease or resection.[80] Symptomatic gallbladder disease with cholecystitis or pancreatitis may be a problem because of multiple prior laparotomies and the potential danger when surgical re-exploration is needed.

Another frequent problem is nephrolithiasis due to oxalate stones. Oxalate, absorbed easily by the colon in the presence of bile acids and fat malabsorption, is excessively excreted in the urine. Concomitant hypocitraturia and hypomagnesuria increase the risk for stone formation.[107] Symptoms may remain subclinical, but in one patient renal failure secondary to oxalate stones necessitated renal transplantation.[104]

A special problem that occurs rarely is mental deterioration and encephalopathy resulting from D-lactic acidosis. This condition is characterized by dizziness, ataxia, confusion, headaches, memory loss, lethargy, inappropriate behaviour and aggressiveness which may progress to reversible coma.[114] The putative neurotoxin is D-lactic acid with other organic anions, produced by an overgrowth of lactobacilli in the intestine due to exposure to malabsorbed carbohydrates. In contrast, endogenous lactic acidosis is caused by L-lactic acid, and differentiation is possible from blood or urinary samples by using nuclear magnetic resonance spectroscopy.

Investigations

Impaired absorption of nutrients, vitamins, minerals and trace elements will result in deficiency states that are reflected by appropriate laboratory tests similar to other malabsorptive diseases that reduce the mucosal surface area such as coeliac disease.

Tests should include a complete blood count, coagulation parameters, blood chemistry (potassium, sodium, bicarbonate, calcium, magnesium, albumin, prealbumin, transferrin, immunoglobulins, iron, copper, zinc, and vitamins B_{12} and A), liver and kidney profile and thyroid hormone levels. Measurement of stool weight, electrolytes, osmolality and fat is necessary to demonstrate osmotic (as opposed to secretory) diarrhoea. Determination of urine electrolyte levels should detect secondary hyperaldosteronism with extremely low sodium concentrations in urine (i.e. below 10 mmol/l). Measurement of urinary oxalate (normally less than 40 mg/day) in combination with citrate and magnesium may reveal a disposition for nephrolithiasis. Calcium metabolism can be assessed by determination of the calcium level in urine, serum parathyroid hormone concentration and osteodensitometry.

Morphological findings can be obtained by endoscopy and mucosal biopsy. A small intestinal radiographic series (with or without double contrast) will give information on the length and diameter of the bowel and a barium enema may be needed to assess the colon.

For assessing intestinal function, the spectrum of tests may include oral tolerance tests and breath tests,[135] balance studies and intubation techniques.[73] D-Xylose, lactose and glucose tolerance tests are widely used. A [^{57}Co/^{58}Co]cyanocobalamin urinary excretion test (Schilling test) should also be performed. Breath tests such as the lactose and lactulose–hydrogen test, [^{14}C]D-xylose and glycocholic acid test or [^{14}C]triolein test[135] can be employed, depending on local availability and interest in clinical research. Additional techniques are measurement of absorption of radioactive calcium[46] and a ^{15}N tracer technique to assess nitrogen absorption. Quantification of the degree of intestinal failure can be performed by calculation of energy absorption from a liquid test meal.[106] In special cases, gastric acid secretion studies, small intestinal culture or determination of the oro-anal transit time by radiological methods may be helpful.

CLINICAL COURSE

Three stages are characteristic for the clinical course of patients with short bowel syndrome. The early postoperative period with water and electrolyte imbalance, the adaptive phase, and the period of equilibrium sometimes troubled by metabolic disturbances.

Postoperative period

The early postoperative period takes 4–6 weeks and is characterized by watery diarrhoea, as mentioned above, starting immediately after resection. Up to 20 bowel movements per day are usual and stool frequency is increased by oral nutrition. The daily weight of the faeces may reach 5 kg. This severe situation may be accompanied by vomiting, which may lead to a loss of 10–30% of original body weight.

Adaptive phase

In this period of several months, diarrhoea decreases and patients may gain weight. The radiological findings show slow gastric emptying and prolonged intestinal transit time. The lumen of the remaining bowel is mildly distended and progressive lengthening of the bowel is found.

Equilibrium period

After 6–12 months, bowel movements should be reduced to 2–4 daily. Faeces often stay greasy and the stool weight remains rather high (up to 1 kg daily). The body weight approaches the preoperative level. If adequate nutrition is provided, clinical improvement and normal growth velocity in children is common,[69,75,93] so that normal maturation and puberty can be expected.[34]

In contrast, if nutritional support is lacking, the effects of malabsorption may appear at this time and may severely influence the prognosis. Continuous total parenteral nutrition may be dangerous with regard to sepsis from indwelling catheters,[98] liver and gallbladder disease,[11,80,124] and bone demineralization[18,35,118] as well as various psychological problems.[97]

Prognosis

Before nutrition became a clinical science, the prognosis for patients with short bowel syndrome was poor. The advent of total parenteral nutrition has made survival possible for most patients.[56,61] Overall survival is above 80%, depending primarily on the nature of the disease and the length of the remaining bowel.[19] Five centimetres of length are now thought by some authors to be the limit of survival. Below this limit, patients are likely to die from their disease or from treatment complications, but individual patients have been reported to survive on total parenteral nutrition with no small bowel at all.[58] The recovery may also be age-dependent because infants with massive small bowel resection reach a stage where enteral nutrition suffices earlier than do adults, particularly elderly patients.[16,56,138]

TREATMENT

Early postoperative period

Emphasis is placed on meticulous parenteral fluid and electrolyte replacement to compensate the losses associated with the voluminous watery diarrhoea during the early postoperative period. Hypokalaemia and acid–base imbalances should be treated with care. Intravenous alimentation is of greatest importance. All essential nutrients, dissolved in a well-tolerable fluid volume (2000–3500 ml/day) should be administered slowly into a high-flow vessel, usually the superior vena cava. Adequate energy is provided by carbohydrates (glucose 20–50 g/dl) and fat (soyabean oil 10 g/dl, prepared for intravenous use). Standard amino acid mixtures provide nitrogen requirements. For optimal positive nitrogen balance, each gram of nitrogen needs to be given with 630–1050 kJ (150–250 kcal) in glucose and fat.

Oral nutrition

Enteral feedings should be instituted as soon as the patient stabilizes, usually after 2–4 weeks. Initiation of oral feeding will aggravate the diarrhoea and feeding should be gradually increased to the limit that is tolerated by the patient with regard to stool weight and possibly metabolic acidosis.[3]

Since the rate of gastric emptying is positively correlated with intragastric volume, frequent meals of small size will help to optimally utilize the remaining absorptive capacity of the small bowel. The patient should eat at least every 2 hours. Constant eating at a very slow rate is ideal. Over the following days and weeks the size of the meals should be slowly increased.[3]

Chemically defined liquid diets may be given early in the course of oral feeding.[155] However, the high osmolality of these preparations (often 800–900 mosmol/kg) may cause osmotic diarrhoea, and the bad taste is often poorly tolerated over prolonged periods of time. Formula diets, when made hypo-osmolar, may still provide the required calories and may be tolerated much better by the patients. These elemental diets may be administered at a slow rate via an intraduodenal or jejunal feeding tube, which also has been successfully used in paediatric patients.[113] For adults, nocturnal nasogastric tube feeding has been developed as safe and efficient nutrition if simpler dietary manipulation proves unsuccessful.[78]

Elemental diets of lower osmolality containing oligopeptides (rather than the bad-tasting individual amino acids) are more promising.[125] The peptide chain length affects absorption of nitrogen and individual amino acid residues, because di- and tripeptides do not require brush border hydrolysis prior to absorption as needed in tetra- and pentapeptides.[49] Oligopeptides may also enhance intestinal adaptation more than other nutrients. Protein supplements may be added to the diets. A large number of preparations are commercially available. Patients on unrestricted diets should take 80–100 g of protein daily in order to maintain a positive nitrogen balance with a large margin of safety.[153]

Reduction of fat intake (down to 40 g/day) may significantly lower the stool volume in patients with small bowel resection if diarrhoea is a great problem.[145] Furthermore, high-fat diets seem to have no increasing effect on the amount of fat absorbed, but lead to increased losses of divalent cations (calcium, magnesium, zinc and copper). Altering the polyunsaturated:saturated fatty acid ratio has no effect on divalent cation losses.[95,154] However, not all observations have supported these findings. In contrast, a high-fat diet resulted in less diarrhoea than a carbohydrate diet in a patient with short bowel syndrome.[123] It was suggested that this was due to the osmotic effect of malabsorbed carbohydrates. In other studies the proportion of fat versus carbohydrate calories did not appear to influence stool volume or loss of monovalent cations.[5,60,153] In patients who are stable over a period of at least 1 year and who are able to tolerate an oral diet no restriction for fat should be made in enteral alimentation. In general, dietary restrictions should be very flexible. An oral supplement of calcium, magnesium and zinc to maintain the divalent cation balance should be given. Medium-chain triglyceride supplementation is thought to be a rational dietary manipulation which is quite successful if tolerated by the patient.[151] Unfortunately, many patients will not comply with such a regimen because of the bad taste and the difficulties in cooking appetizing meals using these triglycerides. The latest experimental findings suggest that short-chain triglycerides (triacetin:tributyrin as a 1:1 mixture) improve jejunal and colonic adaptive growth to a significantly higher degree than medium-chain triglycerides or chemically defined diets while maintaining comparable nutritional status.[67]

Lactose intolerance should be excluded, as it may have been latent prior to resection, and may subsequently contribute to osmotic diarrhoea.

Quantification of faecal carbohydrate excretion shows the loss of up to 65% of dietary carbohydrate intake.[5,153] Both the amount and the type of carbohydrate correlate with the diarrhoea seen in short bowel syndrome. It is controversial whether the measured faecal carbohydrate excretion also accounts for significant caloric losses.[5,60] Compared to fat malabsorption, carbohydrate effects are more profound, because they result in fluid and electrolyte imbalance, acidosis and gaseous abdominal distension. Carbohydrate diets cannot be recommended in the treatment of patients with short bowel syndrome.

Sugar and salt solutions such as the World Health Organisation's oral rehydration solution can be used in patients with continuing excess fluid and electrolyte losses as is often found in patients with stomata or fistulas.[79] These isotonic solutions are most readily absorbed, contain 110 mmol/l of sodium chloride and 80 mmol/l of glucose, and are easily prepared by the patient. They may be given as oral supplementation when replacement of fluid and electrolytes is more of a problem than just satisfying the nutritional requirements. In the special case of small bowel stoma patients, one group can be classified as 'secretors' with more sodium loss than oral intake (up to 400 mmol/day), who need parenteral sodium supplementation, whereas 'absorbers', who lose less sodium than they take by mouth (i.e. about 200 mmol/day), may take oral solutions as described above. Lower sodium concentrations, or drinking water, lead to a more pronounced negative balance. If the output exceeds 2 litres daily, oral supplements are not sufficient.[72]

Glucose electrolyte solutions may fail to provide a positive fluid and salt balance.[38] A more promising approach is the use of glucose polymers.[110] These polymers consist of linear chains of 4–10 glucose molecules attached by α-$(1 \rightarrow 4)$-glycosidic bonds (average molecular weight of 1000), and are available as Caloreen in the UK and as Polycose in the USA. Easily hydrolysed in the intestine in healthy subjects, they lead to corresponding plasma glucose levels as if glucose itself was used in an equimolar fashion. While maintaining isotonicity of the solution, large amounts of glucose and salt can be administered. The authors have successfully used the following solution: glucose polymer 40 mmol/l, sodium chloride 90 mmol/l, sodium bicarbonate 30 mmol/l and potassium chloride 15 mmol/l with an osmolality of 290 mosmol/kg.[48,66] Another high-sodium polymeric glucose solution has recently been used via nasogastric tube at 2 ml/min in jejunostomy patients. Glucose absorption was greater than 90% and sodium absorption was significantly greater with this maltodextrine solution (18 g of Glucidex 12/l) than with a standard oral solution.[9]

Another method optimally to use remaining bowel absorption in the setting of an enterostomy is the instillation of electrolyte or nutrient solutions or the reinfusion of chyme in the lower part of the stoma, so that the distal bowel segments – otherwise unused – are able to contribute to fluid and salt repletion and finally benefit from enhanced adaptation. In reinstillation of chyme the distal circuit may be able to absorb up to 70% of the volume reinfused (i.e. about 2.5 litres.[74] In this study, total parenteral nutrition could be discontinued after a mean of 36 days of continuous enteral nutrition with additional high-viscosity tapioca suspension.

The role of fibre in the diet is still controversial.[48,81,121] A pectin-supplemented diet in short gut syndrome may lead to higher nitrogen absorption and prolonged stomach-to-anus transit time. Since pectin had no adverse effects on electrolyte balance or glucose absorption,[33] experimental evidence suggests that more clinical investigations should be conducted using fibre in this special condition.

If hyperoxaluria is present (as shown by repeated analysis of 24-hour collection of urine during follow-up with an upper limit of normal of 40 mg/24 h), high-oxalate foods such as rhubarb, spinach, tea and chocolate need to be avoided.[107] Additional therapy with magnesium and citrate may be important (see below).

It is clear from many observations that patients maintain their body weight only by greatly increasing their energy intake above the normal limits. The calories consumed generally exceed resting energy expenditure regardless of the underlying disease.[25] This was calculated for short bowel syndrome caused by Crohn's disease to be 200% of energy expenditure, and gut failure for other reasons to be about 170% of normal resting energy. The extent of absorption in these cases is nevertheless very variable. When patients are able to tolerate massive protracted diarrhoea under a regimen of unrestricted compensatory enteral hyperalimentation (2000–6000 g/day), they sometimes may rapidly (within 8 days) be weaned from continuous parenteral nutrition[20] and maintain stable body weight because intestinal adaptation is enhanced by this diet. Special attention should be given to maintain adequate calcium and magnesium intake.

In patients with more than 60–80 cm of bowel remaining, refeeding usually will progress until a full oral diet is reached. The type of diet and vitamin supplements are then prescribed according to the site of resection. In general, a low-oxalate diet with calcium supplements is provided for ileal–non-colon resections, with cholestyramine supplements to avoid choleric diarrhoea, depending on the size of ileal resection.

Sometimes patients have difficult periods when introducing oral refeeding because of their poor compliance.[12] The occurrence of metabolic acidosis in such patients whenever there is no strict dietary adherence provides a ready marker for non-compliance.[40] With intensive counselling on an individual basis, compliance may improve and patients are able to maintain good nutritional status with enteral feeding. Although initial survival depends on total parenteral nutrition, it should be followed by an aggressive attempt to use enteral feeding alone.[12]

Specific replacements

Some specific replacements will be required even after adequate energy intake by mouth has been achieved following a prolonged process of adap-

tation. High-calcium and vitamin D replacement is almost always necessary to treat or prevent deficiency.[35,69] Hypocalcaemia may occur because of reduced absorptive area alone, but formation of calcium soaps, accelerated intestinal transit and lack of vitamin D or hypoparathyroid disease have to be considered. These causes are also partially valid for magnesium. Vitamin D_2 may produce metabolic bone disease by itself, requiring prolonged withdrawal for improvement.[118] Osteodensitometry at intervals of 6–12 months is used to assess adequate calcium balance.

Because of deficient renal action of 1,25-dihydroxyvitamin D_3 and possible renal magnesium wasting,[36] a magnesium supplement should always be given with vitamin D_3 in patients with short bowel syndrome. Initial parenteral replacement of calcium and magnesium may be necessary, if deficiency is severe.

The correlation between nephrolithiasis, hypomagnesuria and hypocitraturia discussed above suggests the administration of magnesium and citrate for the prevention of renal stones.[107]

Even if fat intake is sufficient to prevent essential fatty acid deficiency, the absorption of fat-solution vitamins may still not be provided.[31] It may be necessary to supplement vitamins A, E and K, especially if symptoms or laboratory data (e.g. a prolonged prothrombin time) indicate vitamin deficiency. Depending on the extent of ileal resection, vitamin B_{12} must be given parenterally at regular intervals. Intravenous biotin is sometimes required.[65] The need for oral or intravenous application of iron depends on the site of resection. Trace elements such as zinc, manganese, copper and selenium should be monitored, even during replacement therapy, because of the altered bioavailability of trace elements in short bowel syndrome.[109] The importance of zinc on mucosal adaptation has been emphasized.[139]

Specific drug treatment

Antimotility drugs are of great importance because prolongation of the transit time in the shortened bowel will increase the contact time of chyme with the mucosa, and net absorption per unit surface area may be enhanced. Opiates have remained the drug of choice, and initially parenteral administration may be necessary. Oral agents should be tried alone or in combination, each after a baseline period to assess effectiveness. These drugs include codeine, loperamide, diphenoxylate and anticholinergics. If oral anticholinergics are not effective, parenteral self-administration may be successful in selected patients. A beneficial effect of antimotility drugs on the colon flora[126] and a partial inhibition of the absorptive process have been described.[51]

Recently, a role has been suggested for octreotide, a somatostatin analogue. Either intravenous or subcutaneous application reduced intestinal output by 0.5–5 kg, the total daily intestinal losses of sodium and potassium were also reduced and the transit time was markedly prolonged.[91] This allowed reduction of intravenous fluids of 1–1.5 l/day. However, in some patients, there was no improvement or even worsening of symptoms. Octreotide may decrease water and sodium output by reducing secretion of digestive juices rather than by increasing absorptive capacity. It may be useful in patients with high-output jejuno- or ileostomies. In patients with total parenteral nutrition the effect seems to be negligible and does not significantly alter management.[70,101]

In patients with ileal resection in whom diarrhoea induced by bile acids is causing significant problems, cholestyramine may be employed to bind bile acids to prevent their effect on the colon. While this often improves or stops the diarrhoea, steatorrhoea may be enhanced due to further depletion of the bile acid pool. Once bound to the drug, bile acids are not available for micelle formation to subserve fat absorption.

If bacterial overgrowth is found (with a colony count in intestinal aspirate of more than 107/ml) or suspected, antibiotic treatment should be given (e.g. tetracyclines or metronidazole).

On an empirical basis, pancreatic enzymes may be given in an attempt to improve fat absorption. In addition, they might enhance intestinal adaptation as discussed above because of the influence of pancreatic and biliary secretions on the growth and function of the small bowel.

Gastric hypersecretion early after resection with losses of 4–5 litres of gastric juice is not uncommon and needs to be replaced diligently by parenteral therapy. The effect of H_2 receptor blockers has remained controversial.[4,58,59,149] A beneficial effect of H_2 receptor blockers on intestinal adaptation by reversal of lipid malabsorption and a direct trophic effect has been postulated.[42]

Peptic ulcer disease and its complications rarely cause serious problems.[11] Conservative therapy must be preferred in this situation, using H_2 receptor blockers or omeprazole.[58] Ulcer surgery should be avoided, because any of the surgical procedures may reduce the absorptive capacity of the upper small bowel and worsen the diarrhoea because of dumping, motility changes and impaired mixing. Even in the rare situation of a bleeding ulcer, prolonged conservative treatment should be employed.

The administration of drugs for additional disease should be considered with care. The necessity of anticoagulation may be a problem in short bowel syndrome caused by thromboembolic conditions (e.g. mesenteric artery occlusion). Due to heparin incorporation into total parenteral nutrition and vitamin K supplements, adjustment of anticoagulation may be difficult.[96] Lipid-free parenteral nutrition is sometimes necessary to maintain successful warfarin therapy.[77] A prolonged warfarin half-life with normal drug absorption, and an altered drug metabolism have been investigated.[64] The administration of digoxin may also be difficult because the therapeutic index is narrow and the drug is normally absorbed from the duodenum and upper jejunum. Erratic absorption of digoxin may thus be observed in short bowel syndrome unless it is given in liquid form.[68] Similar problems may arise with the administration of antibiotics[83] or psychopharmacological drugs.[13]

Prolonged parenteral nutrition

Transition period

Considering the length of the remaining small bowel and anticipating adaptation, parenteral nutrition may appear necessary for several months or even for a year. In this situation, parenteral hyperalimentation may be planned on an outpatient basis. The patients may come to the hospital to get intravenous hyperalimentation over a period of several hours on alternate days or daily. Solutions are administered via an indwelling catheter, e.g. into the superior vena cava, a port-a-cath system or an arteriovenous fistula. Disadvantages of the artificial shunt are the irritation of the venous wall by the highly concentrated infusates despite the high flow, and the fact that it may be surgically difficult to construct the fistula. On a single visit, some 16 000 kJ (4000 kcal) may be given, consisting of glucose, soyabean oil preparations, and amino acids. Vitamins and trace elements are added as required. Simultaneous insulin administration may be necessary to avoid hyperglycaemia and the loss of calories due to glucosuria.[45] In most patients, the interval between the administration of total parenteral nutrition can be prolonged gradually. Maintenance of normal or near-normal body weight should determine how often total parenteral nutrition is given. This also provides a good challenge for the patient to direct his or her utmost efforts towards improvement of his or her oral intake. If he or she is able to stabilize body weight with oral nutrition and supportive drug therapy, the parenteral feeding programme can be stopped and catheters or arteriovenous fistulas are removed.[152]

Permanent home parenteral nutrition

If a total or almost total enterectomy has been performed, plans for life-long intravenous alimentation should be made soon after surgery. This means a home treatment programme, so that patients can perform normal social activities. Irish and UK registers of home total parenteral nutrition patients showed 52% of them without any complications out of 237 persons monitored between 1977 and 1987.[128]

Patients need a superior vena cava or right atrial catheter with subcutaneous tunnelling, so that care of the catheter entry site is possible. However, a certain degree of intelligence, insight, technical understanding, physical fitness and manual dexterity is necessary and must be present in the patient or in another person constantly at hand. Patients need to undergo careful instruction and must gather sufficient experience under supervision. Procedures and formulas have been extensively described.[6]

Problems with home total parenteral nutrition are thrombosis of the catheter with consequent pulmonary embolism, metabolic problems and severe infections perhaps facilitated by the removal of immunocompetent gut-associated lymphoid tissue.[112] Because of the risk of gallbladder disease, a prophylactic cholecystectomy during a laparotomy for other reasons may help avoid further surgical problems.[80] Besides the high cost (well over US$100 000 per year for a patient on total parenteral nutrition),[142] patients may suffer from impaired quality of life, even if modern techniques allow often near-normal social activities.

Overall, total parenteral nutrition is a safe and effective treatment for patients with acute or chronic gut failure and remains the cornerstone of therapy at present.[100]

Surgical treatment

In patients who fail to regain adequate digestion and absorption after 1 year or more, operations to improve absorption might be considered.[113] Since the authors are internists, they are very reluctant to recommend any of these procedures. The reversed intestinal segment, the colon interposition[14] and the intestinal tapering or lengthening procedures, based on the anatomical division of the intestinal vasculature within two leaves of mesentery,[99,132] have been reported. The rationale is an attempt to preserve all mucosa, slow transit of chyme and 'correct an ineffective peristalsis'. Recirculating loops or intestinal valves have mostly been abandoned because of their risk and disadvantages such as loss of surface, stagnant loop syndrome, and operative mortality

and morbidity, which includes anastomotic leak, complete obstruction and infarction of the operated segment. Pure experimental procedures include growing of new intestinal mucosa on serosal patches,[133] intestinal pacing and small bowel transplantation. With the latter the problems of surgical technique and immunological reactions are still considerable despite the introduction of such agents as cyclosporin A and FK 506. Successful small bowel transplantation in a patient was carried out by the Kiel group for the first time in 1988. A graft which had been removed from a related donor showed complete adaptation after 22 months, so that the patient became independent of parenteral nutrition.[23] The Pittsburgh group has performed several small bowel transplants in 1991 and reports on graft survival can be expected soon.

Thus, for the surgeon, prevention of intestinal resection and preservation of intestinal length whenever possible should be emphasized.[131] Newer surgical procedures that may help to preserve the small bowel are strictureplasty, minimal resection, serosal patching and intestinal tapering.

REFERENCES

1. Aber, G.M., Ashton, E., Carmalt, M.H. and Whitehead, T.P. (1967) Gastric hypersecretion following massive small bowel resection in man. *American Journal of Digestive Diseases*, **12**, 785–794.
2. Adrian, T.E., Ferri, G.L., Bacarese-Hamilton, A.J., Fuessl, H.S., Polak, J.M. and Bloom, S.R. (1985) Human distribution and release of a putative new gut hormone, peptide YY. *Gastroenterology*, **89**, 1070–1077.
3. Allard, J.P. and Jeejeebhoy, K.N. (1989) Nutritional support and therapy in the short bowel syndrome. *Gastroenterology Clinics of North America*, **18**, 589–601.
4. Aly, A., Barany, F., Kollberg, B., Monsen, U., Wisen, O. and Johansson, C. (1980) Effect of an H_2-receptor blocking agent on diarrhoea after extensive small bowel resection in Crohn's disease. *Acta Medica Scandinavica*, **207**, 119–122.
5. Ameen, V.Z., Powell, G.K. and Jones, L.A. (1987) Quantitation of fecal carbohydrate excretion in patients with short bowel syndrome. *Gastroenterology*, **92**, 493–500.
6. American Society for Parenteral and Enteral Nutrition, Board of Directors (1987) Guidelines for use of home TPN. *Journal of Parenteral and Enteral Nutrition*, **11**, 342–344.
7. Ammon, H.V. and Phillips, S.F. (1973) Inhibition of colonic water and electrolyte absorption by fatty acids in man. *Gastroenterology*, **65**, 744–749.
8. Banerjee, A.K., Chadwick, S.J. and Peters, T.J. (1990) Adaptation of jejunal to colonic mucosal

autografts in experimentally induced short bowel syndrome. *Digestive Diseases and Sciences*, **35**, 340–348.

9. Beaugerie, L., Cosnes, J., Verwaerde, F. *et al.* (1991) Isotonic high-sodium oral rehydration solution for increasing sodium absorption in patients with short bowel syndrome. *American Journal of Clinical Nutrition*, **52**, 769–772.

10. Bond, J.H. and Levitt, M.D. (1976) Fate of soluble carbohydrate in the colon of rats and man. *Journal of Clinical Investigation*, **57**, 1158–1164.

11. Bowyer, B.A., Fleming, C.R. and Ludwig, B.A. (1985) Does long-term parenteral nutrition in adult patients cause chronic liver disease? *Journal of Parenteral and Enteral Nutrition*, **9**, 11–17.

12. Brenner, C.J. and Atkinson, R.L. (1989) Short-bowel syndrome: a case report. *Nutritions Review*, **47**, 350–353.

13. Broyles, J.E., Brown, R.O., Self, T.H., Frederick, R.C. and Luther, R.W. (1990) Nortriptyline absorption in short bowel syndrome. *Journal of Parenteral and Enteral Nutrition*, **14**, 326–327.

14. Brolin, R.E. (1986) Colon interposition for extreme short bowel syndrome: a case report. *Surgery*, **100**, 576–580.

15. Buchan, A.M.J., Griffiths, C.J., Morris, J.F. and Polak, J.M. (1985) Enteroglucagon cell hyperfunction in rat small intestine after gut resection. *Gastroenterology*, **81**, 8–12.

16. Caniano, D.A., Starr, J. and Ginn Pease, M.E. (1989) Extensive short-bowel syndrome in neonates: outcome in the 1980s. *Surgery*, **105**, 119–124.

17. Caridis, D.T., Roberts, M. and Smith, G. (1969) The effect of small bowel resection on gastric acid secretion in the rat. *Surgery*, **65**, 292–297.

18. Compston, J.E., Horton, L.W.L., Ayers, A.B., Tighe, J.R. and Creamer, B. (1978) Osteomalacia after small intestinal resection. *The Lancet*, **i**, 9–12.

19. Cooper, A., Floyd, T.F., Ross, A.J., III, Bishop, H.C., Templeton, J.M., Jr and Ziegler, M.M. (1984) Morbidity and Mortality of short bowel syndrome acquired in infancy: an update. *Journal of Pediatric Surgery*, **19**, 711–718.

20. Cosnes, J., Gendre, J.P., Evard, D. and LeQuintrec Y. (1985) Compensatory enteral hyperalimentation for management of patients with severe short bowel syndrome. *American Journal of Clinical Nutrition*, **41**, 1002–1009.

21. Cummings, J.H., James, W.P.T. and Wiggins, H.S. (1973) Role of the colon in ileal-resection diarrhoea. *The Lancet*, **i**, 344–347.

22. Debognie, J.C. and Phillips, S.F. (1978) Capacity of the human colon to absorb fluid. *Gastroenterology*, **74**, 698–703.

23. Deltz, E., Schroeder, P., Gundlach, M., Hansmann, M.L. and Leimenstoll, G. (1990) Successful clinical small-bowel transplantation. *Transplantation Proceedings*, **22**, 2501.

24. Dembinski, A.B. and Johnson, J.R. (1982) Role of gastrin in gastrointestinal adaptation after small bowel resection. *American Journal of Physiology*, **243**, G16–G20.

25. DiCecco, S., Nelson, J., Burnes, J. and Fleming, C.R. (1987) Nutritional intake of gut failure patients on home parenteral nutrition. *Journal of Parenteral and Enteral Nutrition*, **11**, 529–532.

26. Dowling, R.H. (1982) Small bowel adaptation and its regulation. *Scandinavian Journal of Gastroenterology*, **17**(Suppl. 74), 53–74.

27. Dowling, R.H. and Booth, C.C. (1966) Functional compensation after small bowel resection in man. *The Lancet*, **ii**, 146–147.

28. Dowling, R.H. and Booth, C.C. (1967) Structural and functional changes following small intestine resection in the rat. *Clinical Sciences*, **32**, 139–149.

29. Dowling, R.H., Bell, G.D. and White, J. (1972) Lithogenic bile in patients with ileal dysfunction. *Gut*, **13**, 415.

30. Dudrick, S.J. and Ruberg, R.L. (1971) Principles and practice of parenteral nutrition. *Gastroenterology*, **61**, 901–910.

31. Edes, T.E., Walk, B.E., Thornton, W.H., Jr and Fritsche, K.L. (1991) Essential fatty acid sufficiency does not preclude fat-soluble vitamins. *American Journal of Clinical Nutrition*, **53**, 499–502.

32. Feldman, E.J., Dowling, R.H., McNaughton, J. and Peters, T.J. (1976) Effects of oral versus intravenous nutrition on intestinal adaptation after small bowel resection in the dog. *Gastroenterology*, **70**, 712–719.

33. Finkel, Y., Brown, G., Smith, H.L., Buchanan, E. and Booth, I.W. (1990) The effects of a pectin supplemented diet in a boy with short bowel syndrome. *Acta Paediatrica Scandinavica*, **79**, 983–986.

34. Flombaum, C.D. and Berner, Y.N. (1989) TPN-induced catch-up of growth in a 22-y-old male with radiation enteritis. *American Journal of Clinical Nutrition*, **50**, 1341–1347.

35. Foldes, J., Rimon, B., Muggia-Sullam, M. *et al.* (1990) Progressive bone loss during long-term home total parenteral nutrition. *Journal of Parenteral and Enteral Nutrition*, **14**, 139–142.

36. Fukumoto, S., Matsumoto, T., Tanaka, Y., Harada, S. and Ogata, E. (1987) Renal magnesium wasting in a patient with short bowel syndrome with magnesium deficiency: effect of 1-alpha-hydroxy-vitamin D_3 treatment. *Journal of Clinical Endocrinology and Metabolism*, **65**, 1301–1304.

37. Furness, J.B. and Costa, M. (1987) *The Enteric Nervous System*. Edinburgh: Churchill Livingstone.

38. Gerson, C.D. (1972) Failure of oral glucose electrolyte therapy in short bowel syndrome. *The Lancet*, **ii**, 353–355.

39. Gerson, C.D. (1990) Intestinal secretions in short bowel syndrome (letter). *The Lancet*, **336**, 1379.

40. Gilchrist, P.N., Phillips, P.J., Heddle, R. and Harley, H. (1984) dietary compliance in the short bowel syndrome. *Journal of Parenteral and Enteral Nutrition*, **8**, 315–316.

41. Gleeson, M.H., Bloom, S.R., Polak, R.M., Henry, K. and Dowling, R.H. (1971) Endocrine tumor in kidney affecting small bowel structure, motility and absorptive function. *Gut*, **12**, 773–782.

42. Goldmann, S.D., Rudloff, M.A. and Ternberg, J.L. (1987) Cimetidine and neonatal small bowel adaptation: an experimental study. *Journal of Pediatric Surgery*, **22**, 484–487.

43. Goodlad, R.A., Lenton, W., Ghatei, M.A., Adrian, T.E., Bloom, S.R. and Wright, N.A. (1987) Effects of an elemental diet, inert bulk and different types of dietary fibre on the response of the intestinal epithelium to refeeding in the rat and relationship to plasma gastrin, enteroglucagon and PYY concentrations. *Gut*, **28**, 171–180.

44. Goodlad, R.A., Wilson, T.J.G., Lenton, W., Gregory, H., McCullagh, K.G. and Wright, N.A. (1987) Epidermal growth factor. *Gut*, **28**, 573–578.

45. Gouttebel, M.C., Saint-Aubert, B., Astre, C., Joyeux Ph.D. and H. (1986) Total parenteral nutrition needs in different types of short bowel syndrome. *Digestive Diseases and Sciences*, **31**(7), 718–723.

46. Gouttebel, M.C., Saint-Aubert, B., Colette, C., Astre, C., Monnier, L.H. and Joyeux, H. (1989) Intestinal adaptation in patients with short bowel syndrome. Measurement with calcium absorption. *Digestive Diseases and Sciences*, **34**, 709–715.

47. Grey, V.L. and Morin, C.L. (1985) Evidence for a growth-stimulating fraction in the rat proximal intestine after small bowel resection. *Gastroenterology*, **89**, 1305–1312.

48. Griffin, G.E., Fagen, E.F., Hodgson, H.J. and Chadwick, V.S. (1982) Enteral therapy in the management of massive gut resection complicated by chronic fluid and electrolyte depletion. *Digestive Diseases and Sciences*, **27**, 902–908.

49. Grimble, B.K., Rees, R.G., Keohane, P.P., Cartwright, T., Desreumaux, M. and Silk, D.B.A. (1987) Effect of peptide chain length on absorption of egg hydrolysates in the normal human jejunum. *Gastroenterology*, **92**, 136–142.

50. Hancock, B.J. and Wiseman, N.E. (1990) Lethal short-bowel syndrome. *Journal of Pediatric Surgery*, **25**, 1131–1134.

51. Hardcastle, J., Hardcastle, P.T. and Cookson, J. (1986) Inhibitory actions of loperamide on absorptive process in rat small intestine. *Gut*, **27**, 686–694.

52. Hart, M.H., Phares, C.K., Erdman, S.H., Grandjean, C.J., Park, J.H. and Vanderhoof, J.A. (1987) Augmentation of postresection mucosal hyperplasia by plerocercoid growth factor (PGF). Analog of human growth hormone. *Digestive Diseases and Sciences*, **32**, 1275–1280.

53. Haymond, H.E. (1935) Massive resection of small intestine: analysis of 257 collected cases. *Surgery, Gynecology and Obstetrics*, **61**, 693–705.

54. Hofman, A. (1989) The enterohepatic circulation of bile acids in health and disease. In: *Gastrointestinal Disease*, pp. 144–161 (Eds) Sleisenger, M. and Fordtran, J.S. London: W.B. Saunders.

55. Hunt, J.N. (1968) Control of gastric emptying. *American Journal of Digestive Diseases*, **13**, 372–375.

56. Huysman, W.A., Tibboel, D., Bergmeijer, J.H. and Molenaar, J.C. (1991) Long-term survival of a patient with congenital short bowel and malrotation. *Journal of Pediatric Surgery*, **26**, 103–105.

57. Hylander, E., Ladefoged, K. and Jarnum, S. (1980) The importance of the colon in calcium absorption following small-intestinal resection. *Scandinavian Journal of Gastroenterology*, **15**, 55–60.

58. Hyman, P.E., Garvey, T.Q., III and Harada, T. (1985) Effect of ranitidine on gastric acid hypersecretion in an infant with short bowel syndrome. *Journal of Pediatric Gastroenterology and Nutrition*, **4**, 316–319.

59. Hyman, P.E., Everett, S.L. and Harada, T. (1986) Gastric acid hypersecretion in short bowel syndrome in infants: association with extent of resection end enteral feeding. *Journal of Pediatric Gastroenterology and Nutrition*, **5**, 191–197.

60. Jeejeebhoy, K.N. (1987) Fecal carbohydrate excretion in short bowel syndrome. *Gastroenterology*, **93**, 435 (letter).

61. Jeejeebhoy, K.N., Zohrab, W.J., Langer, B., Phillips, M.J., Kuksis, A. and Anderson, G.H. (1973) Total parenteral nutrition at home for 23 months, without complications, and with good rehabilitation. A study for technical and metabolic features. *Gastroenterology*, **65**, 811–820.

62. Johnson, L.R. (1974) Effect of gut hormones on growth of gastrointestinal mucosa. In: *Endocrinology of the Gut*, pp. 163–177 (Eds) Chey, W.Y. and Brooks, F.P. Thorofare: Slack.

63. Johnson, L.R. and Guthrie, P. (1976) Effect of cholecystokinin and 16,16-dimethyl prostaglandin E_2 on RNA and DNA of gastric and duodenal mucosa. *Gastroenterology*, **70**, 59–65.

64. Kearns, P.J. and O'Reilly, R.A. (1986) Bioavailability of warfarin in a patient with severe short bowel syndrome. *Journal of Parenteral and Enteral Nutrition*, **10**, 100–101.

65. Khalidi, N., Wesley, J.R., Thoene, J.G., Whitehouse, W.M., Jr and Baker, W.L. (1984) Biotin deficiency in a patient with short bowel syndrome during home parenteral nutrition. *Journal of Parenteral and Enteral Nutrition*, **8**, 311–314.

66. Krejs, G.J. (1983) Allgemeine Störungen nach Ileostomie. In: *Therapie Postoperative Stoerungen des Gastrointestinaltraktes*, pp. 229–236 (Eds) Domschke, W. and Lux, G. Stuttgart: Thieme.

67. Krupke, S.A., DePaula, J.A., Berman, J.M., Fox, A.D., Rombeau, J.J. and Settle, R.G. (1991) Experimental short-bowel syndrome: effect of an elemental diet supplemented with short-chain triglyceride. *American Journal of Clinical Nutrition*, **53**, 954–962.

68. Kumer, K.P., Nwangwu, J.T. and P.U. (1983) Perspectives on digoxin absorption from small bowel resections. *Drug Intelligence and Clinical Pharmacology*, **17**, 121–123.

69. Kurz, R. and Sauer, H. (1983) Treatment and metabolic findings in extreme short bowel syndrome with 11 cm jejunal remnant. *Journal of Pediatric Surgery*, **18**, 251–263.

70. Ladevoged, K., Christensen, K.C., Hegnhoj, J. and Jarnum, S. (1989) Effect of a long acting somatostatin analogue SMS 201–995 on jejunostomy effluents in patients with severe short bowel syndrome. *Gut*, **30**, 943–949.

71. Lee, D.B.N., Walling, M.W., Gafter, U., Silis, V. and Coburn, J.W. (1980) Calcium and inorganic phosphate transport in rat colon. Dissociated response to 1,25-dihydroxyvitamin D. *Journal of Clinical Investigation*, **65**, 1326–1331.

72. Lennard-Jones, J.E. (1990) Oral rehydration solutions in short bowel syndrome. *Clinical Therapy*, **12**(Suppl. A), 129–137 (discussion 138).

73. Levin, R.J. (1982) Assessing small intestinal function in health and disease *in vivo* and *in vitro*. *Scandinavian Journal of Gastroenterology*, **17**(Suppl. 74), 31–51.

74. Levy, E., Frileux, P., Sandrucci, S. *et al.* (1988) Continuous enteral nutrition during the early adaptive stage of the short bowel syndrome. *British Journal of Surgery*, **75**, 549–553.

75. Lin, C.H., Rossi, T.M., Heitlinger, L.A., Lerner, A., Riddlesberger, M.H. and Lebenthal, E. (1987) Nutritional assessment of children with short bowel syndrome receiving home parenteral nutrition. *American Journal of Diseases of Children*, **141**, 1093–1098.

76. Lucey, M.R. (1986) Endogenous somatostatin and the gut. *Gut*, **27**, 457–467.

77. Lutomski, D.M., Palascak, J.E. and Bower, R.H. (1987) Warfarin resistance associated with intravenous lipid administration. *Journal of Parenteral and Enteral Nutrition*, **11**, 316–318.

78. McIntyre, P.B., Wood, S.R., Powell-Tuck, J. and Lennard Jones, J.E. (1983) Nocturnal nasogastric tube feeding at home. *Postgraduate Medical Journal*, **698**, 767–769.

79. MacMahon, R.A. (1984) The use of the World Health Organisation's oral rehydration solution in patients on home parenteral nutrition. *Journal of Parenteral and Enteral Nutrition*, **8**, 720–721.

80. Manji, N., Bistrian, B.R., Mascioli, E.A., Benotti, P.A. and Blackburn, G.L. (1989) Gallstone disease in patients with severe short bowel syndrome dependent on parenteral nutrition. *Journal of Parenteral and Enteral Nutrition*, **13**, 461–464.

81. Maxton, D.G., Cynk, E.U. and Thompson, R.P.H. (1987) Small intestine response to "elemental" and "complete" liquid feeds in the rat: effect of dietary bulk. *Gut*, **28**, 688–693.

82. Mekjijan, H.S., Phillips, S.F. and Hofman, A.F. (1971) Colonic secretion of water and electrolytes induced by bile acids: perfusion studies in man. *Journal of Clinical Investigation*, **50**, 1569–1577.

83. Menardi, G. and Guggenbichler, J.P. (1984) Bioavailability of oral antibiotics in children with short bowel syndrome. *Journal of Pediatric Surgery*, **19**, 84–86.

84. Miazza, B.M. Al-Mukhtar, M.Y.T. and Salmeron, M. (1985) Hyperenteroglucagonaemia and small intestinal mucosal growth after colonic perfusion of glucose in rats. *Gut*, **26**, 518–524.

85. Mitchell, J., Zuckerman, L. and Breuer, R.I. (1977) The colon influences ileal resection diarrhoea. *Gastroenterology*, **72**, 1103.

86. Mogard, M.H., Maxwell, V., Wong, H., Reedy, T.J., Sytnik, B. and Walsh, J.H. (1988) Somatostatin may not be a hormonal messenger of fat-induced inhibition of gastric functions. *Gastroenterology*, **94**, 405–408.

87. Moosa, A.R., Hall, A.W., Skinner, D.B. and Winans, C.S. (1976) Effect of fifty percent small bowel resection on gastric secretory function in rhesus monkeys. *Surgery*, **80**, 208–213.

88. Murphy, R.F., Chen, M., Herlin, P.M., Gallavan, R.M., Joffe, S.N. and Fischer, J.E. (1985) Glucagon, secretin and vasoactive intestinal polypeptide immunoreactivities in rat gut after jejuno-ileal bypass and resection. *Digestion*, **32**, 106–113.

89. Myrvold, H., Tindel, M.A., Isenberg, H., Stein, T.A., Scherer, J. and Wise L. (1984) The nipple valve as a sphincter substitute for the ileocecal valve: prevention of bacterial overgrowth in the small bowel. *Surgery*, **96**, 42–47.

90. Nightingale, J.M., Lennard-Jones, J.E. (1991) Jejunal secretion in short bowel syndrome. *The Lancet*, **337**, 312 (letter).

91. Nightingale, J.M., Walker, E.R., Burnham, W.R., Farthing, M.J. and Lennard-Jones, J.E. (1990) Short bowel syndrome. *Digestion*, **45**(Suppl. 1), 77–83.

92. Nundy, S., Malamud, D., Opertop, H., Sczerban, J. & Malt, R.A. (1977) Onset of cell proliferation in the shortened gut. Colonic hyperplasia after ileal resection in the dog. *Gastroenterology*, **72**, 263–266.

93. Ohkohchi, N., Igarashi, Y., Tazawa, Y. *et al.* (1986) Evaluation of the nutritional conditions and absorptive capacity of nine infants with short bowel syndrome. *Journal of Pediatric Gastroenterology and Nutrition*, **5**, 198–206.

94. Opertop, H., Nundy, S., Malamud, D. and Malt, R.A. (1977) Onset of cell proliferation in the

shortened gut. Rapid hyperplasia after jejunal resection. *Gastroenterology*, **72**, 267–270.

95. Ovesen, L., Chu, R. and Howard, L. (1983) The influence of dietary fat on jejunostomy output in patients with severe short bowel syndrome. *American Journal of Clinical Nutrition*, **38**, 270–277.

96. Owens, J.P., Mirtallo, J.M. and Murphy, C.C. (1990) Oral anticoagulation in patients with short bowel syndrome. *Drug Intelligence and Clinical Pharmacology*, **24**, 585–589.

97. Perl, M., Hall, R.C.W. and Dudrick, S.J. (1980) Psychological aspects of long-term home hyperalimentation. *Journal of Parenteral and Enteral Nutrition*, **4**, 554.

98. Piedra, P.A., Dryja, D.M. and La Scolea, L., Jr (1989) Incidence of catheter-associated gram-negative bacteraemia in children with short bowel syndrome. *Journal of Clinical Microbiology*, **27**, 1317–1319.

99. Pokorny, W.J. and Fowler, C.L. (1991) Isoperistaltic intestinal lengthening for short bowel syndrome. *Surgery, Gynecology and Obstetrics*, **172**, 39–43.

100. Purdum, P.P., III and Kirby, D.F. (1991) Short-bowel syndrome, a review of the role of nutrition support. *Journal of Parenteral and Enteral Nutrition*, **15**, 93–101.

101. Rambaud, J.C. (1990) Short bowel syndrome and somatostatin. *Gut*, **31**, 124(letter).

102. Read, N.W., McFarlane, A. and Kinsman, R.I. (1984) Effect of infusion of nutrient solutions into the ileum on gastrointestinal transit and plasma levels of neurotensin and enteroglucagon. *Gastroenterology*, **86**, 274–280.

103. Reisenauer, A.M., Halsted, C.H. and Jacobs, L.R. (1985) Human intestinal folate conjugase: adaption after jejunoileal bypass. *American Journal of Clinical Nutrition*, **42**, 660–665.

104. Roberts, R., Sketris, I.S., Abraham, I., Givner, M.L. and MacDonald, A.S. (1988) Cyclosporine absorption in two patients with short-bowel syndrome. *Drug Intelligence and Clinical Pharmacology*, **22**, 570–572.

105. Robinson, J.W.L., Dowling, R.H. and Riecken, E.O. (Eds) (1982) *Mechanisms of Intestinal Adaptation*. Lancaster: MTP Press.

106. Rodrigues, C.A., Lennard-Jones, J.E., Thompson, D.G. and Farthing, M.J. (1989) Energy absorption as a measure of intestinal failure in the short bowel syndrome. *Gut*, **30**, 176–183.

107. Rudman, D., Dedonis, J.L., Fountain, M.T. *et al.* (1980) Hypocitraturia in patients with gastrointestinal malabsorption. *New England Journal of Medicine*, **303**, 657–661.

108. Sagor, C.R., Gathei, M.A., O'Shaughnessy, D.J., Al-Mukhtar, M.Y.T., Wright, N.A. and Bloom, S.R. (1985) Influence of somatostatin and bombesin on plasma enteroglucagon and cell

proliferation after intestinal secretion in the rat. *Gut*, **26**, 89–94.

109. Sandstrom, B., Davidson, L., Bosaeus, I., Eriksson, R. and Alpsten, M. (1990) Selenium status and absorption of zinc, selenium and manganese in patients with short bowel syndrome. *European Journal of Clinical Nutrition*, **44**, 697–703.

110. Saunders, D.R. and Sillery, J.K. (1985) Absorption of carbohydrate–electrolyte solutions in rat duodenojejunum. Implications for the composition of oral electrolyte solutions in man. *Digestive Diseases and Sciences*, **30**, 154–160.

111. Savage, A.P., Matthews, J.L., Ghatei, M.A., Cooke, T. and Bloom, S.R. (1987) Enteroglucagon and experimental intestinal carcinogenesis in the rat. *Gut*, **28**, 33–39.

112. Scherer, L.R., III, Bschorner, W.E. and Colombani, P.M. (1990) The ontogeny of the gut-associated lymphoid tissue in short bowel syndrome. *Journal of Surgery Research*, **48**, 358–362.

113. Schraut, W.H. (1988) Current status of small-bowel-transplantation. *Gastroenterology*, **944**, 525–538.

114. Scully, T.B., Kraft, S.C., Carr, W.C. and Harig, J.M. (1989) D-Lactate-associated encephalopathy after massive small-bowel resection. *Journal of Clinical Gastroenterology*, **11**, 448–451.

115. Seal, A.M., Debas, H.T., Reynolds, C., Said, S.I. and Tailor, I.L. (1982) Gastric and pancreatic hyposecretion following massive small bowel resection. *Digestive Diseases and Sciences*, **27**, 117–123.

116. Seelig, L.L., Winborn, W.B. and Weser, E. (1977) Effect of small Bowel resection on the gastric mucosa in the rat. *Gastroenterology*, **74**, 421–428.

117. Seelig, L.L., Winborn, W.B. and Weser, E. (1978) Changes in gastric glandular cell kinetics after small bowel resection in the rat. *Gastroenterology*, **74**, 1–6.

118. Seligman, J.U., Basi, S.S. and Dietel, M. (1984) Metabolic bone disease in a patient on long-term parenteral nutrition: a case report and review of literature. *Journal of Parenteral and Enteral Nutrition*, **8**, 722–727.

119. Sidhu, G.S., Narashimharao, K.L., Rami, V.U., Sarkar, A.K., Chakracarti, R.N. and Mitra, S.K. (1984) Morphological and functional changes in the gut after massive small bowel resection and colon interposition in rhesus monkeys. *Digestion*, **29**, 47–54.

120. Sidhu, G.S., Narashimharao, K.L., Rani, V.U., Sarkar, A.K. and Mitra, S.K. (1985) Absorption studies after massive small bowel resection and antiperistaltic colon interposition in rhesus monkeys. *Digestive Diseases and Sciences*, **30**, 483–488.

121. Silk, D.B. (1989) Fibre and enteral nutrition. *Gut*, **30**, 246–264.

122. Sigalet, D.L., Lees, G.M., Aherne, F. *et al.* (1990) The physiology of adaptation to small bowel resection in the pig: an integrated study of morphological and functional changes. *Journal of Pediatric Surgery*, 25, 650–657.

123. Simko, V. (1980) Short bowel syndrome. *Gastroenterology*, 78, 190–191.

124. Sorensen, T.I., Anderson, B., Hylander, E., Jensen, L.I., Laursen, K. and Klein, H.C. (1988) Prospective study of malabsorption induced risk of gall stone formation in relation to fall in plasma cholesterol. *Gut*, 29, 108–113.

125. Spiller, R.C., Jones, B.J.M. and Silk, D.B.A. (1987) Jejunal water and electrolyte absorption from two proprietary enteral feeds in man: importance of sodium content. *Gut*, 28, 681–687.

126. Stephen, A.M., Wiggins, H.S. and Cummings, J.H. (1987) Effect of changing transit time on colonic microbial metabolism in main. *Gut*, 28, 601–609.

127. Stock-Damge, C., Aprahamian, M., Lhoste, E. *et al.* (1984) Pancreatic hyperplasia after small bowel resection in the rat: dissociation from endogenous gastrin levels. *Digestion*, 29, 223–230.

128. Stokes, M.A. and Irving, M.H. (1988) How do patients with Crohn's disease fare on home parenteral nutrition? *Diseases of the Colon and Rectum*, 31, 454–458.

129. Straus, E., Gerson, C.D. and Yalow, R.S. (1974) Hypersecretion of gastrin associated with the short bowel syndrome. *Gastroenterology*, 66, 175–180.

130. Taguchi, T., Zorchta, E., Sonnino, R.E. and Guttman, F.M. (1989) Small intestinal transplantation in the rat: effect on physiological properties of smooth muscle and nerves. *Journal of Pediatric Surgery*, 24, 1258–1263.

131. Thompson, J.S. (1987) Strategies for preserving intestinal length in the short bowel syndrome. *Diseases of the Colon and Rectum*, 30, 208–213.

132. Thompson, J.S., Vanderhoof, J.A. and Antonson, D.L. (1985) Intestinal tapering and lengthening for short bowel syndrome. *Journal of Pediatric Gastroenterology and Nutrition*, 4, 495–497.

133. Thompson, J.S., Harty, R.J., Saigh, J.A. and Giger, D.K. (1988) Morphologic and nutritional responses to intestinal patching following intestinal resection. *Surgery*, 103, 79–86.

134. Trier, J.S. and Lipsky, M. (1989) The short bowel syndrome. In: *Gastrointestinal Disease*, pp. 1106–1112 (Eds) Sleisenger, M. and Fordtran, J.S. London: W.B. Saunders.

135. Turner, J.M., Lawrence, S., Fellows, I.W., Johnson, I., Hill, P.G. and Holmes, G.K.T. (1987) ^{14}C-triolein absorption: a useful test in diagnosis of malabsorption. *Gut*, 28, 694–700.

136. Urban, E. (1986) Man is what he eats. *Gastroenterology*, 91, 484–485.

137. Urban, E., Starr, P.E. and Michel, A.M. (1983) Morphologic and functional adaptations of large bowel after small bowel resection in the rat. *Digestive Diseases and Sciences*, 28, 265–272.

138. Vanderhoof, J.A., Burkley, K.T. Antonson, D.L. (1983) Potential for mucosal adaptation following massive small bowel resection in 3-week-old versus 8-week-old rats. *Journal of Pediatric Gastroenterology and Nutrition*, 2, 672–676.

139. Vanderhoof, J.A., Park, J.H.Y. and Grandjean, C.J. (1986) Effect of zinc deficiency on mucosal hyperplasia following 70% bowel resection. *American Journal of Clinical Nutrition*, 44, 670–677.

140. Vanderhoof, J.A., Grandjean, C.J., Baylor, J.M., Baily, J. and Euler, A.R. (1988) Morphological and functional effects of 16,16-dimethyl-prostaglandin-E_2 on mucosal adaptation after massive distal small bowel resection in the rat. *Gut*, 29, 802–808.

141. Vanderhoof, J.A., Park, J.H.Y. and Grandjean, C.J. (1988) Reduced mucosal prostaglandin synthesis after massive small bowel resection. *American Journal of Physiology*, 254, G373–G377.

142. Watestka, L.P., Sattler, L.L. and Steiger, E. (1980) Cost of home parenteral nutrition program. *Journal of the American Medical Association*, 244, 2303–2304.

143. Welch, I.M., Cunningham, K.M. and Read, N.W. (1988) Regulation of gastric emptying by ileal nutrients in humans. *Gastroenterology*, 94, 401–404.

144. Weser, E. (1985) Luminal nutrients and intestinal absorption. *Journal of Pediatric Gastroenterology and Nutrition*, 4, 165–166.

145. Weser, E., Fletcher, J.T. and Urban, E. (1979) Short bowel syndrome. *Gastroenterology*, 77, 572–579.

146. Weser, E., Bell, D. and Tawil, T. (1981) Effects of octapeptide cholecystokinin, secretin, and glucagon on intestinal mucosal growth in parenterally nourished rats. *Digestive Diseases and Sciences*, 26, 409–416.

147. Weser, E., Babbitt, J.J. and Vandeventer, A. (1985) Relationship between enteral glucose load and adaptive mucosal growth in the small bowel. *Digestive Diseases and Sciences*, 30, 675–681.

148. Wickbom, G., Landor, J.H., Bushkin, F.L. and McGuigan, J.E. (1975) Changes in canine gastric acid output and serum gastrin levels following massive small intestinal resection. *Gastroenterology*, 69, 448–452.

149. Williams, N.S., Evans, P. and King, R.F. (1985) Gastric acid secretion and gastrin production in the short bowel syndrome. *Gut*, 26, 914–919.

150. Wilson, J.P. (1967) Surface area of the small intestine in man. *Gut*, 8, 618–621.

151. Winawer, S.J., Broitman, S.A., Wolochow, D.A., Osborne, M.P. and Zamcheck, N. (1966) Successful management of massive small bowel resection based on assessment of absorption defects and nutritional needs. *New England Journal of Medicine*, 274, 72–78.

152. Wolfe, B.M., Beer, W.H., Hayashi, J.T., Halsted,

C.H., Cannon, R.A. and Cos, R.L. (1983) Experience with home hyperalimentation. *American Journal of Surgery*, **146**, 7–14.

153. Woolfe, G.M., Miller, C., Kurian, R. and Jeejeebhoy, K.N. (1983) Diet for patients with a short bowel: high fat or high carbohydrate. *Gastroenterology*, **84**, 823–828.

154. Woolfe, G.M., Miller, C., Kurian, R. and

Jeejeebhoy, K.N. (1987) Nutritional absorption in short bowel syndrome. Evaluation of fluid, calorie, and divalent cation requirements. *Digestive Disease and Sciences*, **32**, 8–15.

155. Young, E.A., Heuler, N., Russell, P. and Weser, E. (1975) Comparative nutritional analysis of chemically defined diets. *Gastroenterology*, **69**, 1338–1345.

RADIATION ENTEROPATHY

L. Morgenstern

Radiation enteropathy, or radiation enteritis, refers to a broad spectrum of structural and functional disturbances seen in the radiation-injured intestine. The critical level of radiation which results in radiation enteropathy is 4500 cgy. The average radiation dosage for therapy of abdominal neoplasms is listed in *Table 3.56*. At these dosages demonstrable enteropathy can be anticipated in up to 15% of patients undergoing therapy. The higher the dosage required for the control of the neoplasm, the higher will be the expected incidence of enteric sequelae. The combination of external beam and intracavitary radiation is especially likely to result in a high incidence of complications. The continuing serious incidence of enteric radiation injury is documented in several recent reviews of this subject.[4,38,50,55]

Dosage levels which induce injury have been quantified in terms of expected morbidity.[48] The minimum tolerance dose $(TD_{5/5})$ is the dose at which up to 5% of patients will manifest radiation-induced damage within 5 years. The comparative sensitivities of different portions of the intestinal tract are listed in *Table 3.57*. The variation in sensitivity is a function of the cellular kinetics of each portion of the intestinal tract. The small intestine, which has the highest cellular turnover rate, is most vulnerable. Although the rectum is comparatively less vulnerable, rectal radiation injury is common because of the higher radiation dosage employed in pelvic neoplasms; the anatomical fixation of the rectum also predisposes it to injury. This section will principally discuss the small intestine, although radiation injury in other portions of the gastrointestinal tract will be briefly described.

Table 3.56 Average dosage schedules for common neoplasms

Neoplasm	Average dosage (cgy)	Organs injured
Oesophageal cancer	5000–6500	Oesophagus
Pancreatic cancer	5000–6000	Stomach, small intestine, colon
Hodgkin's disease	4000–4500	Small intestine, colon
Non-Hodgkin's lymphoma	3000–6500	Small intestine, colon
Retroperitoneal liposarcoma	5500–6500	Small intestine, colon
Testicular cancer		
Seminoma	3000	Small intestine, colon
Embryonal	4500–5000	Small intestine, colon
Ovarian cancer	4000–5500	Small intestine, colon
Uterine cancer		
Cervix	4500–8000	Small intestine, colon, rectum
Endometrium	4000–8000	Small intestine, colon, rectum
Bladder cancer	4000–6000	Small intestine, colon, rectum
Rectal cancer	4500–5500	Small intestine, rectum

Table 3.57 Comparative radiation tolerance

Organ	Injury	Minimum tolerance dose (cgy) ($TD_{5/5}$)	Maximum tolerance dose (cgy) ($TD_{5/5}$)
Oesophagus	Ulcer, stricture	6000	7500
Stomach	Ulcer, perforation	4500	5000
Intestine	Ulcer, stricture	4500	6500
Colon	Ulcer, stricture	4500	6500
Rectum	Ulcer, stricture	5500	8000

Adapted from Rubin and Casarett.[49]

PATHOLOGY

Excellent descriptions of the pathological changes occurring in radiation injury have been published by Warren and Friedman,[61] White,[63] Berthrong[6,7] and Farjardo.[18] A knowledge of these changes is basic to the understanding of the clinical syndromes associated with radiation enteropathy. The pathological changes commence within hours after the inception of radiation and continue throughout the individual's lifetime.

The earliest changes are those which affect the cytokinetics of replication in the intestinal mucosa. Within hours after an average therapeutic dose of irradiation (150–200 cgy), cell necrosis occurs along the crypt walls. Although regeneration occurs rapidly from stem cells at the crypt base, overall cell turnover is diminished, with resultant flattening and blunting of the villi, mucosal atrophy, shortened crypts and focal ulceration (*Figure 3.115*).

Regeneration and repair are impeded with each successive dose of radiation. It is in the initial phases of injury that the inflammatory component of enteropathy is greatest, with large numbers of polymorphonuclear leukocytes forming a surface syncytium with the desquamated mucosal cells. The acute inflammatory reaction subsides when the radiation treatment is stopped, although the inexorable progression of the radiation-induced damage continues. A recent study[44] has demonstrated an increase in intestinal endocrine cells in radiation enteritis, suggesting possible noxious secretory products of such cells and a possible relationship to late malignant change.

Subacute and chronic changes, which are more insidious in their development and more serious from the clinical point of view, affect the submucosa, the blood vessels, the muscularis propria, and the serosa. The submucosa exhibits oedema, progressive hyalinization, and deposition of dense masses of collagen-containing bizarre, abnormal fibroblasts ('radiation fibroblasts') (*Figure 3.116*).

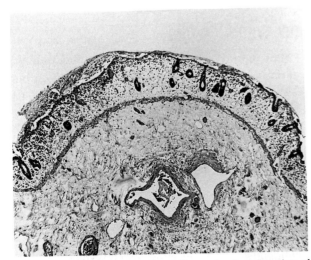

Figure 3.115 Section of irradiated ileum showing distortion of villous architecture, vascular ectasia and perivascular hyalinosis (haematoxylin and eosin).

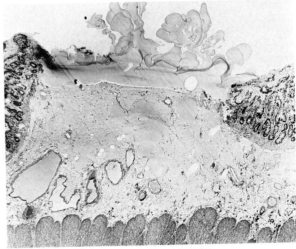

Figure 3.116 Marked oedema of the submocosa in irradiated ileum, with focal ulceration and vascular ectasia (haematoxylin and eosin).

The principal vascular changes are submucosal telangiectasia, hyalinization of vessel walls, alterations in endothelial cells, subendothelial swelling (foam cells), intimal plaque formation, and obliterative endarteritis. Veins show similar intimal and mural changes. The vascular changes in radiation enteropathy have been described in detail by Hasleton et al.[26] The muscularis propria may show focal areas of fibrosis and may be secondarily involved in fissures or deep, penetrating ulcers. Damage to the basic structure of the muscularis, however, is not an important aspect of radiation enteropathy. The serosa exhibits diffuse or patchy hyalinosis with scattered, bizarre fibroblasts, telangiectasia of smaller vessels, and the vascular changes already mentioned in larger vessels (*Figure 3.117*). Grossly, this is manifest as a 'peel' of opaque greyish or grey-white tissue enveloping the intestinal wall (*Figure 3.118*). Dense adhesions between adjacent intestinal loops result in fusion of the abnormal serosal surfaces.

Warren and Friedman[61] have designated the primary criteria of radiation enteropathy as follows: hyalinization of connective tissue, abnormal fibroblasts, telangiectasia, and hyaline degeneration of vessel walls. Secondary criteria include the mucosal changes, endothelial abnormalities, phlebosclerosis, and changes in muscle fibres.

Changes at the microscopic level are reflected

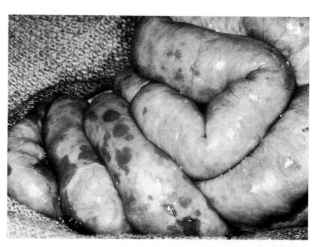

Figure 3.118 Gross appearances at operation of late changes in irradiated obstructed ileum. Loops are oedematous and thick serosal peel over the chronically thickened bowel wall is evident. The haemorrhagic spots are due to handling.

clinically in the occurrence of ulceration, haemorrhage, stricture, infarction and perforation.

CLINICAL SYNDROMES

EARLY

The acute or early effects of therapeutic irradiation are transient and non-specific. They include nausea, vomiting, abdominal cramps, and diarrhoea. Acute ulceration may occur but is rare. Radiographic studies performed at this time show evidence of oedema of bowel loops and hypermotility, but none of the specific features of radiation enteropathy. Signs and symptoms abate shortly after the radiation is stopped.

DELAYED

Following the cessation of irradiation, a quiescent period ensues unless the dosage was unusually high. The average onset of late symptoms is shortly after the first year; primary or recurrent symptoms may then occur at any time thereafter for the lifetime of the individual.

Severe symptoms during the early phases of therapy or shortly following cessation of therapy may be predictors of the development of late sequelae.

LATE SEQUELAE

Functional

Varying degrees of malabsorption are common following therapeutic irradiation. Bile acid absorption

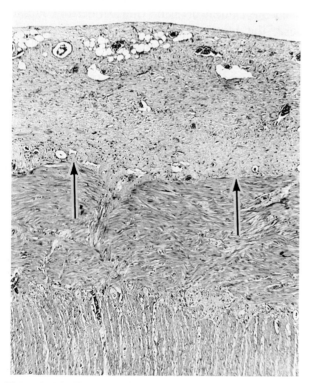

Figure 3.117 Thickened serosa or peel (arrows) over irradiated ileal segment showing hyalinization and telangiectasia (haematoxylin and eosin).

has been shown to be impaired, as demonstrated by abnormal[43] [^{14}C]bile acid breath tests.[29] Excess bile acid excretion in the stool has also been found in patients with radiation-induced diarrhoea.[5] There is also impaired absorption of carbohydrate, fat and vitamin B_{12}. Significant protein loss may occur, particularly in the presence of severe steatorrhoea.

Disturbances in motility, apart from those due to altered absorption patterns, are due to the direct effect of radiation on the muscularis propria. Myofibrillar degeneration, muscle fibre atrophy, and patchy hyalinization are common histological findings. Effects on the intrinsic neural mechanisms are not well documented. Characteristic radiographic findings are hypermotility, delayed segmental motility, 'feathering' of the mucosal pattern, separation of bowel loops, and a generalized distortion of the normal architecture (*Figure 3.119*). 'Pseudo-obstruction' has been reported as a late complication characterized by functional obstruction in the absence of a true obstructing lesion.[11,42]

Structural

The principal late clinical sequelae following radiation are obstruction, ulceration, haemorrhage, fistula formation, infarction and perforation.[13,14,20,45,64]

Obstruction

Acute and subacute intestinal obstruction is perhaps the most common mechanical clinical disorder caused by radiation injury. It is a manifestation of radiation-induced fibrosis, chiefly in the submucosa, as well as adhesion formation between bowel loops due to radiation-induced serositis (*Figure 3.120*). The obstructed bowel loops become heavy with oedema and intraluminal fluid, initiating the cycle of events leading to complete obstruction. The obstructed, distended loops are tender to palpation and may give rise to rebound tenderness even in the absence of infarction or perforation. Volvulus is not as common as is seen in simple adhesive obstruction due to the thickening and foreshortening of the irradiated mesentery. Partial obstruction of varying degrees is more common than complete obstruction, since the obstructive mechanisms are strictures, stenotic segments and multiple adhesions, rather than the single fibrous bands usually seen in adhesive obstruction. Nevertheless, the progression to a picture of complete obstruction, if the partial obstruction is not treated early, is not uncommon.

Ulceration

Ulceration is probably the result of ischaemic changes induced by progressive vascular sclerosis.

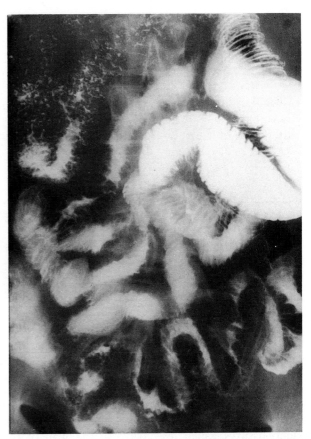

Figure 3.119 Typical radiograph appearance in radiation enteropathy. Note obstructed dilated jejunal loop, distorted architecture, and narrowing and separation of distal loops.

Ulcers may be shallow and scattered (*Figure 3.121*) or deeply penetrating through all layers (*Figure 3.122*). Deep penetrating ulcers may perforate, may cause obstruction by the cicatrical reaction they evoke, or may bleed. Although shallow ulcers heal with a thin layer of regenerative mucosa and a tendency to recurrence, deeper ulcers which traverse all layers rarely heal. If healing does occur, stricture and resultant obstruction are inevitable.

Haemorrhage

Bloody diarrhoea is not uncommon during the initial phases of radiation therapy, particularly in the higher-dosage range, and it reflects diffuse mucosal damage. When bleeding occurs as a late phenomenon, it usually occurs as frank haematochezia due to a solitary ulcer or diffuse ulceration occurring over ectatic submucosal vessels.[59] Exsanguinating haemorrhage is uncommon. Occasionally, mucosal haemorrhage may be exacerbated in the radiation-induced intestine by chemotherapeutic agents which have a radiomimetic action on the intestinal mucosa.

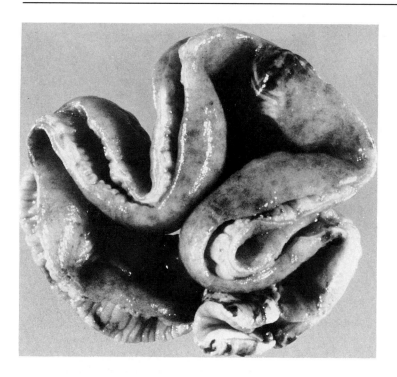

Figure 3.120 Resected, obstructed segment of irradiated small intestine. Note thickness of wall, rigidity, opaque serosal peel, and intersegmental adhesions.

Fistula formation

Fistula formation is probably a late manifestation of a deeply penetrating ulcer or the commonly seen deep fissures which may traverse the wall of the radiation-injured bowel. Sometimes a dense adhesion will have sealed such a fistula at its serosal exit, and an overt fistula results only when the adhesion is severed. Fistulas seek a point of exit; they may do so through an adjoining loop of bowel, recent wounds, drain sites or old scars. Lacking a point of exit, unsealed fistulas result in intra-abdominal abscesses.

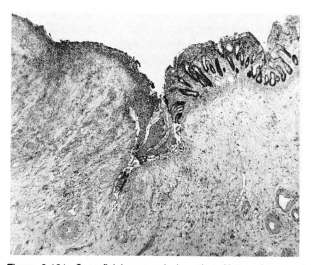

Figure 3.121 Superficial mucosal ulceration. Note submucosal vascular sclerosis underlying ulcerated zone (haematoxylin and eosin).

Infarction

This disastrous and often lethal complication occurs rarely in end-stage enteropathy. It is a consequence of major vessel occlusion due to obliterative endarteritis. The infarction is segmental at times, involving multiple segments of irradiated bowel. The full thickness of intestinal wall is affected. Left unresected, free perforation occurs. The most common site for infarction, sometimes many years after the original injury, is the pelvic ileum. This region of the intestine often receives the brunt of the radiation injury. The usual clinical manifestation of infarction is the acute surgical abdomen, with tenderness, rigidity and rebound tenderness.

Perforation

Free perforation of the intestine into the peritoneal cavity is the ultimate catastrophe. It usually occurs as a consequence of infarction. Generalized peritonitis from free perforation is not as common as with other causes of free perforation since the radiation-injured bowel is enveloped in dense fibrous adhesions.

Malignancy

The late occurrence of malignancy in radiation-injured intestine deserves mention. Sandler and Sandler[49] have recently assessed the risk of radiation-induced cancers of the colon and rectum. They conclude that women who have received pelvic irradiation are more prone to develop colon cancer, the risk factor being 1.2–8 times that of the general population. In addition to other reports of rectal

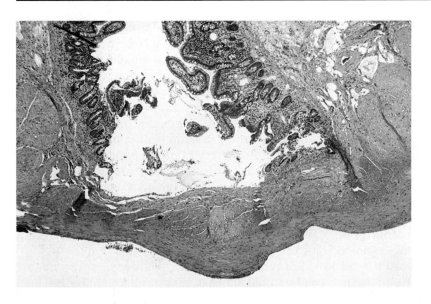

Figure 3.122 Deeply penetrating ulcer in irradiated small intestine. Resection was necessary because of obstruction.

cancer after pelvic irradiation,[27,30] there have also been reports of rectal lymphoma,[54] angiosarcoma of the terminal ileum,[39] and malignant peritoneal mesothelioma.[23]

MANIFESTATIONS OF RADIATION INJURY IN ENTERIC SITES OTHER THAN THE SMALL INTESTINE

OESOPHAGUS

The oesophagus is relatively resistant to radiation injury. During the second or third week of therapy, oesophagitis is common, with dysphagia as the major symptom.

If radiation is given to an extremely radiosensitive neoplasm, acute haemorrhage and ulceration may ensue due to rapid radionecrosis of the neoplasm. Ulceration, abscess formation or even free perforation into adjacent structures or the pleural cavity may also occur.

The principal late complication is stenosis due to fibrosis.

STOMACH

No significant sequelae occur in the irradiated stomach until the dose exceeds 2000 cgy. All of the changes described in the small intestine occur in the stomach, albeit to a lesser degree. Radiation-induced acute gastritis subsides following cessation of therapy, but achlorhydria may persist for years. Purposely induced achlorhydria for the treatment of peptic ulcer with 2000 cgy of external irradiation is an obsolete therapeutic procedure.

The late manifestation of radiation injury to the stomach is atrophic gastritis[62] with attendant dyspepsia. Chronic ulceration may be superimposed on the atrophic gastritis, a situation in which healing is unlikely.

Colon

The transverse colon is vulnerable during irradiation of the upper abdomen. Bleeding, usually secondary to a radiation-induced ulcer, is the principal symptom. Later problems in the colon are related to fibrotic stenosis and partial obstruction.

The rectum is one of the most highly radioresistant portions of the alimentary tract. Some degree of radiation proctitis occurs at all dosages above 4000 cgy and is manifested clinically by cramping, tenesmus and frequent stools. The late sequelae of radiation injury to the rectum are stenosis, ulceration, haemorrhage and fistulas. Rectovaginal fistula at the point of maximum injury on the anterior rectal wall usually results from combined intracavitary and external beam irradiation in excess of 6000 cgy.

FACTORS WHICH ENHANCE RADIATION INJURY

Radiation injury from dosages in the average therapeutic range (around 4500 cgy) is a relatively unpredictable phenomenon in any individual patient. Certain factors, however, are known to predispose to radiation injury. Potish[46,47] has summarized and quantified some of these predisposing factors, alone and in combination. An occasional individual will show an unusual degree of radiation hypersensitivity with no identifiable risk factors.[35] Since certain congenital syndromes such as ataxia telangiectasia, Fanconi's anaemia and Down's syndrome are associated with unusual radiosensitivity, genetics has been implicated as a possible identifiable predictive factor in radiation injury.[40]

A thin physique increases the likelihood of radiation enteropathy, as does malnutrition and lean tissue loss. Diabetes and hypertension predispose to radiation injury due to the structural and functional microvascular abnormalities which exist in these disorders.

Adhesions which result in the abnormal fixation of normally mobile intestinal loops also predispose to radiation enteropathy.[32] Adhesions from prior pelvic infection or prior pelvic surgery are common in women subjected to pelvic irradiation. Prior abdominal surgery is common in patients being irradiated for lymphoma, retroperitoneal neoplasms, pancreatic carcinoma, bladder carcinoma and other miscellaneous neoplasms.

Simultaneous or postirradiation chemotherapy may aggravate radiation injury.[1,43,53,60] Among the principal chemotherapeutic agents which exert a radiomimetic effect on intestinal mucosa, and thus predispose to or aggravate previous radiation damage, are actinomycin D, 5-fluorouracil, methotrexate and adriamycin. A quiescent radiation enteropathy may become actively symptomatic during chemotherapy.

Finally, misjudgements in administration of radiation may result in injury. Unusually high fractionation doses, overlap of portals, excessive total dosage (especially with combined intracavitary and external beam irradiation), and lack of attention to fixed anatomical structures can all be implicated in the induction of radiation injury.

TREATMENT

MEDICAL

Symptoms occurring during the early phases of radiation are treated with simple non-specific measures. The diet should be bland and low-residue. Mild antiemetic, antispasmodic and sedative drugs will relieve the majority of acute radiation symptoms. If radiation proctitis is a problem in early phases of treatment, hydrophilic stool softeners, sitz baths, analgesics and, in more severe cases, steroid retention enemas are effective. More stringent medical measures in the acute treatment phases are rarely necessary.

In the intermediate and late stages of radiation enteropathy, there is a plethora of measures in the medical armamentarium, none of which are universally effective. The bland, lactose-free diet is often used in the management of small intestinal symptoms. In the recovery from an acute bout of intestinal obstruction, or to offset an impending obstruction, elemental diets have been used with some success. Anticholinergics, antispasmodics and analgesics are of minimal value, but none the less may be useful. Prednisone is a lysozomal stabilizing agent and can be useful in small intestinal syndromes where bleeding is a prominent symptom. Cholestyramine, which binds excess bile salts, is useful for the more persistent diarrhoeal syndromes. Nonabsorbed antibiotics, such as sulphasalazine, may also be helpful.

For radiation proctitis, dietary measures, hydrophilic stool softeners, and steroid retention enemas (administered nightly for 10–14 days) may give significant relief. Oral administration of glycosaminoglycans (sodium pentosanpolysulphate) has been reported as an effective agent.[25] Intractable bleeding rarely responds to purely medical measures and ultimately requires operation, although effective local treatment has been reported[2] with both the neodymium–yttrium aluminium garnet (Nd–YAG) laser[3] and the argon laser.[41] Rectal fistulas do not respond to medical measures.

SURGICAL

Surgical intervention in patients with radiation enteropathy is reserved for acute life-threatening complications, such as obstruction, haemorrhage, infarction or perforation, or for chronic morbidity refractory to medical therapy, such as bleeding, fistula formation, ulceration, recurrent obstruction, intractable pain or incontinence. Radiation-induced carcinoma is, of course, an absolute indication for surgical intervention. Approximately 15% of patients with radiation enteropathy ultimately require operation. The indications and guidelines for surgical intervention have been well described by Localio et al.,[31] Morgenstern et al.,[38] Schmitt and Symmonds,[51] and others.[13,21,22,34,36,56] The following principles are applicable to most operations for radiation enteropathy:

1. Avoid operations, if at all possible, in patients with radiation enteropathy.
2. In elective procedures, achieve optimal nutritional status before operation. This may require 7–14 days of total parenteral nutrition. Continue total parenteral nutrition for as long as necessary postoperatively.
3. Avoid incisions in heavily irradiated areas. Skin

necrosis, infection and wound dehiscence may ensue.

4. In elective procedures involving the small intestine, insert a long tube (Cantor, Miller–Abbot) for decompression before operation.

5. Prepare a bowel with antibiotics preoperatively. The irradiated or obstructed bowel is not bacteria-free. Continue broad-spectrum parenteral antibiotics for 5 days postoperatively.

6. Although bypass procedures may be safer and more expeditious in any individual patient, it is generally more effective to resect a diseased segment rather than bypass it. Bypassed segments may bleed, ulcerate, perforate or infarct.

7. Avoid extensive adhesiolysis, which may open sealed perforations. Instillation of methylene blue through the long intestinal tube aids in the detection of occult mural defects.

8. Remember that all anastomoses in irradiated bowel are precarious and require meticulous surgical technique. Avoid multiple anastomoses.

9. Mark anastomoses with identifiable metallic clips at the extremities of each anastomosis.

10. Avoid early postoperative oral feeding and continue long tube decompression for at least 7 days. Study the anastomotic integrity radiographically before removing the tube.

11. Protect low colorectal anastomoses with proximal transverse colostomy, if the anastomotic suture or staple line is at all precarious.

12. In the formation of stomas, avoid using irradiated bowel if possible. If the use of irradiated bowel is unavoidable, exteriorize an ample segment. Sloughing, retraction and ulceration are common.

13. Fistulas do not respond to simple closure or diversion, particularly in the rectum. Resection of the diseased segment is nearly always necessary.

The management of rectal injures requiring resection has been well described in several excellent reviews.[9,10,12]

PREVENTION

Stewart and Gibbs[58] have provided a comprehensive summary of measures to prevent radiation injury in general. Unfortunately, no currently available preparations are radioprotective. Elemental diets during radiotherapy have been described as a prophylactic measure against radiation injury.[8,33] Green et al.[24] have described surgical measures to minimize small intestinal injury during pelvic irradiation. Also proposed as surgical measures to minimize or prevent injury to the small bowel are the use of omentum,[15] and the use of absorbable mesh to exclude the small bowel from the pelvis during radiotherapy.[16,17,28,57] Although encouraging early results have been reported with these techniques, only late evaluation will help assess their true value. Their use is not without complications.[52] Perhaps the most promising measures lie in advances in radiotherapeutic techniques. A technique recently described by Fowler,[19] utilizing hyperfractionated radiotherapy, shows promise, particularly in the prevention of late complications. Modifications in radiation dosage, fractionation and mode of delivery, especially in patients with known predisposition to injury, may possibly reduce the incidence of this condition.

REFERENCES

1. Abrams, R.A., Lichter, A.S., Bromer, R.H. et al. (1985) The hematopoietic toxicity of regional radiation therapy: correlations for combined modality therapy with systemic chemotherapy. Cancer, 55, 1429–1435.

2. Ahlquist, D.A. and Gostout, C.J. (1986) Laser therapy for severe radiation-induced rectal bleeding. Mayo Clinic Proceedings, 61(12), 927–931.

3. Alexander, T.J. and Dwyer, R.M. (1988) Endoscopic Nd:YAG laser treatment of severe radiation injury of the lower gastrointestinal tract: long-term follow-up. Gastrointestinal Endoscopy, 34(5), 407–411.

4. Allen-Mersh, T.G., Wilson, E.J., Hope-Stone, H.F. et al. (1986) Has the incidence of radiation-induced bowel damage following treatment of uterine carcinoma changed in the last 20 years? Journal of the Royal Society of Medicine, 79(7), 387–390.

5. Arlow, F.L., Dekovich, A.A., Priest, R.J. and Beher, W.T. (1987) Bile acids in radiation-induced diarrhea. Southern Medical Journal, 80(10), 1259–1261.

6. Berthrong, M. (1986) Pathologic changes secondary to radiation. World Journal of Surgery, 10(2), 155–170.

7. Berthrong, M. and Fajardo, L.F. (1981) Radiation injury in surgical pathology. Part II. Alimentary tract. American Journal of Surgical Pathology, 5, 153–178.

8. Bounous, G., LeBel, E., Shuster, J. et al. (1975) Dietary protection during radiation therapy. Strahlentherapie, 149, 476–483.

9. Bricker, E.M., Kraybill, W.G. and Lopez, M.J. (1986) Functional results after postirradiation rectal reconstruction. World Journal of Surgery, 10, 249–258.

10. Browning, G.G., Varma, J.S., Smith, A.N., Small, W.P. and Duncan, W. (1987) Late results of mucosal proctectomy and colo-anal sleeve anastomosis for chronic irradiation rectal injury. *British Journal of Surgery*, **74**(1), 31–34.

11. Conklin, J.L. and Anuras, S. (1981) Radiation-induced recurrent intestinal pseudo-obstruction. *American Journal of Gastroenterology*, **75**, 440–444.

12. Cooke, S.A. and Wellsted, M.D. (1986) The radiation-damaged rectum: resection with coloanal anastomosis using the endoanal technique. *World Journal of Surgery*, **10**(2), 220–227.

13. DeCosse, J.J., Rhodes, R.S., Wentz, W.B. *et al.* (1969) The natural history and management of radiation-induced injury of the gastrointestinal tract. *Annals of Surgery*, **170**, 369–384.

14. Deitel, M. and To, T.B. (1987) Major intestinal complications of radiotherapy. Management and nutrition. *Archives of Surgery*, **122**(12), 1421–1424.

15. DeLuca, F.R. and Ragins, H. (1985) Construction of an omental envelope as a method of excluding the small intestine from the field of postoperative irradiation to the pelvis. *Surgery, Gynecology and Obstetrics*, **160**, 365–366.

16. Deutsch, A.A. and Stern, H.S. (1989) Technique of insertion of pelvic Vicryl mesh sling to avoid postradiation enteritis. *Diseases of the Colon and Rectum*, **32**(7), 628–630.

17. Devereux, D.F., Thompson, D., Sandhaus, L. *et al.* (1987) Protection from radiation enteritis by an absorbable polyglycolic acid mesh sling. *Surgery*, **101**(2), 123–129.

18. Fajardo, L.F. (1982) General morphology of radiation injury. In: *Pathology of Radiation Injury*, pp. 6–14. New York: Masson.

19. Fowler, J.F. (1982) Non-standard fractionation in radiotherapy. *International Journal of Radiation Oncology, Biology, Physics*, **8**, 50(abstract).

20. Galland, R.B. and Spencer, J. (1985) Spontaneous postoperative perforation of previously asymptomatic irradiated bowel. *British Journal of Surgery*, **72**(4), 285.

21. Galland, R.B. and Spencer, J. (1986) Surgical management of radiation enteritis. *Surgery*, **99**(2), 133–139.

22. Galland, R.B. and Spencer, J. (1987) Natural history and surgical management of radiation enteritis. *British Journal of Surgery*, **74**, 742–747.

23. Gilks, B., Hegedus, C., Freeman, H. *et al.* (1988) Malignant peritoneal mesothelioma after remote abdominal radiation. *Cancer*, **61**, 2019–2021.

24. Green, N., Iba, G. and Smith, W.R. (1975) Measures to minimize small intestine injury in the irradiated pelvis. *Cancer*, **35**, 1633–1640.

25. Grigsby, P.W., Pilepich, M.V. and Parsons, C.L. (1990) Preliminary results of a phase I/II study of sodium pentosanpolysulfate in the treatment of chronic radiation-induced proctitis. *American Journal of Clinical Oncology*, **13**(1), 28–31.

26. Hasleton, P.S., Carr, N. and Schofield, P.F. (1985) Vascular changes in radiation bowel disease. *Histopathology*, **9**(5), 517–534.

27. Jao, S.W., Beart, R.W. Jr., Reiman, H.M. *et al.* (1987) Colon and anorectal cancer after pelvic irradiation. *Diseases of the Colon and Rectum*, **30**(12), 953–958.

28. Kavanah, M.T., Feldman, M.I., Devereux, D.F. and Kondi, E.S. (1985) New surgical approach to minimize radiation-associated small bowel injury in patients with pelvic malignancies requiring surgery and high-dose irradiation. *Cancer*, **56**(6), 1300–1304.

29. Kinsella, T.J. and Bloomer, W.D. (1980) Tolerance of the intestine to radiation therapy. (Collective review.) *Surgery, Gynecology and Obstetrics*, **151**, 273–284.

30. Levitt, M.D., Millar, D.M. and Stewart, J.O. (1990) Rectal cancer after pelvic irradiation. *Journal of the Royal Society of Medicine*, **83**(3), 152–154.

31. Localio, S.A., Pachter, H.L. and Gouge, T.H. (1979) The radiation-injured bowel. *Surgery Annal*, **11**, 181–205.

32. LoIudice, T., Baxter, D. and Balint, J. (1977) Effects of abdominal surgery on the development of radiation enteropathy. *Gastroenterology*, **73**, 1093–1097.

33. McArdle, A.H., Reid, E.C., Laplante, M.P. and Freeman, C.R. (1986) Prophylaxis against radiation injury: the use of elemental diet. *Archives of Surgery*, **121**(8), 879–885.

34. Mäkelä, J., Nevasaari, K. and Kairaluoma, M.I. (1987) Surgical treatment of intestinal radiation injury. *Journal of Surgical Oncology*, **36**, 93–97.

35. Matsubara, S., Saito, F., Suda, T. *et al.* (1988) Radiation injury in a patient with unusually high sensitivity to radiation. *Acta Oncologica*, **27**, 67–71.

36. Miholic, J., Schlappack, O., Klepetko, W. *et al.* (1987) Surgical therapy of radiation-induced small-bowel lesions. Report of 34 cases with a high share of patients with combined chemotherapy. *Archives of Surgery*, **122**(8), 923–926.

37. Morgenstern, L., Thompson, R. and Friedman, N.B. (1977) The modern enigma of radiation enteropathy: sequelae and solutions. *American Journal of Surgery*, **134**, 166–172.

38. Morgenstern, L., Hart, M., Lugo, D. and Freidman, N.B. (1985) Changing aspects of radiation enteropathy. *Archives of Surgery*, **120**, 1225–1228.

39. Nanus, D.M., Kelsen, D. and Clark, D.G.C. (1987) Radiation-induced angiosarcoma. *Cancer*, **60**, 777–779.

40. Norman, A. *et al.* (1988) The importance of genetics for the optimization of radiation therapy. *American Journal of Clinical Oncology*, **11**(1), 84–88.

41. O'Connor, J.J. (1989) Argon laser treatment of radiation proctitis. *Archives of Surgery*, **124**(6), 749.

42. Perino, L.E., Schuffler, M.D., Mehta, S.J. and

Everson, G.T. (1986) Radiation-induced intestinal pseudoobstruction. *Gastroenterology*, **91**(4), 994–998.

43. Phillips, T.L., Wharam, M.D. and Margolis, L.W. (1975) Modification of radiation injury to normal tissues by chemotherapeutic agents. *Cancer*, **35**, 1678–1684.

44. Pietroletti, R., Blaauwgeers, J.L. and Taat, C.W. (1989) Intestinal endocrine cells in radiation enteritis. *Surgery, Gynecology and Obstetrics*, **169**(2), 127–130.

45. Poddar, P.K., Bauer, J., Gelernt, I. *et al.* (1982) Radiation injury to the small intestine. *Mount Sinai Journal of Medicine*, **49**, 144–149.

46. Potish, R.A. (1980) Prediction of radiation-related small bowel damage. *Radiology*, **135**, 219–221.

47. Potish, R.A. (1982) Importance of predisposing factors in the development of enteric damage. *American Journal of Clinical Oncology: Cancer Clinical Trials*, **5**, 189–194.

48. Rubin, P. and Casarett, G. (1972) A direction for clinical radiation pathology: the tolerance dose. In: *Frontiers of Radiation Therapy and Oncology*, Vol. 6, pp. 1–16 (Ed.) Vaeth, J.M. Baltimore: University Park Press.

49. Sandler, R.S. and Sandler, D.P. (1983) Radiation-induced cancers of the colon and rectum: assessing the risk. *Gastroenterology*, **84**, 51–57.

50. Schellhammer, P.F., Jordan, G.H. and El-Mahdi, A.M. (1986) Pelvic complications after interstitial and external beam irradiation of urologic and gynecologic malignancy. *World Journal of Surgery*, **10**, 259–268.

51. Schmitt III, E.H. and Symmonds, R.E. (1981) Surgical treatment of radiation-induced injuries of the intestine. *Surgery, Gynecology and Obstetrics*, **153**, 896–900.

52. Sener, S.F., Imperato, J.P., Blum, M.D. *et al.* (1989) Technique and complications of reconstruction of the pelvic floor with polyglactin mesh. *Surgery, Gynecology and Obstetrics*, **168**(6), 475–480.

53. Shehata, W.M. and Meyer, R.L. (1980) The enhancement effect of irradiation by methotrexate: report of three complications. *Cancer*, **46**, 1349–1352.

54. Sibly, T.F., Keane, R.M., Lever, J.V. and

Southwood, W.F.W. (1985) Rectal lymphoma in radiation injured bowel. *British Journal of Surgery*, **72**(11), 879–880.

55. Smith, D.H. and DeCosse, J.J. (1986) Radiation damage to the small intestine. *World Journal of Surgery*, **10**(2), 189–194.

56. Smith, S.T., Seski, J.C., Copeland, L.J. *et al.* (1985) Surgical management of irradiation-induced small bowel damage. *Obstetrics and Gynecology*, **65**(4), 563–567.

57. Soper, J.T., Clarke-Pearson, D.L. and Creasman, W.T. (1988) Absorbable synthetic mesh (910-polyglactin) intestinal sling to reduce radiation-induced small bowel injury in patients with pelvic malignancies. *Gynecologic Oncology*, **29**(3), 283–289.

58. Stewart, J.R. and Gibbs, Jr, F.A. (1982) Prevention of radiation injury: predictability and preventability of complications of radiation therapy. *Annual Review of Medicine*, **33**, 385–395.

59. Taverner, D., Talbot, I.C., Carr-Locke, D.L. and Wicks, A.C.B. (1982) Massive bleeding from the ileum: a late complication of pelvic radiotherapy. *American Journal of Gastroenterology*, **77**, 29–31.

60. Thomas, P.R., Lindblad, A.S. and Stablein, D.M. (1986) Toxicity associated with adjuvant postoperative therapy for adenocarcinoma of the rectum. *Cancer*, **57**(6), 1130–1134.

61. Warren, S. and Friedman, N.B. (1942) Pathology and pathologic diagnosis of radiation lesions in the gastrointestinal tract. *American Journal of Pathology*, **18**, 499–513.

62. White, D.C. (1975) Esophagus and stomach. In: *An Atlas of Radiation Histopathology*, pp. 136–140 (Ed.) White, D.C. Washington, DC: Technical Information Center, Office of Public Affairs, US Energy Research and Development Administration.

63. White, D.C. (1975) Intestines. In: *An Atlas of Radiation Histopathology*, pp. 141–160 (Ed.) White, D.C. Washington, DC: Technical Information Center, Office of Public Affairs, US Energy Research and Development Administration.

64. Yoonessi, M., Romney, W. and Dayem, H. (1981) Gastrointestinal tract complications following radiotherapy of uterine cervical cancer: past and present. *Journal of Surgical Oncology*, **18**, 135–142.

CHRONIC DISEASES OF THE SMALL INTESTINE IN CHILDHOOD

J.A. Walker-Smith

Diseases of the small intestine account for the most frequently seen gastroenterological problems that occur in childhood. They can be divided into acute disorders such as gastroenteritis (by far the most important problem worldwide), and chronic disorders such as coeliac disease. In most of these there is some abnormality of the gut mucosa, i.e. a small intestinal enteropathy is present. In all, there is some degree of malabsorption; in the acute diarrhoeal syndromes of gastroenteritis this is principally of salt and water, but in the chronic conditions such as coeliac disease malabsorption of a wide variety of nutrients such as fat and folic acid also occurs. The most important of these chronic disorders occurring in children will be briefly reviewed here. In the past, in these chronic disorders the emphasis in diagnosis was to first establish the existence of malabsorption, e.g. fat malabsorption by faecal fat estimation, and then to consider the possible cause. Now the emphasis in the first instance is often upon diagnosis of the underlying disease process. Thus, if on analysis of the clinical features coeliac disease appears likely, a small intestinal biopsy should be done; if cystic fibrosis is considered possible, sweat electrolytes are estimated first. In practice, the initial clinical assessment of children presenting with gastrointestinal symptoms usually suggests two or three possibilities. Those tests that are most relevant to these possible diagnoses should be performed.

COELIAC DISEASE

The aetiology, incidence and pathogenesis of coeliac disease have been discussed earlier in this chapter.

CLINICAL FEATURES

There is considerable variation in the age of onset of symptoms in children with coeliac disease. As Gee described in 1888,[6,8] symptoms present most often between the ages of 1 and 5 years. There is usually a variable 'latent' interval between the introduction of gluten into the diet and the development of clinical manifestations, the explanation for which remains unknown. In some children the interval may be months and in others many years, as coeliac disease may present for the first time in adult life. Occasionally infants may have symptoms immediately gluten is added to their diets.

Mode of presentation

Classical presentation aged 9–18 months
There is gradual failure to gain weight or loss of weight after introduction of cereals, the child having previously been well. There is also anorexia and chronic diarrhoea; typically the stools are softer, paler, larger, more offensive and more frequent than usual.

Presentation in infants before 9 months
Vomiting is frequent and may be projectile. Diarrhoea may be severe, especially with intercurrent infections (not necessarily gastroenteritis). Abdominal distension may not be marked. With the later introduction of gluten into the diet of infants in the UK this is now an uncommon mode of presentation.

Presentation with constipation
These children are often very hypotonic with marked abdominal distension. This is an uncommon presentation.

Presentation at an older age
Short stature, iron-resistant anaemia, rickets and personality problems all may occur.

Presentation in children originating from the Indian subcontinent now living in Western countries
These present later, often with iron-resistant anaemia or rickets, and/or short stature. Diarrhoea is not a prominent feature.[19]

Presentation in asymptomatic siblings
After a case is positively diagnosed, siblings should have their clinical history and growth checked. If a suspicion of coeliac disease arises, a full blood count, serum folate, red cell folate and gliadin antibody should be performed. A biopsy is then necessary if there is evidence of a deficiency state or the presence of a gliadin or endomysiae antibody.

Physical findings

On physical examination these children characteristically have wasting of the proximal limb girdles with a protuberant abdomen. There may be some ankle oedema due to hypoproteinaemia and occasionally finger clubbing. Typically, the child is very miserable. Measurements of height and weight are valuable, especially when serial observations are available, often showing a slowing of weight gain and then weight loss. If the disease has been present for some time there is also slowing of growth (*Figure 3.123*).

Differential diagnosis

The diagnosis of coeliac disease is based initially upon the demonstration of an abnormal small intestinal mucosa (usually flat) by small intestinal biopsy, and then upon a clinical response to the gluten withdrawal consisting of significant weight gain and relief of symptoms.[16]

The principal differential diagnoses are cystic

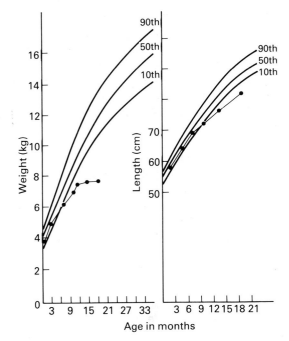

Figure 3.123 Weight and growth chart for an infant with untreated coeliac disease. (Reproduced, with permission, from Walker-Smith, J.A. (1979) *Diseases of the Small Intestine in Childhood*, 2nd edn. Tunbridge Wells: Pitman.)

fibrosis, giardiasis, toddler's diarrhoea, cow's milk protein intolerance, and the postenteritis syndromes. Other causes of a flat mucosa are listed in *Table 3.58*. Reintroduction of gluten into the child's diet at a later date when the small intestinal mucosa has been shown to return to normal, followed by mucosal deterioration with or without a clinical relapse, is necessary before the diagnosis of coeliac disease may be said to have been definitely established[18] (*Figure 3.124*). These diagnostic criteria are known as the ESPGAN criteria.[16] This diagnostic approach is recommended for children presenting under 2 years of age, for those who have not had an initial diagnostic biopsy or where the initial biopsy is unsatisfactory or in some way non-characteristic and also for those teenagers who wish to depart from their gluten-free diet. The relapse in mucosal

appearance may not occur for up to 2 years or sometimes even longer after the reintroduction of gluten into the child's diet (gluten challenge).

Complications

Most of these are due to malabsorption.

Growth retardation
Some children with coeliac disease may be asymptomatic apart from severe growth retardation. Out of 13 children, 9 had reduced levels of plasma growth hormone.[25] Thus, coeliac disease should be considered whenever a child with short stature has evidence of impairment of the release of growth hormone.

Anaemia
The incidence of anaemia in children with coeliac disease is variable. The most common type is hypochromic microcytic anaemia due to iron deficiency. Megaloblastic anaemia only rarely occurs.[5] Despite this, serum folate and red cell folate levels are often reduced in children with untreated coeliac disease. Folate levels rapidly rise on a gluten-free diet and tend to fall, although not always to a pathological level, after a gluten challenge. Estimation of folate levels is thus a useful way to evaluate progress on a gluten-free diet of a child with coeliac disease.

Hypoproteinaemia
Hypoproteinaemia due to protein-losing enteropathy is a common complication of coeliac disease. When there is severe hypoproteinaemia, the child may present with generalized oedema mimicking the nephrotic syndrome. The oedema is relieved by treatment with a gluten-free diet.

Hypogammaglobulinaemia
Low levels of serum IgA and IgM have been described in some children with coeliac disease.[12] The IgA deficiency is not reversible with a gluten-free diet, whereas IgM levels rise to normal. It is

Table 3.58 Reported causes of a flat small intestinal mucosa in childhood

Coeliac disease, i.e. permanent gluten intolerance
Transient gluten intolerance ⎫
Cow's milk sensitive enteropathy ⎬ Temporary food-sensitive enteropathies
Soya protein intolerance ⎭
Gastroenteritis and postenteritis syndromes
Giardiasis
Autoimmune enteropathy
Acquired hypogammaglobulinaemia
Tropical sprue
Protein energy malnutrition

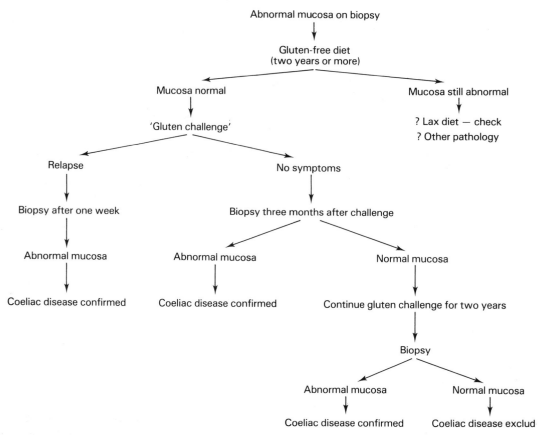

Figure 3.124 Diagnostic criteria and investigation regimen for coeliac disease. (Reproduced, with permission, from Walker-Smith, J.A. (1979) *Diseases of the Small Intestine in Childhood*, 2nd edn. Tunbridge Wells: Pitman.)

possible that pre-existing IgA deficiency predisposes to coeliac disease. On the other hand, serum IgA levels are more commonly elevated in coeliac disease.

Hypoprothrombinaemia

An abnormal prothrombin time due to malabsorption of vitamin K may occur in coeliac disease, and estimation of prothrombin time and other parameters of coagulation before small intestinal biopsy has been recommended. Hypoprothrombinaemia is rapidly corrected by intramuscular vitamin K_1.

Treatment

Elimination of gluten from the child's diet usually leads to a dramatic and rapid clinical response,[4] but this may sometimes be delayed. Weight gain and relief of emotional symptoms in the mother as well as the child usually occur first, before cessation of diarrhoea and other signs of improvement. There is some disagreement as to precisely what constitutes a gluten-free diet. All authorities agree that wheat and rye should be eliminated from the diet, but some also recommend elimination of barley and oats,

although it is still uncertain whether these two cereals are also toxic to children with coeliac disease.

Although secondary disaccharidase deficiency has been shown, by assay of small intestinal biopsies, to be present in virtually all children with untreated coeliac disease, clinical lactose intolerance is present in only 5%. Only when there is evidence of such intolerance, i.e. an abnormal amount of reducing substances in the stool and diarrhoea after a lactose load, is elimination of lactose from the diet indicated.

OTHER FOOD-RELATED DISORDERS

Apart from coeliac disease, all other food-related disorders associated with gastrointestinal symptoms in children appear to be transient. Food intolerance comprises a wide range of abnormal reactions to food. An approach to the diagnosis of chronic diarrhoea in infancy which may be food related is given in *Figure 3.125*.

Changes in the structure of the small intestinal mucosa, enteropathy, assessed by biopsy in re-

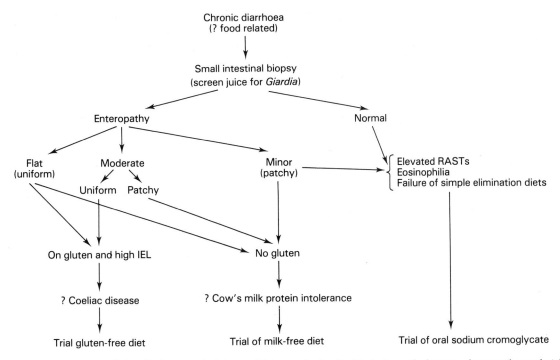

Figure 3.125 The diagnosis of chronic diarrhoea in infancy which may be food related. A practical approach currently used at Queen Elizabeth Hospital for Children, London. High IEL, increased counts of intraepithelial lymphocytes.

sponse to ingestion of particular foods, provide clear objective evidence of food-sensitive disorders. Serial small intestinal biopsies related to dietary elimination and then to challenge have implicated chiefly three foods in the production of small intestinal mucosal damage, probably mediated via a lymphocytic immune reaction. These produce *cow's milk-sensitive enteropathy* as part of cow's milk protein intolerance, *soya protein intolerance* and *transient gluten intolerance*. All are temporary disorders of early life and usually resolve clinically by the third year. In addition, Vitoria *et al*[26] have described an enteropathy related to fish, rice and chicken. Other food allergic disorders may or may not be associated with recognizable small intestinal mucosal damage or enteropathy; it is possible that, in part at least, their clinical manifestations are mediated through structural or functional abnormality of the small intestinal mucosa. These disorders are not yet well defined clinically but include multiple food allergy.

The features of small intestinal mucosa pathology which may provide evidence of local allergic reactions, based upon animal experiments, are illustrated in *Figure 3.126*. Induction of a T-cell-mediated lesion in human fetal small intestine produces a similar lesion.[14]

When a small intestinal biopsy in food allergy shows enteropathy characterized by crypt hyperplasia, villous atrophy and an increased number of intraepithelial lymphocytes, a cell-mediated immune reaction may be present. On the other hand a type I reaction in the gut, due to IgE antibody, is likely to produce virtually no structural abnormality on biopsy apart from oedema.

COW'S MILK PROTEIN INTOLERANCE

Cow's milk protein intolerance is the clinical syndrome or syndromes resulting from the sensitization

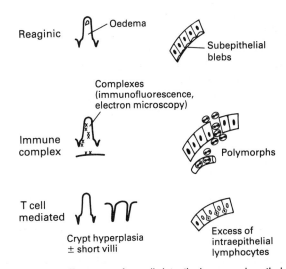

Figure 3.126 Features of small intestinal mucosal pathology which (on the basis of experimental work in animals) may provide evidence of local allergic reactions. (Reproduced, with permission, from Ferguson, A. (1980) Pathogenesis and mechanisms in the gastrointestinal tract. In: *Proceedings of the First Fisons Food Allergy Workshop*, pp. 28–38. Medicine Publishing Foundation.)

of an individual child to one or more proteins in cow's milk, presumably following absorption via a permeable small intestinal mucosa.

Pathogenesis

The pathogenesis of cow's milk protein intolerance is not clear. There appear to be two syndromes: a primary form in which there appears to be no predisposing factors, and a secondary form following acute gastroenteritis.[28] Two factors may be important in both: first, the permeability of the small intestinal mucosa to the antigen and, secondly, the control of the antigen and the immune response to it once it has been absorbed. Primary cow's milk intolerance may be due to primary disturbance of the local immune system for antigen control, particularly antigen exclusion. The secondary syndrome may be a sequel to primary gut damage due to gastroenteritis permitting excess antigen entry, perhaps coupled with a defect of local antigen control. An immunodeficiency state, such as transient IgA deficiency, may be an important predisposing factor for both syndromes. *Figure 3.127* outlines a hypothesis for the pathogenesis of cow's milk protein intolerance and suggests a relationship between gastroenteritis and lactose intolerance.

Pathology

Most children with cow's milk protein intolerance who have gastrointestinal symptoms appear on biopsy to have an abnormal small intestinal mucosa at the time of initial diagnosis. However, unlike coeliac disease, this enteropathy is not an invariable finding on a single proximal biopsy, but is patchy and of variable severity. The mucosa is often thinner than in coeliac disease, although a mucosa indistinguishable from coeliac disease may be found; more often the mucosal abnormality is less severe. When present, the enteropathy can be shown to be sensitive to

cow's milk by serial biopsies related to withdrawal of and challenge with cow's milk. After a positive milk challenge, alteration in the microvilli of the enterocyte may be seen in parallel with a fall in disaccharidase activity. Although the numbers of intraepithelial lymphocytes may rise after a positive milk challenge, the level reached is usually within the normal range.

Some children who are milk intolerant have a colitis which histologically is characterized by an increase in lamina propria eosinophils. This often occurs independently of the small intestinal lesion.

Clinical features

In most children with gastrointestinal symptoms due to cow's milk protein intolerance the symptoms commence within the first 6 months of life, either acutely or insidiously. In some children, there may be a family history of atopy or cow's milk protein intolerance, but often there is not. Such a history is usually absent when the syndrome occurs as a sequel to acute gastroenteritis.

The acute onset syndrome may be characterized by a sudden attack of vomiting and diarrhoea, which then becomes persistent. It may be impossible at first to distinguish such an illness from acute gastroenteritis, which is confusing as cow's milk protein intolerance may itself be a sequel to gastroenteritis. The acute onset syndromes may be subdivided as follows: first, there are those infants who appear to be so sensitive to cow's milk that they develop acute symptoms immediately on weaning on to cow's milk, although they are still being chiefly breast fed; secondly, there are those infants who have an acute attack of symptoms after receiving cow's milk feedings for several months. In this latter group particularly, an attack of acute gastroenteritis is often implicated as a triggering event. Finally, another but fortunately rare acute onset syndrome is characterized by the sudden onset of vomiting, followed by pallor and an acute anaphylactic state of circulatory collapse (hypotension and altered consciousness) or significant upper airway obstruction (swelling of structures in the mouth or throat).

The chronic onset syndrome may manifest as chronic diarrhoea with failure to thrive and clinical features to suggest coeliac disease. It may also present as the intractable diarrhoea syndrome and must always be considered in the differential diagnosis of this condition. The colitis with increased lamina propria eosinophils, referred to above, presents with chronic bloody diarrhoea with many of the features of ulcerative colitis. This syndrome may present in the first days of life and needs to be distinguished from necrotizing enterocolitis as well as chronic inflammatory bowel disease.

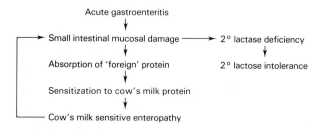

Figure 3.127 A hypothesis for the relationship between gastroenteritis and lactose intolerance with cow's milk-sensitive enteropathy. (Reproduced, with permission, from Walker-Smith, J.A. (1979) *Diseases of the Small Intestine in Childhood*, 2nd edn. Tunbridge Wells: Pitman.)

Investigations

Until recently, the only satisfactory way to make the diagnosis of cow's milk protein intolerance was clinical observation of the effects of repeated withdrawal of and challenge with milk as formulated by Goldman and colleagues in 1963.[9] However, serial small intestinal biopsies at the time of initial presentation, after a clinical response to milk withdrawal, and finally after the return of symptoms following a milk challenge, now permit a firm diagnosis of cow's milk-sensitive enteropathy to be made on the basis of one diagnostic milk challenge. This approach is only usually practical in a paediatric gastroenterology unit but it has clearly established the existence of this syndrome. In practice, a cow's milk challenge is often deferred until about the age of 1 year, both because the risk of anaphylaxis is greater under a year and because of the natural reluctance to prematurely change the feeding when an infant is doing well on a cow's milk-free diet. Often, therefore, by the time of the challenge, the infant has recovered and postchallenge biopsy is not done. An initial biopsy, however, is indicated as part of the diagnostic investigation of an infant with chronic diarrhoea and failure to thrive.

Differential diagnosis

Cow's milk-sensitive enteropathy has to be distinguished from secondary lactose intolerance (occurring as a temporary sequel to acute gastroenteritis), coeliac disease, other forms of food allergy, toddler's diarrhoea, and even at times from normality. Small intestinal biopsy is the most useful diagnostic test to make this distinction, combined with clear knowledge of the child's precise dietary intake; the principal clinical feature is a clear response to a cow's milk-free diet.

Treatment

The obvious treatment for this condition is to eliminate cow's milk and all foods based on cow's milk from the child's diet. This latter point is most important as therapeutic failure is sometimes related to neglect of a restriction of cow's milk-based foods such as ice cream, despite strict avoidance of cow's milk itself. It is usually necessary to provide a cow's milk-based substitute, and it is essential to ensure that the diet is nutritionally adequate.

The need for such dietary restriction of milk is nearly always temporary, although there is little documentation concerning the precise duration of this intolerance. On clinical grounds, most children over 2 years of age are apparently able to tolerate milk without any untoward sequelae. The timing of a rechallenge with cow's milk is arbitrary and varies from paediatrician to paediatrician.

A large number of substitute products are available and vary in nutritional adequacy for different age groups. They fall into three categories based on protein hydrolysates, either casein or whey hydrolysates, soya protein, or goat's milk. A factor of key importance, especially in early infancy, is the osmolality of the formula. High-osmolality feeds draw water into the gut and may increase any diarrhoea that is present. Casein hydrolysate feeds are often preferred for children with cow's milk-sensitive enteropathy, especially as such children can occasionally be sensitive to other proteins used in replacement feeds such as soya protein. Casein hydrolysate formulas appear to be very low in allergenicity. Nutramigen is especially suitable for the young infant because of its nutritional adequacy and the low osmolality of the current formulation. A number of soya 'milks' are available on the market but many are only a social replacement of milk, and do not supply calcium, riboflavin and other nutrients provided by cow's milk. Several new soya infant formulas are available and appear to be safe nutritional alternatives to modified cow's milk feeds, e.g. Formula S, Prosobee and Wysoy. The first two are solely of vegetable origin and so are acceptable to vegetarians and vegans.

SOYA PROTEIN INTOLERANCE

A soya bean food prepared to resemble milk has been used in many countries since it was first recommended by Hill and Stuart in 1929[11] for infants with milk allergy. It has also been suggested that soya bean milk when used as a substitute for cow's milk could play an important role in the prevention of allergy to cow's milk in those who are at risk. Although soya beans have low antigenicity, over the past 10 years there has been an increasing number of reports of intolerance to soya protein. Such reactions have varied from a dramatic anaphylactic response to the onset of respiratory and gastrointestinal symptoms.

In 1972, Ament and Rubin[1] clearly documented soya protein intolerance in an infant by monitoring the clinical and small intestinal mucosal response to a soya protein challenge. Challenge produced a flat small intestinal mucosa indistinguishable from that found in untreated coeliac disease. The lesion was reversible and serial biopsies revealed that it disappeared within 4 days of withdrawal of soya protein, only to recur on further challenge. Varying degrees of small intestinal mucosal abnormality have been recognized by other workers.

Soya-free diets are almost as difficult to maintain

as cow's milk-free diets because of the extensive use of soya protein in manufactured food products.

TRANSIENT GLUTEN INTOLERANCE

Transient gluten intolerance is recognized when a child with gastrointestinal symptoms and an abnormal small intestinal mucosa responds to a gluten-free diet, but subsequently thrives on a normal gluten-containing diet and, after 2 or more years on such a diet, is found to have a normal mucosa. In Holland in 1952, Dicke[4] described a transient wheat sensitivity in pre-school children after enteritis. In 1970, a child with transient gluten intolerance was described in Australia.[20] This child had an abnormal mucosa (a severe degree of partial villous atrophy) and responded clinically to a gluten-free diet. After 1 year, while he was still taking a gluten-free diet, a further biopsy revealed a normal mucosa. He was put back on a normal diet and 16 months later a further biopsy demonstrated a persistently normal mucosa. He has subsequently remained in excellent health.

Although a diagnosis of transient gluten intolerance was made retrospectively in this child, more recent criteria lay down stricter requirements for this diagnosis. These are, first, the need to provide evidence that gluten toxicity was in fact present and that the apparent response to gluten restriction was not fortuitous[14] and, secondly, the need to demonstrate the presence of a normal small intestinal mucosa 2 years or more after the return to a normal diet.[30]

The precise criteria necessary to establish the existence of any form of transient intolerance to a dietary substance associated with small bowel mucosal abnormality have been outlined by McNeish[15] and are indicated in diagrammatic form in *Figure 3.128.*

Pathogenesis

Two explanations have been proposed to explain the development of this syndrome. First, there may be a temporary depression of dipeptidase activity occurring in the small intestinal mucosa secondary to nonspecific mucosal damage, such as may occur after gastroenteritis. Secondly, and more likely, it is possible that a transient 'allergy' to gluten may occur in a similar manner to that suggested earlier in relation to cow's milk protein.

Pathology

The small intestinal mucosa is by definition abnormal, i.e. thickened, ridged mucosa characterized

histologically by partial villous atrophy or, sometimes, a flat mucosa. The demonstration of a flat mucosa is more characteristic of coeliac disease; the mucosal abnormality is usually less severe in transient gluten tolerance than that found in coeliac disease. Only long-term follow-up with subsequent reinvestigation would allow the retrospective diagnosis of transient gluten intolerance to be made in a child with a flat mucosa who earlier had responded clinically to gluten withdrawal, but who is now thriving on a gluten-containing diet.

Clinical features

Transient gluten intolerance may accompany other forms of food intolerance, or occur on its own. The diagnosis should be considered in the infant who develops gastrointestinal symptoms when he or she first encounters wheat protein, especially when he or she appears to be intolerant to other food proteins such as milk and egg. It should also be considered in a child who fails to thrive following gastroenteritis in the presence of an abnormal small intestinal mucosa and the absence of other explanations, such as secondary lactose intolerance or secondary cow's milk protein intolerance.

Treatment

Initial management is as for coeliac disease; the diagnosis is inevitably retrospective after the child has been reinvestigated to establish the presence or absence of permanent gluten intolerance. Early

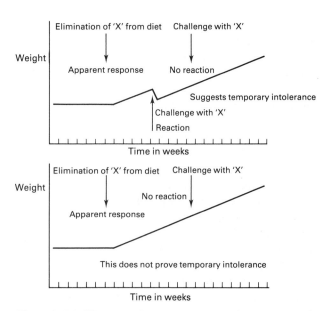

Figure 3.128 Diagrammatic representation of the diagnostic criteria for transient gluten intolerance (Reproduced, with permission, from McNeish.[15])

challenge is not recommended routinely, so in most cases the diagnosis is not only retrospective but provisional as the initial response to a gluten-free diet is not definite proof of gluten sensitivity. Whether any or all such children with transient gluten intolerance will ultimately relapse remains uncertain as there have been reports of intervals as long as 5 years after gluten challenge before relapse occurs.

SUGAR INTOLERANCE

Sugar intolerance is characterized by the development of diarrhoea and/or failure to thrive in infants and children due to ingestion of sugar. Such a syndrome may be primary, for example glucose–galactose malabsorption, or it may be secondary to temporary damage to the small intestinal mucosa, as may occur, for example, following an acute rotavirus gastroenteritis. There are two principal syndromes – monosaccharide and disaccharide intolerance. The latter is often more severe and persistent. Causes of secondary lactose intolerance are:

1. Gastroenteritis
2. Coeliac disease
3. Giardiasis
4. Protein-energy malnutrition
5. Following neonatal surgery
6. Cow's milk protein intolerance
7. Immunodeficiency syndrome
8. Massive small intestinal resection.

Investigations

The simplest clinical way to make the diagnosis of sugar intolerance is to demonstrate the presence of excess amounts of reducing substances in diarrhoeal stools. The stools are typically watery and contain 1–5% reducing substances, less than 1% being found normally. The importance of proper stool collections cannot be overstressed. If there is some doubt about which feed may be responsible for the child's continuing diarrhoea (as may be the case when there has been a recent change of feed) stool chromatography may help identify the sugar present. The hydrogen breath test has also been used in the diagnosis of both monosaccharide and disaccharide intolerance. An increasing concentration of breath hydrogen reflects bacterial fermentation of carbohydrate reaching the colon. This test is most viable in epidemiological studies.

The second aspect of clinical diagnosis is the demonstration of a clinical response to the removal of the offending sugar from the diet. The formulas discussed earlier as being appropriate for cow's milk protein intolerance are also lactose-free, and so can be used in sugar intolerance.

POSTENTERITIS SYNDROME

The postenteritis syndrome describes the child who has had an attack of acute gastroenteritis followed by intermittent or chronic diarrhoea. There may or may not be failure to gain weight following the return to a normal diet.

Two main groups of problems cause delayed recovery after acute gastroenteritis in infancy. First, there may be an acute coexistent intolerance to the increasing concentrations of milk and, secondly, there may be a more chronic problem with persistent diarrhoea and failure to thrive. An acute intolerance to milk leads to diarrhoea, which is often watery and copious and sometimes accompanied by vomiting. This is most often due to malabsorption of lactose and sometimes also of sucrose, but there may be intolerance to cow's milk protein. Sometimes, in addition, there may be temporary monosaccharide intolerance. The acute problem of sugar intolerance is usually easily dealt with, but the more chronic problem of persistent diarrhoea and failure to gain weight following gastroenteritis is more difficult to solve. The differential diagnosis of, for example, a child under 2 years of age in this state is as follows: postenteritis syndrome, coeliac disease, cystic fibrosis, giardiasis, and cow's milk protein intolerance, as well as an anatomical abnormality of the small intestine producing partial obstruction. These also need to be distinguished from toddler's diarrhoea, in which there is chronic diarrhoea but no failure to thrive.

Sometimes long-term follow-up is the only way to establish the diagnosis definitively. In view of this, when symptoms have been present for 3 weeks or more after gastroenteritis, if there is any doubt about the diagnosis, a small intestinal biopsy should be performed to demonstrate whether there is any structural abnormality of the small intestinal mucosa. When the mucosa is flat, the diagnosis of coeliac disease must be considered if the child is eating gluten, even though it is known that gastroenteritis *per se* may rarely cause a flat mucosa. However, unlike coeliac disease, intraepithelial lymphocytes are not increased in the postenteritis syndrome. More often a characteristic less severe patch enteropathy is present. Why such persistent mucosal damage occurs in only a minority of children after gastroenteritis is uncertain but, in some children at least, it appears to be due to cow's milk-sensitive enteropathy or other food-sensitive enteropathy.

TODDLER'S DIARRHOEA

This disorder, variously known as toddler's diarrhoea, chronic non-specific diarrhoea, or the irritable colon syndrome,[3] is one of the commonest causes of chronic diarrhoea in childhood.

PATHOGENESIS

It seems most probable that this is a motility disorder. When small intestinal motility has been studied in normal individuals, there is a fasting pattern characterized by recurring migrating complexes which is disrupted within 2 minutes of eating and replaced by random segmenting activity known as the postprandial pattern. In children with toddler's diarrhoea, intraduodenal dextrose fails to disrupt the migrating motor complex. This could play a major role in the pathogenesis of this condition.[7] The small intestinal mucosa in these children is morphologically normal, although there is a significant increase in the specific enzyme activity of adenyl cyclase, and also of Na^+/K^+ – ATPase in small intestinal tissue.[23] This increase could be the response of normal villous cells to crypt cell secretion, which in turn may be mediated via prostaglandins, as high plasma prostaglandin F levels have been reported in children with this syndrome.[10] Whether the colon is also functionally abnormal is not yet clear.

CLINICAL FEATURES

Toddler's diarrhoea usually begins between the age of 6 and 24 months. Often, the child has previously been constipated and sometimes has had infantile colic. It may also be a sequel to acute gastroenteritis. In most children the diarrhoea ceases spontaneously between the ages of 2 and 4 years, sometimes earlier. The stool pattern is, typically, a large stool early in the day, formed or partly formed, followed by the passage of smaller looser stools containing undigested vegetable material and mucus. The passage of undigested food is characteristic; indeed, one popular name for the syndrome stemming from this observation is 'the peas and carrots syndrome'. A severe napkin rash may accompany the diarrhoea. Despite the diarrhoea, the child grows and develops completely normally. Psychosomatic factors may be important, as suggested by the higher proportion of children coming from families of the professional classes. Often the mother may become preoccupied with every stool the child passes, the loose stools causing severe anxiety despite the child's evident general well-being. Sometimes these children are given complicated elimination diets which may even lead to weight loss and unnecessarily add to maternal anxiety.[2]

DIFFERENTIAL DIAGNOSIS

Detailed investigation such as small intestinal biopsies are indicated only when there is some doubt about the child's nutritional status or the presence of other symptoms. There is no evidence of malabsorption of enteric infection. However, giardiasis and sucrase–isomaltase deficiency can sometimes be confused with this disorder, and then biopsy and examination of duodenal juice is helpful. It is also important to differentiate toddler's diarrhoea from cow's milk-sensitive enteropathy, where the small intestinal mucosa is characteristically abnormal, and also from multiple food allergy, where the mucosa may be normal or show only minor abnormality. In this disorder the serum immunoglobulin E level is typically raised, specific radioallergosorbent (RAST) tests are positive, indicating the presence of immunoglobulin E antibodies against specific foodstuffs, and there is often an eosinophilia.[22]

Toddler's diarrhoea should only be considered as the diagnosis when the child is otherwise thriving and in good general health. In some children this diarrhoea may be part of a spectrum of familial functional bowel disorders with continuing gastrointestinal complaints presenting later in life.

TREATMENT

Treatment at the moment ranges from reassurance and explanation to the prescription of drugs. Hamdi and Dodge[10] showed that loperamide gave symptomatic benefit to some children with this syndrome and was as effective in those with raised prostaglandin levels as those without. The widespread use of antidiarrhoeal drugs in paediatrics is to be deplored, but occasionally a child with a severe form of this syndrome benefits from a course of loperamide (although it may be the mother who benefits the most). Such therapy should be given for a limited period only. Elimination diets of any kind are not indicated and their use in this syndrome is to be discouraged. As fruit and vegetables are recognizable in stools these are sometimes excluded, but restriction of these, or of total fat intake, is of no value.[13] Cessation of excess fruit juice ingestion may help produce symptomatic relief.

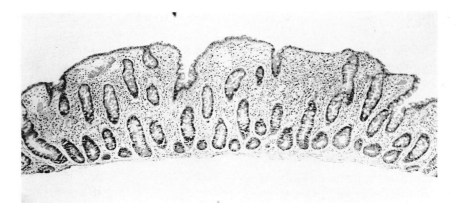

Figure 3.129 Small intestinal mucosa in microvillous atrophy. Light microscope. (From A.D. Phillips, with permission.)

MICROVILLOUS ATROPHY

Microvillous atrophy may be defined as a specific disorder within the syndrome of intractable diarrhoea in infancy which presents shortly after birth and is characterized by a hypoplastic villous atrophy of the small intestinal mucosa and the specific ultrastructural abnormalities of microvillous involutions and increased secretory granules.[20]

PATHOLOGY

Light microscopy of small intestinal biopsies from infants with this disorder demonstrates hypoplastic villous atrophy, i.e. villous atrophy without crypt hypertrophy producing a thin mucosa (*Figure 3.129*). Periodic acid–Schiff staining of the mucosa reveals an abnormal accumulation of periodic acid–Schiff-positive material in upper crypt and villous epithelium with an absence of the usual brush border staining. Any goblet cells present stain normally.

Transmission electron microscopy shows a severely abnormal exposed surface epithelium with the general appearance of short and depleted microvilli. In some instances, microvilli are seen within involutions of the apical membrane, the hallmark of this disease. Large lysosomal bodies are also present, which in some instances contain obvious microvillous fragments. The periodic acid–Schiff-staining material corresponds to the increased numbers of electron-dense secretory granules in the epithelium.

In summary, the ultrastructural features of microvillous atrophy are the following:
1. Enterocyte:
   (a) Severely abnormal exposed surface epithelium
   (b) Short and depleted microvilli
   (c) Microvilli within involutions of apical membrane (*Figure 3.130*).
2. Crypt epithelium:
   (a) Well-preserved microvilli
   (b) Increased electron-dense membrane-bound secretory granules in upper crypt.

Similar changes may also be seen in the colonic mucosa. Thus, both small and large bowel mucosa are affected.

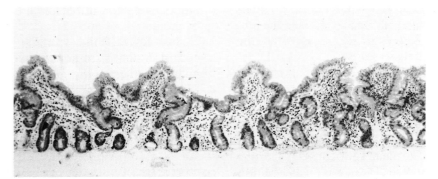

Figure 3.130 Small intestinal mucosa in microvillous atrophy. Characteristic involutions of microvilli within the enterocytes are shown. Electron microscope. (From A.D. Phillips, with permission.)

CLINICAL FEATURES

Typically there is chronic diarrhoea which begins a few days after birth and becomes intractable. At first it may seem that the child has acute gastroenteritis; however, no pathogen is found and the diarrhoea persists. It is often associated with severe dehydration. Frequently there are features of secretory diarrhoea, i.e. the diarrhoea persists when the infant is given intravenous fluids and nil by mouth. Vomiting may occur. Severe malnutrition results from chronic diarrhoea and death occurs in most cases, usually as a result of septicaemia complicating the use of parenteral nutrition.

PROGNOSIS

This disorder is usually fatal but survival is possible with total parenteral alimentation, and this can be carried out at home. Only the distant prospect of small bowel transplant offers any more favourable prognosis.

TREATMENT

Total intravenous alimentation is the only possible therapy. Other measures such as steroids and somatostatin have been unsuccessful.

AUTOIMMUNE ENTEROPATHY

Autoimmune enteropathy is a syndrome of intractable diarrhoea associated with a severe proximal small intestinal enteropathy and the production of specific autoantibodies against gut epithelium.

PATHOLOGY

There is typically a severe enteropathy, sometimes flat, as in coeliac disease and with features of hyperplastic villous atrophy. Like coeliac disease the mucosa is not thin (*Figure 3.131*). Less often the enteropathy may not be so severe.

CLINICAL FEATURES

Fourteen such children with protracted diarrhoea and enterocyte autoantibodies have been reported by Mirakian *et al.*[17] The mean age of onset of chronic diarrhoea was 6.6 months. There was an association with endocrine disorders, namely insulin-dependent diabetes and hypothyroidism. There was also an association with interstitial nephropathy and Still's

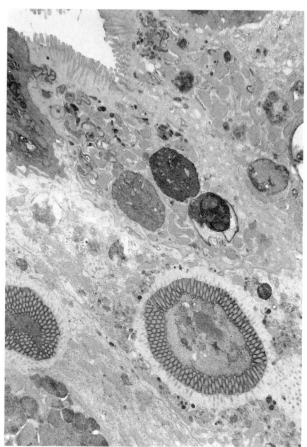

Figure 3.131 Small intestinal mucosa in autoimmune enteropathy. Light microscope. (From A.D. Phillips, with permission.)

disease. There was a family history of a similar syndrome in some cases. This has been a feature of previous reports.

DIAGNOSIS

This is based upon four criteria:

1. Presentation with intractable diarrhoea and a severe small intestinal enteropathy.
2. No clinical response to an exclusion diet or, indeed, a period of complete bowel rest and nil by mouth.
3. No histological response of the enteropathy to an exclusion diet or total parenteral nutrition with nil by mouth.
4. Evidence of autoimmune disease, i.e. circulating gut and other autoantibodies and association with other diseases considered to be autoimmune.

TREATMENT

A milk-free, gluten-free and egg-free diet is recommended in the first instance, but parenteral nutrition may be required. Steroids have been successful in some cases but not in others. A persistently high titre of autoantibodies with complement-fixing ability indicates a poor prognosis. Death may sometimes be the outcome.

REFERENCES

1. Ament, M.E. and Rubin, C.E. (1972) Soy protein – another cause of the flat intestinal lesion. *Gastroenterology*, **62**, 227.

2. Cohen, S.A., Hendricks, K.M., Mathias, R.K. *et al.* (1979) Chronic non-specific diarrhoea: dietary relationships. *Pediatrics*, **64**, 402–407.

3. Davidson, M. and Wasserman, R. (1966) The irritable colon of childhood (chronic non-specific diarrhoea syndrome). *Journal of Pediatrics*, **69**, 1027–1038.

4. Dicke, W.K. (1952) De subactue, chronische en recidiverende darmstoornis van de kleuter. *Nederlandsch Tijdschrift voor Geneeskunde*, **96**, 860.

5. Dormandy, K.M., Waters, A.H. and Mollin, D.L. (1963) Folic acid deficiency coeliac disease. *The Lancet*, **i**, 632.

6. Dowd, B.D. and Walker-Smith, J.A. (1974) Samuel Gee, Aretaeus and the coeliac affection. *British Medical Journal*, **ii**, 45.

7. Fenton, T.R., Harries, J.T. and Milla, P.J. (1988) Disordered small intestinal motility: a rational basis for toddler's diarrhoea. *Gut*,

8. Gee, S.J. (1888) On the coeliac affection. *St Bartholomew's Hospital Reports*, **24**, 17.

9. Goldman, A.S., Anderson, D.W., Sellers, W. *et al.* (1963) Milk allergy. *Pediatrics*, **32**, 425.

10. Hamdi, I. and Dodge, J.A. (1978) Prostaglandins in non-specific diarrhoea. *Acta Paediatrica Belgica*, **31**, 106.

11. Hill, L.W. and Stuart, H.C. (1929) A soy-bean food preparation for feeding infants with milk allergy. *Journal of the American Medical Association*, **93**, 986.

12. Kenrick, K.G. and Walker-Smith, J.A. (1970) Immunoglobulins and dietary protein antibodies in childhood coeliac disease. *Gut*, **11**, 635.

13. Lloyd-Still, J.D. (1979) Chronic diarrhoea of childhood and the misuse of elimination diets. *Journal of Paediatrics*, **95**, 10–13.

14. MacDonald, T.T. and Spencer, J. (1977) Evidence that activated mucosal T cells play a role in the pathogenesis of enteropathy in human small intestine. *Journal of Experimental Medicine*, **167**, 1341–1349.

15. McNeish, A.S., Rolles, C.J. and Arthur, L.J.H. (1976) Criteria for diagnosis of temporary gluten intolerance. *Archives of Disease in Childhood*, **51**, 275.

16. Meeuwisse, G.W. (1970) Diagnostic criteria in coeliac disease. *Acta Paediatrica Scandinavica*, **59**, 461.

17. Mirakiam, R., Richardson, A., Mills, P.J., Walker-Smith, J.A., Unsworth, J., Savage, M.O. and Bottazzo, G.F. (1986) Protracted diarrhoea of infancy: evidence in support of an autoimmune variant. *British Medical Journal*, **293**, 1132–1137.

18. Mortimer, P.E., Stewart, J.S., Norman, A.P. and Booth, C.C. (1968) Follow-up of coeliac disease. *British Medical Journal*, **ii**, 17.

19. Nelson, R., McNeish, A.S. and Anderson, C.M. (1973) Coeliac disease in children of Asian immigrants. *The Lancet*, 348.

20. Phillips, A.D., Jenkins, P., Raafat, F. and Walker-Smith, J.A. (1985) Congenital Microvillous Atrophy. *Archives of Disease in Childhood*, **60**, 135–140.

21. Rudd, P., Manuel, P. and Walker-Smith, J.A. (1981) Anaphylactic shock in infant after feeding with a wheat rusk. A transient phenomenon. *Postgraduate Medical Journal*, **57**, 794–795.

22. Syme, J. (1979) Investigation and treatment of multiple intestinal food allergy in childhood. In: *The Mast Cell*, pp. 438–443 (Eds) Pepys, J. and Edwards, A.M. Tunbridge Wells: Pitman.

23. Tripp, J.H., Manning, J.A., Muller, D.P.P. *et al.* (1978) Abnormalities of intestinal transport systems in the postenteritis syndrome (PES) and toddler 'non-specific' diarrhoea. *Acta Paediatrica Belgica*, **31**, 257.

24. Unsworth, D.J. and Walker-Smith, J.A. (1985) Autoimmunity in diarrhoeal disease. *Journal of Pediatric Gastroenterology and Nutrition*, **4**, 375–381.

25. Vanderschueren-Lodeweyckx, M., Wolter, R., Molla, A. *et al.* (1973) Plasma growth hormone in coeliac disease. *Helvetica Paediatrica Acta*, **28**, 349.

26. Vitoria, J.A., Camarero, C., Sojo, A. *et al.* (1982) Enteropathy related fish, rice and chicken. *Archives of Disease in Childhood*, **57**, 44–48.

27. Walker-Smith, J.A. (1970) Transient gluten intolerance. *Archives of Disease in Childhood*, **45**, 523.

28. Walker-Smith, J.A. (1982) Cow's milk intolerance as a cause of postenteritis diarrhoea. *Journal of Pediatric Gastroenterology and Nutrition*, **1**, 163–175.

29. Walker-Smith, J.A. (1987) Transient gluten intolerance: does it exist? *Netherlands Journal of Medicine*, **92**, 1356–1362.

30. Walker-Smith, J.A., Kilby, A. and France, N.E. (1978) Reinvestigation of children previously diagnosed as coeliac disease. In: Perspectives in Coeliac Disease, pp. 267–277 (Eds) McNicholl, B., McCarthy, C.F. and Fottrell, P.F. Lancaster: MTP Press.

31. Walker-Smith, J.A., Guandalini, S., Schmitz, J., Shmerling, D.H. and Visakorpi, J.K. (1990) Revised criteria for diagnosis of coeliac disease. *Archives of Disease in Childhood*, **65**, 909–911.

DRUG ABSORPTION AND BIOAVAILABILITY

C.W. Howden and M.J. Brodie

THERAPEUTIC CONSIDERATIONS

The small intestine plays a vital role in the absorption of nutrients, minerals and therapeutic drugs. Its mucosa contains metabolic enzymes and its lumen bacteria which may alter the structure and function of a number of exogenous substances, presumably acting as a protective mechanism for the organism. Biliary secretion represents a major route of elimination for some drugs and is particularly important for metabolites. Local hydrolysis in the gut lumen then leads to the enterohepatic cycling of these drugs. All these processes can be altered in the presence of small bowel disease.

DRUG ABSORPTION

The factors influencing the absorption of drugs from the upper gastrointestinal tract are complex (*Table 3.59*) and are governed by the physicochemical properties of the drug.[64]

Although absorption can take place throughout the gastrointestinal tract, all drugs are substantially absorbed in the upper small intestine; the absorptive area has been calculated to be equivalent to two full-size tennis courts. The pH at the mucosal surface varies widely. Lipid-soluble drugs are rapidly absorbed across the mucosal cells by passive diffusion. Absorption of water-soluble drugs is slower and often incomplete. Acidic drugs such as aspirin, phenobarbitone and warfarin might be expected to be ionized in the alkaline contents of the small intestine and therefore be less well absorbed (the un-ionized form will cross biological membranes more readily) but this is compensated for by the enormous absorptive area available. Strong acids or bases (e.g. neostigmine) are completely ionized in aqueous solution and therefore poorly absorbed from all areas of the gut.

The two most important factors affecting drug absorption are the surface area of the small intestine and the rate of gastric emptying. The latter dictates the speed with which a drug reaches the major absorptive surface of the upper jejunum, which influences the time to, and the level of, the peak concentration. Absolute bioavailability is unaffected unless the drug is also metabolized or degraded in the intestinal lumen or wall (*Figure 3.132*).

Table 3.59 Factors influencing drug absorption

Drug characteristics
    Molecular size
    Lipid–water partition coefficient
    Degree of ionization
    Formulation
    Gut metabolism

Patient characteristics
    pH at absorptive site
    Gastric emptying time
    Intestinal motility
    Surface area of small intestine
    Mesenteric blood flow
    Gastrointestinal disease

Other factors
    Large meal
    Interacting drugs

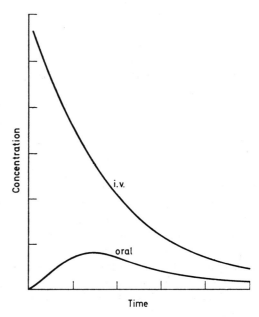

Figure 3.132 A typical concentration time curve for a well-absorbed drug given orally. The time to, and extent of, the peak concentration can be decreased by reducing gastric emptying time and increased by accelerating gastric emptying. The absolute bioavailability of the drugs remains unaltered unless the drug is metabolized or degraded in the gastric wall or lumen.

Table 3.60 Factors affecting drug absorption in disease states

Factor	Disease state	Drug absorption
Reduced gastric acid secretion	Pernicious anaemia	Normal or reduced
Prolonged gastric emptying	Gastric ulcer Migraine Myocardial infarction Chronic pain (Labour)	Normal or reduced
Accelerated gastric emptying	Duodenal ulcer Gastrointestinal surgery	Normal, reduced or increased
Accelerated intestinal transit	Gastroenteritis Crohn's disease	Normal or reduced
Reduced intestinal surface area	Coeliac disease Crohn's disease	Normal, reduced or increased
Steatorrhoea	Coeliac disease Chronic pancreatitis	Normal or reduced
Bacterial colonization	Blind loop syndrome Crohn's disease	Normal or increased
Reduced splanchnic blood flow	Congestive cardiac failure Mesenteric ischaemia	Normal or reduced
Reduced secretion of bile	Obstructive jaundice Primary biliary cirrhosis	Normal or reduced

A number of disease states have been reported to affect drug absorption. As can be seen from *Table 3.60*, the amount of drug absorbed is simultaneously affected by many factors. Upper small bowel disease may change the pattern of absorption, so that more drug is absorbed further down the gastrointestinal tract.[63] This only has clinical relevance if a rapid high peak plasma concentration is important, such as with an antibiotic or analgesic. Gut oedema in patients in congestive cardiac failure may also reduce absorption. In general terms, lipid-soluble drugs continue to be well absorbed even in the face of extensive gastrointestinal disease, whereas the absorption of water-soluble substances is more likely to be impaired.

In a group of patients with treated coeliac disease, plasma levels of propranolol following oral administration were higher than in controls.[54] This was attributed to an increased rate of absorption of propranolol together with saturation of its first-pass metabolism (see below). The absorption of practolol, a more water-soluble compound, was delayed. The absorption of methyldopa was similar in patients with coeliac disease and in controls although absorption was decreased in patients with Crohn's disease.[60]

Because of variability in the physicochemical properties of drugs and in the extent of small intestinal disease in patients, it is difficult to predict the degree of drug malabsorption; in practice it is not usually necessary to alter drug dosage if absorption might be impaired. However, if a patient with gastrointestinal disease does not respond in the expected manner to oral medication, drug malabsorption should be considered.

METABOLISM IN THE GASTROINTESTINAL TRACT

The gut provides protection as well as fulfilling digestive and absorptive functions, with a substantial capacity for metabolism and detoxification of exogenous compounds. Degrading enzymes are present in the gut lumen, in intestinal secretions, and within intestinal microorganisms. The intestine contains a large number of metabolic enzymes responsible for a wide range of chemical biotransformation reactions. Intestinal enzymes can metabolize potentially toxic substances and drugs given therapeutically. The extent of enzyme activity for a particular reaction can approach that of the liver on a weight for weight basis. For most drugs, gastrointestinal metabolism is apparent only when they are given orally.

Intestinal lumen

Enzymes in the gut lumen originate either from exocrine glands or shed mucosal cells. Many enzyme reactions, such as the hydrolysis of pivampicillin, can take place to some extent in the gut lumen.[68]

Intestinal flora

The intestinal microorganisms represent a potent, diverse and adaptable metabolizing force for environmental xenobiotics and drugs. These are capable of performing a number of chemical functions such as hydrolysis, reduction and deconjugation. Gut organisms are responsible for the breakdown of the now banned sweetener cyclamate to cyclohexylamine and the metabolism of the dubious anticancer agent laetrile, with the release of cyanide.[59] Sulphasalazine, which is used principally to maintain remission in ulcerative colitis, undergoes azo reduction by bacteria in the gut lumen (*Figure 3.133*) to sulphapyridine and 5-aminosalicylic acid. It is the latter which is thought to be the active moiety of the drug.[3] Bacterial metabolism is also involved in the breakdown of a number of other drugs, including metronidazole, chloramphenicol and digoxin. This metabolism can be reduced by treatment with a broad-spectrum antibiotic.[39]

Gut wall

Drug metabolism is classically divided into phase 1 and phase 2 reactions involving, respectively, oxidation and conjugating enzymes (*Figure 3.134*). Phase 1 reactions, responsible for oxidation, hydroxylation, dealkylation, reduction and hydrolysis, are present in the intestine[32] although the oxidative metabolic capacity in this site is less than that of the liver on a weight for weight basis. However, when conjugating mechanisms are considered, the activity of the gut wall may even exceed that of the liver for some reactions. Conjugation with glucuronide, sulphate, glutathione and glycine all take place.[13] *N*-Acetylation and *O*-methylation reactions also occur, the latter being an important metabolic pathway for catecholamines.

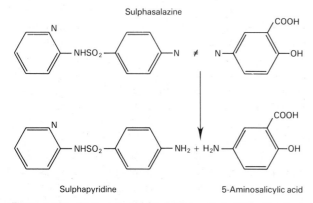

Sulphasalazine

Sulphapyridine   5-Aminosalicylic acid

Figure 3.133 Bacterial azo reduction of sulphasalazine to sulphapyridine and 5-aminosalicylic acid.

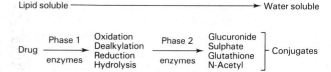

Figure 3.134 Stages of drug metabolism. The gut wall is particularly rich in conjugating enzymes.

The activity of these mucosal enzymes is not static but can be induced by substances in natural foodstuffs such as indoles in vegetables of the genus *Brassica* (e.g. brussels sprouts, cabbage and kale) and polycyclic hydrocarbons produced by cooking procedures such as the charcoal broiling of meat. Cigarette smoke and enzyme-inducing drugs such as phenobarbitone may also increase the synthesis, and hence activity, of gastrointestinal enzymes.

The ability of the gut to perform some metabolic functions, particularly sulphation and glucuronidation, can be saturated by excess substrate since the availability of certain cofactors for these reactions is low in the enterocyte. Inhibition of conjugation can also occur due to competition from other substrates utilizing the same metabolic route. Dose-dependent metabolism can, therefore, occur and this may be responsible for the marked variability of the first-pass metabolism of some drugs.

First-pass metabolism

For oral absorption a drug must pass through the gut wall, largely in the upper jejunum, and from there traverse the liver via the portal circulation. A number of drugs undergo substantial biotransformation on this 'first pass' through to the systemic circulation. For most of these drugs, this presystemic elimination takes place in the liver but for a minority it occurs primarily in the gut wall. Some drugs are metabolized at both sites.[35] Aspirin is rapidly hydrolyzed by esterases to salicylic acid in both the gut wall and liver. The *O*-dealkylation of phenacetin to paracetamol can also take place in the gut wall and this may be accelerated by polycyclic hydrocarbons in charcoal-broiled beef and cigarette smoke.[52] Conjugation of the opioid analgesics morphine and pentazocine, and the oxidation of lignocaine, also appear to have an intestinal component. The phase 2 metabolism of the sympathomimetic amines, such as isoprenaline, salbutamol and terbutaline, occurs largely in the intestinal epithelium[26] and gut wall dopa decarboxylase may be responsible for the high presystemic elimination of levodopa.[2] This peripheral decarboxylation can be inhibited by the concomitant administration of a dopa decarboxylase inhibitor, such as carbidopa or benserazide, which are routinely included in combined preparations used to treat Parkinsonism. Ethinyloestradiol, the most commonly incorporated oestrogenic component of the oral contraceptive pill, is largely sulphated in the small bowel.[5] The dopaminergic antagonist chlorpromazine also undergoes substantial and variable first-pass metabolism in the gut wall.[61]

Tyramine, found in foodstuffs such as cheese, bananas, tomatoes, red wine and yeast extracts, is another substance which is extensively metabolized in the gut. The enzyme involved, monoamine oxidase, can be inhibited by concurrent administration of monoamine oxidase inhibitors including phenelzine and tranylcypromine which are sometimes used as antidepressants. If tyramine is ingested by a patient on a monoamine oxidase inhibitor, large quantities may be absorbed into the general circulation, stimulating noradrenaline release and causing severe hypertension. This was described as the 'cheese reaction'.[55]

The synthesis of 'pro-drugs', which are rapidly converted to the active parent compound within the body, is a pharmacologically attractive concept. Pivampicillin is one such compound which is rapidly hydrolysed to ampicillin largely in the intestinal mucosa.[40] This drug is then absorbed as ampicillin. Other similar 'pro-antibiotics' include talampicillin, bacampicillin and pivmecillinam.

BILIARY EXCRETION OF DRUGS

Excretion in bile plays a relatively minor role in the elimination of unmetabolized drugs, but is a major route for drug metabolites, particularly water-soluble conjugates. Small molecules can passively diffuse into bile and this may account for the elimination of 5–10% of the dose. An active transport system into the bile exists for substances of molecular weight greater than 300 which possess an ionic polar group. Conjugated drug metabolites tend to fulfil both these criteria.

Drugs which have substantial biliary excretion include digitoxin, doxorubicin, steroids and spironolactone.[62] Biliary excretion is an important alternative route for drug elimination in patients with renal failure. The biliary secretion of only a few drugs has been actively studied and recent advances in the methods of bile collection will undoubtedly increase the amount of available information.

A number of conjugated drug metabolites, on entering the alimentary tract in bile, undergo hydrolysis or deconjugation by gut wall enzymes or bacteria to reform the parent compound. The reconstituted drug can then be reabsorbed. A drug

for which such a cycle operates will persist in the body for longer than would have been predicted from single-dose kinetic studies. This phenomenon will produce postabsorption peaks in concentration. This has been described for benzodiazepines, phenothiazines and some of the β-adrenoceptor antagonists.[19] Depending on the concentration gradient and membrane permeability, drugs can also diffuse from the general circulation back into the gastrointestinal lumen.

The effect of blocking the biliary excretion of a drug which is predominantly eliminated by this route will lead to drug accumulation. Interruption of the enterohepatic cycle of a drug may markedly reduce its biological half-life. This is the mechanism by which activated charcoal increases phenobarbitone, carbamazepine and phenylbutazone elimination, suggesting a role for this substance in the management of patients poisoned with these drugs.[38] Similarly, cholestyramine will substantially increase digitoxin clearance by binding in the gut and preventing its enterohepatic circulation.[14] Biliary excretion of drugs will, of course, be impaired if the liver is diseased, particularly in cirrhosis.[34]

UNDESIRABLE EFFECTS OF DRUGS ON THE SMALL BOWEL

Drugs can produce unwanted effects in the small intestine. This may result in interference with the normal processes of absorption of nutrients or of other drugs. Structural as well as functional abnormalities of the intestinal mucosa may be produced.

DRUG-INDUCED MALABSORPTION

Drugs may affect small intestinal function in a number of ways but severe malabsorption only rarely occurs.[22] Colchicine and methotrexate can arrest mitotic activity and hence cell renewal, and may produce a malabsorption syndrome associated with morphological changes of partial villous atrophy. Milder abnormalities in fat and carbohydrate absorption can also be found in patients taking these drugs. Neomycin, methyldopa and p-aminosalicylic acid may damage the intestinal epithelium producing variable degrees of malabsorption.[26,57]

Other drugs implicated in causing malabsorption and steatorrhoea include phenindione, anthraquinone cathartics, tetracycline[46] and allopurinol.[16] The anion exchange resin cholestyramine can bind fat-soluble vitamins as well as bile salts, and deficiency syndromes involving vitamins D and K have been reported.[43]

The fenamates, including mefenamic acid and meclofenamate sodium, have been reported to cause an inflammatory enteritis associated with malabsorption and steatorrhoea,[31,47,56] although they are probably more likely to have adverse effects on the colon. Sulindac may cause small intestinal villous atrophy, anaemia and diarrhoea.[25]

Alcohol, anticonvulsant drugs (particularly phenytoin and primidone), oral contraceptives and methyldopa can all reduce the absorption of folic acid. The mechanism of these effects is complex and not fully understood.[17] Since folic acid is not stored to any appreciable extent, its malabsorption rapidly produces megaloblastic changes in the bone marrow. The biguanides, metformin and phenformin, can interfere with the ileal absorption of vitamin B_{12}.[22]

Aluminium-containing antacids and sucralfate can bind phosphate in the gut. Antacids are given therapeutically to limit phosphate absorption in patients with hyperphosphataemia complicating chronic renal failure as part of the treatment of renal osteodystrophy.

INTESTINAL ULCERATION

Ulceration and perforation of the intestine have been associated with the use of slow-release preparations in which a drug, most notably a formulation of potassium or iron, is incorporated into a wax or plastic matrix. Patients with small bowel strictures such as in Crohn's disease seem particularly at risk.[65]

Non-steroidal anti-inflammatory drugs (NSAIDs) have been heavily implicated in causing damage to the small intestine. There are a number of case reports of small intestinal ulceration or perforation attributed to NSAIDs. In addition to ulceration and fibrous stricture, there are reports of delicate diaphragm-like obstructions narrowing the lumen. Individual drugs which have been implicated include slow-release indomethacin,[15,18,20] conventional preparations of indomethacin[70] and naproxen.[42] Phenylbutazone, little used nowadays, can also produce recurrent ulceration and stricture of the small bowel.[48]

A case–control study of 268 patients admitted to hospital with small or large bowel bleeding or perforation showed a positive association with NSAID ingestion.[37] Patients were more than twice as likely to have taken NSAIDs than controls. However, in a series of 54 patients with small bowel perforation,[21] only five were receiving NSAIDs.

The topic of small intestinal ulceration due to NSAIDs has recently been comprehensively reviewed.[45]

Although truly anti-inflammatory, NSAIDs have paradoxically been reported to induce small intestinal inflammation in some patients.[9] This is represented by an increased uptake of indium-labelled leukocytes in the distal small bowel in up to two-thirds of treated patients. Increased blood and protein loss from the small intestine and small diaphragmatic strictures have been documented in patients on NSAIDs.[10,11] The apparent inflammatory changes in the small intestine appear to be preceded by an increase in the mucosal permeability to normally poorly absorbed marker substances.[8] This defect may be secondary to inhibition of local prostaglandin synthesis by NSAIDs since it is at least partly prevented by pretreating with the prostaglandin E_1 analogue misoprostol.[12] Interestingly, sulphasalazine also reduces the increase in permeability produced by NSAIDs.[6]

SMALL INTESTINAL ISCHAEMIA

Among the many cardiovascular complications of the contraceptive pill, small intestinal ischaemia is one of the least familiar. This condition is associated with a high morbidity and mortality.[23] Although a high oestrogen content is probably the major determinant in causing thrombosis, the progesterone component may also play a part.[44]

DRUG BIOAVAILABILITY INTERACTIONS

Drug absorption interactions are most likely to occur with drugs which are relatively poorly absorbed, particularly if they have a narrow therapeutic index such as digoxin or phenytoin. There are three mechanisms by which such interactions can take place: luminal effects, changes in gastric emptying time, and damage to the gut wall.[41] Interference with the bioavailability of a drug can also be produced by modification of its intestinal first-pass metabolism.

Luminal effects

Chemical reactions between drugs in the upper gastrointestinal tract resulting in treatment failure are probably more common than is appreciated. The best known example is the mutual interaction between ferrous salts and tetracycline, with the absorption of both being reduced.[49]

Antacids can bind a number of different drugs in the gut lumen and so reduce their systemic absorption.[29,33] These include captopril, chlorpromazine, cimetidine, ciprofloxacin, diflunisal, digoxin, isoniazid, ketoconazole, ofloxacin, phenytoin, prednisolone, ranitidine, rifampicin and tetracyclines. Cimetidine has been reported to reduce the absorption of some drugs. By raising intragastric pH, there will be increased dissolution of weak acids and decreased dissolution of weak bases. Drugs whose absorption has been reported to have been affected by this mechanism include ketoconazole, mexiletine, chlormethiazole, tolbutamide and indomethacin.[69] If these effects, which seem slight in any case, are due solely to alteration in intragastric pH, similar though quantitatively greater effects should be seen with other drugs which raise intragastric pH by a greater degree, e.g. omeprazole.

The basic anion exchange resin cholestyramine binds a number of drugs including digoxin, warfarin, paracetamol, penicillin, trimethoprim, tetracyclines, thyroxine and thiazides.[33] Significant reduction of drug absorption can also occur with kaolin–pectin mixtures and neomycin.[1] These interactions only occur when the interacting drugs are given simultaneously and can generally be avoided by separating the doses by at least 2 hours.

Sucralfate, which binds bile salts and phosphate in the gut lumen, also binds other drugs and may reduce their absorption if given concomitantly. These include cimetidine, digoxin, phenytoin and tetracyclines.[33]

Motility effects

A number of drugs including anticholinergics, phenothiazines, tricyclic antidepressants and narcotic analgesics, can slow the rate of gastric emptying. This has been shown to modify the concentration–time profile of a single dose of a number of drugs, producing delayed and attenuated peak concentrations.[51] The total amount of drug absorbed is usually unaltered. This type of interaction has most relevance for therapeutic situations where an early high peak concentration is important, e.g. with analgesics and antibiotics.

Conversely, if gastric emptying is accelerated pharmacologically, earlier and higher peak concentrations of drugs can be produced. The antidopaminergic agents metoclopramide and domperidone, and the indirect cholinomimetic cisapride all accelerate gastric emptying.

Metoclopramide, the most extensively studied, has been shown to accelerate the absorption of paracetamol, levodopa, ethanol and some antibiotics from the upper small intestine.[33] Parenteral metoclopramide rapidly reverses the gastric stasis in severe migraine, restoring acceptable absorption of simple analgesics such as aspirin and paracetamol. Oral metoclopramide is less effective as it must first

reach the upper small bowel to be absorbed. Metoclopramide may reduce the bioavailability of cimetidine although the mechanism has not been fully elucidated.[30]

The effect of both slowing and accelerating the gastric emptying time on the absorption of paracetamol in a single patient is demonstrated in *Figure 3.135*.

Enterotoxic effects

A number of drugs may themselves cause damage to the absorptive surface of the small intestine and thus reduce the bioavailability of other drugs. Although reported interactions are few, this may be an underestimate, particularly in patients receiving chemotherapy for malignant disease. Cancer at various sites may cause villous atrophy in the jejunum, and this will be exacerbated by additional chemotherapy or radiotherapy.[67] Malabsorption of orally administered drugs probably occurs in this situation and has been documented for phenytoin.[24]

Neomycin, colchicine and the now superseded antituberculous agent *p*-aminosalicylic acid have also been implicated in this form of drug interaction.[26]

First-pass metabolism interactions

There is some evidence that drugs employing the same route of presystemic metabolism will compete for binding sites on the enzymes involved.[28] Thus, salicylamide has been found to inhibit isoprenaline conjugation in the canine gut wall, increasing its systemic bioavailability.[7] Similarly in humans,

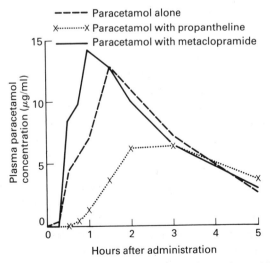

Figure 3.135 The effect of propantheline and metoclopramide on paracetamol absorption in a 22-year-old man. (Reproduced, with permission, from Nimmo *et al.*[50])

presystemic elimination of ethinyloestradiol by sulphate conjugation is inhibited by concomitant ascorbic acid administration[4] so that plasma levels of ethinyloestradiol are increased. Care, therefore, should be taken if combining two drugs metabolized by the same enzymes in the gut wall.

DIFFICULTIES IN DRUG ADMINISTRATION CONSEQUENT UPON GASTROINTESTINAL DISEASE

Chronic, often painful, conditions such as Crohn's disease are associated with a disinclination to eat, particularly since food may precipitate pain or diarrhoea. This may be extended to oral medications and so compliance with complicated drug schedules may be erratic. This will be further compounded if the patient is experiencing nausea or vomiting.

Drug absorption may be unpredictable in Crohn's disease due to inflammatory activity or to one of the complications of the disease such as enteroenteric fistula, stricture formation or secondary bacterial overgrowth. Surgical resection will limit the surface area available for drug absorption although, in practice, this is not usually a problem. Involvement of the terminal ileum in the inflammatory process or its previous surgical resection will interrupt the enterohepatic recirculation of drugs normally eliminated by that route.

The absorption of prednisolone is reduced in some patients with Crohn's disease affecting the small intestine.[66] This may contribute to the variability in favourable response to oral steroids seen in this condition and to the apparent unpredictability of steroid-related adverse effects.

Patients with bowel strictures, as in Crohn's disease, should not be prescribed slow-release preparations of potassium salts or NSAIDs because of the dangers, as mentioned above, of small intestinal ulceration and perforation. In addition, there is growing evidence that NSAIDs may induce relapse in inflammatory bowel disease[36,58,71] and so should probably be avoided in such patients.

Drug absorption may be delayed or reduced in patients with coeliac disease. However, the situation is complex since some drugs, including various antibiotics such as fusidic acid, trimethoprim and sulphamethoxazole, are better absorbed in patients with coeliac disease.[53] This has been attributed to a generalized increase in small intestinal permeability in coeliac disease.

Some patients with ulcerative colitis are genuinely intolerant to oral iron supplements, which can cause severe diarrhoea or even disease relapse. If such patients are found to be iron-deficient, parenteral iron administration may be an appropriate option if oral iron is not tolerated.

REFERENCES

1. Aarons, L. (1981) Kinetics of drug–drug interactions. *Pharmacology and Therapeutics*, **14**, 321–344.
2. Abrams, W.B., Coutinho, C.B., Leon, A.S. and Spiegal, H.E. (1971) Absorption and metabolism of levodopa. *Journal of the American Medical Association*, **218**, 1912–1914.
3. Azad Khan, A.K., Piris, J. and Truelove, S.C. (1977) An experiment to determine the active therapeutic moiety of sulphasalazine. *The Lancet*, **ii**, 892–895.
4. Back, D.J., Breckenridge, A.M., MacIver, M. *et al.* (1981) Interaction with ethinyloestradiol with ascorbic acid in man. *British Medical Journal*, **282**, 1516.
5. Back, D.J., Breckenridge, A.M., MacIver, M. *et al.* (1982) The gut wall metabolism of ethinyloestradiol in humans. *British Journal of Clinical Pharmacology*, **13**, 325–337.
6. Banerjee, A.K., Sherwood, R., Rennie, J.A. and Peters, T.J. (1990) Sulphasalazine reduces indomethacin induced changes in small intestinal permeability in man. *Gut*, **31**, A593(Abstract).
7. Bennett, P.N., Blackwell, E.W. and Davies, D.S. (1975) Competition for sulphate during detoxification in the gut. *Nature*, **258**, 247–248.
8. Bjarnason, I., Williams, P., So, A. *et al.* (1984) Intestinal permeability and inflammation in rheumatoid arthritis: effects of non-steroidal anti-inflammatory drugs. *The Lancet*, **ii**, 1171–1174.
9. Bjarnason, I., Zanelli, G., Smith, T. *et al.* (1987) Non-steroidal anti-inflammatory drug-induced intestinal inflammation in humans. *Gastroenterology*, **93**, 480–489.
10. Bjarnason, I., Zanelli, G., Prouse, P. *et al.* (1987) Blood and protein loss via intestinal inflammation induced by non-steroidal anti-inflammatory drugs. *The Lancet*, **ii**, 711–714.
11. Bjarnason, I., Price, A.B., Zanelli, G. *et al.* (1988) Clinicopathological features of non-steroidal anti-inflammatory drug-induced small intestinal strictures. *Gastroenterology*, **94**, 1070–1074.
12. Bjarnason, I., Smethurst, P., Fenn, G., *et al.* (1989) Misoprostol reduces indomethacin-induced changes in human small intestinal permeability. *Digestive Diseases and Sciences*, **34**, 407–411.
13. Caldwell, I. and Marsh, M.V. (1982) Metabolism of drugs by the gastrointestinal tract. In: *Presystemic Drug Elimination*, pp. 29–42 (Eds) George, C.F., Shand, D.G. and Renwick, A.G. London: Butterworth.
14. Caldwell, J.H., Bush, C.A. and Greenberger, N.J. (1971) Interruption of the enterohepatic circulation

of digitoxin by cholestyramine. *Journal of Clinical Investigation*, **50**, 2638–2644.

15. Calin, A. (1984) Intestinal perforation associated with osmotic slow release indomethacin capsules. *British Medical Journal*, **288**, 240–241.

16. Chen, B., Shapira, J., Ravid, M. and Lang, R. (1982) Steatorrhoea induced by allopurinol. *British Medical Journal*, **284**, 1914.

17. Clark, F. (1981) Disorders of metabolism II. In: *Textbook of Adverse Drug Reactions*, pp. 330–405 (Ed.) Davies, D.M. Oxford: Oxford University Press.

18. Cree, I.A., Walker, M.A., Wright, M. and Forrester, J.C. (1985) Osmosin and ileal ulceration: a case report. *Scottish Medical Journal*, **30**, 40–41.

19. Curry, S. (1977) Disposition and fate. In: *Drug Disposition and Pharmacokinetics*, pp. 62–64. Oxford: Oxford University Press.

20. Day, T.K. (1983) Intestinal perforation associated with osmotic slow release indomethacin capsules. *British Medical Journal*, **287**, 1671–1672.

21. Dixon, J.M. and Lumsden, A.B. (1985) Anti-inflammatory drugs and bowel perforations and haemorrhage. *British Medical Journal*, **290**, 788.

22. Douglas, A.P. and Bateman, D.N. (1981) Gastrointestinal disorders. In: *Textbook of Adverse Drug Reactions*, pp. 202–215 (Ed.) Davies, D.M. Oxford: Oxford University Press.

23. Editorial (1978) Small-bowel ischaemia and the contraceptive pill. *British Medical Journal*, **i**, 4.

24. Fincham, R.W. and Schottelius, D.D. (1979) Decreased phenytoin levels in antineoplastic therapy. *Therapeutic Drug Monitoring*, **1**, 277–283.

25. Freeman, H.J. (1986) Sulindac associated small bowel lesion. *Journal of Clinical Gastroenterology*, **8**, 569–571.

26. George, C.F. and Holdstock, G.E. (1985) Drug-induced disorders. In: *Drugs of the Small Intestine*, pp. 398–412 (Eds) Booth, C.C. and Neale, G. London: Blackwell.

27. George, C.F., Blackwell, E.W. and Davies, D.S. (1974) Metabolism of isoprenaline in the intestine. *Journal of Pharmacy and Pharmacology*, **26**, 265–267.

28. Grimmer, M. (1984) Gut wall metabolism. In: *Clinical Pharmacology and the Gut. Proceedings of the Fifth BSG.SK&F International Workshop*, pp. 1–4 (Ed.) Langman, M.J.S. Welwyn Garden City: Smith Kline & French.

29. Gugler, R. and Allgayer, H. (1990) Effects of antacids on the clinical pharmacokinetics of drugs: an update. *Clinical Pharmacokinetics*, **18**, 210–219.

30. Gugler, R., Brand, M. and Somogyi, A. (1981) Impaired cimetidine absorption due to antacids and metoclopramide. *European Journal of Clinical Pharmacology*, **20**, 225–228.

31. Hall, R.I., Petty, A.H., Cobden, I. and Lendrum, R. (1983) Enteritis and colitis associated with mefenamic acid. *British Medical Journal*, **287**, 1182.

32. Hartiala, K. (1973) Metabolism of hormones, drugs and other substances by the gut. *Physiological Reviews*, **53**, 496–534.

33. Howden, C.W. (1990) Drug interactions and the gastroenterologist. *GI Futures and Clinical Practice* Reviewed by C.W. Howden and M.J. Brodie, 1989.

34. Howden, C.W., Birnie, G.G. and Brodie, M.J. (1989) Drug metabolism in liver disease. *Pharmacology and Therapeutics*, **40**, 439–474.

35. Ilett, K.F. and Davies, D.S. (1982) In vivo studies of gut wall metabolism. In: *Presystemic Drug Elimination*, pp. 43–65 (Eds) George, C.F., Shand, D.G. and Renwick, A.G. London: Butterworth.

36. Kaufmann, H.J. and Taubin, H.L. (1987) Non-steroidal anti-inflammatory drugs activate quiescent inflammatory bowel disease. *Annals of Internal Medicine*, **107**, 513–516.

37. Langman, M.J.S., Morgan, L. and Worrall, A. (1985) Use of anti-inflammatory drugs by patients admitted with small or large bowel perforations and haemorrhage. *British Medical Journal*, **290**, 347–349.

38. Levy, G. (1982) Gastrointestinal clearance of drugs with activated charcoal. *New England Journal of Medicine*, **307**, 676–678.

39. Lindenbaum, J., Rund, D., Butler, V.P., Tse-Eng, D. and Saha, J.R. (1981) Inactivation of digoxin by the gut flora: reversal by antibiotic therapy. *New England Journal of Medicine*, **305**, 789–794.

40. Lund, B., Lampmann, J.P., Lindahl, F. and Hansen, J.M. (1976) Pivampicillin and ampicillin in bile, portal and peripheral blood. *Clinical Pharmacology and Therapeutics*, **19**, 587–591.

41. McInnes, G.T. and Brodie, M.J. (1988) Drug interactions that matter – a critical reappraisal. *Drugs*, **36**, 83–110.

42. Madhok, R., Mackenzie, J.A., Lee, F.D. *et al.* (1986) Small bowel ulceration and perforation in patients receiving non-steroidal anti-inflammatory drugs for rheumatoid arthritis. *Quarterly Journal of Medicine*, **58**, 53–58.

43. Matsui, M.S. and Rosovski, S.J. (1982) Drug-nutrient interaction. *Clinical Therapeutics*, **4**, 423–440.

44. Meade, T.W., Greenberg, G. and Thompson, S.G. (1980) Progestogens and cardiovascular reactions associated with oral contraceptives. *British Medical Journal*, **280**, 1157–1161.

45. Mills, P.R. (1988) Small intestinal ulceration. *Current Opinion in Gastroenterology*, **4**, 260–276.

46. Mitchell, T.H., Stamp, T.C.B. and Jenkins, M.V. (1982) Steatorrhoea after tetracycline. *British Medical Journal*, **285**, 780.

47. Moeller, D.D. (1987) Steatorrhoea associated with meclofenamate sodium therapy. *American Journal of Gastroenterology*, **82**, 1320–1321.

48. Neoptolemos, J.P. and Locke, T.J. (1983) Recurrent small bowel obstruction associated with phenylbutazone. *British Journal of Surgery*, **70**, 244–245.

49. Neuvonen, P.J., Pentikainen, P.J. and Gothoni, G.

(1975) Inhibition of iron absorption by tetracycline. *British Journal of Clinical Pharmacology*, **2**, 94–96.

50. Nimmo, J., Heading, R.C., Tothill, P. and Prescott, L.H. (1973) Pharmacological modification of gastric emptying: effects of propantheline and metoclopramide on paracetamol absorption. *British Medical Journal*, i, 587–589.

51. Nimmo, W.S. (1976) Drugs, diseases and altered gastro emptying. *Clinical Pharmacokinetics*, **1**, 189–203.

52. Pantuck, E.J., Hsaio, K.-C., Conney, A.H. *et al.* (1976) Effect of charcoal-broiled beef on phenacetin metabolism in man. *Science*, **194**, 1055–1057.

53. Parsons, R.L., Hossack, G.A. and Paddock (1975) The absorption of antibiotics in adult patients with coeliac disease. *Journal of Antimicrobial Chemotherapy*, **1**, 39–50.

54. Parsons, R.L, Kaye, C.M., Raymond, K., Trounce, J.R. and Turner, P. (1976) Absorption of propranolol and practolol in coeliac disease. *Gut*, **17**, 139–143.

55. Pettinger, W.A. and Oates, J.A. (1968) Supersensitivity to tyramine during monoamine oxidase inhibition in man. *Clinical Pharmacology and Therapeutics*, **9**, 341–344.

56. Phillips, M.S., Fehilly, B., Stewart, S. and Dronfield, M.W. (1983) Enteritis and colitis associated with mefenamic acid. *British Medical Journal*, **287**, 1626.

57. Race, T.F., Paes, K. and Faloon, W.W. (1970) Intestinal malabsorption induced by oral colchicine. Comparison with neomycin and cathartic agents. *American Journal of Medical Sciences*, **259**, 32.

58. Rampton, D.S. and Sladen, G.E. (1981) Relapse of protocolitis during treatment with non-steroidal anti-inflammatory drugs. *Postgraduate Medical Journal*, **57**, 297–299.

59. Renwick, A.G. (1982) First-pass metabolism within the lumen of the gastrointestinal tract. In: *Presystemic Drug Elimination*, pp. 3–28 (Eds) George, C.F., Shand, D.G. and Renwick, A.G. London: Butterworth.

60. Renwick, A.G., Higgins, V., Powers, K., Smith, C.L. and George, C.F. (1983) The absorption and conjugation of methyldopa in patients with coeliac and Crohn's disease during treatment. *British Journal of Clinical Pharmacology*, **16**, 77–83.

61. Rivera-Calimlim, L., Castenada, L. and Lasagna, L. (1973) Effect of mode of management on plasma chlorpromazine in psychiatric patients. *Clinical Pharmacology and Therapeutics*, **14**, 978–986.

62. Rollins, D.E. and Klaassen, C.D. (1979) Biliary excretion of drugs in man. *Clinical Pharmacokinetics*, **4**, 368–379.

63. Sandle, G.I., Ward, A., Rawlins, M.D. and Record, C.O. (1982) Propranolol absorption in untreated coeliac disease. *Clinical Science*, **63**, 81–85.

64. Scott, A.K. and Hawksworth, G.M. (1981) Drug absorption. *British Medical Journal*, **282**, 462–463.

65. Shaffer, J.A., Higham, C. and Turnberg, L.A. (1980) Hazards of slow-release preparations in patients with bowel strictures. *The Lancet*, **ii**, 487.

66. Shaffer, J.A., Williams, S.E., Turnberg, L.A., Houston, J.B. and Rowland, M. (1983) Absorption of prednisolone in patients with Crohn's disease. *Gut*, **24**, 182–186.

67. Shaw, M.T., Spector, M.H. and Ladman, A.J. (1979) Effect of cancer, radiotherapy and cytotoxic drugs on intestinal structure and function. *Cancer Treatment Reviews*, **6**, 141–151.

68. Shindo, H., Fukuda, K., Kawai, K. and Tanaka, K. (1978) Studies on intestinal absorption of pivampicillin and species differences in the intestinal esterase activity. *Journal of Pharmacobiodynamics*, **1**, 310–323.

69. Somogyi, A. and Muirhead, M. (1987) Pharmacokinetic interactions of cimetidine 1987. *Clinical Pharmacokinetics*, **12**, 321–366.

70. Stewart, J.T., Pennington, C.R. and Pringle, R. (1985) Anti-inflammatory drugs and bowel perforations and haemorrhage. *British Medical Journal*, **290**, 787–788.

71. Walt, R.P., Hawkey, C.J. and Langman, M.J.S. (1984) Colitis associated with non-steroidal anti-inflammatory drugs. *British Medical Journal*, **288**, 238.

THERAPEUTIC NUTRITION

G.L. Hill

Since the introduction of total parenteral nutrition as a safe form of therapy for the restoration and maintenance of protein and energy stores of patients with gastroenterological disease, the relevance and importance of nutrition has become increasingly recognized. Nutritional disorders resulting from severe gastrointestinal pathology can now be effectively treated and there is growing awareness of the prevalence and prognostic implications of malnutrition in hospital patients.

NORMAL DIETARY REQUIREMENTS

ENERGY

A basic requirement of living organisms is for energy to maintain cellular function and structure. Energy is stored as chemical energy inherent in the covalent bonding structure of the terminal phosphate group of the ATP molecule. ATP is free to diffuse to sites where energy is required in the cell. Although some ATP is formed from glycolytic pathways outside the mitochondria, most is formed within the mitochondria in the tricarboxylic cycle. The major body store of energy is fat, with a limited amount of carbohydrate stored as glycogen. Protein is not an energy store as such, but structural–cellular proteins are used as an energy source through gluconeogenesis in some situations.

Energy requirements

A patient's total daily requirement for energy is the sum of his or her resting metabolic expenditure, his or her dietary-induced energy expenditure, and his or her activity energy expenditure.

Resting metabolic expenditure is closely related to the fat-free body mass and represents the energy necessary for the work of the heart and lungs, work for the synthesis of new chemical bondings and work to maintain electrochemical gradients in cells. Approximately 97 kJ/(kg/day) (23 kcal(kg/day)) is usually required by normal adults for basal energy expenditure.[51]

Activity energy expenditure depends on the amount of physical work performed, and varies in active people from 2 MJ (500 kcal) per day in sedentary individuals to 13 MJ (3000 kcal) per day for manual labourers. In hospital patients spending much of the day lying in bed it is less than 2 MJ per day, although this will be increased if the patients are restless or hypoxic. In addition, there is energy expended in the assimilation of nutrients, whether given by mouth or vein. This is called *dietary-induced thermogenesis*, and it varies with the type of food ingested and the metabolic state of the patient. For example, protein sufficient to provide 1 MJ increases the basal metabolic rate by 300 kJ, whereas 1 MJ of glucose increases it by 60 kJ and 1 MJ of fat increases it by 40 kJ. In very septic patients, a high glucose intake may induce a significant rise in dietary-induced thermogenesis, an effect which is not seen with similar intakes of fat. Sick gastroenterological patients may have additional energy requirements due to fever, major surgery, sepsis and disseminated carcinoma.[53]

Generally speaking, gastroenterological patients having intravenous feeding require about 170 kJ/(kg/day) (40 kcal/(kg/day)) to reach energy balance.[74] Depleted patients have a lesser requirement for energy but if there is extensive sepsis or widespread inflammatory bowel disease, energy requirements will be around 170 kJ/(kg/day).[26] It is important to remember that it can be quite difficult to administer high-energy intakes to very sick patients. In particular, glucose is not oxidized at high rates of energy intake and fat may be needed as a substitute if energy balance is to be attained.[7,54]

Increasingly, nutrition support teams are measuring resting energy expenditure (REE) directly using some form of indirect calorimetry (metabolic carts) and this makes the process much simpler. For tissue preservation multiply REE by 1.3; for tissue repletion multiply REE by 1.5.

Energy sources

Carbohydrate

Carbohydrate is an essential energy source for the brain, erythrocytes, neural tissue, renal medulla and cells involved in inflammation and repair. Sixty per cent of ingested glucose is phosphorylated in the liver to glucose 6-phosphate and is then converted to glycogen, fatty acids or blood glucose. Carbohydrate is stored as glycogen in the liver (1.3 MJ or 300 kcal) and in muscle (2.5 MJ or 600 kcal) but these stores are rapidly depleted in fasting (in 18 hours) and exercise (in minutes). Carbohydrate sources provided in commercially available enteral diets include sucrose, liquid glucose (corn syrup), lactose, maltodextrins and starch. For intravenous use glucose is the safest and most widely used energy source in therapeutic nutrition, but alternative carbohydrate energy sources are fructose, maltose and the polyols sorbitol, xylitol and glycerol.

Fat

Fat is the main energy store of the body, accounting for over 400 MJ (100 000 kcal). Besides insulating and protective functions, its main reason for existence is as an energy store. Some fat is stored as triglyceride in adipose tissue and transported in various forms (lipoprotein complexes) to sites where energy is required. In fasting states, fat is metabolized by the liver to ketone bodies, and this decreases the glucose requirements of neural tissue.[4]

There is a group of fats with unsaturated bonds in their carbon chains which are precursors of prostaglandins and are considered essential fatty acids.

About 4% of the total energy intake should consist of such polyunsaturated fats from vegetable sources, according to recommended dietary allowances. Normal ratios of fatty acids in the blood are maintained if 1–2% of energy is supplied as linoleic acid.[26] For clinical use, fat is supplied in commercially available enteral preparations as whole-milk fat, vegetable oil, coconut oil or hydrogenated soya oil. Medium-chain triglycerides are indicated for some malabsorption states and when long-chain fatty acids are contraindicated. For intravenous use, fat is supplied as soya bean or safflower oil emulsions, which have the same properties as chylomicrons.

PROTEIN

Protein forms 16% of the body mass and forms its major structural component, being an integral part of cell walls, cytoplasm, nuclei and intracellular matrix. Any breakdown of protein as an energy source, therefore, will have an effect on structure and compromise body function. Collagen is the main extracellular protein of the body, while actin and myosin form a large part of intracellular total body protein. Plasma proteins play an important part in immunological and transport functions and have effects in processes of inflammation and repair.

Protein requirements

Because body protein is constantly being broken down and remodelled, a certain amount of nitrogen from the pool of amino acids is excreted as urea and needs to be replaced. About 50 g/day (100 mg N/(kg/day)) of good-quality protein is required to balance this loss.[16] Quality of protein, however, is important and, while a Western diet may contain more than twice the amount of protein required, the biological value of that protein may only be 50%.

There are eight essential amino acids (isoleucine, leucine, lysine, methionine, phenylalanine, threonine, tryptophan and valine), which cannot be synthesized from other amino acids in the body. Amino acids absorbed from the intestine are used by the liver for manufacture of export proteins and to maintain constant turnover in peripheral tissues. The process of gluconeogenesis occurs to supply essential glucose requirements in starvation. It also occurs in catabolic states such as trauma and sepsis.[7] With excess protein, the liver can eliminate amino acids, form urea, and feed the remaining carbon chains into the Krebs cycle for energy production. When the liver is damaged, urea synthesis may stop and free ammonia ions are formed.

The protein requirements of gastroenterological patients on parenteral feeding regimens vary according to their nutritional and metabolic state. Gastroenterological patients require 1.0–1.5 g protein/(kg/day) of good-quality protein and, unless very septic, there is no improvement in protein sparing with increased amounts.[69]

This greatly exceeds recommended dietary allowances for normal subjects.[16] With adequate intakes of protein all gastroenterological patients will have increases in whole body protein synthesis. In non septic protein depleted patients this leads to gains in whole body protein but those who are septic, particularly those who are not depleted cannot be repleted of body protein.[43] The best that can be expected is a reduction in the loss that would have otherwise occurred[69]

Protein sources

From a therapeutic point of view, protein can be given either enterally or by the intravenous route. Enteral protein sources are supplied as calcium or sodium caseinates, soy protein isolate, whey protein and lactalbumin. The form of protein can influence absorption in gastroenterological patients. Peptide based diets may be better absorbed than amino acid diets.[56,72,73] Intravenous protein requirements can be supplied either as protein hydrolysates or as synthetic crystalline amino acid solutions. Although protein hydrolysates may produce a positive nitrogen balance, they are less effective than crystalline amino acids and have more often been associated with adverse effects.[52] Special amino acid mixtures may be required in renal failure[33] and hepatic failure,[44,57] although indications for their use have not yet been clearly defined.

INTERRELATIONSHIPS OF PROTEIN AND ENERGY

Within certain limits of energy and protein intake there is a region where increases in either will result in protein retention.[26] Normally-nourished patients lay down protein only when energy requirements are met but depleted patients retain protein at lesser energy intakes. In this respect depleted patients behave as growing children.[43] Nevertheless, authorities agree that high rates of restoration of lean body mass require high protein intake and that by proper manipulation of energy and protein intake it is possible to increase lean body mass or body fat in proportions appropriate to the individual.[26,40]

Table 3.61 Recommended daily allowances of vitamins

Vitamin	Action	Effect of deficiency	Dietary[a]	Intravenous[b]
Water-soluble				
Thiamine (B_1)	Glucose metabolism	Beriberi	1.4 mg	3 mg
Riboflavine (B_2)	Energy transfer	Glossitis, chelosis	1.6 mg	3.6 mg
Nicotinic acid (niacin) (B_3)	Energy transfer	Pellagra	18 mg	40 mg
Pyridoxine (B_6)	Decarboxylation and transamination	Convulsions	2.2 mg	4 mg
Pantothenic acid	Part of coenzyme A	Dermatitis, enteritis	NR	15 mg
Folate	Coenzyme with B_{12}	Anaemia	400 μg	400 μg
B_{12}	Coenzyme in nucleic acid synthesis	Pernicious anaemia	3 μg	5 μg
C	Collagen synthesis	Scurvy	60 mg	100 mg
Fat-soluble				
A	Visual pigments	Night blindness	1000 μg RE[c]	1135 μg RE[c]
D	Calcium and phosphate utilization	Rickets	5 μg	5 μg
E	Energy transfer	?	10 mg[d]	210 mg[d]
K	Prothrombin synthesis	Bleeding disorder	NR	500 μg

NR, no recommendation.
[a] Committee on Dietary Allowances (1980) (males 23–50 years old).[16]
[b] Nutrition Advisory Group (1979a).[60]
[c] Retinol equivalents: 1 μg of retinol equivalent corresponds to 1 μg of retinol or 6 μg of betacarotene.
[d] α-tocopherol equivalents: 1 mg of α-tocopherol equivalent has the same activity as 1 mg of $(+)$-α-tocopherol.

VITAMINS AND TRACE ELEMENTS

Vitamins

Vitamins are organic substances required to maintain normal cellular activity. Deficiency states do not usually single out a particular vitamin and the clinical syndromes observed often combine deficiencies of protein, energy and multiple vitamins. *Table 3.61* shows the major vitamins, their normal action, the effects of deficiency, and the recommended daily allowances. Recommended intravenous allowances are based on dietary allowances in healthy individuals and patients with deficiencies will need more.[60]

Trace elements

Trace elements are found in micromolar amounts in the tissues and are essential for normal cellular function. The place of iron in haem, cobalt in vitamin B_{12} and iodine in thyroid metabolism has been known for some time. Deficiencies of zinc, copper, selenium and chromium have also been described and these are listed along with other elements considered essential in *Table 3.62*.[61]

Zinc is one important element which often needs to be given in increased amounts in gastroenterological patients.[80] About 2 mg/day of elemental zinc is lost in the urine and this increases with sepsis or injury. Patients with diarrhoea or ileostomies lose about 17 mg/l, but with a high small bowel fistula the losses are less (12 mg/l). If zinc is given as zinc sulphate, the elemental requirement needs to be multiplied by 2.5. As only 20% of orally administered zinc is absorbed, a further multiplication by 5 is required if given orally. Zinc levels in the blood reflect zinc ingestion rather than balance. While 4 mg of elemental zinc is sufficient for parenteral regimens to maintain most patients in zinc balance, many gastroenterological patients will require more than this, and 10 mg as a basic requirement is suggested.

Copper requirements are not increased in gastroenterological patients above 300–500 μg/day.[71]

Other elements listed in *Table 3.62* have not been specifically studied in gastroenterological patients.

ASSESSMENT OF NUTRITIONAL STATUS

Surveys of hospital patients in Western countries have revealed a high incidence of protein-energy malnutrition.[42] Nutritional assessment should make it possible to select patients whose nutritional status adversely affects the outcome of their illness. Clinically significant malnutrition which may also be called nutritional depletion may be defined as that

Table 3.62 Recommended daily allowances of trace elements

Element	Effect of deficiency	Dietary[a]	Intravenous
Zinc	Impaired wound healing and growth, dermatitis, alopecia	15 mg	2.5–4 mg[b] 4–14 mg
Copper	Anaemia, neutropenia, bone demineralization	2–3 mg	0.5–1.5 mg[b]
Chromium	Impaired glucose handling	0.05–0.2 mg	10–15 μg[b]
Iodine	Goitre, hypothyroidism	150 μg	150 μg
Iron	Anaemia	10–30 mg	1–4 mg
Fluorine	Dental susceptibility to caries	1.5–4 mg	0.4 mg
Manganese	Vitamin K deficiency	2.5–5.0 mg	0.15–0.8 mg[b]
Molybdenum	?	0.15–0.5 μg	20 μg
Selenium	Muscle weakness and pain	0.05–0.2 mg	40–120 μg

[a] Committee on Dietary Allowances (1980).[16]
[b] Nutrition Advisory Group (1979b).[61]

degree of tissue loss which results in physiological impairment. Patients with more than 20% weight loss almost always have a number of physiological impairments, and those with less than 10% weight loss almost never. Those with losses of weight in between usually have some measure of physiological impairment, but it may be of no significance clinically.[79] For this reason, broadly based nutritional syndromes are suggested here to aid assessment and give guidance in the management of patients with nutritional disorders.[40]

NUTRITIONAL SYNDROMES

Gastroenterological patients can be affected by two metabolic and nutritional processes. Semi-starvation in patients with anorexia, vomiting or a partial obstruction results in gradual wasting of muscle and fat stores, with lowered metabolic rate. Compensatory mechanisms are designed to conserve energy and body protein. Sepsis or other severe types of stress result in rapid breakdown of protein for gluconeogenesis with raised metabolic rate. Compensatory mechanisms are designed to provide essential protein and energy components for healing and repair. From the combination of these two processes, semi-starvation and stress, four nutritional syndromes can be identified.

The normal state

The majority of gastroenterological patients do not have a clinically relevant nutritional problem. Food intake has been normal, they are not septic and clinically they have normal stores of subcutaneous fat and muscle. Such patients can be maintained on an adequate oral diet unless the pathology of their disorder requires a specific therapeutic measure

(such as a gluten-free diet in coeliac disease). After surgery there is a loss of body weight (about 6%) and a temporary fall in plasma protein levels. These plasma protein levels return to normal when normal oral intake resumes, usually during the second post-operative week.

Nutritional depletion

Patients with this syndrome have an overall deficit in their intake or utilization of food or both. Weight loss is marked, with clinical evidence of sub-cutaneous fat loss and wasting of muscles. Metabolic rate is low and urinary nitrogen loss is small. Plasma proteins remain normal. There will also be loss of physiological function which has occurred over the same time period as the loss of weight, there may be difficulties with wound healing, or a history of easy tiredness or change in exercise tolerance. Grip strength and respiratory muscle function will usually be clinically impaired.[14] Examples of this syndrome include cachexia seen in patients with strictures of the oesophagus or cancer of the stomach. The patient, if the condition is severe, looks like a 'walking skeleton'.

Normal with sepsis

These patients are usually quite easily picked out, for they either are septic or have recently been so. In gastroenterological patients the classic causes of this syndrome are acute attacks of inflammatory bowel disease and pancreatic abscess. Clinically, such patients may have normal stores of muscle and fat, but there are clear signs of sepsis and plasma albumin levels are low. If this situation persists muscle wasting follows, although fat stores are preserved (see below). Nutritional therapy will be required in these patients if the acute disease lasts more than 5–7 days, for after this time there is increasing incidence of nutritional depletion and physiological impairment.

Nutritional depletion and sepsis

This occurs in two situations: (1) in depleted patients who have a metabolic insult such as sepsis, or a major operation; or (2) in normally nourished patients who have a severe metabolic stress and rapidly become depleted of their nutritional reserves. Examples of the first situation are depleted patients with carcinoma of the oesophagus or stomach who develop septic complications after oesophagectomy or gastrectomy. Examples of the second situation are normally nourished patients with prolonged severe pancreatitis with sepsis, or prolonged exacerbations of colitis. These patients are obviously unwell, with tachycardia, fever and low intravascular volume. However, the degree of depletion may not be apparent from the history and may be masked on physical examination by preservation of body fat stores or oedema. However, muscle wasting is a constant feature of all these patients, along with a low plasma albumin level and clinically obvious physiological impairment.[14] While treatment must be aimed at identifying the septic source and controlling the hypermetabolic stimulus, these patients need early nutritional support.

PRIMARY ASSESSMENT

The identification of these nutritional syndromes relies on a good history and a physical examination supported by a few basic measurements.

History

The history should determine the energy balance of the patient, and consider his energy intake and energy output to arrive at an estimate of nutritional depletion and the time scale over which this has occurred. Particular attention should be paid to a clinical history of anorexia, vomiting, nausea, diarrhoea and abnormal losses from diarrhoea or fistulas. A detailed dietary history may be helpful in identifying the patient's food fads, proportions of fat, carbohydrate and proteins in the diet, use of dietary supplements and vitamins, and additional calories from alcohol which may be associated with other nutritional deficiencies. Dietary recall beyond 24 hours, however, is not very accurate, and dietetic assessment has been shown to be of little help in the classification of patients.

Weight loss is of major importance in the clinical history. Changes in weight over very short periods of time reflect fluid balance, but changes over a period of weeks or months indicate loss of body tissue. Excluding fluid balance problems, rapid changes in weight are associated with hypermetabolism and sepsis while long-term changes in weight are associated with depletion syndromes. With severe sepsis up to 1 kg of wet lean tissue may be lost each day, whereas in total starvation only half of this amount is lost. Assessment of weight loss relies on an accurate recall of well weight, but this may be difficult in very sick or elderly patients. However, using recalled well weight is more accurate than using standard tables of predicted weight for height.[59]

Physical examination

Physical examination should aim to estimate the nutritional reserves of the patient, look for signs of physiological impairment and hypermetabolism and assess the state of hydration. Fat stores are estimated by gently pinching the skinfolds on the arms, back and abdomen to feel the amount of subcutaneous fat present. Muscle wasting is best observed in muscles around the scapulae and in the temporalis fossae, the interossei and the muscle bellies on the upper arm. Hydration needs to be assessed by looking for oedema in the lower legs and sacral area. If oedema is present, weight loss may be greater than that estimated from the history. Unlike childhood kwashiorkor, oedema is seldom observed in malnourished adult patients unless other factors such as cardiac, renal or hepatic dysfunction are present. Subtle skin and hair changes are described in association with different vitamin and trace metal deficiencies, but these are not usually specific in gastroenterological patients in whom protein–energy malnutrition has complex manifestations. The evaluation of functional impairment secondary to loss of body protein is the most important part of the clinical assessment of nutritional state. Weight loss without evidence of physiological impairment is probably of no clinical importance.[79] Function is observed whilst performing the physical examination and by watching the patient's activity around the ward. Grip strength is assessed by asking the patient to squeeze the examiner's index and middle fingers for at least 10 seconds. Impairment is judged in the light of the patient's age, sex and body habitus. Respiratory muscle function is assessed by asking the patient to cough, holding a strip of paper 8 cm from the lips, which should normally be blown away with some force. Unhealed wounds or scratches are also looked for.

Basic measurements

A nutritional assessment is incomplete without a few basic measurements. The patient's weight should be recorded, and weight loss estimated by subtracting this from the recalled well weight.[59] Apart from clinical evidence of sepsis the most useful measurement associated with the hypermetabolic and stress syndromes is a low level of plasma albumin. Low plasma albumin reflects protein losses into inflamed tissues, alterations in protein turnover and changes in intravascular/extravascular distribution of albumin and water.[36] Important clinically is the fact that in these circumstances a low level of plasma albumin almost always indicates an expanded extracellular fluid with bodily hypotonicity and intolerance to excessive salt and water administration. From this primary assessment the nutritional syndromes categorized above are identified.

In the clinical setting it will be found that there is considerable overlap in the clinical picture of these syndromes: they form a spectrum of nutritional disorders rather than defined categories.

SECONDARY ASSESSMENT TECHNIQUES

Further information may be gained by more detailed measurements using anthropometry, immunology, calorimetry, body composition and biochemistry.

Anthropometry

This includes the measurement of weight, height, skinfold thickness (by calipers) and upper arm circumference.[9] Various ratios of weight to height have been suggested to indicate obesity and depleted states (weight/height, weight/height^2, weight/height^3). Recent population-based studies have made anthropometric measurements more meaningful, especially if age-, sex- and race-specific standards are based on large studies. Probably, where good local standards are available weight/height^2 is the best of these estimates.

Skinfold thickness measurements are usually taken at the midpoint of the upper arm over the biceps and triceps. Other skinfolds that may be measured include the subscapular skinfold and the suprailiac skinfold. From the triceps skinfold and arm circumference measurements, mid-arm muscle circumference can be derived as an index of muscle wasting. There are large random errors in the measurement of skin folds and they have little meaning in the individual patient. They are useful, however, in evaluating groups of patients.[15]

Immunological assessment

Protein–energy malnutrition is associated with impaired immunological responses.[17] Defects in B- and T-cell function as well as impaired inflammatory responses have been described. In clinical practice, total lymphocyte count and delayed hypersensitivity skin tests have been routinely used. While a total lymphocyte count below 10^9/l has been observed in groups of patients with severe nutritional depletion, the association is tenuous and does not help to distinguish nutritional syndromes.

Cell-mediated immunity as tested by the delayed hypersensitivity skin test is impaired in depleted states.[17] A battery of recall antigens (purified protein derivative, mumps, candida, trichophyton, streptokinase/streptodornase) are injected intradermally on the forearm and read at 24 and 48 hours. Reactions are scored according to the diameter of induration produced at the injection sites. Problems are recognized in standardizing the administration, recording and interpretation of the results.[3] There are many conditions apart from disorders of nutritional state associated with absent skin test reactions (anergy): these include sepsis, advanced cancer, trauma, old age, diabetes mellitus, steroid administration and immunosuppressive disorders.

CALORIMETRY

Energy requirements should be tailored to the energy needs of individual patients. Of the methods available for measurement of metabolic expenditure at rest, the only practical method for clinical practice is indirect calorimetry. Expired gases are collected and analysed to determine oxygen consumption and carbon dioxide output of fasting patients at rest. This is referred to as resting metabolic expenditure. Variations occur with body build, age, sex and physical activity. Estimates of total energy expenditure can also be made from equations which have been derived for males and females, using weight, height and age with additional factors added for activity and injury. *Table 3.63* shows the components of energy expenditure and total energy requirements of gastroenterological patients according to the nutritional syndromes detailed above.

Body composition analysis

Most body composition analysis methods use the dilution of administered radioisotopes to measure various body spaces or compartments. Assessment of total body water is made using deuterated or

Table 3.63 Energy expenditure in gastroenterological patients. (kJ/(kg/ day); kcal/(kg/day) in parentheses)

Nutritional syndromes	Resting energy expenditure	Activity energy expenditure	Total energy expenditure
Normal: operative	109 (26)	42 (10)	151 (36)
Normal: postoperative	122 (29)	29 (7)	151 (36)
Nutritional depletion	92 (22)	42 (10)	134 (32)
Nutritional depletion and sepsis	147 (35)	29 (7)	176 (42)
Septic (not depleted)	189 (45)	29 (7)	218 (52)

tritiated water. Total exchangeable sodium and potassium are estimated from the rapid dilution in the body of the appropriate isotope. Total body potassium can also be measured in a whole body counter and this can be used as an estimate of body cell mass. In vivo neutron activation analysis is a method of measuring total body nitrogen that can be used in sick patients.[5] Two techniques of measuring total body nitrogen have been developed. With the delayed technique, the patient is irradiated with fast neutrons, then moved to a whole body counter and the resulting radiation decay measured. With the prompt γ technique the patient is irradiated with neutrons and the resulting radiation is counted at the same time. In combination with total body water measurements, the total body content of protein, water, fat and minerals can be determined. These methods are currently research tools and have been used to detect changes in body nitrogen in groups of patients undergoing specific nutritional regimens.[43]

Plasma proteins

There are four plasma proteins synthesized in the liver which are currently used in assessment of nutritional status.

Albumin

Within 24 hours of protein being eliminated from the diet, albumin synthesis is halved. However, this dramatic fall in synthesis is not reflected in the plasma albumin level for many weeks. Studies in primates indicate that unless the protein content of the diet is less than 3%, plasma albumin levels do not fall even after several months.[36] The reasons why plasma albumin levels are maintained are related to the shifts of extravascular albumin (comprising 50% of total albumin) into the intravascular compartment, contraction of the albumin pool and a lowered albumin breakdown rate. Furthermore, albumin has a long half-life of about 21 days. Changes in plasma albumin levels, therefore, do not reflect a patient's total protein status.[36] Low plasma albumin levels seen in gastroenterological patients

are most often associated with leakage of albumin in inflammatory conditions of the gastrointestinal tract and increased capillary permeability, which occurs in trauma (including operations) and sepsis.[21,76]

Transferrin

Transferrin has a short half-life of 7 days and responds more rapidly than albumin to nutritional changes. Although transferrin is less affected by fluid changes than albumin, its plasma level is greatly influenced by iron deficiency, which can be associated with malnutrition. While a low level of plasma transferrin present before surgery is an adverse prognostic factor,[62] its association with total body protein status is uncertain.[36]

Prealbumin and retinol-binding protein

Prealbumin is the transport protein for thyroxine and is linked in a constant molar ratio with retinol-binding protein, which transports retinol (vitamin A). Retinol-binding protein is metabolized by the kidney and may be markedly elevated in chronic renal failure.[36] Because the half-lives of these proteins are much shorter than those of albumin and transferrin (2 days for prealbumin, 12 hours for retinol-binding protein) they more accurately reflect acute changes in nutritional status.[70] There is some confusion, however, about whether these proteins are markers of energy status or protein status.[36]

DYNAMIC NUTRITIONAL ASSESSMENT

The problem with the nutritional measurements outlined so far is that as single static measurements they cannot give information on the dynamics of the nutritional state. Most markers change so slowly that it can be many weeks before repeated measurements will show a clear indication of change in nutritional stores. Nitrogen balance studies can determine whether positive nitrogen balance is being achieved but need repetitive and time-consuming nitrogen analyses of urine and faeces and other secretions. In ordinary clinical care nitrogen balance studies are often inaccurate and misleading.

Recently, the short half-life plasma proteins transferrin and prealbumin protein have been suggested as indicating dynamic nutritional state.[13] It was found that in patients requiring intravenous nutrition for 2 weeks, a positive nitrogen balance was reflected by a rise in the prealbumin level in 90% of cases, whereas a negative nitrogen balance was associated with a falling prealbumin level in 70%. Predictive values in the group indicated that 93% of patients with a rising prealbumin level had a positive nitrogen balance.

PREOPERATIVE ASSESSMENT OF SURGICAL RISK

It has been suggested that gastroenterological patients who are nutritionally depleted have a higher risk of major complications after surgery than patients who are not depleted. Various formulas, all of which reflect low levels of plasma proteins, are available for use in individual patients to assess risk from a surgical operation.[2,11] It is now realized that most of these risk factors are associated with manifest or occult sepsis rather than nutritional depletion alone, and that a careful clinical appraisal along the lines set out above may be just as effective in identifying patients at risk from major surgery.[62]

The question of which patients will benefit from specific nutritional therapy before their operation has not been answered. A recent formal prospective trial has helped to identify those particularly at risk.[79] It was found that only those patients who had preoperative loss of body weight *plus* clinically obvious physiological impairments had significantly more postoperative complications and a longer hospital stay. It is this group who should be identified as candidates for nutritional support, especially if major surgery with a fair probability of postoperative complications is anticipated. A short course of nutritional therapy of 4–7 days is probably all that is required.[14]

NUTRITION AND INFECTION

The metabolic and nutritional consequences of sepsis have important implications in the planning of nutritional therapy. In many gastroenterological patients, metabolism may change from the low protein turnover, low-energy requirement of nutritional depletion, to the high protein turnover, high-energy requirement of sepsis. The extent of these changes will depend on the source of infection, the virulence of the organism and the host response. It is the host response (particularly immunological defence mechanisms) that is affected by nutritional status.

EVIDENCE FOR INCREASED SUSCEPTIBILITY IN MALNUTRITION

Nutritional depletion is known to affect the structure and function of the immune system.[12] There are marked histomorphological changes in the thymus, with depletion of lymphocytes, reduction in size and loss of corticomedullary differentiation. Similar changes occur in the spleen and lymph nodes. More important, however, are the functional changes. T-cell function, assessed by delayed hypersensitivity skin testing, blast transformation of lymphocytes to mitogens and lymphokine production, is reduced, while B-cell function is not affected to the same extent. Polymorphonuclear leukocytes ingest bacteria normally, but their intercellular killing is reduced in depleted patients. Lower liver synthesis of some complement components has been noted, and lysozyme production is reduced in plasma, tears, saliva and other secretions.

These impaired responses, which can be observed in nutritionally depleted patients, are complex.[17] Iron deficiency has been shown to affect lymphocyte distribution by complex mechanisms, while zinc deficiency is known to alter the delayed hypersensitivity skin test results and impair thymic development and *in vitro* lymphocyte activation. Deficiencies of the vitamins pyridoxine, folate and vitamins A, C and E affect lymphocyte function. Polyunsaturated fatty acids and the amino acid arginine have immunostimulatory effects which may be of clinical benefit in some sick patients.[18,48] Among these factors, the place of protein and energy depletion is difficult to ascertain. There is evidence that children with kwashiorkor are more susceptible to infection than those with marasmus.[68] Rats fed a protein-depleted diet succumb to infections more readily than rats fed a normal diet.[45] The clinical impression is that malnourished patients are more susceptible to septic complications, but a clear association between protein–energy malnutrition and susceptibility to infection has been difficult to show.

THE PATIENT'S RESPONSE TO SEPSIS

The challenge of sepsis sets in motion a series of cellular, metabolic and hormonal effects leading to a catabolic state which, if left unchecked, rapidly exhausts the nutritional reserves of the patient, particularly those of protein.

Cellular responses

Much recent research has focused on the possible role of substances released from inflamed tissues. Many different cell types release *cytokines*, which not only have local effects but systemic effects as well. These systemic effects contribute to the metabolic response to sepsis and infectious disease. Thus, the cytokines appear to be links between inflamed tissues, wounds and inflammatory masses and metabolic and immunological responses. Interleukins-1, -2 and -6, tumour necrosis factor and γ-interferon may have important roles in this regard.[49,58,78]

Endocrine responses

The metabolic response to infection is to some extent mediated by hormones released by the changes in circulating blood volume and the metabolites released from damaged tissues which affect the neuroendocrine system. The catecholamines adrenaline and noradrenaline, released from the adrenal medulla, are essential for survival during stress. Their effects on cardiac function and respiration are well known, but they also affect glucose metabolism in liver and muscle and mobilize free fatty acids. Adrenocorticotrophic hormone acts on the adrenal cortex to release glucocorticoids which may increase tenfold in sepsis, stimulating gluconeogenesis in conjunction with peripheral breakdown of protein in muscle and augmenting lipolysis.[7] The increased insulin observed in septic states is counteracted by a greater increase in glucagon with a resultant fall in the insulin:glucagon ratio. This interaction between the catecholamines and pancreatic endocrine hormones is fundamental to the regulation of substrates during infection. Growth hormone also increases in sepsis.

Metabolic responses

The main metabolic changes in severe sepsis are an increase in protein breakdown, a smaller increase in protein synthesis and an alteration in glucose metabolism.[7] The increased requirement for energy of cellular metabolism (ATP) is seen as a rise in whole body oxygen consumption and resting metabolic expenditure. The magnitude of increase in energy expenditure and acceleration of the flux of substrates through organ systems is small in mild infections, but up to 50% above resting expenditure in septicaemic patients. In sick patients, the extra energy requirement cannot be met by increasing energy intake. Clinically, the results are early weight loss from loss of muscle and fat and hypoproteinae-

mia. The major change in energy metabolism in septic patients is an acceleration of gluconeogenesis.[7] Both glucagon and the catecholamines stimulate the accelerated hepatic production of glucose. In many of the rapidly healing tissues of the inflammatory process the metabolism of glucose to lactate provides the main energy source. However, for other energy needs in the body fat is still the principal energy source. The protein for gluconeogenesis comes from muscle catabolism. Alanine, the main amino acid released from muscle, is the principal gluconeogenic precursor. The branched-chain amino acids released by muscle catabolism can become a fuel source for the remaining muscle. The nitrogen residues are processed to urea in the liver and excreted in the urine. The amount of nitrogen lost in the urine can be up to 40 g/day in severe sepsis. Most of this nitrogen loss is from muscle, which also contributes to an increased urinary loss of potassium, phosphate, magnesium and zinc.

The metabolic events change with time following infection. The earliest response to sepsis may be a transient depression of physiological responses (ebb phase) followed by the increase in metabolic reactions just described (flow phase). This phase depends on the severity of the sepsis and the host's ability to deal with it successfully. It is followed by a convalescent phase in which muscle protein and fat are resynthesized over a period of months.

IMPLICATIONS FOR THE MANAGEMENT OF THE SEPTIC PATIENT

The different hormonal and metabolic environment of the septic patient compared with that of the non-septic patient means that nutritional requirements are different. The aim should be to remove the source of the sepsis, with nutritional therapy providing a supportive role as other therapeutic measures take effect. Because positive nitrogen balance is very difficult, if not impossible, to achieve in the hormonal and metabolic environment of uncontrolled sepsis, the nutritional goals in the septic patient are to prevent or minimize tissue losses. However, as the patient recovers, there is not only a need to maintain the patient's nutritional state, but to replenish the deficits that have occurred during the septic insult.

Currently there is no consensus as to the optimal energy source for septic patients. Because of the impaired glucose metabolism in septic patients, infusions of glucose are handled poorly, often requiring large amounts of insulin to prevent glycosuria.[8] Such glucose may be deposited as excess glycogen and constitute a metabolic stress rather than effective nutrient support.[26] Most energy sources containing fat are carnitine-dependent, and in septic conditions carnitine may be reduced in the mitochondria. However, combinations of fat and glucose are recommended in septic patients as a compromise, though not optimal regimen.[54]

In septic patients, vitamins and trace metals may need to be given in increasing amounts. Hypermetabolic patients receiving maintenance amounts of zinc[80] and folate[4] have been shown to become deficient in these nutrients, particularly when moving into an anabolic phase.

NUTRITIONAL SUPPORT

ORAL INTAKE

There is no doubt that the natural route for the ingestion and assimilation of nutrients is the cheapest, most efficient, and preferred route. For an adequate oral intake, an intact gastrointestinal tract, an ability to absorb nutrients, a favourable metabolic environment and a motivated patient are required. There are many gastroenterological disorders where modification of the diet is an essential part of therapy. Removal of gluten from the diet in coeliac disease, and of lactose in disaccharidase deficiency are such situations. However, the benefits of other dietary modifications are not so easily demonstrated. The use of bland diets in peptic ulcer disease has shown no advantage over normal diets in clinical trials.[10] Symptomatic relief of diverticular disease has been demonstrated to follow the addition of fibre to the diet. Chronic hepatic encephalopathy, usually treated with protein restriction, has shown improvement with diets containing high proportions of branched-chain amino acids.[34] Low-protein diets enriched with essential amino acids have been given orally in chronic renal failure patients with benefit.[35] Patients with steatorrhoea may benefit from the use of medium-chain triglycerides, available as an oil for cooking, or baking, or as a drink. Medium-chain triglycerides do not require bile acids or pancreatic lipase for absorption and pass into the portal circulation for oxidation in the liver. Dietary modification for patients with dumping after gastric surgery is often successful with low-carbohydrate and high-fat diets[64] or by adding pectin to the diet.[47]

There are other gastroenterological disorders where modification of the diet cannot overcome problems of ingestion and absorption of nutrients. Anorexia, nausea and vomiting affect the ability of the patient to take an adequate oral diet.

Despite good dietetic services and ingenious manipulation of the presentation of food, many patients fail to increase energy intake sufficiently to maintain body weight. The causes are many. Alterations in taste and sensation of satiety have been shown in cancer patients:[20] 30% have an elevation in the recognition threshold for sweetness, and in patients with upper gastrointestinal carcinoma meat aversion has been correlated with altered sensations of bitterness. Catecholamine release in response to stress depresses eating by neuroendocrine changes in hypothalamic centres. In advanced carcinoma, patients also complain of fullness, further decreasing their motivation to eat. The ability of dietary manipulation to meet the requirements of patients with these gastrointestinal disorders is therefore limited and other therapeutic measures are required.

Postoperative patients do not usually require specific nutritional therapy. Usually, oral fluids can be commenced within a few days of surgery and the patient progresses to a light diet. The loss of body weight (about 6% after the average major operation) and the deficit of nitrogen and energy occurring during this time are replenished over the next few months. It must be remembered, however, that it takes at least 10–14 days after commencing oral intake for a patient to reach normal energy requirements, even with careful dietary manipulation and supplemental feeding.[38] While this deficit can be tolerated reasonably well in properly nourished patients, those malnourished prior to surgery may not be able to cope with this degree of weight loss. Furthermore, postoperative complications, especially sepsis, magnify the deficit and may further extend the convalescence of the patient. In such circumstance the early use of an alternative nutritional therapy must be considered.

ENTERAL THERAPY

Enteral feeding can be used to supplement oral intake or as a method of using the gastrointestinal tract where disorders of the mouth, oesophagus or stomach prevent natural delivery of food to the absorptive areas. There is growing awareness of the importance of enteral nutrition – in its absence there is rapid atrophy of the intestine due mainly to lack of blood flow but also because specific nutrients required by the enterocytes may not be available. Absent or inadequate enteral nutrition also results in failure of gut barrier function, leading to translocation of endotoxin and microorganisms from the intestine. When translocation occurs it is associated with activation of macrophages both in the mesenteric lymph nodes and the liver with release of interleukins-1 and -6 and tumour necrosis factor.[1]

Recently new technologies have been developed not only for efficient and comfortable nasogastric feeding but also direct feeding into the stomach or intestine. The number of commercially available enteral diets is nearing 100.[25]

Indications

There are three conditions which need to be fulfilled before nutritional therapy via the enteral route should be considered.

1. Spontaneous oral intake must be inadequate for nutritional requirements. A careful dietary assessment is needed to determine if energy and protein intake meet estimated requirements.
2. The proximal small intestine needs to be functional. Often fine-bore tubes can be fed past obstructions in the oesophagus or stomach to the functional area of the digestive tract.
3. The gastrointestinal tract needs to be an appropriate route for administration of nutrients for the patient's condition. This particularly applies in conditions where gut rest is considered part of management despite a functional gastrointestinal tract. Such conditions as pancreatitis or high small bowel fistulas are not appropriately treated by enteral therapy.

Conditions which particularly fulfil these criteria include non-gastrointestinal problems such as severe head injury, central nervous system disorders, burns and major trauma. Among the gastroenterological disorders which may be treated with enteral diets are ileal or colonic fistulas, non-obstructive problems in the large bowel, and obstructive lesions in the upper gastroenterological tract.

Methods

Nasogastric tube

There is no indication for the use of wide-bore nasogastric tubes in enteral feeding. They are uncomfortable for the patient and increase the incidence of aspiration and ulceration. There are many fine-bore tubes on the market, with variations of weighted ends, side and end holes, and adaptations to aid placement. As these tubes do not permit aspiration, the position needs to be checked by radiography before feeding commences. Feeding tubes, which may become blocked when the consistency of the nutrient is too thick for the size of the tube, can be irrigated with water to overcome the obstruction. Regurgitation may still occur with fine-bore tubes, particularly at night, and patients should be encouraged to sleep semi-recumbent to avoid this

potentially serious problem. Nasogastric tubes are indicated when the patient is to be fed for up to a month or 6 weeks. If there is a risk of aspiration the tube should be passed into the jejunum.

Tube enterostomy

With the development of percutaneous endoscopic techniques for gastrostomy and jejunostomy there is growing popularity for tube enterostomy.[63] These techniques are required when enteral feeding is to be prolonged for more than 4–6 weeks. Percutaneous endoscopic jejunostomy or surgical jejunostomy is used when there is risk of aspiration, otherwise percutaneous endoscopic gastrostomy or surgical gastrostomy is used. The techniques for tube insertion are still being evolved, with the 'pull method' being the most popular. Here, after the endoscope is passed and the stomach fully inflated, the room lights are dimmed, allowing transillumination of the stomach. An intravenous cannula is then passed percutaneously into the transluminated stomach to lie within a snare loop which is then tightened around the cannula, where the needle is removed and then replaced with a thread of nylon about 150 cm in length. The scope, snare and nylon are then pulled up through the oesophagus and out of the patient's mouth. The nylon is then attached to the pointed end of a specially constructed gastrostomy tube which is then drawn through into the stomach and out through its wall and through the abdominal wall. Some tubes are made of polyurethane and the balloon maintains its natural expanded shape by a compressible/expandable polyurethane foam. In this way, pressure necrosis of the stomach wall is less likely when the tube is anchored. Those patients requiring jejunostomy have another tube which passes into the stomach via the gastrostomy tube and out of the pylorus to lie in the upper jejunum.

Fine-needle catheter jejunostomy

Recently, the technique of fine-needle catheter jejunostomy has been re-evaluated as a method of infusing nutrients directly into the jejunum postoperatively. The catheter is inserted by a needle tunnelled submucosally along a 10-cm length of the jejunum at the time of operation, and the bowel segment is secured to the anterior abdominal wall. This catheter can then be used for early postoperative feeding.[82] The catheters may leak into the abdominal cavity. However, for those who do not have access to safe parenteral nutrition, this technique, if used properly, can be a valuable aid.

Administration

With fine-bore tubes, continuous infusion of nutrients is preferable because nursing care is easier, and there is less diarrhoea and fewer problems with nausea and vomiting. Although three litres of nutrient solution can quite easily be administered by gravity feeding over a 24-hour period, the use of a pump enables a more constant infusion to be maintained.

Enteral feeding should be commenced gradually, usually at full strength at around 25 ml/h, progressing 10 ml/h every 6 hours as tolerated until full intake is reached. As with all forms of nutritional therapy, there is need for careful monitoring of the patient with regard to fluid and electrolytes, watching for fluid retention, hyperglycaemia and electrolyte imbalances. Diarrhoea, which is a common complication, is usually corrected by slowing the rate of delivery or reducing the osmotic load.

Types of enteral diets

There are many types of liquid feeding formulas available and to the uninitiated the choice seems overwhelming. The ideal complete formula should have about 4 MJ (1000 kcal) per litre, with a nitrogen:energy ratio (gram:kilojoule) of about 1:840 (a gram:kilocalorie ratio of about 1:200).

Formulas can be classified into four groups, each with particular indications as shown in *Table 3.64*.

Elemental diets

Elemental diets were developed in the 1960s for astronauts, to eliminate problems of storage, ingestion and waste disposal. They are composed of amino acids or small peptides as the nitrogen source, with up to 30% of the energy supplied as fat. They have no lactose or digestive residues and have added to them recommended daily allowances of trace metals and vitamins. They have been demonstrated to maintain nitrogen and energy balance in normal subjects for up to 6 months. However, they are unpalatable, expensive, and their indications for use in gastroenterological patients have been seriously questioned.[50]

The clinical application of elemental diets has been based on the premise that they are more easily absorbed, do not stimulate gastrointestinal secretions and have low residue. While the last premise is unquestioned, the first two have not found support in experimental or clinical situations. Particular situations where these diets may be indicated include the short bowel syndrome, gastrointestinal fistulas, inflammatory bowel disease, pancreatic disease, chronic intestinal obstruction, diverticulitis and various diarrhoeas. While most trials of elemental diets have a satisfactory outcome, one cannot be certain that other less expensive and more palatable diets might have been as effective. One study comparing the effectiveness of elemental diets with total parenteral nutrition in gastroenterological patients showed that nitrogen retention was equivalent.[81]

A number of side-effects have been reported with these diets, including gastric retention, altered bowel habits, fluid balance problems, hyperglycae-

Table 3.64 Enteral nutrition formulas

Classification	Constituents	Use	Examples
Meal replacements	Balanced proportions of protein, carbohydrate and fat with electrolytes	Provide complete and balanced means	Ensure, Isocal, Osmolite, Clinifeed
Supplements	Proportions of protein, carbohydrate and fat with particular emphasis on either protein or carbohydrate	Added to regular meals to provide the extra calories or protein	Sustacal (extra calories) Sustagen (extra protein)
Feeding components	Only one or two components	Used to make up specific diets for specific purposes	Caloreen (carbohydrate) Polycose (carbohydrate) MCT oil (fat) Casec (protein)
Elemental diets	No-residue balanced diets with protein components reduced to basic elements (amino acids, simple sugars)	Suggested for malabsorption, pancreatic insufficiency (see text)	Flexical Vivonex Aminaid (essential amino acids) Hepaticaid (branched-chain-enriched amino acids)

mia and deficiencies of vitamins or fatty acids. Most can be corrected by careful attention to the composition of the diet or by slowing delivery to the gut.

After initial enthusiasm, elemental diets have only a limited role in gastroenterological patients.[50] Patients with malabsorption problems such as exocrine pancreatic insufficiency or the short gut syndrome, who have failed on conventional dietary manipulation, should be tried on an elemental diet.

PARENTERAL THERAPY

In the early decades of this century, the feasibility of using nutritional therapy by intravenous routes was established. In 1937 Elman showed that a protein hydrolysate of casein could be given intravenously to humans.

Isotonic dextrose solutions were used in the 1920s, but fat solutions initially produced in the 1930s were found to be unstable. The major problem in developing effective nutritional therapy, however, was related to administration of the hypertonic nutrient solutions. The successful development in the late 1960s of central venous catheterization techniques enabled hypertonic solutions to be infused safely, which led to the successful management of patients who previously would have died of the nutritional consequences of their disease.

Indications

The indications for using the parenteral route for feeding patients are related to the inability of the intestine to absorb adequately sufficient nutrients for the patient's needs. Thus, intravenous nutrition is indicated when the intestinal tract is blocked, too short, inflamed or simply cannot cope.

When the gastrointestinal tract is blocked
Although acute obstruction of the intestine is usually treated as a surgical emergency regardless of the nutritional state of the patient, conditions which gradually produce obstruction of the pharynx, oesophagus, stomach or duodenum may first require intravenous nutrition to treat the insidious and often far advanced protein–energy malnutrition that has occurred. Available evidence suggests that weight loss must be large (probably more than 20%) and plasma proteins very low (albumin less than 30 g/l) before it can be said that the patient has a 'dangerous' level of malnutrition. Nevertheless, it must be remembered that if an already malnourished patient should sustain a postoperative complication, his nutritional reserves may be unable to withstand the consequent nutritional assault. Thus although

patients with weight loss of more than 20% and those with very low concentrations of plasma proteins should be fed intravenously for 2 weeks before a major operation, others, who on physical examination have depleted reserves of protein and fat yet do not fulfil these criteria, should be considered carefully for intravenous nutrition. This is particularly so if it is considered that the postoperative course may be complicated.

When the gastrointestinal tract is too short
This category includes not only those patients who have had massive small bowel resections but also those with fistulas where the effective length of the gut is reduced. Intravenous nutrition is particularly effective in high-output small intestinal fistulas, where oral feeding produces an increase in fistula output and greater morbidity and mortality.[39] In patients with a short gut syndrome, parenteral therapy is necessary to maintain nutrition until it is possible to gradually introduce enteral feeding.[31]

When the gastrointestinal tract is inflamed
Nutritional depletion is a common feature of inflammatory bowel disease. More than 50% of patients requiring urgent surgery for acute colitis suffer from protein–energy malnutrition.[41] There is some evidence that postoperative parenteral nutrition may be beneficial in such patients.[83]

Although some patients with intractable Crohn's enteritis go into remission when the gut is rested and vigorous nutritional therapy is instituted,[23] there does not appear to be any primary effect of total bowel rest and intravenous nutrition on acute colitis.[22] Thus, even though no primary effect of total gut rest in inflammatory bowel disease can be observed there is no question that a short course of intravenous nutrition – perhaps no longer than 4–7 days – results in clinically obvious improvement in physiological function in patients with acute attacks of inflammatory bowel disease.[14]

In summary, intravenous nutrition is indicated in severely malnourished patients about to undergo major surgery for inflammatory bowel disease. It should also be used in some patients with Crohn's disease of the small intestine, particularly where there is evidence of obstruction. Here, nutritional integrity can be preserved while the gut is rested and time is gained which may allow spontaneous remission. Other patients with intestinal inflammation may also receive benefit from gut rest and parenteral nutrition, particularly if awaiting major surgery. There is some evidence that fluorouracil toxicity is less when the gut is rested, and patients with radiation enteritis and protein–energy malnutrition may also be helped by a period of such treatment.[6]

When the gastrointestinal tract cannot cope

Whenever there is an intra-abdominal abscess or septic focus, it is difficult to administer nutrients via the enteral route. Patients with complications of pancreatitis, in particular, come into this category. Prolonged attacks of acute pancreatitis can be associated with rapid deterioration in nutritional state and treatment with total gut rest and intravenous nutrition appears to be effective.[37]

Prolonged postoperative ileus, pseudo-obstruction of the colon and idiopathic pseudo-obstruction of the intestine may all require intravenous nutrition for varying periods while awaiting spontaneous remission. In idiopathic pseudo-obstruction of the intestine[67] very prolonged periods of feeding may be required and some patients may need to be fed intravenously permanently.

Methods

There are three forms of parenteral nutritional support currently used. While each has a place in the nutritional support of patients, central venous administration of adequate energy and nitrogen remains the standard method for providing total balance nutritional support.

Protein-sparing therapy

Dextrose-free amino acid solutions have been shown to have a nitrogen-sparing effect. The concept is to promote low glucose and low insulin concentrations in plasma, allow mobilization of endogenous fat stores and satisfy the energy deficit by ketogenesis. Some workers believe that if additional glucose is given nitrogen-sparing is less and that elevation of insulin impairs visceral protein synthesis. After many studies it is now clear that amino acids alone are protein-sparing, can be given via peripheral veins and are associated with fewer side-effects than when dextrose is given. Nevertheless, the provision of an energy supply with the amino acids has marked clinical and metabolic advantages[83] and there are very few indications for isotonic dextrose-free amino acid solutions in gastroenterological patients.

Peripheral total parenteral nutrition

The early attempts to give glucose in sufficient quantity for energy needs were limited by the inability of the peripheral veins to accept hypertonic solutions. With the development of isotonic fat solutions, energy needs can be met more easily when the sole access is by the peripheral route. By combining amino acids and fat with a small quantity of isotonic glucose for essential cellular metabolism, the nutritional needs of an average patient can be met. There are, however, disadvantages in this approach. Peripheral lines are more cumbersome for the patient than central lines, and despite meticulous care, they do need changing frequently as phlebitis and venous occlusion occurs with these solutions. The place of peripheral total parenteral nutrition is therefore limited to those occasional patients in whom a central line is contraindicated or is impossible to insert.

Central total parenteral nutrition

The development of central venous catheterization has enabled the delivery of hypertonic solutions to be given safely. The glucose, fat and amino acids are given simultaneously through a central venous line with its tip in the superior vena cava. On such therapy, patients gain weight and may be put into positive nitrogen balance.

There are a number of techniques for placement of central venous catheters, with the infraclavicular puncture being recommended. The use of long catheters from the antecubital fossa is not recommended because they are associated with a high rate of catheter tip misplacement and the patient's movements may be restricted. Complications of insertion include arterial puncture, air embolism, pneumothorax and misplaced tip. Air embolism is reduced if the catheter is inserted with the patient tilted head-down. A chest radiograph after the procedure is important to check for pneumothorax and the position of the catheter tip. The incidence of venous thrombosis increases if the tip is in any other vessel than the superior vena cava.

The most important complication of central parenteral nutrition is catheter tip sepsis. The main source of organisms contaminating central venous catheters is the skin puncture site. However, with meticulous nursing care a central line may be maintained for many months without adverse effects. Catheter sepsis has an incidence of 3–10%, much higher rates occurring in units dealing with major complicated gastrointestinal patients.[55] It is clear, however, that the colonization of central catheters is very much more common than the reported clinical sepsis rate. The potential for septic problems is therefore great. When a patient with a central venous line develops clinical signs of sepsis, the catheter must be suspected. If no other source of infection is found, the catheter is removed. About 75% of catheters removed for suspected catheter sepsis, however, are eventually exonerated as the source of sepsis.[66]

Administration and monitoring

Ideally, administration of the nutrient solution should be managed by a team of clinicians, nursing staff, pharmacists and technicians. The incidence of complications and catheter sepsis increases in situations where only an occasional patient is treated. Solutions need to be prepared under aseptic conditions, preferably in the pharmacy under a laminar flow hood. The attending physician each day evaluates the patient's clinical situation, and appropriate amounts of glucose, amino acids and electrolytes are prescribed. Vitamins and trace metals are added and the solution is infused over a 24-hour period. Fat is added to the nutrient solution. Delivery of the nutrient solution is best carried out by a modern intravenous pump with microprocessor control which will administer solutions at specified volume rates very accurately. This not only reduces the problems of nursing care in adjusting drip flow rates but ensures that solutions are administered evenly over 24-hour periods, minimizing problems of hyperglycaemia and glycosuria.

When starting parenteral nutrition, it is important to commence with less than half the glucose load intended and gradually increase the glucose over the first 24–48 hours, to prevent hyperglycaemia and glycosuria. Similarly, when stopping parenteral nutrition, a solution of 10% dextrose should be give for 12–24 hours after finishing to prevent rebound hypoglycaemia.

Patients receiving parenteral nutrition need to be monitored daily with clinical and biochemical assessments. Daily weighing is important to indicate hydration and is more accurate than fluid balance records. Urine testing for glycosuria is required to check that prescribed glucose is not being lost, and the regular recording of body temperature is an essential part of monitoring for catheter sepsis. Daily biochemistry monitoring should include electrolytes, urea, chloride and phosphate, and 2–3 times a week liver function tests need to be checked. Other ions such as zinc, copper and magnesium should be monitored weekly. If fat is being used, the blood should be centrifuged and the plasma assessed for opalescence.

Prescribing

The basis for prescribing parenteral nutritional therapy when the patient is not oedematous is the weight of the patient. Weight is used to calculate energy requirements for maintenance of body protein and further increments allowed for depleted patients and hypermetabolic patients.

Energy

Glucose and fat remain the most commonly used source of energy for most parenteral nutrition regimens. For most gastroenterological patients 170 kJ/(kg/day) (40 kcal/(kg/day)) is sufficient. Infusion rates of energy above 170 kJ/(kg/day) result in fat synthesis and occasionally may be harmful.[74] A 50:50 mixture of fat and glucose is recommended, although much less fat is possible. One litre of 10% fat solution per week is sufficient to prevent fatty acid deficiency.[26]

Other energy sources such as fructose, sorbitol, xylitol and ethanol have been used but advantages over dextrose and fat solutions have not been demonstrated.

Protein

Hydrolysates of casein have been superseded by crystalline amino acids in balanced proportions.[53] There are many commercial preparations, some with electrolytes and energy added. Protein should be given in proportion to the energy: the nitrogen:energy ratio (grams:kilojoules) should be between 1:420 and 1:630 (a gram:kilocalorie ratio between 1:100 and 1:150).[74]

The requirement for protein varies according to the state of depletion. Generally, most gastroenterological patients will go into positive balance when 1.0–1.5 g/kg/day. Depleted patients will readily utilize protein even when less than optimal energy is supplied.[26] Hypermetabolic patients have an increased nitrogen and energy requirement as most of the losses are from the protein compartment. *Table 3.65*, which outlines the energy and protein requirements of patients with the nutritional syndromes, is a fair guide suitable for use in gastroenterological patients.[40]

Fluid and electrolytes

In patients receiving total parenteral nutrition, deficiencies of sodium, phosphate, or potassium will cause a fall in nitrogen retention while fat accumulation still occurs.[65] Adequate replacement of electrolyte losses and continued maintenance are therefore critical to successful nutritional therapy.

The protein and energy are supplied in a fluid load which is appropriate to the patient's needs. Usually two to three litres are required, but losses from fistulas, diarrhoea and nasogastric tubes and extra renal losses all need to be accounted for. Elderly patients in particular are easy to overload with total parenteral nutrition and some restriction of the sodium is usually necessary. Large increases in weight due to water in any patient may be countered by sodium restriction.

Table 3.65 Guidelines for intravenous administration of energy (kJ/(kg/day); kcal/(kg/day) in parentheses) and protein (kg/(kg/day)) in different categories of gastroenterological patients

Nutritional syndrome	Energy	Protein	Remarks
Normal: preoperative	170 (40)	1.0	Glucose intake above this level is not oxidized
Normal: postoperative	170 (40)	1.0	Energy requirements do not increase significantly but increased nitrogen loss occurs owing to decrease in protein synthesis
Nutritional depletion	170 (40)	1.0	The aim is to replenish body fat stores and lean body mass. Energy needs are low with nutritional depletion and moderate gains in fat and protein will occur
Nutritional depletion and sepsis	190 (45)	1.5	Energy stores and protein compartment are depleted, but energy requirements and protein loss are high. There is a need to match losses and provide extra protein for repletion. Part of the energy load should be given as fat (42 kJ/(kg/day)
Septic	210 (50)	1.5	This group has the highest requirements for energy and protein, although the aim is to prevent loss, not to replete. At least 42 kJ/(kg/day) should be given as fat

Malnourished patients starting parenteral nutritional therapy have a marked avidity for potassium. As cells are turned from catabolism to anabolism, extra potassium is required for glycogen storage and increased cell growth. Phosphate is another ion which may fall precipitously in malnourished patients starting intravenous nutrition. About 15 mmol/l per day is required and blood levels should be carefully monitored.

Magnesium is given at 4 mmol/l per day. Most of the anion is given as chloride, but if hyperchloraemic metabolic acidosis becomes a problem some should be substituted by acetate in the formula, acetate being metabolized to bicarbonate. Gastroenterological patients with acid loss from fistulas, nasogastric tubes or vomiting usually do not require acetate.

Vitamins and trace elements
A suitable preparation of fat- and water-soluble vitamins should be added daily to the nutrient solution. Of the many preparations available, none supply all vitamins, and vitamins B_{12} and K need to be given intramuscularly as injections usually once a week. Folic acid should be given also at 1 mg/day to the intravenous solution. This should be increased to 5 mg/day in trauma or septic patients as megaloblastic anaemias have been demonstrated in these circumstances on smaller doses of folate.[4]

Ideally, trace elements should be given daily, especially in children and debilitated patients. With fistulas and in inflammatory conditions increased losses of zinc occur in the bowel as well as in the urine. The daily requirement of about 10 mg of zinc may need to be increased in these situations. Other elements given daily are copper (1.5 mg/day), manganese (0.5 mg/day), chromium (20 μg/day), iodine (100 μg/day) and selenium (50 μg/day). Such solutions need to be made up for intravenous administration. A weekly infusion of fresh plasma, suggested by some to supply trace elements, will not compensate for increased losses or make up deficits that have occurred.

Other additives
In general, the central venous line used for parenteral nutrients should not be used for any other additives. However, insulin may be added by the pharmacy if required. H_2 blockers have also been given in nutrient solutions, but other drugs such as antibiotics should be given through separate intravenous lines as compatibility with nutrients is not known.

Complications

Complications of parenteral nutrition are either metabolic or related to the catheter. The most important catheter complication is sepsis, and meticulous nursing care is essential to minimize this. Other catheter complications occur at insertion (pneumothorax, arterial puncture etc.), from disconnection of the line (air embolus) or from thrombosis of a large vein, almost always because the nutrients were infused into a vein other than the superior vena cava.

Metabolic complications are uncommon if the

patient is monitored carefully each day. Hyperosmolar crises usually occur with too rapid infusion of glucose. Hypoglycaemia may occur if the infusion is stopped suddenly. Other metabolic complications occur with deficiencies of vitamins, trace metals or electrolytes.

Special conditions

Hepatic failure

In patients with fulminant hepatic failure, administration of conventional amino acid solutions may worsen encephalopathy. Hepatic encephalopathy has been related to the high levels of aromatic amino acids (phenylalanine, tyrosine and tryptophan) in the plasma acting as precursors of false neurotransmitter amines in the central and peripheral nervous systems.[29] Administration of branched-chain amino acid solutions (enriched with leucine, isoleucine and valine) will normalize the plasma aminogram and possibly reverse the coma in patients with chronic hepatic encephalopathy.[30] There have in fact been a number of branched-chain amino acid trials but the results have been rather conflicting. Nevertheless, they improve hepatic protein synthesis and to some extent reverse the catabolic state which is characteristic of cirrhosis. Thus it seems reasonable to give amino acid solutions enriched with up to 45% branched-chain amino acids when the protein intake is restricted, at least for nutritional reasons if not for neurological ones. Glucose should be used as the energy source in hepatic failure, but it needs careful monitoring. Blood levels may fluctuate widely because carbohydrate tolerance is impaired as a result of peripheral insulin resistance. Intravenous lipid infusions are contraindicated as they have a synergistic effect in producing coma, particularly with ammonia and they may exacerbate coma by displacing tryptophan from plasma protein binding sites.[19] Patients with chronic hepatic failure should also receive increased amounts of vitamins.

Renal failure

Patients with acute renal failure are usually hypercatabolic and have increased requirements for energy and nitrogen.[75] Because of limited fluid volumes and the increased blood urea from protein administration, modified nutritional regimens have been suggested in such patients. However, with the early use of dialysis, many of these problems can be overcome and a full nutritional regimen prescribed. It has been suggested that the use of essential amino acids only may improve survival as well as improving blood urea levels.[33] Others have shown that the administration of adequate amounts of protein and energy with haemodialysis is more important in improving survival than the use of essential or non-essential amino acids.[28] Careful monitoring of potassium, phosphate, hydrogen, magnesium and calcium ions in patients with renal failure on parenteral nutrition is essential.

Respiratory failure

Administration of high doses of glucose to patients with borderline respiratory function may increase their carbon dioxide production to the point of compromising respiratory function.[26] Such patients in intensive care may benefit from the replacement of some glucose energy intake with fat. High rates of infusion of amino acids may increase respiratory drive in some patients: this may be important therapeutically.[27]

Home parenteral nutrition

There are a small number of gastroenterological patients who are unable to survive without prolonged intravenous nutrition. Most of these patients have had massive small bowel resections for vascular problems or Crohn's disease, and are left with insufficient absorptive surface to maintain protein and energy balance. The development of regimens and equipment suitable for long-term intravenous administration outside the hospital setting has vastly improved the lifestyle of these patients and some have been maintained on such therapy for up to 20 years.[32,77]

Solutions are prepared in the pharmacy and given intermittently, usually overnight so the patient is free of the infusion apparatus during the day.[46] A vest with a small pump has been devised to enable continuous infusion of nutrients throughout the day if required.[24]

REFERENCES

1. Alexander, J.W., Boyce, S.T., Babcock, G.F. *et al.* (1990) The process of microbial translocation. *Annals of Surgery*, **212**, 496–512.
2. Baker, J.P., Detsky, A.S., Whitwell, J. *et al.* (1982) A comparison of the predictive value of nutritional assessment techniques. *Human Nutrition: Clinical Nutrition*, **36**, 233–241.
3. Bates, S.E., Suen, J.Y and Tranum, B.L. (1979) Immunological skin testing and interpretation – a plea for uniformity. *Cancer*, **43**, 2306–2314.
4. Beard, M.E.J., Hatipov, C.S. and Hamer, J.W. (1980) Acute onset of folate deficiency in patients under intensive care. *Critical Care Medicine*, **8**, 500–503.
5. Beddoe, A.H. and Hill, G.L. (1985) Clinical measurement of body composition using *in vivo* neutron activation analysis. *Journal of Parenteral and Enteral Nutrition*, **9**, 504–520.

6. Beer, W.H., Fan, A. and Halstead, C.H. (1985) Clinical and nutritional implications of radiation enteritis. *American Journal of Clinical Nutrition*, **41**, 85–91.

7. Beisel, W.R. and Wannemacher, R.W. (1980) Gluconeogenesis, ureagenesis and ketogenesis during sepsis. *Journal of Parenteral and Enteral Nutrition*, **4**, 277–285.

8. Black, P.R., Brooks, D.C., Bessey, P.Q. *et al.* (1982) Mechanisms of insulin resistance following injury. *Annals of Surgery*, **196**, 420–435.

9. Blackburn, G.L., Bistrian, B.R., Maini, B.S. *et al.* (1977) Nutritional and metabolic assessment of the hospitalised patient. *Journal of Parenteral and Enteral Nutrition*, **1**, 11–22.

10. Buchman, E., Kaung, D.T., Dolan, K. and Knapp, R.N. (1969) Unrestricted diet in the treatment of duodenal ulcer. *Gastroenterology*, **56**, 1016–1020.

11. Buzby, G.P., Mullen, J.L., Matthews, D.C. *et al.* (1980) Prognostic nutritional index in gastrointestinal surgery. *American Journal of Surgery*, **139**, 159–167.

12. Chandra, R.K. (1981) Immunocompetence as a functional index of nutritional status. *British Medical Bulletin*, **37**, 89–94.

13. Church, J.M. and Hill, G.L. (1987) Assessing the efficiency of intravenous nutrition in general surgical patients – dynamic nutritional assessment using plasma proteins. *Journal of Parenteral and Enteral Nutrition*, **11**, 135–139.

14. Christie, P.M. and Hill, G.L. (1990) Effect of intravenous nutrition on nutrition and function in acute attacks of inflammatory bowel disease. *Gastroenterology*, **99**, 730–736.

15. Collins, J.P., McCarthy, I.D. and Hill, G.I. (1979) Assessment of protein nutrition in surgical patients – the value of anthropometrics. *American Journal of Clinical Nutrition*, **32**, 1527–1530.

16. Committee on Dietary Allowances (1980) *Recommended Dietary Allowances*, 9th edn. Washington DC: National Academy of Sciences.

17. Cunningham-Rundles, S. (1982) Effects of nutritional status on immunological function. *American Journal of Clinical Nutrition*, **35**, 1202–1210.

18. Daly, J.M., Reynolds, J., Thom, A. *et al.* (1988) Immune and metabolic effects of arginine in the surgical patient. *Annals of Surgery*, **208**, 512–523.

19. Davis, M. and Williams, R. (1977) Nutritional problems in fulminant hepatic failure. In: *Nutritional Aspects of Care of the Critically Ill*, pp. 487–498 (Eds) Richards, J.R. and Kinney, J.M. Edinburgh: Churchill Livingstone.

20. DeWys, W.D. (1978) Changes in taste sensation and feeding behavior in cancer patients: a review. *Journal of Human Nutrition*, **32**, 447–453.

21. Deysine, M. and Stein, S. (1980) Albumin shifts across the extracellular space secondary to experimental infections. *Surgery, Gynecology and Obstetrics*, **151**, 617–620.

22. Dickinson, R.J., Ashton, M.G., Axon, A.T.R. *et al.* (1980) Controlled trial of intravenous hyperalimentation and total bowel rest as an adjunct to the routine therapy of acute colitis. *Gastroenterology*, **79**, 1199–1204.

23. Driscoll, R.H. and Rosenberg, I.H. (1978) Total parenteral nutrition in inflammatory bowel disease. *Medical Clinics of North America*, **62**, 185–201.

24. Dudrick, S.J., Englert, D.M., Van Buren, C.T. *et al.* (1979) New concepts of ambulatory home hyperalimentation. *Journal of Parenteral and Enteral Nutrition*, **3**, 72–76.

25. Eisenberg, P. (1989) Enteral nutrition: indications, formulas and delivery techniques. *Nursing Clinics of North America*, **24**, 315–338.

26. Elwyn, D.H. (1980) Nutritional requirements of adult surgical patients. *Critical Care Medicine*, **8**, 9–20.

27. Elwyn, D.H., Askanazi, J., Kinney, J.M. and Gump, F.E. (1980) Kinetics of energy substrates. *Acta Chirurgica Scandinavica Supplementum*, **507**, 209–219.

28. Feinstein, E.I., Blumenkrantz, M.J., Healy, M. *et al.* (1981) Clinical and metabolic responses to parenteral nutrition in acute renal failure – a controlled double-blind study. *Medicine*, **60**, 124–137.

29. Fischer, J.E. and Baldessarini, R.J. (1971) False neurotransmitters and hepatic failure. *The Lancet*, **ii**, 75.

30. Fischer, J.E., Rosen, H.M., Ebeid, A.M. *et al.* (1976) The effect of normalization of plasma aminoacids on hepatic encephalopathy in man. *Surgery*, **80**, 77–91.

31. Fleming, C.R. and Remington, M. (1981) Intestinal failure. In: *Nutrition and the Surgical Patient*, pp. 219–235 (Ed.) Hill, G.L. Edinburgh: Churchill Livingstone.

32. Fleming, C.R., Beart, R.W., Berkner, S. *et al.* (1980) Home parenteral nutrition for management of the severely malnourished adult patient. *Gastroenterology*, **79**, 11–18.

33. Freund, H. and Fischer, J. (1980) Comparative study of parenteral nutrition in renal failure using essential and non essential aminoacid containing solutions. *Surgery, Gynecology and Obstetrics*, **151**, 652–656.

34. Freund, H., Yoshimura, N. and Fischer, J.F. (1979) Chronic hepatic encephalopathy – long term therapy with a branched-chain aminoacid enriched elemental diet. *Journal of American Medical Association*, **242**, 347–349.

35. Giovannetti, S. and Maggiore, Q. (1964) A low-nitrogen diet with proteins of high biological value for severe chronic uraemia. *The Lancet*, **i**, 1000–1003.

36. Golden, M.H.N. (1982) Transport proteins as indices of protein status. *American Journal of Clinical Nutrition*, **35**, 1159–1165.

37. Grant, J.P., James, S., Grabowski, V. and Trexler, K.M. (1984) Total parenteral nutrition in pancreatic disease. *Annals of Surgery*, **200**, 627–631.

38. Hackett, A.F., Yeung, C.K. and Hill, G.L. (1979) Eating patterns in patients recovering from major surgery – a study of voluntary food intake and energy balance. *British Journal of Surgery*, **66**, 415–418.

39. Hill, G.L. (1983) Operative strategy in the treatment of enterocutaneous fistulas. *World Journal of Surgery*, **1**, 495–501.

40. Hill, G.L. and Church, J.M. (1983) Energy and protein requirements of general surgical patients requiring intravenous nutrition. *British Journal of Surgery*, **70**.

41. Hill, G.L., Blackett, R.L., Pickford, I.R. and Bradley, J.A. (1977) A survey of protein nutrition in patients with inflammatory bowel disease. A rational basis for nutritional therapy. *British Journal of Surgery*, **64**, 894–896.

42. Hill, G.L., Blackett, R.L., Pickford, I. *et al.*(1977) Malnutrition in surgical patients: an unrecognised problem. *The Lancet*, **i**, 689–692.

43. Hill, G.L., Witney, G.B., Christie, P.M. and Church, J.M. (1991) Protein status and metabolic expenditure determine the response to intravenous nutrition – a new classification of surgical malnutrition. *British Journal of Surgery*, **78**, 109–113.

44. Horst, D., Grace, N.D., Conn, H.O. *et al.* (1984) Comparison of dietary protein with an oral branched chain enriched amino acid supplement in chronic portal-systemic encephalopathy: a randomised controlled trial. *Hepatology*, **4**, 279.

45. Ing, A.F.M., Meakins, J.L., McLean, A.P.H. and Christou, N.V. (1982) Determinants of susceptibility to sepsis and mortality: malnutrition *vs* anergy. *Journal of Surgical Research*, **32**, 249–255.

46. Jeejeebhoy, K.N., Langer, B., Tsalla, G. *et al.* (1976) Total parenteral nutrition at home: studies in patients surviving 4 months to 5 years. *Gastroenterology*, **71**, 943–953.

47. Jenkins, D.J.A., Gassull, M.A., Leeds, A.R. *et al.* (1977) Effect of dietary fibre on complications of gastric surgery: prevention of post-prandial hypoglycaemia by pectin. *Gastroenterology*, **73**, 215–217.

48. Kinsella, J.E., Lokes, H.B., Broughton, S. and Whelan, J. (1990) Dietary polyunsaturated fatty acids and eicosanoids: potential effects of the modulation of inflammatory and immune cells: an overview. *Nutrition*, **6**, 24–44.

49. Koji, A. (1989) The role of interleukin-6 as the hepatocyte stimulating factor in the network of inflammatory cytokines. *Annals of the New York Academy of Sciences*, **557**, 1–8.

50. Koretz, R.L. and Meyer, J.H. (1980) Elemental diets – facts and fantasies. *Gastroenterology*, **78**, 393–410.

51. Long, C.L. and Blakemore, W.S. (1980) Energy and protein requirements in the hospitalized patient. *Journal of Parenteral and Enteral Nutrition*, **3**, 69–71.

52. Long, C.L., Zikria, B.A., Kinney, J.M. and Geiger, J.W. (1974) Comparison of fibrin hydrolysates and crystalline amino acid solutions in parenteral nutrition. *American Journal of Clinical Nutrition*, **27**, 163–174.

53. Long, C.L., Schaffel, N., Geiger, J.W. *et al.* (1979) Metabolic response to injury and illness: estimation of energy and protein needs from indirect calorimetry and nitrogen balance. *Journal of Parenteral and Enteral Nutrition*, **3**, 452–456.

54. MacFie, J., Smith, R.C. and Hill, G.L. (1981) Glucose or fat as a nonprotein energy source? *Gastroenterology*, **80**, 103–107.

55. Maki, D.G. (1982) Infections associated with intravascular lines. In: *Current Topics in Infectious Diseases*, pp. 309–363 (Eds) Remington, J.S. and Swartz, M.N. New York: McGraw Hill.

56. Mathews, D.M. and Adibi, S.A. (1976) Peptide absorption. *Gastroenterology*, **71**, 151–161.

57. McGhee, A., Henderson, M., Millikan, J.W. *et al.* (1983) Comparison of the effects of hepatic-aid and a casein modular diet on encephalopathy, plasma amino acids and nitrogen balance in cirrhotic patients. *Annals of Surgery*, **197**, 288.

58. Michie, H.R., Spriggs, D.R., Manogue, K.R. *et al.* (1988) Tumour necrosis factor and endotoxin induce similar metabolic responses in human beings. *Surgery*, **104**, 280–286.

59. Morgan, D.B., Hill, G.L. and Burkinshaw, L. (1980) The assessment of weight loss from a single measurement of body weight: the problems and limitations. *American Journal of Clinical Nutrition*, **33**, 2101–2105.

60. Nutrition Advisory Group (1979a) Multivitamin preparations for parenteral use – a statement by the Nutrition Advisory Group (AMA). *Journal of Parenteral and Enteral Nutrition*, **3**, 258–262.

61. Nutrition Advisory Group (1979b) Guidelines for essential trace element preparations for parenteral use. *Journal of the American Medical Association*, **241**, 2051–2054.

62. Pettigrew, R.A. and Hill, G.L. (1986) Indicators of surgical risk and clinical judgement. *British Journal of Surgery*, **73**, 47–51.

63. Ponsky, J.L. and Gauderer, M.W.L. (1989) Percutaneous endoscopic gastrostomy: indications, limitations, techniques and results. *World Journal of Surgery*, **13**, 165–170.

64. Robinson, F.W. and Pittman, A.C. (1957) Dietary management of postgastrectomy dumping syndrome. *Surgery, Gynecology and Obstetrics*, **104**, 529–534.

65. Rudman, D., Millikan, W.J., Richardson, J. *et al.* (1975) Elemental balances during intravenous hyperalimentation of underweight adult subjects. *Journal of Clinical Investigation*, **55**, 94–101.

66. Ryan, J.A., Abel, R.M., Abbott, W.M. *et al.* (1974) Catheter complications in total parenteral nutrition – a prospective study of 200 consecutive patients. *New England Journal of Medicine*, **290**, 757–761.

67. Schufflers, M.D., Lowe, M.C. and Bill, A.H. (1977) Studies of idiopathic intestinal pseudoobstruction. Hereditary hollow visceral myopathy: clinical pathological studies. *Gastroenterology*, **73**, 327–338.

68. Scrimshaw, N.S., Taylor, C.E. and Gordon, J.F. (1968) *Interactions of Nutrition and Infection*. World Health Organisation Monograph Series, No. 57.

69. Shaw, J.H.F., Wildbore, M. and Wolfe, R.R. (1987) Whole body protein kinetics in severely septic patients. *Annals of Surgery*, **205**, 288–294.

70. Shetty, P.S., Watrasiewicz, K.E., Jung, R.T. and James, W.P.T. (1979) Rapid-turnover transport proteins: an index of subclinical protein energy malnutrition. *The Lancet*, **ii**, 230–232.

71. Shike, M., Roulet, M., Kurian, R. *et al.* (1981) Copper metabolism and requirements in total parenteral nutrition. *Gastroenterology*, **81**, 290–297.

72. Silk, D.B.A., Kumar, P.J. and Perret, D. (1974) Amino acid and peptide absorption in patients with coeliac disease and dermatitis herpetiformis. *Gut*, **15**, 1–8.

73. Smith, J.L., Arteaga, C. and Heymsfield, S.B. (1982) Increasd ureagenesis and impaired nitrogen use during infusion of a synthetic amino acid formula. *New England Journal of Medicine*, **306**, 1013–1018.

74. Smith, R.C., Burkinshaw, L. and Hill, G.L. (1982) Optimal energy and nitrogen intake for gastroenterological patients requiring intravenous nutrition. *Gastroenterology*, **82**, 445–452.

75. Spreiter, S.C., Myers, B.D. and Swenson, R.S. (1980) Protein-energy requirements in subjects with acute renal failure receiving intermittent haemodialysis. *American Journal of Clinical Nutrition*, **33**, 1433–1437.

76. Starker, P.M., Gump, F.E., Askanazi, J. *et al.* (1982) Serum albumin levels as an index of nutritional support. *Surgery*, **91**, 194–199.

77. Steiger, E. and SRP, F. (1983) Morbidity and mortality related to home parenteral nutrition in patients with gut failure. *American Journal of Surgery*, **145**, 102–105.

78. Watters, J.M., Bessey, P.Q., Dinarello, C.A. *et al.* (1985) Both inflammatory and endocrine mediators stimulate host response to sepsis. *Archives of Surgery*, **121**, 179–190.

79. Windsor, J.A. and Hill, G.L. (1988) Weight loss with physiological impairment – a basic indicator of surgical risk. *Annals of Surgery*, **207**, 290–296.

80. Wolman, S.L., Anderson, H., Marliss, E.B. and Jeejeebhoy, K.N. (1979) Zinc in total parenteral nutrition requirements and metabolic effects. *Gastroenterology*, **76**, 458–467.

81. Yeung, C.K., Smith, R.C. and Hill, G.L. (1979) Effect of an elemental diet on body composition: a comparison with intravenous nutrition. *Gastroenterology*, **77**, 652–657.

82. Yeung, C.K., Young, G.A., Hackett, A.F. and Hill, G.L. (1979) Fine needle catheter jejunostomy – an assessment of a new method of nutritional support after major gastrointestinal surgery. *British Journal of Surgery*, **66**, 727–732.

83. Young, G.A. and Hill, G.L. (1980) A controlled study of protein sparing therapy after excision of the rectum. Effects of intravenous aminoacids and hyperalimentation on body composition and plasma amino acids. *Annals of Surgery*, **192**, 183–191.

MALNUTRITION IN DEVELOPING COUNTRIES

P.S.E.G. Harland

STARVATION

When dietary intake ceases totally, rapid adaptation occurs.[7] Liver glycogen is consumed and fat breakdown increases, supplying ketones as alternatives to glucose for brain metabolism. Insulin levels fall, and cortisol, glucagon and growth hormone levels rise. The inhibitory effect of insulin on lipolysis decreases and fat is broken down into fatty acids and glycerol. Gluconeogenesis from protein increases and muscle wasting occurs through the alanine gluconeogenesis cycle. There are rapid decreases in basal metabolic rate and body temperature, mediated through a fall in T_3 and an increase in reverse T_3 (rT_3) levels, while T_4 levels are unchanged. The increased energy supply from fat conserves glucose and prevents hypoglycaemia. Protein catabolism is slowed and serum albumin levels are maintained, at least initially.

The absence of nutrients in the gut results in a very rapid loss of cellular mass, even when nutrition is maintained by parenteral feeding. The rate of DNA synthesis falls, cellularity declines and disacchari-dase levels fall. The pancreas loses cell mass and exocrine secretions decrease.[14]

PROTEIN–ENERGY MALNUTRITION

In contrast to starvation, which is acute, protein–energy malnutrition is a chronic state resulting from the interaction of dietary deficiencies and infection[6] (*Figure 3.136*). *Marasmus* resembles starvation: there is severe wasting of fat and muscle, but physiological adaption is good. When provided with energy, the children recover quickly. In *kwashiorkor* there is malabsorption: fat stores are increased even when energy deficiency is acute and low levels of important proteins such as albumin lead to clinical problems such as oedema.[2]

FACTORS DETERMINING THE DEVELOPMENT OF KWASHIORKOR OR MARASMUS

The factors which determine the type of protein–energy malnutrition a given child develops are not clear. Originally it was thought that children who developed kwashiorkor suffered from protein deficiency in the face of excess carbohydrate, while marasmus resulted from lack of energy. However, dietary analysis shows that protein deficiency when measured as the proportion of energy intake derived from protein rarely falls below calculated requirements even in places where kwashiorkor is common. In Nigeria, children with kwashiorkor were found to

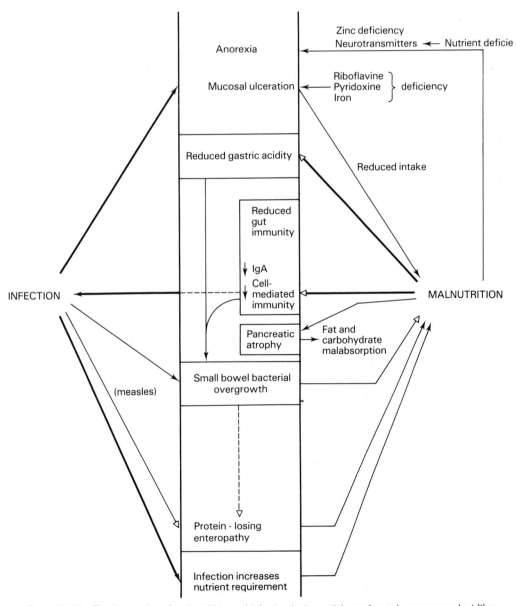

Figure 3.136 The interaction of malnutrition and infection in the aetiology of protein–energy malnutrition.

have consumed 7% of their diet as protein but had only taken 25% of their energy requirement.[28] Unless energy requirements are satisfied, protein is broken down to supply the energy deficit and thus is not available for protein synthesis. Efforts to prevent kwashiorkor solely by increasing the protein in the diet are doomed to failure unless energy requirements are satisfied. The protein content of most Third World diets is adequate but energy requirements are not.[27]

The importance of imbalance in nutrient deficiency as a factor is suggested by the epidemiological data: kwashiorkor is less common where a wide variety of foods is consumed, for example among the Sandawe of Tanzania.[30] Recent evidence implicates zinc deficiency as a critical factor responsible for immune deficiency and the skin lesions which are characteristic of the disease.[18] Sodium pump abnormalities, perhaps mediated through deficiencies of vanadium or other trace elements,[16] may contribute to the oedema.

Protein–energy malnutrition is usually precipitated by infection. Cortisol levels tend to be higher as a result of infection and this might favour the wasting of muscle and preservation of serum albumin, leading to a marasmic type of protein–energy malnutrition.[45] Infection can lead to malnutrition if repeated episodes of diarrhoea or pneumonia diminish food intake. The weight loss is not fully recovered because of the high bulk and low energy density of the diet.[26,37] Conversely, whilst infection can lead to malnutrition, malnutrition impairs the immune response and predisposes to more severe infection. Thus, in developing countries, these two are inextricably intertwined.

THE ECOLOGY OF DEFICIENCY DISEASES

Our ancestors were probably hunter-gatherers whose way of life was similar to the Bushmen of Africa. The diet would have been of great variety – traditional diets of the !Kung Bushmen include 40 different plants, besides insects and animals – rich in 'fibre', lacking refined carbohydrate and low in fat. Leafy vegetables and berries would have a high content of folic acid, ascorbic acid and trace elements, and the animal protein would be rich in essential amino acids and fats. Because of frequent droughts, however, such populations would often be subject to famine.

With the development of agriculture, dietary patterns changed. Storage carbohydrates of manioc (cassava or yucca) became the chief energy sources. Such diets contain less protein and trace elements and the amino acid and vitamin pattern is often imbalanced.

With industrialization, food consumption changed yet again, with the introduction of 'junk food', further refinement of staples, removing fibre and vitamins, and the introduction of chemicals to prevent decay and enhance flavour and appearance.

These changes are reflected in the type of deficiency diseases seen in these communities. In hunter-gatherer or pastoral societies, gross starvation is frequent; however, specific syndromes such as kwashiorkor and vitamin deficiencies are uncommon. In agricultural societies, specific deficiencies may occur. With colonization, the East African staple food changed from millet to maize and pellagra appeared. The habit of polishing rice appeared in Malaysia and caused beri-beri.

In societies with a long stable history, methods have evolved to maximize the utilization of diets. For example, in Central America, cooking maize with ash increases the availability of tryptophan and niacin, thus preventing pellagra. In the Indian subcontinent an adequate protein intake is provided, with little or no animal protein, by mixing foods of complementary amino acid composition.

In the Third World, the process of industrialization changes the patterns of deficiency disease. Urbanization is associated with more marasmus and infection owing to crowding and lack of sanitation. As infection and malnutrition nearly always go together it is often difficult to distinguish their individual effects. The diet of the urban poor tends to be based on one or two foods such as flour or rice and hence lacks micronutrients as well as being energy-deficient. When the general level of nutrition is suboptimal, the syndrome of marasmus or general wasting is seen but, as the intake level falls, deficiencies of micronutrients are exposed.

The availability of nutrients in many diets is also reduced because of the high content of fibre and phytates. The fibre satiates appetite because of its bulk and water content. Zinc, iron and calcium may be bound by the high phytate content.

CLINICAL SYNDROMES OF PROTEIN–ENERGY MALNUTRITION

The classical syndromes of marasmus and kwashiorkor are the tip of the iceberg. The prevalence is only 1–2%, although 10–50% of children in the non-industrial world suffer from growth failure. This is measured by comparing their weight and height against standards from adequately nourished communities.

Protein–energy malnutrition can be classified by comparing the child's weight with the 50th centile of weight for his or her age according to World Health

Organisation (WHO) or Stuart standards. By using the 'Wellcome criteria'[15] children can be classified according to severity as under-nourished, marasmus, marasmic kwashiorkor or kwashiorkor (*Table 3.66*).

The Wellcome classification does not take failure to grow into account. Children with chronic malnutrition may be stunted (below 90% height for age). If their body weight loss is in proportion to their height deficit they are perfectly proportioned dwarfs.

Waterlow has proposed a classification in which weight-for-height is used as an indication of current nutritional status and height-for-age as an indication of past nutritional history.[44] In a population, children can be divided into broad categories: normal, wasted but not stunted (acute malnutrition), wasted and stunted (acute or chronic), and stunted but not wasted (chronic).

Infant and child mortality rates in developing countries range from 170–20 per 1000 live births. A high proportion of those who survive fail to attain their full genetic potential for either intelligence or growth. The main reason for this is subclinical protein–energy malnutrition. The functional value of these criteria in terms of the quality of adult performance is poorly understood. The final adult height in developing countries is reduced, but the delay in skeletal maturation allows some catch-up in height, providing that the nutritional insult was not too early in development.

Table 3.67 summarizes the clinical differences between kwashiorkor and marasmus, while *Tables 3.68, 3.69* and *3.70* summarize the effects of protein–energy malnutrition on biochemical values, blood constituents and hormones, respectively.

Marasmus

The marasmic child has the classical appearance of starvation. There is gross wasting of muscle and fat but skin and hair are usually normal. There is no oedema and the child is alert and hungry if fed. The patient usually sits immobile, the limbs are flexed and permanent flexion deformities of the hips may result. The temperature may be reduced, even in tropical countries. The intercostal muscles are

Table 3.66 A classification of protein–energy malnutrition[15]

	Percentage of expected weight for age	
	<60%	60–80%
Oedema	Marasmic kwashiorkor	Kwashiorkor
No oedema	Marasmus	Underweight

Table 3.67 Clinical differences between kwashiorkor and marasmus

	Kwashiorkor	*Marasmus*
Oedema	Yes	No
Hair	Pale/easily pluckable	Normal
Skin	Flaky-paint rash	Normal
Muscle wasting	Moderate	Severe
Appetite	Poor	Good
Mental state	Apathy/irritability	Alert
Hypothermia	Moderate	Severe
Liver	Enlarged	Normal
Tonsils/spleen	Reduced	Reduced
Face	Moon-shaped	Wasted

Table 3.68 Biochemical changes in protein–energy malnutrition

Electrolytes	*Plasma*	*Intracellular*
Na^+	Normal	↑
K^+	Normal	↓
Mg^{2+}	Normal or ↓	↓
Ca^{2+} (serum)	Normal	?
Zn^{2+}	Normal or ↓	↓
Water	—	↑
Serum protein		
Albumin	Reduced	
Immunoglobulin	Increased	
Transferrin	Reduced	
Transcortin (cortisol-binding protein)	Reduced	
Retinol-binding protein	Reduced	
Lipids		
Lipoprotein	Reduced	
Cholesterol	Reduced	
Glucose	Often reduced	

↑, increased; ↓, reduced

Table 3.69 Blood constituents in protein–energy malnutrition

	Marasmus	*Kwashiorkor*
Total protein	Normal	↑ ↓
Albumin	Normal	↓
Transferrin	?	↓
Transcortin (cortisol-binding protein)	Normal	↓
Immunoglobulins	↑	↑
Lipoprotein	Normal	↓
Complement C3	?	↓

Table 3.70 Endocrine changes in protein–energy malnutrition

	Kwashiorkor	*Marasmus*
Adrenocortical axis		
Cortisol: total	↑	↑
free	↑	?
Diurnal rhythm	Abolished	Normal
ACTH response	↓	↑
Dexamethasone suppression	Normal	?
Thyroid function		
Protein-bound iodine	↓	Normal
T_4	↑ or normal	↓ or normal
Thyroid-stimulating hormone	↓ or normal or ↑	↓ or normal or ↑
^{131}I uptake	Normal	↓ or normal
Glucose metabolism		
Insulin	↓ or normal	↓
Glucose	↓ or normal	↓ or normal
Glucose tolerance	↓	Normal
Glucagon response	↓ or normal	?
Growth hormone	↑	?
Growth		
Somatomedin	↓	?

Data from Pimstone.[34] ↑, increased; ↓, reduced.

wasted and coughing is weak. Clinical signs are often absent even in the presence of infection. The pulse is normal, the heart may be small and cardiac sounds muffled. The abdomen is usually distended but, in contrast to kwashiorkor, the liver is not enlarged. The rectum is sometimes prolapsed. The stools are usually soft, and chronic diarrhoea may occur. Careful palpation may reveal enlarged abdominal nodes suggestive of tuberculosis. The tonsils are small because of wasting of the lymphoreticular system. Splenic enlargement is usually the consequence of malaria or sickle cell anaemia.

This condition arises during famines when there is a general reduction in energy intake, in children of 6 months or less whose mothers fail to breast-feed, and in children with chronic infection (such as tuberculosis), severe mental retardation or congenital heart disease.

Kwashiorkor

The characteristic features of kwashiorkor have been summarized by Trowell *et al.*[41] The early changes in the skin are hyperkeratotic; it then flakes, leaving a weeping dermatosis characteristically distributed in the flexures. In mild cases, hypopigmentation of the face and flexor surfaces is seen. The hair shows dyspigmentation, especially at the hair line. The hairs themselves are atrophic and brittle and are easily plucked without pain. Curiously, the eyelashes are often luxuriant and thick. The face is 'moon-shaped' and body fat is normal or increased. Muscle wasting is concealed and the appearance of the body suggests Cushing's disease.

Hypothermia occurs but is less marked than in marasmus. The blood pressure may be reduced and the heart sounds are soft. In severe cases the extremities are cold and peripheral perfusion is reduced. During refeeding, cardiac failure with gallop rhythm may develop if excessive energy is given too early.

Many cases are precipitated by diarrhoea, which leads to dehydration. This may be masked by oedema and it is not uncommon to find both oedema and dehydration in the same patient. The abdomen is distended and the liver markedly enlarged with a soft smooth edge. The mucous membranes usually show chronic ulceration, especially at the corner of the mouth. Candidiasis is usual, especially after measles, and may also be seen at the anus.

The patient's behaviour is characterized by lethargy and lack of interest in the surroundings. On stimulation, the child is intensely irritable and peevish. There is muscular weakness and hypotonia, the reflexes often showing markedly prolonged relaxation. Severe anorexia occurs and tube feeding is often necessary.

INFECTION IN THE AETIOLOGY OF PROTEIN–ENERGY MALNUTRITION

The environment of children in developing countries is highly contaminated with pathogens. The climate favours the transmission of malaria, poor sanitation results in contamination of water with faecal organisms, the humidity and constant warmth encourages bacteria and flies, and lack of water discourages hygiene. Consequently, children and adults are infected most of the time.

In Uganda the incidence of protein–energy malnutrition increased after the rains and the rise in malaria and respiratory infections rather than at times of drought or food shortage.[35] Children attending a 'well child clinic' were almost always colonized by enteroviruses and respiratory viruses.[13]

Guatemalan children are infected almost constantly and longitudinal studies have demonstrated that recurrent infections result in anorexia, loss of weight and, eventually, in frank protein–energy malnutrition.[26] These frequent bouts of gastroenteritis are thought to result from infection with specific enteroviruses such as rotavirus or from infection with enterotoxigenic bacteria.

Staple foods in the tropical setting show very heavy bacterial contamination. Ingestion of these diets may contribute to small bowel overgrowth.

BREAST-FEEDING AND PROTEIN–ENERGY MALNUTRITION

The traditional pattern of breast-feeding in developing countries is rapidly being eroded. Breast-feeding protects infants from protein–energy malnutrition by providing immunological factors such as virus- and bacteria-specific serum IgA and cell-mediated immunity as well as non-specific antiviral and antibacterial factors. Artificial feeds are usually contaminated and prepared wrongly and contribute to malnutrition.

MALNUTRITION AND THE GUT

Diarrhoea is a common complication of protein–energy malnutrition. Between the ages of 7 and 13 months, children in the Gambia have diarrhoea on 6 days in each month on average. The main aetiological factor is very heavy bacterial colonization of the upper bowel and reduced concentration of bile salts.[36] Rotavirus infection is the commonest aetiological factor in Guatemala, while in the crowded cities enterotoxinogenic *Escherichia coli*, *Salmonella* and *Shigella* are prevalent. Acute secretory diarrhoea causes death by electrolyte depletion. It may also be followed by prolonged chronic diarrhoea in the survivors.

In children with protein–energy malnutrition, measles presents with severe diarrhoea caused by 'Koplik's' lesions throughout the intestine. Measles is often followed by *Candida* infection of the mouth and gastrointestinal tract.

Enteric bacterial infections are frequent because faeces contaminate the drinking water, personal hygiene is poor owing to lack of water, and flies and the warm weather encourage bacterial growth and dispersion. In addition, indigenous methods of preparing food often involve leaving warm foods overnight, thus encouraging bacterial growth.[26]

The effect of diarrhoea is often worsened by incorrect attempts at treatment: very often the children are starved or put on clear fluids for long periods. During recovery, prolonged hypokalaemia results in anorexia, intestinal ileus and weakness. The introduction of WHO oral rehydration fluid as the first line of treatment has greatly reduced these complications and the decline in the practice of 'resting' the bowel and the early reintroduction of food reduces the risk of malnutrition and promotes mucosal healing.

Clinical effects of diarrhoea

The anorexia associated with gastroenteritis significantly decreases intake. Repeated attacks of gastroenteritis produce significant weight loss, especially in children already malnourished. Viral infections complicated by vitamin deficiencies lead to a painful mouth, which inhibits eating. The associated fever, mobilization of immune mechanisms, increased basal metabolic rate and the losses due to diarrhoea, sweating and vomiting increase nutrient requirements.[5] Changes in function of the gut interfere with absorption. Reduced D-xylose absorption accompanies systemic infection.[10]

After the episode of infection, failure to replace potassium leads to prolonged weakness, atonia of the gut and anorexia. In 10% of cases chronic diarrhoea may follow an acute episode. This may be due to damage to the intestinal mucosa, reduction in brush border lactase or contamination of the small bowel. The child's ability to catch up when he or she regains his or her appetite is hampered by the very low energy density and high bulk of many tropical staple foods.[37]

GASTROINTESTINAL ABNORMALITIES

The mouth

The mucosa of the mouth and tongue is atrophic in protein–energy malnutrition, the sign of 'sordes' resulting from chronic infection with bacteria, virus such as herpes, or thrush; such infection commonly occurs as a result of depression of local immunity and the resulting sore mouth is an important cause of anorexia. In severe malnutrition, infection with *Leptotrichea buccalis (Fusiformis fusiformis)* can lead to cancrum oris, a necrotic lesion which exposes underlying bone.

The tongue is smooth, with papillary atrophy and fissuring, which is also typical of associated dietary deficiencies such as iron deficiency and vitamin B_{12} deficiency.

The stomach

Gastric hypochlorhydria and gastric mucosal atrophy are reported and may predispose to small intestinal bacterial contamination as occurs in other achlorhydric conditions.[42]

The small intestine

Structural changes

In early protein–energy malnutrition the villus and crypt cellularity is equally affected but, in more severe cases, villous atrophy occurs. The normal finger villi are replaced by ridges and convolutions and the surface area is markedly reduced.[39] As villous cells predominantly subserve absorption and crypt cells secretion, this may contribute to the frequency with which diarrhoea occurs. The bowel wall is more permeable to dietary peptides, giving rise to elevated levels of food antibodies.[8,9]

Absorption tests

Brush border lactase levels are diminished and xylose tolerance is impaired. Reduced absorption of sucrose and glucose can be detected when these sugars are given in hypertonic solutions. When administered isotonically in small boluses absorption is satisfactory.[22] Reduced absorption of fat and vitamin A has also been demonstrated but amino acid absorption is only affected in severe cases.[1]

Follow-up studies after treatment of protein–energy malnutrition show that these changes persist for years. Similar changes occur in adults in the tropics. It seems likely that chronic infection may be responsible for these changes, perhaps through immune damage caused by T-cell cytolysis.

The significance of the malabsorption documented is controversial: the bowel reserve capacity is such that treatment of protein–energy malnutrition with high-fat, lactose-containing diets can be initiated within a few days of commencing therapy.[3]

The contaminated bowel syndrome in protein–energy malnutrition

Bacterial counts in the small intestine show an increase in *E. coli* and anaerobes such as *Bacteroides* spp., anaerobic lactobacilli and clostridia which are able to deconjugate bile salts to form free bile salts. *Candida* overgrowth may be prominent.[42] A high proportion of people living in these contaminated environments have elevated levels of breath hydrogen. As a result of bacterial contamination, a spectrum of absorptive defects occurs – in absorption of fat,[19] carbohydrate, vitamin B_{12}, water and electrolytes. It has been suggested that this causes the chronic diarrhoea seen so frequently in protein–energy malnutrition. Why this contamination occurs is unknown; decreased gastric acidity, high levels of environmental contamination and reduced gut immunity are all possible causes.

The large intestine

The large intestine is usually dilated, giving rise to the pot belly of protein–energy malnutrition. Intestinal transit times are accelerated but fluid absorption is probably unaffected. Prolapse of the rectum is often found, especially in children with heavy *Trichuris* infection.

The exocrine pancreas

In protein–energy malnutrition the pancreas is atrophic with loss of cellularity, reduced levels of lipase, trypsin and amylase and an impaired response to pancreozymin stimulation. There is a little evidence that chronic pancreatitis may follow protein–energy malnutrition.[12]

The liver in protein–energy malnutrition

Fatty infiltration of the liver is a cardinal feature of kwashiorkor. Liver failure, with jaundice, clotting defects and raised transaminase levels, has been described in very severe cases in Jamaica. Jamaican cases of kwashiorkor also tend to have more fat infiltration in the liver. In a baboon model of kwashiorkor, the addition of sucrose to the protein-deficient diet increased fat deposition.[11] This observation may be relevant since Jamaican children have a very high sucrose intake. The fat deposition starts in the portal tracts and spreads towards the centre. It results from impaired hepatic synthesis of very low-density lipoproteins,[2] which prevent fat from being transported or utilized. The protein matrix is wasted, cell atrophy occurs and the endoplasmic reticulum disappears. Liver glycogen stores are increased; the release by glucagon is not significantly reduced. Bile production is also diminished.

Albumin levels are reduced in kwashiorkor, especially in African children, but not in marasmus. The rate of synthesis is depressed and despite a slower catabolic rate serum levels are low (10–20 g/l). This may play a role in the aetiology of the characteristic oedema. It results from a reduction in the pool of amino acids available for synthesis.[43]

The endocrine pancreas

The effects of the endocrine adaptations (*Table 3.70*) in protein–energy malnutrition are to maintain blood glucose. Insulin levels are low and the response to intravenous glucose is blunted. When children are supplemented with potassium the insulin response improves.[24] An additional factor may be chromium deficiency. Persistence of low insulin levels after treatment has been reported; its significance is uncertain.

The blood glucose level is low in protein–energy malnutrition. The adrenergic response is defective. Blood glucagon levels are reduced in fasting, hypoglycaemic children. Hypoglycaemia contributes to hypothermia and increased death rates occur in children allowed to get cold or fed at infrequent intervals. The normal shivering and sweating effect of adrenal secretion does not occur.[21]

IMPAIRED IMMUNE RESPONSE IN PROTEIN–ENERGY MALNUTRITION

Deficiency of the immune response is an important complication of protein–energy malnutrition.

Delayed hypersensitivity

Skin reactions to both *Candida* and tuberculin are impaired. This is associated with reduced T-cell populations and diminished mitogen-stimulated transformation.[8,9] In the gut, protein-deficient young animals have reduction of absolute and relative numbers of intraepithelial lymphocytes. It has been postulated that the villous atrophy in protein–energy malnutrition could be the result of T-cell-induced damage from the immunostimulation caused by chronic infection.

Humoral immunity

In general, serum immunoglobulin levels are increased in protein–energy malnutrition. The response to antibody stimulation is also normal. However, IgA levels are reduced: young rats have reduced IgA in colostrum and the response of secretory IgA to immunization with measles is reduced.[8,9]

Structural changes in the cysternae of B lymphocytes have been reported.[25]

The immune response to polio immunization is diminished in children in developing countries but this does not appear to be related to their nutritional state but rather to the frequency of competing enterovirus infection and by the presence in saliva of an inhibitor which can be neutralized with horse antihuman globulin.

Macrophage function

Clearance of PVP and antibody affinity are diminished in children with protein–energy malnutrition and in protein-deficient rats. However, the numbers and appearance of macrophages in the gut and liver are normal.

Iron deficiency

This almost invariably accompanies protein–energy malnutrition and contributes to the immunodepression.

The role of iron is complex. It is a component of the cytochrome system and necessary for the integrity of cell function; excess free iron is, however, required for the multiplication of bacteria. When the binding capacity of transferrin is exceeded, free iron enhances bacterial multiplication, and exacerbation of bacterial infection and malaria has been suggested. Excess Fe^{++} may contribute to free radical damage, especially when there are deficiencies of free radical quenchers such as tocopherol, β carotene and selenium. Lack of iron impairs the delayed hypersensitivity response and, more specifically, reduces the capacity of neutrophils to kill bacteria.

Zinc deficiency

Zinc seems to play a crucial role in the immune depression associated with protein–energy malnutrition. The atrophy of the thymus is reversed by zinc supplementation. Zinc also influences T-cell function because local application of zinc sulphate can repair the depressed cutaneous delayed hypersensitivity response to *Candida* antigen.[18] Zinc is also necessary for *in vitro* lymphocyte transformation. The presence of zinc transferrin is a critical factor.

Other vitamins

Other vitamins, notably B vitamins such as pyridoxine, are required for DNA synthesis and their deficiency reduces the ability to mount an immune response. Interference with fat absorption can result in vitamin A deficiency, which is an important cofactor in the immune response. Mass community treatment with vitamin A has been shown to improve infant survival rates.

TREATMENT OF DIARRHOEA WITH ORAL REHYDRATION IN PROTEIN–ENERGY MALNUTRITION

The development of a balanced oral electrolyte solution – WHO oral rehydration fluid[29] – has revolutionized treatment of diarrhoea in the developing world. Treatment can be given to moderately dehydrated children orally at a rate of 100 ml/kg over 4 hours. Because of the low glucose concentration (110 mmol/l), it is adequately absorbed despite the suboptimal function of the small gut and facilitates the absorption of sodium and potassium. The added potassium is important because deficiency causes ileus. The newer oral rehydration solutions, which contain complex carbohydrate as rice powder, enable restoration of energy deficit without the added osmolar load inherent in sucrose- or glucose-based formulas. Rehydration occurs rapidly and breast or weaning feed is commenced after 4 hours. Rapid provision of nutrients in the gut encourages early healing of the gut mucosa. The rapid replacement of potassium leads to resolution of hypotonia, improved appetite and recovery of weight loss. Field trials have confirmed the value and practicality of this method of treatment. The early refeeding does not lead to prolongation of diarrhoea, provided that small boluses of isosmotic feeds are given frequently.

Electrolyte replacement is fully discussed in the context of cholera in Chapter 9.

TREATMENT OF PROTEIN–ENERGY MALNUTRITION

Mortality rates in the 1960s were between 5 and 10% but in the 1970s the rate fell to less than 1% in many units. The almost universal use of WHO oral rehydration techniques throughout the Third World has resulted in decreased infant mortality from acute gastroenteritis. The problem of nutritional rehabilitation and repair of the immune system remains because of the lack of high-energy, -protein and -micronutrient diets at the community level. The principles of treatment are:

1. Initiation of cure by giving only basal energy requirements as frequent small boluses of a diet containing 0.7 g/(kg/day) of protein and 380 kJ/(kg/day) (90 kcal/(kg/day)).
2. Correction of electrolyte disturbances using oral rehydration fluid.
3. Prevention of hypoglycaemia by frequent feeding and by giving a porridge feed at night to cover the long night and cold dawn.
4. Enteral feeding if the patient is anorexic.
5. Gradual increase of energy from basal (see (1) above) to 630–840 kJ/(kg/day) (150–200 kcal/(kg/day)) and protein to 2.5 g/(kg/day) using a milk- and vegetable-oil-reinforced diet.
6. Replacement of potassium and magnesium deficits.
7. Replacement of trace elements and vitamins during the period of rapid weight gain.

Despite the impaired absorption of lactose and fat, providing small boluses of isotonic feed are offered, absorption and then weight gain are usually very fast and should exceed 10 g/kg. A nutritional replacement diet following an acute episode has not yet been codified, but the usual village diet – with a sauce made from beans, groundnuts and other locally available complex carbohydrates/proteins – has been shown to be as good as casein-based 'formulas'.

During refeeding the voluntary appetite is enormous. When feeds containing energy reinforcement in the form of added fat to bring the energy content up to 6.3 MJ/l (1500 kcal/l) are offered, weight increases rapidly, then falls as the child attains his or her expected weight-for-height.[3] During this phase of rapid growth, balanced vitamin and trace element supplementation is vital.

Treatment of associated intestinal parasites, and also the family carriers, is essential. Antibiotics may only be used with extreme caution. They are only indicated where an adherent *E. coli* or an invasive pathogen is present, as interference with the natural flora of the gut is itself a cause of chronic malabsorption through bacterial overgrowth.

During recovery, feeding with excess energy can lead to cardiac failure and massive fluid secretion into the gut due to excessive sodium pump action.[31]

LONG-TERM GOALS

The increasing population pressure, and the breakdown of the traditional communal behaviour pattern inherent in the Westernization of the world, provide more problems than solutions. However, the emphasis on community level health intervention and improved nutrition through mass campaigns such as vitamin A supplementation, increasing immunization rates for measles, control of parasitic disease and improved health education remain essential priorities. Prevention of gastrointestinal disease by improving sanitation, providing clean water and promoting breast-feeding remain the best long-term solutions.

REFERENCES

1. Abidi, S.A. and Mercer, D.W. (1973) Protein digestion in human intestine as reflected in luminal mucosal and plasma amino acids concentrations after meals. *Journal of Clinical Investigation*, **52**, 1586–1594.
2. Alleyne, G.A.O., Hay, R.W., Picou, D.I. *et al.* (1977) *Protein Energy Malnutrition*. London: Edward Arnold.
3. Ashworth, A. (1979) Progress in the treatment of protein energy malnutrition. *Proceedings of the Nutrition Society*, **38**, 89–97.
4. Ball, P.C. (1975) The effect on oral tissues of dietary deficiencies and hormonal imbalance. In: *Applied Physiology of the Mouth* (Ed.) Lavalle, C.L.B. Bristol: John Wright.
5. Beisel, W.R. (1982) Single nutrients and immunity. *American Journal of Clinical Nutrition*, **35**(Suppl.), 417–468.
6. Bhattacharya, A.K. (1986) Protein–energy malnutrition (Kwashiorkor–marasmus syndrome). Terminology, classification and evolution. *World Review of Nutrition and Dietetics*, **47**, 80.
7. Cahill, G.F. (1966) Starvation in man. *New England Journal of Medicine*, **282**, 668–675.
8. Chandra, R.K. (1980) Food antibodies in malnutrition. *Archives of Disease in Childhood*, **50**, 532.
9. Chandra, R.K. (1980) *Immunology of Nutritional Disorders*. London: Edward Arnold.
10. Cook, G. (1972) Impairment of D-xylose absorption in Zambian patients with systemic infection. *American Journal of Clinical Nutrition*, **25**, 490.
11. Coward, W.A. and Lunn, P.G. (1981) The biochemistry and physiology of kwashiorkor and marasmus. *British Medical Bulletin*, **37**(1), 19–24.
12. Dani, R., Penna, F.J. and Rogueira, C.E. (1986) Etiology of chronic calcifying pancreatitis in Brazil: a report of 329 consecutive cases. *International Journal of Pancreatology*, **1**, 399.
13. Domok, I., Fayinka, D.A., Skritic, N. *et al.* (1974) Factors affecting the efficacy of live polio vaccine in warm climates. *Bulletin of the World Health Organisation*, **51**, 347.
14. Duthie, H.L. and Wormsley, K.G. (1979) *Scientific Basis of Gastroenterology*. Edinburgh: Churchill Livingstone.
15. Editorial (1970) Classification of infantile malnutrition. *The Lancet*, **ii**, 302–303.
16. Golden, M.H.N. (1982) Protein deficiency, energy deficiency and the oedema of malnutrition. *The Lancet*, **i**, 1261–1265.
17. Golden, M.H.N. and Golden, B.E. (1981) *American Journal of Clinical Nutrition*, **34**, 892–899.
18. Golden, M.H.N., Harland, P.S.E.G., Golden, B.E. and Jackson, A.A. (1978) Zinc and immunocompetence in protein energy malnutrition. *The Lancet*, **i**, 1226–1228.
19. Gracey, M. (1979) The contaminated small bowel syndrome: pathogenesis, diagnosis and treatment. *American Journal of Clinical Nutrition*, **32**, 234–243.
20. Harris, W.S., Kottke, B.A. and Subbiah, M.T.R. (1979) Bile acid metabolism in ascorbic-acid-deficient guinea pigs. *American Journal of Clinical Nutrition*, **32**, 837–841.
21. Heard, C.R.C. (1978) The effects of protein energy malnutrition on blood glucose homeostasis. *World Review of Nutrition and Dietetics*, **30**, 107–147.
22. James, W.P.T. (1970) Sugar absorption and intestinal motility in children when malnourished and after treatment. *Clinical Science*, **38**, 305–318.
23. Lunn, P.G., Whitehead, R.G., Cole, T.J. and Austin, S. (1979) The relationship between hormonal balance and growth in malnourished children and rats. *British Journal of Nutrition*, **41**(1), 73–84.
24. Mann, M.D., Becker, B.L., Pimstone, B.L. and Hanson, J.D.L. (1975) Total body potassium, serum immuno-reactive insulin concentration and glucose tolerance in protein energy malnutrition. *British Journal of Nutrition*, **33**, 55–61.
25. Martins Campos, J.V., Fagundes Neto, U., Patricio, F.R.S. *et al.* (1979) Jejunal mucosa in marasmus children. *American Journal of Clinical Nutrition*, **32**, 1575–1591.
26. Mata, L., Kromal, R.A., Urrutia, J.J. and Garcia, B. (1977) Effect of infection on food intake and the nutritional state: perspectives as viewed from the village. *American Journal of Clinical Nutrition*, **30**, 1215–1227.
27. McLaren, D.S. (1974) The great protein fiasco. *The Lancet*, **ii**, 93.
28. Naismith, D.J. (1973) Kwashiorkor in western Nigeria: a study of traditional weaning foods with particular reference to energy and linoleic acid. *British Journal of Nutrition*, **30**, 567.
29. Nalin, D.R., Cash, R.A., Islam, R. *et al.* (1968) Oral maintenance therapy for cholera in adults. *The Lancet*, **ii**, 370–373.
30. Newman, J.L. (1970) Dimensions of the Sandawe diet. *Ecology of Food and Nutrition*, **4**, 33–39.
31. Patrick, J. (1977) Death during recovery from severe malnutrition and its possible relationship to sodium pump activity in the leucocyte. *British Medical Journal*, **i**, 1051–1054.
32. Patrick, R.S., Mackays, A.M., Coward, D.G. and Whithead, R.G. (1979) Experimental protein energy malnutrition in baby baboons. 2. Liver pathology. *British Journal of Nutrition*, **30**, 171.
33. Peto, R., Doll, R., Buckley, J.D. and Sporn, M.B.

(1981) Can dietary beta-carotene materially reduce human cancer rates? *Nature*, **290**, 201–208.

34. Pimstone, B. (1976) Endocrine function in protein-calorie malnutrition. *Clinical Endocrinology*, **5**, 79–95.

35. Poskitt, E.M.E. (1971) Seasonal variation in infection and malnutrition at a rural paediatric clinic in Uganda. *The Lancet*, **ii**, 517.

36. Rowland, M.G.H. and McCollum, J.P.K. (1977) Malnutrition and gastroenteritis in the Gambia. *Transactions of the Royal Society of Tropical Medicine and Hygiene*, **71**(3), 199–203.

37. Rustihauser, I.H.E. and Frood, J.D.L. (1973) The effect of a traditional low fat diet. *British Journal of Nutrition*, **29**, 261.

38. Sporn, M.M., Dunlop, N.M., Newton, D.L. and Smith, J.M. (1976) Prevention of chemical carcinogenesis by vitamin A and its chemical analogs. *Federation Proceedings*, **35**, 1332–1338.

39. Stanfield, J.P., Hutt, M.S.R. and Tunnicliffe, R. (1965) Intestinal biopsy in kwashiorkor. *The Lancet*, **ii**, 519–523.

40. Stuart, H.C. and Stevenson, S.S. (1954) In: *Textbook of Pediatrics* (Ed.) Nelson, W.E. Philadelphia: Saunders.

41. Trowell, H.C., Davies, J.N.P. and Dean, R.F.A. (1954) *Kwashiorkor*. London: Edward Arnold.

42. Vikeri, F.E. and Schneider, R.E. (1974) Gastrointestinal alterations in protein–calorie malnutrition. *Medical Clinics of North America*, **58**, 1467.

43. Waterlow, J.C. and Jackson, A.A. (1981) Nutrition and protein turnover in a man. *British Medical Bulletin*, **37**(1), 5–10.

44. Waterlow, J.V. (1976) Classification and definition of protein energy malnutrition. *World Health Organisation Monograph Series*, **62**, 52.

45. Whitehead, R.G. and Lunn, P.G. (1979) Endocrines in protein–energy malnutrition. *Proceedings of the Nutrition Society*, **38**, 69.

46. Van Rensburg, S.J. (1981) Epidemiologic and dietary evidence for a specific nutritional predisposition to esophageal cancer. *Journal of the National Cancer Institute*, **67**, 243–250.

CHAPTER 4

COLON, RECTUM AND ANUS

COLON

EMBRYOLOGY AND ANATOMY

M.H. Lyall

EMBRYOLOGY

By the third week of intrauterine life, the alimentary canal is a simple tube suspended from the dorsal wall of the embryo by a dorsal mesentery. Three vessels leave the aorta and pass ventrally through this dorsal mesentery to supply the fore-gut, mid-gut and hind-gut of the digestive tube, respectively. As the digestive tube elongates it forms a mid-gut loop which at its apex communicates with the yolk sac through the vitello-intestinal duct. The part of the mid-gut loop distal to this duct eventually becomes the terminal ileum and large intestine from the caecum to the splenic flexure. The remainder of the large intestine develops from the hind-gut. During the 6th week of intrauterine life, the mid-gut loop herniates through the poorly developed abdominal wall into the umbilical cord. It remains in this position until, by the 10th week of intrauterine life, the abdominal wall has grown enough to accommodate the abdominal contents. As the mid-gut loop returns to the abdominal cavity, it rotates in an anticlockwise direction so that the distal limb goes upwards and to the left, whereas the proximal limb passes downwards to the right. The last part of the mid-gut loop to return is the caecum, which at first lies high up in the midline. It then grows to the right and descends to its definitive position in the right iliac fossa. As the mid-gut loop returns to the abdominal cavity, the hind-gut swings to the left on its dorsal mesentery. The layers of peritoneum behind the ascending colon and the descending colon fuse with the abdominal wall, leaving these two parts retroperitoneal. The dorsal mesentery of the transverse and sigmoid colon persist as the transverse and sigmoid mesocolon.

ANATOMY

The large intestine extends from the caecum to the anorectal junction and is approximately 135 cm in length. It consists of the caecum and appendix, the ascending, transverse, descending and sigmoid colon, and the rectum (*Figure 4.1*). The calibre of the large bowel is greatest at the caecum and dimi-

nishes distally towards the sigmoid colon. At the rectosigmoid junction it again dilates to become the rectum.

The general structure of the large intestine resembles that of the small intestine but there are several important differences in its external appearance. Throughout the greater part of the large intestine, the outer longitudinal layer of muscle is incomplete and takes the form of longitudinal bands known as taeniae coli. These are shorter than the colon itself giving rise to a sacculated appearance. These sacculations or haustrations can be readily seen at operation or during radiological examination. The taeniae coli coalesce in the appendix and lower sigmoid colon and rectum to give these areas a complete outer longitudinal coat. The large intestine can also be identified by the presence of the appendices epiploicae, which are small peritoneal sacs filled with fat and are most numerous in the sigmoid colon.

The caecum is a blind sac projecting downwards from the level of the ileocaecal junction. It is

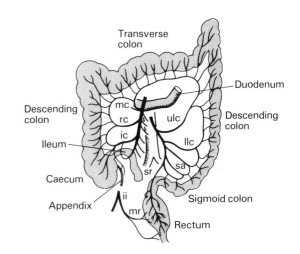

Figure 4.1 The colon: divisions and arterial blood supply. The major branches of the superior mesenteric artery are the middle colic (mc); the right colic (rc); and the ileocolic (ic). The major branches of the inferior mesenteric artery are the upper left colic (ulc); the lower left colic (llc); the sigmoidal arteries (sa); and the superior rectal (sr). The rectal wall muscle is also supplied by the middle rectal branches (mr) of the internal iliac artery (ii). Modified from Hanbrich (1976) The anatomy of the colon. In *Gastroenterology*, vol. 2, 3rd edn (Ed.) H.L. Bockus, with permission.

covered by peritoneum on its anterior and lateral surfaces. This peritoneal coat continues up behind the caecum for a variable distance before being reflected on to the floor of the right iliac fossa, thus forming the retrocaecal recess. If the three taeniae coli are traced downwards on the caecum, they will be seen to coalesce at the base of the appendix. In infancy, the appendix lies at the apex of the caecum, but during growth the lateral wall of the caecum outgrows the medial wall, so that the base of the appendix comes to lie on the posteromedial wall of the caecum about 2 cm below the ileocaecal junction. The appendix is attached to the small intestinal mesentery by the peritoneal fold – the mesoappendix. The appendicular artery passes through this fold to supply the appendix. The position of the tip of the appendix is very variable, the most common sites being behind the caecum, in the pelvis and behind the ileum.

The ileocaecal valve opens into the medial wall of the colon at the junction of the caecum with the ascending colon. It consists of upper and lower lips which project into the lumen of the bowel. It has no true valve and is controlled by a thickening of the circular muscle in the terminal 3 cm of the ileum.

The ascending colon extends from the ileocaecal junction to the hepatic flexure of the colon. It is retroperitoneal and lies in close contact with the ureter and gonadal vessels anteriorly and the inferior pole of the right kidney and the second part of the duodenum posteriorly.

The transverse colon lies between the hepatic and splenic flexures of the colon in a loop which is convex downwards. It is mobile, being suspended from the posterior abdominal wall by the transverse mesocolon. The greater omentum, a fatty apron rich in lymphatics, is attached to the convex surface and is particularly important in the adult in its capacity to localize intraperitoneal infection. In infants, the greater omentum is poorly developed, resulting in an increased susceptibility of infants to develop generalized peritonitis from an infected intraperitoneal focus, for example, in appendicitis.

The descending colon, is also retroperitoneal, passes directly downwards from the splenic flexure to the pelvic brim. The sigmoid colon extends from the pelvic brim to the upper margin of the rectum. It is mobile, of variable length and completely invested in peritoneum. It is attached to the posterior wall of the pelvis by a mesentery – the sigmoid mesocolon. It is in the form of an inverted V, the apex of which is at the bifurcations of the left common iliac artery. This is a surgically important landmark as the left ureter can always be identified in this area.

The rectum is a continuation of the sigmoid colon and starts at the level of the third sacral vertebra. It is about 12 cm long and curves downwards and forwards to the pelvic floor where it bends sharply downwards and backwards to form the anal canal. In its upper third it is covered with peritoneum on its anterior surface and both sides. The middle third is in contact with peritoneum only on its anterior surface, whereas the lower third lies below the peritoneal reflection. The interior of the rectum is divided into compartments by three crescentic horizontal shelves of circular muscle covered by mucosa. These are the rectal valves which can be seen easily at sigmoidoscopy.

BLOOD SUPPLY

Arterial blood to the large intestine is supplied by branches of the superior and inferior mesenteric arteries (see *Figure 4.1*). Close to the intestine these branches anastomose with each other in such a way that they form a continuous anastomotic channel from ascending colon to the sigmoid colon. This is often termed the marginal artery.

The *superior mesenteric artery* arises from the front of the aorta at the level of the first lumbar vertebra. It passes downwards between the layers of the small intestinal mesentery to end at the ileum, approximately 50 cm from the ileocaecal junction. Three main branches arise from the right side of the superior mesenteric artery – the ileocolic, right colic and middle colic arteries. The ileocolic artery supplies the caecum, appendix and the lower ascending colon. The right colic branch supplies the ascending colon and hepatic flexure, whilst the middle celic artery passes through the transverse mesocolon to supply the transverse colon.

The *inferior mesenteric artery* supplies the left side of the colon from the splenic flexure to the anorectal junction. It arises from the aorta at the level of the third lumbar vertebra and passes to the left and enters the apex of the sigmoid mesocolon. It gives off upper and lower left colic branches which supply the descending colon with sigmoid branches to the sigmoid colon. After it enters the sigmoid mesocolon, the inferior mesenteric artery crosses the pelvic brim and enters the pelvis as the superior rectal artery to supply the rectum. The muscle of the rectal wall has an additional blood supply from the middle rectal branches of the internal iliac artery.

LYMPHATIC DRAINAGE

The lymphatic drainage of the large intestine follows the main vessels. Lymphatic vessels in the wall of the intestine pass first to the epicolic lymph nodes. These are situated on the wall of the intestine often closely related to the appendices epiploicae. From these nodes, efferent lymphatics pass to the paracolic lymph nodes which lie on the medial side of the colon, and hence to the intermediate lymph nodes alongside the main branches of the superior and inferior mesenteric arteries. These in turn drain to the preaortic lymph nodes around the origins of the main arteries.

NERVE SUPPLY

The large intestine is supplied by sympathetic and parasympathetic fibres of the autonomic system.

The sympathetic fibres enter the abdomen in the splanchnic nerves. These relay in the coeliac ganglion and then pass along the blood vessels to supply the whole of the large intestine. The source of parasympathetic fibres to the mid-gut and hind-gut differ. The mid-gut is supplied by parasympathetic fibres from the vagus nerve, whereas the hind-gut is supplied by the pelvic parasympathetic nerves. These preganglionic fibres also pass along the blood vessels to relay in the wall of the intestine in cell bodies of the myenteric and submucosal plexuses.

HIRSCHSPRUNG'S DISEASE, 'CONGENITAL MEGACOLON'

J.O.N. Lawson

HISTORICAL

In 1691, Fredricus Ruysch described the postmortem findings, of an enormous megacolon, in a child aged 5 years.[100] C.H. Parry in 1825 reported the case of a doctor with a long history of constipation, who failed to respond to treatment, and who has found at postmortem to have a grossly dilated colon 'which extended to the beginning of the sigmoid flexure, where it resumed almost its normal size.[90] In 1886, Harald Hirschsprung demonstrated the postmortem findings of two infants, dying at the ages of 11 and 8

months, at the Gesellschaft für Kinderhielkunde in Berlin.[46] Both infants had given a similar history of inability to open their bowels. This inability was associated with marked abdominal distention, dating back to birth (*Figure 4.2*). Any response to the treatments available at the time had only given temporary relief. Both, just before their death, suffered from severe diarrhoea. At postmortem, they were found to have enormous dilatation of their intestines, including the colon. Hirschsprung showed, in one child, that the rectum was not enlarged. He described, in detail, the changes in the proximal bowel. As the symptoms dated from birth,

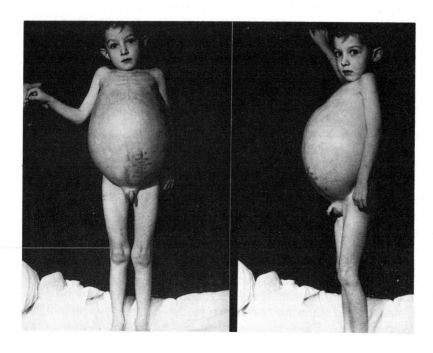

Figure 4.2 Classic case of Hirschsprung's disease (1947).

he suggested that the cause was to be found in a developmental anomaly, or a disease process, occurring in utero. In later accounts he and Mya[84] termed the condition 'megacolon congenitum'. The wide acceptance of this concept of congenital megacolon resulted in operative treatment being largely directed at the hypertrophied segment, rather than the distal segment. Although the idea that the faults lay in the distal segment, and the changes in the proximal bowel were secondary to obstruction, did not become generally accepted until 1946, Treves[122] in 1898 thought that the cause for the megacolon was 'a congenital narrowing of the lower extremity of the bowel' and treated a 5-year-old girl by proximal decompression and abdominoperineal resection. Others also suspected distal obstruction: Fenwick[34] in 1900 and Hawksley[44] in 1944 suggested a congenital spasm in the distal bowel; and Arthur Hurst[48] in 1934 described an 'anal achalasia'.

That the fault, in the distal segment, might lie in an abnormality in the innervation of the bowel was also suspected in 1901 and 1904 respectively by Tittel[118] and Brentano[15], who described a poorly developed myenteric plexus. Dalla Valla in 1920, 1924 and Tiffin, Chandler and Faber[117] in 1940 reported an absence of ganglion cells in the distal bowel in Hirschsprung's disease. Wade and Royle[125], Judd and Adson[52] in 1928, and Learmont and Markowitz[69] in 1929 considered that the changes in the distal bowel resulted from sympathetic overactivity and treated cases of Hirschprung's disease with sympathectomy but it was not until 1946–47 that the concept of distal segment obstruction became widely accepted. In 1946, Ehrenpreis[28] carried out serial barium enemas on 10 neonates, which he thought might be developing Hirschsprung's disease, and showed that the massive dilatation and hypertrophy, considered to be characteristic of 'megacolon congenitum', developed over a period of weeks. In 1948, Swenson and Bill[111] showing normal motility in the proximal dilated bowel, which was not present in the distal segment, established the concept of function obstruction in the narrow distal segment. Established histological criteria for the diagnosis of Hirschsprung's disease came in 1948 with the confirmation of the absence of ganglion cells,[10,25,26,131] and the description of abnormal, tortuous, hypertrophied nerve trunks in myenteric plexuses of the distal segment.[127] A decrease in adrenergic fibres in the myenteric plexus,[29,31,85] and a marked increase in adrenergic innervation of the muscle layers has been observed.[39,41,47] The severity of the disease may correlate with the degree of abnormal adrenergic innervation of the smooth muscle wall in the distal segment.[40,47] But the technical difficulties in

the immunofluorescent staining techniques, required to demonstrate adrenergic fibres, has not lead to a wide acceptance of these stains for the diagnosis of Hirschsprung's disease. Histochemical staining has shown a marked increase in the acetylcholinesterase content of the hypertrophied nerve bundles in the myenteric plexus, of the distal segment,[53] which has aided their identification. A marked excess of acetylcholinesterase staining fibres in the mucosa and submucosal plexuses has been noted in Hirschsprung's disease.[60,62,77]

Harald Hirschsprung's interest in the bowel proximal to the narrow segment was not entirely misplaced; apart from the mucosal changes and muscle hypertrophy in the proximal segment, a number of reports suggest an abnormal innervation, extending from a varying distance into the bowel proximal to the Hirschsprung's segment. These include hyperganglionosis, neuronal colonic or neuronal intestinal dysplasia.[16,32,41,56,58,59,82,84,91–94,99,103]

Swenson, Nenhauset and Pickett,[112] in 1949, using intraluminal balloons to measure pressure in the distal bowel, showed that normal peristalsis which passed down from the colon into the rectum and anal canal, was absent in the narrow segment of Hirschsprung's disease. They noted that the peristalsis was replaced by a 'low rhythmical series of segmental waves'. Bacon and Sherman,[3] confirming the peristaltic waves in the proximal bowel in 1951, reported rhythmical mass contractions of the distal segment. It was on this concept, that there was a functional obstruction in the distal segment, that Swenson and Bill[111] based their operation to resect the distal segment, preserving the anus and its sphincters. Hypertrophied stimulated rectal waves, of otherwise normal configurations, have been noted in the rectum, proximal to a Hirschsprung's segment. Prominent rhythmical activity was noted in the Hirschsprung's segment and the internal anal sphincter zone, but no organized contraction wave occurs in the rectum and there is no rectoanal inhibitory response. In some cases, a rise in pressure in the internal sphincter zone indicates a more severe form of the disease.[65–67] A consistent loss of the rectoanal reflex in the presence of a prominent rhythmical contractions, in the internal sphincter zone, forms the basis of a test for Hirschsprung's disease.[67]

AETIOLOGY

The aetiology of Hirschsprung's disease is unknown. The many factors involved appear to have their effect on the development of the neural crest, the basal ganglia in particular. The current concept of a 'neurocristopathy' is well supported by experimental, biological and clinical studies.[70,74,97,130] Yntema and Hammond[130] showed that extirpation of the vagal neural crest in chicken embryos, at the 5th–14th somite stage, resulted in a total absence of ganglion cells from the heart, oesophagus, stomach and intestines. If the destruction was limited to the chordal end of the vagal crest, ganglion cells failed to appear in the most distal part of the bowel. They noted that extirpation of the trunk neural crest was required to interrupt the neurones destined to pass, via the lumbar and pelvic plexuses and the mesenteric vessels, to the intestine distal to the ampulla of Vater. They noted that 'if any part of the tract contained intrinsic ganglia, parts located orally also contained ganglia' and, in addition, 'if any level lacked intrinsic ganglia, those following that also do not have them'. Limb reduction defects can be produced by disrupting the neural crest of chick embryos.[74] A developmental anomaly of the neural crest may explain the occurrence of males with brachydactyly in a family with Hirschsprung's disease.[97] Okamoto and Ueda[86] showed that neuroblasts appear in the head end of the gut tube during the 5th week of intrauterine life. These neuroblasts, destined to form the ganglion cells of the myenteric plexus, migrate down the length of the intestinal tract to reach the developing anus by the 12th week. They postulated that the origin of these neuroblasts was from the vagal nuclei, and that the ganglion cells of the developing myenteric plexuses obtained secondary connections from the sympathetic and parasympathetic systems. Failure of these connections, they thought, accounted for the tortuous hypertrophied nerve trunks found in the distal bowel of patients with Hirschsprung's disease. In long segment disease, the density of nerve fibres, stained for acetylcholinesterase, increases exponentially distal to the splenic flexure, to reach a maximum just above the anal sphincter. This observation suggests that the tortuous, hypertrophied, nerve trunks are derived from the pelvic parasympathetic outflow.[81]

There is an association with Hirschsprung's disease and abnormalities of other structures derived from the neural crest. Concomitant phaeochromocytoma, neurofibroma and neuroblastoma are reported.[19,21,38] An associated megaureter has been attributed to an autonomic abnormality. The association with failure of automatic control of ventilation and heart rate, with extensive aganglionosis, is well documented.[12,42,50,68,110] Concurrent Hirschsprung's disease with Waardenberg's syndrome, is also well documented.[2,13,33,53,75,87,95,129].

If the hold-up of migration of ganglion cell precursors is considered to be the mechanism for the production of Hirschsprung's disease, a cause for this failure should be sought. There is increasing evidence for genetic factors with the strong family histories, particularly with long segment disease; occurrences in progeny of first-cousin marriages and the association with familial conditions such as Waardenberg's syndrome. There is also the association with Down's syndrome.[91] Any environmental factors could be expected to act on the embryo between the 5th and 12th week of intrauterine life. The theory of arrested migration of ganglion cell precursors would not explain the very rare demonstration of skip lesions.

Degeneration of ganglion cells has been noted in the distal colon, following gastrointestinal ischaemia, resulting from both clinical and experimental occlusion of vessels, or injection of neurotoxic substances into these vessels. The resulting macroscopic and clinical changes bear little resemblance to Hirschsprung's disease, the affected segment becoming distended. Macroscopically a similar appearance has been produced experimentally in rats, with distention of an isolated segment of distal bowel, by corrosive sublimate.[50] This resulted in the destruction of all neural elements and also the mucosa in the segment but, as in Hirschsprung's disease, the segment remained contracted, whereas the proximal bowel hypertrophied and became dilated. Some support for the theory of vascular insufficiency is given by reported cases showing vascular abnormalities in the transitional zone and in the muscle wall of the vessel[114] attributed to fibromuscular hyperplasia.[63] Disappearance of previously noted ganglion cells, or the presence of eosinophils around ganglion cells, are quoted as further evidence of ischaemic reaction.[119,121]

Aganglionosis has been described in children with anorectal anomalies.[3,14,89,123] In the region of the fistula, as in the region of the anal canal, the distribution of ganglion cells varies. Hyperganglionosis and NID have been observed in two of the author's cases of imperforate anus. Colonic atresia, in association with Hirschsprung's disease, has been reported.[24,43,49,128]

PREVALENCE

An increasing frequency has been noted since the end of the last century, when it was thought to be rare. By 1951 the frequency was 1 : 20 000 live births and in 1967 it was thought to be 1 : 5000 live births. It is certainly more common than this, if ultrashort segment disease is included, as it accounts for about

10% of children presenting with chronic constipation and soiling.[22]

SEX RATIO

An overall male preponderance is noted in Hirschsprung's disease. Recent reports suggest a 3.8:1 ratio.[56] The male preponderance is most marked in the distal colonic disease, the ratio increasing to 11.7:1, when the cone lies in the rectum. The preponderance becomes less marked in longer segment disease (2.8:1), in disease extending up beyond the sigmoid colon, and the ratio is 2.2:1 where the whole colon is involved. The figures for ultrashort segment disease suggest approximately equal frequency (1.5:1).[22] There is a 3:1 ratio when there is a family history of Hirschsprung's disease.

RACE

Early reports of preponderance among Caucasian patients in the USA[113] has not been confirmed by a large series (1196 cases)[56] where the frequency was almost the same in black people as in white.

ASSOCIATED ANOMALIES

In most studies there has been a low incidence of associated anomalies. The most consistent association has been with Down's syndrome, 3.2%[113] to 3.7%.[90] The two reports suggested that the overall frequency of other congenital anomalies was 13.5% and 4.4%; the former excludes 2% with megaureters. An association with Waardenburg's syndrome (white forelock, wide epicanthic distance, broad root of nose and congenital deafness) has been reported.[33,74,86,94,104]

FAMILY HISTORY

A family history of Hirschsprung's disease is now generally accepted.[8,9,10,23,25,26,30,71,91,131] The incidence varies with different accounts, early reports suggest a frequency of 3.6% (7.2% in families of female cases and 2.6% in families of male cases). A recent American Academy of Paediatrics study shows an overall frequency of 11%, with 8% for female and 6% for male patients.[56] The mode of inheritance is thought to be sex modified by multifactorial, one of these multiple factors appears to be the length of the segment. If the whole colon is involved, the family incidence increases to 21%, the inheritance pattern now appears to be recessive.[18,73] In one Menonite family, with cosanginous marriages, diagnosed presumptive cases were followed back through nine generations and recorded an instance of 57%. A number of monozygotic twins, concordant for Hirschsprung's disease, are reported.[8,9,91] Others report monozygotic twins which have not been concordant for Hirschsprung's disease. There are no records of dizygotic twins concordant for Hirschsprung's disease. The reported risk for siblings with usual length Hirschsprung's disease is 1 in 20 for brothers, 1 in 100 for sisters; with long segment disease, the risk increase to 1 in 10, irrespective of sex.[20]

PHYSIOLOGY: ANORECTAL PRESSURE STUDIES (*Figure 4.3*)

Disordered peristalsis has long been recognized in Hirschsprung's disease.[112] Since 1967, anorectal pressure studies have been used both as an aid to

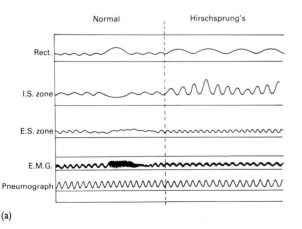

(a)

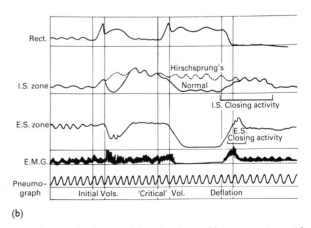

(b)

Figure 4.3 Squeeze pressure changes in the normal anorectum and in Hirschsprung's disease: (a) resting trace; (b) response to rectal distension. Rect. = rectum; IS = 'internal sphincter; ES = external sphincter. From Lawson and Nixon (1967)[38] (with permission).

diagnosis and for the measurement of residual segment and ultrashort segment disease.[65-67] The diagnosis of Hirschsprung's disease depends on:

1. The enhancement of rhythmical contraction waves seen in the smooth muscle of the anal canal and rectum, particularly in the former.
2. Loss of normal spontaneous contraction waves recorded from the rectum, where the recording balloon lies in the aganglionic segment.
3. The abnormal configuration of the rectal pressure trace when air is introduced into a rectal balloon lying in the aganglionic segment, or a hypertrophied stimulated wave recorded where the balloon lies above the segment.
4. The absence of the normal fall in pressure in the internal sphincter zone ('rectoanal reflex'). An actual increase in baseline pressure suggesting the more severe form of the disease; seen usually in the ultrashort segment disease or in cases with obstructive symptoms after definitive treatment (residual segment obstruction).[65] Occasional grossly abnormal mass contractions, with superimposed rhythmical waves, which may been seen in the affected segment, can force the rectal balloon into the anal canal.

LENGTH OF AGANGLIONIC SEGMENT

In the majority of cases the 'transitional zone' or cone lies in the rectum or sigmoid colon (73-82%) in most large series (*Figure 4.4a*). Where the rectum has been reported separately the cone lies in the rectum in 45%. (*Figure 4.4b*).

These figures exclude ultrashort segment disease (segments under 5 cm long). Longer segments occur, with transitional zones demonstrated in the descending colon and splenic flexure in 13.5-15%, transverse colon 2-2.4%, ascending colon and caecum 0.16-4% and extending into the small bowel in 3-8%. Fortunately total aganglionosis is rare,[18] with an incidence of none to 1.4% of reported cases.

PATHOLOGY (*Figure 4.5*)

MACROSCOPIC

The distal bowel
The distal bowel is either small (newborn) or normal in external appearance and calibre.

The proximal bowel (*Figures 4.6* and *4.7*).
The proximal bowel is dilated. The dilatation varies, from that associated with acute obstruction in the newborn to the massive hypertrophy and dilatation of the classic long-standing case.

The cone (see *Figure 4.7*).
Where the disease is confined to the bowel distal to the transverse colon, there will usually be a tapering from the dilated proximal bowel to the affected distal bowel. This is known clinically as the cone. It can be demonstrated radiologically and at operation, and usually corresponds to the 'transitional zone' histologically. Variants occur where there is a long 'transitional zone' and, in a few long-standing cases, where the dilatation may extend into the aganglionic segment (see *Figure 4.7*). No proper cone is formed if the aganglionic bowel extends proximal to the transverse colon.

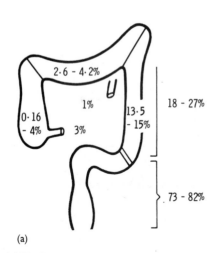

(a)

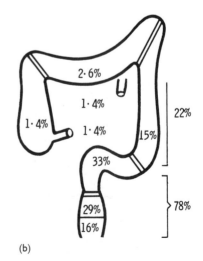

(b)

Figure 4.4 (a) Distribution of transitional zone in 1175 cases of Hirschsprung's disease; (b) distribution of transitional zone (75 cases) including breakdown of distribution in pelvic colon and rectum.

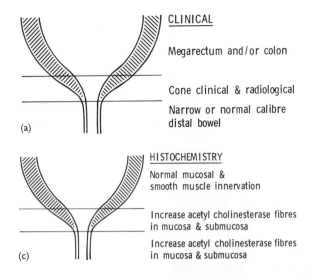

CLINICAL

Megarectum and / or colon

Cone clinical & radiological

Narrow or normal calibre
distal bowel

(a)

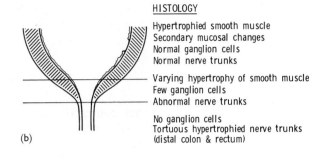

HISTOLOGY

Hypertrophied smooth muscle
Secondary mucosal changes
Normal ganglion cells
Normal nerve trunks

Varying hypertrophy of smooth muscle
Few ganglion cells
Abnormal nerve trunks

No ganglion cells
Tortuous hypertrophied nerve trunks
(distal colon & rectum)

(b)

HISTOCHEMISTRY

Normal mucosal &
smooth muscle innervation

Increase acetyl cholinesterase fibres
in mucosa & submucosa

Increase acetyl cholinesterase fibres
in mucosa & submucosa

(c)

Figure 4.5 (a) Clinical; (b) histological; and (c) histochemical findings in Hirschsprung's disease.

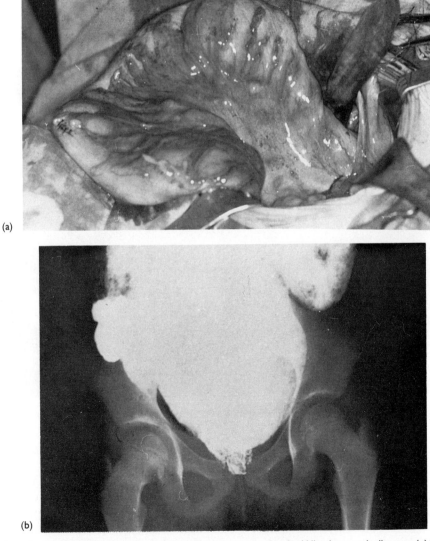

(a)

(b)

Figure 4.6 Cone in rectum with massive dilatation and hypertrophy seen in classical Hirschsprung's disease: (a) bowel at operation (after decompression); (b) barium enema (dilatation extending into aganglionic segment).

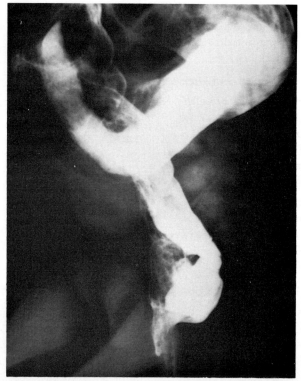

(a)

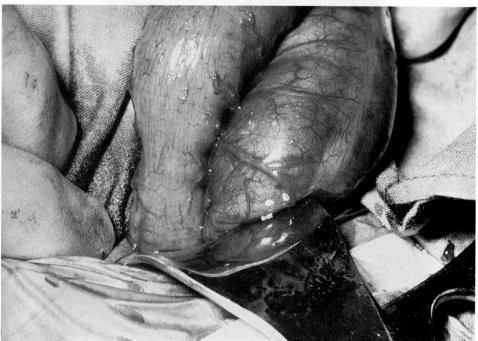

(b)

Figure 4.7 Cone in pelvic colon in Hirschsprung's disease; (a) barium enema; (b) at operation.

Secondary changes

1. Colitic changes, stercoral ulcers and melanosis coli may be seen in the mucosa of the proximal bowel.
2. Areas of necrotizing enterocolitis and perforation may occur either in the bowel just proximal to the cone or in the caecum and ascending colon.
3. Diffuse superficial mucosal loss, widely distributed in the proximal and distal segment, can occur resulting in catastrophic diarrhoea with fluid and protein loss.[35] Rarely, a more protracted form results in mucosal changes very similar to ulcerative colitis.

HISTOLOGY

The histological diagnosis of Hirschsprung's disease is based on the absence of ganglion cells and the presence of abnormal tortuous and hypertrophied nerve trunks in the myenteric plexus of a distal segment, on routine staining. For routine stains biopsies need to be deep mucosal or full thickness, if an accurate diagnosis is to be obtained using these criteria. Examination of the proximal bowel, using haematoxylin and eosin, confirms the hypertrophy of the muscle layers, the mucosal changes and normal innervation in most cases. Some degenerative changes may occur in ganglion cells. The 'transitional zone' is characterized by fewer ganglion cells, which may be abnormal, and abnormal nerve trunks. The transitional zone usually extends for a few centimetres proximal to the Hirschsprung's segment, but the characteristic histological changes may extend proximally for a considerable distance. Excess ganglion cells, in the myenteric and submucus plexuses, the presence of large ganglion cells, extending into the lamina propria and musculase mucosa, confirm the diagnosis of associated neuronal intestinal dysplasia.[78] In long segment disease, as in total colonic aganglionosis (Zeulzer Wilson syndrome),[131] there is a reduction in the nerve fibre diameter and an increase in extra mural parasympathetic fibres.[80]

HISTOCHEMISTRY

Acetylcholinesterase stains[53]
Acetylcholinesterase stains demonstrate an excess of acetylcholinesterase staining nerve fibres in the mucosa and submucosa of the distal bowel in both Hirschsprung's disease and neuronal intestinal dysplasia although, in the latter, the increase is moderate in degree.[82] Neuronal intestinal dysplasia is seen in association with Hirschsprung's disease.[94] It is the availability of these histochemical staining techniques that has made rectal suction biopsy,[17] rather than full thickness biopsy, practicable for the diagnosis of Hirschsprung's disease and neuronal intestinal dysplasia.

Lactate and succinate dehydrogenase (LDH, SDH) and non-specific esterase stains
These stains facilitate the rapid identification of ganglion cells, by staining nerve filaments in close relationship to the cells. These stains are particularly useful for staining the perioperative frozen section biopsies, providing a rapid, reliable method of identifying the normally innervated bowel.

Immunocytochemical techniques
These techniques are now well established in the examination of the Hirschsprung's segment. Their importance lies in the assessment of the bowel proximal to the aganglionic segment and the diagnosis of other neurogenic abnormalities of the distal bowel. Neurone-specific enolase,[124] glycolytic enzymes found in the cytoplasm, neurones and other neuro-endocrine tissue cells, are used to demonstrate the normal ganglion cells in the proximal bowel, and abnormal nerve trunks in the affected segment.

S100
Antibody stains can be produced to protein found in neuroglial and Schwann's cells and malanocytes. These stains can be used to identify ganglion cells, immature cells and to demonstrate intramural fibres.

Protein Gene Product 9.5 (PGP9.5)
The use of PGP9.5 is gaining wide acceptance in the diagnosis of Hirschsprung's disease, neuronal intestinal dysplasia and related disorders. That formalin fixed is required is an obvious advantage. It reliably stains mucosal and submucosal plexus, nerve fibres and ganglion cells. An increased accuracy, in staining the abnormal submucosal fibres in Hirschsprung's disease, is obtained if the sections are counter stained with S100.[102] Clinical results suggest that these stains are a satisfactory substitute for the acetylcholinesterase stains.

CLINICAL FEATURES

Hirschsprung's disease presents as intestinal obstruction of varying intensity. The degree of obstruction varies not only from patient to patient but also, in some cases, from time to time. It can be best understood if considered as a disorder of the balance between propulsive forces, active above the aganglionic segment, and resistance, afforded by the segment and the consistency of the bowel content.

The age at presentation can be subdivided broadly into those presenting: (a) in the neonatal period (first month of life); (b) in infancy (1 month to 1 year) and early childhood; (c) in later childhood; and (d) in adult life.

NEONATAL PERIOD (*Figure 4.8*)

In the neonatal period, unremitting intestinal obstruction may be present until definitive colos-

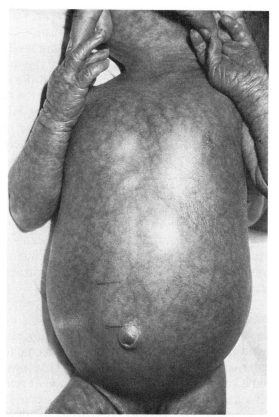

tomy or ileostomy is performed. However, obstructive symptoms and signs may settle temporarily, following rectal examination or rectal washout, or may remit spontaneously. In the latter situation the remission is usually temporary (often occurring after an explosive passage of gas and fluid stool) and obstruction recurs within hours or days. On examination apart from abdominal distension and increased bowel sounds, the anus and lower rectum may feel smaller than normal and may even present with anal stenosis.

INFANCY AND EARLY CHILDHOOD
(*Figure 4.9*)

Patients in this age group present either with subacute or remitting symptoms, which have persisted from the neonatal period, or who have had little in

---

Figure 4.8 (left) Neonatal intestinal obstruction caused by Hirschsprung's disease.

Figure 4.9 (below) (a) Hirschsprung's disease in infancy; (b) Hirschsprung's disease in early childhood.

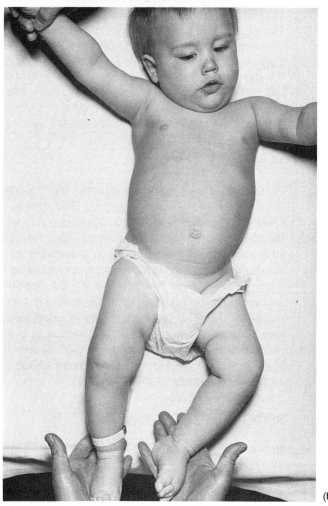

(a)

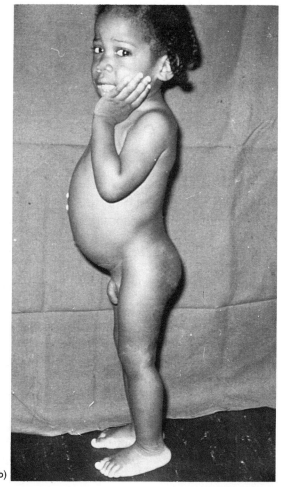

(b)

the way of symptoms, initially, but present later with increasing difficulty in defecation, accompanied by increasing abdominal distension. The symptoms usually commence at about the 6th month of age or at the end of the first year. The onset appears to be related to changes in consistency of the stool, associated with weaning or increased physical activity. The distension may be intermittent. There may be episodes of diarrhoea and soiling, with semi-solid stool. There is often a marked failure to thrive, poor appetite and listlessness. On examination, varying degrees of emaciation and abdominal distension are noted; distension is often gross, with flaring of the ribs and visible loops of bowel. Rectal examination may be characteristic; the examining fingers enter a dilated bowel through what seems to be a long anal canal. The content is usually semi-solid or liquid and withdrawal of the finger may be followed by an explosive discharge of fluid stool and gas. The anal tone appears normal. The symptoms persist until definitive treatment, or colostomy, is carried out.

LATER CHILDHOOD

These include those patients with symptoms persisting from an earlier age and those presenting primarily with a history of refractory 'constipation'. The complaint is one of difficulty in defecation, the child often experiencing difficulty in passing even soft or semi-solid stool. There is usually a history of failure to thrive, poor appetite and a poor school record. On examination the abdomen is distended, usually in excess of what would have been expected from the degree of faecal loading. Large loops of bowel may be seen through the abdominal wall. On rectal examination, in short segment disease, the dilated rectum above the segment can sometimes be identified.

ADULT LIFE

Cases are noted into adult life even up to 65–75 years of age.

DIARRHOEA AND ENTEROCOLITIS IN HIRSCHSPRUNG'S DISEASE

Diarrhoea, as a terminal event, was first noted by Hirschsprung in his original presentation.[46] It appears to have been the terminal event in 50–90% of the cases described in early reports. There are five main causes of diarrhoea in children suffering from Hirschsprung's disease:

1. Loose stools resulting from the relief of obstruction, spontaneous or induced. The clinical presentation and management is that for uncomplicated Hirschsprung's disease.
2. Bloody diarrhoea associated with ischaemic enterocolitis. This condition is indistinguishable from the neonatal ischaemic necrotizing enterocolitis resulting from other causes. In the neonatal period or early infancy, the child presents with abdominal distention, vomiting, and passage of bloody diarrhoea. The child becomes listless, then shocked and collapsed, with a marked metabolic acidosis. The abdomen becomes progressively more distended and there may be redness of the abdominal wall, particularly around the umbilicus and in the suprapubic region. Plain films of the abdomen show dilated loops of bowel, separated by oedema or fluid. Pneumotosis intestinalis and perforation may be present. At operation, full thickness ischaemic necrosis and perforation may be found. In Hirschsprung's disease, the necrosis may be of segmental distribution and seen predominantly in the ileacaecal region. Pathological changes in the bowel proximal to the Hirschsprung's segment are indistinguishable from ischaemic enterocolitis of other causes. Treatment should include appropriate resection of the gangrenous segment,[115] and should include exteriorization of the bowel proximal to the Hirschsprung's segment. Definitive treatment of the outflow obstruction should precede re-anastomosis. Hirschsprung's disease should be suspected and excluded in infants presenting with necrotizing enterocolitis.
3. The fulminating bloody diarrhoea of entercolitis of Hirschsprung's disease is one of the most dreaded complications of Hirschsprung's disease. It has been seen before and after colostomy, before and after definitive treatment. The reported incidence of up to 13% may be an underestimate, as some of these children may die, from their diarrhoea, undiagnosed. These children present with high fever, prostation and hypovolaemic shock associated with the fulminating bloody diarrhoea, proceeding rapidly to death. Histological examination of the bowel demonstrates a very superficial mucosal necrosis, with little in the way of inflammatory response. The condition has been attributed to a Schwartzman sensitization phenomenon, resulting in a vascular shut-down of superficial vessels in the mucosa and diversion of blood through submucosal shunts.[5,6,35]
4. Chronic diarrhoea prior to definitive treatment. Chronic diarrhoea may occur, prior to definitive treatment, and may be related to chronic colitic changes and stercoral ulceration.[46] This colitis

may be characterized by marked lymphoid hyperplasia. Similar changes may be seen in the distal bowel after colostomy.

5. Chronic loose stools and soiling after definitive treatment. Chronic loose stools and soiling may indicate a 'residual segment' of untreated neuronal intestinal abnormalities (neuronal intestinal dysplasia) in the proximal bowel.[6,115]

AETIOLOGY OF HIRSCHSPRUNG'S ENTEROCOLITIS

The following theories have been proposed:

1. Mucosal ischaemia resulting from distention of bowel initiating bacterial invasion of mucosa.[7]
2. Hypersensitivity reaction to bacterial content of bowel.[6,35]
3. High levels of prostaglandin, observed in enterocolitis.[72]
4. The role of *Clostridium difficile*, and its production of cytopathic toxins, reported in Hirschsprung's enterocolitis.[116]
5. Experimental work, using the piebald lethal mouse model for Hirschsprung's disease, identifies two types of enterocolitis. One occurs early, exhibiting a more acute inflammatory response. The other occurs late, showing a different pathological profile, with changes suggesting that a gut-derived infection is a significant factor.[36,37]

INVESTIGATIONS

RADIOLOGY (*Figures 4.6* and *4.10*)

Plain film of abdomen

Supine and erect (or lateral decubitus in a sick child). To diagnose lower intestinal obstruction or to assess the degree of faecal retention.

Barium enema 'on unprepared bowel'

Introducing hypotonic solution into an enlarged bowel is a hazard.[3] Tap water enemas, or insoluble barium suspended in tap water,[109] have resulted in nausea, vomiting, fits and even death from water intoxication. This complication can be avoided by suspending barium in normal saline and by the technique of introducing very small quantities of barium into the unprepared bowel.[112] This technique also reduces the risk of proximal distension and risk of perforation.

Running small quantities of barium up the distal segment, until it spills into the distended proximal segment, facilitates the demonstration of the aganglionic segment and the cone. Lateral films of the pelvis are important to demonstrate short or ultrashort segment disease.

ANORECTAL PHYSIOLOGY STUDIES

The trace in Hirschsprung's disease is diagnostic. Traces can also be used to measure the segment in short and ultrashort segment disease.[65–67]

BIOPSY

The definitive diagnosis of Hirschsprung's disease depends on the histological and histochemical criteria, so the taking of satisfactory biopsies is essential. The satisfactory treatment depends not only on identifying the upper limit of the Hirschsprung's segment and transitional zone, but also the exclusion of neuronal intestinal disorders in the bowel proximal to that segment. The following biopsies are recommended at laparotomy:

1. For immediate perioperative frozen section examination
    (a) from below clinical cone to establish diagnosis.
    (b) From above cone, with (a) to establish the level of the transitional zone.
    (c) At proposed colostomy site, to ensure that the colostomy is established in normally innervated bowel.
2. For subsequent detailed examination (a–c) as above.
    (b) Biopsies taken at intervals, between the clinical cone and the colostomy site.

Rectal biopsy

Mucosal or full thickness biopsy can be taken to establish the diagnosis. If histochemical stains are available, the initial diagnosis can be made reliably by demonstrating an excess of acetylcholinesterase staining nerve fibres in the mucosa and submucosa. This enables serial suction biopsies to be carried out per annum without anaesthesia. Otherwise deep mucosal (to include muscularis mucosa) or full thickness biopsies are required to demonstrate the absence of ganglion cells and abnormal nerve trunks. If ultrashort segment disease is to be excluded, biopsy should extend down below 5 cm, and the lowest suction biopsy should be taken 2–3 cm from the anal verge.

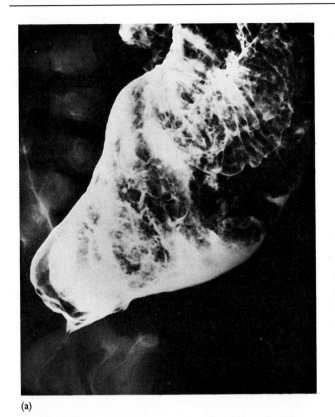

(a)

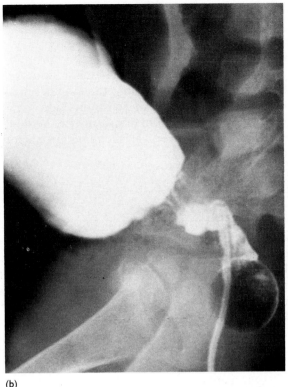

(b)

Figure 4.10 Barium enema in Hirschsprung's disease: (a) ultrashort segment; (b) short segment. (c) Long segment: the transitional zone extended 14 cm above the ileocaecal valve. There is apparent cone dilatation of the proximal colon and there are irregular contractions in the distal colon.

(c)

TREATMENT

The clinical presentation varies widely. Treatment will therefore vary with the mode and time of presentation. In general, the more severe disease presents in the neonatal period, or early infancy, and will require more urgent treatment. A later presentation may allow for a fuller preoperative assessment.

Neonatal presentation

Laparotomy and colostomy (or ileostomy)

Preoperative decompression of intestinal obstruction, with saline rectal washouts, is advisable where possible. At laparotomy a cone is identified, if present. The level of transition from normal to abnormal innervation should be confirmed by frozen section biopsies. The latter is particularly important in the longer segment disease where a cone may not be apparent.

A defunctioning stoma is established proximal to the 'transitional zone'. In cases with a normal length segment this may be either a pelvic or transverse colostomy, the author favouring the latter. In the longer segment disease, an ileostomy may be necessary.

Most paediatric surgeons favour a skin-bridge defunctioning loop colostomy; the loop is retained over a bridge of skin. An ileostomy loop may be retained by a similar skin bridge or may be double ended, if resection of bowel is required for necrotizing enterocolitis.

Later presentation

In older children and adults, if the bowel can be adequately prepared, a single stage definitive operation may be considered. In general, as most of these cases will have massive dilatation and hypertrophy of the bowel proximal to the affected segment, it is advisable to establish a preliminary defunctioning transverse colostomy.

DEFINITIVE OPERATIONS

Four main resection and pull-through procedures are currently in favour. In addition, short and ultra-short, segment disease may be treated per annum.

Rectosigmoidectomy, pull-through and coloanal anastomosis with preservation of sphincters

Modification of the operation originally described by Swenson and Bill[111] (*Figure 4.11*).

Retro-rectal pull-through with coloanal or ileoanal anastomosis

Modification of the original operation described by Duhamel[27] (currently that described by Martin and Caudill[76] and Steichen, Talbert and Ravitch[108] using a stapler of the gastrointestinal autosuture type (*Figure 4.12*).

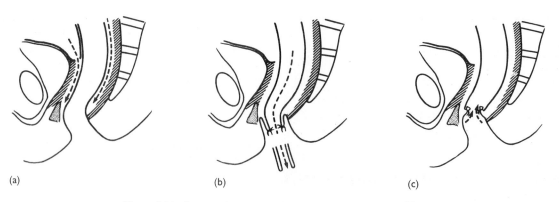

(a)   (b)   (c)

Figure 4.11 Swenson's operation for Hirschsprung's disease.[67]

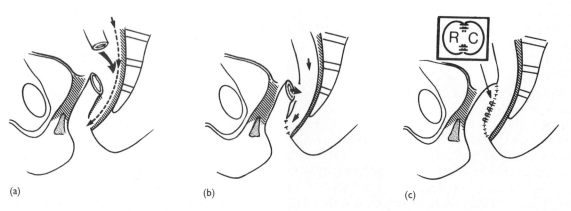

(a)   (b)   (c)

Figure 4.12 Duhamel's operation for Hirschsprung's disease.[14,42]

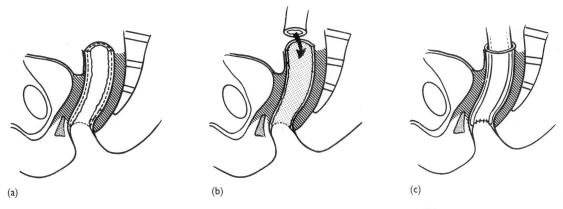

(a)   (b)   (c)

Figure 4.13   Soave's operation for Hirschsprung's disease.[5,64]

Endorectal pull-through

The operation as described by Soave[106] or its modification[11] (*Figure 4.13*).

Anterior resection to include dilated hypertrophied bowel[107]

This operation should include either forcible dilatation of the distal segment[96] or extended sphincterotomy (myotomy).[88] A very low anastomosis can be made with an intraluminal circular stapler.

Extended upper partial sphincterotomy (myotomy)

In short or ultrashort segment disease, or in the residual segment disease, where the segment can be approached per annum, an extended upper partial sphincterotomy, preserving only the lowermost fibres of the internal sphincter ani, can be carried out.[66]

Complications of pull-through for Hirschsprung's disease

1. Anastamotic leak
   Commoner after rectosigmoidectomy, anterior resection and endorectal pull-through. Leak is minimized by colostomy cover.
2. Anastomotic stricture
   Commoner after rectosigmoidectomy, anterior resection and, particularly, endorectal pull-through. Often follows anastomotic leak or cuff abscess.
3. Cuff abscess
   Abscesses may occur between the pulled-through bowel and muscle cuff in endorectal pull-through.
4. 'Residual segment obstruction'
   Inadequate resection of distal aganglionic bowel is uncommon. Even 1.5–2 cm of internal anal sphincter may be obstructive. In the severe form of the disease, the segment may respond to vigorous anal dilatation, or require internal anal sphincterotomy.[66]

ABNORMALITIES OF INTRINSIC NERVE SUPPLY OF THE BOWEL, OTHER THAN HIRSCHSPRUNG'S DISEASE: HYPERGANGLIONOSIS, NEURONAL INTESTINAL OR NEURONAL COLONIC DYSPLASIA

A number of children, presenting with varying manifestations of lower intestinal obstruction, can be shown to have abnormalities of the intrinsic nerve supply to the bowel. But, unlike Hirschsprung's disease, ganglion cells are present in the myenteric plexuses. The intestinal obstruction in these children results from disordered motility, interfering with the propulsion of the bowel content. In most reported cases, the condition is characterized by an increase in ganglion cells, abnormal ganglia and neurones in the myenteric and submucus plexuses, and the abnormal presence of ganglion cells in the lamina propria. Although there is an abnormal increase in acetylcholine staining fibres in the lamina propria, it is said not to be as prominent as that seen in Hirschsprung's disease. There may be a marked reduction in sympathetic innervation of the bowel.[32,79] Fadda *et al.*,[32] in their Type A neuronal intestinal dysplasia, relate the paucity of sympathetic fibres and the dysplasia of the submucus plexus to a clinical parasympathetic overactivity, resulting in intestinal spasticity and ulcerative colitis. In their Type B neuronal intestinal dysplasia they place those cases where, though the ganglion cell hyperplasia and dysplasia are prominent, there is no reduction in sympathetic innervation to the muscle. In this type they attribute the Megacolon to 'adynamia'. In Type A, occurring predominantly in neonates, Fadda *et al.*[32] thought that spontaneous improvement of symptoms could take place. Lake *et al.*[60] stress the difficulties in diagnosis, unless the pathologist had considerable experience. The diagnosis of these abnormalities in small bowel, where acetylcholinesterase staining fibres are normally prominent, has not been possible to date with the histological and histochemical stains generally available.

Hypoganglionosis, associated with an increase in acetylcholine esterase staining fibres, can involve bowel segments of varying lengths.[29,82] Where it occurs in association with Hirschsprung's disease it has in the past been thought to represent a long 'transitional' zone.

CLINICAL PRESENTATION

There appears to have been a degree of selection in the larger published series of clinical cases,[83,99] depending on the pattern of referral; whether increases are mainly neonatal or whether mainly older children and secondary referrals. Most of the clinical cases fall into one of two groups:

1. Those presenting in the neonatal period.
2. Those presenting in later childhood, or with symptoms persisting into adult life.

Neonatal and infant disease

Most cases present with intestinal obstruction and perforation, the perforation usually occurring in the ileocaecal region. This type of disease may be found incidently in biopsies taken above the segment in Hirschsprung's Disease or during the treatment of a child with imperforate anus.[99]

This diagnosis should be considered in cases of unexplained intestinal obstruction and as a differential diagnosis to Hirschsprung's disease, particularly where the obstruction occurs in the distal large bowel, and in those cases complicated by localized necrosis and perforation in the ileocaecal region. At laparotomy, a small distal colon will be the usual finding.

Investigation

The differentiation from Hirschsprung's disease may be initially difficult. Contrast studies may show a similar distal undilated segment (four out of five cases reported by Munakata).[83] In this group, Munakata reports an absent rectoanal inhibitory response in six out of eight cases. In one the reflex returned, although the child still needed retrorectal pull-through. Loss of this response is not uncommon as a transient finding in neonates presenting with obstructive symptoms in the first 48 hours of life, although the prominent rhythmical activity, seen in

the resting trace of a child with Hirschsprung's disease, is not observed.

Treatment

Treatment will initially be dictated by any complicating factors. Where laparotomy is required for necrosis and perforation, the finding of a small distal colon would suggest that an enterostomy is preferable to an attempted primary anastomosis. This allows full histochemical assessment to be carried out before the enterostomy is closed.

Alternatively the condition may be diagnosed on biopsy material, obtained from the bowel proximal to a segment showing the changes of Hirschsprung's disease,[56,92–94,99] also where biopsies are taken incidentally, during the treatment of a high or intermediate anorectal anomaly.[99]

Spontaneous clinical recovery has been reported in neonates.[83,99] 'Normalisation of histology' has been observed in type A cases.[32,99] The improvement has been attributed to 'maturation of the myenteric plexus'.

Later childhood

The older child will usually present with persistent refractory constipation and soiling, the symptoms dating back to infancy. The diagnosis should be suspected in any case presenting with gross megarectum, megarectum associated with megacolon, or unexplained colonic or intermittent low bowel obstruction.[83,92] Most of these children fall into histochemical (Fadda) type B neuronal intestinal dysplasia; clinically they have persistent symptoms after conservative treatment, vigorous anal dilatation and extended upper partial sphincterotomy (myotomy).[92] An association with proctitis has been reported.[99] Proctocolitis has been seen after defunctioning colostomy, in the author's cases, with an excessive production of mucus. Identical histological and histochemical findings are seen in the bowel of children with multiple endocrine neoplasia syndrome, type 2B,[99] presenting with constipation and moderate megacolon. Where the disease extends into small bowel, the child may present with failure to thrive and malabsorption caused by intestinal hurry and vomiting. In 26 children treated in my department, presenting with disabling persistent symptoms after failure of conservative treatment, vigorous anal dilatation and extended upper partial sphincterotomy (myotomy), it was found that the causes fell into one of three main groups:

1. Enormous hypertrophic megarectum where colonic dilatation and abdominal distention, in excess of faecal retention, was not a prominent feature.

2. Marked megarectum and megacolon, resulting in prominent abdominal distension.
3. High bowel obstruction, malabsorption and failure to thrive.

Four of five reported cases in this third group died. Two children had dysfunction extending up to the stomach.[16,83,92] Apart from the one death, in a child with whole gut involvement, five of the author's cases, where the disease extends into small bowel, survive with ileostomies.

ASSOCIATION OF NEURONAL ANOMALIES WITH HIRSCHSPRUNG'S DISEASE

The association of neuronal intestinal dysplasia with Hirschsprung's disease is now well documented,[16,32,41,56,59,64,82,94,99,103] the Hirschsprung's and dysplasia segments being of varying length. Out of 28 of the author's cases presenting with neuronal intestinal dysplasia, 10 had associated Hirschsprung's disease.[93] Six have been of 'the usual length aganglionic segment with cones in the proximal rectum and pelvic colon', the diagnosis of associated neuronal intestinal dysplasia being made on resected material or investigation for persistent symptoms following the definitive treatment of Hirschsprung's disease. Where the dysplasia segment has been completely excised, the children are asymptomatic (three cases). Kluck et al.[59] report neuronal anomalies in the bowel, proximal to the treated Hirschsprung's disease, in 11 of 13 cases where symptoms persist after definitive operation for Hirschsprung's segment.

NEURONAL INTESTINAL DYSPLASIA AND IMPERFORATE ANUS

Cases of neuronal intestinal dysplasia in children with imperforate anus are less well documented. Rintala[99] reports the finding of the histological changes of type B in seven cases with anorectal malformations. In five of these, the abnormality was identified on examination of biopsies taken during the pull-through procedure. In one, the abnormality was detected on full investigation of subsequent proctitis and one had persistent constipation and megacolon. In the author's two cases,[92] one child had a low anomaly and sacral agenesis and the other a high lesion and segmental neuronal intestinal dysplasia. These reports would suggest that investi-

gation of persistent symptoms after treatment for imperforate anus should include rectal biopsy.

INCIDENCE

The incidence of neuronal intestinal dysplasia is difficult to ascertain because of a degree of selection in most reports. The reported incidence varies from 'neuronal intestinal dysplasia is equal to that of Hirschsprung's Disease'[32] to 20% of disturbances of innervation of the gut.[16] Type A accounts for 15%, type B 75%, combined 15%.[32] In 2500 children, investigated between 1990 and 1992 for refractory low bowel obstruction in the author's units, approximately 14% have been diagnosed as Hirschsprung's disease, and compared with 28 children diagnosed neuronal intestinal dysplasia, but most of these presented in the last 8 years.

SEX RATIO

Rintala[99] reports a male preponderance with a ratio of 15:6, and Munakata[83] reports 6:4. In the author's cases, the ratio was 7:3.

INVESTIGATIONS

Contrast enema (in type B)

Contrast studies may demonstrate dilatation and hypertrophy confined to the rectum. The enlargement may be massive, the rectum extending up to the costal margin. The colon may be surprisingly normal in size. Alternatively, the rectum and colon are both involved in the dilatation and hypertrophy. In the long segment type of the disease, the distal bowel may be of normal calibre and show changes similar to a long Hirschsprung's segment.

Histological and histochemical status

Routine rectal suction biopsies, stained for acetylcholinesterase, and haematoxylin and eosin, will usually identify cases of Hirschsprung's disease and neuronal intestinal dysplasia, but they may not differentiate between the two, unless ganglion cells are present in the biopsy. In general, the excess of acetylcholinesterase staining fibres is less prominent in neuronal intestinal dysplasia. Full thickness biopsies, which may be taken at the time of sphincterotomy (myotomy) or at laparotomy, should be diagnostic. Unfortunately a perioperative diagnosis of neuronal intestinal dysplasia, or the rarer hypoganglionosis, and those cases with a paucity of adrenergic innervation, is rarely practicable.

Anorectal manometry

Munakata et al.[83] reports normal rectoanal response in six out of eight cases, mostly histologically type A. Scharli and Meier-Ruge[103] report the absence in their two cases. In the author's cases, the following changes have been noted in type B cases.

Rectal distension

The rectal trace was similar to that seen in Hirschsprung's Disease[67] with a peak rise of pressure on inflation and a rapid fall off to a raised baseline pressure with superimposed slow rhythmical waves. In the anal canal the normal rectoanal inhibitory response was not seen. The upper anal canal mimicked the rectal trace but a fall in the lower anal canal pressure mirrored the rise of tension in the rectum, with distension.

Closing activity

No internal sphincter closing activity was noted. It is suggested that combining anorectal manometry with mucosal biopsy would enhance the chance of diagnosing NID at the initial assessment.

TREATMENT

The optimum treatment of children presenting with the gross changes of neuronal intestinal dysplasia type B, requires resection of the affected segment. An endorectal pull-through anastomosis is desirable. Where the segment extends proximal to the ileocaecal valve, complete resection may not be practicable and pull-through of the ascending colon may be satisfactory. Where NID is associated with Hirschsprung's disease, retrorectal pull-through is satisfactory. If the dysplasia segment is excised, resection is curative.[92,93] Symptomatic improvement has been reported in neonates[82] and in an infant.[99] Only one child in our series has shown a very slow improvement, over a period of 7 years, after incomplete resection.[92] Residual disease, after resection of megarectum or Hirschsprung's segment has usually been followed by intractable loose stools and soiling, with rapid transit of radio-opaque markers. Contrast studies show a 'spastic' residual segment, with loss of haustrations in the colon and a 'saw tooth' appearance similar to that seen in longer segment Hirschsprung's disease. The symptoms have been particularly distressing in four cases where the dysplasia segment extended proximal to the ileocaecal valve.

A permanent ileostomy may be required in total colonic involvement, where intractable loose stools have followed pull-through procedures.

REFERENCES

1. Akklar, S., Sahwy, E., Kandil, W. and Handy, M.H. (1981) A histochemical study of the mucosubstance of the colon in cases of Hirschsprung's disease with and without enterocolitis. *Journal of Pediatric Surgery*, **16**, 664–668.
2. Ambani, L.M. (1983) Waadenberg and Hirschsprung's syndromes. *Journal of Pediatrics*, **102**(5), 802.
3. Bacon, H.E. and Sherman, L.F. (1952) Surgical management of congenital malformations of the anus and rectum: Report of 111 cases. *AMA Archives of Surgery*, **64**, 331.
4. Bennett, A., Garrett, J.R. and Howard, E.R. (1986). Adrenergic myenteric nerves in Hirschsprung's disease. *British Medical Journal*, **i**, 487.
5. Berry, C.L. (1969) Persistent changes in the large bowel following the enterocolitis associated with Hirschsprung's disease. *Journal of Pathology*, **97**, 731–732.
6. Berry, C.L. and Fraser, G.C. (1968). The experimental production of colitis in the rabbit with particular reference to Hirschsprung's Disease. *Journal of Pediatric Surgery*, **3**(1), 36–41.
7. Bill, A.H. and Chapman, N.D. (1962) The enterocolitis of Hirschsprung's disease. *American Journal of Surgery*, **103**, 70–74.
8. Bodian, M. and Carter, C.O. (1963) A family study of Hirschsprung's disease. *Annals of Human Genetics*, **26**, 261–277.
9. Bodian, M., Carter, C.O. and Ward, B.C.H. (1951) Hirschsprung's disease. *The Lancet*, **i**, 302–309.
10. Bodian, M., Stephens, F.D. and Ward, B.C.H. (1949) Hirschsprung's disease and idiopathic megacolon. *The Lancet*, **i**, 6.
11. Boley, S.J., Lafter, D.J., Kleinhaus, S. *et al.* (1968) Endorectal pull-through procedure for Hirschsprung's disease, with and without primary anastomosis. *Journal of Pediatric Surgery*, **3**, 258–262.
12. Bower, R.J. and Adkins, J.C. (1980) Ondine's curse and neurocristopathy. *Clinical Pediatrics*, **19**(10), 665–668.
13. Braski, D., Dennis, N.R. and Neal, J.M. (1980) Hirschsprung's disease and Waadenberg's syndrome. *Pediatrics*, **63**, 803.
14. Brayton, D. and Norris, W.J. (1958) Further experience with the treatment of imperforate anus. *Surgery Gynecology and Obstetrics*, **107**, 719–726.
15. Brentano, A. (1904) Uber einen Fall von Hirschsprunger krankenheit. *Verhandlungen der Deutschen Gesellschaft Chirurgie*, **1**, 265.
16. Briner, J., Oswald, H.W., Hirsig, J. and Lehner, M. (1986) Neuronal intestinal dysplasia – clinical and histochemical findings and its association with Hirschsprung's disease. *Zeitschrift für Kinderchirurgie*, **41**, 282–286.

17. Campbell, P.E. and Noblett, H.R. (1969) Experience with rectal suction biopsy in the diagnosis of Hirschsprung's disease. *Journal of Pediatric Surgery*, **4**, 410–415.

18. Caniano, D.A., Nishijima, E., Muraji, T., Tsugawa, C. and Matsutmo, Y. (1985) Total intestinal aganglionosis. *Journal of Pediatric Surgery*, **20**(4), 456–460.

19. Carachi, R., Auldist, A.W. and Chow, C.W. (1982) Neuroblastoma and Hirschsprung's disease. *Zeitschrift für Kinderchirurgie*, **35**, 24–25.

20. Carter, C.O., Evans, K. and Hickman, V. (1981) Children of those treated surgically for Hirschsprung's Disease. *Medical Genetics*, **18**, 87–90.

21. Clausen, N., Anderson, P. and Tommerup, N. (1989) Familial occurrence of neuroblastoma, von Recklinghausen's neurofibromatosis, Hirschsprung's aganglionis and jaw-winking syndrome. *Acta Paediatr Scandinavica*, **78**, 736–741.

22. Clayden, G. and Lawson, J.O.N. (1976) Investigation and management of long standing constipation in childhood. *Archives of Diseases in Childhood*, **51**, 918–923.

23. Cohen, I.T. and Gadd, M.A. (1982) Hirschsprung's disease in kindred: a possible clue to the genetics of the disease. *Journal of Paediatric Surgery*, **17**, 632–634.

24. Currie, A.B.M., Hemalatha, A.H., Doraiswamy, N.V. and Cox, S.A. (1983) Colonic atresia associated with Hirschsprung's disease. *Journal of the Royal College of Edinburgh*, **28**(1), 31–34.

25. Dalla Valla, A. (1920) Ricerche Istologiche su di un Caso di Megacolon Congenito. *Paediatria*, **28**, 740–752.

26. Dalla valla, A. (1924) Contributo Alla Conoscenza Della Forma Famigliare del Megacolon Congenito. *Paediatria*, **32**(10), 569–599.

27. Duhamel, B. (1956) Une nouvelle operation pour le megacolon congenital: l'abaissement retro-rectal et trans-anal du colon, et sone application possible au traitement de quelques autres malformations. *Presse Medical*, **64**, 2249.

28. Ehrenpreis, Th. (1946) Megacolon in the newborn. A clinical and roentgenological study with special regard to the pathogenesis. *Acta Chirurgica Scandinavica*. 94 (suppl.) 112.

29. Ehrenpreis, Th. (1966) Some newer aspects on Hirschsprung's disease and allied disorders. *Journal of Pediatric Surgery*, **1**, 329–337.

30. Ehrenpreis, Th. (1970) Hirschsprung's disease. Chicago: Year Book Medical Publishers.

31. Ehrenpreis, Th., Norberg, K.A. and Wirsen, C. (1968) Sympathetic innervation of the colon in Hirschsprung's disease: a histochemical study. *Journal of Pediatric Surgery*, **3**, 43–49.

32. Fadda, B., Maier, W.A., Meier-Ruge, W., Scharli, A. and Daum, R. (1983) Neuronal Intestinal Dysplasia – a critical 10 year analysis of clinical and bioptic results. *Zeitschrift für Kinderchirurgie*, **38**, 305–311.

33. Farndon, P.A. and Bianchi, A. (1983) Waadenberg's Syndrome associated with total aganglionosis. *Archives Diseases in Childhood*, **58**(2), 932–933.

34. Fenwick, W. (1900) Hypertrophy and dilatation of the colon in infancy. *British Medical Journal*, **ii**, 564.

35. Fraser, G.C. and Berry, C. (1967) Mortality in neonatal Hirschsprung's disease: with particular reference to enterocolitis. *Journal of Pediatric Surgery*, **2**, 205–211.

36. Fujimoto, T. (1988) Natural history and pathophysiology of enterocolitis in the piebald lethal mouse model of Hirschsprung's disease. *Journal of Pediatric Surgery*, **23**(3), 237–242.

37. Fujimoto, T., Reen, D.J. and Puri, P. (1988) Inflammatory response in enterocolitis in the piebald lethal mouse model of Hirschsprung's disease. *Pediatric Research*, **24**(2), 152–155.

38. Gaisie, G., Kook Sang, O.H. and Young, L.W. (1979) Co-existant neuroblastoma and Hirschsprung's disease – another manifestation of neurocrystopathy? *Paediatric Radiology*, **8**, 161.

39. Gannon, B.J., Noblett, H.R. and Burnstock, G. (1969) Adrenergic innervation of bowel in Hirschsprung's disease. *British Medical Journal*, **iii**, 338.

40. Garrett, J.R., Howard, E.R. and Nixon, H.H. (1969) Autonomic nerves in rectum and colon in Hirschsprung's disease. *Archives of Diseases in Childhood*, **44**, 406–417.

41. Gullotta, F. and Straaten, G. (1977) Hirschsprungsche krankheit mit gleichzeitiger aganglionose und sogenannter neuronaler colondysplasie (Dysganglionosis Colica) *Zeitschrift für Kinderchirurgie*, **20**, 42–47.

42. Hadhad, G.G., Mazza, N.M., Defendini, R. *et al.* (1978) Congenital failure of automatic control of ventilation, gastrointestinal motility and heart rate. *Medicine*, **57**(6), 517–526.

43. Haffner, J.F.W. and Schistad, G. (1969) Atresia of the colon combined with Hirschsprung's Disease. *Journal of Pediatric Surgery*, **4**(5), 560–562.

44. Hawksley, M. (1944) Spinal anaesthesia in the treatment of Hirschsprung's Disease (with reports of 12 cases). *British Journal of Surgery*, **31**, 245.

45. Hiatt, R.B. (1951) Pathology and physiology of congenital megacolon. *Annals of Surgery*, **133**, 313.

46. Hirschsprung, H. (1887) Stuhltragheit neugeborener in folge von dilatation und hypertrophie des colons. *Jahresbuch Kinderheilkd*, **27**, 1.

47. Howard, E.R. and Garrett, J.R. (1970) Histochemistry and electron microscopy of rectum and colon in Hirschsprung's disease. *Proceedings of the Royal Society of Medicine*, **63**, 20.

48. Hurst, A. (1934) Anal achalasia and megacolon. Hirschsprung's disease: idiopathic dilatation of the colon. *Guy's Hospital Report*, **84**, 317–350.

49. Hyde, G.A. and De Lorimier, A.A. (1968) Colon atresia and Hirschsprung's disease. *Surgery*, **64**(5), 976–978.

50. Imamura, K., Yamamoto, M., Sato, A. *et al.* (1975) Pathophysiology of aganglionic colon segment: an experimental study on aganglionosis produced by a new method in the rat. *Journal of Pediatric Surgery*, **10**, 865.

51. Johnston, M.C., Vig, K.W.L. and Ambrose, L.J.H. (1981) Neurocristopathy a unifying concept: clinical correlations. In *Advances in Neurology. Neurofibromatosis (von Recklinghausen Disease),* vol. 29, pp. 97–104. (Eds) Riccadi, V.M. and Mulvihill, J.J. New York: Raven Press.

52. Judd, S. and Adson, A.W. (1928) Lumbar sympathetic ganglionectomy and ramisection, for congenital idiopathic dilatation of the colon. *Annals of Surgery*, **88**, 479–498.

53. Kamijo, K., Hiatt, R.B. and Koelle, G.B. (1953) Congenital megacolon. A comparison of the spastic and hypertrophied segments with respect to cholinesterase activities and sensitivities to acetylcholine, DFP and the barium ion. *Gastroenterology*, **24**, 173.

54. Karnovsky, M.J. and Roots, L. (1964) A 'direct-coloring' thiocholine method for cholinesterase. *Journal of Histochemistry and Cytochemistry*, **12**, 219–221.

55. Kelley, R.I. and Zackai, E.H. (1981) Congenital deafness, Hirschsprung's and Waandenberg syndrome. *American Journal of Human Genetics*, **33**, 65A.

56. Kessler, S. and Campbell, J.R. (1985) Neuronal colonic dysplasia associated with short segment Hirschsprung's disease. *Archives of Pathological Laboratory Medicine*, **109**, 532–533.

57. Kleinhaus, S., Boley, S.J., Sheran, M. and Sieber, W.K. (1979) Hirschsprung's disease. A survey of the members of the Surgical Section of the American Academy of Pediatrics. *Journal of Pediatric Surgery*, **14**, 588–597.

58. Klück, P., Van Muijen, G.N.P., Van der Kamp, A.W.M. *et al.* (1984) Hirschsprung's disease studied with monoclonal anti-neurofilament antibodies on tissue sections. *The Lancet*, **1**, 652–653.

59. Kluck, D., Tibboel, K., Leendertse-Verloop, A.W.M. *et al.* (1986) Diagnosis of congenital neurogenic abnormalities of the bowel with monoclonal anti-neurofilament antibodies. *Journal of Pediatric Surgery*, **21**(2), 132–135.

60. Lake, B.D. (1976) A cholinesterase method for light and electron microscopy. *Proceedings of the Royal Microscopic Society*, **11**, 77.

61. Lake, B., Malone, M.T. and Risdon, R.A. (1989) The use of acetylcholinesterase (AchE) in the diagnosis of Hirschsprung's disease and neuronal intestinal dysplasia. *Pediatric Pathology*, **9**(30), 351–354.

62. Lassman, G. (1974) The clinical relevance of neurohistological investigations of intestinal

biopsies. *Journal of Neural Transmission II* (suppl. XI) 255–280.

63. Lassman, G. (1988) Vascular dysplasia of arteries in neurocrystopathies; a lesson for neurofibromatosis. In *Neurofibromatosis*, (Riccardi, V.M., ed) **1**, 281–293. Basle. Karger.

64. Lassman, G. and Wurnig, P. (1973) Lokale Ganglienzell Hyperplasie in der submucosa am Oralen Ende des Aganglionaren segmentes bei Morbes Hirschsprung. *Zeitschrift für Kinderchirurgie*, **12**, 236–243.

65. Lawson, J.O.N. (1970) Structure and function of the internal anal sphincter. *Proceedings of the Royal Society of Medicine*, **63**, 84–89.

66. Lawson, J.O.N. (1972) Observations on 'residual segment obstruction' in treated Hirschsprung's disease. *Progress in Pediatric Surgery*, **4**, 129–164.

67. Lawson, J.O.N. and Nixon, H.H. (1967) Anal canal pressures in the diagnosis of Hirschsprung's disease. *Journal of Pediatric Surgery*, **2**, 544–552.

68. Lawson, J.O.N., Harding, B. and Singer, J.D. (1992) Total aganglionosis of the gastrointestinal tract associated with congenital failure of automatic control of ventilation. A clinical and neuropathological study (in press).

69. Learmont, J.R. and Markowitz, J. (1929) Studies on the function of the lumbar sympathetic outflow. The relation of the lumbar sympathetic outflow to the sphincter anii internus. *American Journal of Physiology*, **89**, 686–691.

70. le Dourin, N. and Teillet, M.A. (1973) The migration of the neural crest cells to the wall of the digestive tract in avian embryo. *Journal of Embryology and Experimental Morphology*, **30**, 31–48.

71. Lipson, A.H. and Harvey, J. (1987) A three generation transmission of Hirschsprung's disease. *Clinical Genetics*, **32**, 175–178.

72. Lloyd-Still, J.D. and Demers, L.M. (1978) Hirschsprung's enterocolitis, prostaglandins, and response to cholestyramine. *Journal of Pediatric Surgery*, **13**(4), 417–418.

73. MacKinnon, A.E. and Cohen, S.J. (1977) Total intestinal aganglionosis: an autosomal recessive condition? *Archives of Diseases in Children*, **52**, 898–899.

74. McCredie, J., Cameron, J. and Shoobridge, R. (1978) Congenital malformations and the neural crest. *The Lancet*, **ii**, 761–763.

75. McKusick, V.A. (1973) Congenital deafness and Hirschsprung's disease. *New England Journal of Medicine*, **288**, 691.

76. Martin, L.W. and Caudill, D.R. (1967) A method for elimination of the blind rectal pouch in the Duhamel operation for Hirschsprung's disease. *Surgery*, **62**, 951–953.

77. Meier-Ruge, W. (1972) Fortschritte in der Diagnostik des Aganglionären Segmentes. *Padiatrie und Padologie*. Suppl 2, 55.

78. Meier-Ruge, W. (1974) Hirschsprung's disease: it's aetiology pathogenesis and differential diagnosis. *Current Topics in Pathology,* Ergb. Pathol Volume

59, pp. 131–179. Berlin, Heidelberg, New York: Springer-Verlag.

79. Meier-Ruge, W. (1974) Hirschsprung's disease: etiology, pathogenesis and differential diagnosis. *Current topics in Pathology*, **59**, 131–179. Berlin: Springer-Verlag.

80. Meier-Ruge, W. (1982) In *Hirschsprung's Disease*, chapter X,1.10.3., (Ed.) Holschneider, Stuttgart: Hippokrates Verlag; New York: Thieme-Stratton, Inc.

81. Meier-Ruge, W., Butterbeck, P., Herzog, B. and Scharli, A. (1972) Acetylcholinesterase activity in suction biopsies of the rectum in the diagnosis of Hirschsprung's disease. *Journal of Pediatric Surgery*, **7**, 11–17.

82. Munakata, K., Okabe, I. and Morita, K. (1978) Histologic studies of recto-colic aganglionosis and allied diseases. *Journal of Pediatric Surgery*, **13**(i), 67–75.

83. Munakata, K., Morita, K., Okabe, I. and Sueka, H. (1985) Clinical and histologic studies of Neuronal Intestinal Dysplasia. *Journal of Pediatric Surgery*, **20**(3), 231–235.

84. Mya, G. (1894) Due osservazioni di dilatazione ed ipertrofia congenita del colon. *Sperimentale*, **48**, 215.

85. Okamoto, E. (1961) Neuropathological and embryological studies on aetiology of aganglionic megacolon. *Medical Journal of Osaka Univesity*, **13**, 285.

86. Okamoto, E. and Ueda, T. (1967) Embryogenesis of intramural ganglia of the gut and it's relation to Hirschsprung's disease. *Journal of Pediatric Surgery*, **14**, 58.

87. Omenn, G.S. and McKusick, V.A. (1979) Association of Waardenberg's Syndrome and Hirschsprung's megacolon. *American Journal of Medical Genetics*, **3**, 217–223.

88. Orr, J.D. and Scobie, W.G. (1979) Anterior resection combined with anorectal myectomy in the treatment of Hirschsprung's disease. *Journal of Pediatric Surgery*, **14**, 58–61.

89. Parkkulainen, K.V., Hjelt, L. and Sulamaa, M. (1959/1960). Anal atresia combined with aganglionic megacolon. *Acta Chirurgica Scandinavica*, **118**, 252–256.

90. Parry, C.H. (1825) Singular and fatal accumulation of faeces. In *Selections from Unpublished Writings of the Late C.H. Parry*, Vol 2, pp. 380–387, Underwoods.

91. Passarge, E. (1967) The genetics of Hirschsprung's disease. Evidence for heterogeneous etiology and a study of sixty-three families. *New England Journal of Medicine*, **276**, 138–143.

92. Pradhan, G.N., Siddiqui, M. and Lawson, J.O.N. (1989) *Severe refractory constipation in association with neuronal intestinal disorders*. Paper given to the British Association of Paediatric Surgeon's meeting, Edinburgh.

93. Pradhan, G., Lawson, J.O.N., Pambakian, H. and Hosie, G. (1991) *Association of colonic neuronal intestinal dysplasia (NID) with Hirschsprung's disease*. Paper read at B.A.P.S. International Meeting Budapest.

94. Puri, P., Lake, B.D., Nixon, H.H. *et al.* (1977) Neuronal colonic dysplasia: an unusual association of Hirschsprung's disease. *Journal of Pediatric Surgery*, **12**, 681–685.

95. Rarey, K.E. and Davis, L.E. (1984) Inner ear anomalies in Waadenberg's syndrome associated with Hirschsprung's disease. *International Journal of Pediatric Otorhinolaryngology*, **8**, 181–189.

96. Rehbein, F. (1958) Intraabdominelle resektion oder recto-sigmoidektomic (Swenson) hei der Hirschsprungschen Krankheit? *Chirurgie*, **29**, 366.

97. Reynolds, J.F., Barber, J.C., Alford, B.A., Chandler, J.G. and Kelly, T.E. (1983) Familial Hirschsprung's disease and Type D brachydactyl: a report of four affected males in two generations. *Pediatrics*, **71**(2), 246–249.

98. Riker, W.L. (1957) Diagnosis and treatment of aganglionosis of the myenteric plexus. *Archives of Surgery*, **75**, 362–376.

99. Rintala, R., Rapola, J. and Louhimo, I. (1989) Neuronal intestinal dysplasia. *Progress in Pediatric Surgery*, **24**, 186–192.

100. Ruysch, F. (1691) Observationem anatomica–chirurgicarum centuria, Amsterdammen. (Quoted) *Journal of Pediatric Surgery*, **5**(i), 1–3 (1970).

101. Saing, H., Lee, J.M. and Tam, P.K.H. (1986) The use of intraluminal stapler in the definitive management of Hirschsprung's disease. *Diseases of the Colon and Rectum*, **29**(3), 211–215.

102. Samu, V.A., Bobrow, L.G., Happerfield, L. and Keeling, J. (1992) Evaluation of PGP9.5 in the diagnosis of Hirschsprung's disease. *Journal of Pathology*, **168**, 55–58.

103. Scharli, A.G. and Meier-Ruge, W. (1981) Localized and disseminated forms of neuronal intestinal dysplasia mimicking Hirschsprung's disease. *Journal of Pediatric Surgery*, **16**(2), 164–170.

104. Shah, K.N., Dalal, S.J., Dasai, M.P. and Seth, P.N. (1981) White forelock, pigmentary disorder of the irides, and long segment Hirschsprung's disease. *Journal of Pediatrics*, **99**, 432–435.

105. Sikaniwa, A.F. *et al.* (1981) Association of anorectal malformation and aganglionosis. *Japanese Journal of Paediatric Surgery*, **13**, 895–900.

106. Soave, F. (1963) Die nahtiose colon-anastomose nach extramucoser Mobilierung und Herabzielhung des Rectosigmoids zur chirurgischen Behandlung des M. Hirschsprung. *Zentralblan für Chirurgie*, **88**, 31.

107. State, D. (1952) Surgical treatment for idiopathic congenital megacolon (Hirschsprung's disease). *Surgery, Gynecology and Obstetrics*, **95**, 201–202.

108. Steichen, F.M., Talbert, J.L. and Ravitch, M.M. (1968) Primary side to side colorectal anastomosis in the Duhamel operation for Hirschsprung's disease. *Surgery*, **64**, 475–483.

109. Steinbach, H.L., Rosenberg, R.H., Grossman, M. and Nelson, T.L. (1955) The potential hazard of

enemas in patients with Hirschsprung's disease. *Radiology*, **64**, 45.

110. Stern, M., Hellwege, I., Gravinghoff, L. and Lambrecht, W. (1981) A total aganglionosis of the colon (Hirschsprung's disease) and congenital failure of automatic control of ventilation (Ondine's curse). *Acta Paediatrica. Scandinavica*, **70**, 121–124.

111. Swenson, O. and Bill, A.H. (1948) Resection of rectum and rectosigmoid with preservation of the sphincter for benign spastic lesions producing megacolon: an experimental study. *Surgery*, **24**, 212.

112. Swenson, O., Neuhauser, E.B.D. and Pickett, L.K. (1949) New concept of aetiology, diagnosis and treatment of congenital megacolon (Hirschsprung's disease). *Paediatrics*, **4**, 201–206.

113. Swenson, O., Sherman, J.O. and Fisher, J.H. (1973) Diagnosis of congenital megacolon. Analysis of 501 patients. *Journal of Pediatric Surgery*, **8**, 587–594.

114. Taguchi, T., Tanaka, K. and Ikeda, K. (1985) Fibromuscular dysplasia of arteries in Hirschsprung's disease. *Gastroenterology*, **88**, 1099–1103.

115. Teich, S., Schisgall, R.M. and Anderson, K.D. (1986). Ischemic Enterocolitis as a complication of Hirschsprung's disease. *Journal of Pediatric Surgery*, **21**(2), 143–145.

116. Thomas, D.F.M., Fernie, D.S., Bayston, R., Spitz, L. and Nixon, H.H. (1986) Enterocolitis in Hirschsprung's disease: a controlled study of the etiologic role of *Clostridium Difficile. Journal of Pediatric Surgery*, **21**(1), 22–25.

117. Tiffin, M.E., Chandler, L.R. and Faber, H.K. (1940) Localized absence of ganglion cells of the myenteric plexus in congenital megacolon. *American Journal of Diseases of Childhood*, **59**, 1071.

118. Tittel, K. (1901) Uber eine angerborene Missbildung des Dickdarmes. *Wiener Klinische Wochenscrift*, **14**, 903.

119. Touloukian, R.J. and Duncan, R. (1975) Acquired aganglionic megacolon in a premature infant. Report of a case. *Pediatrics*, **56**, 459–462.

120. Touloukian, R.J., Aghajanian, G. and Roth, R.H. (1973) Adrenergic hyperactivity of the aganglionic colon. *Journal of Pediatric Surgery*, **8**, 191.

121. Towne, B.H., Stocker, J.Th, Thompson, H.E. and Chang, J.H. (1979) Acquired aganglionosis. *Journal of Paediatric Surgery*, **14**, 688.

122. Treves, F. (1898) Idiopathic dilation of the colon. *The Lancet*, **i**, 276–279.

123. Vanhoutte, J.J. (1969) Primary aganglionosis associated with imperforate anus. Review of the literature pertinent to one observation. *Journal of Pediatric Surgery*, **4**(4), 468–472.

124. Vinores, S.A. and May, E. (1985) Neuron-specific enolase as an immuno-histochemical tool for the diagnosis of Hirschsprung's disease. *American Journal of Surgical Pathology*, **9**(4), 281–285.

125. Wade, R.B and Royle, N.D. (1927) The operative treatment of Hirschsprung's disease: a new method. *Medical Journal of Australia*, **14**(i), 137.

126. Webster. W. (1973) Embryogenesis of the enteric ganglia in normal mice and mice that develop congenital aganglionic megacolon. *Journal of Embryology and Experimental Morphology*, **30**, 573–585.

127. Whitehouse, F.R. and Kernohan, J.W. (1948) Myenteric plexus in congenital megacolon. *Archives of Internal Medicine*, **82**, 75.

128. Wolloch, Y. and Dintsman, M. (1976) Colonic atresia associated with Hirschsprung's disease. *Israel Journal of Medical Science*, **13**(3), 202–207.

129. Woodyear, L., Boulesteix, J., Rutkowski, J. and Dumdenstock, R. (1980) Waardenberg Syndrome associated with Hirschsprung's disease and other abnormalities. *Pediatrics*, **65**(2), 368–369.

130. Yntema, C.L. and Hammond, W.S. (1954) The origin of intrinsic ganglia of the trunk visera from vagal neural crest in the chick embryo. *Journal of Comparative Neurology*, **101**, 515–542.

131. Zuelzer, W.W. and Wilson, J.L. (1948) Functional intestinal obstruction on a congenital neurogenic basis in infancy. *American Journal of Diseases in Childhood*, **75**, 40–64.

ANORECTAL MALFORMATION

J.O.N. Lawson

HISTORY

Anorectal malformations were noted in ancient times.[74] Accounts appear in Egyptian papyri (papyrus ebers 1600 BC) and in cuneiform tablets in the library of King Assurbanipal (650 BC) at Nineva. Dempedocles of Agrigent (484–424 BC) and Democritos Abdera (460–470 BC) looked for a cause in the appearance of the fathers. Aristotle (384–322 BC) noted the male preponderance. Laurentius Heister (1718 AD) differentiated between high and low abnormalities, also describing recto- or anovaginal fistulas. He recommended incision and dilatation of low lesions but stated that there was no treatment for those cases where the bowel could not be entered from below. From 1640 on, there are numerous accounts of the early treatment of identifiable types of abnormality, but progress towards a definitive treatment of intermediate and high lesions awaited the ability to successfully establish a colostomy (Dubois in 1783,[23] Duret in 1798[24] and Amussat in 1839[1] and 1843[2]). The perineal approach gained increasing popularity towards the end of the 19th century, with perineal incisions becoming more extensive, demonstrated by Matas in 1897[47] and Heinecke and Kocher in 1888.[30,40] Until 1948, the perineal approach continued to be the most widely used. In all but the low lesions this approach had considerable disadvantages. Attempts to reach the rectourethral or rectovaginal fistulas resulted in considerable damage to the pelvic floor muscles and pelvic nerves and plexuses. Kronlein in 1879[43] and Hadra in 1880[28] mobilized the rectal pouch from above, bringing the stump of the rectum down to the perineal dissection, without the cover of a colostomy.

With the improvement of anaesthetic techniques, abdominal dissection was facilitated, so that by 1948 the abdominoperineal approach had become an established procedure.[52,65,66] Mortality, which was still in the region of 73% in 1934[44] had fallen to 5% by 1952.[69] The next 30 years saw further development of the abdominoperineal approach, with techniques aimed at preserving the pelvic floor muscle, slings, sphincters and nerves.[51,59–61,77,86,88,93] Unfortunately many of these involved an extensive dissection of the rectum impairing rectal sensation. The last decade has shown a return to the largely perineal approach (posterior saggital anorectoplasty).[21,57] Division of pelvic floor muscles and sphincters is again involved but gives good access to rectum and fistula where present.

AETIOLOGY

Current theories of production of this malformation are based on the studies of Wood-Jones.[99,100] He attributed failure of formation of a permanent anus to a failure of communication between the postallantoic gut and the proctodaeum and attributed the fistulas to failure of separation of the hind-gut from the allantois.[11]

INCIDENCE

An incidence of 1 in 5000 live births is the generally accepted figure, although reports indicate a wide variation from 1 in 2500 to 1 in 6000 live births with a male preponderance of between 57% and 66%. In a series where anal stenosis was included, the incidence increases markedly (13.8% to 39%).[3,13,16,25,29,34,46,48,55,69,78,96] The breakdown of the incidence between high, intermediate and low anomalies is difficult to ascertain, as the most recent figures antedate the international classification. There seems general agreement that the high abnormalities represent about 40%. It would appear that these figures also fail to take into account all the cases of anal stenosis, many of whom will present later in childhood with chronic constipation.[17]

There is a high incidence of other congenital anomalies in cases of anorectal malformation. Prominent among these will be abnormalities of the genital and urinary tract, cardiovascular system and oesophagus.

GEOGRAPHICAL VARIATIONS

From the reported series, there may be geographical variations. An incidence of 1 in 4500 to 1 in 5000 live births is reported from the USA, Australia, UK, Canada, Belgium, Finland.[3,13,48,51,54,55,65,66,69,96] A low incidence of 1 in 6000 live births is reported from India[78] and a higher instance of 1 in 2000 to 1 in 2500 live births from British Colombia, South Africa, Pakistan and Israel.[46,58,72,85]

RACE

A lower incidence has been reported among American blacks in Pittsburgh, Pennsylvania,[38] but higher in South African Bantu.[46] There appears to be a higher incidence in areas where cosanguinous (first cousin) marriages are common.

SEX

There is general agreement that there is overall a male preponderance with 55.9% in a collected series of 5454 cases.[81] In this series, the abnormalities were divided into 'high' (supra levator) or 'low' (infra levator). The male preponderance persists in both groups but the relative incidence varies. In the male, the high abnormality predominates (52.9%) but in the female, the low (64.6%), whilst the figures for the female are weighed in favour of the less severe anomalies. These figures compare with other reported series. Otte reports a more marked female preponderance of 'low' lesions (86%).[54] The sex differentiation is lost in anal stenosis.[16,25,29]

CLASSIFICATION

Early attempts were made to classify imperforate anus: Amussat[1] described five anomalies in 1835.

Bodenhammer[12] produced a classification in 1860, based on the postmortem findings of 287 cases, which was later extended by Ball in 1887.[6] This classification divided anomalies into nine types and included most of the cases recognized today. Further detailed and accurate classifications, stressing the sites of fistulae, followed.[19,92]

In the period up to 1970, the adoption of two main classifications made comparison between published series difficult. In the first an attempt was made to give an embryological explanation for the observed anomalies[39,99,100] and this classification, which was more generally accepted in Europe and Australasia, was further developed by Dennis Brown (1951 and 1955),[14,15] Stephens (1953),[86] Nixon (1959 and 1961)[50,51] and Partridge and Gough (1961).[56] Anomalies were subdivided into high and low, depending on whether the bowel passed down through

Table 4.1   International classification of anorectal anomalies (1970)[40]

				Male	*Female*
Low deformities (translevator)					
1	At normal anal site				
	Covered anus – complete			2	13
	Anal stenosis			1	12
2	At perineal site				
	Anterior perineal anus			4	15
	Anocutaneous fistula (covered anus – incomplete)			3	14
3	At vulvar site				
	Female	vestibular anus			18
		anovulvar fistula			16
		anovestibular fistula			17
Intermediate deformities					
1	Anal agensis:				
	Male	*without fistula:*	anal agenesis	5	
		with fistula:	rectobulbar	6	
	Female	*without fistula:*	anal agensis		19
		with fistula:	rectovaginal – low		20
			rectovestibular		21
2	Anorectal stenosis			7	22
High deformities (supralevator)					
1	Anorectal agenesis				
	Male	*without fistula:*	anorectal agenesis	8	
		with fistula:	rectourethral	9	
			rectovesical	10	
	Female	*without fistula:*	anorectal agenesis		23
		with fistula:	rectovesical		26
			rectocloacal		25
			rectovaginal – high		24
2	Rectal atresia			11	27
Miscellaneous deformities, including:					
1	Imperforate anal membrane				
2	(a) Covered anal stenosis				
	(b) Anal membrane stenosis				
3	Vesico-intestinal fissure (cloacal exstrophy)				
4	Duplications of anus, rectum and genitourinary tract				
5	Combination of deformities from the basic list				
6	Perineal groove				
7	Perineal canal				

Table 4.2 Wingspread classification (1984) of anorectal malformations

Female		Male

1   Anorectal agensis
    (a)   with rectovaginal fistula
    (b)   without fistula
2   Rectal atresia
	High	1 Anorectal agenesis
		    (a) with rectoprostatic urethral fistula
		    (b) without fistula
		2 Rectal atresia

1 Rectovestibular fistula 2 Rectovaginal fistula 3 Anal agenesis without fistula	**Intermediate**	1 Rectobulbar urethral fistula 2 Anal agenesis without fistula
1 Anovestibular fistula 2 Anocutaneous fistula 3 Anal stenosis	**Low**	1 Anocutaneous fistula 2 Anal stenosis
	Cloacal malformations	
Rare		Rare

the levator ani or not. In the second, which was based on clinical and anatomical observations, classifications became increasingly complex and detailed.[4,5,13,18,26,27] In view of this complexity, Ladd and Gross[44] introduced the following simplified version was generally accepted in the USA.[44]

Type 1: Anal stenosis and anorectal stenosis.
Type 2: Imperforate anal membrane.
Type 3: Imperforate anus, with blind rectal pouch or associated with fistula into bladder, urethra, vagina or perineum.
Type 4: Rectal atresia.

Bill (1964)[9] recommended that the classification should be standardized. In 1970 a meeting was convened in Melbourne, to produce a unified international classification. Although this largely followed the Wood-Jones/Arthur Keith premise, it included some of Ladd and Gross' sub-divisions. In this international classification (*Table 4.1*) the anomalies are divided into three main groups, high (where the bowel is held up above the pelvic floor), intermediate (where the bowel enters the pelvic floor muscles), and low (where the bowel passes down through the pelvic floor muscles).

Comprehensive as these sub-divisions are there still remains a long list of types of anomaly which do not fit comfortably under the main headings ('miscellaneous') (*Table 4.1*).

Two accounts of this classification, with minor variations, appeared shortly after the meeting.[70,90]

Since 1970, the international classification has been widely accepted, with a few reservations. Although many would be concerned with the in-

creasing number of abnormalities, which do not fall readily into the main classifications, there are some who feel that it is too detailed for common use and for teaching. It was a group of such-minded paediatric surgeons that met, at the Wingspread Community Centre, Racine, Wisconsin in 1984, to produce a simplified version.[81,82,89] Their main classification included types of anomaly most commonly encountered. They listed under separate headings the 'rare' and 'super rarities', and male and female anomalies. The concept of high, intermediate and low lesions was retained (*Table 4.2*).

CLINICAL FEATURES AND TREATMENT

LOW ABNORMALITIES

In these the bowel extends below the levator ani, into or through voluntary sphincters.

Abnormalities in which the bowel extends along normal line of anorectum towards normal site

Covered anus (male *2* and female *13*)
The bowel extends down to its normal site, but is covered by an operculum (*Figure 4.14*). This covering consists of a layer of skin and a layer of mucosa (stratified cuboidal epithelium). Clinically, the membrane presents as a bulge at the normal anal site. There may be an anteroposterior bar or raphe with a thin membrane on either side.

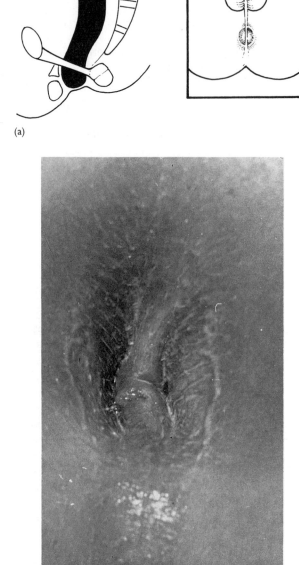

(a)

(c)

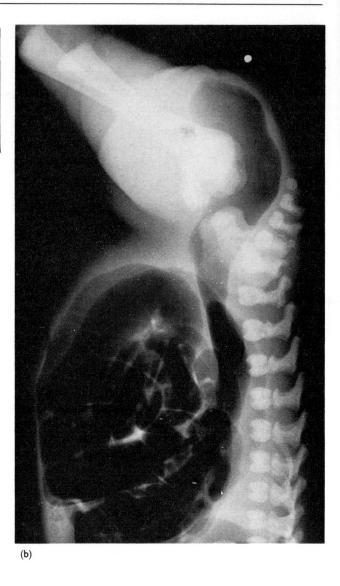

(b)

Figure 4.14 Covered anus, complete (male *2* and female *13* – low anomaly). (a) Diagram; (b) inversion film; (c) clinical appearance.

TREATMENT

Treatment consists of uncovering the anus by excising the membrane and anal dilatation. Some mucocutaneous sutures may be required, the suture line requiring digital dilatation for up to 3 months postoperatively.

Anal stenosis (male *1* and female *12*)

There is a small opening at the normal site (*Figure 4.15*). The size varies between that of an intravenous catheter and that of the distal phalanx of the fifth finger (in a full-term mature baby). Structurally this may consist of a thin mucocutaneous stricture or a stenotic segment, usually in the region of 0.5–1.0 cm in length. Histological study of the latter shows

absence of the internal sphincter from the lower canal. The muscle fibres between the mucosa and the voluntary muscle are predominantly arranged vertically.

Anal stenosis, caused by narrowing of the mucocutaneous junction, is common in the neonatal period. It should be suspected in a new born who persistently strains (*Figure 4.15b*). The straining may wake the mother at night. When a stool is passed it is usually liquid. It should be excluded when a child has multiple hernias, particularly if a tense umbilical hernia has a narrow neck. It should also be excluded where there is persistent vomiting and a diagnosis of gastro-oesophageal reflux is entertained.

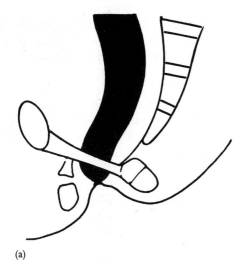

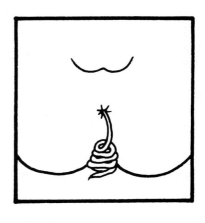

(a)

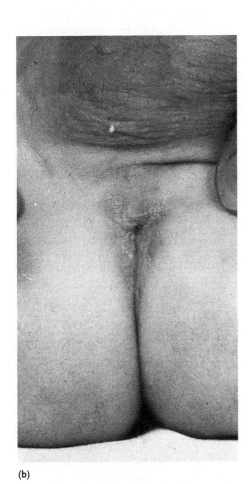

(b)

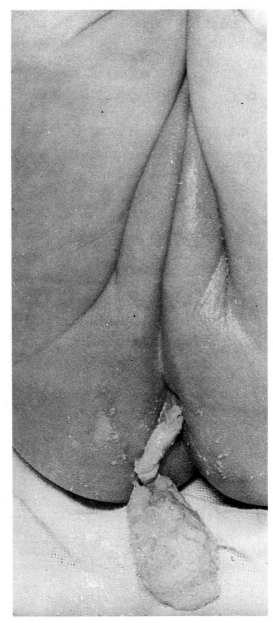

(c)

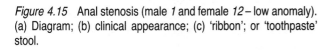

Figure 4.15 Anal stenosis (male *1* and female *12* – low anomaly). (a) Diagram; (b) clinical appearance; (c) 'ribbon'; or 'toothpaste' stool.

Even severe stenosis may not be diagnosed before the age of 2–3 months, when there is a history of much straining and crying to pass a soft milk stool. Bright blood may have been noted on the nappy. Defaecation may take a long time, and the extrusion of a 'toothpaste' or 'ribbon' stool may have been observed (*Figure 4.15c*). It is significant that the parent's complaint, that the child strains to defaecate, is often dismissed. Further, these children are liable to fulminating enterocolitis, comparable with that of Hirschsprung's disease, which may culminate in collapse and early death.

TREATMENT

Treatment is gentle, graded, dilatation. In the severe form, preliminary dilatation may be under general anaesthetic with Hegar's dilators, may be required, but subsequent progressive digital dilatation should continue until the anus takes the index finger readily. It should then be continued for up to 3 months. In the severe form, too vigorous dilatation may result in rupture of the stenosed segment. If this occurs, subsequent dilatation will be into soft tissue, without dilating the stenosed segment. These children tend, later, to soil. Delayed diagnosis of anal stenosis is associated with megarectum, which may be gross, in the severe form, with resulting long-term problems with constipation.

Openings on the perineum other than the normal site

These openings vary in size; if adequate or near adequate, they are termed anuses, narrower openings being termed fistulas (numbers *4, 3, 15* and *14*).

Anterior perineal anus (male *4* and female *15*)

This is an anteriorly placed anus, the canal usually passing down in front of the annulus of the deep sphincter. There may be a dimple at the normal site, with or without a median raphe, with a palpable, contracting, voluntary sphincter around it. Even where the anus appears adequate, there may be a moderate mucocutaneous stenosis and, if associated with megarectum, a probe or finger passes back over a 'shelf' containing the voluntary sphincters. Histologically, the internal sphincter can usually be shown to retain its normal relation to the bowel, which passes in front of the pelvic floor slings.

In males the abnormally placed anus, if not stenosed, may give little or no symptoms other than minimal incontinence with loose stools. If stenosed, it will present in the same way as anal stenosis.

In females clinical presentation will be similar to

that in males, but in addition severe third-degree tears of the thin anovaginal septum (perineal body) may occur later during parturition.

TREATMENT

When there is no stenosis, no treatment is required, except careful management of pregnancy and delivery in the female. Those presenting early with stenosis will require progressive anal dilatation but, if the presentation is delayed, additional long-term management of constipation may be required. Some surgeons consider 'cut-back' to the 'shelf', but this may result in diminished continence.

Anocutaneous fistula (covered anus, incomplete) (male *3* and female *14*)

Here the bowel passes down through the external sphincter ani (*Figure 4.16a*), but then turns forward, being continued subcutaneously, as a fistulous track deep to the median raphe, to open anywhere from a point just in front of the normal anal site to the tip of the penis (*Figure 4.16b*) in males, and as far as the fourchette in females. If the fistula opens in front of the fourchette, it is termed an anovulvar fistula (*Figure 4.17*) (number *16*; compare with anovestibular fistulas, considered below).

The abnormality appears to be associated with an over-migration of the internal sphincter. The thickened covering at the normal site usually contains the internal sphincter, which may be cut during the classic cut-back operation.

Clinically, most of the cases present as 'imperforate anus' in the newborn period. A few, with larger openings, present much later, usually with an associated gross megarectum. On examination there may be an appearance of an inverted 'V' of skin over the normal anal site, and anterior to this a very superficial thin-walled tract extending forwards, coloured by the contained meconium, which discharges at the fistulous opening along the line of the median raphe.

TREATMENT

The superficial part of the fistula is laid open, an inverted 'V' flap is raised over the normal anal site, to expose the underlying internal sphincter fibres. The fistula is then dilated, pushing the internal sphincter fibres back. Dilatation is augmented by a small mucosal incision up the back of the anal canal. The inverted 'V' skin flap is then advanced into this incision and secured with an apical stitch, the repair being completed with interrupted mucocutaneous stitches to the flap and to the edges of the new anus.

Once the wound is healed, progressive gentle and then 3 months anal dilatation is required.

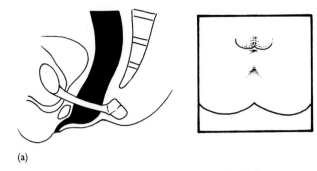

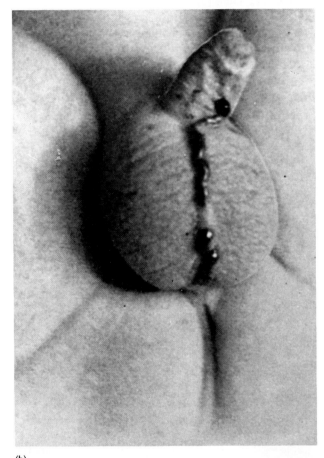

Figure 4.16 Anocutaneous fistula (covered anus, incomplete) (male *3* – low anomaly). (a) Diagram; (b) Clinical appearance: fistula extending forwards to tip of penis.

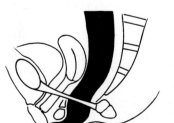

Opening in front of Forchette

Figure 4.17 Covered anus, incomplete, with anovulvar fistula (female *16* – low anomaly).

Openings at vestibular sites (below the hymen, but in the vestibule or introitus)

Vestibular anus (*18*) and anovestibular fistula (*17*)

Here the lumen tracks more obliquely downwards and forwards, and may pass through the external sphincter to reach a vestibular opening (*Figure 4.18*). Where the opening is adequate the anus may contain an internal anal sphincter, but where it is fistulous the sphincter, if present, is attenuated.

Clinically, it is unusual for the diagnosis to be delayed, the abnormal appearance being noted at birth. Straining, abdominal distension and passage of 'toothpaste' or 'ribbon' stool may be noted. On examination the opening lies in front of the fourchette but below and behind the hymen. A finger or silver probe passes backwards and upwards from the abnormal opening. A varying degree of stenosis is usually present.

TREATMENT

Although, occasionally, a vestibular anus may be missed and present in later life, most will require treatment. If a vestibular anus is stenosed, anal dilatation may be required initially. A preliminary colostomy is advisable, before formal transplantation of the anus back to a more normal position. An early colostomy will usually be required for anovestibular fistula. Anal transposition using a modified sacroperineal dissection and cruciate skin incision, at the normal anal site, allows accurate identification of voluntary sphincters and slings, anal transposition and anoplasty. It also aids accurate mobilization of the vestibular anus or fistula. The new anus will require progressive gentle dilatation.

Anovulvar fistula (*16*)

This lesion is very similar to anocutaneous fistula (covered anus, incomplete) (see above). A probe introduced passes directly back to the normal anal site.

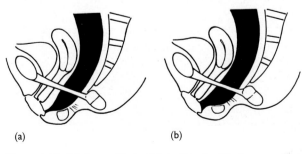

(a)   (b)

Figure 4.18 (a) Anovestibular fistula (female *17* – low anomaly). (b) Vestibular anus (female *18* – low anomaly).

INTERMEDIATE ABNORMALITIES

Here the bowel extends into the levator ani but not through it.

Anal agenesis

Anal agenesis without fistula (male *5* and female *19*)

Here the stump of the rectum extends into the pelvic floor and the blind end is lined with stratified cuboidal epithelium (*Figure 4.19*). Macroscopically it is thrown into folds resembling anal columns. Simple tubular glands extend out into, or through, the internal anal sphincter.

On the initial examination this abnormality is indistinguishable from the high variants. Inversion (Wagenstein) films suggest the abnormality, and the expression cystoloopogram, in the male, and expression loopogram, in the female, will give the diagnosis.

TREATMENT

Sacral and perineal approach gives adequate exposure for anoplasty.

Anal agenesis with fistula (male):
Rectobulbar fistula (*6*)

This abnormality was considered intermediate at the Melbourne meeting. In many, the fistula extends forwards, below the deep anal sphincter and perineal body and above the external sphincter and scrotum, to open into the bulb of the urethra (*Figure 4.20*).

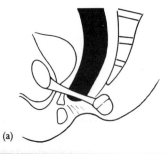

(a)

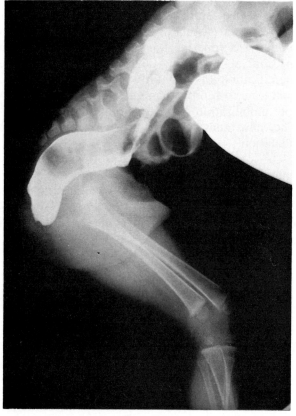

(b)

Figure 4.19   Anal agenesis (male *5* and female *19* – intermediate anomaly. (a) Diagram; (b) distal loop barium study.

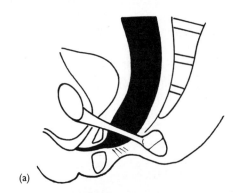

(a)

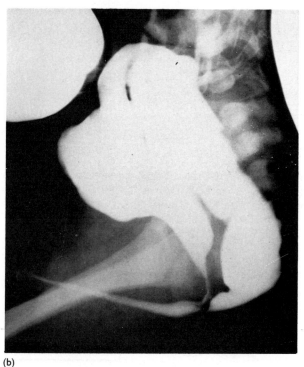

(b)

Figure 4.20   Anal agenesis with retrobulbar fistula (male *6* – intermediate anomaly). (a) Diagram; (b) cystoloopogram contrast studies.

Initially, this abnormality is clinically indistinguishable from the high variants. The passage of gas or meconium through the urethra may confirm the presence of a rectourethral fistula. Inversion films may indicate that this is an intermediate, rather than a high variant.

TREATMENT

Initial treatment is colostomy. Later, assessment with a cystoloopogram and cytourethroscopy is required to confirm bulbar fistulas (*Figure 4.20b*).

Usually these boys will have had a defunctioning colostomy before the diagnosis of this abnormality has been made. For the definitive procedure an anterior perineal approach is appropriate. After cystourethroscopy, to confirm the level of the fistula, a urethral catheter or sound should be inserted, to identify the urethra during dissection. The fistula divided and transposed to a four flap anoplasty at the normal anal site.

Anal agenesis with fistula (female):
Rectovaginal fistula (*21*)
Rectovestibular fistula (*20*)

In both of these the bowel extends into the pelvic floor, but in the former the fistula tracks horizontally forward and opens just above the hymen and in the latter it passes downwards and forwards obliquely through the perineal body to open below the hymen (*Figure 4.21*).

Diagnosis is usually made soon after birth, and is usually associated with a discharge of meconium from the vagina or vulva. The diagnosis is confirmed by probing the fistulous opening. In rectovaginal fistulas, the probe passes into the fistula just above the hymen and passes almost directly backwards into the rectal stump. In rectovestibular fistulas, entry is made below the hymen, and the probe passes obliquely upwards through the perineal body. Inversion films may suggest the diagnosis but, as a result of the escape of gas, may not be helpful.

Subsequent investigations, with expression loopogram, confirm the anatomical arrangement.

TREATMENT

Most of these children will require an initial colostomy and proper assessment before definitive treatment by sacroperineal or posterior saggital, anorectoplasty procedures to be discussed later.

Anorectal stenosis atresia (male *7* and female *22*). Rectal stenosis atresia (male *11*, female *27*)

These abnormalities consist of either a fibrous narrowing or atresia, either at the level of the pelvic floor (*Figure 4.22a*) or higher in the rectum (*Figure 4.22b,c*). The anus is of normal appearance, opening at the normal site, but a finger cannot be advanced up into the rectum. In my experience this is an extremely rare variant. The majority of cases referred to me with this diagnosis turn out to have Hirschsprung's disease, spasm of the affected segment preventing the advancement of the examining finger into the rectum of a newborn.

TREATMENT

Although it may be possible to dilate a stenosis, a preliminary colostomy is usually required. Subsequent treatment will depend on the severity of the abnormality. A septum may be resected or an anastomosis carried out, through a sacral approach.

HIGH ABNORMALITIES

These are abnormalities in which the bowel ends above the levator ani.

Anorectal agenesis

Anorectal agenesis without fistula (male *8* and female *23*)

In this abnormality the bowel ends above the pelvic floor (*Figure 4.23*). This group represents lesions of

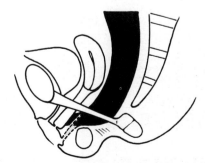

Figure 4.21 Anal agenesis with retrovaginal (*21*) or rectovestibular (*20*) fistula (female – intermediate anomaly).

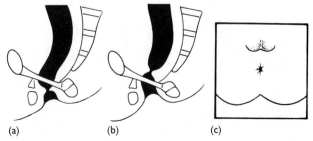

Figure 4.22 (a,c) Anorectal stenosis or atresia (male *7* and female *22* – intermediate anomaly). (b,c) Rectal stenosis or atresia without fistulas (male *11* and female *27* – high anomaly).

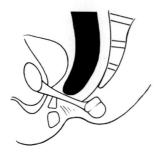

Figure 4.23 Anorectal agenesis without fistulas (male *8* and female *23* – high anomaly).

varying severity; in the most common the bowel extends down to the pelvic floor, to a position comparable with those cases with a rectourethral or rectovaginal fistula. Where the bowel is held up at a much higher level, even as high as the splenic flexure, it is usually associated with other severe congenital anomalies. The stump may be connected to the pelvic floor or to the back of the bladder by a fibrous cord.

Clinically, these are usually indistinguishable from the other intermediate and high variants. Meconium is not discharged through the urethra or vagina.

TREATMENT
This condition will required colostomy in the newborn period and careful assessment with expression cystoloopogram or loopogram, before definitive treatment. Lower lesions can be treated by sacroperineal or posterior saggital anorectoplasty. Adequate mobilization may rarely require an abdominal as well as sacroperineal approach to gain adequate length of bowel, for pull-through to the perineum.

Rectal agenesis with fistula (male *9/10*)
Here the rectal stump lies above the levator ani, and is connected by the fistula with the posterior urethra (*9*) or, higher, with the bladder (usually the bladder

neck) (*10*) (*Figure 4.24*). Those fistulas that open into the membranous urethra pass forwards below the apex of the prostate. Those opening at a slightly higher level may pass obliquely down through prostatic tissue, to open most commonly just below the verumontanum. Structurally these fistulas appear to represent the upper anal canal, with its lining of stratified cuboidal epithelium and circular smooth muscle, with the appearance of the upper internal anal sphincter. The author has not seen a fistula entering the urinary tract higher than the bladder neck.

Clinically, these cases are indistinguishable from other high or intermediate cases until subsequent cystoloopogram and urethroscopy. Gas and meconium may be passed via the urethra.

Anorectal agenesis with fistula (female[24,25])

With rectovaginal fistula (24). This is the commonest female high variant. The bowel ends above the levator ani and is connected to the vagina by a fistula which opens into the posterior wall, anywhere from the insertion of the pelvic floor, to as far up as the fornix of the vagina (*Figure 4.25*).

This abnormality presents in the newborn period with a variable degree of abdominal distension and

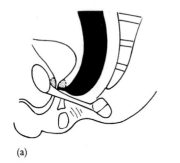

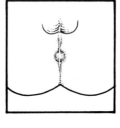

(a)

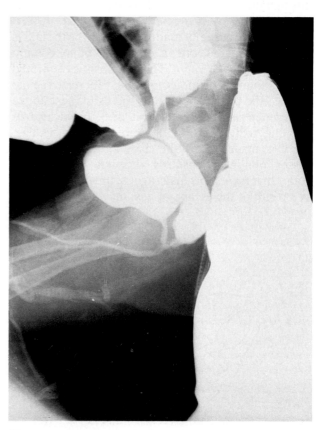

Figure 4.24 Anorectal agenesis with recto-urinary fistula (male – high anomaly) recto-urethral *9* (membranous or prostatic) or rectovesical *10*. (a) Diagram; (b) cystoloopogram contrast study showing recto-urethral fistula.

(b)

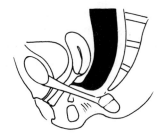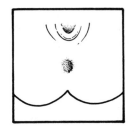

Figure 4.25 Anorectal agenesis with rectovaginal fistula *24* (female – high anomaly).

usually discharge of gas or meconium from the vagina. It can be distinguished from the intermediate variant if a silver probe can be passed into the fistula. Inversion films may assist by indicating the level of air in the rectal stump.

With rectovesical fistula (26). Rectovesical fistulas in the female are very rare. In general, for a rectovesical fistula to be present in the female, there must be splitting of the mullerian cord and duplication of the resulting structures – the vagina and uterus.

Rectocloacal fistula (25). Where there is an anorectal agenesis and fistula, and a urethra opening ectopically, high up, the cavity into which both open is known as a cloaca.

These lesions vary in severity. In the less severe variant, the appearance may be similar to any other female with a high or intermediate variant except, on closer examination, the introitus looks narrower and the urethra opens at a higher level. In the more severe variant, there may be a small opening behind the clitoris. A narrow genitourinary canal extends back and up. The urethra, the vagina (or, more usually two) and a rectal fistula open into the common channel or cloaca.

TREATMENT
Initially these children will require a transverse colostomy in the newborn period, with full assessment before definitive operation. A sacroperineal or posterior saggital anorectoplasty will be required, with division of rectocloacal fistula. Management of the cloaca, similar to that required for the genitourinary sinus anomalies requires V-flap advancement or a pull-through vaginoplasty.[31,80]

Rectal atresia (male 11 and female 27)

The findings in rectal atresia are comparable with those in anorectal atresia but the atresia is at a higher level (see 'anorectal stenosis/atresia' above and *Figure 4.22*).

MISCELLANEOUS

There are numerous rare variants. Some form recognizable syndromes, such as vesicointestinal fissure (ectopia cloacae). Some of these anomalies are listed in *Table 4.1*.

INVESTIGATIONS

INITIAL ASSESSMENT OF A CHILD WITH ANORECTAL ANOMALY

The assessment of a child with an anorectal anomaly should identify the type and severity of the abnormality. It should also diagnose any associated anomaly. The initial assessment should obtain as much information as possible, particularly of the low abnormalities, to determine the nature of early treatment. It will also aim to confirm or exclude other life-threatening abnormalities and to give them their appropriate priority. Subsequent investigations aim to give much more detailed information, which will be required to reach a decision on the most appropriate definitive operation.

Clinical assessment should take note of the presence or absence of abdominal distention. The absence of sacral segments and coccyx, or other obvious spinal anomalies, should be noted. The abnormal discharge of meconium from urethra, vagina or fistula may be observed. Meconium may be passed through the urethra, separate or mixed with urine. On examination of the perineum, note should be made of the presence or absence of a dimple at the normal anal site. If present, the nature of the skin lining it, the presence of a raphe, or triangle of skin crossing it, should be noted. Contractions of the voluntary sphincter, or retraction of a dimple, with crying or following gentle stimulation of the perineal skin may be observed. In the male, the appearance of the scrotum should be noted: it may be bifid. There may be an anteriorly placed anus or fistula. A fistula may extend along the scrotal raphe, even onto the shaft of the penis. If a probe can be passed into the fistula, the direction of the fistula can be noted. An abnormally placed anus should be examined to exclude stenosis.

In the female, perineal, vulval and vestibular openings can be readily assessed. An absent or septate vagina should be noted. The level of a vaginal fistula can be assessed by probing the posterior wall of the vagina. The position of the external urinary meatus should be noted. Although the more severe cloacal anomaly will be obvious, the urethra and fistula may open in what would appear to be a vagina.

RADIOGRAPHY

As well as plain abdominal films in supine, erect or lateral decubitus positions (*Figure 4.26*), lateral inversion (Wagensteen) films[97] should be included, although the appearances should be interpreted with caution (*Figures 4.14b* and *4.27*) The distance from a lead-shot marker on the perineum to the gas in the rectum is no longer considered reliable: the gas is now related either to a line drawn on the lateral film from the upper border of the pubis to the last ossified spinal segment (Stephen's line)[86] or to the distance the gas extends around the ossified ilium (Santulli's criterion).[71] Meconium adherent to the stump and air escaping through a large rectourethral or rectovaginal fistula or the distal end of the rectal stump gripped in the pelvic floor may give the appearance that the lesion is higher than it is.

ULTRASOUND

There are a number of papers reporting ultrasonic examination of the rectal stump with measurement of the distance between perineal skin and rectal gas (perineal pouch distance). This examination suffers the same disadvantage as the Wagensteen inversion films, the only advantage being that meconium in the distal pouch can be identified.[22,53,75,98]

INVESTIGATIONS BEFORE DEFINITIVE OPERATION

In view of the large number of variants, and the incidence of associated anomalies, careful preoperative assessment is essential.

Investigations of associated anomalies

Careful examination and investigation should exclude genetic, cardiac, urinary,[94] mullarian cord and gastrointestinal tract anomalies. Spinal anomalies, particularly sacral, should be investigated, as should any resulting neurological deficit.

Investigation of the anal, rectal, vaginal and lower urinary tract anomalies in anorectal agenesis

These investigations should determine the relationship of the distal bowel to the pelvic floor and its

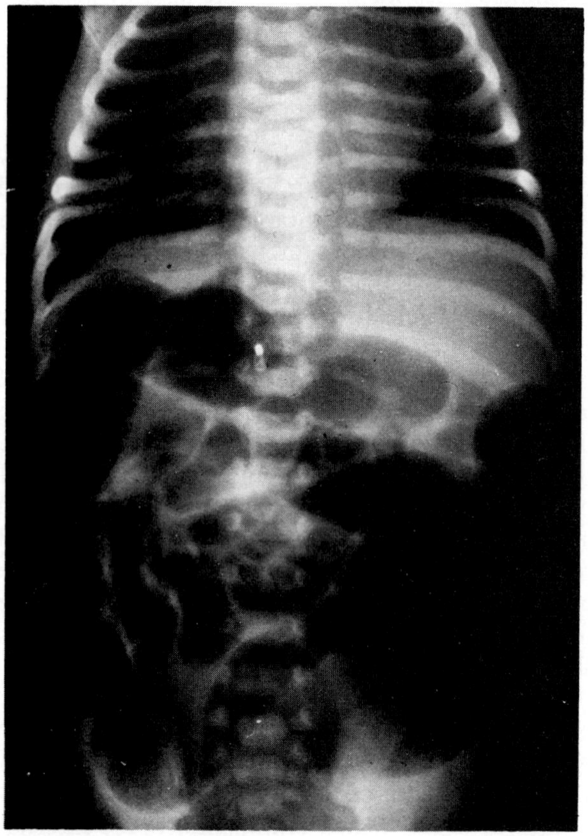

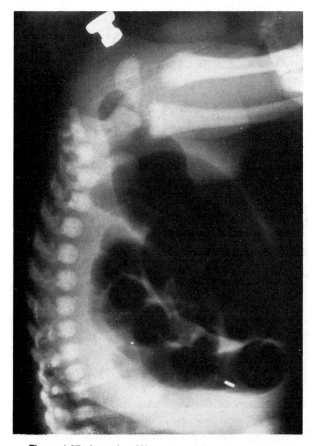

Figure 4.26 Plain, supine film of abdomen in imperforate anus, showing gaseous distension.

Figure 4.27 Inversion (Wagensteen) film in low anomaly.

associated sphincters and slings, as well as its relationship to the bladder, urethra, vagina, vulva and perineum, where appropriate.

CT and MRI imaging (saggital, transverse and coronal projections)

The increasing use of these modalities has contributed to the more detailed investigation of anorectal anomalies. Detailed knowledge of the normal appearance, as well as the abnormal, is required to interpret the images of the pelvic floor muscles, the sphincters and slings. Cuts at 1 cm intervals from the base of the bladder to the perineum, parallel to the pubacoccygeal line, show the pubanalis and anal sphincters and slings well.[32,41,83] The interpretation of the appearance of the distal bowel, urinary tract and fistulas are more straightforward, in the saggital sections.

It is from the more detailed information of the pelvic floor, slings and sphincters that operative management can be planned preoperatively.

'Distal loopogram'

Water-soluble contrast medium, instilled via a catheter into the distal loop of the colostomy, passes readily down into the left colon and rectum. Lateral views, centred on the greater trochanter, demonstrate contrast medium in the rectum. Contrast medium may pass via a fistula into the lower urinary tract in the male, and the vagina in the female. Misleading information in intermediate and lower variants may be obtained where the lower rectum and anal canal, or fistula, are gripped in the pelvic floor and therefore may not fill. The appearance may then suggest a higher anomaly or that no fistula exists (*Figure 4.28*).

'Cystoloopogram'

To overcome the disadvantages of the distal loopagram, the author, over the past 23 years, has combined an expression cystogram with a contrast medium-filled distal loop[45] (see *Figures 4.20* and *4.24*) in the male, and loop alone in the female (*Figure 4.29*).[45] Image intensifier views and films are obtained with the tube centred on the greater trochanter and the hips flexed to a right angle.

In the male, the investigation commences with an expression cystogram. The distal loop is then filled with water-soluble contrast medium and the bladder

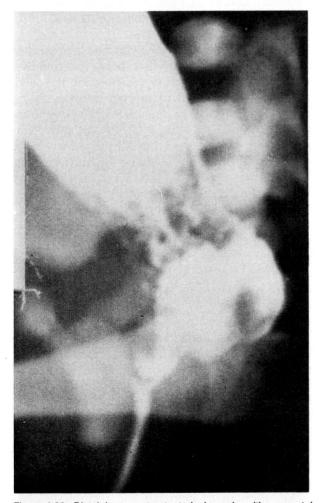

Figure 4.28 Distal loop contrast study in male with anorectal agenesis and fistula to posterior urethra, barium being passed through the urethra.

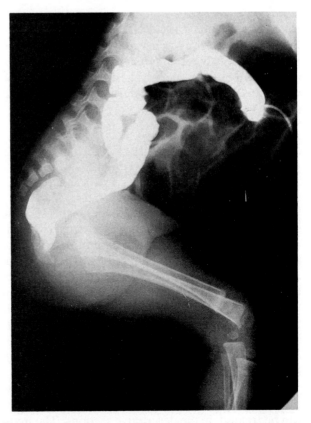

Figure 4.29 Distal loop contrast study in female with anal agenesis without fistulous connection.

and rectum expressed together. This technique opens up any bowel extending into the pelvic floor.

Contrast medium is more likely to outline a fistula, and the relationship of the fistula to the urethra and vagina is well demonstrated.

Cystourethroscopy and vaginoscopy

With the advent of the small cystourethroscopes (7 and 8 ch) all but the smallest infant can be examined to determine the point of entry of an ano- or rectourinary fistula. In the female, the urethroscope can be used to examine the vagina or vaginas, cervix or cervices and any recto- or anovaginal fistulas.

Laparoscopy

Laparoscopy may be indicated, usually at a later stage, in girls with mullarian cord anomalies and where inter-sex problems are suspected.

Endoscopy of distal loop

Where a pelvic colostomy has been established, the rectal stump can be examined using a urethroscope. Later, in salvage or delayed procedures, a flexible endoscope may be passed via the colostomy to visualize the stump and fistula. The author does not believe that the advantage of this examination outweighs the disadvantage of a pelvic colostomy in the routine treatment of imperforate anus.

Electromyography and electrical muscle stimulation

Preoperative electromyographic records may be used to identify external sphincter and slings.[101] Pre- and perioperative electrical stimulation is now widely used to identify external sphincters and slings.

SUMMARY OF TREATMENT

As we have seen, anorectal anomalies include a wide spectrum of abnormalities, the treatment of which is further complicated by anomalies of the sacrum and urinary tract. It would therefore be difficult to visualize a single operative approach that would satisfactorily treat all the variants. A detailed knowledge of the disorganized anatomy and physiology is required to determine the best operative treatment. The recent tendency to recommend a single procedure as a panacea for all the intermediate and high lesions should be treated with caution.

The author has made some suggestions as to how the low anomalies and some intermediate anomalies can be treated, in the descriptive sections. The main challenge lies in the more severe intermediate and high anomalies, particularly where they are associated with rectourinary or rectovaginal fistulas.

HISTORY OF THE TREATMENT OF ANORECTAL ANOMALIES

The improvement of anaesthetic techniques facilitated the abdominoperineal approach to anorectal anomalies in the 1940s.[52,65,66] A mortality of 73% reported in 1934[44] had fallen to 5% by 1952.[69] These abdominoperineal procedures were carried out either as a single or a two-stage operation. If a single stage, the rectal stump was mobilized from above, dividing a rectourinary or rectovaginal fistula if present, and the stump brought down to a perineal incision. If the procedure was carried out in two stages, the mobilized rectal stump was brought onto the anterior abdominal wall, usually the left iliac fossa, as an end stoma.[44] At the second stage, the mobilized stoma was brought down to the proposed anal site where usually a disc of skin had been excised. These procedures, involving a blind dissection through the pelvis, resulted in damage to the pelvic floor muscles and nerves.

Improved techniques involved careful dissection from above, into the curve of the sacrum and over the pelvic floor, to identify and preserve the pelvic muscle slings[51,77] and to meet a perineal dissection.[93] In an attempt to minimize the damage to the pelvic floor nerves, Rehbein[59–61] divided the rectum above the pelvic floor, coring out the mucosa of the stump and ligating and dividing the mucosa of the fistula from within. A dissection, carried down through the dependent part of the stump, brought the operator and the proximal bowel to the perineal incision. Stephens[86,88] stressed the importance of preserving the puborectalis sling, described a 'sacroperineal rectoplasty'. Through a vertical sacrococcyxgeal incision, the coccyx is disarticulated to enter the pelvis above the pelvic floor, thus facilitating the dissection forward over the pelvic floor, muscles and slings to meet the incision at the proposed anal site. This approach enabled the operator to assess the level of the rectal pouch, and either complete the mobilization from below, or combine the sacroperineal dissection with an abdominal approach to mobilize the distal bowel through the abdomen. Kiesewetter[35,36] combined the sacroperineal approach with Rehbein's abdominal approach, coring the mucosa from the divided rectal stump and ligating the mucosa of the fistula to bring the proximal bowel down to the sacroperineal dissection.

An alternative approach for rectoplasty[73] involved a 'buttock-reflecting incision', an incision curving laterally around the perineal incision to expose and identify the voluntary sphincter and sling complex and accurately route the bowel through the pelvic floor. This procedure was combined with an anoplasty, fashioning a skin lining to the lower canal from four skin flaps.

During a clinical and physiological review of over 100 children treated by abdominoperineal procedures at the Hospital for Sick Children, London, before 1970, the author noted that few 'high' lesions obtained satisfactory continence.[20,21,57] Anorectal manometry confirmed the importance of rectal sensation, where anal sensation had been lost. Careful dissection to preserve the pelvic floor muscles and sphincters had not given the improvement in continence expected. In fact, in the procedures involving the Rehbein approach, rectal sensation was further diminished. The practice of excising a disc of skin at the proposed anal site removed physiologically active skin and skin less prone to scar. The resulting pouting rectal mucosa produce mucous soiling. The physiological findings in the patients managed by abdominoperineal pull-through contrasted with children treated by perineal dissection without preservation of pelvic floor sphincters and slings. Here the limited rectal dissection and the consequent preservation of rectal sensation allowed sufficient warning for these patients to contract their gluteal muscles and obtain reasonable continence where the stool was formed.

The current vogue for a posterior saggital rectoplasty[20,21,57] (see below) marked a return to the earlier perineal dissection[11,42] dividing the pelvic floor muscles to give a wide exposure of the rectal stump, rectourethral and rectovaginal fistulas. Twenty years experience of a modified sacroperineal approach with anoplasty has convinced the author that few anomalies require an additional abdominal mobilization.

SURGICAL MANAGEMENT OF INTERMEDIATE AND HIGH ANOMALIES

The aim of treatment of the intermediate and high anomalies must be early and adequate faecal continence. This will be attained, not only by preservation of the anal sphincters and pelvic floor slings, but the retention of sensation. Sensatory nerves reach the rectal stump and fistula via branches of the pelvic floor nerves and from the pelvic and lumbar autonomic outflow, via the hypogastric and pelvic plexuses and along the branches of the inferior mesenteric vessels. Although branches of the pelvic floor nerves can sometimes be seen passing to the fistula, they are not usually preserved. It is therefore important, where possible, to avoid an abdominal dissection and division of superior rectal vessels. Fortunately, in most cases, adequate mobilization of the stump and fistula can be obtained from below, with preservation of proximal nervous connections.

There are two widely accepted approaches to the problem.

Posterior saggital rectoplasty

This much publicized procedure[20,21,57] marks a return to the earlier perineal dissection.[11,42] In this procedure, wide access to the pelvic cavity is obtained through an extensive saggital incision, extending forwards across the sacrum, coccyx and perineum, as far as the scrotum or labial frenulum. The incision is deepened to divide the anal sphincters, pelvic floor muscles and slings, which gives wide access to the rectal stump and fistula, which is mobilized and brought down to suture in the anterior part of the wound. The pelvic floor muscles are sutured behind the pull-through bowel and an attempt is made to repair sphincters and slings.

Sacroperineal anorectoplasty (modified Stephens approach[86,88])

Through a median sacrococcygeal skin incision, the coccyx is disarticulated, the pelvic floor muscles, the anococcygeal raphe and pelvic fascia incised laterally to gain access to the pelvic cavity. The dissection is continued forward over the anococcygeal raphe and downwards into the 'V' of the puboanalis insertion, into the anal dimple, which brings the dissector down to a cruciate perineal incision at the proposed anal site. Access to the rectal stump, and fistula, though adequate, is not as good as that of the posterior saggital approach. The rectoanal or vaginal fistula is divided and the rectal stump mobilized. The track through the voluntary sphincters and slings is gently dilated so that the rectal stump can be brought down to the perineal incision. The bowel is tacked to the sphincters before completing the interdigitating anoplasty. Preservation of the voluntary sphincters results in earlier and better continence than that of the posterior saggital rectoplasty.

REFERENCES

1. Amusat, J.Z. (1835) Histoir d'une opération d'anus artificiel practiqué avec succès par un nouveau procédé, dans un cas d'absence congenital de l'anus: suive de quelques réflexions sur les obturation du rectum. *Gazette Médical de Paris*, **3**, 735–758.

2. Amusat, J.Z. (1843) Troisième mémoire sur la possibilité d'etablir une ouverture artificielle sur le colon lombaires gauche sans ouvrir le péritoine, chez les enfans imperforés. *L'Examinateur Medical de Paris*, **18**.

3. Anderson, R.C. and Reed, S.C. (1954) Likelihood of recurrence of congenital malformations. *The Lancet*, **74**, 175.

4. Bacon, H.E. (1949) Anus, rectum and sigmoid colon: modern operative procedures. *Trans American Surgical Association*, **15**, 453.

5. Bacon, H.E. and Sherman, L.F. (1952) Surgical management of congenital malformations of the anus and rectum: report of 111 cases. *American Medical Association Archives of Surgery*, **64**, 331.

6. Ball, C.B. (1887) *The Rectum and Anus. Their Diseases and Treatment*. London: Cassel and Company.

7. Ball, C.B. (1887) *The Rectum and Anus*. Philadelphia: Lea.

8. Bell, B. (1887) *A System of Surgery, Third Edition*, Vol 2, chap 19, pp. 275–282, Edinburgh 1787.

9. Bill, A.H. (1964) Common denominators in rectal anomalies on both sides of the Atlantic. *Archives of the Diseases of Childhood*, **39**, 149–152.

10. Bill, A.H. and Johnson, R.J. (1953) Congenital median band of the anus. *Surgery, Gynecology and Obstetrics*, **97**, 307–311.

11. Bill, A.H. and Johnson, R.J. (1958) Failure of migration of the rectal opening as a cause of most cases of imperforate anus. *Surgery, Gynecology and Obstetrics*, Vol 106, 643–651.

12. Bodenhamer, W.A. (1860) A practical treatise on the aetiology, pathology and treatment of the congenital malformation of the rectum and anus. New York: Samuel S. and William Wood.

13. Brenner, E.C. (1915) Congenital defects of the anus and rectum. *Surgery, Gynecology and Obstetrics,* Vol 20, 579–588.

14. Browne, D. (1951) Some congenital deformities of the rectum, anus, vagina and urethra. *Annals of the Royal College of Surgeons of England*, **8**, 173.

15. Browne, D. (1955) Congenital deformities of the anus and rectum. *Archives of the Diseases of Childhood*, **30**, 42.

16. Brown, S.S. and Schoen, A.H. (1950) Congenital anorectal stricture. *Journal of Paediatrics*, **36**, 746.

17. Clayden, G.S. and Lawson, J.O.N. (1976) Investigation and management of long standing chronic constipation in childhood. *Archives of Disease in Childhood*, **51**, 918–923.

18. Crowell, E.A. and Dulin, J.W. (1940) Congenital anomalies of the anus and rectum. *Surgery*, **7**, 529–539.

19. Delbet, P. and Brechot   (1916) *Maladies de l'Anus et du Rectum*. Paris: J.B. Baillière et fils.

20. de Vreis, P.A. (1984) The surgery of anorectal anomalies: Its evolution, with evaluations of procedures. *Current Problems in Surgery*, **21**, 1.

21. De Vreis, P.A. and Peña, A. (1982) Posterior saggital anorectoplasty. *Journal of Pediatric Surgery*, **17**,(5), 638–643.

22. Donaldson, J.S., Black, C.T., Reynolds, M., Kerman, J.O. and Shkonik, A. (1989) Ultrasound of the distal pouch in infants with imperforate anus. *Journal of Pediatric Surgery*, **24**(5) 465–468.

23. Dubois, A. (1783) *Receuil Periodique de la Société de Médicine de Paris*, **3**, 125.

24. Duret, C. (1798) Observation sur un enfant né sans anus, et auquel il été fait un ouverture pour y suppléer. *Receuil Periodique de le Société de Médicine de Paris*, **4**, 45.

25. Eckerle, W.J. (1951) Congenital anomalies of the anus, rectum and sigmoid colon and their surgical management. *American Journal of Surgery*, **82**, 651.

26. Fitchett, S.M. (1926) Imperforate anus. *Boston Medical and Surgical Journal*, Vol 195, 25.

27. Fraser, J. (1926) *Surgery of Childhood,* Volume 2. New York: William Wood and Company.

28. Hadra, (1880) *Berlin Klinische Wochenschrift*. No. 7.

29. Harris, L.E., Corbin, H.P.F. and Hill, J.R. (1954) Anorectal rings in infancy; instance and significance. *Paediatrics*, **13**, 59.

30. Heinecke, (1888) *Müchen medizinische Wochenschrift*, 37.

31. Henderen, H. (1986) Repair of cloacal anomalies. Current Techniques. *Journal of Pediatric Surgery*, **21**(12), 1159–1176.

32. Ikawa, H., Yokoyama, J., Sanbonmatsu, T., Hagane, K., Endo, M., Katsumata, K. and Kohda, E. (1985) The use of computerised tomography to evaluate anorectal anomalies. *Journal of Pediatric Surgery*, **20**(6), 640–644.

33. Jones, F.W. (1915) Explanation of recto-urethral anomalies and some points in a normal anatomy.

34. Jones, P.G. (1967) *Clinical Paediatric Surgery (Diagnosis and Management),* pp. 67–99. London: Blackwell Scientific Publications.

35. Kiesewetter, W.B. (1966) Imperforate anus: the role and results of the sacro-abdomino-perineal operation. *Annals of Surgery*, **164**, 655.

36. Kieswetter, W.B. (1967) Imperforate anus. II. The rationale and technique of the sacro-abdomino-perineal operation. *Journal of Pediatric Surgery*, **2**, 60.

37. Kiesewetter, W.B. (1980) Imperforate anus. In *Paediatric Surgery* (Eds) Holder, T.M. and Ashcraft, K.W. pp. 401–417. Philadelphia: W. B. Saunders and Co.

38. Kiesewetter, J.M., Turner, C.R. and Sieber, W.K. (1964) Imperforate anus: a review of a 16 year experience with 146 patients with imperforate anus. *American Journal of Surgery*, **107**, 412.

39. Keith, A. (1908) Malformation of the hind end of the body. *British Medical Journal*, **2**, 1736–1741.

40. Kocher, (1888) Deutscher Zeitscrift fur Chirurgie. Bd. XIII.

41. Kohda, E., Fujioka, M., Ikawa, H. and Yokoyama, J. (1985) Congenital anorectal anomaly – CT evaluation. *Radiology*, **157**, 349–352.

42. Kraske, P. (1885) Zur Exstirpation Hochsitzender

Mastdarmkrebse. *Deutsche Geselisch. für chirurgie* XIV. congr.II., pp. 464–474.

43. Kronlein, (1879) Casuistische Beiträge zur operativen Chirurgie des Digestionstractus. *Berlin Klin. Wchnschr*, **16**, 507 und 526.

44. Ladd, W.E. and Gross, R.E. (1934) Congenital malformations of the anus and rectum. *American Journal of Surgery*, Vol 23, 167–183.

45. Lawson, J.O.N. (1978) Surgical Conditions in Paediatrics In (Nixon, H.H., ed), p. 86. London: Butterworth.

46. Louw, J.H. (1965) Congenital abnormalities of the rectum and anus. Chicago: Yearbook Medical Publishers.

47. Matas, R. (1897) The surgical treatment of congenital ano-rectal imperforation considered in the light of modern operative procedures. *Trans American Surgical Association*, **15**, 453.

48. Moore, T.C. and Lawrence, E.A. (1952) Congenital malformations of the rectum and anus; associated anomalies in a series of 120 cases. *Surgery, Gynecology and Obstetrics*, **95**, 281.

49. Murkien, J.D. and Albert, A. (1976) Genetic counselling in cases of anal and rectal atresia. *Progress in Paediatric Surgery*, **9**, 115–118.

50. Nixon, H.H. (1959) Anorectal anomalies. *Post-graduate Medical Journal*, Vol 35, 80–85.

51. Nixon, H.H. (1961) *Imperforate Anus: British Surgical Practice. Surgical Progress*. London: Butterworth.

52. Norris, N.J., Brophy, T.W. and Brayton, D. (1949) Imperforate anus: a case series and preliminary report of the one stage abdomino perineal operation. *Surgery, Gynecology and Obstetrics*, **88**, 623.

53. Oppenheimer, D.A., Carroll, B.A. and Chochat, S.J. (1983) Sonography of imperforate anus. *Radiology*, **148**, 127–128.

54. Otte, J.B. (1983) L'imperforation anale. *Acta Chirurgica Belgica*, **83**(3), 158–162.

55. Parkkulainen, K.V. (1957) Sacral, cocxygeal and urological anomalies in connection with congenital malformation of the anus and rectum: a preliminary report. *Annals of Paediatrics Finnige*, **3**, 51–57.

56. Partridge, J.P. and Gough, M.H. (1961) Congenital abnormalities of the anus and rectum. *British Journal of Surgery*, Vol 49, 37.

57. Peña, A. and de Vries, P.A. (1982) Posterior sagittal anorectoplasty: important technical considerations and new applications. *Journal of Pediatric Surgery*, **17**(6), 796–809.

58. Rathore, A.H. and Raynaud, E. (1979) Imperforate anus. *Journal of the Pakistani Medical Association*, **29**(1), 150–153.

59. Rehbein, F. (1959) Operation der Anal- und rectumatreie mit Recto-urethralfistel. *Der Chirurg.*, **30**(9), 417–418.

60. Rehbein, F. (1965) Zur Operation der hohen Rectumatresie mit Recto-Urethral-Fistel. Abdomino-sacro-perinealer Durchzug. *Zeitschrift für Kinderchirurgie*, **2**, 503.

61. Rehbein, F. (1967) Imperforate anus: experience with abdomino-perineal and abdomino-sacro-perineal pullthrough procedures. *Journal of Pediatric Surgery*, **2**(2), 99–105.

62. Rhodes, R.L. (1933) Imperforate anus: a suggested mode of handling. *Transactions of the Southers Surgical Association*, pp. 634–637.

63. Rhodes, R.L. (1934) Imperforate anus: a suggested mode of handling. *American Journal of Surgery (New Series)*, **24**(3), 828–831.

64. Rhodes, R.L. (1946) Further observations upon imperforate anus. *Annals of Surgery*, **123**(5), 877–883.

65. Rhoads, J.E. and Koop, C.E. (1955) The surgical management of imperforate anus. *Surgical Clinics of North America*, **35**, 1251–1257.

66. Rhoads, J.E., Pipes, R.L. and Randall, J.P. (1948) A simultaneous abdominal and perineal approach in operations for imperforate anus with atresia of the rectum and rectosigmoid. *Annals of Surgery*, **127**(3), 552–556.

67. Ricardi, V.M., Hassler, L. and Lubinsky, M.S. (1978) The F G Syndrome; Further characterisation, report of a third family, and of a sporadic case. *American Journal of Medical Genetics*, **1**, 58–67.

68. Roux, J. (1835) Observation d'imperforation de l'anus et de l'uretre. *Memoires de l'Academie Royale de Medicine*, **4**, 183–190.

69. Santulli, T.V. (1952) Treatment of imperforate anus and associated fistulas. *Surgery, Gynecology and Obstetrics*, **95**, 601.

70. Santulli, T.V., Kiesewetter, W.B. and Bill, A.H. (1970) Ano-rectal anomalies; A suggested international classification. *Journal of Pediatric Surgery*, Vol 5 (3), 281–287.

71. Santulli, T.V., Schullinger, J.N. and Amoury, R.A. (1965) Malformations of the anus and rectum. *Surgical Clinics of North America*, Vol 5, 1253–1271.

72. Sarah, N., Barma, R. and Nissens, J.A. (1983) Heredity in anal atresia. *Zeitschrift für Kinderchirurgie*, **38**, 105–107.

73. Sauvage, L.R. and Bill, A.H. (1965) Imperforate anus repair through a buttock reflecting incision. *Surgery*, **57**, 448.

74. Scharli, A.F. (1978) Malformations of the anus and rectum and their treatment in medical history. *Progress in Pediatric Surgery*, **11**, 141–172.

75. Schuster and Teele (1979) An analysis of the ultrasound scanning as a guide to the determination of "high" or "low" imperforate anus. *Journal of Pediatric Surgery 14*, **6**, 798–800.

76. Schwoebe, I.M.G., Hirsig, J., Schinrel, A. and Stauffer, U.G. (1984) Familial incidence of congenital anorectal anomalies. *Journal of Pediatric Surgery*, **19**, 179–182.

77. Scott, J.E.S. and Swenson, O. (1959) Imperforate anus, results in 63 cases and some anatomical considerations. *Annals of Surgery*, **150**, 477.

78. Shahi, U.N. and Misra, S.N. (1961) Congenital anorectal anomalies: a study of 100 cases. *Indian Journal of Surgery*, **5**, 269.

79. Shapiro, S. (1960) Proctological problems in children. *The Lancet*, **84**, 134.

80. Simmer, K. and Lawson, J.O.N. (1989) Neonatal Hydrometrocolpos. *Zeitschrift für Kinderchirurgie*, **44**, 124–125.

81. Smith, E.D. (1988) Incidence, Frequency of Types, and Etiology of Anorectal Malformations. *Birth Defects (Original Article Series)*, **24**(4), 231–246.

82. Smith, E.D. (1988) Classification. In *Anorectal Malformations in Children (Update 1988)*, **24**, 211–222.

83. Smith, E.D. and Cywes, S. (1988) Diagnosis and Investigations. *Birth Defects (Original Article Series)*, **24**(4), 247–299.

84. Solowiejczyk, M. (1961) Suggested aid to the surgical treatment of imperforate anus and congenital malformations of the rectum. *Journal of the International College of Surgeons*, **35**, 371.

85. Spouge, D. and Baird, P.A. (1986) Imperforate anus in 700,000 live born infants. *American Journal of Medical Genetics* (suppl. 2), 151–161.

86. Stephens, F.D. (1953) Congenital imperforate rectum, recto-urethral and recto-vaginal fistulae. *Australian and New Zealand Journal of Surgery*, Vol 22, 161–172.

87. Stephens, F.D. (1961) Congenital malformations of the rectum and anus in female children. *Australian and New Zealand Journal of Surgery*, Vol 31, 90.

88. Stephens, F.D. (1963) *Congenital Malformations of the Rectum, Anus and Genitourinary Tracts*. Edinburgh and London: E & S Livingstone.

89. Stephens, F.D. (1988) Wingspread Anomalies, Rarities, and Super Rarities of the Anorectum and Cloaca. *Birth Defects (Original Article Series)*, **24**, 581–585.

90. Stephens, F.D. and Smith, E.D. (1971) *Anorectal Malformation in Children*. Chicago, Philadelphia: Chicago Yearbook Medical Publishers.

91. Stephens, F.D. and Smith, E.D. (1986) Classification, identification and assessment of surgical treatment of anorectal anomalies. *Paediatric Surgery International*, Vol 1, 200.

92. Stieda, A. (1903) Uber atresia ani congenita und die damit verbundenen miss bildungen. *Langenbeck's Archive für Klinische Chirurgie*, Vol 70, 555–583.

93. Swenson, O. and Donellan, W.L. (1967) Preservation of the puborectalis sling in imperforate anus repair. *Surgical Clinics of North America*, **47**, 173–193.

94. Teixeira, O.H.P., Malhotia, K., Sellers, J. and Mercer, S. (1983) Cardiovascular anomalies with imperforate anus. *Archives of the Diseases of Childhood*, **58**(9), 747–749.

95. Touloukian, R.J. (1973) Anorectal malformations. In *Birth Defects – Atlas and Compendium* (Ed) Bergsma, D. Baltimore: Williams and Wilkins Company.

96. Trusler, G.A. and Wilkinson, R.H. (1962) Imperforate anus; a review of 147 cases. *Canadian Journal of Surgery*, **5**, 269.

97. Wagensteen, O.H. and Rice, C.O. (1930) Imperforate anus: A method of determining the surgical approach. *Annals of Surgery*, **92**, 77–81.

98. Willital, G.H. (1971) Advances in the diagnosis of anal and rectal atresia by ultrasonic echo examination. *Journal of Pediatric Surgery 6*, **4**, 454–457.

99. Wood-Jones, F. (1904) Nature of the malformations of the rectum and uro-genital passages. *British Medical Journal*, Vol 2, 1630.

100. Wood-Jones, F. (1915) The explanation of a recto-urethral anomaly and some points of normal anatomy. *The Lancet*, **2**, 860.

101. Yokoyama, J., Ikawa, H. and Katsumata, K. (1985) Abdomino-extended sacral perineal approach in high type anorectal malformation – a new operative method. *Z Kinderchirurgie*, **40**, 151–157.

102. Zoehner. Quoted in: Matusoveski: A – Einfall von Anus Urethralis in Zeitum. *Entralb. gynak*, **52**, 496.

CONSTIPATION, FAECAL IMPACTION AND LAXATIVES

M.A. Kamm and C.T.M. Speakman

Constipation is a symptom, not a specific diagnosis or disease. Although it may seem trivial to the clinician, it may indicate significant underlying disease if it is of recent onset, or, if long standing, it may indicate a serious disorder of motility which interferes with a patient's well-being. When describing constipation, a patient may mean that defaecation is infrequent, stools are hard or difficult to evacuate, the patient may have a sensation of incomplete evacuation, or even just a sensation of bloating. A generally accepted definition is a bowel frequency of less than twice per week, or straining at stool for more than 25% of the time.[30]

EPIDEMIOLOGY

Constipation is of similar incidence in most Western countries. In one study of British factory workers, less than 1% had less than two stools per week, although 16% took laxatives.[21] Those with infrequent bowel actions were all women. Less than a quarter of those who took laxatives considered themselves constipated. However about 10–20% of the British and North American adult population often strain at stool.[152] In an Australian study of the general population, 19% reported a feeling of incomplete rectal evacuation, 17% took laxatives, 11% needed to strain at stool at least once every 2 weeks, 4% had a bowel motion only every 3 or 4 days, and 1% even less.[26] In another Australian study, 30% of a population surveyed reported subjective 'constipation', although only 2% reported infrequent bowel actions and 22% used laxatives.[90]

In childhood, constipation is more common in boys.[24] In adults with a normal diameter colon, constipation is much more common in women,[89,115,125,126,138] and more common with increasing age: in one study it affected 2.9% of young adults compared with 8% of the middle-aged and 20% of elderly subjects.[152] In adults with an idiopathic megacolon the proportion of males and females affected is similar.[7]

PATHOPHYSIOLOGY

Many different pathophysiological processes may result in constipation. For example, the pathogenic mechanism producing constipation in children is unlikely to be the same as that in women of reproductive age or patients with a megacolon. Attempts to subdivide patients into distinct clinical syndromes allows different pathophysiological processes to be identified.

Factors that affect the function of the large bowel and stool formation include dietary intake, drugs, bile acids, circulating and local hormones, intrinsic and extrinsic neural pathways, mechanical obstruction, mucosal absorption and pelvic floor function. The colon may be the site of primary abnormalities, such as those found in Hirschsprung's disease, or affected as part of some other systemic condition, such as myxoedema.

THE MOTILITY DISTURBANCE

Early motility studies of the colon were confined to the rectosigmoid region and appeared to demonstrate an increase in segmenting activity in constipated patients.

Subsequent studies of colonic motility in man have involved the use of colonoscopically inserted manometric tubes which measure pressure changes along the entire length of the colon.[106] These extensive and prolonged studies have resulted in a clearer understanding of the pattern of normal and abnormal colonic function. The normal colonic activity is characterized by irregular segmenting activity which is not coordinated between different colonic segments. Several times a day there is a high pressure peristaltic wave (mass movement) which traverses a large part of the length of the colon and is responsible for the transport of colonic contents. Some of these mass movements progress distally and are associated with defaecation.[79]

In severely constipated women with a normal diameter colon, there is a reduction in the frequency and duration of these movements.[9] In one study of 14 such patients and 18 healthy volunteers, the mean number of mass movements observed over a 24-hour period was 6.1 in the healthy subjects, but only 2.6 in the constipated patients. Four of the patients had no recorded mass movements in 24 hours. This lack of propulsive activity is likely to be the most important motility disturbance in these constipated patients.

FIBRE

The fibre content of the diet is thought to have a major influence on colonic function. This group of carbohydrates contains a diverse group of substances which vary in their physical properties and possibly in their effect on the colon. Fibre can be regarded as mixed cell-wall material, non-starch polysaccharide or whole vegetable food with the cell walls intact.[61]

There is a relationship between dietary fibre intake and bowel function. The mean transit time is shorter, and the frequency of defaecation and wet weight of faeces is greater in those with a higher fibre intake.[25] Vegans hava a greater bowel frequency than omnivores and pass a larger wet weight of stool.[25] In addition to the increased water, the mass of colonic bacteria in the stool is increased.

Dietary fibre may act on the bowel by several different mechanisms. Some types of fibre may draw water into the colonic lumen, whilst others may indirectly increase the faecal bacterial mass. Fermentation of fibre produces short-chain fatty acids which may stimulate colonic activity; fermentation may also allow for the release of absorbed bile acids which also stimulate the colon. The irritating effect of insoluble particles may also act to increase motility – larger particles of the same fibre type have a greater effect on transit time.

What role does dietary fibre have in the causation of constipation? A deficiency of fibre in the diet is not the cause of constipation in patients with the irritable bowel syndrome–their fibre intake is no different from asymptomatic controls. Nevertheless, the administration of fibre does relieve their constipation and shorten their gut transit time.[22] Similarly, in young women with severe idiopathic constipation, the diet is not lacking in fibre.[115] Fibre does not relieve constipation in these particular patients, however, and often worsens their symptom of bloating, perhaps by providing an increased fermentable substrate while not affecting colonic motility.

If the diet is deficient in fibre, and the stools are low in water content, then constipation may result. Small hard stools are more difficult to pass, even in normal individuals.[4] The differences in normal daily stool output between rural Ugandans (approx 500 g) and Westerners (approx 100–200 g) may be largely due to the amount of dietary fibre, but even a large increase in the fibre intake does not increase a Westerner's output to the level of the African counterpart. Genetic or local factors may therefore also play a role in determining stool output.

GENETIC FACTORS

Constipation is so common in the community that it is to be expected that some relatives of patients with constipation will also be affected, even if there is no genetic component to the causation of the condition. Nevertheless, some constipated patients have a striking family history. There is some evidence from a study of fingerprint patterns, which are a genetic marker, that there may be a genetic factor involved in some cases of idiopathic constipation.[54] Of those patients with the onset of constipation before the age of 10, together with abdominal pain, 64% had one or more digital arches. This was in contrast to healthy controls in the population without constipation, or abdominal pain, in whom this was found in only 10%.

In about a third of patients with chronic idiopathic intestinal pseudo-obstruction caused by a visceral myopathy or neuropathy, there is clearly an inherited basis – often autosomal dominant or recessive.

SEX HORMONES

The possibility that hormonal factors influence gut transit time is suggested by the fact that men have a faster transit time than women, and a greater proportion of adult women than men are constipated. Relaxation of gastrointestinal smooth muscle by progesterone may be the reason for the increased incidence of constipation during pregnancy, although changes in other hormones such as motilin may also be important.[20] Experimentally, female sex hormones slow the intestinal transit time of male laboratory animals.[41,46,131]

Patients with severe idiopathic constipation and a colon of normal diameter are almost exclusively women, usually of reproductive age. A study comparing the range of sex hormones during the follicular and luteal phases in 23 healthy women and 26 women with severe idiopathic constipation demonstrated a consistent reduction in adrenal and ovarian steroid hormones in the patient.[72] These changes did not appear to be large enough to account for the constipation, and may have been caused by changes in the steroid hormone enterohepatic circulation.

Other differences in anatomy and physiology may also play a role in the different incidence of constipation between the sexes.

PSYCHOLOGICAL FACTORS

There is substantial evidence linking psychological disturbance and bowel function. Personality profiles have been shown to correlate with stool weight in healthy subjects, and individuals with higher self-esteem and more extrovert personalities produce heavier more frequent stools.[153] Normal healthy subjects can suppress defaecation and thereby slow colonic transit voluntarily[84] providing direct evidence of cerebral control over colonic function.

In young women with severe constipation there appears to be a high incidence of psychosexual problems, adverse early life events, and personality difficulties.[120] In a group of patients having surgery for severe constipation, there was a higher depression score on psychometric testing compared to a control group with other surgical conditions.[37] Furthermore, those patients who did not benefit from surgery had significantly higher anxiety and depression scores than those who did well.

Another study compared two groups of severely constipated women – those with a measured slow intestinal transit time and those with a normal transit time. Those with a normal transit time demonstrated the most psychopathology on psychometric testing whereas those with slow transit resembled healthy controls.[161]

There are several possible mechanisms by which gastrointestinal function might be affected by psychological factors:

1. Efferent autonomic pathways exert an effect on colonic motility[47] and this may be affected by stress.
2. Neurotransmitters that are common to both the enteric nervous system and the brain may be abnormal.
3. Psychological problems may disturb the regulation of hormones which affect colonic motility.

Alternatively, the persistent symptoms of severe constipation and abdominal pain may lead to depression and other neurotic symptoms.

ABNORMALITIES OF EXTRINSIC INNERVATION

Although the enteric nervous system demonstrates a large degree of physiological independence from the central nervous system,[11] injury to its extrinsic innervation at any level may result in constipation. The integrity of the extrinsic autonomic supply to the large intestine appears to be necessary for normal function.

The constipation observed in patients with spinal cord lesions is likely to be related to an absent sacral parasympathetic supply to the large bowel. Animal studies have shown that lesions of the *spinal cord* effect colonic transit[12,102] and patients with complete lesions of the thoracic spinal cord show decreased colonic compliance and an abnormal rectosigmoid motility response to a meal.[49]

Certain *surgical procedures* may result in damage to the extrinsic innervation of the bowel leading to constipation. Pelvic surgery that affects the sacral nerves has been shown to cause intractable constipation.[49,55] Hysterectomy produces constipation in a small proportion of patients, although the exact mechanism is not clear – the effect may be via extrinsic nerve damage, or it may be via altered local pelvic reflexes.[142] Rarely, the same symptoms follow difficult childbirth, also presumably caused by pelvic nerve damage.

Patients undergoing abdominal rectal mobilization and fixation (rectopexy) for rectal prolapse often have an abnormal bowel habit preoperatively, but as many as half who were not constipated before surgery become so after the operation. Division of the lateral rectal ligaments, which may carry some of the autonomic innervation to the distal bowel, leads to a higher incidence of this complication.[146] Constipation developing after sacral *trauma* is believed to be due to damage to the parasympathetic innervation to the left colon.[48]

ABNORMALITIES OF THE ENTERIC NERVOUS SYSTEM

The enteric nervous system within the wall of the bowel contains a numerous and complex array of more than 10^{125} ganglion cells[40] and is responsible for most of the coordinated motility throughout the gut. The enteric circuitry is capable of organizing patterns of colonic motility, and the brain and spinal cord modify this activity. Processes that directly affect the intramural plexuses of the bowel may result in constipation.

Aganglionosis of the distal bowel occurs as a congenital defect in *Hirschsprung's disease*.[16] Although the intrinsic nerves are absent, extrinsic innervation[110] by adrenergic[42,44] and cholinergic[70] nerves is still present. Biopsies of the bowel wall show an absence of nerve ganglia in the submucosal and myenteric plexuses, and staining of fresh tissue demonstrates an increase in acetylcholinesterase due to hypertrophy of the extrinsic nerves. There is a reduction in the nerves in the bowel wall staining for substance P and vasoactive intestinal polypeptide. In patients with *severe idiopathic constipation*, there is both morphological and functional evidence for an abnormality of the intrinsic colonic innervation. In a study in vivo, in which internal anal sphincter relaxation was induced by electrical stimulation of the rectal wall, a larger current was required to produce maximal sphincter relaxation in constipated patients compared with healthy controls.[71,73,76] Silver staining of the myenteric plexus in these patients reveals a decrease in the number, and morphological abnormalities of, argyrophilic neurons[89] (*Figure 4.30*). Oral laxatives, however, have been shown to induce changes in the myenteric plexus in animal experiments[145] – it is therefore not clear whether these changes are primary or secondary to these drugs.

Enteric neurotransmitters are responsible for coordinating and mediating colonic motility. In two studies the concentration of vasoactive intestinal peptide in the descending[85] and sigmoid colon[104] of patients with idiopathic constipation was found to be reduced. Decreased levels of this inhibitory neurotransmitter may relate to the decrease in propulsive mass movements seen in this condition. Levels of serotonin have also been found to be raised in the circular muscle and mucosa of the sigmoid colon in patients with severe idiopathic constipation;[96] this increase in serotonin may correlate with the manometrically observed increase in non-propulsive segmenting activity found in this condition.

A study of mucosal biopsies from severely constipated subjects found a decreased concentration of substance P,[52] but this was not found in a study of resected colons from constipated patients.[85] One study, using immunohistochemistry, found an increase in the number of nerve fibres immunoreactive to calcitonin gene-related peptide (CGRP) but no difference in the number of vasoactive intestinal peptide staining fibres.[29]

The extrinsic cholinergic nerves provide an important motor innervation to the bowel, but there may be an abnormality which also involves intrinsic cholinergic nerves. Studies in vitro of the taenia coli from constipated patients[17] have shown reduced activity of cholinergic nerves in response to electrical field stimulation.

An abnormality of endogenous central, circulat-

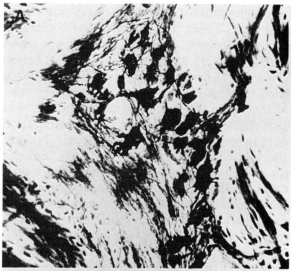

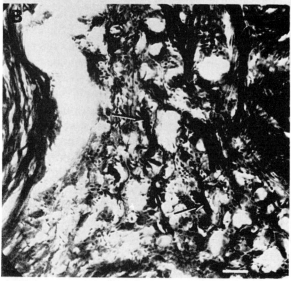

Figure 4.30 (a) Myenteric plexus ganglia from a normal colon showing numerous normal argyrophilic neurones with multiple nerve processes and nerve fibres. (b) Nerve ganglia from a woman with severe idiopathic constipation showing lack of argyrophilic neurones, paucity of nerve fibres, and multiple nuclei. Arrows denote muscle fibres. [Both × 149, silver stain, bar = 50 μm]. (From Krishnamurthy *et al.*[26])

ing or local gut opiates or enkephalins may affect gastrointestinal motility. Opioid receptors and enkephalin receptors are found in the brain and throughout the gastrointestinal tract in endocrine cells,[112] extrinsic nerves[97,104] and the myenteric plexus.[85] In a study of healthy volunteers, morphine was shown to decrease the frequency of bowel movements and decrease proximal colonic transit. Naloxone, an opioid antagonist, accelerated transit in the transverse and rectosigmoid colon, without affecting bowel movements.[81] Evidence for a colonic wall abnormality involving opioid receptors comes from *in vitro* sucrose gap studies which show

reduced activity of enkephalin receptors in colon from constipated patients.[68] Constipated patients treated with naloxone or nalmefene, a well-absorbed opioid antagonist, showed no improvement in transit time.

CIRCULATING HORMONES

The plasma levels of the peptides β-endorphin, neurotensin, somatostatin, substance P and motilin were assessed in constipated patients – apart from reduced levels of motilin, there was no difference from controls.[140] The measured plasma levels may be normal, however, in spite of marked abnormalities of the myenteric plexus.

Some regulatory circulating gastrointestinal peptides are thought to modify colonic motor activity. Preston *et al.*[116] demonstrated a smaller than normal rise in serum gastrin and pancreatic polypeptide in severely constipated subjects following an oral water stimulus. Motilin also rises less than normal in these subjects postprandially.[116,140]

CHRONIC INTESTINAL PSEUDO-OBSTRUCTION

In patients with chronic idiopathic intestinal pseudo-obstruction, careful examination of the gut wall using special stains and electron microscopy will usually reveal an abnormality of either the nerve plexuses (visceral neuropathy), or one or both of the muscle coats (visceral myopathy).[88]

A similar clinical, radiological and motility disorder can be seen with other chronic abnormalities of the nerve plexuses or muscle coats. Systemic sclerosis produces fibrous tissue replacement of one or both of the muscle coats, rendering propulsion ineffective. Inflammation of the nerve plexuses is seen in Chagas' disease, and as a non-metastatic effect in some tumours, especially small-cell tumours of the lung.

PELVIC FLOOR ABNORMALITIES

Using neurophysiological and radiological techniques, it has been possible to demonstrate that patients with constipation have abnormalities of the pelvic floor. Inability to expel a water-filled balloon, slow and incomplete evacuation of radio-opaque contrast medium[154] and poor evacuation of saline placed in the rectum[155] have all been demonstrated in severely constipated subjects.

Rectal evacuation may be abnormal in patients with slow colonic transit, or may occur in patients with difficulty in defaecation but normal transit time. The latter group are often older women and, in some, there is a history of suspected damage to the pelvic nerves.

Electromyography of the striated sphincter muscles has shown that some patients with constipation inappropriately contract the puborectalis and external sphincter during defaecation,[113,125] and it has been postulated that this plays a role in causing difficult rectal evacuation by increasing the anal canal pressure during attempted evacuation. This abnormality has also been demonstrated in normal individuals and other patients without constipation, however.[69] A recent ambulatory electromyographic and pressure study of the anal sphincter of constipated subjects in their own home suggested that laboratory tests overestimate the incidence of paradoxical striated muscle contraction.[33]

It is possible that in some cases the paradoxical contraction is a learned response to the inability to evacuate the rectum. A similar increase in activity during straining in other voluntary striated muscles, such as the gluteal muscles, has also been demonstrated, suggesting that it is a form of dystonia.[101] If this is a learned phenomenon then biofeedback conditioning may help in treatment.

Although it is unlikely that paradoxical activity of the sphincter muscles is the primary pathogenic abnormality, it is possible that it is responsible for some of the patients symptoms and may result in development of further pathological changes.

INTERNAL ANAL SPHINCTER

Although it has been postulated that the internal anal sphincter may be abnormal in some patients with constipation, there is little evidence to support this. Although the resting pressure and rectosphincteric reflex have been reported as normal in constipation,[76,125] it has been difficult to assess the activity of the sphincter during defaecation.

There has been one clearly defined hereditary myopathy affecting the internal anal sphincter, which causes both proctalgia fugax and constipation. In this condition there is gross thickening and dysfunction of the internal sphincter. Light and electron microscopy have shown abnormal polyglucosan inclusion bodies, and the condition responds to an internal anal sphincter strip myectomy.[75]

NON-COLONIC ABNORMALITIES IN CONSTIPATED PATIENTS

Even in patients with a disorder that appears to be confined to the colon, there is often an abnormality of the upper gastrointestinal tract, and sometimes other systems. Nausea is common in women with severe constipation[115] and these same patients have demonstrable abnormalities of oesophageal motility, gastric emptying and small bowel motility.[126,139,166]

Women with severe constipation also have an increased incidence of urogynaecological symptoms. Some studies have suggested an abnormality in the spinal control of pelvic function.[83,160]

Women with severe constipation also have a mild reduction in many of their steroid hormones[72] but whether this is primary or secondary to an altered enterohepatic circulation of those hormones remains to be determined.

AETIOLOGY AND CLINICAL PRESENTATIONS

CONSTIPATION OF UNKNOWN CAUSE

Asymptomatic but low bowel frequency

Many people who have infrequent bowel actions are otherwise asymptomatic and do not seek medical attention; they are part of the normal range. Most of these are women. Some may have an inadequate intake of fluids or dietary fibre; in others the factors responsible may be their sex hormone environment, mental state or personality. Others may just be at the 'slow' end of the physiological spectrum. A patient who has always had infrequent bowel actions and is otherwise asymptomatic does not require investigation or treatment.

The irritable bowel syndrome

Patients who experience constipation alternating with diarrhoea, which is accompanied by bloating and abdominal pain, are regarded as having the 'irritable bowel syndrome' in the absence of identifiable gut pathology. Other symptoms in these patients include excessive straining at stool, unsatisfied defaecation, passage of mucus, and numerous non-gastrointestinal symptoms such as general malaise, backache, and urinary symptoms. They usually have a normal measured intestinal transit time. The constipation is usually easily treated by an increase in dietary fibre or simple symptomatic measures, although the patient's diet is not necessarily deficient in fibre content. The abdominal pain and bloating is often more resistant to treatment than the constipation.

Anorectal problems

Some patients with various anorectal problems, such as a solitary rectal ulcer, rectal prolapse and anterior mucosal prolapse,[1] may have constipation as their primary problem. These anorectal 'functional' disorders are part of the same poorly understood disorder of colonic and anorectal myoneural function that causes their constipation, but the constipation is often overshadowed by other more prominent symptoms. The underlying motility disturbance should not be ignored, as it may be worsened by treatment of the pelvic floor disorder. Patients with complete rectal prolapse often have underlying constipation, for example; treatment by abdominal rectopexy may worsen this constipation.[146]

Some patients have a normal bowel frequency and measured transit time but are distressed by a great difficulty with rectal evacuation. These patients, who are almost exclusively women and often middle-aged, can spend several hours a day in total on the toilet. Many patients aid defaecation by the insertion of a digit into the rectum. In some the onset is gradual with no obvious precipitating cause, whereas in others the condition follows or is worsened by hysterectomy, abdominal rectopexy, or other pelvic or anorectal surgery. Examination is usually normal. A study of the rate of evacuation may show slow incomplete rectal emptying.[71] Proctography may also show incomplete emptying or failure of anal relaxation, whilst in some there is evidence of a large 'rectocele', an anterior bulging of the rectal wall. The relationship of this radiological or anatomical change to symptoms is not clear – the same radiological 'abnormalities' can be seen in normal individuals.[8,137]

The elderly

Constipation is common in the elderly. In one study 42% of all acute geriatric patients admitted to hospital had faecal impaction.[122] In another series faecal impaction was the main reason for hospital admission in 18% of acutely ill and 27% of chronically ill geriatric patients.[45] The pathogenesis of this problem is likely to be multifactorial. Depression or confusion may lead to the call to stool being ignored. Immobility, weakness or lack of physical activity may also contribute; colonic motor activity is related to the extent of somatic activity – the propulsive colonic movements seen after meals are much more frequent in subjects who are physically active.[65] Another important factor is the frequent use of drugs in the elderly, many with anticholinergic or other constipating side-effects.[121]

Faecal impaction in the elderly affects both sexes in similar proportion.[122] About half the elderly patients with faecal impaction have been taking laxatives, and about half have taken drugs that could contribute to constipation, including atropine-like antiparkinsonian drugs, tricyclic antidepressants, dextropropoxyphene, codeine phosphate, and phenothiazines. Patients with faecal impaction demonstrate impaired rectal sensory function, assessed using distension of an intrarectal balloon, with higher balloon volumes required to elicit initial sensation of balloon presence, a desire to defaecate, and pain.[122] Anal canal sensation is also impaired. Rectal expulsion and sphincter relaxation appear to be relatively normal. The disturbance of sensory function may be a primary problem, or related to medications or previous laxative nerve damage.

Pregnancy

Constipation is common in pregnancy, as are other disturbances of gastrointestinal motility such as gastro-oesophageal reflux, delayed gastric emptying, and reduced gall bladder contraction. The slowing of colonic transit is thought to be related to the large increase in concentration of circulating female sex hormones, especially progesterone, but other changes may also be important, such as the decrease in the propulsive hormone motilin.[20]

Severe idiopathic constipation

Young adults with a grossly decreased bowel frequency and a colon of normal diameter are almost exclusively women.[89,115,125,126,138] Some of these patients have been constipated since birth, whereas in others, the onset is in adolescence or young adulthood.[115] Whether each of these groups has the same aetiology is not known, although they appear to be clinically identical. In most of these patients, there was no obvious precipitating cause for their symptoms.[115] They complain of infrequent bowel actions, sometimes only every 2–4 weeks, difficulty with rectal evacuation, abdominal pain and bloating. They do not give a history of soiling, and usually have an empty rectum on examination.[162] They have a high incidence of previous gynaecological surgery, appendicectomy and laparotomy; this probably relates to previous misdiagnosis of their lower abdominal pain, as their reproductive organs appear to be normal.[77] These patients are usually resistant to increased dietary fibre and large doses of oral laxatives.[115]

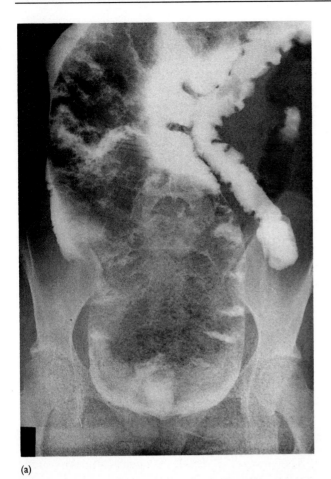
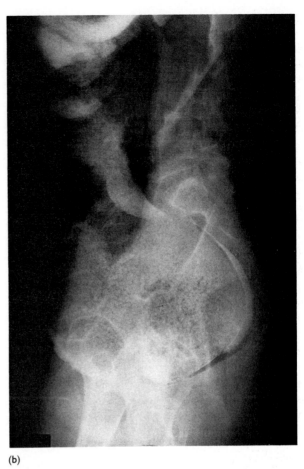

(a)   (b)

Figure 4.31 Gastrografin enema on a young woman with idiopathic megacolon. (a) The gross faecal retention and dilatation of the rectosigmoid is outlined by the contrast. (b) On the lateral view, this dilatation is seen to extend down to the anal margin.

Idiopathic megarectum or megacolon

Patients with severe constipation may be subdivided on the basis of the rectal and colonic diameter, assessed by contrast studies,[94] into those with a normal diameter bowel and those with an idiopathically dilated rectum (with or without dilated colon). Those with an idiopathically dilated rectum, or rectum and colon, appear to form part of a characteristic clinical group (*Figure 4.31*). Both sexes are affected equally. Those with the onset of symptoms in childhood often have faecal soiling secondary to their impaction, a clinical feature that distinguishes them from patients with Hirschsprung's disease who very rarely soil. Other patients have the onset of symptoms in adulthood – it is not known whether they acquire a megacolon or if it only becomes symptomatic later in life.[7]

SECONDARY CAUSES OF CONSTIPATION

Constipation may be related to a local colonic or anorectal cause, or may be secondary to some metabolic disorder, systemic illness or neurological lesion (*Table 4.3*).

Gastrointestinal myopathy or neuropathy

Patients with an abnormality of the muscle coats or the nerve plexuses in the gut may present with constipation. The best defined is *Hirschsprung's disease,* a congenital condition characterized by absent neurones within the bowel wall. The abnormal bowel extends for a variable proximal length from the anorectal junction, with proximal dilated normal bowel leading into the relatively narrow aganglionic segment (*Figure 4.32*). The affected segment ranges from very short, to involving the whole colon. The most common presentation is during infancy, but occasionally patients may present for the first time even into old age, although the symptoms have been present since birth.

The intramural nerve plexuses may be damaged in *Chagas' disease,* caused by infection with *Trypanosoma cruzi.* Inflammation around the nerve ganglia

Table 4.3 Causes of constipation

Idiopathic
Dietary abnormality
Pregnancy
Old age
Irritable bowel syndrome
Severe idiopathic constipation ('slow transit') in women

Structural disease of the colon, rectum or anus
Colonic or rectal stricture
    Tumour
    Inflammation
    Chronic infection
    Ischaemia
    Diverticular disease
Distal ulcerative colitis
Colonic neuromuscular abnormality
    Hirschsprung's disease (congenital aglanglionosis)
    Chagas' disease
    Intestinal pseudo-obstruction
    Idiopathic megarectum ± megacolon
    Segmental megacolon
    Myotonic dystrophy
    Systemic sclerosis
    Dermatomyositis
    Ganglioneuromatosis
        Primary
        Von Recklinghausen's disease
        Multiple endocrine neoplasia type 2B
Anal lesion
    Tumour
    Infection
    Anal fissure
    Ectopic anus
    Internal anal sphincter myopathy

Abnormality outside the colon
Neurological
    Central nervous system disorders
    Damage to the spinal cord or sacral outflow
    Autonomic neuropathy: primary, paraneoplastic
Psychological
    Anorexia nervosa
    Depression
Metabolic disorders
    Hypothyroidism
    Glucagonoma
    Hypercalcaemia
    Diabetic autonomic neuropathy
    Porphyria
    Amyloidosis
    Uraemia
    Hypokalaemia
    Lead poisoning
Drug induced

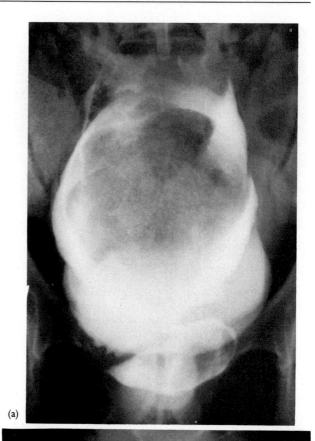

(a)

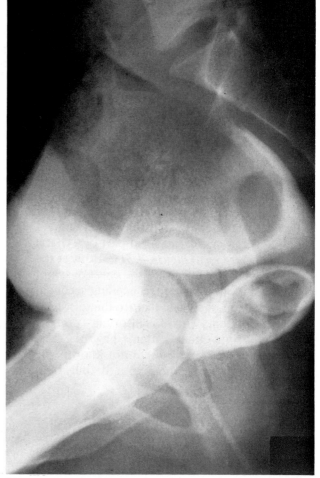

(b)

Figure 4.32 Gastrografin enema on a young man with constipation caused by a short segment of aganglionosis in the rectum (Hirschsprung's disease). (a) Dilatation of the rectum is apparent but only the lateral view (b) demonstrated that this does not extend as far as the anal margin and that there is a distal narrowing.

and neurone degeneration leads to bowel dilatation and constipation.

Patients with *chronic intestinal pseudo-obstruction* may have prominent colonic disease with colonic dilatation and constipation. The underlying disorder is one that affects either the gastrointestinal smooth muscle, that is, a visceral myopathy, or one that affects the nerve plexuses, that is, a visceral neuropathy. Those patients with a visceral myopathy often have just one of the two gut wall muscle coats affected. The conditions may be inherited in an autosomal recessive or autosomal dominant way, or may occur sporadically. When the condition is inherited, different family members with a pathologically similar condition can have different severity of symptoms and degree of disability. Upper gastrointestinal symptoms are common, as the condition may affect segments of the entire gastrointestinal tract. Some of these inherited syndromes have associated non-gastrointestinal abnormalities.[88]

A recently described myopathy of the internal anal sphincter can cause constipation, in particular, difficulty with rectal evacuation, in association with proctalgia fugax. The internal anal sphincter in these patients is thickened and shows abnormalities of function and morphology.[75]

Extrinsic neurological lesions

A neurological lesion at different levels from the cerebrum to the extrinsic pelvic nerves can cause constipation. Patients with a cerebrovascular accident, including those who have had a subarachnoid haemorrhage, experience constipation in the early period after their stroke but this resolves with time. Some patients with Parkinson's disease have constipation that fluctuates with their general motor function.[101] Either anterior or posterior pontine lesions may be associated with delayed colonic transit.[167] A study in dogs has highlighted the important role that pontine centres play in defaecatory activity.[39]

Constipation is common in patients with multiple sclerosis, occurring in 43% of affected individuals in one study.[63] It is more common in patients with moderate or severe disability, and correlates strongly with the duration of disease and the presence of genitourinary symptoms. Abnormalities of rectal compliance and absence of the normal postprandial colonic motor and myoelectrical response have been demonstrated in patients with advanced multiple sclerosis, suggesting a disturbance of the autonomic outflow to the gut.[50]

Constipation is common after spinal cord lesions. The constipation may occur soon after the injury, or even years later. It is thought to occur as a result of decreased extrinsic autonomic supply to the gut. The colonic compliance is markedly decreased, and there is a failure of postprandial increase in colonic motility.[48]

In some patients, constipation immediately follows either pelvic surgery or presumed trauma to the sacral outflow.[74] This can follow abdominal rectopexy, hysterectomy, or other pelvic surgery. The symptoms are of slow colonic transit with abdominal pain and bloating indistinguishable from those in young women with idiopathic constipation, or of normal bowel frequency and colonic transit time, but marked difficulty with rectal evacuation causing prolonged straining at stool. In one study, all the patients who related the onset of their constipation to a previous hysterectomy had absent sacral reflexes and impaired urodynamics, suggesting extensive pelvic nerve trauma.[83]

Some patients experience profound constipation after sacral trauma, caused by car accidents, spinal surgery, or even a simple fall onto the sacrum.[28,55] The presumed mechanism is damage to the sacral parasympathetic supply to the left colon, and occasionally this is accompanied by damage to the somatic voluntary muscles innervated by sacral motor roots. A similar syndrome of left colonic inertia may be produced by deliberate division of the nervi erigentes.[27] Pathological examination of the resected colon in such cases demonstrates similar abnormalities of argyrophilic neurones in the myenteric plexus to those seen in severe idiopathic constipation.[27,28,89,117]

Metabolic causes

Patients with hypothyroidism may present with constipation. In most cases this is related to the effect of thyroid hormone deficiency on the colonic muscle or neural control, without a change in colonic dimensions, but severe myxoedema can be associated with infiltration of the colon and subsequent megacolon.[18]

Abnormalities of calcium and potassium metabolism probably affect the bowel by interference with intramural neural conduction, or a direct effect on smooth muscle. They are reversible.

The autonomic neuropathy seen in some patients with diabetes mellitus may result in constipation. These patients often give a history of several years of alternating diarrhoea and constipation, followed by intractable unresponsive constipation. Diabetic patients with severe constipation have an absent gastrocolonic response to feeding.[10] The colonic response to neostigmine is normal, suggesting that cholinergic postganglionic neurons are intact and that the colonic smooth muscle is capable of a normal motor response. Histological abnormalities involving the myenteric plexus and parasympathetic nerve fibres have been described in the upper gastro-intestinal tract of diabetic patients.[144]

ASSESSMENT AND INVESTIGATIONS

A careful history and precise definition of the patient's main complaints are essential. Some estimate of the amount and type of dietary intake is important. A drug history is important with particular attention to drugs that may have constipation as a side-effect, and to laxatives. The age of onset of symptoms may give an important clue to the diagnosis. Constipation from birth in the absence of perianal soiling suggests congenital aganglionosis. Soiling from early childhood suggests a congenital megarectum or anorectal malformation. Symptoms developing in adolescence, or as a young adult, suggest a motility disorder. Neoplasm should be excluded in a middle-aged or elderly patient developing new symptoms.

EXAMINATION

During the physical examination, general causes such as hypothyroidism should be considered. Abdominal palpation may reveal faecal retention in those with a dilated or impacted bowel. Urinary retention may be present in those with a neurological lesion. Rectal examination and sigmoidoscopy are mandatory and in patients with pain preventing defaecation, a fissure, abscess or haemorrhoids should be excluded. Digital examination of the lower rectum will show if there is faecal impaction or a rectal or pelvic tumour. Sigmoidoscopy is helpful in excluding a tumour or proctitis, and in confirming melanosis coli. The rectal size can also be appreciated. Reproduction of pain using air insufflation may suggest the irritable bowel syndrome.

Which patients require further investigations? Most young patients with mild long-standing symptoms do not require investigation. Those with severe symptoms of any age, or constipation of recent onset, require further investigation.

RADIOLOGICAL STUDIES

In patients with a megarectum or megacolon, a plain abdominal radiograph will often demonstrate the colonic dimension as well as faecal retention. In patients without megacolon, a double contrast barium enema after bowel preparation will exclude a primary colonic cause such as diverticular stricture or carcinoma. In patients with a megarectum or megacolon, including those with faecal impaction, a contrast study without preparation, using a water-soluble contrast medium, will provide a more useful picture of colonic size and morphology. Bowel preparation in patients with megarectum or megacolon may reduce the bowel to normal size, giving a misleading impression about the extent of bowel dilatation. A further advantage is that, unlike barium, a water-soluble contrast medium does not solidify. The maximum normal rectal diameter in a lateral radiograph at the pelvic brim is 6.5 cm – a greater diameter suggests that the rectum is enlarged.[119]

A contrast study may also show a distal narrow segment with proximal dilatation, which is suggestive of Hirschsprung's disease.

BOWEL TRANSIT STUDIES

In patients with severe constipation, it is useful to confirm the presence of delayed gastrointestinal transit. As most of the gut transit time is spent in the colon, studies measuring the time for passage of an ingested substance is largely a reflection of colonic transit time. The most convenient way to measure transit is by the ingestion of radio-opaque markers and a subsequent plain abdominal radiograph to determine the proportion of retained markers. Retention of more than 20% of markers 96 hours after ingestion reflects slow transit.[64] The test should be conducted while the patient is on an adequate dietary fibre intake, and laxatives should be discontinued before the study. The simplest method involves the ingestion of 20 radio-opaque markers and taking a plain abdominal radiograph 96 hours later.[64] Severe constipation will usually be reflected by the retention of an excessive number of markers; however, patients can have similar symptoms of abdominal pain, bloating and difficult defaecation, but demonstrate a normal intestinal transit time.[94] Similarly, patients can have a normal bowel frequency but still have symptoms of difficult defaecation and a slow measured intestinal transit time.[99]

Radiographs can be taken at other times and the number of retained markers compared to a normal range.[34] The method can be further refined by ingesting three different radiologically distinguishable markers on three successive days and taking a radiograph at 120 hours – this provides three transit studies (*Figure 4.33*).[34] These techniques can also be used to study the site of delay within the colon[103] although, in patients with slow transit, a daily radiograph would be required. More recently, radioactive isotopes have been used to determine

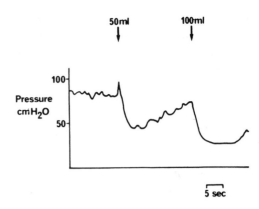

Figure 4.34 Anorectal inhibitory reflex. Anal canal pressure 1.5 cm from the anal verge measured by distension of the lower rectum by an air-filled balloon (1 cmH$_2$O ≈ 98 Pa). Distension of the rectum causes an immediate reflex inhibition of the internal anal sphincter resulting in a fall in anal canal pressure.

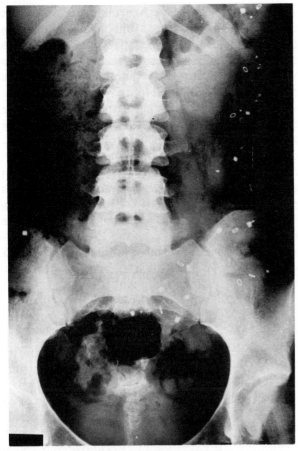

Figure 4.33 Transit study using three, radiologically distinct, radio-opaque markers taken 72 hours (rings), 48 hours (rods) and 24 hours (squares) previously. There is an excessive retention of markers, indicating slow colonic transit. Most of the markers are in the left colon, suggesting that this may be the main site of delayed transit.

regional delay – they allow frequent imaging with a lower radiation dose.[159] The usefulness of determining the site of regional delay in choosing a form of medical or surgical treatment remains to be determined.

COLONIC MOTILITY STUDIES

Whilst these are useful in a research context to characterize the motility disturbance, so far, they do not provide information which influences the management.

STUDIES OF DEFAECATION AND ANORECTAL PHYSIOLOGY

Most studies of anorectal physiological function are of research interest and do not help directly with management. Patients with severe constipation may fail to relax their pelvic floor on defaecation strain-

ing: this can be demonstrated as a failure of relaxation or striated sphincter muscle, accompanied by a failure of the anal canal pressure to fall.[113] It is likely that this paradoxical pelvic floor contraction, or 'anismus', is secondary to disturbed rectal and pelvic floor function. In a model of rectal evacuation, patients may be unable to expel a balloon from the rectum.[5] Evacuation proctography may demonstrate a reduced or absent ability to empty the rectum, or may show a large rectocele or rectal–anal intussusception. Unfortunately these radiological changes often correlate poorly with symptoms, may be seen in normal individuals without a defaecatory disturbance,[137] and are not helpful in predicting the outcome of surgery for constipation.

In those patients with a dilated distal bowel, the presence of the rectoanal inhibitory reflex should be sought, to distinguish idiopathic megarectum from Hirschsprung's disease. Balloon distension in the rectum causes a fall in anal pressure, which can be monitored by an anal pressure probe (*Figure 4.34*). This reflex is caused by a descending inhibitory neural pathway within the wall of the bowel.[76] It is absent in Hirschsprung's disease, because of the absence of distal myenteric plexus. A false-negative study may be obtained in some patients with idiopathic megarectum caused by the difficulty in distending a large rectum.

RECTAL BIOPSY

Patients with a megarectum or megacolon and an absent rectoanal reflex should have a full thickness rectal biopsy performed under anaesthesia. This should be taken from the low rectum, but not within 2 cm of the dentate line, which can have an absence of ganglia in the normal rectum. Aganglionosis is diagnostic of Hirschsprung's disease. Staining with acetylcholinesterase demonstrates increased tissue levels in the affected aganglionic segment, due to hypertrophied extrinsic nerves. This stain needs to be performed on fresh unfixed tissue.

Other conditions occasionally identifiable on biopsy include systemic sclerosis and amyloidosis. The conditions of hypoganglionosis and hyperganglionosis remain poorly defined, in the absence of accurate quantitative data on neuronal numbers in the distal bowel.

TREATMENT: MEDICAL

Most patients with constipation can be managed on a symptomatic basis without investigations. This is especially true if the constipation is mild, there are no severe associated symptoms and the condition is long standing without recent changes.

DIETARY FIBRE

The first step in treatment is a dietary assessment, and addition of fibre to the diet. Bringing the fibre intake up to 30 g per day will relieve mild constipation in many. Unprocessed bran, composed of particles of large size, can be added to breakfast cereal and is the most effective fibre supplement. Particle size as well as the type of fibre appears to be important. For patients who do not tolerate the addition of bran to the diet, commercial fibre preparations, such as ispaghula or sterculia, are often effective. Although the addition of fibre to the diet helps the constipation, it will cause increased wind and bloating and usually does not relieve abdominal discomfort.

MEDICAL PREPARATIONS

If laxatives are to be used, they should be employed on a temporary basis if possible. If used long term, they should be used as infrequently as necessary. Osmotic laxatives such as magnesium sulphate or lactulose, are satisfactory first choices. They are gentler in their action than many of the stimulant laxatives and avoid the theoretical problem of nerve plexus damage. If a stronger laxative is required, bisacodyl by mouth is often satisfactory. Senna may cause bowel nerve plexus damage but is an effective stimulant. A more detailed discussion of the mode of action of laxatives is given below.

Suppositories or enemas are a good alternative to oral laxatives. Glycerine suppositories are gentle in their action whilst bisacodyl suppositories are

stronger, but leave some patients with cramps after defaecation. Enemas are available as microenemas (sodium citrate) or larger phosphate enemas of 100 ml. Even in patients with severe constipation in whom oral laxatives are ineffective, per rectal preparations are often helpful.

For the most severely constipated patients, stronger medications may be required intermittently. Oral stimulants include sodium picosulphate, or even electrolyte solutions in large quantity, which are used for colonoscopy or radiography preparation. These should be used with caution in patients who are extremely constipated or who may have bowel obstruction. Strong enemas include the use of a stimulant in water of a larger volume, for example, bisacodyl rectal solution, or oxyphenisatin. For the most intractable constipation, an enema consisting of 200 ml of one part treacle to two parts milk, warmed, is usually effective.

Patients with faecal impaction must be disimpacted before starting laxatives. Occasionally this can be done with sedation only, but often a general anaesthetic is required. A plain abdominal radiograph is useful to confirm that the bowel has been adequately emptied.

Patients with an indiopathic megarectum or megacolon must be disimpacted initially. They can then usually prevent further impaction by keeping the stool semiliquid, using magnesium sulphate or lactulose each day. This is usually necessary for life.

BIOFEEDBACK

Biofeedback conditioning for constipation has been employed in the belief that abnormal pelvic floor contraction is a learned phenomenon which causes constipation. Bleijenberg and Kuijpers (1987) used an intensive inpatient regimen to treat 10 patients with both delayed colonic transit and abnormal pelvic floor activity.[15] Seven of these patients had a normal defaecation frequency and feeling of urgency after treatment. It is not known whether the response to such treatment is due to an effect on the pelvic floor or to improved general relaxation with a subsequent effect on the cerebral control of colonic motility. In support of the latter are two studies which have shown that biofeedback, combined with relaxation training or other psychotherapeutic techniques, provide a greater success rate than biofeedback alone.[86,156]

BOTULINUM A TOXIN

Botulinum A toxin has been used in the treatment of disorders of the ocular muscles such as blepharospasm and strabismus, and in torticollis. It is a neurotoxin produced by *Clostridium botulinum*, which causes irreversible neuromuscular blockade and a flaccid paralysis. Patients with inappropriate puborectalis contraction have been treated with injections into the muscle.[56] The treatment is successful in decreasing the voluntary anal contraction pressure, the amount of straining and abdominal pain, but it does not improve patients' bowel frequency.

LAXATIVES

Laxatives are agents used in the treatment of constipation to promote defaecation. In 1989 in the UK, £17.4 million was spent on 6.2 million prescriptions, comprising 1.5% of the total number of prescriptions. A much greater number of laxatives are sold over the counter. In addition to their use in constipation, laxatives are used to prepare the colon for colonoscopy and radiological investigations.

Although laxatives are usually divided into bulk-forming agents, osmotic laxatives, stimulant laxatives and stool-softening preparations (*Table 4.4*), the exact mode of action of many of these substances is poorly understood. Some drugs may act by more than one mechanism. The overall effect of these substances is a complex combination of an increase of faecal water content, an acceleration of intestinal transit and other alterations of intestinal motility. The change seen with acute use are different from those seen with chronic use, due partly to tolerance, induced changes in colonic flora, and possible neuromyogenic gut damage.

EFFECT OF LAXATIVES ON INTESTINAL MOTILITY

Colonic motility

When taken orally, bisacodyl is absorbed to a variable degree, most being excreted in the faeces. When introduced directly into the colon, bisacodyl induces propagated pressure waves within 2–3 minute.[57,114] This local colonic response can be prevented by prior application of lignocaine to the mucosa, suggesting a neurally mediated mechanism.[106] Another polyphenolic drug, oxyphenisatin, which is the active aperient principle of prunes, produces peristalsis affecting mainly the proximal colon when given by the rectum.[129] Sennosides are broken down by colonic bacterial enzymes to form the active component rheinanthrone. Introduction of sennosides incubated with faeces or *Escherichia coli* into the colon through a colostomy has been

Table 4.4 Types of laxative

Bulk-forming (fibre preparations)

Methyl cellulose
Bran
Psyllium
Ispaghula husk
Sterculia
Guar gum

Osmotic

Magnesium sulphate or magnesium hydroxide
Magnesium citrate or magnesium carbonate
Sodium sulphate and sodium-potassium tartrate
Alcohols: sorbitol, mannitol
Glycerol
Lactulose

Stimulant laxatives

Polyphenolic drugs
  Phenolphthalein
  Bisacodyl
  Sodium picosulphate (bisacodyl disulphate)
Anthranoid derivatives
  Naturally occurring: senna, cascara, aloe, rhubarb
  Sennosides (glycosides of rhein dianthrone)
Castor oil

Prokinetic drugs

Cisapride

Stool softeners

Liquid paraffin
Dioctyl sodium sulphosuccinate
Arachis oil

Suppositories and enemas

Glycerine, bisacodyl, sodium citrate

shown to induce colonic peristalsis.[58] Studies of the effect of oral sennosides using prolonged myoelectrical recordings from the descending and sigmoid colon, showed a marked increase in the number of rapidly propagated spike bursts which correspond to peristaltic pressure waves.[38] This effect was seen 6–8 hours after taking the sennoside, which would correspond with the time taken for orocaecal transit and breakdown of the sennoside. Other studies suggested that certain patterns of colonic activity may be depressed after administration of sennosides – orally administered senna extract was found to reduce segmenting pressure activity[164] and, in animal studies, colonic myoelectrical activity was inhibited by oral sennosides after a 6–10 hour delay.[43] One study that employed strain-gauge transducers in dogs found a similar reduction in segmenting activity but the induction of giant contractions of short duration.[151] These colonic giant contractions can also be produced by magnesium citrate and castor oil.[80]

Laxatives can exert their effect on intestinal motility by either a direct action on the intestinal neuromuscular activity or secondary to an increase in intraluminal contents brought about by changes in fluid and electrolyte movement.

Sennosides appear to have a direct action on intestinal motility. A study looking at both colonic transit and net colonic fluid absorption following oral sennosides showed that maximum acceleration of transit occurred 2 hours before the maximum effect on water and electrolyte movements.[93] In dogs the changes in colonic motility induced by duodenal infusion of a hypertonic mannitol solution were very different from those seen after sennoside, although diarrhoea was produced by both.[36] Mannitol produced an increase in the number of contractions with a disruption of the cyclical pattern of contractions, whereas sennosides inhibited basal colonic motility but giant contractions were recorded.[151]

Gastric and small intestine

Although the major problem in constipation is the delay in colonic transit, delays in gastric emptying and small bowel transit are also present.[123,139] It is of interest, therefore, that certain laxatives have an effect on gastric and small intestinal transit. Lactulose, an osmotic laxative, is broken down by colonic bacterial enzymes to produce unabsorbed organic acids which acidify the stool. A study of intestinal transit of healthy human patients demonstrated that incorporation of lactulose into a standard meal significantly shortened the transit of a meal through the small intestine but had no effect on the rate of transit through the whole gut.[124] Bisacodyl, the polyphenolic compound that does not require bacterial metabolism, also increases the human jejunal transit rate.[35]

Laxatives may act on the small intestine indirectly. Ricinoleic acid produces a pattern of contractions occurring at one-minute intervals.[3] A similar pattern of contractions, called 'minute rhythm', is seen in healthy humans and increases in diarrhoeal disease[157] suggesting that the action of ricinoleic acid may be a result of increased volume of intestinal content.

Prokinetic drugs

Cisapride has been shown to accelerate upper gastrointestinal transit.[136] Animal studies suggest that by facilitating cholinergic neurotransmission in the gastric wall, it selectively improves motor function and accelerates delayed gastric emptying.[135] In the human colon, studies in vitro indicate that cisapride has no direct effect on the smooth muscle or its inhibitory innervation, but it antagonizes responses mediated by serotonin receptors and adrenoceptors in the circular muscle.[67] In children with chronic idiopathic constipation it has been reported to increase stool frequency and decrease total gastrointestinal transit time.[150] In this study, anorectal tests showed that cisapride decreased the rectoanal inhibitory reflex threshold and the conscious rectal sensitivity volume. In constipated patients, cisapride has been shown to accelerate colonic transit.[87] It has some effect in mild constipation but is not effective in most patients with severe constipation.

Mediators

Little is known about the mediators involved in the action of laxatives. Magnesium sulphate causes release of cholecystokinin from the duodenal mucosa which then stimulates colonic motility.[59] Prostaglandins are probably involved in the action of a number of laxatives. Prostaglandin synthesis inhibitors, such as indomethacin or aspirin, and prostaglandin receptor antagonists have been shown to prevent the laxative action of a phenolphthalein,[19] sennosides,[92] and rhein anthrone.[168] Indomethacin infusion into canine right colonic artery abolished the giant contractions produced by sennoside[151] and sennoside-induced changes in colonic motility were reproduced by prostaglandin E_2 administered into the colonic lumen as a gel or infused into the colonic artery.

TOXICOLOGY

A number of laxatives have serious side-effects or toxicity. Oxyphenisatin causes hepatitis and cirrhosis.[109,127] Danthron, a synthetic anthraquinone, may be hepatotoxic[51] and chronic administration of high doses has produced liver and intestinal tumours in rats and mice.[100] Phenolphthalein can cause allergic skin reactions[141] and rarely encephalitis.[82] Liquid paraffin may cause lipoid pneumonia and interfere with absorption of fat-soluble vitamins if taken chronically in high doses.

In view of their widespread use, it is important to ask whether long-term laxative use might result in damage to the nerve plexuses or muscle. Smith studied the myenteric plexus in mice after intraperitoneal and oral senna[145] and found impaired peristalsis. After four months of oral senna there was axonal fragmentation and dendritic swelling within the myenteric plexus. In those mice in which the senna was administered intraperitoneally, this damage was present after 2 weeks. The histological findings in the colon of a patient with longstanding constipation were also reported. There was a vast increase in the number of Schwann cells which filled the plexus region and a reduction in the number of neurones and axons. Ultrastructural studies of the mouse and rat colon after long-term treatment with sennosides have not shown damage to intramural nerve tissue.[31,130]

In humans, it is difficult to determine whether observed gut nerve changes are the underlying primary disorder, or secondary to long-term laxative use. Biopsies from the descending colon, sigmoid and rectum from patients with chronic idiopathic constipation were compared with similar biopsies from control subjects and patients with irritable bowel syndrome.[128] The histological features in the submucosal plexus in those with constipation and laxative use were ballooning of axons, reduction of nerve-specific cell organelles and a decrease of neurosecretory granules in nerve endings. A decrease in the number of argyrophilic neurones and morphological abnormalities of the neurones within the myenteric plexus of severely constipated patients have been demonstrated using Smith's silver staining.[89,115] In one study monoclonal antibodies raised against neurofilament showed abnormalities in the submucosal and myenteric plexuses of constipated patients.[132]

LAXATIVE ABUSE

Laxative abuse can range from a habitual weekly purge, more commonly in the elderly, to the addictive consumption of over 50 senna tablets a day. Laxative abuse can occur in the absence of constipation, caused in part by the widespread erroneous belief that a daily bowel action is essential for good health. Most patients with addictive consumption are reported to be women and commonly have associated psychiatric disorders such as depression, anorexia nervosa or a personality problem. In patients with anorexia nervosa, the use of laxatives along with self-induced vomiting is a bad prognostic indicator. In patients presenting with unexplained diarrhoea, laxatives abuse should be considered.

Clinical features

Laxative abuse is much more common in women. Patients may present with diarrhoea, abdominal pain, weakness, weight loss and occasionally vomiting. The features of malabsorption may be present with hypoproteinaemia, amenorrhoea, hypokalae-

mia and iron deficiency anaemia. Hypocalcaemia and hypomagnesaemia may also occur. Severe metabolic disturbance may be associated with a frank psychosis, hallucinations, ataxia and epileptic seizures. Previous investigations may have shown steatorrhoea, increased gastrointestinal protein loss, abnormal renal function, abnormal gastric and pancreatic function tests or a diabetic glucose tolerance curve. Laparotomy may have been performed in some cases.[23]

Investigation

Urine can be analyzed for products of anthraquinone-type laxatives, and phenolphthalein in the stool may be detected by alkalization (sodium hydroxide) which produces a red colour. Rectal biopsy may show melanosis coli which is diagnostic of recent and prolonged intake of laxatives, usually anthraquinones.

Melanosis coli, in which the abnormal pigment is probably derived from lipofuscin[74] or degenerated mitochondria[133] is seen in patients taking laxatives long term, usually anthraquinones. In patients who stop laxatives, the melanosis disappears 4–12 months later. In addition to melanosis coli, the changes seen in cathartic colon are mucosal inflammation, hypertrophy of the muscularis mucosae and thinning or atrophy of the muscle layers.[105]

SURGERY

The indications for surgical intervention in the management of patients without a clear organic cause for their constipation are poorly defined and remain controversial. In organic conditions such as Hirschsprung's disease the treatment is better defined (and described in the previous section). The surgical treatment of patients with a clearly defined organic abnormality is not discussed here.

Comprehensive evaluation over a prolonged period is essential before making a decision to operate. Surgery should be restricted to those with intractable symptoms referable to the large bowel, who remain incapacitated despite intense conservative treatment, and in whom there are no adverse psychological factors present.

PSYCHOLOGICAL ASPECTS

Psychological problems are common among those operated on for constipation and are prominent in many surgical series.[37,74] These problems may be present preoperatively or may become more obvious postoperatively. Severely constipated patients with the greatest psychological problems often tolerate their symptoms least well and seek a surgical solution. In one series of patients who had a colectomy for idiopathic constipation, 9 out of 44 patients had a serious psychiatric disorder requiring treatment.[74] In another series, a comparison of patients having surgery for constipation with patients undergoing surgery for faecal incontinence and another group matched for age and sex, found that those requiring surgical treatment for constipation had a significantly higher depression score than the control patients.[37] Those constipated patients who had a poor surgical result had a higher anxiety and depression score compared with both the control group and those patients who did well.

SURGERY FOR SEVERE IDIOPATHIC SLOW TRANSIT CONSTIPATION

Colectomy

Colectomy with ileorectal anastomosis for constipation was first described at the beginning of the century by Sir William Arbuthnot Lane.[2] Subsequent operative series have demonstrated that the outcome of this operation is variable and unpredictable.[74,45,118,170]

Although many patients are generally improved with a better quality of life, postoperative problems included re-admission with abdominal pain, further surgical procedures, recurrent constipation, intractable diarrhoea and faecal incontinence. Abdominal pain is a prominent symptom in these patients and may be a major indication for surgery, but two-thirds still have some pain postoperatively.[74]

Categorization of patients with severe constipation into those with delayed transit due to a colonic disorder and those with abnormalities of 'outlet obstruction' is now commonly performed before surgery. It has been suggested that colectomy in someone with features of abnormal evacuation is doomed to failure,[13] but those with evacuation abnormalities, as measured by electromyography and balloon expulsion, have as good an outcome as those without, when treated by colectomy.[74]

Partial colonic resections, such as sigmoid resection or left hemicolectomy, have in the past resulted in recurrent constipation.[115] The use of colonic scintigraphy or radio-opaque markers to define segmental delayed colonic transit may lead to better patient selection for limited resections[78](*Figure 4.35*). Retention of the caecum in the belief that the ileocaecal valve may prevent postoperative diarrhoea has been reported, but subsequent caecal

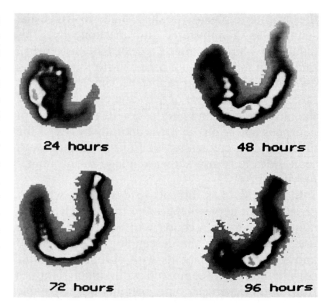

Figure 4.35 Colonic radioisotope scan taken after the ingestion of a meal labelled with ^{111}In, in a 29-year-old woman with severe idiopathic constipation. Transit is held up in the transverse colon, indicating that at least this part of the colon has deficient propulsive activity. Scans such as this allow more detailed studies of regional colonic transit than radio-opaque marker studies, partly because the radioisotope can be incorporated more physiologically into a meal and partly because more frequent observations are possible. Regional transit studies may allow more specific treatment of severe constipation, both medically and surgically (see reference [150]).

dilatation and recurrent constipation is more common after caecorectal anastomosis than after ileorectal anastomosis.[118]

Postoperative symptoms after colectomy with ileorectal anastomosis may relate to a defective sphincter mechanism, leaving in situ an abnormal rectum, or alternatively, impaired small bowel function.

Operations on the internal anal sphincter

A strip myectomy of the internal anal sphincter has been performed in patients with constipation, including those with slow transit, in the belief that the sphincter behaves abnormally and obstructs emptying. Early reports on the results of this operation were favourable[99,169] but the long-term results are disappointing, with poor results in 70% after 30 months median follow up.[111]

In children, the procedure produced good results in half of 53 cases, and, in over half, significant abnormalities of the nerve plexuses were detected.[62]

Internal anal sphincter strip myectomy has also been used to treat a recently identified internal sphincter myopathy. In this group of patients with severe proctalgia fugax and constipation, the internal sphincter was non-compliant with a high resting anal canal pressure.[75]

Puborectalis division

Initial series of puborectalis division reported encouraging results,[163,165] but these have not been sustained.[16,73]

Other procedures

When the results of colectomy are unsatisfactory, what are the alternatives? A primary colostomy for severe constipation produces satisfactory symptomatic relief.[158] For patients after a failed colectomy, an alternative to ileostomy is the creation of an ileal reservoir with ileoanal anastomosis.[107] Although only a small number of patients have undergone this procedure for constipation and the follow up is short, the initial results have been satisfactory.[66,91]

SURGERY FOR MEGARECTUM AND MEGACOLON

Many patients with this condition can be adequately managed in the long term with laxatives but a small group of patients will require surgical treatment.

Colectomy

Subtotal colectomy has been the most widely performed operation for idiopathic megarectum or megacolon.[14,91,98,108] In two series, sigmoid resection alone produces poor results.[91,108] In one series of 40 patients, 83% had a normal bowel frequency after surgery. Only those who had had an ileorectal anastomosis did not have recurrent constipation.[148] Most patients did not require laxatives postoperatively but abdominal pain was still present in about a third of patients. There was no difference in the outcome between those with dilatation of the whole colon and those with dilatation of the rectosigmoid.[148]

Duhamel procedure

Although the Duhamel procedure was originally designed for Hirschsprung's disease,[32] it has subsequently been used for patients with idiopathic megarectum or megacolon. The operation is usually reserved for patients with a grossly dilated rectum in whom it is felt that a colectomy and end-to-end anastomosis would not be feasible. Only half the patients develop a normal postoperative bowel frequency.[147]

Restorative proctocolectomy

Only five patients having this operation for idiopathic megarectum have been reported, with good functional results.[166]

Stoma

Formation of a colostomy using normal calibre colon above the dilated rectum relieves constipation.[149] Formation of a colostomy in patients with dilatation of the whole colon is not successful.[53,149]

Pelvic floor operations

Internal anal sphincter strip myectomy has a variable outcome in this condition, although there are few detailed studies. In one study, nine adolescents were improved[60] but, in another study, three of five adults had a poor outcome.[14]

Although patients with idiopathic megarectum paradoxically contract their pelvic floor during straining, puborectalis division does not appear to be beneficial.[73]

REFERENCES

1. Allen-Mersh, T.G., Henry, M.M. and Nicholls, R.J. (1987) Natural history of anterior mucosal prolapse. *British Journal of Surgery*, **74**, 679–682.
2. Arbuthnot Lane, W. (1908) The results of the operative treatment of chronic constipation. *British Medical Journal*, **1**, 126–130.
3. Atchison W.D., Stewart, J.J. and Bass, P. (1978) A unique distribution of laxative-induced spike potentials from the small intestine of the dog. *American Journal of Digestive Diseases*, **23**, 513–520.
4. Bannister, J.J., Davison, P., Timms, J.M., Gibbons, C. and Read, N.W. (1987) Effect of stool size and consistency on defaecation. *Gut*, **28**, 1246–1250.
5. Barnes, P.R.H. and Lennard-Jones, J. E. (1985) Balloon expulsion from the rectum in constipation of different types. *Gut*, **26**, 1049–1052.
6. Barnes, P.R.H., Hawley, P.R., Preston, D.M. and Lennard-Jones, J.E. (1985) Experience of posterior division of the puborectalis muscle in the management of chronic constipation. *British Journal of Surgery*, **72**, 475–477.
7. Barnes, P.R.H., Lennard-Jones, J.E., Hawley, P.R. and Todd, I.P. (1986) Hirschsprung's disease and idiopathic megacolon in adults and adolescents. *Gut*, **27**, 534–541.
8. Bartram, C.L., Turnbull, G.K. and Lennard-Jones, J.E. (1988) Evacuation proctography: an investigation of rectal expulsion in 20 subjects without defecatory disturbance. *Gastrointestinal Radiology*, **13**, 72–80.

9. Bassotti, G., Gaburri, M., Imbimbo, B.P., Rossi, L., Farroni, F. and Pelli, M.A. *et al.* (1988) Colonic mass movements in idiopathic chronic constipation. *Gut*, **29**, 1173–1179.

10. Battle, W.M., Snape, W.J., Alavi, A., Cohen, S. and Braunstein, S. (1980) Colonic dysfunction in diabetes mellitus. *Gastroenterology*, **79**, 1217–1221.

11. Bayliss, W.M. and Starling, E.H. (1889) The movements and innervation of the small intestine. *Journal of Physiology (Lond)*, **24**, 99–143.

12. Bayliss, W.M. and Starling E.H. (1900) The movements and innervation of the large intestine. *Journal of Physiology (Lond)*, **26**, 107–118.

13. Beck, D.E., Jagelman, D.G. and Fazio, V.W. The surgery of idiopathic constipation. *Gastroenterology Clinics of North America*, **16**, 143–156.

14. Belliveau, P., Goldberg, S.M., Rothenberger, D.A. and Nivatvongs, S. (1982) Idiopathic acquired megacolon: the value of subtotal colectomy. *Diseases of the Colon and Rectum*, **25**, 118–121.

15. Bleijenberg, G. and Kuijpers, H. C. (1987) Treatment of the spastic pelvic floor syndrome with biofeedback. *Diseases of the Colon and Rectum*, **30**, 108–111.

16. Bodian, M., Stephens, F.D. and Ward, B.C.H. (1949) Hirschsprung's disease and idiopathic megacolon. *Lancet*, **i**, 6–11.

17. Burleigh, D.E. (1988) Evidence for a functional cholinergic deficit in human colonic tissue resected for constipation. *Journal of Pharmacy and Pharmacology*, **40**, 55–57.

18. Burrell, M., Cronan, J., Megna, D. and Toffler, R. (1980) Myxedema megacolon. *Gastrointestinal Radiology*, **5**, 181–186.

19. Capasso, F., Mascolo, N., Autore, G. and Duraccio, M.R. (1984) Suppression of laxative action of phenolphthalein by orally-administered indomethacin or aspirin. *Journal of Pharmacy and Pharmacology*, **36**, 132–133.

20. Christofides, N.D., Ghatei, M.A., Bloom, S.R., Borberg, C. and Gillmer, M.D.G. (1982) Decreased plasma motilin concentrations in pregnancy. *British Medical Journal*, **285**, 1453–1454.

21. Connell, A.M., Hilton, C., Irvine, G., Lennard-Jones, J.E. and Misiewicz, J.J. (1965) Variation of bowel habit in two population samples. *British Medical Journal*, **2**, 1095–1099.

22. Cook, I.J., Irvine, G.J., Campbell, D., Shannon, S., Reddy, S.N. and Collins, S.M. (1990) Effect of dietary fiber on symptoms and rectosigmoid motility in patients with irritable bowel syndrome. A controlled, crossover study. *Gastroenterology*, **98**, 66–72.

23. Cummings, J.H. (1974) Progress report. Laxative abuse. *Gut*, **15**, 758–766.

24. Davidson, M., Kugler, M.M. and Bauer, C.H. (1963) Diagnosis and management in children with severe and protracted constipation and obstipation. *Journal of Pediatrics*, **62**, 261.

25. Davies, G.J., Crowder, M., Reid, B. and Dickerson, J.W.T. (1986) Bowel function measurements of individuals with different eating patterns. *Gut*, **27**, 164–169.

26. Dent, O.F., Goulston, K.J., Kubrzycki, J. and Chapuis P.H. (1986) Bowel symptoms in an apparently well population. *Diseases of the Colon and Rectum*, **29**, 243–247.

27. Devroede, G. and Lamarche, J. (1974) Functional importance of extrinsic parasympathetic innervation to the distal colon and rectum in man. *Gastroenterology*, **66**, 273–280.

28. Devroede, G., Arhan, P., Duguay, C., Tetreault, L., Akoury, H. and Perey, B. (1979) Traumatic constipation. *Gastroenterology*, **77**, 1258–1267.

29. Dolk, A., Brodén, G., Holmström, B., Johansson, C. and Schultzberg, M. (1990) Slow transit chronic constipation. An immunohistochemical study of neuropeptide-containing nerves in resected specimens from the large bowel. *International Journal of Colorectal Disease*, **5**, 181–187.

30. Drossman, D.A., Sandler, R.S., McKee, D.C. and Lovitz, A.J. (1982) Bowel patterns among subjects not seeking health care. *Gastroenterology*, **83**, 529–534.

31. Dufour, P. and Gendre, P. (1984) Ultrastructure of mouse intestinal mucosa and changes observed after long-term anthraquinone administration. *Gut*, **25**, 1358–1363.

32. Duhamel, B. (1964) Retrorectal and transanal pull-through procedure for the treatment of Hirschsprung's disease. *Diseases of the Colon and Rectum*, **7**, 455–458.

33. Duthie, G.S., Bartolo, D.C.C. and Miller, R. (1991) Estimation of the incidence of anismus by laboratory tests. *British Journal of Surgery*, **78**, A747.

34. Evans, R.G., Kamm, M.A., Hinton, J.M. and Lennard-Jones, J.E. The normal range and a simple diagram for recording whole gut transit time. *International Journal of Colorectal Disease* (in press).

35. Ewe, K. (1987) Effect of bisacodyl on intestinal electrolyte and water net transport and transit. Perfusion studies in men. *Digestion*, **37**, 247–253.

36. Fioramonti, J., Droy-Lefaix, M.T. and Buéno, L. (1987) Changes in gastrointestinal motility induced by cholera toxin and experimental osmotic diarrhoea in dogs: effects of treatment with an argillaceous compound. *Digestion*, **36**: 230–237.

37. Fisher, S.E., Brecon, K., Andrews, H.A. and Keighley, M.R.B. (1989) Psychiatric screening for patients with faecal incontinence or chronic constipation referred for surgical treatment. *British Journal of Surgery*, **76**, 352–355.

38. Frexinos, J., Staumont, G., Fioramonti, J. and Buéno, L. (1989) Effects of sennosides on colonic myoelectrical activity in man. *Digestive Diseases and Sciences*, **34**, 214–219.

39. Fukuda, H., Fukai, K., Yamane, M. and Okada, H. (1981) Pontine reticular unit responses to pelvic nerve and colonic mechanical stimulation in the dog. *Brain Research*, **207**, 59–71.

40. Furness, J.B. and Costa, M. (1980) Types of nerves in the enteric nervous system. *Neuroscience*, **5**: 1–20.

41. Ganiban, G., Besselman, D., Harcelrode, J. and Murthy, S.N.S. (1985) Effect of sex steroids on total gastrointestinal transit in male rats. *Gastroenterology*, **88**, 1713.

42. Gannon, B.J., Noblett, H.R. and Burnstock, G. (1969) Adrenergic innervation of bowel in Hirschsprung's disease. *British Journal of Medicine*, **3**, 338–340.

43. Garcia-Villar, R., Leng-Peschlow, E. and Ruckebusch, Y. (1980) Effects of anthraquinone derivatives on canine and rat intestinal motility. *Journal of Pharmacy and Pharmacology*, **32**, 323–329.

44. Garrett, J.R., Howard, E.R. and Nixon, H.H. (1969) Autonomic nerves in the rectum and colon in Hirschsprung's disease. *Archives of Disease in Childhood*, **44**, 406–417.

45. Geboes, K. and Bossaert, H. (1977) Gastrointestinal disorders in old age. *Age and Ageing*, **6**, 197–200.

46. Gill, R.C., Bowes, K.L. and Kingma, Y.J. (1985) Effect of progesterone on canine colonic smooth muscle. *Gastroenterology*, **88**, 1941–1947.

47. Gillis, R.A., Souza, J.D., Hicks, K.A., Mangel, A.W., Pagani, F.D., Hamilton, B.L., Garvey, T.Q., Pace, D.G., Browne, R.K. and Norman, W.P. (1987) Inhibitory control of proximal colonic motility by the sympathetic nervous system. *American Journal of Physiology*, **253**, G531–539.

48. Glick, M.E., Haldeman, S. and Meshkinpour, H. (1986) The neurovisceral and electrodiagnostic evaluation of patients with thoracic spinal cord injury. *Paraplegia*, **24**, 129–137.

49. Glick, M.E., Haldeman, S. and Meshkinpour, H. (1986) The neurovisceral and electrodiagnostic evaluation of patients with thoracic spinal cord injury. *Paraplegia*, **24**, 129–137.

50. Glick, M.E., Meshkinpour, H., Haldeman, S., Narender B.N. and Bradley, W.E. (1982) Colonic dysfunction in multiple sclerosis. *Gastroenterology*, **83**, 1002–1007.

51. Godding, E.W. (1984) Bowel function and dysfunction. 4. Chemical laxatives. *Pharmacology Journal*, **232**, 168–169

52. Goldin, E., Karmeli, F., Selinger, Z. and Rachmilewitz, D. (1989) Colonic substance P levels are increased in ulcerative colitis and decreased in chronic severe constipation. *Digestive Diseases and Sciences*, **34**, 754–757.

53. Goligher, J. (1961) In discussion on megacolon and megarectum with emphasis on conditions other than Hirschsprung's disease. *Proceedings of the Royal Society of Medicine*, **54**, 1053–1055.

54. Gottlieb, S.H. and Schuster, M.M. (1986) Dermatoglyphic (fingerprint) evidence for a congenital syndrome of early onset constipation and abdominal pain. *Gastroenterology*, **91**, 428–432.

55. Gunterberg, B., Kewenter, J., Peterson, I. and Stener, B. (1976) Anorectal function after major resections of the sacrum with bilateral or unilateral sacrifice of sacral nerves. *British Journal of Surgery*, **63**, 546–554.

56. Hallan, R.I., Williams, N.S., Melling, J., Waldron, D.J., Womack, N.R. and Morrison, J.F.B. (1988) Treatment of anismus in intractable constipation with Botulinum A toxin. *Lancet*, **ii**, 714–716.

57. Hardcastle, J.D. and Mann, C.V. Study of large bowel peristalsis. *Gut*, **9**, 512–520.

58. Hardcastle, J.D. and Wilkins, J.L. (1970) The action of sennosides and related compounds on human colon and rectum. *Gut*, **11**, 1038–1042.

59. Harvey, R.F., Dowsett, L., Hartog, M. and Read, A.E. (1973) A radioimmunoassay for cholecystokinin-pancreozymin. *Lancet*, **ii**, 826–829.

60. Hata, Y., Sasaki, F. and Uchino, J. (1988) Sphincteromyectomy and sphincteroplasty in chronic constipation with megarectum. *Journal of Paediatric Surgery*, **23**, 141–142.

61. Heaton, K.W. (1991) Fibre and bulk preparations. In *Gastrointestinal Transit. Pathophysiology and Pharmacology* (Eds) Kamm, M.A. and Lennard-Jones, J.E. pp. 209–218. Wrightson Biomedical Publishing.

62. Heaton, N. D. and Howard, E.R. (1985) Anorectal myectomy: a valuable treatment for chronic constipation. *Gut*, **26**, A1130.

63. Hinds, J.P., Eidelman, B.H. and Wald, A. (1990) Prevalence of bowel dysfunction in a multiple sclerosis. A population survey. *Gastroenterology*, **98**, 1538–1542.

64. Hinton, J.M., Lennard-Jones, J.E. and Young, A.C. (1969) A new method for studying gut transit times using radio-opaque markers. *Gut*, **10**, 842–847.

65. Holdstock, D.J., Misiewicz, J.J., Smith, T. and Rowlands, E.N. (1970) Propulsion (mass movements) in the human colon and its relationship to meals and somatic activity. *Gut*, **11**, 91–99.

66. Hosie, K.B., Kmiot, W.A. and Keighley, M.R.B. (1990) Constipation: another indication for restorative proctocolectomy. *British Journal of Surgery*, **77**, 801–802.

67. Hoyle, C.H.V., Kamm, M.A., Burnstock, G. and Lennard-Jones, J.E. (1991) Effects of cisapride on the circular muscle of the human sigmoid colon in vitro. *British Journal of Surgery*, **78**: A757.

68. Hoyle C.H.V., Kamma, M.A., Lennard-Jones, J.E. and Burnstock, G. (1989) Reduced activity of enkephalins in the colon of patients with idiopathic constipation. *Gut*, **30**, A706.

69. Jones, P.N., Lubowski, D.Z., Henry, M.M. and

Swash, M. (1987) Is paradoxical contraction of puborectalis muscle of functional importance? *Diseases of the Colon and Rectum*, **30**, 667–670.

70. Kamijo, K., Hiatt, R.B. and Koelle, G.B. (1953) Congenital megacolon. A comparison of the spastic and hypertrophied segments with respect to cholinesterase activities and sensitivities to acetylcholine, DFP, and barium ion. *Gastroenterology*, **24**, 173–185.

71. Kamm, M.A., Bartram, C.I. and Lennard-Jones, J.E. (1989) Rectodynamics – quantifying rectal evacuation. *International Journal of Colorectal Disease*, **4**, 161–163.

72. Kamm, M.A., Farthing, M.J.G., Lennard-Jones, J.E., Perry, L.A. and Chard, T. (1991) Steroid hormone abnormalities in women with severe idiopathic constipation. *Gut*, **32**, 80–84.

73. Kamm, M.A., Hawley, P.R. and Lennard-Jones, J.E. (1988) Lateral puborectalis division in the management of severe constipation. *British Journal of Surgery*, **75**, 661–663.

74. Kamm, M.A., Hawley, P.R. and Lennard-Jones, J.E. (1988). Outcome of colectomy for severe idiopathic constipation. *Gut*, **29**, 969–973.

75. Kamm, M.A., Hoyle, C.H.V., Burleigh, D.E., Law, P.J., Swash, M., Martin, J.E., Nicholls, R.J. and Northover, J.M.A. (1991) Hereditary internal anal sphincter myopathy causing proctalgia fugax and constipation. *Gastroenterology*, **100**, 805–810.

76. Kamm, M.A., Lennard-Jones, J.E. and Nicholls, R.J. (1989) Evaluation of the intrinsic innervation of the internal anal sphincter using electrical stimulation. *Gut*, **30**, 935–938.

77. Kamm, M.A., McLean, A., Farthing, M.J.G. and Lennard-Jones, J.E. (1989) Ultrasonography demonstrates no abnormality of pelvic structures in women with severe idiopathic constipation. *Gut*, **30**, 1241–1243.

78. Kamm, M.A., van der Sijp, J.R.M., Hawley, P.R., Phillips, R.K.S. and Lennard-Jones, J.E. (1991) Left hemicolectomy with rectal excision for severe idiopathic constipation. *International Journal of Colorectal Disease*, **6**, 49–51.

79. Karaus, M. and Sarna, S.K. (1987) Giant migrating contractions during defecation in the dog colon. *Gastroenterology,* **92**, 925–933.

80. Karaus, M., Sarna, S.K., Ammon, H.V. and Wienbeck, M. (1987) Effects of oral laxatives on colonic motor complexes in dogs. *Gut*, **28**, 1112–1119.

81. Kaufman, P.N., Krevsky, B., Malmud, L.S., Maurer, A.H., Somers, M.B., Siegel, J.A. and Fisher, R.S. (1988) Role of opiate receptors in the regulation of colonic transit. *Gastroenterology*, **94**, 1351–1356.

82. Kendall, A.C. (1954) Fatal case of encephalitis after phenolphthalein ingestion. *British Medical Journal*, **2**, 1461–1462.

83. Kerrigan, D.D., Lucas, M.G., Sun, W.M., Donnelly, T.C. and Read, N.W. (1988) Manometric and electrophysiological investigation

of anorectal and urethrovesical function in constipated females. *Gastroenterology*, **94**, A223.

84. Klauser, A.G., Voderholzer, W.A., Heinrich, C.A., Schindlbeck, N.E. and Müller-Lissner, S.A. (1990) Behavioral modification of colonic function. Can constipation be learned? *Digestive Diseases and Sciences*, **35**, 1271–1275.

85. Koch, T.R., Carney, J.A., Go, L. and Go, V.L.W. (1988) Idiopathic chronic constipation is associated with decreased colonic vasoactive intestinal peptide. *Gastroenterology*, **94**, 300–310.

86. Koutsamanis, D., Jabbour, R. and Benaisson, F. (1990) Evaluation of biofeedback and autogenous training (AT) in the treatment of anismus (A). A preliminary report. The World Congress of Gastroenterology, Sydney, Australia, Aug 1990 pp. 687.

87. Krevsky, B., Maurer, A.H., Malmud, L.S. and Fisher, R.S. (1989) Cisapride accelerates colonic transit in constipated patients with colonic inertia. *Gastroenterology*, **84**, 882–887.

88. Krishnamurthy, S. and Schuffler, M.D. (1987) Pathology of neuromuscular disorders of the small intestine and colon. *Gastroenterology*, **93**, 610–639.

89. Krishnamurthy, S., Schuffler, M.D., Rohrmann, C.A. and Pope, C.E. II. (1985) Severe idiopathic constipation is associated with a distinctive abnormality of the colonic myenteric plexus. *Gastroenterology*, **88**, 26–34.

90. Kune, G.A., Kune, S., Field, B. and Watson, L.F. (1988) The role of chronic constipation, diarrhoea and laxative use in the etiology of large-bowel cancer. *Diseases of the Colon and Rectum*, **31**, 507–512.

91. Lane, R.H.S. and Todd, I.P. (1977) Idiopathic megacolon: a review of 42 cases. *British Journal of Surgery*, **64**, 305–310.

92. Leng-Peschlow, E. (1986) Acceleration of large intestine transit time in rats by sennosides and related compounds. *Journal of Pharmacy and Pharmacology*, **38**, 369–373.

93. Leng-Peschlow, E. (1986) Dual effect of orally administered sennosides on large intestine transit and fluid absorption in the rat. *Journal of Pharmacy and Pharmacology*, **38**, 606–610.

94. Lennard-Jones, J.E. (1985) Constipation: pathophysiology, clinical features and treatment. In *Coloproctology and the Pelvic Floor*. (Eds) Henry, M.M. and Swash, M. London: Butterworth.

95. Leon, S.H., Krishnamurthy, S. and Schuffler, M.D. (1987). Subtotal colectomy for severe idiopathic constipation. A follow-up study of 13 patients. *Digestive Diseases and Sciences*, 1249–1254.

96. Lincoln, J., Crowe, R., Kamm, M.A., Burnstock, G. and Lennard-Jones, J.E. (1990) Serotonin and 5-hydroxyindoleacetic acid are increased in the sigmoid colon in severe idiopathic constipation. *Gastroenterology*, **98**: 1219–1225.

97. Lundberg, J.M., Hokelt, T. and Nilsson, G. *et al.*

(1978) Peptide neurons in the vagus splanchnic and sciatic nerves. *Acta Physiologica Scandinavia*, **104**, 499–502.

98. McReady, R.A. and Beart, R.W. (1979) The surgical treatment of incapacitating constipation associated with idiopathic megacolon. *Mayo Clinic Proceedings*, **54**, 779–783.

99. Martelli, H., Devroede, G., Ahran, P. and Duguay, C. (1978) Mechanisms of idiopathic constipation: outlet obstruction. *Gastroenterology*, **75**, 623–631.

100. Martindale (1989) The extra pharmacopoeia. (Eds) Reynolds, J.E.F. and Parfitt, K. 29th Edition p1087. London: The Pharmaceutical Press.

101. Mathers, S.E., Kempster, P.A., Swash, M. and Lees, A.J. (1988) Constipation and paradoxical puborectalis contraction in anismus and Parkinson's disease: a dystonic phenomenon? *Journal of Neurology, Neurosurgery and Psychiatry*, **51**, 1503–1507.

102. Meshkinpour, H., Harmon, D., Thompson, R. and Yu, J. (1985) Effects of thoracic spinal transection on the colonic motor activity in rats. *Paraplegia*, **25**, 272–276.

103. Metcalf, A.M., Phillips, S.F., Zinsmeister, A.R., MacCarty, R.L., Beart, R.W. and Wolff, B.G. (1987) Simplified assessment of segmental colonic transit. *Gastroenterology*, **92**, 40–47.

104. Milner, P, Lincoln, J., Crowe, R., Kamm, M.A., Lennard-Jones, J.E. and Burnstock, G. (1987) Serotonin is increased and VIP decreased in the sigmoid colon in idiopathic constipation. *Gut*, **30**, A715.

105. Morson, B.C. (1971) Histopathology of carthartic colon (Abstr.) *Gut*, **12**, 867–868.

106. Narducci, F., Bassotti, G., Gaburri, M. and Morelli, A. (1987) Twenty four hour manometric recording of colonic motor activity in healthy man. *Gut*, **28**, 17–25.

107. Nicholls, R.J. and Kamm, M.A. (1988) Proctocolectomy with restorative ileoanal reservoir for severe idiopathic constipation. *Diseases of the Colon and Rectum*, **31**, 968–969.

108. Parc, R., Berrod, J.L., Tussiot, J. and Loygue, J. (1984) Le megacolon de l'adulte. A propos de 76 cas. *Ánnales De Gastroentorologie et d'Hepatologie*, **20**, 133–141.

109. Pearson, A.J.G., Grainger, J.M., Scheur, P.J. and McIntyre, N. (1971) Jaundice due to oxyphenisatin. *Lancet*, **i**, 994–996.

110. Penninckx, F. and Kerremans, R. (1975) Pharmacological characteristics of the ganglionic and aganglionic colon in Hirschsprung's disease. *Life Sciences*, **17**, 1387–1394.

111. Pinho, M., Yoshioka, K. and Keighley, M.R.B. (1989) Long term results of anorectal myectomy for chronic constipation. *British Journal of Surgery*, **76**, 1163–1164.

112. Polak, J.M., Bloom, S.R. and Sullivan, S.N. (1977) Enkephalin-like immunoreactivity in the human gastrointestinal tract. *Lancet*, **i**, 972–974.

113. Preston, D.M. and Lennard-Jones, J.E. (1985) Anismus in chronic constipation. *Digestive Diseases and Sciences*, **30**, 413–418.

114. Preston, D.M. and Lennard-Jones, J.E. (1985) Pelvic motility and response to intraluminal bisacodyl in slow transit constipation. *Digestive Diseases and Sciences*, **30**, 289–294.

115. Preston, D.M. and Lennard-Jones, J.E. (1986) Severe chronic constipation of young women: 'idiopathic slow transit constipation'. *Gut*, **27**, 41–48.

116. Preton, D.M., Adrian, T.E., Christofies, N.D., Lennard-Jones, J.E. and Bloom, S.R. (1985) Positive correlation between symptoms and circulating motilin, pancreatic polypeptide and gastrin concentrations in functional bowel disorders. *Gut*, **26**, 1059–1064.

117. Preston, D.M., Butler, M.G., Smith, B. and Lennard-Jones, J.E. (1983) Neuropathology of slow transit constipation. *Gut*, **24**, A997.

118. Preston, D.M., Hawley, P.R., Lennard-Jones, J.E. and Todd, I.P. (1984) Results of colectomy for severe idiopathic constipation in women (Arbuthnot Lane's disease). *British Journal of Surgery*, **71**, 547–552.

119. Preston, D.M., Lennard-Jones, J.E. and Thomas, B.M. (1985) Towards a radiologic definition of idiopathic megacolon. *Gastrointestinal Radiology*, **10**, 167–169.

120. Preston, D.M. Pfeffer, J. and Lennard-Jones, J.E. (1984) Psychiatric assessment of patients with severe constipation. *Gut*, **25**, A582–583.

121. Read, N.W. (1983) Drug induced constipation. *Mims Magazine*, 19–21.

122. Read, N.W., Abouzekry, L., Read, M.G., Howell, P., Ottewell D. and Donnelly T.C. (1985) Anorectal function in elderly patients with faecal impaction. *Gastroenterology*, **89**, 959–966.

123. Read, N.W., Al-Janabi, M.N., Holgate, A.M., Barber, D.C. and Edwards, C.A. (1986) Simultaneous measurement of gastric emptying, small bowel residence and colonic filling of a solid meal by the use of the gamma camera. *Gut*, **27**, 300–308.

124. Read, N.W., Miles, C.A., Fisher, D., Holgate, A.M., Kime, N.D., Mitchell, M.A., Reeve, A.M., Roche, T.B. and Walker, M. (1980) Transit of a meal through the stomach, small intestine, and colon in normal subjects and its role in the pathogenesis of diarrhea. *Gastroenterology*, **79**, 1276–1282.

125. Read, N.W., Timms, J.M., Barfield, L.J., Donnelly, T.C. and Bannister, J.J. (1986) Impairment of defaecation in young women with severe constipation. *Gastroenterology*, **90**, 53–60.

126. Reynolds, J.C., Ouyang, A., Lee, C.A., Baker, L., Sunshine, A.G. and Cohen, S. (1987) Chronic severe constipation. Prospective motility studies in 25 consecutive patients. *Gastroenterology*, **92**, 414–420.

127. Reynolds, T.B., Peters, R.L. and Yamada, S.

(1971) Chronic active and lupoid hepatitis caused by a laxative, oxyphenisatin. *New England Journal of Medicine*, **285**, 813–820.

128. Riemann, J.F., Schmidt, H. and Zimmermann, W. (1980) The fine structure of colonic submucosal nerves in patients with chronic laxative abuse. *Scandinavian Journal of Gastroenterology*, **15**, 761–768.

129. Ritchie, J. (1972) Mass peristalsis in the human colon after contact with oxyphenisatin. *Gut*, **13**, 212–219.

130. Rudolph, R.L. and Mengs, U. (1988) Electron microscopical studies on rat intestine after long-term treatment with sennosides. *Pharmacology*, **36**, (Suppl 1) 188–193.

131. Ryan, J.P. and Bhojwani, A. (1985) Effect of ovariectomy and sex steroid hormone pretreatment on colonic transit in the rat. *Gastroenterology*, **88**, 1564.

132. Schouten W.R., Kluck, P., ten Kate F.J.W. and van Blankenstein, M. (1988) Visceral neuropathy in slow transit constipation. An immunohistochemical investigation with monoclonal antibodies. *Gastroenterology*, **94**, A411.

133. Schrodt, G.R. (1963) Melanosis coli: a study with the electron microscope. *Diseases of the Colon and Rectum*, **6**, 277.

134. Schultzberg, M., Dreyfus, C. and Gershon, M.D. *et al.* (1978) VIP, enkephalin substance-P and somatostatin-like immunoreactivity in neurons intrinsic to the intestine: immunohistochemical evidence from organotypic tissue cultures. *Brain Research*, **155**, 239–248.

135. Schuurkes, J. (1990) Effect of *cisapride* on gastric motility. *Zeitschrift Fur Gastroentrologie*, **28(1)**, 27–30 discussion 44.

136. Schuurkes, J. (1991) Pharmacotherapy of gastrointestinal transit. In *Gastrointestinal Transit. Pathophysiology and Pharmacology* (Eds) Kamm, M.A. and Lennard-Jones, J.E. pp. 171–178. Wrightson Biomedical Publishing.

137. Shorvon, P.J., McHugh, S., Diamant, N.E., Somers, S. and Stevenson, G.W. (1989) Defecography in normal volunteers: results and implications. *Gut*, **30**, 1737–1749.

138. Shouler, P. and Keighley, M.R.B. (1986) Changes in colorectal function in severe idiopathic constipation. *Gastroenterology*, **90**, 414–420.

139. Sijp van der J.R.M., Kamm, M.A., Nightingale, J.M.D., Walker, E., Granowska, M., Britton, K., Akkermans, L.M.A. and Lennard-Jones, J.E. (1991) Evidence for disturbed gastric and panenteric transit in patients with severe idiopathic constipation. *Gastroenterology*, **100**, A503.

140. Sjölund, K., Ekman, R., Akre, F. and Lindner, P. (1986) Motilin in chronic idiopathic constipation. *Scandinavian Journal of Gastroenterology*, **21**, 914–918.

141. Slavin, J.A. (1970) Current causes of fixed drug eruptions. *British Journal of Dermatology*, **83**, 546–549.

142. Smith, A.N., Varma, J.S., Binnie, N.R. and Papachrysostomou, M. (1990) Disordered colorectal motility in intractable constipation following hysterectomy. *British Journal of Surgery*, **77**, 1361–1366.

143. Smith, B. (1973) Pathologic changes in the colon produced by anthraquinone purgatives. *Diseases of the Colon and Rectum*, **16**, 455.

144. Smith, B. (1974) Neuropathology of the esophagus in diabetes mellitus. *Journal of Neurology, Neurosurgery and Psychiatry*, **37**, 1151–1154.

145. Smith, B. (1986) Effect of purgatives on the myenteric plexus of man and the mouse. *Gut*, **9**, 139–143.

146. Speakman, C.T.M., Madden, M.V., Nicholls, R.J. and Kamm, M.A. (1991) Lateral ligament division during rectopexy causes constipation but prevents recurrence. *British Journal of Surgery*, **78**, 1431–1433.

147. Stabile, G., Kamm, M.A., Hawley, P.R. and Lennard-Jones, J.E. (1991) Results of the Duhamel operation in the treatment of idiopathic megarectum and megacolon. *British Journal of Surgery*, **78**, 661–663.

148. Stabile, G., Kamm, M.A., Hawley, P.R. and Lennard-Jones, J.E. (1991) Colectomy for idiopathic megarectum and megacolon. *Gut*.

149. Stabile, G., Kamm, M.A., Hawley, P.R., Phillips, R.K.S. and Lennard-Jones, J.E. (1991) Alternative surgery for idiopathic megarectum and megacolon. *Gut*.

150. Staiano, A., Cucchiara S., Andreotti, M.R., Minella, R. and Manzi, G. (1991) Effect of cisapride on chronic idiopathic constipation in children. *Digestive Diseases and Sciences*, **36**, 733–736.

151. Staumont, G., Fioramonti, J., Frexinos, J. and Buéno, L. (1988) Changes in colonic motility induced by sennosides in dogs: evidence of prostaglandin mediation. *Gut*, **29**, 1180–1187.

152. Thompson, W.G. and Heaton, K.W. (1980) Functional bowel disorders in apparently healthy people. *Gastroenterology*, **79**, 283–288.

153. Tucker, D.M., Sanstead, H.H., Logan, G.M., Klevay, L.M., Kahalko, J., Johnson, L.K., Inman, L. and Inglett, G.E. (1981) Dietary fibre and personality factors as determinants of stool output. *Gastroenterology*, **81**, 879–883.

154. Turnbull, G.K., Bartram, C.I. and Lennard-Jones, J.E. (1988) Radiological studies of rectal evacuation in adults with idiopathic constipation. *Diseases of the Colon and Rectum*, **31**, 190–197.

155. Turnbull, G.K., Lennard-Jones, J.E. and Bartram, C.I. (1986) Failure of rectal expulsion as a cause of constipation: why fibre and laxatives sometimes fail. *Lancet*, **i**, 767–769.

156. Turnbull, G.K., Ritvo, P.G. and Woolnough, J.

(1991) Biofeedback treatment for constipation: is "sham" biofeedback as effective? *Gastroenterology*, **100**, A503.

157. Vantrappen, G., Janssens, J., Coremans, G. and Jian, R. (1986) Gastrointestinal motility disorders. *Digestive Diseases and Sciences*, **31** (Suppl 9), 5S–25S.

158. Van der Sijp, J.R., Kamm, M.A., Evans, R. and Lennard-Jones, J.E. (1990) Does a stoma benefit patients with severe idiopathic constipation. *Gut*, **31**, A1173.

159. Van der Sijp, J.R.M., Kamm, M.A., Nightingale, J.M.D., Walker, E., Granowska, M., Morris, G.P., Lennard-Jones, J.E. and Akkermans, L.M.A. (1991) Regional colonic transit: radioisotope resin demonstrates invalidity of plastic radioopaque markers in patients with severe idiopathic constipation. *Gastroenterology*, **100**, A503.

160. Varma, J.S. and Smith, A.N. (1988) Neurophysiology dysfunction in young women with intractable constipation. *Gut*, **29**, 963–968.

161. Wald, A., Hinds, J.P. and Caruana, B.J. (1989) Psychological and physiological characteristics of patients with severe idiopathic constipation. *Gastroenterology*, **97**, 932–937.

162. Waldron, D., Bowes, K.L., Kingma, Y.J. and Cote, K.R. (1988) Colonic and anorectal motility in young women with severe idiopathic constipation. *Gastroenterology*, **95**, 1388–1394.

163. Wallace, W.C. and Madden, W.M. (1969) Experience with partial resection of the puborectalis muscle. *Diseases of the Colon and Rectum*, **12**, 196–200.

164. Waller, S.L. (1975) Comparative effects of codeine and senna on the motor activity of the left colon. *Gut*, **16**, 407–408.

165. Wasserman, I.F. (1964) Puborectalis syndrome (rectal stenosis due to anorectal spasm). *Diseases of the Colon and Rectum*, **7**, 87–98.

166. Watier, A., Devroede, G., Duranceau, A., Abdel-Rahman, M., Duguay, C., Forand, M.D., Terteault, L., Ahran, P., Lamarche, J. and Elhilali, M. (1983) Constipation with colonic inertia. A manifestation of systemic disease? *Digestive Diseases and Sciences*, **28**, 1025–1033.

167. Weber, J., Denis, P., Mihout, B., Muller, J.M., Blanquart, F., Galmiche, J.P., Simon, P. and Pasquis, P. (1985) Effect of brain-stem lesion on colonic and anorectal motility. Study of three patients. *Digestive Diseases and Sciences*, **30**, 419–425.

168. Yagi, T., Migrawaki, Y., Nishikawa, T., Yamauchi, K. and Kuwano, S. (1988) Involvement of prostaglandin E-like material in the purgative action of rhein anthrone, the intraluminal active metabolite of sennosides A and B in mice. *Journal of Pharmacy and Pharmacology*, **40**, 27–30.

169. Yoshioka, K. and Keighley, M.R.B. (1987) Anorectal myectomy for outlet obstruction. *British Journal of Surgery*, **74**, 373–376.

170. Yoshioka, K. and Keighley, M.R.B. (1989) Clinical results of colectomy for severe idiopathic constipation. *British Journal of Surgery*, **76**, 600–604.

DIVERTICULAR DISEASE

M. Killingback

INCIDENCE

Diverticular disease may have been first described by Voigtel in 1804.[53] It was also described by Cruveilhier in 1849,[11] who appreciated the risk of infective sequelae of the disease. There probably has been a true increase in the incidence of the disease over the past 100 years, which may have been related to the wider adoption of a western diet. Diverticular disease is common in the UK, North America, northern Europe, Australia and New Zealand, but is uncommon throughout black Africa, the Middle East, India, the Far East and the Pacific islands. It was formerly uncommon in Japan, but Sato *et al.*[48] recently reported an increase in the Japanese community, and related this to the consumption of a more Westernized diet. Stemmerman[55] emphasizes that the incidence of diverticular disease in the Japanese community in Hawaii now approaches that of the white population of North America. In the USA, the Negro population has now developed an incidence of diverticular disease similar to that of the white population. Segal, Solomon and Hunt[45] have also indicated an increasing incidence of diverticular disease in the urban black South African community. These reports therefore support the concept that the disease is not racially determined, but related to changes in the environment and to dietary factors.

Postmortem studies within the Western community have reported an incidence of diverticular disease from 36% (Parks)[33] to 45% (Hughes).[18] A radiological study by Petrie, Needham and

Gillenders[38] reported an incidence of 59.1% from 2650 barium enema examinations performed in the north-east of Scotland from 1967 to 1970. Kyle and Davidson[24] reported on the numbers of patients admitted to hospital for diverticular disease in the north-east of Scotland in two 4-year periods, 10 years apart (1958–1961 and 1968–1971). Despite a slight increase in the population, the admissions to hospital rose from 12.8 per 100 000 to 23.5 per 100 000. The actual numbers increased from 206 to 366, which was an increase of 77%. Chalmers et al.[9] examined the incidence of diverticular disease in Scottish hospital inpatient statistics from 1968 to 1977. There was a progressive increase in the total number of cases seen throughout the entire decade under consideration. The increase was greater for females. Admissions were classified as emergencies in 33% and the highest operation rates occurred at the younger end of the age range.

Diverticular disease is rare before 30 years of age. Painter and Burkitt[30] found that the incidence in patients over 60 was 33%. In a clinical study, Parks[36] found that the maximum incidence of diverticular disease was in the sixth, seventh and eighth decades. In a postmortem study, Parks[33] found that the incidence of diverticular disease was 50% in patients between 80 and 90 years of age. This study also indicated that the ratio of females to males affected was 3:2. Similarly, Kyle and Davidson[24] found that in the two periods of their study, the incidence in females was greater, 64% (1958–1961) and 62% (1968–1971) than in males.

AETIOLOGY

DIETARY FACTORS

The geographical distribution of diverticular disease reported by Painter and Burkitt[30] link it to a Western diet, in particular, a lack of residue and cereal. They suggest it is related to the milling of flour which has effectively removed much of the fibre content from bread. Coincidentally, there has been an increasing ingestion of over-refined, low-residue diets. Eastwood et al.[12] challenged the significance of bran, as the high fibre content in the diet of developing countries is derived mainly from fruit and vegetables, and not wheat products. Whilst there may be other factors in the Western diet that may affect the intraluminal pressures of the colon, there is considerable support for the concept that a low-residue diet is important in the aetiology of diverticular diseases. Carlson and Hoelzel[8] produced diverticular disease in rats fed on a low-

residue diet, and Hodgson[17] observed similar changes in rabbits fed on a low-residue diet. Gear et al.[16] studied the incidence of symptomless diverticular disease in the vegetarian and non-vegetarian population. Vegetarians consumed an average of 41.5 g of fibre per day, and had an incidence of symptomless diverticular disease of 12%. Non-vegetarians consumed an average of 21.4 g of fibre per day with a 33% incidence of symptomless diverticular disease. This difference was even more apparent among older, female patients. Cereal is probably the most important fibre, as it is not influenced by colonic bacteria, and appears to increase stool weight and decrease transit time.

Much slower intestinal transit times have been demonstrated in the Western communities compared with rural Africans taking their normal diet (Burkitt, Walker and Painter[7]). Sixth-form British schoolboys were found to have an average transit time of 76.2 hours, compared with that of African Ugandan villagers, who had a transit time of 35.7 hours. Ingestion of unprocessed bran decreased the intestinal transit time of normal subjects with diverticular disease (Findlay et al.)[14] McCance and Widdowson[26] demonstrated that the transit time was 24 hours longer in patients eating white bread compared with brown. They also demonstrated that the transit time was inversely proportional to the weight of the stool, and directly related to the fibre content of the diet.

INTRALUMINAL PRESSURE

Painter and Truelove[31] did not show any difference in the basal pressure, or the type of pressure waves between normal subjects and those with diverticular disease. By contrast, Arfwidsson[2] has demonstrated higher resting pressures and an increased frequency of high-pressure waves in patients with diverticulosis. Food increased the intraluminal pressure, and the incidence of high-pressure waves in both normal subjects and those with diverticular disease. Painter and Truelove[31] recorded greater increases in intraluminal pressure with the injection of morphine and prostigmine, an observation later confirmed by Parks and Connell.[36] Parks[35] also recorded that abnormal resting and stimulated pressures still existed in those patients who had undergone resection of diverticular disease 6 months before, indicating some intrinsic abnormality of the colon after resection of diverticular disease. This finding supports the concept of a functional muscle abnormality which precedes the development of diverticulosis. However, because patients undergoing resection for diverticular disease rarely develop further diverticula, in spite of a continuing muscle abnormality, the vulnerability of the sigmoid colon in this disease is also apparent. Eastwood et al[13] have drawn a distinction between studies on inpatient and outpatient subjects, and failed to demonstrate high pressures in patients with diverticular disease who were attending outpatient departments. Smith, Shepherd and Eastwood,[49] studying pressure changes after balloon distension of the colon wall in diverticular disease, demonstrated an altered compliance of the colon. They found that this reduced compliance did not change after successful bran treatment and, although it was altered initially by resection, it later reverted to its former response. They concluded that there was a degenerative component in diverticular disease, in which the intrinsic mechanical properties of the intestine wall are altered. This being so, dietary fibre is unlikely to correct this abnormality.

SEGMENTATION

Faecal material is propagated through the colon by mass peristalsis. Movement and water absorption is facilitated by the process of segmentation, which is non-expulsive. Faeces can pass through the colon without any change in intraluminal pressure (Painter et al.)[32] Segmentation can also occur without any change in intraluminal pressure. However, using combined pressure measurements and cineradiography, Painter[28] related episodes of high pressures in diverticular disease to the excessive effects of segmentation. It is interesting to postulate whether this excessive segmentation may be the mechanism of pain in patients with chronic non-inflammatory diverticular disease. Pressure within these segments rises with contraction of the circular muscle, both in and between the closed segments. These contraction rings are frequently seen by endoscopists during colonoscopy. Radiologists find that it can be impossible to introduce barium in a retrograde fashion for a radiographical study of patients with diverticular disease without the parenteral administration of a smooth muscle relaxant such as hyoscine (Buscopan). Painter[28] suggests that the pressure within these closed segments is sufficiently high to induce mucosal herniation and hence an area of diverticulosis. Painter and Burkitt[30] suggest that a lack of dietary fibre produces a stool transit time which is slower than normal, allowing more water absorption with the production of smaller, firmer stools. It is postulated that this facilitates excessive segmentation which, being associated with higher pressures, will induce the formation of diverticulosis.

SITE OF COLON AFFECTED

No evidence has been produced to explain why diverticular disease is usually confined to the sigmoid colon, although it has been suggested that because the diameter of the colon is smallest at this site, intraluminal pressures would be higher. The tensile strength in the large bowel, in descending order is: rectum; ascending colon; descending colon; and transverse colon[6] and this factor may be related to the more common occurrence of diverticular disease in the sigmoid colon. In a postmortem study, Hughes[18] showed that the sigmoid colon was involved in 95% of cases of diverticular disease. In 16% the disease involved the whole colon. Parks,[34] in a study of 461 patients given barium enemas, reported a 96% incidence of diverticular disease in the sigmoid colon and involving the whole colon in 7%. Diverticular disease in the rectum is rare.

VASCULAR SUPPLY

The circumferential distribution of diverticula is constant and is related to the sites of vascular entry, having been precisely defined by Slack[45] and Watt and Marcus.[54] They demonstrated two rows of diverticula between the mesenteric and antimesenteric taenia. Hughes,[18] while agreeing that these diverticula occur at the entry points of the vessels, also found areas of muscle atrophy and early diverticula formation not related to vascular anatomy. The small arteries are closely associated with the fundus of the diverticulum, with the smaller vessels cascading over it before entry through the muscle layer. Diverticula vary in size from 1 mm to 10 cm when they are then classified as giant diverticula. Many, but not all, diverticula contain faecoliths. These diverticula emerge within the appendices epiploicae and therefore may not be seen easily at operation. Diverticula which are close to the mesenteric taenia may be completely obscured within the fat of the mesentery, particularly in obese patients. Such diverticula consist only of mucosa and serosa if they project into the peritoneal cavity, although the necks of the diverticula may have attenuated muscle fibres association with them. Watt and Marcus[54] have drawn attention to the smaller and less common diverticula which can occur in the intertaenial part of the circular muscle on the antimesenteric border which may be intramural and usually contain more muscle in their wall.

SMOOTH MUSCLE ABNORMALITY

The smooth muscle thickening in diverticular disease is of great interest, and it is likely to be related to the pathogenesis of the disease, but a final explanation of this abnormality has not been provided. Morson[27] first drew attention to the fact that diverticular disease accompanied by a muscle abnormality could produce symptoms sufficient to warrant surgical treatment. Of 173 resected specimens for 'diverticulitis' at St Mark's Hospital, 112 specimens (64.7%) were found to have focal or extensive inflammatory changes, whereas 56 (32.4%) had no inflammatory changes on histological examination, but marked abnormal muscle thickening.

Williams[56] studied the pathological changes of diverticular disease in relation to its radiological appearance following a barium enema and demonstrated that areas of muscle thickening occupied two-thirds of the circumference of the lumen, fading out in the wall of the bowel near its antimesenteric border. Marked smooth-muscle thickening was present in 74% of patients with diverticular disease, but it was also found in 8% of those patients without diverticula (Hughes).[18] Such thickening, usually greater than 1.8 mm, corresponded to the area of maximum diverticulosis. Diverticula were present both proximal and distal to this abnormality, however. It is also usual in specimens resected for the severe inflammatory complications of diverticular disease to find the maximum thickening of the muscle layer of the bowel at the point of maximum inflammation. Longitudinal taenia in diverticular disease are also shortened and thickened. The changes in the distribution of muscle fibres in diverticular disease probably represents shortening by contraction of the taenia, so there is a 'concertina' effect on the circular muscle.

Arfwidsson[2] found evidence of true circular muscle hypertrophy. It is still not known for certain whether diverticulosis occurs before or after this muscle hypertrophy. A few postmortem specimens contain these muscular changes without diverticula, but most specimens with diverticula also exhibit these muscle changes. Painter and Burkitt[30] believe that these muscle changes occur first and precede the development of diverticulosis.

Whiteway and Morson[55] have thrown further light on the muscle abnormality in diverticular disease with electron microscope morphometry. In their view the thickening of the circular muscle and taenia is neither hyperplasia nor hypertrophy. Increase in elastin fibres (elastosis) is demonstrable within the longitudinal taenia but not within the circular muscle. It is thought that this elastosis may be responsible for shortening of the colon, which in turn produces the "concertina" thickening of the circular muscle.

NATURAL HISTORY

There are a number of clinical patterns affecting patients with diverticular disease. Most patients are symptomless; others suffer chronic pain, and have a chronic inflammatory focus which produces continuous symptoms. Recurrent inflammatory episodes of a mild nature may also be a feature in some patients. Interestingly, the patients who appear to suffer the most florid disease such as acute diverticulitis with abscess or perforation, or severe inflammatory changes of a more chronic nature, have no preceding history. This lack of antecedent history argues against elective and prophylactic surgical treatment.

Boles and Jordan[4] followed up 294 patients with diverticular disease for periods of 10–30 years. They found that 40% of the patients suffered one episode of acute diverticulitis, 6% of patients had multiple episodes, and 5.5% of patients came to surgical treatment. Parks and Connell[37] surveyed 455 patients who were admitted to hospital with a diagnosis of acute diverticulitis. Of these, 30% came to surgical treatment during that admission. Of the 70% of patients who were discharged from hospital without an operation, 26.5% remained well, 19.5% continued with symptoms, 19% died of other causes, and only 4.5% had an operation for diverticular disease.

ACUTE DIVERTICULITIS

PATHOGENESIS

Acute and later chronic inflammation may occur in a diverticulum without any breach of the mucosa. It is likely that this is the case in patients with mild, recurring attacks of diverticulitis. In almost all cases where the clinical features are severe, there will be some evidence of a perforation in the wall of the diverticulum. It is not certain whether this perforation is a mechanical rupture of a diverticulum, or an erosion of the diverticulum wall by an abscess within it. Hughes[18] has referred to the absence of faecoliths in areas of diverticulitis that are most severe. Ryan[42] supports this view and emphasizes that faecoliths are not usually found in resected specimens of acute diverticulitis treated as an emergency. Ryan's study indicated that inflammatory changes were more extrinsic rather than affecting the mucosa of the diverticulum. It also seems possible that a faecolith might obstruct the neck of a diverticulum, analogous to appendicitis, and cause a diverticula abscess, but this explanation is also hypothetical. Nevertheless, a faecolith within a diverticulum might mechanically erode the thin fundus wall and cause perforation, initiating inflammatory changes in the mesentery or in the peritoneal cavity.

ACUTE MILD DIVERTICULITIS

This entity is usually managed by the patient's family practitioner, and many patients, particularly the elderly, are treated for mild recurring attacks without admission to hospital. It is therefore difficult to assess the incidence of this clinical group. The patients usually experience pain in the left lower quadrant of the abdomen, feel unwell, possibly with a fever. Tenderness is noted in the left iliac fossa and there may be tenderness in the pelvis on digital examination of the rectum. Restriction of diet and treatment with metronidazole and a cephalosporin for 5 days will usually settle the episode. Some of these patients develop an abdominal or pelvic mass with constitutional symptoms, indicating the need for hospital care.

SURGICAL PATHOLOGY AT OPERATION

At operation for acute diverticulitis, the pathology encountered is one of three types.[20] Surprisingly, an abscess or a perforation in this situation can be overlooked.

The sigmoid colon may be the site of an *acutely inflamed phlegmon,* including the colon and mesentery, without an obvious abscess or free perforation. There may be a concealed abscess within a diverticulum, or in the mesentery, but the appearances are those of a non-perforated phlegmon. The peritoneal exudate may be serious or purulent, but not usually faecal.

There may be a *pericolic abscess* with purulent exudate leaking from it into the peritoneal cavity. This abscess is often in the pelvis related to the sigmoid loop which lies above it, concealing the abscess from view. These abscesses will usually have a connection to the diverticulum where the perforative inflammatory process has originated.

If the perforative process is rapid, and possibly if it occurs in a diverticulum less protected by the retroperitoneal position or juxtamesenteric site, then a free, non-localised *purulent or faecal perforation* can occur. It is in this situation that faecal peritonitis is most likely to occur. The perforation may be small or large, and this may be the determining factor in the extent of the peritoneal contamination and infection.

ACUTE DIVERTICULITIS AND PERITONITIS

Between 1967 and 1970, the Royal Australasian College of Surgeons conducted a prospective survey accruing 246 patients with acute diverticulitis and peritonitis undergoing emergency surgery.[20] The age range was 32–87 years (average 59.9 years).

There were 127 males and 119 females. In 64% this was the initial manifestation with no previous history. Faecal peritonitis was found in 13.1%. The mid-sigmoid colon was most frequently involved in 37.4%, proximal sigmoid in 27.5%, distal sigmoid in 19.8%, descending colon in 5.4% and the rectosigmoid area in 5.0%.

Undoubtedly most of these patients had at least a microperforation in a diverticulum but a macroscopic perforation was only identified in 95. A paracolic or pelvic abscess without identification of a perforation in the wall of the bowel occurred in 76, and 77 had an acute phlegmon without perforation communication with the peritoneal cavity. Disease mortality was 22 (8.8%), 13 patients succumbing to infection in either the acute phase of the disease or during the hospital admission.

CLINICAL FEATURES

Patients may present in a dramatic manner, with sudden onset of severe abdominal pain and clinical signs of peritonitis. If there is faecal contamination of the peritoneal cavity, septic shock rapidly develops and, after resuscitation, early laparotomy is mandatory. By contrast, some patients may be clearly unwell with fever, tachycardia and abdominal tenderness, and the indications for laparotomy may not be so obvious. There may be a tender mass in the left iliac fossa or in the pelvis on rectal examination. Assessment is made more difficult in the obese patient.

RADIOGRAPHIC INVESTIGATIONS

Abdominal radiographs show free gas in the peritoneum in 32% of patients (RACS Survey)[20] hence there are many patients with a free perforation in whom no gas can be demonstrated.

A limited Gastrograffin enema may be helpful in identifying localized extravasation, or even a free perforation into the peritoneal cavity, clarifying the indications for surgical treatment. A barium enema in this situation is not advisable, as the barium may extravasate into the peritoneal cavity, aggravating the inflammatory process and complicating management. Kourtesis, Williams and Wilson[22] report the use of a water-soluble contrast enema in 48 patients with acute diverticulitis. In 30 patients, spasm and diverticulosis were present, and this was an indication for conservative treatment. In two patients the findings were normal. In 16 there was evidence of a leak of definite diverticulitis. In the presence of pericolic extravasation, surgical treatment was indicated. There were no complications from this investigative procedure.

Computed tomography has been gaining acceptance in recent years in the diagnosis and management of acute diverticulitis, particularly in the presence of an abscess. Saini et al.[43] were able to institute percutaneous catheter drainage in 8 of 11 patients with acute diverticulitis, 7 of whom went on to one-stage resection. Stabile et al.[50] managed 19 patients with a diverticulitis by percutaneous drainage guided by computed tomography. In all patients, sepsis was controlled and in most the drainage ceased within 3 weeks. There was a communication with the colon, demonstrated on sinogram, in 47%. Fourteen (74%) were treated by single-stage resection and anastomosis with a satisfactory outcome. Labs et al.[25] found that computed tomography correctly diagnosed abscesses in all of 10 patients examined, whereas air-contrast enema diagnosed only two abscesses in eight patients suffering this complication. However, Balthazar et al.[3] pointed out some of the shortcomings of computed tomography diagnosis in acute diverticulitis, where small collections and intramural abscesses were not detected. Contrast enema used in this study was useful in excluding carcinoma and confirming acute diverticulitis.

ENDOSCOPY

Flexible endoscopy of the rectum and sigmoid colon may be indicated in a patient in whom laparotomy is not necessarily indicated. Endoscopy is the only reliable means of differentiating diverticulitis from carcinoma, but it may be a difficult examination in the acutely ill patient without sedation or anaesthesia, and would only be indicated if it was regarded as a helpful investigation to assist in the decision for laparotomy. It would also be useful during laparotomy to know, for instance, if there was a carcinoma at the 'centre' of a large inflammatory mass in the colon. In a patient with a free perforation into the peritoneal cavity, the insufflation of air under positive pressure would obviously be undesirable.

TREATMENT

Medical

In the Parks and Connell[37] series, 70% of patients admitted to hospital with a diagnosis of acute diverticulitis were managed without operation. Restriction of oral intake, intravenous therapy and appropriate antibiotics for aerobic and anaerobic bacteria for some days will usually settle the inflammatory process. Indications for emergency oper-

ation are clinical signs for peritonitis, evidence of septic shock, free gas on a plane radiograph of the abdomen, and an intraperitoneal leak demonstrated on air-contrast enema.

SURGERY

As with much emergency abdominal surgery, there are options that exist for the various pathological circumstances found at laparotomy. Surgical management should vary according to the type of pathology, the extent of the peritoneal infection, the general condition of the patient, and the experience of the operating theatre team.

No resection

If at operation there is no obviously perforated colon or related pericolic abscess, then resection of the colon is not obligatory unless other factors apply,[20] nor is there a need for a defunctioning stoma. Krukowski, Koruth and Matheson[23] agree with this viewpoint.

Resection without anastomosis (Hartmann procedure)

In the presence of an acute abscess or a free perforation, must surgeons would now advocate immediate resection to remove the focus of infection from the abdomen (*Figure 4.36*). The most established

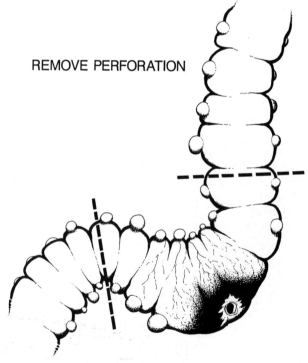

REMOVE PERFORATION

Figure 4.36 Limited resection is indicated for acute diverticulitis with perforation.

current practice is not to perform an anastomosis in these patients, who are often elderly and have coexistent medical problems.

Resection and primary anastomosis

In recent years, however, there has been an increasing interest in immediate anastomosis after resection in these patients. Alanis *et al.*,[1] in dividing the severity of patient disease into four stages, advocate resection and anastomosis in stages 1–3 and a resection without anastomosis in stage 4. Krukowski *et al.*[23] also advocate resection with anastomosis in carefully selected patients when treated by experienced surgeons. This policy certainly overcomes the problems of the morbidity of a second operation to restore intestinal continuity. It remains to be proven whether resection with anastomosis is a safe policy to apply widely to the emergency treatment of acute diverticular disease as experienced surgeons are not always available for these emergencies. Ravo *et al.*[41] have introduced the intracolonic bypass tube which protects the anastomosis, reporting success in 28 patients treated for acute diverticulitis as emergencies, with no anastomotic leaks and no mortality. Wider experience with this technique will be awaited with interest.

CHRONIC UNCOMPLICATED DIVERTICULAR DISEASE

DEFINITION

Non-inflammatory diverticular disease undoubtedly can induce symptoms as indicated by Morson.[27] These patients have a variable disturbance of bowel habit, the most prominent sympton being abdominal pain situated in the left lower quadrant of the abdomen. The cause of this pain is not fully understood, and it may be spasm from excessive segmentation in the sigmoid colon, or an element of obstruction also related to the spasm, or to the thickened muscle abnormality. Although fewer of these patients now come to elective resection, in some the symptoms can be so persistent and disabling in the presence of demonstrable diverticulosis, that the patients are prepared to undergo operation to obtain relief.

Other patients with diverticular disease do have foci of inflammation within one (usually) or more diverticula, and there may be a small abscess within the sigmoid mesentery (with or without a microperforation.) But more usually in this form of the disease, there is a non-purulent chronic phlegmon referred to by Pheils, Duraiappah and Newland[39] as chronic phlegmonous diverticulitis. This can produce swelling in the pericolic and mesenteric tissues, and it is surprising on dissecting the mesentery of such a resected specimen, to find no abscess but a proliferation of fat and fibrous tissue. Histologically there is chronic inflammatory cell infiltration without pus formation (*Figure 4.37*).

CLINICAL FEATURES

It is frequently clinically difficult to separate these two pathological entities, which constitute chronic uncomplicated diverticular disease as radiological and endoscopic findings may be identical. Tenderness or a palpable sigmoid colon in the left lower quadrant or on digital examination of the rectum may be present in non-inflammatory chronic diverticular disease. In the younger patient with diarrhoea it is well recognized that the symptoms of irritable bowel syndrome are indistinguishable from those of

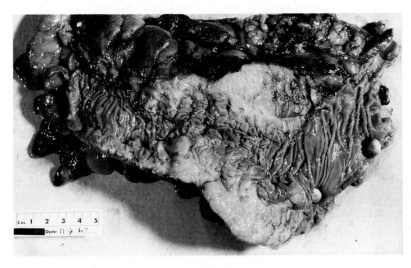

Figure 4.37 Chronic phlegmonous diverticulitis without an obvious abscess in the mesentery, which is infiltrated with chronic inflammatory reaction and adipose tissue.

mild diverticular disease. Patients with a fever during their attacks, persistent tenderness, and a palpable mass either in the abdomen or in the pelvis, are obviously more likely to have inflammatory changes supervening on the chronic disease.

TREATMENT

Antispasmodics may be anticholinergic, affecting the autonomic nervous system, or musculotropic, acting directly on the smooth muscle wall. Both, however, appear to have little effect in diverticular disease and probably have no real place in treatment. Although there is no evidence that increasing the fibre intake reverses the process in a patient with established diverticular disease, there seems no question that symptoms can be relieved in many patients. Increasing faecal bulk by ingestion of a high roughage diet containing cereal, bran, fruit and vegetables or with added pharmaceutical fibre, as occurs in gums and mucillage, may benefit the patient by increasing the water content of the stool, thereby producing a larger volume, and softer consistency.[40] Fibre appears to accelerate the transit time in all parts of the colon (Kirwan and Smith)[21] and bran has also been shown to reduce the pressure in the sigmoid colon and the rectum, this effect being more marked with the ingestion of coarse bran.[40] Beneficial effects in diverticular disease are also obtained with sterculia and methylcellulose.

Hyland and Taylor[19] found that 91% of patients were symptom-free after the ingestion of bran and Painter[31] similarly reported that 70% of patients lost their symptoms. Smith, Shepherd and Eastwood,[48] studying the motility effects of operations for diverticular disease, found that bran ingestion after surgery maintained lower intraluminal pressures compared with controls.

SURGICAL

There may be a place for elective surgical treatment in patients with chronic uncomplicated diverticular disease, but the decision to operate must be taken carefully. Operation should be avoided if there are features of the irritable bowel syndrome and probably only indicated in patients with persistent, long- term symptoms whose general health is otherwise satisfactory.

The author has performed 170 elective resections, and, in spite of a bias to avoid surgery in noninflammatory uncomplicated diverticular disease, no inflammation was found in 26 of 170 resected specimens (15.3%) (*Table 4.5*).

In patients complaining only of chronic pain in the left iliac fossa, and in the absence of objective

Table 4.5 Pathology findings in 170 resected specimens in diverticular disease

	No. of patients	*Percentage*
Non-inflammatory	26	15.3
Localized diverticulitis	55	32.4
Extracolic (complicated) diverticulitis	89	52.3
Total	170	

criteria (radiological and endoscopic), results of resection are variable. Charnock *et al.*[10] examined 71 patients undergoing resection for diverticular disease in a 7-year period, 22 of whom were regarded as having uncomplicated diverticular disease. In 38% of these patients the pain was unchanged after operation, and the authors therefore advise strict criteria in this group of patients to avoid disappointing results of surgical resection. There are patients whose recurring episodes of left iliac fossa pain with tenderness and some fever, with or without pelvic tenderness, can be accepted on clinical grounds as evidence of diverticulitis, even in the absence of endoscopic and radiological confirmation (*Figure 4.38*). If these attacks are mild, of brief duration, and respond quickly to antibiotics, then the patient's conservative management may continue almost indefinitely. There is no evidence that these patients will necessarily develop complications in the future. Conservative management particularly applies to elderly patients. If, however, the episode is severe, possibly needing hospital care, then the patient must subsequently be monitored carefully to see that the inflammatory process resolves adequately without the formation of a permanent inflammatory mass or colonic stricture, when surgical treatment would be indicated.

How many attacks of significant diverticulitis should a patient sustain before being advised to undergo elective surgery? This is a difficult question to answer, and the decision must be finely tuned to the circumstances of any given patient. Veidenheimer[56] emphasizes that almost 50% of patients who recover from their first attack of acute diverticulitis will have a recurrence of their acute disease, and that the risk of complications increases with each ensuing attack. Further, those patients requiring operation for complications have a higher risk of more serious postoperative complications and mortality.

The author believes that if a patient makes a complete recovery from a first attack of acute diverticulitis, then elective surgical treatment is not

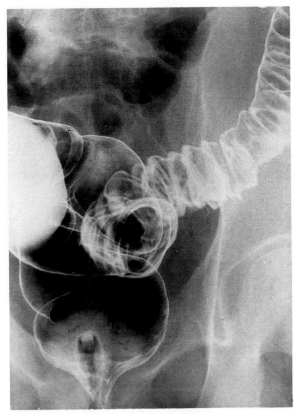

Figure 4.38 This patient's radiograph shows minimal radiological evidence of diverticular disease. Prolonged symptoms were treated by resection revealing a significant focus of diverticulitis. (From *Colorectal Surgery*, 1983, p. 299, Edinburgh: Churchill Livingstone, with permission. Sir Edward Hughes, Alan Cuthbertson, Mark Killingback).

usually necessary. If a second severe attack occurs, however, then surgical treatment should be recommended in most patients who are fit enough for major abdominal surgery.

CHRONIC COMPLICATED DIVERTICULAR DISEASE

PATHOLOGY

Chronic abscess

Uncomplicated diverticulitis is contained within a diverticulum (or diverticula) or the mesentery, and therefore is confined to the anatomical structures of the colon. When the inflammatory process extends beyond these structures and becomes 'extracolic', then it is classified as complicated disease (*Figure 4.39*). The inflammatory process may adhere to adjacent viscera such as bladder, uterus, ovaries or

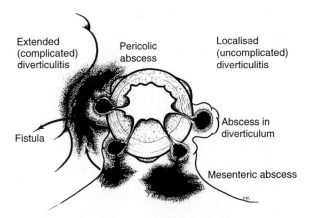

Figure 4.39 Classification of chronic complicated diverticular disease.

small bowel, or be complicated by a fistula to the bladder or the small bowel. The sigmoid colon becomes densely adherent to these structures and to the upper third of the rectum, making surgical treatment more complex. The colon is frequently kinked by this process and associated with pericolic fibrosis, so that chronic large bowel obstruction may occur. A chronic pericolic or pelvic abscess may develop as a result of a slow perforation of a diverticulum or diverticular abscess. This scenario may complicate surgical treatment, because of dense fibrosis at the left pelvic brim obscuring the ureter, and in the pouch of Douglas, producing rigidity that can resemble a 'frozen pelvis'.

Enteroenteric, enterouterine, enterovaginal and enterovesical fistula

The chronic abscess may erode an adjacent viscus to form a fistula and, when it does, the abscess may drain effectively into this 'recipient' organ diminishing the size of the intervening abscess so that the track may be short and direct between the colon and the involved viscus. Most fistulas from the sigmoid into the bladder are small and require very little surgical attention during resection of the disease. Woods *et al.*[57] have reviewed the internal fistulas in diverticular disease at the Cleveland Clinic Foundation. The distribution of these fistulas were colovesical (65%), colovaginal (25%), coloenteric (7%) and colouterine (3%). Eight of the 84 patients had two fistulas each. Although unusual, spontaneous fistulas from diverticular disease may involve the anterior abdominal wall, ureter, hip joint, thigh and perianal region. Pollard *et al.*,[40] in a collected series of 66 colovesical fistulas, recorded that diverticular disease was the cause in 47 patients (71%). In reviewing the methods of diagnosis they report successful demonstration of a fistula by

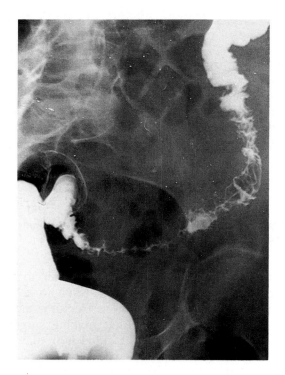
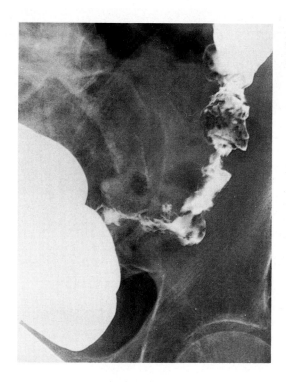
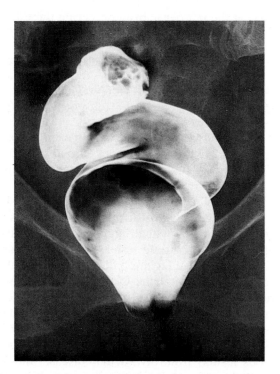
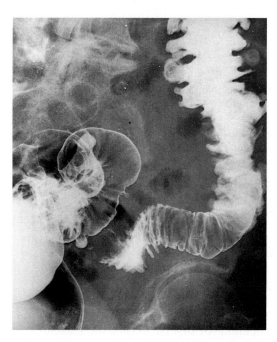

Figure 4.40 These radiographs show four varieties of stricture caused by diverticular disease which are consistent with carcinoma. Endoscopy was unhelpful in each case. (From *Colorectal Surgery*, 1983, p. 300, Edinburgh: Churchill Livingstone, with permission. Sir Edward Hughes, Alan Cuthbertson, Mark Killingback.)

barium enema in 57%, cystoscopy in 35%, cystogram in two of five patients, and a fluid level in the bladder on plane radiograph of the abdomen in 29%. Pneumaturia was present in 85% of the patients.

Mucosal pseudopolyps

In areas of muscle thickening and pericolic fibrosis, with shortening of the colon, the mucosal lining is thrown up into redundant folds with small, red, polypoid projections on the mucosa. Biopsy shows a hyperaemic, congested mucosa. These pseudopolyps are probably a phenomenon of traction as the redundant mucosa is dragged distally with the stool through the narrow segment. At times they can be mistaken for adenomatous polyps. They indicate a significant degree of chronic obstruction. This finding may assist surgeons in their assessment of patients' symptoms, when considering surgical treatment.

Giant diverticulum

A large, solitary diverticulum may occur in the sigmoid colon in association with sigmoid diverticulosis. These diverticula are generally 7–15 cm in size, and Foster and Ross[15] report such a diverticulum measuring 29 cm in diameter. Although the mucosa may be identified in the wall of the diverticulum, it is often destroyed by a chronic inflammatory reaction. The diverticulum may be mobile or densely adherent to surrounding structures. It is unusual for a stricture to be associated in the adjacent colon.

These diverticula may be clinically silent, but may perforate, obstruct or cause a torsion of the sigmoid colon.

Plane radiographs may demonstrate a large gas shadow in the abdomen, with or without a fluid level. Barium does not always enter the diverticulum, and associated diverticulosis is common. Because of the risks of complications a giant diverticulum is an indication for surgical treatment.

CAN CANCER BE EXCLUDED?

The symptoms caused by complicated diverticulitis are often not as typical as one would expect. The onset of bowel symptoms may be insidious, and the initial symptoms of colovesical fistula, for example, may be a sudden pneumaturia not preceded by a clinically recognizable episode of lower abdominal or pelvic inflammation. If this presentation is associated with a palpable mass and stricture of the colon, exclusion of cancer may be very difficult. Furthermore, the association of an inflammatory reaction around a carcinoma is well known and may lead to diagnostic difficulties.

Flexible sigmoidoscopy or colonoscopy may exclude the presence of a carcinoma if the instrument can be passed through the sigmoid colon into the descending colon. However, if there is an abscess, pericolic fibrosis, stricture or kinking of the colon, then the instrument may not pass beyond the narrow segment of bowel, and the examination will remain inconclusive. Oedema of the mucosa, narrowing of, and pus in the lumen, without obvious neoplastic tissue usually favours a diagnosis of diverticulitis.

In some patients, good quality, double-contrast radiographs following barium enemas may help to distinguish diverticulitis from carcinoma, but in many patients it is radiologically impossible to exclude carcinoma (*Figure 4.40*). In others, a stricture that maintains identifiable mucosal continuity will be suggestive of diverticular disease and may assist the surgeon in deciding upon a more limited resection (*Figure 4.41*) than would be practical for malignant stricture.

There is considerable enthusiasm for computed tomography examination of intra-abdominal masses but, at the present time, this investigation has not established itself as superior to high-quality, double-contrast barium enema in distinguishing an inflammatory mass from a malignant one. Although computed tomography is superior in the diagnosis of a pericolic abscess, it does not give as much information about the mucosal surface of the colon as a barium enema examination. Often the surgeon can distinguish between diverticulitis and cancer at operation but, if not, the colon pathology will need to be resected as if it were malignant.

INDICATIONS FOR OPERATION

In the management of chronic complicated diverticular disease, indications for operation are a persistent mass, persistent stricture, chronic large bowel obstruction, colonic fistula, giant diverticulum and the possibility of carcinoma. Once an extracolonic infection becomes established, the pericolic fibrosis is progressive, and intractable and obstructive symptoms will eventually supervene. A chronic pericolic abscess (*Figure 4.42*) cannot be permanently sterilized by antibiotic therapy and will continue to stimulate proliferative fibrous tissue reaction in the surrounding area. If neglected, this may progress even to a retroperitoneal fibrosis with ureteric obstruction (Siminovitch and Fazio).[46] Colovesical fistula is an indication for surgical treatment in almost all patients. Occasionally this complication can be managed conservatively in a frail patient if

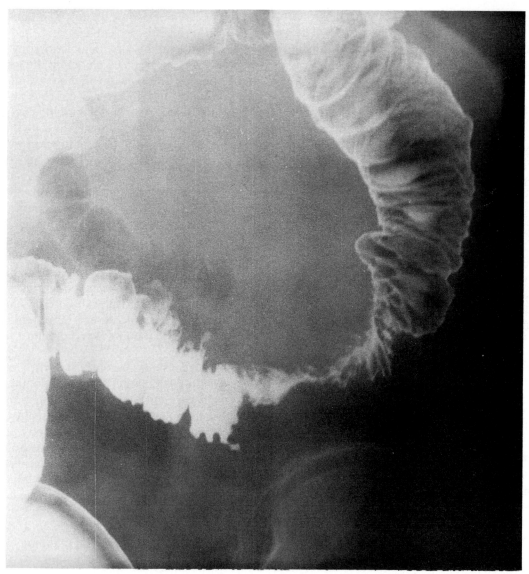

Figure 4.41 This stricture shows the continuity of mucosal pattern which is consistent with diverticular disease, helping to exclude carcinoma.

lower tract symptoms can be controlled by anti-biotics, and there is no bladder neck obstruction which would promote ascending urinary tract infection. Similarly, colovaginal fistula may also be managed without an operation, if not accompanied by obstructive bowel symptoms, an active pelvic abscess, or profuse vaginal faecal discharge, particularly if the patient is a poor operative risk. Usually, however, if there is any faecal discharge from the vagina this is poorly tolerated by the patient and most will want to be considered for surgical treatment. Fistulas affecting the bladder or vagina in diverticular disease contrast with those seen in Crohn's disease where surgery is often not obligatory. The difference is probably due to the pathology of the fistula track, which is usually larger and direct in diverticular disease, whereas in the ileove-

sical or ileovaginal fistulas found in Crohn's disease, the track may be of very small calibre, tortuous and not so direct, so that faecal debris does not so readily contaminate the bladder or vagina.

ELECTIVE SURGICAL TREATMENT

Table 4.6 summarizes the author's experience from 1962 to 1990 of 170 patients undergoing initial elective resection of sigmoid and left colon for diverticular disease. It is now less usual for patients to undergo three-stage operations with a preliminary stoma to manage peritonitis or abscess without resection. A preliminary stoma may still be appropriate in patients presenting with large bowel obstruction rather than immediate resection, with or

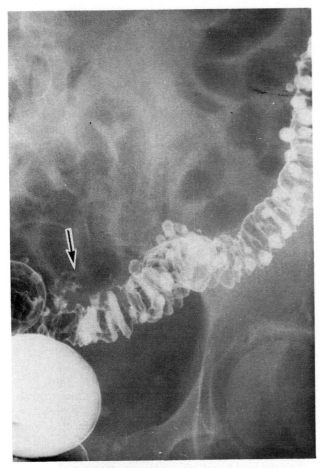

Figure 4.42 A localized, chronic abscess is indicated by a focus of extravasated barium. (From *Colorectal Surgery*, 1983, p. 299, Edinburgh: Churchill Livingstone, with permission.)

without anastomosis. Two-stage operations, that is, a protecting stoma at the time of resection, still has an important role in selected patients, but is used less commonly today. In the author's series, it was used in 12 of 43 patients (28%) between 1962 and 1978 whereas in the period 1979–1990 it was used in only 10 of 107 patients (9%).

The two-stage Hartmann (or modified Hartmann) operation, where resection is performed without anastomosis, was performed only once in this series. Although it has been advocated for elective surgery in complicated diverticulitis with abscess formation, the patient is then required to undergo a major and, at times, quite difficult reconstruction operation at a later date. By contrast, closure of a proximal stoma which has protected an anastomosis is a much simpler procedure for both patient and surgeon.

With improved surgical techniques and bowel preparation, one-stage resection is now the operation of choice in elective surgery of diverticular disease. This policy is particularly indicated in entero-vaginal or enterovesical fistula or for stricture. The

Table 4.6 Elective resections for sigmoid and left colon diverticular disease 1962–1990

Type of operation	No. of patients
3-stage	18
2-stage	22
2-stage (Hartmann)	1
1-stage	128
1-stage (no anastomosis)	1
Total	170

Ages 38–85 years (average 61.4).

amount of resected colon will vary with each patient, but must include the entire sigmoid colon with the rectosigmoid junction taking all distal diverticula and a variable amount of the descending colon. The amount of descending colon will depend on the extent of the thickened muscle segment and density of the diverticula.

MORBIDITY AND MORTALITY OF SURGICAL TREATMENT

In the author's series of 170 resections, 95 (56%) of the patients were 60 years of age or older, and 45 (26%) were 70 years or older, many of whom had coexisting cardiovascular disease. *Table 4.7* shows that 33 patients suffered significant morbidity from cardiopulmonary and/or abdominal complication. Two patients died in the postoperative period, a mortality rate of 1.2%.

The incidence of specific complications (some patients with more than one complication) is shown in *Table 4.8*. The mortality for the surgical treatment of benign disease should be low but, unfortunately, complex pathology needing complicated surgery occurs principally in elderly patients with coexisting diseases. It is in this group, Veidenheimer[52] reported a mortality rate of 9% for resection of complicated diverticulitis.

Table 4.7 Postoperative complications: elective surgery for diverticular disease

Complication	No. of patients	Percentage
Cardiopulmonary only	12	7
Cardiopulmonary and abdominal	4	2.4
Abdominal only	17	10
Total	33	

Table 4.8 Specific complications after elective surgery for diverticular disease in 33 patients*

Complication	No. of patients	Percentage
Pelvic sepsis	9	5.3
Pulmonary infection	8	4.7
Atelactasis	8	4.7
Cardiac complication	6	3.5
Significant prolonged ileus	6	3.5
Intrapelvic bleeding	5	2.9
Major anastomotic leak	4	2.4
Intestinal obstruction	4	2.4
Septicaemia	4	2.4
GI bleeding	2	1.2
Pulmonary embolism	2	1.2
Deep vein thrombosis	2	1.2

*Some patients had more than one complication.

ACUTE COLONIC OBSTRUCTION

Retrograde obstruction to a barium enema in diverticular disease is quite common. When it occurs, distinction between diverticulitis and cancer can be difficult. Chronic obstruction with a stricture or acute angulation caused by pericolic fibrosis, may cause acute large bowel obstruction and may require an emergency operation. In these circumstances, endoscopy and radiology usually fails to identify the diagnosis, although these investigations are appropriate and may be diagnostic. As the obstruction is due to marked deformity of the bowel lumen, associated with muscle thickening and pericolic fibrosis, possibly with a chronic abscess, this will not resolve with conservative measures, and laparotomy is indicated. The pathology in diverticular disease is associated with dense fibrosis, unlike carcinoma, where the obstruction is usually mobile and nonadherent to the left pelvic brim. Diverticulitis causing acute large bowel obstruction is usually complex, and therefore best treated by proximal stoma and later by an interval resection. If the surgeon is unable to exclude carcinoma on the basis of preoperative investigation and the operative findings, then it would be preferable to manage the obstruction as if it were carcinoma.

PROFUSE LARGE BOWEL BLEEDING

Until 1977, when Boley, Samartano and Adams[5] indicated the importance of acquired, degenerative vascular ectasia as a cause of colonic haemorrhage, most profuse bleeding from the colon was regarded as arising in diverticula, with other causes such as polyps, carcinoma and colitis less frequently. It is now accepted that most profuse bleeding is from vascular ectasia. Occasionally bleeding may occur from a small vessel near the 'summit' of the diverticulum which was probably eroded by a faecolith. The defect in this artery has been demonstrated in resected specimens. Most patients will stop bleeding spontaneously, but a few patients (estimated at 5%) will continue with bleeding that can be life threatening. The patients are often elderly and at poor risk, and management may have to be modified because of coexisting medical problems, the rate of blood loss and the facilities available.

REFERENCES

1. Alanis, A., Papanicolaou, C.K., Tadros, R.R., Fielding, L.P. (1989) Primary resection and anastomosis for treatment of acute diverticulitis. *Diseases of the Colon and Rectum*, **32**, 933–939.
2. Arfwidsson, S. (1964) Pathogenesis of multiple diverticula of the colon in diverticular disease. *Acta Chirurgica Scandinavica Supplement*, **342**, 1–68.
3. Balthazar, E.J., Megibow, A., Schinella, R.A. and Gordon, R. (1990) Limitations in the CT diagnosis of acute diverticulitis: comparison of CT, contrast enema and pathologic findings in 16 patients. *American Journal of Roentgenology*, **154**, 281–285.
4. Boles, R.S. and Jordan, S.M. (1958) *Gastroenterology*, **35**, 579–581.
5. Boley, S.J., Samartano, R. and Adams, A. (1977) On the nature and aetiology of vascular ectasia of the colon. Degenerative lesions of aging. *Gastroenterology*, **72**, 650–660.
6. Bouchier, I.A.D., Allan, R.N., Hodgson, H.J.F. and Keighley, M.R.B. (1984) *Textbook of Gastroenterology*, p. 814. London: Baillière Tindall.
7. Burkitt, D.P., Walker, A.R. and Painter, N.S. (1972) The effect of dietary fibre on stools and transit-times and its role in the causation of disease. *The Lancet*, **ii**, 1408–1412.
8. Carlson, A.J. and Hoelzel, F. (1949) Relation of diet to diverticulosis of the colon in rats. *Gastroenterology*, **12**, 108–115.
9. Chalmers, K., Wilson, J.M.G., Smith, A.N. and Eastwood, M.A. (1983) Diverticular disease of the colon in Scottish hospitals over a decade. *Health Bulletin*, **41**(1), 147–153.
10. Charnock, F.M., Rennie, J.R., Wellwood, J.M. and Todd, I.P. (1977) Results of colectomy for diverticular disease of the colon. *British Journal of Surgery*, **64**, 417–419.
11. Cruveilhier, J. (1849) *Traite d'Anatomie Pathologique*, 1: 593. Paris: J. B. Baillière.
12. Eastwood, M.A., Fisher, N., Greenwood, C.T. and Hutchinson, J.B. (1974) Perspectives on the bran hypothesis. *The Lancet*, **i**, 1029–1033.

13. Eastwood, M.A., Smith, A.N., Brydon, W.G. and Pritchard, J. (1978) Colonic function in patients with diverticular disease. *The Lancet*, **i**, 1181–1182.

14. Findlay, J.M., Smith, A.N., Mitchell, W.D., Anderson, A.J.B. and Eastwood, M.A. (1974) Effects of unprocessed bran on colon function in normal subjects and in diverticular disease. *The Lancet*, **i**, 146–149.

15. Foster, D.R. and Ross, B. (1977) Giant diverticulum: clinical and radiological features. *Gut*, **18**, 1051–1053.

16. Gear, J.S.S., Fursdon, P., Nolan, D.J., Ware, A., Mann, J.I. and Brodribb, A.J.M. (1979) Symptomless diverticular disease and intake of dietary fibre. *The Lancet*, **i**, 511–514.

17. Hodgson, W.J.B. (1972) An interim report on the production of colonic diverticula in the rabbit. *Gut*, **13**, 802–804.

18. Hughes, L.E. (1969) Post-mortem survey of diverticular disease of the colon. *Gut*, **10**, 336–351.

19. Hyland, J.M.P. and Taylor, I. (1979) Diverticular disease of the colon. *Gut*, **20**, 441–442.

20. Killingback, M.J. (1983) Management of perforative diverticulitis. *Surgical Clinics of North America* (Ed.) V.W. Fazio. **63**, 97–115.

21. Kirwan, W.O. and Smith, A.N. (1974) Gastrointestinal transit estimated by an isotope capsule. *American Journal of Clinical Nutrition*, **30**, 659–661.

22. Kourtesis, G.J., Williams, R.A. and Wilson, S.E. (1988) Acute diverticulitis: safety and value of contrast studies in predicting need for operation. *Australian and New Zealand Journal of Surgery*, **58**, 801–804.

23. Krukowski, Z.H., Koruth, N.M. and Matheson, N.A. (1985) Evolving practice in acute diverticulitis. *British Journal of Surgery*, **72**, 684–686.

24. Kyle, J. and Davidson, A.I. (1975) The changing pattern of hospital admission for diverticular disease of the colon. *British Journal of Surgery*, **62**, 537–541.

25. Labs, J.D., Sarr, M.G., Fishman, E.K., Siegelman, S.S. and Cameron, J.L. (1988) Complications of acute diverticulitis of the colon: improved early diagnosis with computerised tomography. *American Journal of Surgery*, **155**, 331–336.

26. McCance, R.A. and Widdowson, E.M. (1956) *Breads White and Brown and Their Place in Thought and Social History*. London: Pitman.

27. Morson, B.C. (1963) The muscle abnormality in diverticular disease of the colon. *Proceedings of Royal Society of Medicine*, **56**, 798–803.

28. Painter, N.S. (1964) The aetiology of diverticulosis of the colon with special reference to the action of certain drugs on the behaviour of the colon. *Annals of the Royal College of Surgeons of England*, **34**, 98–119.

29. Painter, N.S. (1975) *Diverticular Disease of the Colon*. London: William Heinemann.

30. Painter, N.S. and Burkitt, D.P. (1975) Diverticular disease of the colon: a 20th century problem. *Clinics in Gastroenterology*, **3**, 4–21.

31. Painter, N.S. and Truelove, S.C. (1964) The intraluminal pressure patterns in diverticulosis of the colon. *Gut*, **5**, 201–213.

32. Painter, N.S., Truelove, S.C., Andram, G.M. and Tuckey, M. (1965) Segmentation and the localisation of intraluminal pressures in the human colon with special reference to the pathogenesis of the colonic diverticula. *Gastroenterology*, **49**, 169–177.

33. Parks, T.G. (1968) Post-mortem studies on the colon with special reference to diverticular disease. *Proceedings of the Royal Society of Medicine*, **61**, 932–934.

34. Parks, T.G. (1969) Natural history of diverticular disease of the colon: a review of 521 cases. *British Medical Journal*, **4**, 639–642.

35. Parks, T.G. (1970) Rectal and colonic studies after resection of the sigmoid for diverticular disease. *Gut*, **11**, 121–125.

36. Parks, T.G. and Connell, A.M. (1968) Motility studies after resection of the sigmoid colon for diverticular disease. *British Journal of Surgery*, **55**, 867.

37. Parks, T.G. and Connell, A.M. (1970) The outcome in 455 patients admitted for treatment of diverticular disease of the colon. *British Journal of Surgery*, **57**, 775–778.

38. Petrie, J.C., Needham, C.D. and Gillanders, L.A. (1972) Survey of alimentary radiology findings in the North East of Scotland region 1967–1970. *British Medical Journal*, **2**, 78–80.

39. Pheils, M.T., Duraiappah, B. and Newland, R.C. (1973) Chronic phlegmonous diverticulitis. *Australian and New Zealand Journal of Surgery*, **42**, 337–341.

40. Pollard, S.G., MacFarlane, R., Greatorex, R., Everett, W.G. and Hartfall, W.G. (1987) Colovesical fistula. *Annals of the Royal College of Surgeons of England*, **69**, 163–165.

41. Ravo, B., Mishrick, A., Addei, K. *et al.* (1987) The treatment of perforated diverticulitis by one-stage intracolonic bypass procedure. *Surgery*, **102**, 771–776.

42. Ryan, P. (1965) Solitary sigmoid diverticulitis. *British Journal of Surgery*, **52**, 85–89.

43. Saini, S., Mueller, P.R., Wittenberg, J., Butch, R.J., Rodkey, G.V. and Welch, C.E. (1986) Percutaneous drainage of diverticular abscess. An adjunct to surgical therapy. *Archives of Surgery*, **121**, 475–478.

44. Sato, T., Matsuzakis, S., Fujiwara, Y., Takahashi, J. and Suguro, T. (1970) Case of multiple colonic diverticulosis. *Nuika*, **25**, 563–566.

45. Segal, I., Solomon, A. and Hunt, J.A. (1977) Emergence of diverticular disease in the urban South African black. *Gastroenterology*, **72**, 215–219.

46. Siminovitch, J.M.P. and Fazio, V.W. (1980) Obstructive uropathy secondary to sigmoid

diverticulitis. *Diseases of the Colon and Rectum*, **23**, 504–507.

47. Slack, W.W. (1962) The anatomy pathology and some clinical features of diverticulitis of the colon. *British Journal of Surgery*, **50**, 185–190.

48. Smith, A.N., Shepherd, J. and Eastwood, M.A. (1974) Motility effects of operations performed for diverticular disease. *Proceedings of the Royal Society of Medicine*, **67**, 1041–1043.

49. Smith, A.N., Shepherd, J. and Eastwood, M.A. (1981) Pressure changes after balloon distension of the colon wall in diverticular disease. *Gut*, **22**, 841–844.

50. Stabile, B.E., Puccio, E., van Sonnenberg, E. and Neff, C.C. (1990) Preoperative percutaneous drainage of diverticular abscesses. *American Journal of Surgery*, **159**, 99–104.

51. Stemmermann, G.M. (1970) Patterns of disease among Japanese living in Hawaii. *Archives of Environmental Health*, **20**, 266–273.

52. Veidenheimer, M.C. (1983) Clinical presentation

and surgical treatment of complicated diverticular disease. *Inflammatory Bowel Disease* (Eds) Allan, R.N., Keighley, M.R.B., Alexander-Williams, J., Hawkins, Clifford. pp. 519–528. Edinburgh: Churchill Livingstone.

53. Voigtel, F.G. (1804) *Handboch der Pathologischen. Anatomie,* volume 2. Halle.

54. Watt, J. and Marcus, R. (1964) The pre-diverticular state, its relationship to diverticula in the anti-mesenteric intertaenia area of the pelvic colon. *British Journal of Surgery*, **51**, 676–682.

55. Whiteway, J. and Morson, B.C. (1985). Elastosis in diverticular disease of the sigmoid colon. *Gut*, **26**, 258–266.

56. Williams, I. (1963) Changing emphasis in diverticular disease of the colon. *British Journal of Radiology*, **36**, 393–406.

57. Woods, R.J., Lavery, I.C., Fazio, V.W., Jagelman, D.G. and Weakley, F.L. (1988) Internal fistulas in diverticular disease. *Diseases of the Colon and Rectum*, **31**, 591–596.

TUMOURS

BENIGN TUMOURS: POLYPS AND POLYPOSIS   *(C.B. Williams and A.B. Price)*

The world polyp is derived from the Latin *polypus* (literally 'manyfooted') and is used in colloquial Greek and Italian to mean an octopus, which a stalked polyp resembles. A 'polyp' is the vernacular description of any elevation above the mucosal surface of the intestine and lacks precision unless qualified by its histological variety, for example, metaplastic or adenomatous. It may be used to

describe any lesion from a small tag of normal epithelium to a protuberant cancer. A polyp is nevertheless often the clinician's diagnosis and its histological nature is decided thereafter by the pathologist, except in the case of those few polyps with characteristic shapes such as worm-like post-inflammatory polyps and carpet-like villous adenomas. Polyps range in appearance from tiny, translucent and almost invisible 1–2 mm mucosal bumps, through stalked lesions with a diameter of 3–5 cm (*Figure 4.43*), to sessile growths which may reach 10–20 cm in extent. Polyps may be single, occur

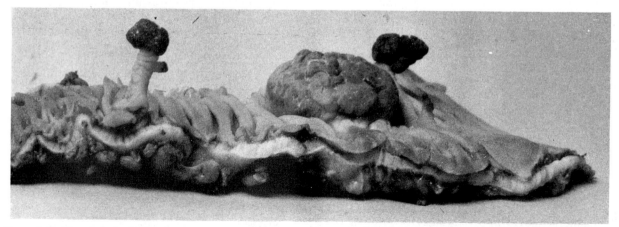

Figure 4.43 Two stalked adenomas and a larger sessile adenoma in the sigmoid colon. A focus of carcinoma was present in the large polyp.

together in small numbers or carpet the colon in hundreds or even thousands, as seen in some of the polyposis syndromes.

Many larger polyps, regardless of histological type, are stalked, particularly in the distal colon, where buffeting by formed stool and the activity of colonic musculature combines to exert traction. By contrast, polyps such as lipomas or villous adenomas growing in the caecum or the fluid-filled ascending colon are seldom stalked. The stalk of a polyp is composed of normal epithelium overlying a core of connective tissue containing arteries and veins drawn up from the vascular plexus in the submucosa; this makes snare polypectomy of the head easy and without risk of damage to the bowel wall.

THE HISTOPATHOLOGY AND CLINICAL FEATURES OF POLYPS

Although tumours can arise from any of the histological constituents of the intestine, less than 1% derive from connective or lymphoid tissue and more than 95% from the epithelium, presumably because of its rapid cell turnover. The majority of developmental polyps (hamartomas) are found in childhood or young adult life when neoplastic polyps (adenomas) are almost unknown. Careful necropsy studies show that almost half of the colons of elderly people contain one or more adenomas.[66] A classification of polyps and polyposis is given in *Table 4.9*. It is worth emphasizing that much of the older literature on polyps is confused by failure to differentiate between histological types, particularly between the common non-neoplastic metaplastic (hyperplastic) polyps and the adenomatous or neoplastic varieties. Occasionally, careful histological assessment can demonstrate that small foci of neoplastic (adenomatous) tissue do occur in non-neoplastic polyps and, in a few patients, there may be a chance coincidence of different polyp types.

NON-NEOPLASTIC POLYPS

Most non-neoplastic polyps are found coincidentally in the process of screening or diagnostic examinations for neoplastic or cancerous tumours. The exceptions are hamartomatous polyposis syndromes, post-inflammatory polyps and bleeding polyps in childhood. Non-neoplastic polyps are frequently covered by normal mucosa and thus often look paler and more shiny than the larger neoplastic polyps, which have a reddened, matt epithelium. Visual differentiation is uncertain, however, and representative polyps must always be submitted for a histopathological diagnosis.

Polypoid mucosa may also be the end result of mechanical stress producing prolapse (*Table 4.9*).[16] This is believed to be the explanation for inflammatory cloacogenic polyps,[34] the polyps seen on the redundant mucosa in diverticular disease and for the

Table 4.9 Classification of colorectal polyps

	Solitary	*Multiple (polyposis syndromes)*

Neoplastic	Adenoma
	  Tubular
	  Tubulovillous
	  Villous
	Carcinoid
		Familial adenomatous polyposis
		
		Malignant lymphoid polyposis

Non-neoplastic hamartomas	Peutz-Jeghers Juvenile	Peutz-Jeghers syndrome Juvenile polyposis
Inflammatory	Lymphoid Inflammatory	Benign lymphoid polyposis

Mechanical stress	Mucosal prolapse syndrome
	  Inflammatory 'cap' polyps
	  Solitary ulcer syndrome
	  Large intestinal prolapse
	  Inflammatory cloacogenic polyp
		'Cap' polyposis

Miscellaneous	Metaplastic (hyperplastic) Connective tissue polyps, e.g. fibroma, leiomyoma and lipoma	Metaplastic polyposis Cronkhite-Canada syndrome

rare occurrence of 'cap' polyps and 'cap' polyposis.[72] Similarly the solitary ulcer syndrome can present, not as an ulcer, but a localized mucosal polypoid lesion.

Individual hyperplastic polyps are not thought to have any cancer potential although both 'mixed' polyps[61] combining hyperplastic and adenomatous tissues and rare intermediate forms[35] have been described. In the rectum 50% or more of small polyps up to 5 mm diameter are found to be hyperplastic.

METAPLASTIC (HYPERPLASTIC) POLYPS

The commonest polyp in the rectum is the 2–5 mm, pale or glistening, metaplastic polyp which is almost a normal finding on sigmoidoscopy in the elderly, during which a score or more of these tiny polyps may be noticed in the distal 15 cm of the bowel (*Figure 4.44*). The incidence of metaplastic polyps increases with age, which partly explains the suggestion in some accounts that they are associated with cancer. In the colon, however, only 20–25% of small polyps prove to be metaplastic and most of even 2–5 mm polyps turn out to be adenomas[65,46] Larger

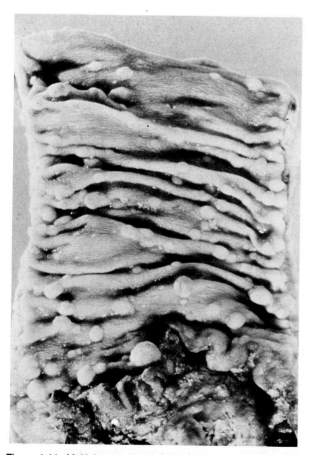

Figure 4.44 Multiple metaplastic polyps clustered close to a rectal carcinoma.

metaplastic polyps are occasionally found in the colon, either semipedunculated or as a sessile mound of shiny tissue. Multiple metaplastic polyposis[71] is rare and can be indistinguishable to the naked eye from adenomatous polyposis. Histologically the differentiation is easy and important, as the former requires only conventional polypectomy and follow-up as it has only moderate malignant potential (probably due to coexisting adenomas), whereas the latter requires surgical treatment because it carries 100% cancer risk by middle age.

Microscopically the mucosal crypts within a metaplastic polyp are elongated with reduced numbers of goblet cells and characteristic saw-toothing of the lining epithelial cells producing a shallow papillary outline (*Figure 4.45*). There is no nuclear dysplasia and no malignant potential. The description metaplastic, implying altered growth, has been encouraged instead of the commonly used term 'hyperplastic' which wrongly suggests abnormal nuclear activity and cellular regeneration.[71] Unlike the disorderly maturation and dedifferentiation in an adenomatous polyp, maturation is maintained but its regulation is disturbed. Immature forms are thus found deep within the crypts and 'hyper-mature' cells at the surface. The immature epithelium can be more darkly staining and should not be mistaken for dysplasia. Such confusion might account for the intermediate forms mentioned above. Metaplastic polyps are commonly seen clustered around carcinomas, especially in the rectum. They share certain mucins with adenomas[28] suggesting they may be induced by common factors in susceptible individuals.

INFLAMMATORY POLYPS AND LYMPHOID POLYPS

Post-inflammatory polyps may be found as scattered worm-like or thread-like (filiform) tags of essentially normal mucosa and imply a previous severe attack of any form of colitis (ulcerative, Crohn's, amoebic, schistosomal or ischaemic) (*Figures 4.46* and *4.47a*). They are usually not inflamed, although some may show superficial ulceration of the tip with a characteristic covering of white slough at endoscopy. Larger inflammatory polyps occur which are composed mainly of granulation tissue (*Figure 4.47*) and may have a misleadingly sinister irregular appearance although their histology is entirely benign. Occasionally, especially after schistosomal colitis, the exudation from the numerous large inflammatory polyps may be sufficient to cause hypoproteinaemia. The description of post-inflammatory polyps as 'pseudo-polyps' seems unnecessary and

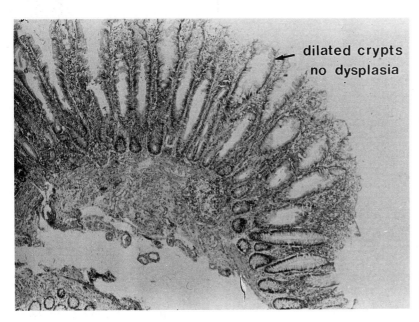

Figure 4.45 A typical sessile metaplastic polyp. The absence of dysplasia is the important feature. Haematoxylin and eosin.

arises only from the need to distinguish them from the neoplastic group. The post-colitic inflammatory polyps must not be confused with the 'plaque-like' raised areas of high-grade epithelial dysplasia (pre-cancer) which, although rare, can occur 8–10 years or more after the onset of ulcerative colitis. Post-inflammatory polyps themselves have no tendency to malignant change but representative biopsies may be needed to prove that adenomas are not present

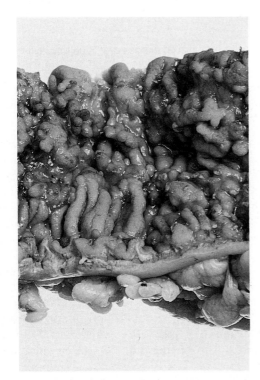

Figure 4.46 A segment of transverse colon from a patient with Crohn's disease showing multiple worm-like inflammatory polyps.

and those of 1 cm or greater are usually snared off to avoid anxiety. Sporadic adenomas can occur in colitis patients and become inflamed and are visually indistinguishable from other inflammatory polyps.

Benign enlargement of lymphoid tissue encompasses an entire spectrum of change from isolated polypoid follicular lesions (*Figure 4.48*) to diffuse lymphoid hyperplasia of the whole intestinal tract. The solitary benign lymphoid polyp of the rectum occurring in young adults is the commonest clinical entity.[51] Multiple benign lymphoid polyposis of the colon exists, but whether it is an exaggerated physiological reaction or a pathological entity is not clear. Minor degrees of diffuse lymphoid hyperplasia are well recognized in children as part of the normal pattern and in adults exposed to infective colitis. The importance of these changes is that they must not be confused with familial adenomatosis polyposis.

A malignant form of lymphoid polyposis termed malignant lymphomatous polyposis[54] occurs in adults and represents about 15% of all gut lymphomas, and is a tumour of adults. Monomorphic collections of centrocyte-like lymphocytes infiltrate the mucosa and submucosa, producing multiple polypoid mucosal projections which may affect several areas of the gut. There is a poor prognosis.

ENDOMETRIOSIS

Endometriosis, classified as heterotopic or misplaced tissue, is exceedingly rare in polypoid form; if the colon is involved, the endometrial tissue is usually in the muscle layers or forms a submucosal mass mimicking cancer.

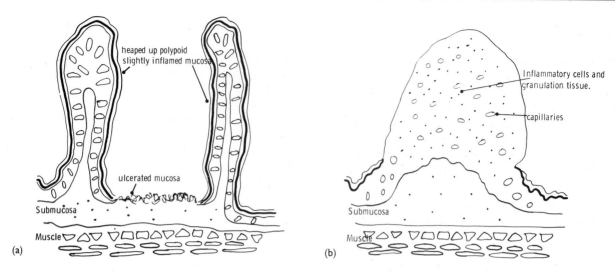

Figure 4.47 The two patterns of inflammatory polyp: (a) a tag of almost normal mucosa, or (b) a polypoid excrescence of granulation tissue.

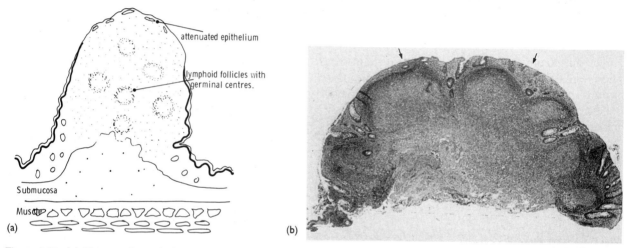

Figure 4.48 (a) Diagram of a typical benign lymphoid polyp. (b) A lymphoid polyp with thinned mucosa over large lymphoid follicles (arrows) with germinal centres. Haematoxylin and eosin.

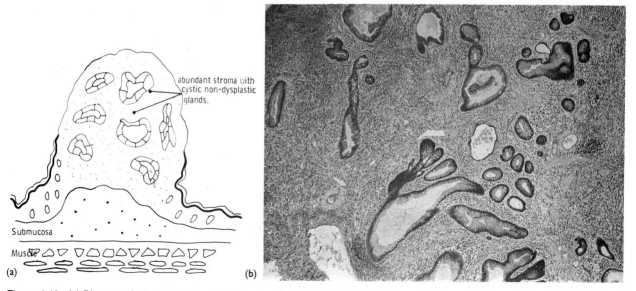

Figure 4.49 (a) Diagram of a juvenile polyp. Note the absence of a stalk. (b) Detail from part of a juvenile polyp showing the abundant stroma and enlarged non-dysplastic cystic glands. Haematoxylin and eosin.

HAMARTOMAS

Hamartomas are localized tumour-like proliferations of normal tissues arranged in an abnormal and disorganized fashion. In the colon the juvenile and Peutz-Jeghers polyps fit this description.

Juvenile polyps are the characteristic polyps of children although they may not present until adult life.[39] They are sometimes referred to as mucus retention polyps because of the cystic inclusions of entrapped mucus (*Figure 4.49a*) which present a 'Swiss cheese' appearance on histological section. Typically they have a smooth surface and are 1–2 cm across. They may intussuscept or present at the anus. The stalk of a juvenile polyp characteristically contains no muscular tissue and so is thin and may twist and auto-amputate – sometimes with massive haemorrhage. Several large polyps may occur in a small child and may be distributed anywhere in the colon, so that examination of the whole colon is desirable if one is found distally.[15]

On histological examination, the crypts and cysts of juvenile polyps are lined by tall, but otherwise normal, cells (*Figure 4.49b*) and the polyp is covered by a single layer of normal colonic epithelium with mucus-secreting goblet cells. The surface is frequently ulcerated. A loose and abundant stroma that may show marked inflammatory changes is characteristic. A second atypical form of juvenile polyp exists. This has a papillary configuration, lacks the abundant stroma and shows a more crowded glandular pattern which can invaginate the underlying muscularis. This variety is more common in juvenile polyposis (defined to include one of the following).

1. More than 5–10 polyps.
2. Juvenile polyps throughout the gut.
3. Any number but with a family history.[29]

Multiple polyps, similar to juvenile polyps, are part of the Cronkhite-Canada syndrome associated with alopecia, nail dystrophy and skin pigmentation.

Individual juvenile polyps have no malignant potential but there is an increased risk of cancer associated with juvenile polyposis. The exact magnitude is unknown but is low and lies between the high risk of adenomatous polyposis and the slightly increased risk associated with Peutz-Jeghers polyposis. When dysplasia has been identified in a juvenile polyp, or when residual elements of a juvenile polyp have been identified within a cancer, the pattern is more commonly that of the atypical form.[29]

Endoscopic polypectomy is adequate treatment for individuals with juvenile polyps. There is insufficient data available for a clear statement on the role of surgery in juvenile polyposis but endoscopic polypectomy and regular surveillance would seem mandatory.

Peutz-Jeghers polyps of the colon occur in most of those affected by the syndrome (mucocutaneous pigmentation, gastrointestinal polyposis and a Mendelian dominant inheritance). They can be a cause of blood loss and anaemia but are of secondary importance to those in the gastroduodenal region (which have malignant potential)[22,57] or the small intestine (which can cause intussusception or even infarction and 'short bowel syndrome'). Isolated Peutz-Jeghers polyps also occur without other features of the syndrome. In the colon, Peutz-Jeghers polyps appear to have negligible malignant potential although 'mixed' hamartomatous polyps also containing adenomatous/dysplastic tissue have been described and probably account for the rare reports of colonic malignancy, as does misplaced epithelium. The larger ones are removed at about 2-yearly intervals in affected subjects, mainly to prevent blood loss.[68] Many of the smaller polyps disappear spontaneously and the tendency to polyp formation declines progressively after 25–30 years of age. There remains a significant risk of extra-intestinal cancers, however, most notably in the ovary, breast and pancreas.[57]

Histologically, Peutz-Jeghers hamartomas do not have the mucus cysts of juvenile polyps but show a branching framework of muscle fibres derived from the muscularis mucosa radiating between disorganized but otherwise normal mucosal crypts (*Figure 4.50*). As with any other colonic polyp liable to growth, ulceration or local haemorrhage, foci of epithelium can become misplaced into the stroma of the head and cause bizarre appearances (pseudo-invasion), but no dysplasia or true neoplastic tissue is present except in the 'mixed' polyps rarely reported.[55]

OTHER MESODERMAL POLYPS

Lipomas are for some reason commonest in the right colon, sometimes as a fatty enlargement of the ileocaecal valve but usually as submucosal rounded elevations and are only rarely pedunculated. The shiny surface and the soft, cystic and pliable nature of the tumour is virtually diagnostic endoscopically.[14,49] Under the surface, yellowish fat may be visible after repeated biopsy but the fat, being loculated, will not run out. Polypectomy is not indicated (even contraindicated because of the difficulty of electrocoagulation and risk of complications) once the diagnosis is made, as lipomas are benign and symptomless, except in rare cases of bleeding from surface ulceration or of intussusception.

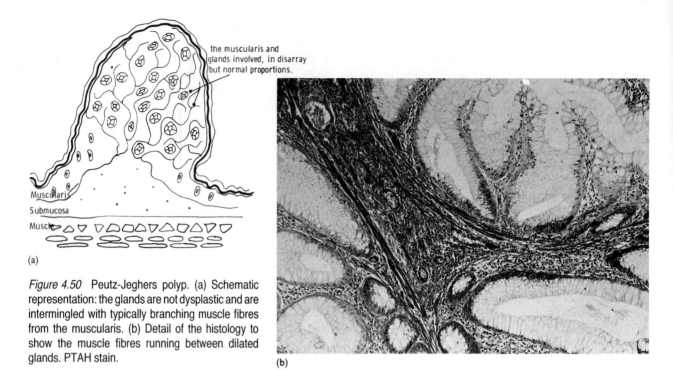

Figure 4.50 Peutz-Jeghers polyp. (a) Schematic representation: the glands are not dysplastic and are intermingled with typically branching muscle fibres from the muscularis. (b) Detail of the histology to show the muscle fibres running between dilated glands. PTAH stain.

Other tissue elements can rarely produce polyps, the exact diagnosis coming as a histological surprise after snare polypectomy. They include polypoid haemangiomas, neurofibromas and leiomyomas.

NEOPLASTIC POLYPS – THE ADENOMAS

The 'adenoma' is the commonest colorectal neoplastic polyp and is the family name for polyps having a common and distinctive dysplastic epithelium but different architectural arrangements (*Figures 4.51* and *4.52*). Each type of adenoma may show varying degrees of epithelial dysplasia, which will influence the likelihood of malignant change. Dysplasia is classified as mild, moderate or severe according to the degree of cytological and architectural abnormality.

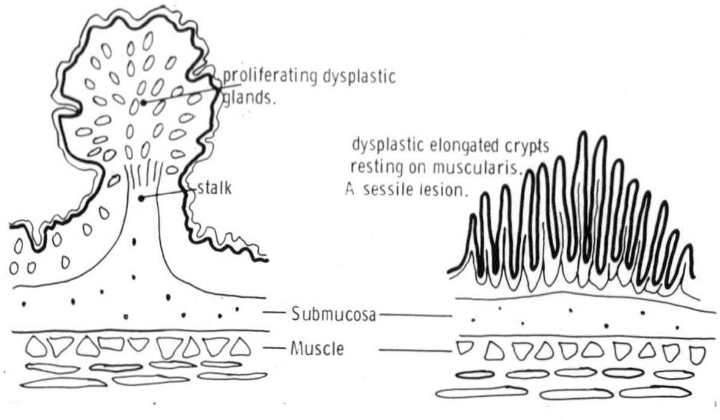

The most frequent adenoma is the tubular variety, which is usually stalked. It has a relatively solid head divided into incomplete lobules which give a fissured appearance on gross inspection (*Figure 4.53a*). Histology demonstrates branching tubules most commonly lined by mildly dysplastic epithelium (*Figure 4.53b*). At the other end of the architectural spectrum is the villous adenoma (villous papilloma), which is often larger, sessile, and has a frond-like stroma covered usually by more severely dysplastic epithelium than the tubular variety (*Figure 4.54*). Between these types comes the tubulovillous (or villoglandular) adenoma, about 20–30% of most series, in which the structure is intermediate with both branching fronds and tubular elements.[24,56]

Histological allocation of a particular polyp to one or other adenoma type is to some extent subjective. The accuracy of classification will depend on the care with which it is examined and the number of histological sections taken as, if more than 20–25% of villous elements are present, the polyp will be termed tubulovillous, whereas with only 15% present it will be called tubular;[41] conversely more than 80% villous structures cause a polyp to be designated a villous adenoma, whereas if it is judged to have under 75% villous it is called 'tubulovillous' – clearly a fairly subjective judgement. The tendency for tubular adenomas to be small and villous adenomas to be larger, and the intermediate position of tubulovillous adenomas is shown in *Table 4.10*.

Figure 4.51 The two main patterns of adenoma: tubular (left) and villous (right). The tubulovillous adenoma has a structure combining both patterns or intermediate between them.

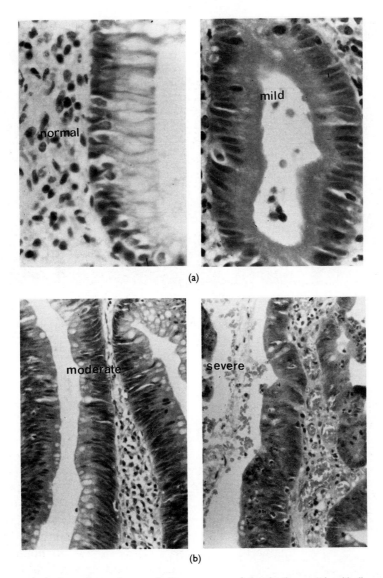

(a)

(b)

Figure 4.52 The pathognomonic feature of an adenoma is the presence of dysplastic cryptal epithelium. The cytological grades of dysplasia are seen here. They are invariably accompanied by increasing architectural disorganization. Haematoxylin and eosin.

Table 4.10 Colorectal adenomas: relationship between histological type, size and frequency of carcinoma. Note the lower frequency of malignancy characteristic of all endoscopic series, compared with the (probably biased) surgical figures often quoted

| | *Proportion of adenomas with carcinoma (%)* | | | | | | | |
| | *Surgical series*[42] | | | | *Colonoscopic series*[24] | | | |
Histological type	*<1 cm*	*1–2 cm*	*>2 cm*	*Total*	*<1 cm*	*1–2 cm*	*>2 cm*	*Total*
Tubular (75%)	1%	10%	35%	5%	1%	3%	10%	2%
Tubulovillous (20%)	4%	7%	46%	23%	0%	4%	11%	6%
Villous (5%)	10%	10%	53%	4%	0%	5%	38%	18%
Overall proportion with carcinoma				10%				5%

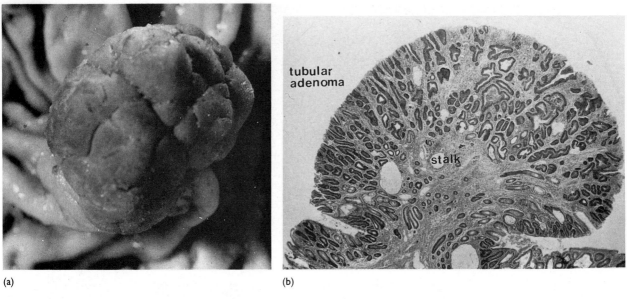

(a) (b)

Figure 4.53 (a) A typical stalked, lobulated, tubular adenoma. (b) A tubular adenoma showing the dysplastic tubular epithelial pattern. Haematoxylin and eosin.

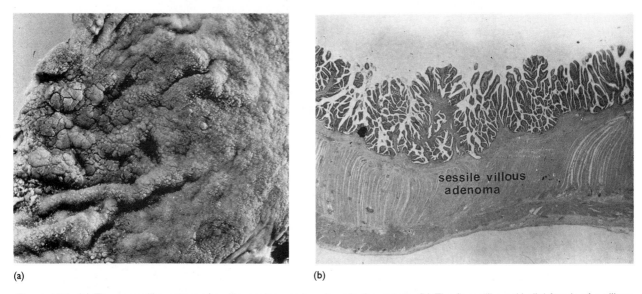

(a) (b)

Figure 4.54 (a) The carpet-like pattern of a villous adenoma low down in the rectum. (b) The finger-like epithelial fronds of a villous adenoma. It is a sessile growth resting directly on the muscularis mucosae and deeper layers. Haematoxylin and eosin.

ADENOMAS, DYSPLASIA AND THE ADENOMA–CARCINOMA SEQUENCE

Histologically an area of severely dysplastic epithelium on the surface of an adenoma is very similar to the appearance of an infiltrating carcinoma and the cells of either will behave similarly in tissue culture; such severely dysplastic areas are thus sometimes referred to as 'carcinoma in situ', 'superficial' or 'focal carcinoma'. These terms should be avoided as they are clinically misleading, however attractive they may seem to the experimental pathologist. The point at issue is that until the dysplastic cells invade across the muscularis mucosae which divides the adenomatous epithelium of the head of the polyp from the submucosa and the lymphatic drainage in the stalk, the likelihood of distant metastasis is so remote that it can be ignored.[40] The diagnosis of carcinoma in the adenoma thus depends on the pathological demonstration of invasion across the muscularis mucosae (*Figure 4.55*). The benign phenomenon of 'misplaced epithelium' or

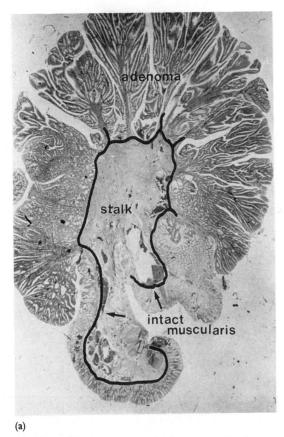

(a)

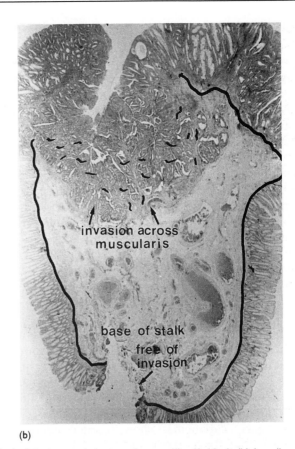

(b)

Figure 4.55 (a) A *benign* tubulovillous adenoma. The feature to note is the intact muscularis musculosae outlined in black. (b) A *malignant* polyp which, in contrast to (a), shows the muscularis musculosae invaded by malignant epithelium. The broken black lines represent the disrupted muscularis, the arrows, the infiltrating epithelium. Haematoxylin and eosin.

'pseudo-invasion' following local ulceration or infarction (which also occurs in hamartomatous polyps) may cause confusion; the misplaced epithelium is non-dysplastic and is surrounded by normal lamina propria rather than the fibrous (desmoplastic) reaction which occurs around carcinomatous tissue.

The risk of malignancy in adenomas is influenced not only by the severity of dysplasia (*Table 4.11*) and its morphological type but also by the size of the lesion (*Table 4.10*).[24,56] The influence of size probably represents a statistical relationship between the mass of the polyp and the number of potentially cancerous cells present. Study of operation specimens from patients with familial adenomatous poly-

posis gives insight into the growth of adenomas from single dysplastic crypts to tiny polyps (*Figure 4.56*) which contain so few neoplastic cells that the likelihood of initiating carcinoma, although possible,

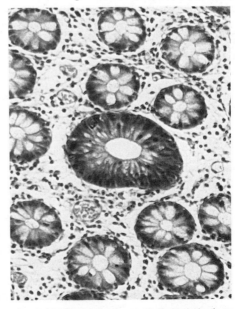

Figure 4.56 A single dysplastic crypt, the seed of a potential adenoma, is seen in the centre. Haematoxylin and eosin.

Table 4.11 Colorectal adenomas: grade of dysplasia and risk of carcinoma[24]

Grade of dysplasia	Percentage with carcinoma
Mild	6%
Moderate	18%
Severe	35%

must be extremely small. Malignancy is very rarely observed in tiny adenomas, although any adenomatous tissue would naturally be engulfed and destroyed by carcinoma at an early stage. This might explain the reports of 'de novo' carcinoma claimed to represent 20–25% of colorectal cancers. The disparity between the malignancy rate reported in adenomas removed from surgical series[42] compared with an endoscopic series from the same department[24] may reflect selection bias. One explanation may be the inclusion of adenomas removed from cancer patients and the pre-endoscopic policy of delaying removal of colonic polyps until they showed suspicious appearances on serial barium enema examinations. Whatever the reason, endoscopic series uniformly find an overall 10% malignancy rate for adenomas (and nearer 20% for those over 2 cm diameter), about half the quoted figure for surgical series.[24,56]

There is much other direct and indirect evidence to support the concept of an adenoma–carcinoma sequence in the large bowel.[42] Cell culture lines from adenomas and carcinomas behave similarly and adenomatous cells show similar histochemical and genetic aberrations to those of cancer cells. Many early carcinomas show residual adenoma tissue within them, the percentage falling in the more advanced cancers where the initiating adenoma is presumed to have been destroyed. The distribution of adenomas and cancers is identical, predominantly in the left colon but with a small increased incidence in the caecum; the latter is explained by an association with an increased incidence of sessile villous adenomas in the caecum.[56] The worldwide geographical influence of adenomas and carcinomas is also similar, both being rare in Africans and indigenous Japanese, but both common in whites and 'Westernized' Japanese such as those living in Hawaii.

Synchronous adenomas are present in many patients with colorectal cancer and adenoma-bearing patients have a higher risk of developing colorectal cancer on follow-up than matched controls.[3] The risk of coexistent (synchronous) or subsequent (metachronous) cancer rises as the number of adenomas increases, with an incidence of 100% in familial adenomatous polyposis patients. Destruction of adenomas reduces the expected cancer incidence in the rectal stump of patients with familial adenomatous polyposis treated by colectomy[42] and the same is claimed for the rectum of normal subjects.[23]

The disparity between the 30% of older Western subjects found to have adenomas and the 2–3% dying of colorectal cancer suggests that 90% of adenomas will not progress to carcinoma.

The time taken to develop a 'significant size' of adenoma and the interval to cancer formation is merely conjectural, although figures have been given for the growth rate or doubling-time of polyps and cancers based on radiological observation.[19] Even cruder estimates have been based on anecdotal clinical data or the difference between the average age of clinical diagnosis of adenomas and colorectal cancer.[42] Morson[40] has suggested an average 5–7-year interval between an adenoma reaching 1 cm and the development of malignancy although the range is likely to be considerable. Colorectal cancer can occasionally be diagnosed in patients apparently normal when examined only a year or two previously, whereas most small adenomas, and even the large adenomas found unexpectedly in some elderly patients, may never become cancerous in the lifetime of the patient.[40]

AETIOLOGY AND GENETICS OF ADENOMA FORMATION

It seems that the aetiology of adenomas and colonic cancer are likely to be at least inter-related.[27,30] Some of the geographical and epidemiological evidence has been discussed. Dietary factors are probably also important. Increased intake of meat and fat have been implicated and low dietary fibre and calcium are other possible factors. Dietary factors may mediate their effect by modifying biliary metabolism with the production of toxic or carcinogenic promoting substances by bacterial action in the colon. It is of interest that, after 10 years, patients in whom the urinary stream has been diverted by ureteric implantation into the sigmoid colon (often because of congenital bladder defects) have an increased incidence of both adenomas and cancers in the colonic mucosa adjacent to the ureter.[2] The risk remains even if the urine flow is subsequently removed from the colon. This phenomenon could be explained by the production of nitrosamines (by bacterial action on urinary nitrites) which are known to be carcinogenic to intestinal mucosa.

In addition to environmental, and particularly dietary, factors there are also important genetic factors which are associated with colorectal cancer development.[62] There are several familial conditions which are dominantly inherited and predispose to the development of colorectal cancer at an early age. These colorectal cancer syndromes (HNPCC) are usually divided into the polyposis syndromes, in which hundreds of adenomatous polyps develop in the colon, and the hereditary non-polyposis, in which a smaller number of polyps develop but cancer is frequent. The gene responsible for familial adenomatous polyposis, designated APC, has been cloned and this will allow presymptomatic diagnosis of affected individuals.

In an atypical non-polyposis kindred with a high incidence of early onset colorectal cancer and a highly variable number of colonic polyps, linkage has been reported to markers in the APC region of chromosome 5.[32] This raises the possibility that different mutants of the APC gene may be responsible for some non-polyposis syndromes.

There is also some evidence from genetic epidemiological studies to suggest that there may be an inherited predisposition to common, apparently sporadic, colorectal cancer.[6] The identification of candidate genes, such as APC, will allow this hypothesis to be tested.

Advances in molecular biology have also revealed the important genetic mutations that occur during colorectal tumourigenesis. The progression from normal colonic mucosa to adenomatous polyp to carcinoma is associated with the accumulation of genetic changes and several of the genes affected have been cloned. These changes involve both the loss of tumour suppressor genes and the activation of proto-oncogenes.

Loss of genetic material on chromosome 5, in the region of the APC gene, is the earliest event commonly detected. This occurs in small polyps, as does activation of the k-ras oncogene. In larger adenomas, loss of genetic material on chromosome 18 in the region of the DCC (Deleted in Colorectal Carcinomas) gene is commonly found. Finally, mutations of the P53 tumour suppressor gene are often associated with the transition from adenoma to carcinoma. P53 mutations have subsequently been shown to be the commonest mutations in human neoplasia.[18]

The clinician makes a diagnosis of 'polyps' and although in most adults these will prove to be adenomatous, it is incorrect to assume this without histological examination. Even on endoscopy or radiology, the different types of polyps can be indistinguishable. Polyps in general are therefore considered next, although the management is described based on the presumption that they will prove to be adenomas.

CLINICAL FEATURES

Colonic polyps only infrequently cause symptoms. The larger ones (1 cm or over) may bleed intermittently and if multiple (20 or more) may cause anaemia. Patients presenting with colorectal bleeding, however, often have obvious local causes for haemorrhage such as haemorrhoids, as well as the polyps found with further investigation. Since both lesions are promptly treated it is sometimes uncertain whether the polyps contributed to the bleeding or were a chance finding. In the authors' experience 60% of colonoscopically removed polyps occur in patients presenting with bleeding, 20% are found on follow-up examinations of symptomless patients and 20% in patients presenting with pain. Except for the remote possibility of traction or intussusception by a very large polyp, there is no mechanism by which a polyp can cause pain, which is usually due to coexisting functional bowel problems which precipitated the colonic examination.

Very large, usually sessile, villous adenomas may cause altered bowel habit, especially because of the production of copious quantities of mucus. Some may even cause mucoid diarrhoea and hypokalaemia but these are rare compared to the numbers of villous adenomas presenting without electrolyte disturbance.

INVESTIGATIONS

Rigid sigmoidoscopy

Rigid sigmoidoscopy or flexible sigmoidoscopy should diagnose a high percentage of colonic polyps[43] since at least 30% occur within 25 cm of the anal canal and about 60% in the rectum and sigmoid colon, including most of the large or malignant lesions. It was previously thought that an even higher percentage of polyps were within range of the rigid sigmoidoscope but this was simply because clinicians did not know what they were missing proximally.[10,60,37] Flexible sigmoidoscopy should replace rigid tube examinations in screening for polyps since by visualizing more bowel the yield is about three times as high, and furthermore, the examination may take only 5 minutes.[38] The relative ease and accuracy of sigmoidoscopy is particularly important since this is the least accurate area for the barium enema. Except for reasons of size, or when there are multiple small polyps, the colonoscopist should aim to provide the pathologist with an 'excision biopsy'. Forceps biopsies do not allow an assessment of the polyp stalk, the crucial area required for the exclusion of malignancy (*Figure 4.56*). Since rigid or flexible sigmoidoscopy are usually performed after only limited bowel preparation, there is a serious explosion hazard during polypectomy and electrocoagulation from residual methane or hydrogen. Therefore an uninflammable gas such as carbon dioxide should be used if polypectomy is intended.

Double contrast barium enema

Double-contrast barium enema examination was the traditional investigation to identify polyps beyond the reach of the sigmoidoscope. This requires thorough bowel preparation and uncomfortable distension of the colon but should demonstrate 70–80% of significant sized polyps compared[20] with the 50% seen on single-contrast enema (and over 90% on colonoscopy).[69] Barium enema is cheaper and safer than colonoscopy and can be the initial screening investigation in low-risk subjects, such as elderly patients with altered bowel habit and pain. It is, however, relatively inaccurate in the sigmoid colon (because of overlapping folds or diverticular disease), in the caecum (because of faecal residue) and for small lesions.

Colonoscopy

Colonoscopy[11] is the 'gold standard' with the advantage of offering the option of immediate polypectomy. It is more accurate, particularly in the left colon which is the site of most polyps, and can identify, biopsy and destroy lesions down to 1–2 mm in diameter which are invisible to the radiologist – giving a reasonable guarantee of a 'clean colon' and allowing long intervals between examinations. Unfortunately, the colons of some patients, either because of fixation or undue mobility, are exceedingly difficult to intubate, so it is unrealistic to suggest total colonoscopy as the only diagnostic procedure for all patients in all countries. Colonoscopy is the logical procedure for high-risk patients, such as those with a previous family history of colon cancer.[31]

TREATMENT

Polypectomy

Once a polyp is found it must be removed,[9,1,67,48,58] allowing for the exceptions already mentioned, such as typical post-inflammatory polyps or lipomas. Even polyps within 10 cm of the anal verge (except for those that are large and sessile) can be removed by the expedient of retroverting the instrument tip so as to see the lower part of the rectal ampulla. Larger sessile polyps in the rectum are better managed with the sphincters relaxed by anaesthesia to permit local proctological techniques, preferably 'floating' them off the rectal wall by submucosal injection of adrenaline–saline solution, to facilitate local scissor excision. Laser photocoagulation may

sometimes be indicated. Over 95% of polyps proximal to the rectum are suitable for colonoscopic excision since few are too large or sessile.[64] Surgery should never be resorted to without first attempting colonoscopic polypectomy, as some lesions that look sessile or malignant on radiography prove to be on small stalks endoscopically. The colon is, except for its outer covering, devoid of sensory innervation and polypectomy is therefore painless and can be performed without sedation on an out-patient basis. Only stalked polyps with a head diameter of 2 cm or greater have any significant risk of haemorrhage and this is negligible if sufficient lower power coagulating current (15–30 watts equivalent) is used to cause heating and coagulation of the stalk before transaction with the snare loop.[11,44] Very large stalks, with an increased likelihood of bleeding, can be pre-injected with 1 ml of adrenaline or an adrenaline/sclerosant mixture before snaring. Polypectomy anywhere in the colon is usually quick and easy because 90% of polyps are under 2 cm diameter and have relatively thin stalks. Recovery of snared polyps means withdrawing the colonoscope with each one, if necessary using a split overtube through which the instrument is easily withdrawn and re-inserted. Small snared polyps can be aspirated through the biopsy channel with a trap placed in the suction line.

Very small polyps (2–5 mm) can be snared but are usually biopsied and simultaneously destroyed by the so-called 'hot-biopsy' technique in which an electrocoagulating current is passed down insulated biopsy forceps. Large sessile polyps up to 3–4 cm diameter can usually be removed endoscopically by piecemeal snare polypectomy, repeated at several sessions if necessary.[7] Whether this is justified depends on the operative risk in the individual and the configuration of the particular polyp.

MULTIPLE POLYPS, POLYPOSIS SYNDROMES AND CANCER FAMILY SYNDROMES

A patient with a known diagnosis of Peutz-Jeghers syndrome, schistosomiasis or other non-neoplastic causes of polyposis can have 50 or more polyps snared in a single session as only one or two need be retrieved for histological review. Sporadic cases of unsuspected adenomatous polyposis occur, presumably by mutation, but multiple biopsies are sufficient to make this diagnosis and to exclude other forms of polyposis (such as metaplastic or lymphomatous polyps). The situation occasionally arises where, for example, a patient is found to have one or two

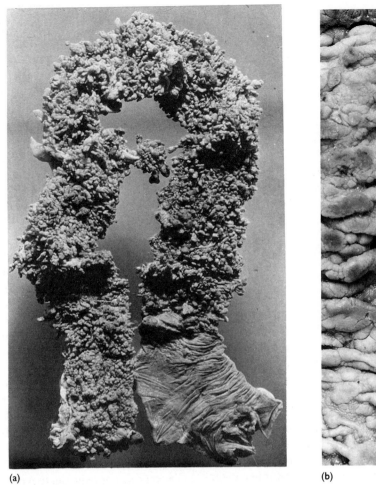

(a)

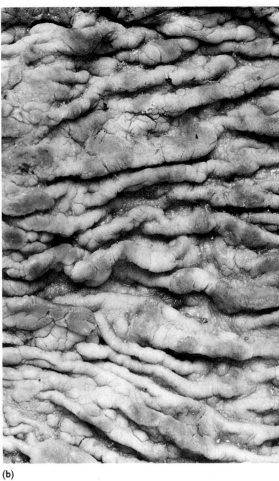

(b)

Figure 4.57 Two patterns of familial adenomatous polyposis. (a) The whole of the colon except the caecum and proximal ascending colon is covered by adenomatous polyps. (b) Here the change is more subtle. Hundreds of tiny sessile polyps cover the mucosa giving it a cobblestone appearance. They resemble metaplastic polyps macroscopically.

polyps with sigmoidoscopy and barium enema examination and 10–15 additional smaller probable adenomas at endoscopy; before attempting multiple polypectomies it is logical to check first for the presence of other minute polyps because, in such cases, surgery might be considered as the first line of management. Visualization of polyps only 1–2 mm in diameter is much enhanced by the 'dye-spray technique' in which blue dye (0.3% indigo carmine or diluted writing ink) is sprayed on to the surface, causing any small polyps to protrude as pink islands against the blue background.[59] The idenitification of 20 or more additional polyps may tip the balance towards surgery, if biopsy shows them to be adenomas.

Familial adenomatous polyposis was often previously termed 'polyposis coli' but it is now recognized that it also involves the gastroduodenal region in over 90% of subjects. Strictly speaking, there must be at least 100 colonic adenomas to justify the

diagnosis but cases with fewer adenomas occur (*Figures 4.57* and *4.58*). Much of the dogma of the past is likely to require re-writing as precise understanding of the gene defect(s) permits gene probe analysis of polyposis and 'hereditary non-polyposis colonic cancer' families.

Treatment of malignant polyps

Endoscopically or radiologically it is often impossible to determine which polyps will be malignant. Signs of possible malignancy include a thick stalk and an ulcerated or indurated polyp head, but soft rounded polyps on thin stalks may contain cancer.[70] The histological diagnosis of malignancy may therefore come as a surprise several days after polypectomy. Providing the endoscopist is satisfied that polypectomy satisfactorily removed the whole lesion, the principal of subsequent management depend entirely on the pathologist's assessment of

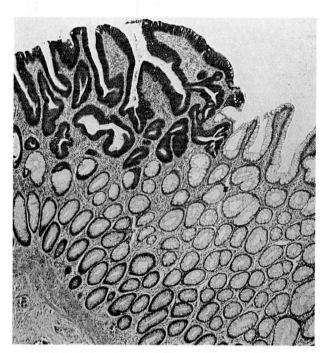

Figure 4.58 The darker dysplastic epithelium is well seen in contrast to the normal mucosa of, in this case, adenomatous polyposis. The change is only producing a minor alteration in the surface contour and, as seen in *Figure 4.57b*, it is easy to overlook macroscopically. Haematoxylin and eosin.

the risk of spread to local lymph nodes. Well- or moderately well-differentiated carcinoma that has not invaded as far as the resection line in the polyp stalk (*Figure 4.55*) and which does not involve veins or lymphatics is exceedingly unlikely to have spread.[70,8,13,26,12,45] The risk of early spread is much higher in the rare circumstances of poorly differentiated (anaplastic) carcinoma, or if involvement extends up to the resection line and indicates surgery unless the patient is very infirm. There is controversy over outcome with local resection if vascular and/or lymphatic invasion of the stalk is identified.[12] Much of this is caused by the difficulty of distinguishing lymphatic invasion from retraction artefact.

If the policy of conservative management is strictly confined to a confident and complete excision in one piece of pedunculated and sessile polyps of about 35 and 15 mm respectively, then vascular and lymphatic involvement does not influence management.[21] Outside these strict limitations, lymphatic and vascular invasion have been shown to be indications for subsequent surgery.[11]

By local resection in these at-risk patients the intention is to remove any local tumour extension or draining lymph nodes before distant metastases occur. The relatively high mortality of colonic surgery means that the patients at lower risk are likely to have a better prognosis by not proceeding to

surgery, the locally malignant lesions being managed by endoscopic local excision alone.[8,70] Clinical experience of endoscopists worldwide and several series of patients followed for 5 years after polypectomy support this policy which can be applied equally to polypoid carcinomas meeting the same criteria.

Endoscopically, it is wise, if in doubt, to re-examine and biopsy the polypectomy site within days of the diagnosis of the malignancy being made, as once healed, it may be impossible to locate. A marker tattoo of 2 ml Indian ink can be injected submucosally to identify the site for subsequent follow-up or to assist the surgeon in the event of resection.[50,33]

Follow-up of adenoma patients

The exact future risk for a patient having had a previous adenoma removed must be re-defined now that more accurate diagnostic methods are available; some of the adenomas and cancers found in reported follow-up studies may simply represent lesions missed at the time of the first polypectomy.[63] Nevertheless, the evidence suggests that there is a significantly increased subsequent risk in patients with previous adenoma or carcinoma and that they represent a high-risk group for the development of colonic cancer.[3,25,47]

After a follow-up interval of about 10 years, further adenomas (mostly small) can be expected in at least 30–40% of patients and carcinomas in 2–4%;[25] the only study with an age-matched control group of non-adenoma patients demonstrated only 7% with polyps and none with cancers at a similar follow-up interval.[3]

Follow-up examinations must include the whole colon, because many of the polyps and cancers occur proximal to the sigmoid colon.[53] Occult blood tests also have no real role in follow-up, as only some of the larger polyps bleed, and then only intermittently.[36] Conventional practice is to advise colonoscopy or barium enema examination one year after the initial polypectomy,[63] with 3-yearly total colonoscopy thereafter. Flexible sigmoidoscopy and double-contrast barium enema radiography is an acceptable alternative but may miss some polyps in the right colon. There is good evidence that patients with more than one adenoma originally, especially if large or numerous, have an increased risk of recurrent polyps and colorectal cancer, whereas after destruction of a few small adenomas in an elderly subject there may be little long-term risk. It is unlikely that routine follow-up is indicated over 75 years of age, as the contribution of colorectal cancer to mortality in old age is under 2% of all causes.

Whatever follow-up routine is adopted, there will always be some surprises; patients should thus be urged to attend earlier if suspicious symptoms occur, particularly bleeding. The problem of adenoma follow-up is essentially one of logistics;[17,52] too frequent follow-up of the enormous numbers of adenoma-bearing patients can easily make unreasonable demands on available diagnostic services. On the other hand, suitably managed, such patients present an opportunity for prevention or early diagnosis of colorectal cancer.

REFERENCES

1. Achkar, E. and Carey, W.D. (1988) Small polyps found during fiberoptic sigmoidoscopy in asymptomatic patients. *Annals of Internal Medicine*, **109**, 880–883.
2. Berg, N.O. (1987) Surveillance colonoscopy and biopsy in patients with uretero-sigmoidostomy. *Endoscopy*, **19**, 60–63.
3. Brahme, F., Ekelund, G.R., Norden, J.G. and Wenckert, A. (1974) Metachronous colorectal polyps: comparison of development of colo-rectal polyps and carcinomas in persons with or without histories of polyps. *Diseases of the Colon and Rectum*, **17**, 166–171.
4. Brunetaud, J.M., Maunoury, V., Cochelard, D. *et al.* (1990) Lasers in rectosigmoid cancers: factors affecting immediate and long-term results. In *Clinical Gastroenterology,* pp. 615–625. London: Baillière Tindall.
5. Brunetaud, J.M., Maunoury, V., Cochelard, D., Boniface, B., Cortot, A. and Paris, J.C. (1989) Endoscopic laser treatment for rectosigmoid villous adenoma: factors affecting the results. *Gastrotenterology*, **97**, 272–277.
6. Cannon-Albright, L.A., Skolnick, M.H., Bishop, T., Lee, R.G. and Burt, R.W. (1988) Common inheritance of susceptibility to colonic adenomatous polyps and associated colorectal cancers. *New England Journal of Medicine*, **319**, 533–537.
7. Christie, J.P. (1978) Colonoscopic removal of sessile colonic lesions. *Diseases of the Colon and Rectum*, **21**, 11–14.
8. Christie, J.P. (1988) Polypectomy or colectomy? Management of 106 consecutively encountered colorectal polyps. *American Journal of Surgery*, **54**, 93–99.
9. Church, J.M., Fazio, V.W. and Jones, I.T. (1988) Small colorectal polyps: are they worth treating? *Diseases of the Colon and Rectum*, **31**, 50–53.
10. Coller, J.A., Corman, M.L. and Veidenheimer, M.C. (1975) Colonic polypoid disease: need for total colonoscopy. *American Journal of Surgery*, **131**, 490–494.
11. Cotton, P.B. and Williams, C.B. (1990) Practical Gastrointestinal Endoscopy. Third Edition. Scientific Publications. Oxford: Blackwell.
12. Coverlizza, S., Risio, M., Ferrari, A., Fenoglio-Proiser, C.M. and Rossini, F.P. (1989) Colorectal adenomas containing invasive carcinoma. Pathologic assessment of lymph node metastatic potential. *Cancer*, **64**, 1937–1947.
13. Cranley, J.P., Petras, R.E., Carey, W.D., Paradis, K. and Sivak, M.V. (1986) When is endoscopic polypectomy adequate therapy for colonic polyps containing invasive carcinoma? *Gastroenterology*, **91**, 419–427.
14. de Beer, R.A. and Shinya, H. (1975) Colonic lipomas: an endoscopic analysis. *Gastrointestinal Endoscopy*, **22**, 90–91.
15. Douglas, J.R., Campbell, C.A., Salisbury, D.M., Walker-Smith, J.A. and Williams, C.B. (1981) Colonoscopic polypectomy in children, *British Medical Journal*, **28**, 1386–1387.
16. Du Boulay, C.E.H., Fairbrother, J. and Isaacson, P.G. (1983) Mucosal prolapse syndrome – a unifying concept for solitary ulcer and related disorders. *Journal of Clinical Pathology*, **36**, 1264–1268.
17. Eddy, D.M. (1990) Screening for colorectal cancer. *Annals of Internal Medicine*, **113**, 373–384.
18. Fearon, E.R. and Vogelstein, B. (1990) A genetic model of colorectal tumorigenesis. *Cell.*, **61**, 759–767.
19. Figiel, L.S., Figiel, S.J. and Wietersen, F.K. (1965) Roentologic observations of growth rates of colonic polyps and carcinoma. *Acta Radiology*, **3**, 417–429.
20. Fork, F.T. (1983) Reliability of routine double contrast examination of the large bowel: a prospective study of 2590 patients. *Gut*, **24**, 672–67?.
21. Geraghty, J.M., Williams, C.B. and Talbot, I.C. (1991) Malignant colorectal polyps: venous invasion and successful treatment by endoscopic polypectomy. *Gut*, **32**, 774–778.
22. Giardiello, F.M., Welsh, S.B. and Hamilton, S.R. (1987) Peutz-Jeghers syndrome: perhaps not so benign. *New England Journal of Medicine*, **316**, 1511–1514.
23. Gilbertson, V.A., McHugh, R., Schumann, L. and Williams, S.E. (1980) The earlier detection of colorectal cancers: a preliminary report of the results of the occult blood study. *Cancer*, **45**, 2899–2901.
24. Gillespie, P.E., Chambers, T.J., Chan, K.W., Doronzo, F., Morson, B.C. and Williams, C.B. (1979) Colonic adenomas – a colonoscopic survey. *Gut*, **20**, 240–245.
25. Grossman, S., Milos, M.L., Tekawa, I.S. and Jewell, N.P. (1989) Colonoscopic screening of persons with suspected risk factors for colon cancer:

II. Past history of colorectal neoplasms. *Gastroenterology*, **96**, 299–306.

26. Haggitt, R.C., Glotzbach, R.E., Soffer, E.E. and Wruble, J.D. (1985) Prognostic factors in colorectal carcinomas arising in adenomas: implications for lesions removed by endoscopic polypectomy. *Gastroenterology*, **89**, 328–336.

27. Hoff, G. (1987) Colorectal Polyps. Clinical implications: screening and cancer prevention. *Scandinavian Journal of Gastroenterology*, **22**, 769–775.

28. Jass, J.R. (1989) Do all colorectal carcinomas arise in preexisting adenomas? *World Journal of Surgery*, **13**, 45–51.

29. Jass, J.R., Williams, C.B., Bussey, H.J.R. and Morson, B.C. (1988) Juvenile polyposis – a precancerous condition. *Histopathology*, **13**, 619–630.

30. Kronborg, O. (1980) Polyps of the colon and rectum. *Scandinavian Journal of Gastroenterology*, **15**, 1–5.

31. Lanspa, S.J., Smyrk, T.C. and Lynch, H.T. (1990) The colonoscopist and the Lynch syndromes. *Gastrointestinal Endoscopy*, **36**, 156–158.

32. Leppert, M., Burt, R., Hughes, J.P., Samovitz, W., Nakamura, Y., Woodward, S., Gardner, E., Lalouel, J.-M, and White, R. (1990) Genetic analysis of an inherited predisposition to colonic adenomatous polyps and associated colorectal cancers. *New England Journal of Medicine*, **322**, 904–908.

33. Lightdale, C.J. (1991) India ink colonic tattoo: blots on the record. *Gastrointestinal Endoscopy*, **37**, 99–100.

34. Lobert, P.F. and Appelman, H.D. (1991) Inflammatory cloacogenic polyps. A unique inflammatory lesion of the anal transition zone. *American Journal of Surgical Pathology*, **5**, 761–766.

35. Longacre, T.A. and Fenoglio-Preiser, C.M. (1990) Mixed hyperplastic adenomatous polyps/serrated adenomas. A distinct form of colorectal neoplasia. *American Journal of Surgical Pathology*, **14**, 524–537.

36. Macrae, F.A. and St John, D.J.B. (1982) Relationship of patterns of bleeding and haemoccult sensitivity in patients with colorectal cancers or adenomas. *Gastroenterology*, **82**, 891–898.

37. Madigan, M.R. and Halls, J.M. (1968) The extent of sigmoidoscopy shown on radiographs with special reference to the recto-sigmoid junction. *Gut*, **9**, 355–362.

38. Marks, G., Boggs, H.W., Castro, A.S., Gathright, J.B., Ray, J.E. and Salvati, E. (1979) Sigmoidoscopic examinations with rigid and flexible fiberoptic sigmoidoscopes in the surgeon's office. *Diseases of the Colon and Rectum*, **22**, 162–168.

39. Mazier, W.P., Bowman, H.E., Sun, K.M. and Muldoon, J.P. (1974) Juvenile polyps of the colon and rectum. *Diseases of the Colon and Rectum*, **17**, 523–528.

40. Morson, B.C. (1978) The pathogenesis of colorectal cancer. In *Major Problems in Pathology No. 10*, (Ed.) Morson, B.C. Philadephia: W.B. Saunders.

41. Morson, B.C., Dawson, I.M.P., Day, D.W., Jass, J.R., Price, A.B. and Williams, G.T. (1990) *Morson and Dawson's Gastrointestinal Pathology (3rd Edition)*. Oxford: Blackwell Scientific Publications.

42. Muto, T., Bussey, H.J.R. and Morson, B.C. (1975) The evolution of cancer of the colon and rectum. *Cancer*, **36**, 2251–2270.

43. Neugut, A.J. and Pita, S. (1988) Role of sigmoidoscopy in screening for colorectal cancer: a critical review. *Gastroenterology*, **95**, 492–499.

44. Nivatvongs, S. (1988) Complications in colonoscopic polypectomy: lessons to learn from an experience with 1576 polyps. *American Journal of Surgery*, **54**, 61–63.

45. Nivatvongs, S., Rojanasakul, A., Reiman, H.M. *et al.* (1991) The risk of lymph node metastasis in colorectal polyps with invasive adenocarcinoma. *Diseases of the Colon and Rectum*, **34**, 323–328.

46. Norfleet, R.G., Ryan, M.E. and Wyman, J.B. (1988) Adenomatous and hyperplastic polyps cannot be reliably distinguished by their appearance through the fiberoptic sigmoidoscope. *Digestive Diseases and Sciences*, **33**, 1175–1177.

47. O'Brien, M.J., Winawer, S.J., Zauber, A.G. *et al.* (1990) The National Polyp Study: patient and polyp characteristics associated with high-grade dysplasia in colorectal adenomas. *Gastroenterology*, **98**, 371–379.

48. Panish, J.F. (1979) State of the art: management of patients with polypoid lesions of the colon: current concepts and controversies. *American Journal of Gastroenterology*, **71**, 315–324.

49. Pfeil, S.A., Weaver, M.G., Abdul-Karim, F.W. and Yang, P. (1990) Colonic Lipomas: outcome of endoscopic removal. *Gastrointestinal Endoscopy*, **36**, 435–438.

50. Ponsky, J.L. and King, J.F. (1975) Endoscopic marking of colonic lesions. *Gastrointestinal Endoscopy*, **22**, 42–43.

51. Price, A.B. (1978) Benign lymphoid polyps and polyposis. In *The Pathogenesis of Colorectal Cancer*, pp. 33–42. Philadephia: W.B. Saunders.

52. Ransohoff, D.F., Lang, C.A. and Kuo, H.S. (1991) Colonoscopic surveillance after polypectomy: considerations of cost effectiveness. *Annals of Internal Medicine*, **114**, 177–181.

53. Rhodes, J.B., Holmes, F.F. and Clark, G.M. (1977) Changing distribution of primary cancers in the large bowel. *Journal of American Medical Association*, **238**, 1641–1653.

54. Shepherd, N.A. and Bussey, H.J.R. (1990) Polyposis syndromes – an update. In *Current Topics in Pathology: Gastrointestinal Pathology*, (Ed.)

Williams, G.T. pp. 323–351. Berlin: Springer Verlag.

55. Shepherd, N.A., Bussey, H.J.R. and Jass, J.R. (1987) Epithelial misplacement in Peutz-Jeghers polyps: a diagnostic pitfall. *American Journal of Surgical Pathology*, **11**, 743–749.

56. Shinya, H. and Wolff, W.I. (1979) Morphology, anatomic distribution and cancer potential of colonic polyps. Analysis of 7000 polyps endoscopically removed. *Annals of Surgery*, **190**, 679–683.

57. Spigelman, A.D., Murday, V. and Phillips, R.K.S. (1989) Cancer and Peutz-Jeghers syndrome. *Gut*, **30**, 1588–1590.

58. Stryker, S.J., Wolff, B.G., Culp, C.E., Libbe, S.D., Ilstrup, D.M. and MacCarthy, R.L. (1987) Natural history of untreated colonic polyps. *Gastroenterology*, **93**, 1009–1013.

59. Tada, M., Katoh, S., Kohli, Y. and Kawai, K. (1976) On the dye spraying method in colonofiberoscopy. *Endoscopy*, **8**, 70–74.

60. Tedesco, F.J., Waye, J.D., Avella, J.R. and Villalobos, M.M. (1980) Diagnostic implications of the spatial distribution of colonic mass lesions (polyps and cancers): a prospective colonoscopic study. *Gastrointestinal Endoscopy*, **26**, 95–97.

61. Teoh, H.H., Delahunt, B. and Isbister, W.H. (1989) Dysplastic and malignant areas in hyperplastic polyps of the large intestine. *Pathology*, **21**, 138–142.

62. Vogelstein, B., Fearon, E.R., Hamilton, S.R., Kern, S.E., Preisinger, A.C., Leppert, M., Nakamura, Y., White, R., Smits, A.M.M. and Bos, J.L. (1988) Genetic alterations during colorectal turmour development. *New England Journal of Medicine*, **319**, 525–532.

63. Waye, J. and Braunfeld, S. (1982) Surveillance intervals after polypectomy. *Endoscopy*, **14**, 79–81.

64. Waye, J.D. (1991) Endoscopic Treatment of Adenomas. *World Journal of Surgery*, **15**, 14–19.

65. Waye, J.D., Lewis, B.S., Frankel, A. and Geller, S.A. (1988) Small colon polyps. *American Journal of Gastroenterology*, **83**, 120–122.

66. Williams, A.R., Balasooriya, B.A.W. and Day, D.W. (1982) Polyps and cancer of the large bowel: a necroscopy study in Liverpool. *Gut*, **23**, 835–842.

67. Williams, C.B. and Bedenne, L. (1990) Quadrennial review: management of colonic polyps – is all the effort worthwhile? *Hepatology and Gastroenterology*.

68. Williams, C.B., Goldblatt, M. and Delaney, P. (1982) Top and tail endoscopy and follow-up in Peutz-Jeghers syndrome. *Endoscopy*, **14**, 82–84.

69. Williams, C.B., Macrae, F.A. and Bartram, C.I. (1982) A prospective study of diagnostic methods in polyp follow-up. *Endoscopy*, **14**, 74–78.

70. Williams, C.B., Whiteway, J.E. and Jass, J.R. (1987) Practical aspects of endoscopic management of malignant polyps. *Endoscopy*, **19**, 31–37.

71. Williams, G.T., Arthur, J.F., Bussey, H.J.R. and Morson, B.C. (1980) Metaplastic polyps and polyposis. *Histopathology*, **4**, 155–170.

72. Williams, G.T., Bussey, H.J.R. and Morson, B.C. (1985) Inflammatory cap polyps of the large intestine. *British Journal of Surgery*, **72** (suppl.), S133.

HEREDITARY NEOPLASTIC DISEASES OF THE INTESTINE (J.M.A. Northover and S. Hodgson)

At least 5% of cases of colorectal cancer arise in individuals with genetic predisposition to colorectal neoplasia. Familial adenomatous polyposis (FAP) is the best characterized of the inherited conditions predisposing to colon cancer, but is less common than the so-called 'non-polyposis' syndromes, the 'cancer family syndromes', in which intestinal adenomata occur, but are much fewer in number. There are several other syndromes, in which hamartomas may develop in the bowel and which may predispose to malignancy. These comprise Peutz-Jeghers' syndrome, juvenile polyposis, Ruvalcaba-Myhre syndrome, Gorlin's syndrome and Cowden's disease (*Table 4.12*).

Apart from those families cited above in which there is a clear dominant inheritance of predisposition to colorectal cancer, close relatives of sporadic cancer sufferers have an increased risk of this condition. Here it may be difficult to make a distinction between multifactorial inheritance of cancer susceptibility, and inheritance of a dominant gene of reduced penetrance predisposing to cancer.

FAMILIAL ADENOMATOUS POLYPOSIS (FAP)

Previously referred to as 'familial polyposis coli' or 'adenomatosis coli', this condition is now known as 'familial adenomatous polyposis'.[16] In the 1950s, Gardner described associated extracolonic manifestations – skin cysts and osteomata – in certain patients with FAP, in what came to be known as Gardner's Syndrome.[31] It is now apparent that most patients with FAP harbour some extracolonic manifestations, so this distinction of FAP from Gardner's syndrome is no longer made.

Calculations of the prevalence of the condition vary between 1:7000 and 1:30 000.[1,84]

Undetected FAP or new mutations present late with symptoms of rectal bleeding, diarrhoea or obstructive symptoms, if the polyps become malig-

Table 4.12 Inheritance and clinical features of hereditary intestinal neoplastic diseases

Condition	Inheritance	Sites of cancer	Sites of polyps	Histological type	Other features
FAP Gardner's syndrome	AD	Colorectal Adrenal Thyroid Ampulla of Vater (Fibrosarcoma) (Osteogenic sarcoma)	Colon Stomach Duodenum	Adenomas	Dental abnormalities Fibromatosis Sebaceous cysts, lipomas Fibromas Osteomas Neurofibromata Skin lesions – café au lait
Turcot syndrome	AR	Colon CNS ?Thyroid	Rectosigmoid Colonic		
Peutz-Jeghers syndrome	AD	Colon Stomach Duodenum Ovarian (Bladder and bronchial)	Small intestinal Stomach Duodenal Colonic (Respiratory and urinary tract)	Hamartomata and adenomata	Mucocutaneous pigmented lesions
Juvenile polyposis	AD	Gastric Duodenal Colonic	Stomach Small intestine Colon	Adenomata and hamartomata	Sometimes macrocephaly Congenital heart disease Bowel structural abnormalities Mental retardation
Gorlin's syndrome	AD	Basal cell carcinoma (Medulloblastoma) Colorectal	Colorectal	Juvenile polyps	Broad facies Ectopic falx calcification Bony abnormalities Dyskeratotic mandibular and maxillary cysts
Ruvalcaba-Myhre	?AD	Mucoepidermoid parotid	Colon	Hamartomatous juvenile polyposis	Myopathy Macrocephaly Café-au-lait spots on penis and skin
Cowden's disease	AD	Breast Thyroid (Ovarian, uterine, lung) (Melanoma, squamous cell)	Gastrointestinal	Few juvenile polyps Melanomata Lipomata Fibromata Fibrocystic breast disease	Sebaceous cysts (esp. scalp) Skin hamartomata Mucocutaneous lesions Macrocephaly Skin hyperkeratoses and papillomata
Neurofibromatosis	AD	Optic gliomas (and other CNS tumours) GI sarcomata Fibrosarcomata and other peripheral neutrogenic tumours		25% have GI hamartomata and neurofibromata especially small intestinal (single or multiple)	Café-au-lait patches Axillary freckling Lisch nodules in eyes Bony abnormalities Skin neurofibromata
Cronkhite-Canada syndrome	ND	Colon	Small bowel Stomach and colon	Inflammatory polyps	Skin pigmentation Alopecia Onychotrophia
MEN IIB	AD	Medullary thyroid Phaeochromocytoma Parathyroid adenoma	Diffuse GI tract	Ganglioneuromatosis	Mucosal neuromas

AD = Autosomal dominance; AR = autosomal recessive; ND = no data.

nant. Every effort is now being made to ensure cases are detected before symptoms and the risk of malignancy develop.

Genetics of FAP and colon cancer

The locus for the FAP gene has been assigned to the long arm of chromosome 5(5 q 21) by linkage analysis,[8,76,83] following the serendipitous report of a mentally retarded man who had Gardner's syndrome and was found to have a constitutional deletion of chromosome 5.[40] Flanking markers, that is, markers identifying loci on either side of the FAP gene, are now available, clearly localizing the FAP locus to 5 q 21[101] and these can be used as described on page 849 for linkage analysis for predictive testing and prenatal diagnosis for FAP. A 'candidate' for the FAP gene, MCC, which is frequently mutated in colon cancer has recently been identified in the 5 q 21 region.[55] The finding of allelic losses relative to genomic DNA at 5 q 21 in carcinomata, detected by markers identifying loci closely linked to FAP, suggests that the normal FAP gene may be a tumour suppressor gene, similar to those described as being aetiologically significant in Wilms' tumour and retinoblastoma. This conforms to Knudson's hypothesis[56] which was based upon the observation that retinoblastoma, which may occur sporadically but also occurs in a hereditary form, has an earlier age at onset and is more often bilateral in the familial type. He proposed that the tumour was initiated by two mutational events. In the hereditary form, one mutation is inherited in the germ line and the second occurs in somatic cells, whereas in sporadic cases the mutations are both somatic. Statistical analysis appears to bear this out, and the theory also appears to hold true for other hereditary tumours. The finding that the wild-type (normal) allele on chromosome 5 q (inherited from the normal parent) is often demonstrated to be lost in colonic carcinomata in FAP is further evidence in favour of this theory. In sporadic colon cancers, 5 q alleles are also lost.

A number of other non-random genetic changes may be observed in colonic carcinomata (both in familial and sporadic types), and the number of changes seems to be related to the stage of malignancy.[25,96,110] These changes include loss of alleles (or deletions) at 18 q 21.3, and 17 p12-p13, and amplification of K ras and N ras oncogenes. The gene that is involved at 17 p12-13 is the p53 tumour suppressor gene – mutations in the gene can cause the transformation of cultured cells, whilst the normal protein is a DNA binding protein which could act as a tumour suppressor.[4] In colonic cancers, if a 17 p12-13 allele is lost, the remaining allele may be

shown to have a point mutation which is assumed to change it to an oncogene. The gene on 18 q 21 (DCC) specifies a protein homologous to neural cell adhesion proteins. Loss or alteration of function of this molecule may potentiate the process of carcinogenesis.[25]

Clinical pathology

Large bowel disease

Typically in patients with FAP, the mucosa of the colon and rectum remain macroscopically normal until the teenage years, when adenomata begin to appear.[12] There is variation in the numbers of adenomata, ranging from 100 to many thousands.[15] At first there may be only a few, but the rectum is involved early, making diagnosis straightforward.[48] Progression to malignancy is inevitable in the untreated individual, developing, on average, two or three decades earlier than the sporadic form of colorectal cancer.

Extracolonic manifestations

Benign extracolonic lesions may be present before bowel lesions appear. Osteomata develop most commonly in the facial skeleton (accompanied by dental abnormalities including unerupted supernumerary teeth) detectable by orthopantomography[48,106] and in the long bones. Epidermoid cysts can occur anywhere on the body, but are most readily noticed on the scalp.[63] Areas of retinal pigmentation, usually around 50–200 μm in diameter, known as 'congenital hypertrophy of the retinal pigment epithelium', were first reported quite recently.[3,7,18,46,102] Three or more of these areas, usually bilateral, are found in 80–90% of FAP patients and rarely in normal individuals (but who may occasionally be found to have one or two such lesions). It has not yet been clearly established whether there is intrafamilial variability in FAP with respect to hypertrophy of the retinal pigment epithelium.

UPPER GASTROINTESTINAL POLYPS

Over the past 15 years, there has been increasing evidence of the high incidence and clinical importance of these lesions. There are two distinct lesions, the so-called 'fundic gland polyp' and the true adenoma. Fundic gland polyps are sessile, a few millimetres in diameter, and present in about 80% of FAP patients, predominantly in the fundus of the stomach. They are not neoplastic, consisting of cystically dilated fundic glands.[60,65,87] These lesions should be distinguished from the much less common gastric adenomata which may occur, usually in the antrum. Gastric cancer in childhood and adults has been reported in FAP.[82]

Duodenal polyps are uniformly adenomatous and carry a significant risk of malignant transformation.[105,113] They are present in most FAP patients, and are commonest in the periampullary region. They tend to be sessile, pale, and usually 2–7 mm in diameter.[13,108] The reason for this concentration around and within the duodenal ampulla is unknown, but it has recently been suggested that an inherited abnormality of a bile constituent may be responsible.[94] Some patients have developed adenomata or carcinoma in the biliary tree.[22,52,117] At St Mark's Hospital, London, duodenal cancer has become the leading cause of death in FAP patients[48] with an estimated incidence of about 12%,[14] and a relative risk (compared with the general population) of ×100–200.[86]

DESMOID TUMOURS

Desmoid tumours are non-metastasizing, but often locally infiltrative, tumours, composed predominantly of fibrous tissue, with multiple vascular channels within them; they are probably more common in women.[12,48] Most occur in the small bowel mesentery, peritoneum or abdominal wall, although they can occur at other sites.[66] Incidences reported vary widely – between 4%[15] and 13% in FAP sufferers; they are very rare in people who do not have FAP.[66] There is usually an initiating event, such as a surgical procedure (usually colectomy) or pregnancy. Although usually discrete and encapsulated, they may present as a diffusely infiltrating sheet ('mesenteric fibromatosis'). Their growth rate is variable. They cause problems through pressure on the bowel, its blood supply or the ureters. Infiltration can cause haemorrhage or bowel perforation. These effects, together with severe pain in some cases, can produce major morbidity and death.

OTHER LESIONS

Other less common tumours in this condition include brain tumours (especially medulloblastoma), although there may be overlap with reports of Turcot syndrome.[42,48,58,59,103] Papillary thyroid carcinoma is more common, particularly in female FAP patients (with a relative risk in women with FAP calculated as 160 times that in normal women) and has an earlier age at onset than the sporadic form. Hepatoblastoma,[30] malignant adrenal tumours, and small bowel carcinoid tumours have also been reported in a few cases.

Treatment

Large bowel disease

Surgical prophylaxis in FAP is a balance between decreasing the cancer risk and maintaining bowel function and body image. For many years, total proctocolectomy and ileostomy was the preferred procedure.[78] It removed the large bowel cancer risk completely, although with a permanent ileostomy as the price. Retention of the rectum, by performing total colectomy and ileorectal anastomosis (TC + IRA), is a popular compromise – it offers good anorectal function, but with a residual rectal cancer risk of around 2–7%.[34,92,99] The most recent surgical alternative is the restorative proctocolectomy, in which the anal canal is preserved and an ileal pouch–anal anastomosis made. Initially viewed with scepticism by some,[47] for other surgeons this is the operation of choice in FAP.[115,116]

As in most therapeutic situations, the choice of operation depends on circumstances. In the patient who has already developed bowel cancer, total proctocolectomy may be the right procedure.[39] In those with very extensive rectal adenomata, the pouch procedure may be the best; many surgeons feel that for other cases, the balance of advantage lies with total colectomy and ileorectal anastomosis.

After primary prophylactic surgery, surveillance is aimed at continued examination of the upper gastrointestinal tract and the rectum, if still present; the patient who has undergone an ileoanal pouch procedure must continue to be followed up, to check for extracolonic disease, and also because of the theoretical risk of cancer arising in the pouch. Careful surveillance of the retained rectum is vital after total colectomy and ileorectal anastomosis; the rectum should be inspected carefully by outpatient sigmoidoscopy every 6–12 months.[17,47] Fulguration is not necessary for all rectal polyps – it is restricted to larger lesions, or those which, by their numbers, make adequate surveillance difficult.[17]

Desmoid tumours

Although these lesions may feel well circumscribed on examination, involvement of mesenteric vessels may make excision impossible;[66] moreover, they are very likely to recur.[48] Surgical results vary,[37,48,53,66,72,89] so operation should be reserved for those with severe symptoms or life-threatening complications. Incision into desmoid tumours can produce uncontrollable bleeding, so only *complete* resection should be attempted, sometimes requiring considerable small bowel resection because of irretrievable involvement of its vessels.

Radiotherapy and chemotherapy have not been effective in the treatment of desmoid disease, though there have been claims for tamoxifen,[112] sulindac[5] and indomethacin.[111] More recently there have been spectacular reports of the results of treatment with toremifene, an analogue of tamoxifen.[11,117]

Treatment of families

Treatment must be of the family as well as the individual. The FAP Registry maintains an up-to-date record of index cases and their extended families, enabling surveillance of patients to be co-ordinated and facilitating the counselling and screening of relatives who are at risk. There is good evidence that prophylactic treatment of affected individuals substantially reduces mortality from colorectal cancer.[6]

Surveillance in 'call-up cases'

The treatment of heriditary polyposis disorders demands the expertise of many individuals – patients and their families need a multidisciplinary approach to help them deal with their problem with its many physical, social and psychological facets.

Surveillance of relatives at risk generally begins in the early to mid-teens. Simple rigid sigmoidoscopy and biopsy is sufficient as a routine method, as the rectum contains adenomata at an early stage.[1,12,15] A normal sigmoidoscopy result is of increasing value for excluding FAP as the age of the person at risk increases. By the age of 35 years, the chance of an individual (at a 50% prior risk of FAP) with a normal sigmoidoscopy being affected has reduced to about 5%.[81] These age-specific risks of being affected with FAP in the absence of polyps on screening can be combined with linkage information (analysed on blood samples) with DNA markers identifying loci close to the FAP gene, using Bayesian methods, to increase the accuracy of the estimate of risk that a relative of an affected person has of having inherited the gene. In this way, the inheritance from an affected parent of a marker allele close to the FAP gene which in turn had been inherited from the affected grandparent, indicates a high risk to the grandchild that they have inherited the FAP gene. Conversely, inheritance of the opposite allele (from the unaffected grandparents) indicates a low risk.

There is a small risk of inaccuracy of prediction by this method due to the possibility of meiotic recombination between the FAP and marker loci (the frequency of such recombination is measured by the recombination fraction, θ). Predictive accuracy is increased by using marker loci very close to the FAP gene, and using informative loci on both sides of the gene (flanking). Family studies are needed for this type of analysis, as blood is needed from affected relatives to identify which marker is in phase with the disease in each family. Some families are uninformative for certain marker loci if these are not detectably different (heterozygous) on the two chromosomes 5 of key individuals. Hence it is necessary to have several available markers to try in each family. Since the FAP was identified, it has been possible to identify mutations within it in some cases, so that a direct test is available which need not rely on linkage analysis in these families. The effect of combining information from linkage analysis with the sigmoidoscopy findings and examination for retinal pigment epithelium hypertrophy, for the presymptomatic diagnosis of FAP, is shown in *Table 4.13* using markers identifying loci linked to FAP at a recombination fraction of 0.05 with FAP. A similar analysis of the effect of linkage analysis on risk estimation is graphically shown by Murday and Slack.[81]

Most screening regimens discontinue screening by sigmoidoscopy at about 30 years when the risk of FAP is still about 5%. When the above calculations indicate a very low risk – say 1% – to an individual under 30 years of age that they have inherited FAP, it would seem reasonable to screen very infrequently – and to reassure the individual regarding their low risk of having affected children. Individuals at high risk would be screened more vigilantly and advised of their high risk (approaching 50%) of having affected children. Prenatal tests, based on the detection of which linked alleles had been inherited by the unborn baby from its affected parent, could be offered to affected individuals and those at high risk, if blood from other affected relatives in the family is available in order to identify which marker alleles are travelling with the disease gene in the family.

Table 4.13 Risk of FAP to offspring of an affected person

Age (years)	Prior risk (%)	Risk if sigmoidoscopy normal (%)	In addition if linkage indicates low risk ($\theta = 0.05$) (%)	In addition if no CHRPE seen (+ve in 80% FAP) (%)
15	50	30	2.2	0.56
20	50	20	1.3	0.33
25	50	10	0.6	0.15
30	50	5	0.3	0.07

CHRPE = Congenital hypertrophy of the retinal pigment epithelium.

Such tests are done by analysis of fetal DNA samples obtained by chorionic villus biopsy, this now being a fairly safe and routine procedure. The result gives a percentage risk to the fetus of having inherited the disease gene (eg 95% or 5% risk). No information can be given as to the severity of disease in an affected child diagnosed prenatally. The acceptability of prenatal testing for FAP is a very personal question and whether to opt for such testing should be the decision of the family alone.

Screening for affected individuals

Regular upper gastrointestinal endoscopy should be performed in affected individuals in the hope that monitoring of duodenal adenomata will allow early detection and treatment of malignant change – as yet, however, there is no definite evidence that upper gastrointestinal endoscopy prevents cancer deaths. Suggested regimens include initiation of screening at 20 or 30 years, repeating at 1–5 year intervals, as appropriate, and removal of larger adenomata.[49,105,113,114]

Screening for thyroid cancer in affected females should be considered, by palpation and possibly also regular ultrasound examination of the neck.

HEREDITARY NON-POLYPOSIS COLORECTAL CANCER SYNDROMES

Familial adenomatous polyposis has a striking phenotype. However, there are other families in which there appears to be a dominantly inherited predisposition to cancer, the non-polyposis colorectal cancer syndromes, which predispose to colorectal cancer, but show few phenotypic abnormalities, and are therefore difficult to distinguish from sporadic cancers. They appear to be much more common causes of colorectal cancer than FAP, responsible perhaps for 3–5% of all cases compared with 0.5–1% for FAP.[68,74] There are two main recognized types – the so-called site-specific colon cancer syndrome, and the cancer family syndrome, also known as Lynch type I and II syndromes respectively.[69] Members of families with these syndromes develop bowel cancers on average two decades earlier than the mean age for 'sporadic' cancers, and there is a greater proportion of right-sided cancers (65% compared with 25%),[104] of multiple colorectal primaries (25% compared with 5%), and of cancers at other primary sites in the Lynch II syndrome. These include malignancies of other gastrointestinal organs, breast and gynaecological organs, including stomach, skin, lung and bladder, the commonest being gynaecological cancers.[50,75,100,109] The Muir-Torre syndrome may

overlap with Lynch II syndrome. None of this may be obvious when examining the individual case, but gastrointestinal adenomatous polyps (characteristically fewer than 100) are often found in such families, and these may be the premalignant lesions in these conditions;[91] flat adenomata have also been described. Thirty per cent of Lynch syndrome patients have been found to have at least one adenoma, and 20% had multiple lesions compared with 11% and in 4% respectively in age and sex-matched controls.[9,61] The cumulative risk of cancer in people carrying the Lynch II gene has been estimated to be 0.5–0.9.[74]

Genetics

The absence of a characteristic phenotype in affected individuals with the Lynch I syndrome makes linkage analysis difficult in this condition. Linkage between the Kidd blood group on chromosome 18, and Lynch I has been suggested (but not confirmed); this is of particular interest in view of the reported loss of alleles on chromosome 18 (18 q 21) in many colorectal carcinomata.[25] An exciting development recently has been the isolation of a gene (DCC, 'deleted in colon cancer') located at 18 q 21 which is expressed in many tissues, whose expression is greatly reduced or absent in many colorectal carcinomas.[93] Somatic mutations in the DCC gene are demonstrable in some colon cancers; the normal gene product shows homology to neural cell adhesion molecules. Loss of alleles at 18 q is also described in other cancers, implying a possible common pathway in tumorigenesis, and the involvement of loss of normal cell contact growth inhibition in cancer development is an interesting theoretical mechanism for this. Linkage to the chromosome 5 locus for FAP has been found in some families with variable numbers of colonic polyps in affected individuals.[64]

Treatment

Where there is a clear dominant pedigree, offspring of affected individuals with Lynch II syndrome may be taken to be at 50% risk of inheriting the gene for this condition and can be offered screening. As with FAP, the maintenance of genetic registers greatly facilitates the tracing and screening of relatives at risk.[27,67,71] A proportion of the general population have single adenomata, so that the finding of a solitary adenoma in a person at risk is suspicious but not certain evidence of the presence of one non-polyposis colorectal cancer syndromes gene. Clearly, the discovery of markers linked to the syndromes should allow more accurate genetic risk

Table 4.14 Empiric risk of colon cancer

	Relative risk	Counselling risk
Population risk	×1	1:50
One 1st degree relative affected, aged 45 years and under	×5	1:10
Same, over 45 years of age	×3	1:17
Two relatives affected, including related cancers:		
one 1st and one 2nd degree		1:12
two 1st degree relatives affected		1:6
Dominant pedigree (1:2 risk of gene)		1:3

estimation in such families, but when dealing with this type of condition, where the clinical pattern is not always clear-cut, caution must be exercized before using linkage analysis for presymptomatic testing because of the possibility of genetic heterogeneity – that is, that changes at different genetic loci may produce a similar clinical picture.

Recommended guidelines for surveillance of individuals at risk for Lynch II include 6-monthly faecal occult blood testing for individuals at less than a 1 in 10 risk of colon cancer. Where the lifetime risk for colon cancer is greater than that, colonoscopic examination at 25 years followed by colonoscopy at 5-year intervals, until at least 65 years of age, has been recommended in the UK; more frequent examinations are practised in the USA.[71] Total colectomy has been suggested for individuals at high risk. In Lynch II families, surveillance should include yearly clinical review, and in women, pelvic ultrasound and breast examination including mammography at regular, possibly yearly intervals, from about 35 years of age (or from 5 years younger than the earliest cancer in a near relative) as appropriate.[26] The question of how to screen individuals at a less than 50% risk of CFS is difficult.[80] Screening procedures are always less reliable in individuals at a smaller prior risk, with the possibility of false-positive tests increasing as the prior risk decreases. Where no clear autosomal dominant pedigree of CFS is seen, but familial clustering of colon (and other) cancers is observed, empiric lifetime risks of cancer in relatives have been calculated, and screening offered as appropriate.

In practice, individuals with up to a 10% risk of CFS are often offered screening (*Table 4.14*).

OTHER POLYPOSIS SYNDROMES

Peutz-Jeghers syndrome (*See also* Benign tumours, p. 698 and skin disease p. 1328)

This was first described in 1896 and subsequently in 1921 and 1949 by Peutz and Jeghers. It is inherited as

an autosomal dominant trait with high penetrance. The characteristic lesions are dark mucocutaneous pigmentation (melanin flecks) especially on the lips and buccal mucosa and less commonly on the fingers, toes and perianal skin. These lesions develop in childhood and may fade later in adult life. Hamartomas occur in the large and small bowel[24,107] in about 90% of patients, particularly the latter, and there is a significantly increased risk of malignancy[33,57,62] not only of the gastrointestinal tract (relative risk × 13) but also at other sites. Bladder and nasal polyps may occur. Small bowel polyps may declare themselves by causing obstruction (because of intussusception) or by bleeding. As with juvenile polyposis, adenomatous change has been described in the polyps and there is an increased risk of gastrointestinal carcinomas in this condition.[28,33] Cancers have been reported in the thryoid, uterus, ovary, testis, pancreas, breast, lung and liver. A cumulative cancer risk of 22% is reported for these patients, with a 48% chance of dying of cancer by 57 years of age. Management should therefore include mammograms, pelvic ultrasound examinations and cervical smears for women, as well as surveillance of the intestinal polyps by upper gastrointestinal endoscopy, at 2-year intervals, and colonoscopy and removal of polyps.[95] Small bowel contrast studies could be included in this regimen. The children of affected individuals, who have a 50:50 risk of being affected, should be examined for the dermatological features of the condition and the gastrointestinal tract examined if skin changes are present. It is rare for the dermatological features to be absent in an affected person, but this can occur.[36,57] Polyps may develop before the dermatological features. Markers linked to Peutz-Jeghers syndrome are not yet available for predictive (or prenatal) testing.

Juvenile polyposis

This condition, probably inherited as an autosomal dominant trait in some families, was described by McColl *et al.* in 1964.[73] Juvenile polyps often occur sporadically as solitary lesions, but in juvenile polyposis they are usually found in large numbers in the colon (from a few to several hundred), and to a lesser extent in the stomach and small bowel.[23] Clinical presentation is usually within the first decade,[54] with rectal bleeding, diarrhoea, abdominal pain, intussusception and protein-losing enteropathy. Associated abnormalities have been described in affected individuals, including mental retardation, macrocephaly, congenital heart disease, Meckel's diverticulum and gut malrotation, and pulmonary atrioventricular anastomoses.[2,20,54] Juvenile polyps are smooth, pedunculated and hamartomatous, and are composed of epithelial and connective tissue elements but without any muscularis mucosae. Dysplastic changes have been observed histologically in some juvenile polyps, and heterogenity of polyp type may occur, with some adenomata.[90] Initially, juvenile polyposis was not regarded as a premalignant condition, but now an increased cancer risk is recognized, reaching a 68% risk by 60 years of age.[35,51,54,90,98] Recent estimates have shown a relative risk of gastrointestinal cancer of 13 and for other cancers of 9 in this condition.

Some authors have suggested that prophylactic colectomy or regular colonoscopic surveillance should be considered in this condition, with postoperative gastroduodenoscopy and regular rectal inspection.[51]

Muir-Torre syndrome

In 1967 Muir[79] described a patient with multiple benign sebaceous adenomata and keratoacanthomata of the skin, especially of the face, who also developed multiple internal carcinomata. The tumours developed in the large bowel, duodenum and larynx. Subsequent reports of this condition have included familial cases showing an autosomal dominant mode of inheritance.[88] The tumours appear to be of low-grade malignancy and broad spectrum, including cancers of the breast, ovary, uterus, oesophagus and bladder. The syndrome overlaps clinically with the cancer family syndrome,[70] and screening for colon and other cancers should be instituted in those members of such families at risk, as for families demonstrating the Lynch II syndrome.

Turcot syndrome

This is a rare condition in which gastrointestinal adenomata may occur in combination with malignant tumours of the nervous system (usually astrocytomas) which usually prove fatal in early adult life.[10,103] The gastrointestinal polyps are larger than in FAP and fewer in number. The inheritance is

thought to be autosomal recessive because the condition is described in siblings with consanguinity in two families.[19,44,45] Other features of the disease include multiple skin lesions, including seborrhoeic keratoses, café-au-lait patches, and basal cell naevi and carcinomata.[77] It is important to differentiate this syndrome from FAP with central nervous system tumours, particularly because of the difference in inheritance.[77,118]

Gorlin's syndrome

Hamartomatous polyps have been reported in occasional cases of the Gorlin's syndrome, an autosomal dominant syndrome characterized by multiple basal cell carcinomata and other abnormalities, particularly of the skeleton.[77]

Ruvalcaba-Myhre syndrome

This is a rare, probably autosomal dominant syndrome comprising juvenile polyposis with mental retardation, fits, macrocephaly, lipomas and penile freckling.[21]

Cowden's syndrome

Cowden's syndrome is a rare autosomal dominant trait of high, but variable penetrance, characterized by multiple hamartomas of the skin, mucous membranes, breast and thyroid gland, associated with multiple hamartomatous polyps of the gastrointestinal and urinary tracts.[32] There is a high incidence of breast cancer and thyroid abnormalities, and colon adenocarcinoma has been described.[85,97]

Neurofibromata are found in the gastrointestinal tract in up to 25% of cases of neurofibromatosis type I.[41] There are also occasional reports of autosomal dominant inheritance of intestinal neurofibromatosis.[38] Multiple endocrine neoplasia type IIb may also be associated with hyperplasia of the intestinal ganglion cells.[29]

CONCLUSION

Identification of the gene for familial adenomatous polyposis was a significant advance, leading to an acceleration of our research into the molecular basis for colorectal cancer, and advancing our knowledge of the genetic basis of carcinogenesis in gastrointestinal disorders. Similar genetic mechanisms may be involved in both polyposis and nonpolyposis colorectal cancer syndromes, and a search for mutations in the FAP gene in the latter may provide interesting insights into these mechanisms, when the gene has been identified. Linkage analysis should soon locate the genes for Peutz-Jeghers syndrome, Gorlin's syndrome and others, and this information can be applied to genetic counselling in these conditions in due course.

References

1. Alm, T. and Licznerski, G. (1973) The intestinal polyposes. *Clinical Gastroenterology*, **2**, 577–602.
2. Baert, A., Casteels-Van-Dael, M., Broeckx, J., Wijndaele, L., Wilms, G. and Eggermont, E. (1983) Generalized juvenile polyposis with pulmonary arteriovenous malformations and hypertrophic osteoarthropathy. *American Journal of Roentgenology*, **141**, 661–662.
3. Baker, R., Heinemman, M-H., Elston, R. and Schuelke, G. (1988) Hyperpigmented lesions of the retinal pigment epithelium in familial adenomatous polyposis. *American Journal of Medical Genetics*, **31**, 427–435.
4. Baker, S., Fearon, E., Nigro, J. *et al.* (1989) Chromosome 17 deletions and p53 gene mutations in colorectal carcinomas. *Science*, **244**, 217–221.
5. Belliveau, P. and Graham, A. (1984) Mesenteric desmoid tumor in Gardner's syndrome treated by sulindac. *Diseases of the Colon and Rectum*, **27**, 53.
6. Berk, T., Cohen, Z., McLeod, R. and Cullen, J. (1987) Surveillance in relatives of patients with adenomatous polyposis. *Seminars in Surgical Oncology*, **3**, 105–108.
7. Blaire, N. and Trempe, C. (1980) Hypertrophy of the retinal epithelium associated with Gardner's syndrome. *American Journal of Ophthalmology*, **90**, 661–667.
8. Bodmer, W., Bailey, C. and Bodmer, J. (1987) Localization of the gene for familial adenomatous polyposis on chromosome 5. *Nature*, **328**, 614–619.
9. Bonelli, L. (1988) Family history of colorectal cancer as a risk factor for benign and malignant tumours of the large bowel. *International Journal of Cancer*, **41**, 513–517.
10. Braughman, F., List, C., Williams, J., Muldoon, J., Segarra, J. and Volkel, J. (1969) The glioma-polyposis syndrome. *New England Journal of Medicine*, **281**, 1345–1346.
11. Brooks, M., Colletta, A. and Baum, M. (1990) Abstracts from the third meeting of the Leeds Castle Polyposis Group. The use of triphenylethylene drugs with desmoid tumours. *International Journal of Colorectal Disease*, **5**, 53–54.
12. Bulow, S. (1986) Familial polyposis coli. A clinical and epidemiological study. Denmark: Laegeforeningens Forlag.
13. Bulow, S., Lauritsen, K. and Johansen, A. (1985) Gastroduodenal polyps in familial polyposis coli. *Diseases of the Colon and Rectum*, **28**, 90–93.
14. Bussey, H. (1972) Extracolonic lesions associated with polyposis coli. *Proceedings of the Royal Society of Medicine*, **65**, 294.
15. Bussey, H. (1975) Familial polyposis coli. Family studies, histopathology, differential diagnosis and results of treatment. pp. 59–63. Baltimore: Johns Hopkins University Press.
16. Bussey, H. (1987) Historical developments in familial polyposis coli. *Seminars in Surgical Oncology*, **3**, 67–70.
17. Bussey, H., Ayers, A., Ritchie, S. and Thomson, J. (1985) The rectum in adenomatous polyposis. The St Mark's policy. *British Journal of Surgery suppl*, **72**, S29–S35.
18. Chapman, P., Church, W., Burn, J. and Gunn, A. (1989) Congenital hypertrophy of retinal pigment epithelium: a sign of familial adenomatous polyposis. *British Medical Journal*, **298**, 353–354.
19. Costa, O., Silva, D., Colnago, F., Vieira, M. and Musso, C. (1987) Turcot syndrome. Autosomal dominant or recessive transmission? *Diseases of the Colon and Rectum*, **30**, 391–394.
20. Cox, K., Frates, R., Wang, A. and Gandhi, G. (1980) Hereditary juvenile polyposis associated with pulmonary a-v malformation. *Gastroenterology*, **78**, 1566–1570.
21. Di Liberti, J., D'Agostino, A., Ruvalcaba, R. and Schimschock, J. (1984) A new lipid storage myopathy observed in individuals with the Ruvalcaba-Myhre-Smith syndrome. *American Journal of Medical Genetics*, **18**, 163–167.
22. Ekelund, G. and Carlsson, U. (1986) Duodenal and jejunal carcinomas in familial adenomatosis of the large bowel. *Digestive Diseases and Sciences*, **31**, 35S.
23. Erbe, R. (1976) Inherited gastrointestinal syndromes. *Annals of Internal Medicine*, **83**, 639–644.
24. Estrada, R. and Spjut, H. (1983) Hamartomatous polyps in Peutz-Jeghers syndrome. *American Journal of Surgical Pathology*, **7**, 747–754.
25. Fearon, E., Cho, K., Nigro, J., Kern, S., Simons, J. and Ruppert, J. (1990) Identification of a chromosome 18q gene that is altered in colorectal cancers. *Science*, **247**, 49.
26. Fitzgibbons, R. (1990) Surgical strategies for management of the Lynch Syndromes. In *Hereditary Colorectal Cancer* (Eds) Utsunomiya, J., Lynch, H.T. pp. 211–217. Springer-Verlag.
27. Fitzgibbons, R., Lynch, H. and Stanislav, G. (1987) Recognition and treatment of patients with hereditary non-polyposis colon cancer (Lynch syndromes I and II). *Annals of Surgery*, **206**, 289–295.
28. Foley, T. and McGarrity, T.A.A. (1988) Peutz Jeghers syndrome. A clinicopathological survey of the "Harrisburg family" with a 49 year follow-up. *Gastroenterology*, **95**, 1535–1540.
29. Fryns, J. and Chrzanowska, Z. (1988) Mucosal neuromata syndrome. *Journal of Medical Genetics*, **25**, 703–706.
30. Garber, J., Li, F., Kingston, J. *et al.* (1988)

Hepatoblastoma and familial adenomatous polyposis. *Journal of the National Cancer Institute*, **80**, 1626–1628.

31. Gardner, E. (1962) Follow-up study of a family group exhibiting dominant inheritance for a syndrome including intestinal polyps and osteomatosis. *American Journal of Human Genetics*, **14**, 376–390.

32. Gentry, W., Eskritt, N. and Gorlin, R. (1978) Multiple hamartoma syndrome (Cowden's disease). *Archives of Dermatology*, **114**, 743–746.

33. Giardello, F., Welsh, S., Hamilton, S. *et al.* (1987) Increased risk of cancer in the Peutz-Jeghers syndrome. *New England Journal of Medicine*, **316**, 1511–1514.

34. Gingold, B., Jagelman, D. and Turnbull, R. (1979) Surgical management of familial polyposis and Gardner's syndrome. *American Journal of Surgery*, **137**, 54.

35. Grotsky, H., Rickert, R., Smith, W. and Newsome, J. (1982) Familial juvenile polyposis coli. *Gastroenterology*, **82**, 494–501.

36. Haggitt, R. and Reid, B. (1986) Hereditary gastrointestinal polyposis syndromes. *American Journal of Surgical Pathology*, **10**, 871–887.

37. Harvey, J., Quan, S. and Fortner, J. (1979) Gardner's syndrome complicated by mesenteric desmoid tumours. *Surgery*, **85**, 475–477.

38. Heiman, E. and Verhost, A. (1988) Intestinal neurofibromatosis. *Neurofibromatosis*, **1**, 26–32.

39. Heimann, T., Bolnick, K. and Aufses, A. (1986) Results of surgical treatment for familial polyposis coli. *American Journal of Surgery*, **152**, 276–278.

40. Herrera, L., Kakatis, S. and Gibas, L. (1986) Gardner syndrome in a man with an intestinal deletion of 5q. *American Journal of Medical Genetics*, **25**, 473–476.

41. Hochberg, F., Da Silva, A, Galdatini, J. and Richardson, E. (1974) Gastrointestinal involvement in Von Recklinghausen's neurofibromatosis. *Neurology*, **24**, 1144–1151.

42. Hoh, H. and Ohsato, K. (1985) Turcot syndrome and its characteristic colonic manifestations. *Diseases of the Colon and Rectum*, **28**, 399–402.

43. Houlston, R., Murday, V., Harocopos, C., Williams, C. and Slack, S. (1990) Screening and genetic counselling for relatives of patients with colorectal cancer in a family cancer clinic. *British Medical Journal*, **301**, 366–368.

44. Itoh, H. and Ohsato, K. (1985) Turcot syndrome and its characteristic colonic manifestations. *Diseases of the Colon and Rectum*, **28**, 399–402.

45. Itoh, H., Ohsato, K., Yao, T., Iida, M. and Watanabe, H. (1979) Turcot's syndrome and its mode of inheritance. *Gut*, **20**, 414–419.

46. Iwama, T., Mishima, Y., Okamoto, N. and Inoue, J. (1990) Association of congenital hypertrophy of the retinal pigment epithelium with familial adenomatous polyposis. *British Journal of Surgery*, **77**, 273–276.

47. Jagelman, D. (1983) Familial polyposis coli. *Surgical Clinics of North America*, **63**, 117–128.

48. Jagelman, D. (1988) The expanding spectrum of familial adenomatous polyposis. *Perspectives in Colon and Rectal Surgery*, **1**, 30–46.

49. Jagelman, D., DeCosse, J. and Bussey, H. (1988) Upper gastrointestinal cancer in familial adenomatous polyposis. *Lancet*, **i**, 1149–1151.

50. Jarvinen, H. (1988) Familial cancer. *Acta Oncologica*, **27**, 783–786.

51. Jarvinen, H. and Fransilla, K. (1984) Familial juvenile polyposis coli: increased risk of colorectal cancer. *Gut*, **25**, 792–800.

52. Jarvinen, H., Nyberg, M. and Peltikallio, P. (1983) Biliary involvement in familial polyposis coli. *Diseases of the Colon and Rectum*, **26**, 525–528.

53. Jarvinen, H., Peltokallio, P., Landtman, M. and Wolf, J. (1982) Gardner's stigmas in patients with familial adenomatous coli. *British Journal of Surgery*, **69**, 718–721.

54. Jass, J., Williams, C., Bussey, H. and Morson, B. (1988) Juvenile polyposis – a precancerous condition. *Histopathology*, **13**, 619–630.

55. Kinzler, K., Nilbert, M., Vogelstein, B. *et al.* (1991) Identification of a gene located at chromosome 5q21 that is mutated in colorectal cancer. *Science*, **251**, 1366–1370.

56. Knudson, A. (1971) Mutation and cancer: statistical study of retinoblastoma. *Proceedings of the National Academy of Science*, **68**, 820–823.

57. Konishi, F., Wyse, N., Muto, T. *et al.* (1987) Peutz-Jeghers polyposis associated with carcinoma of the digestive organs. Report of three cases and review of the literature. *Diseases of the Colon and Rectum*, **30**, 790–799.

58. Kopitak, M., Jagelman, D., Fazio, V., Lavery, I. and McGannon, E. (1988) Brain tumours in familial adenomatous polyposis. *Diseases of the Colon and Rectum*, **32**, 778–782.

59. Kumar, D., Blank, C. and Ponder, B. (1989) A family with Turcot syndrome suggesting autosomal dominant inheritance. *Journal of Medical Genetics*, **26**, 592.

60. Kurtz, R., Sternberg, S., Muller, H. and DeCosse, J. (1987) Upper gastrointestinal neoplasia in familial polyposis. *Digestive Diseases and Sciences*, **32**, 459–465.

61. Lanspa, S., Lynch, H., Smyrk, T. *et al.* (1990) Colorectal adenomas in the Lynch Syndromes. Results of a colonoscopy screening program. *Gastroenterology*, **98**, 1117–1122.

62. Lehur, P., Madarnas, P., Devroede, G., Perey, B., Menard, D. and Hamade, N. (1984) Peutz-Jeghers syndrome. Association of duodenal and bilateral breast cancers in the same patient. *Digestive Diseases and Sciences*, **29**, 178–182.

63. Leppard, B. (1974) Epidermoid cysts and polyposis coli. *Proceedings of the Royal Society of Medicine*, **67**, 1036.

64. Leppert, M., Burt, R., Hughes, J. *et al.* (1990)

Genetic analysis of an inherited predisposition to colon cancer in a family with a variable number of adenomatous polyps. *New England Journal of Medicine*, **322**, 904–908.

65. Lida, M. (1984) Fundic gland polyposis in patients with familial adenomatous polyposis. Its incidence and clinical features. *Gastroenterology*, **86**, 1437–1442.

66. Lotfi, A., Dozois, R. and Gordon, H. (1989) Mesenteric fibromatosis complicating familial adenomatous polyposis: predisposing factors and results of treatment. *International Journal of Colorectal Disease*, **4**, 30–36.

67. Lynch, H. (1985) Hereditary non polyposis colon cancer: epidemiology and clinical genetic features. *Colon Cancer Genetics*, 52–98.

68. Lynch, H. (1986) Frequency of hereditary non-polyposis colorectal carcinoma. *Gastroenterology*, **90**, 486–496.

69. Lynch, H. (1988) Differential diagnosis of hereditary non-polyposis colorectal cancer (Lynch syndrome I and Lynch syndrome II). *Diseases of the Colon and Rectum*, **31**, 372–377.

70. Lynch, H., Fusaro, R., Roberts, L., Voorhees, G. and Lynch, J. (1985) Muir-Torre syndrome in several members of a family with a variant of the cancer family syndrome. *British Journal of Dermatology*, **113**, 295–301.

71. Lynch, P. and Winn, R. (1989) Clinical management of hereditary non polyposis colon cancer. Hematology/Oncology Clinics of North America, **3**, 75–86.

72. McAdam, W. and Goligher, J. (1970) The occurrence of desmoids in patients with FPC. *British Journal of Surgery*, **57**, 618–631.

73. McColl, I., Bussey, H., Veale, A. and Morson, B. (1964) Juvenile polyposis coli. *Proceedings of the Royal Society of Medicine*, **57**, 896–897.

74. Mecklin, J-P. (1987) Frequency of hereditary colorectal carcinoma. *Gastroenterology*, **93**, 1021–1025.

75. Mecklin, J. and Jarvinen, H. (1986) Clinical features of colorectal cancer in Cancer Family Syndrome. *Diseases of the Colon and Rectum*, **29**, 160–164.

76. Meera Khan, P., Tops, C. and c d Broek, M. (1988) Close linkage of a highly polymorphic marker (D5 S37) to familial adenomatous polyposis and confirmation of FAP localisation of chromosome 5q21-11. *Human Genetics*, **79**, 183–185.

77. Michels, V.V. and Stevens, J. (1982) Basal cell carcinomata in a patient with intestinal polyposis. *Clinical Genetics*, **22**, 80–82.

78. Moertel, C., Hill, J. and Adson, M. (1970) Surgical management of multiple polyposis: the problem of cancer in the retain bowel segment. *Archives of Surgery*, **100**, 521–525.

79. Muir, E., Yates-Bell, A. and Barlow, K. (1967) Multiple primary carcinomata of the colon, duodenum and larynx associated with keratoacanthomata of the face. *British Journal of Surgery*, **54**, 191–195.

80. Murday, V. (1990) Screening for Colorectal Cancer. *UKCCCR* (Ed.) Hardcastle, J.D. pp. 9–15. Normed-Verlag.

81. Murday, V. and Slack, J. (1989) Inherited disorders associated with colorectal cancer. *Cancer Surveys*, **8**, 139–157.

82. Murphy, E., Mireles, M. and Beltran, A. (1962) Familial polyposis of the colon and gastric carcinoma. Concurrent conditions in a 16 year old boy. *Journal of the American Medical Association*, **179**, 1026.

83. Nakamura Yea. (1988) Localisation of the genetic defect in FAP within a small region of chromosome 5. *American Journal of Human Genetics*, **43**, 638–644.

84. Neel J. (1954) Problems in the estimation of the frequency of uncommon inherited traits. *American Journal of Human Genetics*, **6**, 51.

85. Nuss, D., Aeling, J., Clemons, D. and Weber, W. (1978) Multiple hamartomata syndrome (Cowden's Disease). *Archives of Dermatology*, **114**, 743–746.

86. Pauli, R., Pauli, M. and Hall, J. (1980) Gardner's syndrome and periampullary malignancy. *American Journal of Medical Genetics*, **6**, 205–219.

87. Ranzi, T., Gastagnone, D., Velio, P., Bianchi, P. and Polli, E. (1981) Gastric and duodenal polyps in familial polyposis coli. *Gut*, **22**, 263–267.

88. Reiffers, J., Laugier, P. and Hunziker, N. (1976) Hyperplasies sebacees keratoacanthomes, epitheliomes du visage et cancer du colon: une nouvelle entite? *Dermatologica*, **153**, 23–33.

89. Richards, R., Rogers, S. and Gardner, E. (1987) Spontaneous mesenteric fibrosis in Gardner's syndrome. *Cancer*, **47**, 597–601.

90. Rozen, P. and Baratz, M. (1982) Familial juvenile polyposis with associated colon cancer. *Cancer*, **49**, 1500–1503.

91. Rozen, P., Fireman, Z., Figer, A., Legum, C., Ron, E. and Lynch, H. (1987) Family history of colorectal cancer as a marker of potential malignancy within a screening program. *Cancer*, **60**, 248–254.

92. Schaupp, W. and Volpe, P. (1972) Management of diffuse colonic polyposis. *American Journal of Surgery*, **124**, 218.

93. Solomon, E. (1990) Colorectal cancer genes. *Nature*, **343**, 412–414.

94. Spigelman, Aea. (1989) Upper GI cancer in patients with familial adenomatous polyposis. *Lancet*, **ii**, 783–785.

95. Spigelman, A. and Phillips, R. (1989) Management of the Peutz-Jeghers patients. *Journal of the Royal Society of Medicine*, **82**, 681.

96. Stanbridge, E. (1990) Identifying tumour suppressor genes in human colorectal cancer. *Science*, **247**, 12–13.

97. Starink, T., Van der Veen, J., Arwert, F. *et al.* (1986) The Cowden syndrome: a clinical and

genetic study in 21 patients. *Clinical Genetics*, **29**, 222–223.

98. Stemper, T., Kent, T. and Summers, R. (1975) Juvenile polyposis and gastrointestinal carcinoma. *Annals of Internal Medicine*, **83**, 639–646.

99. Sugihara, K., Muto, T. and Kamiya, J. (1982) Gardner's syndrome associated with periampullary carcinoma, duodenal and gastric adenomatosis. *Diseases of the Colon and Rectum*, **25**, 766.

100. Swaroop, V., Winawer, S., Kurtz, R. and Lipkin, M. (1987) Multiple primary malignant tumors. *Gastroenterology*, **93**, 779–783.

101. Tops, C., Griffioen, G., Vasen, H. *et al.* (1989) Presymptomatic diagnosis of familial adenomatous polyposis by bridging DNA markers. *Lancet*, **ii**, 1361–1363.

102. Traboulsi, E., Krush, A. and Gardner, E. (1987) Prevalence and importance of pigmented ocular lesions in Gardner's syndrome. *New England Journal of Medicine*, **316**, 661–667.

103. Turcot, J., Despres, J-P. and St Pierre, F. (1959) Malignant tumours of the central nervous system assessed with familial polyposis of the colon. *Diseases of the Colon and Rectum*, **2**, 465–468.

104. Ushio, K. (1990) Hereditary non-polyposis colorectal cancer and tumorigenesis in the human body. In *Hereditary Colorectal Cancer* (Ed.) Utsunomiya, J. and Lynch, H. T. pp. 107–113. Springer-Verlag.

105. Utsunomiya, J.T.I. (1980) Adenomatosis coli in Japan. pp. 83–95. New York: Raven Press.

106. Utsunomiya, J. and Nakamura, T. (1975) The occult osteomatous changes in the mandible in patients with familial polyposis coli. *British Journal of Surgery*, **62**, 45–51.

107. Utsunomiya, J., Gocho, H., Mizanaga, T. *et al.* (1975) Peutz-Jeghers syndrome: its natural course and management. *Johns Hopkins Medical Journal*, **136**, 71–82.

108. van Stolk, R., Sivak, M., Petrini, J., Petras, R., Ferguson, D. and Jagelman, D. (1987) Endoscopic management of upper gastrointestinal polyps and periampullary lesions in familial adenomatous polyposis and Gardner's syndrome. *Endoscopy*, **19**, 19–22.

109. Vasen, H., den Hartog Jager, F. and Menko, F. (1989) Screening for hereditary non-polyposis colorectal cancer: a study of 22 kindreds in the Netherlands. *American Journal of Medicine*, **86**, 278–281.

110. Vogelstein, B., Fearon, E., Hamilton, S. *et al.* (1988) Genetic alterations during colorectal tumor development. *New England Journal of Medicine*, **319**, 525–532.

111. Waddell, W. and Gemer, R. (1980) Indomethacin and ascorbate inhibit desmoid tumours. *Journal of Surgical Oncology*, **15**, 85.

112. Waddell, W., Gemer, R. and Reich, M. (1983). Non-steroid anti-inflammatory drugs and tamoxifen for desmoid tumours and carcinoma of the stomach. *Journal of Surgical Oncology*, **22**, 197.

113. Watanabe, H., Enjoji, M. and Yao, T. (1977) Accompanying gastro-enteric lesions in familial adenomatosis coli. *Acta Pathological Japonica*, **27**, 823–839.

114. Watanabe, H., Enjoji, M., Yao, T. and Ohsato, K. (1978) Gastric lesions in familial adenomatosis coli: their incidence and histological analysis. *Human Pathology*, **9**, 269–283.

115. Welling, D. and Beart, R. (1987) Surgical alternatives in the treatment of polyposis coli. *Seminars in Surgical Oncology*, **3**, 99–104.

116. Williams, N. (moderator). (1986) Restorative proctocolectomy with ileal reservoir. *International Journal of Colorectal Disease*, **1**, 2–19.

117. Wilson, A., Baum, M., Singh, L. and Kangas, L. (1987) Antioestrogen therapy of pure mesenchymal tumour (letter). *Lancet*, **i**, 508.

118. Yaffee, H. (1964) Gastric polyposis and soft tissue tumors. *Archives of Dermatology*, **89**, 806–808.

MALIGNANT TUMOURS *(N.S. Williams)*

Malignant disease of the large bowel was responsible for 17 223 deaths in England and Wales in 1990 and is now second only to lung cancer as a cause of death from malignant disease.[179] The situation is similar in the USA, where colorectal carcinoma is now the commonest solid tumour except for the skin. While progress has been made in aetiology, in improving early diagnosis and in the development of new surgical techniques, the disease still remains a major challenge to physicians, surgeons and scientists alike.

Ninety-eight per cent of all malignant large bowel tumours are adenocarcinomas. The other epithelial tumours are carcinoid or squamous cell carcinoma. The latter nearly always arise from the anorectum and are considered elsewhere in this book. Tumours of mesenchymal origin (sarcomas and malignant melanoma) may also occur in the large bowel.

ADENOCARCINOMA

Geographical distribution

The highest incidences of both colonic and rectal cancer are seen in Western Europe and North America, whereas intermediate rates prevail in Eastern Europe (*Table 4.15*). The lowest rates are seen in Asia, Africa and South America, excluding Argentina.[233] The incidence of rectal carcinoma varies less internationally than does cancer of the colon. Variations in incidence between countries are

Table 4.15 Incidence of colorectal cancer in different countries.*

		Colonic	Rectal	Colorectal
Nigeria		1.3	1.2	2.5
India		4.6	4.4	9.0
Osaka (Japan)		6.3	6.9	13.2
East Germany		13.6	12.0	25.6
Vas (Hungary)		9.1	11.0	20.1
Connecticut (USA)		30.1	18.2	48.3
Detroit (USA)	White	26.2	16.0	42.2
	Black	24.5	13.8	38.3
Birmingham (UK)		16.5	16.1	32.6
Oxford (UK)		15.7	15.4	31.1
Ayrshire (UK)		16.6	14.0	30.0
Denmark		16.2	16.7	32.9
Finland		7.9	7.7	15.6
New Zealand	Maori	7.4	4.6	12.0
	Non-Maori	23.0	15.4	38.4
Hawaii	Japanese	22.4	16.3	38.7
	Caucasian	23.9	13.5	37.4
	Hawaiian	14.1	9.4	23.5

*Per 100 000 age-adjusted to world population.
Adapted from Waterhouse et al. (1976).[224]

much larger than variations within each country, but the disease seems to occur more frequently in urban than in rural areas.[36,233]

Some of the differences in geographical variation may be due to failure of detection in low incidence areas, where techniques for diagnosis are less sophisticated and patient tolerance of symptoms is high. However, this explanation probably only accounts for a small part of the variations and does not explain, for example, the marked differences in incidence between Denmark and Finland or the low rate recorded in Japan.[121]

Aetiology

Although the basic processes underlying the development of large bowel cancer are unknown, considerable strides have been made in understanding the genetic basis of the disease.

The high incidence of colorectal cancer in 'sophisticated' western society suggested that environmental factors were aetiologically more important than genetic factors. Further evidence to support this suggestion came from studies involving migrants; the risk increased among Japanese as they moved from low-incidence Japan to high-risk USA.[98] The incidence of carcinoma among European Jews in Israel was higher than that among Asian and African-born Jews.[163] Similar observations were made in Polish migrants moving to the USA and Australia.[209] It is now realized that, although en-

vironmental factors are very important in the aetiology of the disease, they probably act in many patients on an original genetic defect. If such patients are exposed to certain of these environmental factors throughout their lives, further genetic damage occurs which culminates in the development of cancer.

Dietary factors, bacteria and bile salts

As epidemiological studies point to factors associated with Western society as being of aetiological importance, it is no surprise that diet has received most attention.

There is indirect evidence that a diet rich in animal fat is a major risk factor. The proportion of fat in the Western diet is significantly greater than that in the diet of low-risk populations.[256] Some nutritional statistics on fat and meat consumption correlate positively with the incidence of colonic cancer[6,50] and case-control studies support the association.[45,99] Nevertheless, this view has been challenged. Enström[62] noted that a steady increase in the frequency of beef consumption in the USA from 1940 to 1970 was accompanied by stable or declining rates of incidence and mortality from colorectal disease. No association between fat intake and colorectal cancer was demonstrated when populations in Finland (low risk) and Denmark (high risk) were compared.[120] A carefully conducted case-control study performed as part of the Japan–Hawaii Cancer Study was also unable to confirm an association.[211]

The implication of fat as a possible aetiological factor is linked to the concept that the Western diet favours the development of a bacterial flora containing organisms which are capable of degrading bile salts to carcinogens, possibly related to methylcholanthrene.[255] It has been suggested[113] that *Clostridium paraputrificum* is the responsible organism. Many studies comparing faecal flora in high and low risk populations have now been performed. Although certain organisms have been identified in the high-risk populations, no study has succeeded in linking a specific bacterium with colorectal cancer.[41,42,66,83,150,152,155] It is difficult to draw definite conclusions from studies of this sort since only small numbers of patients have been investigated and any individual may have up to 400 species of bacteria in the gut.

The role that bile acids play in the development of carcinoma is uncertain. Bile acids can promote colorectal cancer in animals.[111,112] Human studies have involved epidemiological surveys which have compared populations at various levels of risk and have implicated bile acids in aetiology.[41,110,112] Case-control studies comparing faecal bile acid concentrations in bowel cancer cases and controls, however, have not shown such a clear relationship.[112] Nevertheless, there does seem to be a relationship between bile acids and benign adenomas, although further corroborative data are awaited.[110,195,236,237]

The increased incidence of right-sided colonic neoplasm in patients who have previously undergone cholecystectomy[137,225,229] is of interest but remains to be established. This operation increases the production and turnover of degraded bile salts.[190]

In summary, therefore, although dietary fat, bacteria and bile salts have all been implicated in colorectal carcinogenesis, proof that any of them is directly involved is lacking.

A low intake of dietary fibre may also predispose the individual to carcinoma. The theory propagated by Burkitt[20] is that lack of fibre reduces faecal bulk, prolongs intestinal transit and allows faecal carcinogens a longer contact time with the mucosa than occurs with a diet rich in fibre. There is substantial indirect evidence to support this theory. Several case-control studies have shown a negative association between colorectal cancer and dietary intake of vegetables; the average weight of faeces is heavier in low-risk groups compared with high-risk groups.[211] Furthermore, higher fibre intake and more rapid intestinal transit have been recorded in high risk groups.[21] These studies can be criticized since the populations compared differed in various respects other than dietary intake. Only one large epidemiological study with adequate control data has demonstrated a low risk of colon cancer for those with a high fibre intake,[164] whereas several international surveys have been unable to do so.[6,50]

Other dietary components have been implicated from time to time. Several authors[30,257] have related high sugar intake to the development of the disease. Similarly, excessive beer consumption has been suggested as a possible risk factor[18] but controlled studies have not confirmed this impression.[119]

Adenomatous polyps

There is a relationship between benign polyps and carcinoma but this is not fully understood. The evidence that adenomas have malignant potential is based on several observations. Examination of operative specimens demonstrate that one or more adenomas are present in nearly one-third of cases with carcinoma.[174] Furthermore, the remaining bowel in these patients is twice as likely to develop a second (or metachronous) tumour compared with patients who have no associated polyp.[23] Adenomas coexist in 75% of cases in which two or more carcinomas are present simultaneously. The finding of benign tissue in a colon carcinoma and vice versa lends weight to the argument.[176] Furthermore, many pathologists have shown a transition from a benign to a malignant neoplastic process on histological examination of polyps [51,58,70,141,171,234,245] and there is now evidence of genetic changes that occur in polyps which result in their transformation to carcinoma (see later). These observations are supported by the invariable development of carcinoma in patients with familial adenomatous polyposis. While benign polyps can undergo malignant change the proportion that will do so and which factors cause this transformation, are unknown. Some pathologists believe that most carcinomas develop from benign adenomatous polyps (the adenoma–carcinoma sequence). This concept is supported by Morson[172] who showed that of tumours confined to the submucosa alone, 60% had contiguous benign adenomatous tissue, whereas with carcinomas that extended into extramural fat this percentage was much reduced. On the other hand, several pathologists have studied many hundred of specimens[27,63,208] and failed to find any benign adenomatous tissue even in carcinomas of less than 2 cm in diameter.[207]

The malignant potential of villous papillomas is not disputed. The frequency of malignant change arising in these tumours varies between 6 and 75%[67,69] with a median incidence of approximately 30%.[94,216]

Inflammatory diseases

The colorectal cancer risk in patients with long-standing ulcerative colitis is well appreciated while the relationship between Crohn's colitis and colonic carcinoma is less certain (see Chapter 7).

Although diverticular disease and carcinoma often coexist and make diagnosis difficult[212] there is no evidence to link the two disorders. Similarly although tumour-like granulomas of amoebiasis, tuberculosis or very rarely syphilis may be confused with a carcinoma, no case has yet been described in which carcinoma has been attributed to the underlying infection.

Schistosomiasis may be a precursor of carcinoma in China. Both diseases are endemic and frequently coexist. In addition the histological changes which precede the development of malignancy are similar to those in ulcerative colitis. Eradication of the infection reduces the incidence of carcinoma. Further studies are eagerly awaited.[28,29]

Genetic factors

Although environment factors play a primary role in colonic carcinogenesis as noted previously, hereditary factors play a greater role than was previously appreciated.

There are three variants of hereditary polyposis coli which eventually lead to the development of carcinoma. Familial polyposis coli, now known as familial adenomatous polyposis is an autosomal dominant disorder characterized by innumerable colonic and rectal adenomas.[40,140] Fifty per cent of children of polyposis families are likely to inherit the disease. Carcinoma most frequently develops about 15 years after the commencement of symptoms at about 35 years of age. The risk of developing carcinoma is approximately 1% by 16 years of age, 50% by 28 to 30 years of age and 90% by 40 to 45 years of age.[22,227,228]

Gardner's syndrome is a variant of familial adenomatous polyposis and involves the same risks.[78] The colonic polyps are associated with sebaceous cysts, dermoid tumours, fibromas, facial bone osteomas and abnormal dentition. There is an increased susceptibility to other carcinomas including those of thyroid, the ampulla of Vater, the duodenum and the adrenal gland. Turcot's syndrome is the third variant in which tumours of the CNS occur with the colonic polyps.[223]

Apart from familial adenomatous polyposis and its variants, there appears to be another group of patients who have a hereditary predisposition to develop large bowel carcinoma. These patients have been classified as suffering from hereditary nonpolyposis colon cancer (HNPCC) so that they can be differentiated from those with hereditary polyposis.

Since the term was originally coined, nonpolyposis cancers have been subdivided into two main syndromes, also named Lynch types I and II.[148] Both are inherited through autosomal dominant genes.

CANCER FAMILY SYNDROME (LYNCH TYPE I)

This is a rare syndrome first noted by Warthin in 1913 who described four families with a remarkable number of multiple cancers. Lynch and Krush[144] at a later date went on to study one of these families and found a malignant neoplasm in 6500 family members. The same authors investigated similar families and coined the term 'cancer family syndrome'.[145]

The criteria for diagnosis are:

1. An increased incidence of adenocarcinoma, primarily in the colon and endometrium.
2. An increased incidence of multiple primary malignant neoplasms.
3. Early stage of onset and autosomal dominant inheritance.[148]

SITE-SPECIFIC COLON CANCER SYNDROME (LYNCH TYPE II)

In this condition the large bowel is the principle site for malignancies. There is a tendency for tumours to occur at a younger age, to be multiple and to be more frequently situated in the right colon.[143]

Individuals who belong to one of these two types of families are difficult to recognize and so, for purposes of screening and risk estimation, an individual can be assumed to be a member of one of these families if they have three first-degree relatives with colorectal cancer and the other commonly occurring adenocarcinomas in CFS cancer family syndrome.[174]

There are individuals who have first-degree relatives with the disease and yet do not necessarily belong to one of these two cancer family syndromes. The incidence with which colorectal carcinoma is found in first-degree relatives of patients with the disease varies between 3.4% and 8.6%.[19,149,251] The risk of developing a colorectal cancer in first-degree relatives has been calculated to be between two and four times the risk in the general population.[4,143,149,251] The risk is similar in relatives of patients with adenomas. There is also a threefold increased risk to the relatives of colorectal cancer patients or probands with adenomas.[17,24]

Lovett[143] calculated the empiric risks to individuals of developing colorectal cancer based on their family trees.

Contributions made by molecular biologists and geneticists over the last decade to our understanding of the genetic basis of colorectal cancer has been of the utmost importance. Changes at the cellular level may well explain the carcinomas that arise in the cancer family syndrome and in patients with a positive family history: whether they are responsible for sporadic cases is less certain. In familial adenomatous polyposis alterations of gene structure and expression have been noted.[8,15] The striking abnormality is an allelic deletion of the long arm of chromosome 5.[15,131,134,231] It has been suggested[15] that the polyposis gene locus may encode a tumour suppressor gene similar to other inherited tumours. Such genes could function recessively, with inactivation of both the alleles required to have an effect (through deletion or mutation). In the progression of colonic cells to adenomas and carcinomas, additional multiple, acquired genetic changes occur.[65,131,206,239] These include mutation in a Ras oncogene and deletion of a segment of chromosomes 17 and 18, but these changes are largely limited to advanced tumours.[131,231] Not every tumour shows all of these genetic alterations or the same sequence of changes. Dominant changes in familial adenomatous polyposis may not explain the recessive changes also occurring in sporadic colonic cancer. Loss of alleles at a single locus is unlikely to explain all the major genetic changes occurring in colon cancer.[131,206,231] The significance of these genetic changes particularly in the sporadic cases is still to be determined but there is little doubt that they hold the key to understanding the aetiology of colorectal cancer.

Pathology

Distribution of carcinoma within the large bowel

Variations in the classification of rectosigmoid growths create difficulties in determining the relative distribution of carcinoma of the colon and rectum. On balance, however, it seems that half the tumours of the large bowel are situated in the rectum. Within the colon approximately 50% occur in the sigmoid colon and 25% occur in the caecum and ascending colon. The remaining 25% are distributed in order of frequency as follows: transverse colon, splenic flexure, descending colon and hepatic flexure.[73,122,127,207] In the rectum approximately 70% occur in the upper and lower thirds in equal proportions.[84]

Multiple carcinomas

About 3% of patients will have two or more tumours present simultaneously, i.e. synchronous tumours.[86] In those patients without concomitant ulcerative colitis or familial adenomatous polyposis, 75% will have associated benign adenomas.[104]

Macroscopic features

There are five varieties of colorectal cancer which can be identified by their gross appearance.

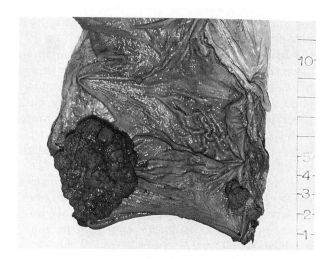

Figure 4.59 Polypoid carcinoma in the upper rectum.

POLYPOID OR CAULIFLOWER LESION

This lesion (*Figure 4.59*) protrudes into the lumen of the bowel, is often ulcerated over part of its surface and usually does not exhibit extensive spread. Some of these tumours have a villous appearance; this occurs in about 7% of all carcinomas.

ULCERATIVE LESION

This lesion (*Figure 4.60*) has a raised rolled everted edge with slough in its base. It tends to deeply infiltrate the bowel wall often distorting the lumen.

ANNULAR LESION

This lesion (*Figure 4.61*) is often referred to as the 'string' carcinoma and usually causes some degree of obstruction to the intestinal lumen.

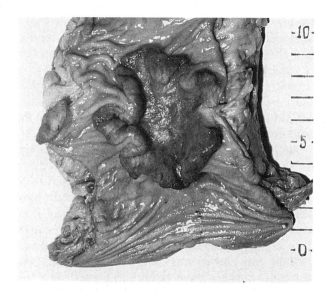

Figure 4.60 Ulcerated carcinoma of the rectum.

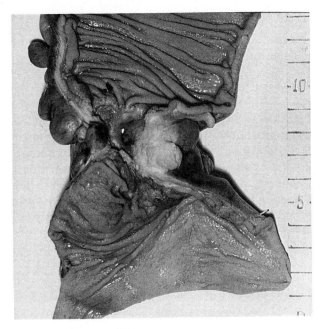

Figure 4.61 Annular carcinoma of the colon.

DIFFUSELY INFILTRATING SCIRRHOUS LESION
This is analogous to the linitis plastica type of gastric cancer but is a rare variant.[202] It is commonly a secondary manifestation of an occult carcinoma of the stomach rather than a true primary carcinoma.

COLLOID CARCINOMA
Approximately 10% of tumours secrete large quantities of mucin which gives them a characteristic gelatinous appearance on their cut surface. They are usually bulky tumours which vary in their extent of infiltration.

Microscopic features and histological grading
The degree of differentiation of colorectal adenocarcinomas is extremely variable. Both Dukes[53] and Grinnell[90] introduced a system in which tumours were graded I to IV according to the relative degree of atypical cells. Grade I was well differentiated and Grade IV was anaplastic. Grade IV also included colloid tumours. The latter represent approximately 10–15% of all tumours and are characterized by the presence of large amounts of mucin either inside (signet ring) or outside the cell. Approximately 20% of tumours are well differentiated (low grade), 60% are moderately differentiated (average grade) and 20% are poorly differentiated (high grade or anaplastic). Grading is subjective and although modifications have been introduced to the original system[14] to obtain uniformity, variations from one pathologist to another are commonplace. In general the histological grade of the tumour is related to the ultimate prognosis, but the variability in reporting the degree of differentiation limits its value. This applies particularly to preoperative biopsies.[221]

DIRECT SPREAD
The commonest mode of spread is in the transverse axis of the bowel wall itself. If allowed to progress, it will eventually become circumferential. Complete encirclement of the rectum takes approximately 2 years.[160] Longitudinal spread within the bowel wall is rare but is important for the surgeon in order to determine the extent of resection. Distal intramural spread is particularly important in rectal carcinoma when the length of resection of macroscopic normal bowel may make the difference between the patient retaining the anal sphincter or being left with a permanent colostomy. Most of the studies suggest that distal spread is rare; when it does occur it is usually less than 1 cm and, in those cases where it exceeds this distance, the tumour is advanced and the patient is very likely to die from widespread metastases.[13,92,194,244]

With extension of the growth, penetration of the bowel wall takes place. The submucosa and muscle coats are first breached and gradually the tumour erodes through the serosa, involving the pericolonic or rectal fat and the peritoneum. If growth is allowed to continue, invasion of local structures will take place. In the rectum, if the growth is situated anteriorly below the peritoneal reflection, the prostrate, seminal vesicles or bladder will be involved in the male and the posterior vaginal wall, cervix or uterus in the female. If the rectal growth is sited posteriorly below the pelvic peritoneum, spread will involve the fascia of Waldeyer and eventually the sacral plexus, sacrum and/or coccyx.

When the tumour lies above the peritoneal reflection, involvement of the ureters may occur in addition to invasion of the bladder, uterus, sigmoid colon or small bowel.

LYMPHATIC SPREAD
Spread in the lymphatic system tends to follow the course of the blood vessels supplying the site of the carcinoma. The carcinoma spreads from node to node and in advanced growths, when the lymphatics are choked with metastases and lymph flow is blocked, metastases may occur in separate lymph node groups. This type of spread is referred to as retrograde lymphatic spread.[93]

When the carcinoma is situated in the colon, the epicolic and the paracolic lymph nodes are first involved, followed by the intermediate glands along either the ileocolic, right colic, middle colic or left colic arteries. Eventually spread reaches the para-aortic glands which surround the origin of the superior and inferior mesenteric vessels.

Carcinoma of the rectum was first thought to spread in three directions, upwards along the superior haemorrhoidal and inferior mesenteric vessels, laterally along the middle rectal vessels in the lateral ligaments to the iliac nodes, and downwards through the sphincter muscles into the ischiorectal fossa and perianal skin and finally to the inguinal nodes. It was considered that these three directions of spread were implicated no matter where the carcinoma was sited within the rectum.[159] This concept led to the adoption of the abdomino-perineal resection for the treatment of carcinoma since only this operation was considered to be radical enough to remove all of the pathways of spread. Careful research has since shown that, although upward spread is most frequent, downward spread is rare and only occurs if the lymph flow along the superior rectal vascular pedicle is obstructed by metastases. Lateral spread is unusual with tumours of the intraperitoneal rectum but is more frequent with carcinomas below the peritoneal reflection.[52,77,230,252] These findings have important implications for both surgeon and patient alike in view of the increasing popularity of sphincter saving resections for the treatment of low rectal cancer.

BLOOD-BORNE SPREAD

Blood-borne spread occurs later than lymphatic spread, primarily to the liver. Pulmonary metastases occur in about 5% of cases[9] and the adrenal glands, kidneys and bones are affected in about 10% of cases.[245] Spread to the liver is via the portal vein and occurs in nearly one half of cases.[245] These data are obtained from postmortem studies. Not surprisingly the incidence of detectable liver metastases present at laparotomy is much lower (10–15%).[84] Recent studies which have performed serial ultrasound and computerized tomography of the liver during the postoperative period have identified 'occult' metastases not found at operation in a higher proportion of patients and the incidence of liver metastases present at the time of diagnosis is probably approximately 30%.[68]

Permeation of the veins draining a carcinoma can be demonstrated on careful section and histological examination of operative specimens. The presence of submucous venous spread has little or no effect on prognosis. Permeation of extramural veins on the other hand reduces the 5-year survival by about 25%.[25,217] The incidence of venous permeation varies between 17 and 38%.[10,54]

Several investigators[168,197] have demonstrated neoplastic cells in the circulation at the time of surgery. The viability of these cells is uncertain. It has not been shown that manipulation of the tumour at the time of operation increases the risk of metastases. It may be that although malignant cells are released they are unable to survive in the circulation.[33,61,71]

TRANSPERITONEAL SPREAD

About 1 in 10 patients after a surgical resection for carcinoma will develop peritoneal deposits. The less differentiated the tumour the more likely the peritoneal involvement.[174] This mode of spread frequently involves the ovaries (so-called Krukenberg tumours). The peritoneal deposits stimulate the excretion of exudate which forms ascites. This form of spread is probably transcoelomic in nature although dissemination may take place via the subperitoneal lymphatics.[160]

SPREAD BY IMPLANTATION

The frequency with which exfoliated malignant cells can become implanted onto a raw surface and lead to a secondary deposit is debatable. There are reports of implantation metastases developing in anal fistulas, haemorrhoidectomy wounds, abdominal incisions and around colostomies.[49,135] The concept that local recurrence at an anastomosis following resection was due to implantation of cells on the suture line is debatable, for although some studies have shown exfoliated cells in the lumen of the bowel to be viable, others have not.[226] Similarly, although free malignant cells can be demonstrated in washings from the peritoneal cavity,[191,192] attempts to grow them in tissue culture have usually failed.[169]

Staging of carcinoma

Staging of colorectal carcinoma has proved of some value in determining prognosis following treatment. The most widely used classification is that of Dukes.[52,54]

STAGE A

The carcinoma has not penetrated through the muscularis propria and there is no involvement of lymph nodes.

STAGE B

The carcinoma has extended through the wall of the bowel and involved the perirectal tissues but has not produced lymph node metastases.

STAGE C

This stage is subdivided into C_1, where nodes in the immediate vicinity of the tumour are involved but the most proximal node nearest the point of transection of the main vascular pedicle is free from tumour, and C_2, where nodes at the proximal margin of the vascular pedicle are involved.

STAGE D

Although Dukes did not originally include this category, it is frequently used to describe patients in whom distant metastases are detected. Several variations in Dukes' classification have been described and these should be taken into account when comparing published data.[7,125] Doubt has recently been cast on Dukes' staging, and its modifications, because they do not take into account the degree of fixity of the tumours at operation. This characteristic is important in determining prognosis. It has been shown[97,253] that Dukes' B tumours, which are fixed or partially fixed, have a similar prognosis to mobile C tumours. In order to obtain some uniformity in staging, it has been suggested that a TNM classification should be introduced, similar to that used for breast carcinoma[12] but this has not been universally adopted yet.

Clinical features

Most patients with colorectal cancer are in the sixth to eighth decades of life. Approximately 200 patients per year in the UK below 35 years of age develop the disease and they tend to have a more favourable outlook than previously thought.[42,180] Colon carcinoma occurs with equal frequency in men and women but rectal cancer seems to be rather more prevalent in men.[180]

In the early stage of development a colonic carcinoma rarely produces symptoms. At a later stage, one or more of the following is usually present:

1. Change in bowel habit, either constipation or diarrhoea or a combination of both.
2. Bleeding per rectum, often dark in colour.
3. Passage of mucus per rectum.
4. Abdominal pain.
5. Abdominal distension.
6. Borborygmi.
7. General malaise with loss of weight.

The site of the carcinoma often dictates the symptom complex. Carcinoma of the caecum and right colon are usually soft friable tumours and bleed easily. Patients complain of a non-specific deterioration in general health and are found to be anaemic. The passage of blood per rectum is unusual although occult blood may be detected by specific tests. Carcinoma in this region is often the cause of 'cryptogenic' iron deficiency anaemia. Some patients complain of abdominal pain and some have a palpable mass in the right iliac fossa.

When the tumour is situated on the left side, the clinical picture is usually different. The faecal contents are more solid, the calibre of the lumen is smaller and the tumours tend to be scirrhous and annular such that obstructive features are common. Constipation occurs in about half of the cases and is often accompanied by abdominal pain. The latter is usually diffuse and vague initially but gradually becomes more griping as the degree of obstruction increases. Bleeding and the passage of mucus per rectum are more common with tumours on the left side.

When the carcinoma is situated in the rectum the characteristic clinical picture is bleeding on defecation which may mimic the bright red bleeding which occurs with haemorrhoids or may be darker and more profuse. The bleeding is nearly always accompanied by a change in bowel habit. Sometimes constipation is present but more classically there is tenesmus in which the patient complains of frequent desire to defecate, with the passage of small amounts of faeces, blood or mucus. These symptoms are worse in the morning and tend to improve during the day.

Anorectal pain is not usually a feature of rectal cancer unless the tumour has invaded locally. Involvement of the sacrum and sacral plexus usually by a tumour on the posterior wall of the rectum will cause back pain and sciatica. Extension downwards into the anal canal can cause severe discomfort on defecation, symptoms which can mimic an anal fissure. Extension of the carcinoma into ureters, bladder or prostate can cause urinary tract symptoms, and involvement of the vagina may lead to a rectovaginal fistula.

Occasionally, rectal carcinoma may be entirely asymptomatic and only detected on routine digital examination.

A complete physical examination is essential and the findings will vary depending on the duration of the illness, the extent of spread and the presence of complications, ranging from a healthy appearance to severe cachexia. Abdominal palpation may detect a nodular enlarged liver suggestive of metastases. Palpation along the course of the colon may reveal the tumour itself. Its mobility will depend on the degree of local spread. If peritoneal metastases are present ascites may be present and, more rarely, a nodule of secondary tumour may be sited at the umbilicus (the so-called Sister Joseph's nodule). It is rare in colorectal cancer to detect enlarged peripheral lymph nodes.

Rectal examination may detect a mass and secondary deposits may be felt in the pelvic peritoneum. The findings in rectal carcinoma will vary depending on the macroscopic type of tumour, its size, its site within the rectum and the degree of spread. About 75% of all rectal cancers are within reach of the examining finger.[33,215] Not all firm masses arising in the rectum are primary neoplasms.

A rectal carcinoma can be confused with a carcinoma or diverticular mass of the sigmoid which becomes adherent to the pelvic floor and is palpable extrarectally. Similarly, a primary tumour of the cervix or prostrate may be palpable outside the rectum. Either of the latter two neoplasms may invade the anterior rectal wall and it then becomes impossible, on digital examination, to differentiate them from a rectal cancer.

Investigations

Proctoscopy and sigmoidoscopy

The appearance of a rectal carcinoma will depend on its macroscopic appearance. Often a polypoid tumour will completely fill the lumen so that its precise attachment cannot be identified. With an ulcerated growth, the observer first notices the lower extremity projecting into the lumen as a congested bleeding protrusion with a dull grey necrotic crater. Sometimes the endoscopist will find that the rectosigmoid junction is unduly fixed and difficult to negotiate due to a proximally adherent lesion. The distance of the lower margin of the tumour from the anal verge should always be noted to assist the surgeon in his decision as to the best operative approach. Although it is useful to examine the bowel lumen beyond the tumour, in practice this is often impossible and certainly so if the growth is of the annular variety. In those cases where a carcinoma is present beyond the reach of the sigmoidoscope, the presence of blood and mucus in the lumen should alert the endoscopist to this possibility.

In most outpatient clinics, the rigid sigmoidoscope is the only type of endoscopic instrument employed. The flexible sigmoidoscope may have considerable benefits. The instrument is 60 cm in length, thus increasing the length of bowel that can be examined. Patients find it more tolerable than the rigid instrument and the complication rate is low.[246] The main disadvantage is that the bowel needs to be prepared before examination. Nevertheless, the instrument is extremely useful in diagnosis, and may reduce the number of patients requiring radiographic or colonoscopic examination.[250]

Radiological examination

Single contrast can be used but the double contrast air inflation technique[235] has significantly improved the diagnostic yield of this investigation. Radiological accuracy diminishes at the extremes of the large bowel (i.e. at the caecum or rectum). Difficulty in the precise delineation of a carcinoma in the caecum may result from unsatisfactory elimination of faecal material, a filling defect produced by an unusually prominent ileocaecal valve, deformity of the caecal

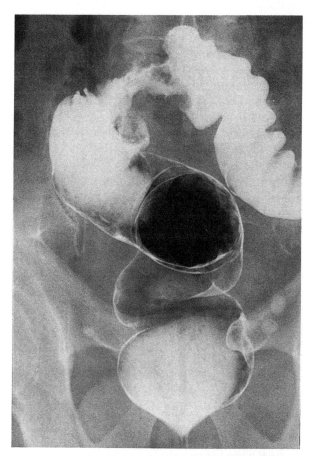

Figure 4.62 Double contrast barium enema showing annular carcinoma in the sigmoid colon – typical 'apple core' deformity.

wall by previous surgical manoeuvres (such as appendicectomy) and also the presence of adjacent disease in the ovary, appendix or terminal ileum. Although demonstration of a rectal carcinoma by radiography is rarely necessary, a barium enema is useful to rule out a synchronous tumour.

A colonic carcinoma is usually seen on barium enema examination as a filling defect and its exact configuration depends upon its size and macroscopic features. In many cases a constant stricture of 3–8 cm in length is seen. Such a stricture with characteristic shouldering is seen as an 'apple core' deformity (Figure 4.62). If the carcinoma is an annular string-type neoplasm the narrowed segment will be much shorter. Another radiological variant is produced by the presence of a bulky polypoid tumour which projects into the lumen and is seen as a filling defect with an irregular edge (Figure 4.63). Although large polypoid carcinomas are clearly evident on barium enema examination, difficulty may be experienced in detection of smaller lesions of this type. Radiological features which suggest possible malignancy in a polyp include indrawing of the outline of the base when the polyp is sessile, an irregular surface, a large size or evidence of growth

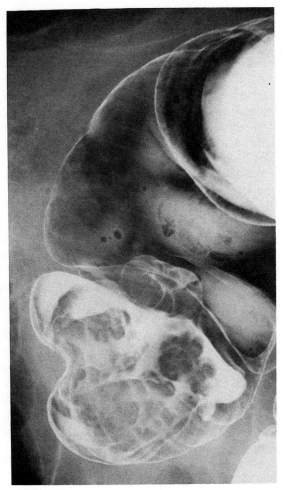

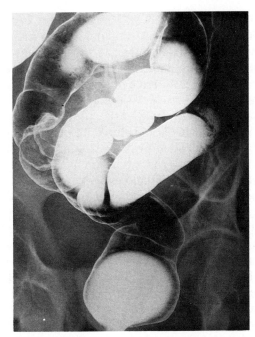

Figure 4.64 Barium enema showing neoplastic polyp in the sigmoid colon. It is 3 cm in diameter and has an irregular base which is drawn in.

Figure 4.63 Barium enema showing large polypoid carcinoma in the caecum.

between consecutive radiological studies (*Figure 4.64*). Any polyp greater than 2 cm in diameter should be regarded as a carcinoma until proved otherwise.[58,258]

Carcinoma may be difficult to detect in loops of redundant colon and where the barium outlines of adjacent loops are superimposed. This particularly applies to the sigmoid segment and to the hepatic and splenic flexures. Oblique views help to overcome this difficulty.

The accuracy of modern radiological techniques is high. The false-positive rate at the Mayo Clinic for example was 0.8% and the false negative rate was 6.9%.[130] Nevertheless, if the study is negative or equivocal and the clinician is still suspicious, there should be no hesitation in proceeding to a colonoscopic examination.

Colonoscopy
Colonoscopy has substantially improved the accuracy of diagnosis in colorectal cancer. It enhances the sensitivity of barium enema throughout the colon but especially in the upper sigmoid, distal descending colon and caecum. A carcinoma of the sigmoid colon may be missed on barium enema in 8% of cases and more frequently if the growth is situated in the caecum.[35] Of 60 lesions missed on barium enema, and detected at colonoscopy, 17 were carcinomas.[220] Some regard colonoscopy as the best investigation for patients with large bowel symptoms.[56] The detractors from this view point out that colonoscopy needs to be performed under sedation, and the presence of adhesions, strictures or diverticular disease may make it impossible. In addition, there is a small risk of perforation even when performed for diagnostic purposes.[75,198] Most clinicians therefore arrange a barium enema first and, if negative and the symptoms persist, go on to order a colonoscopy.

Screening

Because colorectal tumours tend to be slow growing and are often asymptomatic at their onset, early detection depends on population screening. Screening can be divided into selective screening of high-risk groups and general screening of average risk patients. The high-risk group includes patients with long standing ulcerative colitis, a past history of adenoma of the colon or colon cancer, female genital cancer and perhaps those with a strong family history of the disease.[3,47,128,147,246] This group should undergo radiography and/or colonoscopy every one or two years. In patients with ulcerative colitis, multiple biopsies should be taken since the finding of dysplasia, despite a negative colonoscopic investigation, is an important indication of impending carcinoma. Moderate dysplasia is associated with a colorectal cancer risk of approximately 30% and severe dysplasia with a risk of 50%. The presence of dysplasia should be confirmed by repeat biopsy.[48,133] Those individuals who are at average risk of developing a carcinoma are men and women over 40 years of age with no underlying disease, past history or family history of bowel disease. It is in this large group that controversy exists concerning the cost–benefit of screening programmes. It is impractical to use endoscopic methods for detection since patient compliance will be low. Most interest has, therefore, focused on the detection of occult blood in the stool. The development of the impregnated guaiac slide test with stabilized reagent and the use of three to six slides has improved their value.[89] Several studies have now been performed in which the positive rate of detection has varied between 1.5 and 6%. The greater the number of positive tests the less the predictive value for neoplasm. It seems, however, that approximately one-third of patients with positive tests will eventually prove to have a neoplasm, either a polyp or less frequently a carcinoma. The more slides taken the greater the sensitivity.[16,89,247,249] The population to be tested should preferably be on a meat-free diet as an unrestricted diet is associated with a high rate of false positives and negatives.[87]

Measurement of carcinoembryonic antigen both in blood and bowel washings has been used for screening purposes but this antibody has been found to be unreliable due to its lack of specificity.[248] The development of monoclonal antibodies may prove to be a more specific serum marker of the disease.[126]

Screening programmes using faecal occult blood tests are capable of detecting a higher percentage of localized cancer.[101] At present approximately 40% of patients with colorectal cancer have localized disease and because the latter has a better prognosis than non-localized disease, it follows that screening should improve the general outlook. An additional benefit may be derived from the identification and removal of premalignant lesions, i.e. polyps. No screening study has yet demonstrated either a benefit in survival for individual patients or a benefit in mortality for the population.

Complications

Intestinal obstruction

Carcinomas of the left colon are more likely to cause obstruction than those of the right. The intestinal lumen is gradually obliterated by a constricting neoplasm. More rarely, the tumour may cause obstruction by acting as the apex for either an intussusception or volvulus. Most commonly the patient complains of increasing constipation and the obstruction is thus classified as acute or chronic. The constipation gradually becomes worse and abdominal distension supervenes which is associated with discomfort. Although nausea is common vomiting rarely occurs until late in the clinical course.

Occasionally, the clinical presentation is more acute with no preceding symptoms. This picture is seen more commonly with growths of the right colon. The patient complains of sudden acute colicky abdominal pain, absolute constipation, vomiting and abdominal distension. On examination dehydration may be present, the abdomen will be distended and if the ileocaecal valve remains competent a closed loop obstruction will be present; the right colon, particularly the caecum, may be grossly distended and tender on palpation. Visible peristalis may be present and the abdomen is tense on palpation, the degree depending on the extent of distension. Bowel sounds will usually be hyperactive and borborygmi may be heard without recourse to a stethoscope. Rectal examination reveals an empty rectum which is often 'ballooned'. Rarely, a rectal carcinoma which is the cause of the obstruction is palpable. Sigmoidoscopy may be useful since the lower edge of the tumour in the sigmoid colon or upper rectum may be visible.

Erect and supine X-rays of the abdomen will often show gross dilatation of the colon proximal to the tumour with multiple fluid levels (*Figure 4.65*). There may also be fluid levels in the small bowel if the ileocaecal valve is incompetent. If the valve remains competent the distension of the closed loop may become so enormous that the appearances may mimic those of a volvulus of the sigmoid colon.

If time allows, a Gastrografin enema should be obtained to establish the diagnosis (*Figure 4.66*). Barium should not be used in these circumstances, as its removal from the bowel may be difficult and time consuming and may impede the subsequent surgical procedure.

Perforation

The carcinoma may perforate and cause either a generalized faecal peritonitis or a localized abscess. The latter may mimic a diverticular abscess on the left side or an appendix abscess on the right side.[187] Perforation of the colon may occur at a site distant from the carcinoma as a consequence of intestinal obstruction. Classically this occurs in the caecum when a closed loop obstruction exists or it can occur closer to the tumour through a stercoral ulcer.

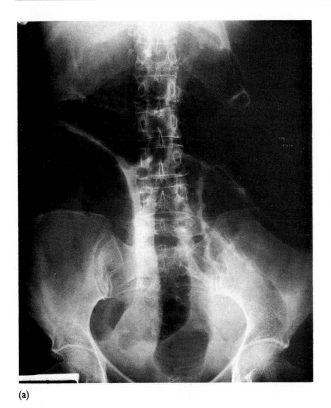

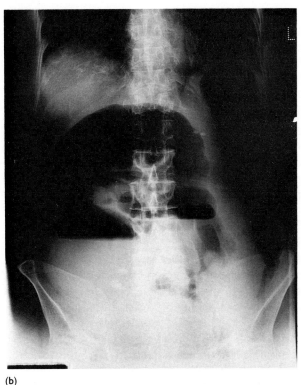

(a)   (b)

Figure 4.65   (a) Supine and (b) erect, straight, abdominal radiographs of a patient with an obstructing carcinoma of the descending colon. The colon is grossly distended with multiple fluid levels.

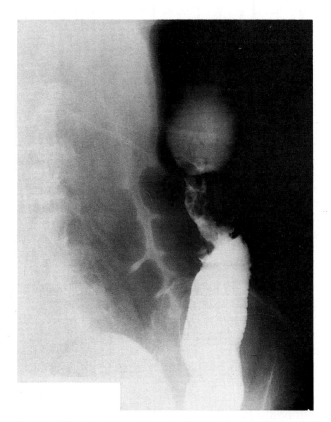

Figure 4.66 Gastrografin enema (the patient in *Figure 4.65* showing that the cause of the obstruction is a carcinoma in the descending colon).

Patients who present with faecal peritonitis are usually in a state of extremis with abdominal distension, diffuse tenderness, vomiting and gross electrolyte disturbance. In this situation mortality rates are high.

Fistula formation

A carcinoma of colon or rectum may adhere to and eventually penetrate any abdominal organ. The bladder is most commonly involved and usually the carcinoma is in the sigmoid colon. The patient with a colovesical fistula may complain of pneumaturia but more often suffers from repeated bouts of cystitis. Men are affected more commonly than women. Diagnosis can be difficult since the fistula is rarely seen on cystoscopy. Carcinoma is second only to diverticular disease as the commonest cause of colovesical fistula.

A rectovaginal fistula may be the presenting feature of a rectal cancer. A fistula may also form between a transverse colon carcinoma and the stomach or duodenum. Rarely a tumour may present as an external spontaneous fistula, thus mimicking Crohn's disease. Initially a fistula may present as a subcutaneous abscess in the abdominal wall, the thigh or the perinephric region.[153,201]

Rarely, a caecal carcinoma obstructs the base of the appendix, and the patient presents with acute appendicitis.[64,161] More than half of all intussusceptions of the large bowel in the adult are due to carcinoma.[199]

Treatment

Excision of the tumour should nearly always be attempted because even if the operation is palliative in nature, intestinal obstruction will be avoided and distressing symptoms alleviated. Many of these patients have coexistent medical problems which need treatment first.

Specific preoperative preparation

Until recently, sepsis was a common problem. The primary source of infection is the endogenous bacteria in the bowel lumen. The bowel cannot be sterilized completely but a complete mechanical clearance of its contents is useful. This is usually achieved by the oral administration of two or three sachets of picosulphate/citrate (Picolax) or the drinking of a balanced electrolyte solution such as GoLytely. Care must be taken in elderly patients or those with a history of cardiovascular or renal disease, or those who have a carcinoma which is causing obstruction.[107] Mannitol should not be used because it can produce explosive mixtures within the bowel.

The introduction of prophylactic antibiotic cover has reduced sepsis rates. Oral antibiotics which are not absorbed by the gut (e.g. neomycin, kanamycin or phthalylsulphathiazole) have some effect, but systemic antibiotics are preferred. A combination of antibiotics which are bactericidal to both aerobic and anaerobic organisms are most effective. Administration of either one dose with the premedication or three doses perioperatively reduces risks of drug resistance and side-effects while achieving maximum efficiency.[106,123]

The nature of the surgery must be fully explained. This is particularly important if a colostomy is necessary. Patients who have needed a stoma often complain that they did not receive adequate counselling before surgery.[46] The best person to supply this information is either the stomatherapist or an experienced ward sister.

Principles and techniques of surgery

THE COLON

The type of operation depends on the site of the tumour. As the lymphatic drainage accompanies the main blood vessels, the length of bowel resected is dependent on the extent of lymphatic clearance that is required. The aim of a radical operation is to remove the tumour with the whole of its appropriate lymphatic drainage. If, however, all tumour cannot

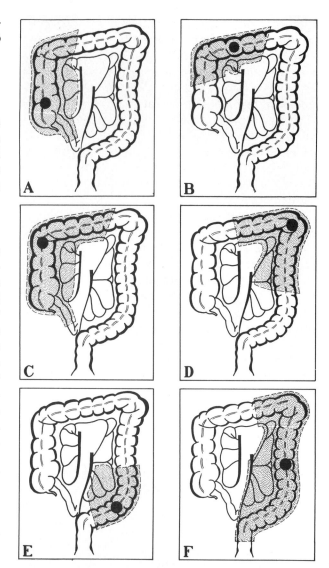

Figure 4.67 Types of colonic resections. A: carcinoma of the caecum – right hemicolectomy; B: carcinoma of the transverse colon – transverse colectomy (this procedure is sometimes extended so as to include the splenic flexure); C: carcinoma of the ascending colon – extended right hemicolectomy; D: carcinoma of the splenic flexure – left hemicolectomy; E: carcinoma of the sigmoid colon – sigmoid colectomy; F: carcinoma of the descending colon – extended left hemicolectomy.

be removed and a palliative procedure is planned it is only necessary to remove the minimum amount of tissue that will ensure relief of symptoms.

For cancer of the right colon (i.e. caecum, ascending colon, hepatic flexure and right half of the transverse colon, which are all supplied by the superior mesenteric artery), resection involves ligation of the appropriate colic branches as close as possible to their origin from their parent vessel. The common types of resection are illustrated in *Figure 4.67A,B,C*.

For cancer of the left colon (i.e. the left half of the transverse colon, splenic flexure, descending and sigmoid colon), radical resection involves ligation of the appropriate colic branches of the inferior mesenteric artery (*Figure 4.67D,E*). Some surgeons believe that an even more radical excision is required for tumours of the left colon in which the inferior mesenteric artery is divided at its origin. The whole of the left colon is excised and an anastomosis is constructed between the distal, transverse colon and upper rectum (*Figure 4.67F*). Colectomy with continuity restored by ileorectal anastomosis may be needed for multiple cancers or the presence of multiple polyps.

If the colonic tumour is invading or adherent to other organis (e.g. a loop of small intestine or uterus), as much of the adherent tissue as possible should be excised *en bloc* with the tumour. The adhesions are often inflammatory and not neoplastic and thus prognosis is better than anticipated.[34,60,118]

THE RECTUM

There are two main types of operation for the treatment of carcinoma of the rectum: the abdominoperineal excision of the rectum (APER) or one form of sphincter-saving resection (SSR). In all these operations the inferior mesenteric artery is divided as close to its origin as possible. In APER the whole of the rectum and sigmoid colon and their mesenteries are excised together with the anal sphincters, the ischiorectal fat and most of the levator ani muscles leaving the patient with a permanent colostomy (*Figure 4.68*). The procedure is usually

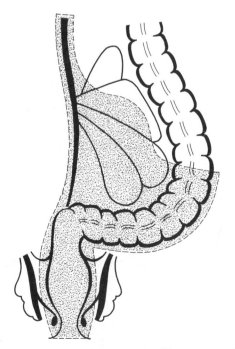

Figure 4.68 Abdominoperineal resection. The structure within the shaded areas are excised. The proximal colon is brought out in the left ioliac fossa as an end colostomy.

conducted by two surgeons working simultaneously via the abdomen and perineum.

There are various types of sphincter-saving procedures but the principles are similar. The rectum containing the carcinoma is mobilized via the abdominal approach as for an APER. It is then divided at least 2 cm below the lower border of the cancer.[85] Once the involved segment of bowel has been removed, an anastomosis between the anorectal stump and the colon, usually the descending part, is constructed. The anastomosis can usually be made via the abdominal approach using a one- or two-layered hand anastomosis. This procedure is referred to as an anterior resection. If the growth is too low or the pelvis too narrow, a conventional anterior resection cannot be performed. The simplest and most popular method to restore continuity is to use a stapling instrument or gun (*Figure 4.69*). The most popular instrument is the Premium (CEEA) gun (American Surgical Corporation) (*Figure 4.70*) which has a detachable head and which has greatly simplified the procedure. Using the instrument, the surgeon is able to construct a low colorectal anastomosis with two rows of staples at levels in the pelvis that are impossible by hand. Occasionally an abdominosacral operation can be used for a low anastomosis.[138] Access to the distal anorectum is achieved via the trans-sacral approach with the patient in the prone position (*Figure 4.70*). Another variation is the abdominotransanal technique[185] in which after rectal excision the colon is drawn down through the anal canal and anastomosed to it via the transanal route (*Figure 4.71*). These techniques are usually associated with complete continence,[102,129,139] although this may take up to 18 months to be achieved.[242] Older methods, such as the abdominoanal pull-through method[44] in which the anorectum is everted and anastomosis constructed externally, are rarely used because they often result in poor anorectal control.

It is generally agreed that carcinomas of the upper third of the rectum (above 13 cm from the anal verge) should be treated by anterior resection. Most surgeons also agree that tumours whose lower edge is 5 cm or less from the anal verge, as measured by sigmoidoscopy, should undergo APER with a permanent colostomy. The treatment of lesions between these two levels is debated. The new sphincter saving techniques result in a better quality of life than can be achieved after APER.[240] Apart from numerous psychological problems related to the colostomy,[46] patients who have undergone APER have a high incidence of bladder and sexual disturbances.[72,240,243] Because, however, less tissue is excised during an SSR than during an APER, the fear is that recurrence and survival rates will be

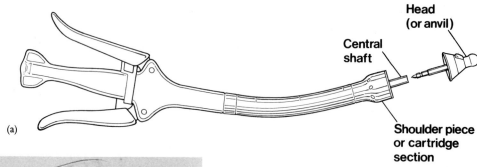

Head
(or anvil)

Central
shaft

Shoulder piece
or cartridge
section

(a)

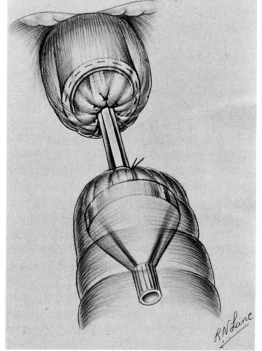

(b)

Figure 4.69 (a) The Premium (EEA) stapling gun with detachable head. (b) After the rectum with the cancer has been excised, the colon is anastomosed to the rectal stump. With the shoulder piece in the rectum and the head in the colon, the two ends of bowel are racked together. When the gun is fired, a circular knife cuts through the infolded bowel contained in a purse string suture. Simultaneously the two ends of bowel are stapled together in two layers.

compromised. There is the theoretical risk that insufficient microscopic distal spread will be removed, and anastomotic recurrence will increase with transection of the rectum with a margin of clearance of less than 5 cm. Retrospective studies, however, suggest that survival and recurrence rates for carcinoma of the middle third of the rectum treated by either type of operation are similar.[157,178,241] Similarly, the incidence of local recurrence is not influenced by the margin of clearance.[189,244]

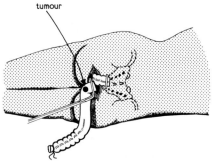

tumour

Figure 4.70 Abdominotrans-sacral anastomosis. The rectum and colon are mobilized via the abdomen and the trans-sacral route. After the tumour-bearing area has been resected, anastomosis is performed via the trans-sacral route.

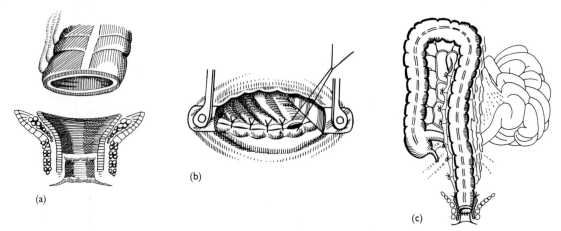

(a)

(b)

(c)

Figure 4.71 (a) After excision of the colon and rectum containing the tumour, the mucosa of the residual rectal stump is removed, and the colon brought down and (b) anastomosed to the anal mucosa (c) via the transanal route.

Table 4.16 Absolute survival rate of patients with carcinoma of rectum

Author	No. of cases	Submitted to rectal excision	Surviving 5 years or more (%)	Corrected 5-year survival rate (%)
Birmingham Regional Cancer Registry (1950–1961)[204]	5800	2900 (50%)	22	29
Bristol Cancer Registry (1961–1964)[232]	1346	857 (65%)	23	ND
Leeds General Infirmary (1955–1965)[238]	550	498 (98.5%)	40	45
St Mark's Hospital (1948–1972)[142]	3163	2948 (93.2%)	47.1	56.6

ND = No data.

If the tumour is well localized and mobile, and if it can be excised with a clearance of not less than 2–3 cm but preferably 5 cm, most surgeons perform a sphincter-saving procedure – an anterior resection with either hand or stapled anastomosis. When the tumour is more extensive, or is too low for either of these techniques, an APER is performed. In a few centres which have acquired special expertise, the ultralow lesions that are not accompanied by local spread are treated by either abdominotransanal or abdominotranssacral techniques.[105,186]

LOCAL TREATMENT OF RECTAL CANCER
The techniques available for patients who are unfit for major surgery include electrocoagulation,[214] contact irradiation[184] or local excision.[39,214] These can relieve symptoms and are associated with very low mortality and morbidity rates. Occasionally, they can result in long-term cure, but there is no general support for their use as primary treatment as suggested by a few enthusiasts.[151]

Results of surgery
CARCINOMA OF COLON
Over the past 30–40 years the proportion of colonic cancers amenable to resection has increased and the operative mortality rate has fallen, now being 70–80% and 5–10%, respectively. The overall crude 5-year survival rate for patients treated by surgery in most centres ranges from 50% to 70%.[80,91,115,194,244] If all patients are included, the 5-year survival rate is much lower (20–25% in the UK).[204,232]

A number of factors influences the results of operative treatment. The most important is the extent of spread. Thus, the corrected 5-year survival for Dukes' C lesions is 30–40%, whereas that for Dukes' A and B lesions is 70–80%.[102] Younger patients may have a worse prognosis than older patients, and the shorter the history the worse the outlook.[37,204] The development of complications, particularly perforation or acute obstruction, considerably decreases survival rates.[79,116]

CARCINOMA OF RECTUM
The results of surgery for rectal carcinoma are similar to those described for colonic carcinoma. In specialized centres the proportion of tumours amenable to resection may be as high as 90%, with an operative mortality of approximately 5%.[142] The rate is much lower in other centres so that survival rates are worse (*Table 4.16*). The most obvious reason for this difference is the higher proportion of advanced and emergency cases which present to district general hospitals. The relationship between Dukes' stage and survival is shown in *Table 4.17*. Other factors which have a specific effect on survival include: the degree of mobility of the tumour;[97,253] the height of the lesion from the anal verge;[81,210] and females do slightly less well then males.[55,156]

Table 4.17 Crude 5-year survival rates after rectal excision for carcinoma according to Dukes' stage

	A (%)	B (%)	C (%)
Whittaker and Goligher (1976)[229]	80	62	33
Slanetz, Herter and Grinnell (1972)[195]	84	55	35
Dukes (1957)[50] Men	80	61	26
Women	82	72	29

Adjuvant therapy

RADIOTHERAPY

Adjuvant radiotherapy has been applied chiefly to patients with carcinomas of the rectum and rectosigmoid region. It may be given either before or after operation. Preoperative therapy aims to decrease the number of viable tumour cells to reduce the risk of dissemination at surgery and reduce the incidence of local recurrence. It may also enhance the immune response.[38] Preoperative therapy may be given in a low dose which allows the surgeon to proceed with the operation quickly and without prejudice to safety but has been proven to be ineffective. A larger dose (about 60% of that normally used for curative radiotherapy) can be given over a 3–6 week period. This technique increases the risk of damage to other organs and delays surgery. High-dose radiation has been used particularly for fixed or partially fixed tumours.

Most studies have shown that, provided the radiation dose is high enough (30–40 Gy), the incidence of local recurrence after rectal excision can be reduced. Although it was believed that adjuvant radiotherapy made no difference to survival, recent metanalysis of the available data suggests a marginal benefit.[88]

Postoperative radiotherapy has the advantage that it can be given after the extent of spread has been accurately defined and can be limited to those at high risk for developing recurrence. Several studies have suggested that, when used in this way, radiotherapy may be beneficial but there is considerable morbidity.[74,158]

CHEMOTHERAPY

Patients with Dukes' A lesions have an excellent prognosis after resection and are unlikely to be helped by adjuvant chemotherapy. The prognosis of patients with obvious metastatic disease at the time of surgery is unlikely to be improved by adjuvant therapy. On the other hand, patients with Dukes' B and C lesions who have undergone 'curative' resection might benefit most. Many of these patients will have circulating cancer cells which may develop into metastases. Indeed some of these patients will already have micrometastases undetected at operation which will lead to a fatal outcome.[68] Adjuvant therapy may intervene in this sequence of events and improve prognosis. There is little evidence so far to show that survival is prolonged in patients without metastases treated by adjuvant chemotherapy. Various drugs such as thiotepa[114] and 5-fluoro-2'-deoxyuridine[57] have been used but only fluorouracil has been comprehensively investigated in randomized controlled trials. Although there are retrospective data to suggest that when fluorouracil is

given systemically prognosis is improved,[136] prospective studies have not borne this out.[108,109,165] The intraluminal route of administration has also been studied, but although this method, in combination with systemic therapy, might be beneficial in patients with Dukes' C lesions,[95] no study has demonstrated a significantly superior overall survival rate.[132] These disappointing results have led to studies using combinations of systemic agents. The most common additional agent is methyl-CCNU (semustine)[124] but mitomycin has also been used. Both these combinations, however, appear to be ineffective.

The most promising technique using adjuvant chemotherapy so far is perfusion of the liver via the portal vein with fluorouracil in patients without macroscopic hepatic metastases. The idea is that, because tumour cells reach the liver via the portal vein,[1,218] perfusion with cytotoxic therapy will prevent the formation of micrometastases. The early results of this technique are encouraging[219] but longer follow up is required.

IMMUNOTHERAPY

Various attempts at non-specific stimulation of the immune system using agents such as *Corynebacterium parvum* and BCG have been abandoned because of their inactivity. Recent data[167] have shown that the non-specific immunostimulant levamisole, when used in combination with fluorouracil as an adjuvant therapy over 1 year, significantly improves survival of patients with Dukes' C carcinoma. Trials with interlukin 2 (IL2) and LAK cell therapy are also being conducted but the results are not available yet. Experimental work also continues with monoclonal antibodies.

Surveillance

Follow up should be regular, at least annually, but more frequent in the first three years. If asymptomatic patients should ideally be colonoscoped every two years to detect metachronous cancer or polyps. Symptoms of general malaise, weight loss, anorexia, abdominal pain, alteration in bowel habit, bleeding or the passage of mucus, either per rectum or per colostomy, are suggestive of recurrence or the development of a metachronous tumour.[23,82] Physical examination may reveal an abdominal mass, ascites, hepatomegaly or perineal nodules. Rectal and sigmoidoscopic examinations may demonstrate local recurrence either at the suture line or extrarectally. Metastatic disease may be detected on barium enema, colonoscopy, ultrasound or CT scan. However, by the time clinical features are apparent the disease is widely disseminated. More sophisticated techniques may detect recurrence at an earlier stage. Recent reports suggest that the CT scan may be very accurate in the detection of hepatic and pelvic recurrence.[68,96,117] Ultrasound may also have a role to play.

Elevated levels of CEA, particularly in combination with abnormal liver function tests, are indicative of widespread metastases,[36] but are not a reliable indicator of early recurrence,[32,166] although some surgeons still regard a rise in CEA as an indication for a second-look laparotomy.[154]

Surgical cure of the patient with recurrence, no matter how early it is detected, is unlikely.[11] Early detection may, however, lead to more effective palliation.

RARE MALIGNANT TUMOURS

Carcinoid

Carcinoid tumour, although only second in frequency to adenocarcinoma, is a rare tumour of the large bowel and only a proportion of these tumours are malignant. They are, like carcinoid tumours elsewhere, derived from the Kulchitsky cells of the crypts of Lieberkühn. Although these cells have the propensity to secrete 5-hydroxytryptamine, carcinoid tumours of the large bowel, even when accompanied by multiple hepatic metastases, are not usually associated with hypersecretion.[76,188]

In their early stage they form polyps, often of a yellowish hue, which enlarge and become ulcerated. They are similar in appearance to adenocarcinomas.

Carcinoid tumours of the colon are more likely to be malignant than those of the rectum.[76,213] The clinical presentation and treatment is identical to that of adenocarcinoma but the prognosis is often better.[183]

Primary malignant lymphoma

This tumour can occur in the large bowel but Goligher reported only two cases in a clinical experience of 1500 cases of malignant tumours.[85] Of 79 primary lymphomas in the gastrointestinal tract, Allen et al.[2] found that nine were in the colon or rectum. They occur more commonly in the caecum than the left colon or rectum[173] and this distribution is probably due to spread into the caecum from tumours arising in the terminal ileum. Primary lymphoma may complicate ulcerative colitis.[196] Their degree of malignancy depends on their cell type. All varieties of non-Hodgkin's lymphoma have been described. Classification is often difficult because of distortion resulting from ulceration and infection. Clinical presentation is usually indistinguishable from that of an adenocarcinoma. Although surgical excision is required, adjuvant chemotherapy and/or radiotherapy may be of particular benefit. The prognosis is rather better than adenocarcinoma.[254]

Secondary lymphoma

The large intestine may be infiltrated secondarily, the colon being more frequently involved than the rectum. The patient usually has obvious evidence of systemic disease.

Malignant lymphomatous polyposis

In this condition, the gastrointestinal tract is diffusely involved with polypoid thickening of the mucosa.[100,201] Although the polyps may be pedunculated, the appearance is usually one of diffuse mucosal nodularity. The patients present with diarrhoea and malabsorption due to small bowel involvement. Splenomegaly and generalized lymphadenopathy are often present. The disease surprisingly tends to run a chronic course.

Leiomyosarcoma

These tumours originate from the muscle coat and project either into the bowel lumen or on the external surface of the bowel. They are usually large, rubbery, lobulated tumours. In about half of them, the overlying mucosa remains intact. The degree of differentiation varies and the pathologist may have difficulty in distinguishing between benign and malignant tumours.[176] They spread both by direct extension or by the blood stream. Lymphatic spread occurs rarely.[222] They are sited more frequently in the rectum than in the colon.[5] Symptoms are usually indistinguishable from other tumours although massive haemorrhage can occasionally occur.[200] Such a tumour should be suspected if on rectal or endoscopic examination the mucosa is intact. Although local excision has been attempted, the tumour usually recurs and a more radical procedure is required. Postoperative radiotherapy may be beneficial.

Fibrosarcoma, rhabdomyosarcoma, haemangiopericytoma, plasmacytoma and endothelioma have all been reported.[170,178,181,183,213] Malignant melanoma and squamous cell carcinoma are tumours which invariably occur in the anorectal region and are described in detail elsewhere.

Acknowledgements

I would like to express my sincere thanks to the following who helped in the preparation of this section: Miss Ruth Bailey, Department of Medical Illustration; Mr Peter Hargreaves, Department of Photography; and Mrs Lorna McQuade, Department of Surgery, Leeds General Infirmary; Miss Janet Mutch, Surgical Unit, The Royal London Hospital. Dr K. Simkins kindly allowed me access to his radiograph collection.

References

1. Ackerman, N.B. (1972) Alteration of intrahepatic circulation due to increased tumour growth. *Proceedings of the VII Congress European Society Experimental Surgery*, 182.
2. Allen, A.W., Donaldson, G., Sniffen, R.C. and Goodale, F., Jr (1954) Primary malignant lymphoma of the gastrointestinal tract. *Annals of Surgery*, **140**, 428–433.
3. Anderson, D.E. and Ramsdahl, M.M. (1977) Family history; a criteria for selective screening. In *Progress in Cancer Research and Therapy. Genetics of Human Cancer* (Ed.) Mulvihill, J.J., Miller, R.W. and Fraumeni, J.F., Jr Volume 3. New York: Raven Press.
4. Anderson, D.E. and Strong, L.C. (1974) Genetics of gastrointestinal tumours. *Proceedings of the XIth International Cancer Congress*, **3**, 267–271.
5. Anderson, P.A., Dockerty, M.B. and Buie, L.A. (1950) Myomatous tumours of the rectum (leiomyomas and myosarcomas). *Surgery*, **68**, 642–647.
6. Armstrong, B.K. and Doll, R. (1975) Environmental factors and cancer incidence and mortality in different countries with special reference to dietary practices. *International Journal of Cancer*, **15**, 167–172.
7. Astler, V.B. and Coller, F.A. (1954) The prognostic significance of direct extension of carcinoma of the colon and rectum. *Annals of Surgery*, **139**, 846–851.
8. Augeninght, L.H., Augeron, C., Yander, G. and Laboisse, C. (1987) Over expression of ras in mucus secreting human colon carcinoma cell of low tumorigenicity. *Cancer Research*, **47**, 3763–3765.
9. Bacon, H.E. and Jackson, C.C. (1953) Visceral metastases from carcinoma of the distal colon and rectum. *Surgery*, **33**, 495–500.
10. Barringer, P.L., Dockerty, M.B., Waugh, J.M. and Bargen, J.A. (1954) Carcinoma of the large intestine: a new approach to the study of venous spread. *Surgery, Gynecology and Obstetrics*, **98**, 62–67.
11. Beart, R.W. and O'Connell, M.J. (1983) Post operative follow up of patients with carcinoma of the colon. *Mayo Clinic Proceedings*, **58**, 361–363.
12. Beart, R.W., Van Heerden, J.A. and Beahrs, O.H. (1978) Evolution in the pathologic staging of carcinoma of the colon. *Surgery, Gynecology and Obstetrics*, **146**, 257–262.
13. Black, W.A. and Waugh, J.M. (1948) The intramural extension of carcinoma of the descending colon, sigmoid and rectosigmoid: a pathologic study. *Surgery, Gynecology and Obstetrics*, **87**, 457–464.
14. Blenkinsopp, W.K., Stewart Brown, S., Blesovsky, K. *et al.* (1981) Histopathology reporting in large bowel cancer. *Journal of Clinical Pathology*, **34**, 509–513.
15. Bodmer, W.F., Bailey, C.J. and Bussey, H.S.R. (1987) Localisation of the gene for familial adenomatous polyposis on Chromosome 5. *Nature*, **328**, 614–616.
16. Bond, J.H. and Gilbertson, V.A. (1977) Early detection of colonic carcinoma by mass screening for occult stool blood. Preliminary Report. *Gastroenterology*, **72**, A-8/1031.
17. Bonelli, L., Martines, H., Conio, M. and Bruzzi, P. (1988) Family history of colorectal cancer as a risk factor for benign and malignant tumours of the large bowel. A case control study. *International Journal of Cancer*, **41**, 513–517.
18. Breslow, N.E. and Enström, J.E. (1974) Geographic correlations between cancer mortality rates and alcohol–tobacco consumption in the United States. *Journal of the National Cancer Institute*, **53**, 631–639.
19. Burdette, W.J. (1970) Hereditable cancer of the colorectum. In *Carcinoma of the Colon and Antecedent Epithelium*, (Ed.) Burdett, W.J. Springfield, MA: C.C. Thomas.
20. Burkitt, D.P. (1971) Epidemiology of cancer of the colon and rectum. *Cancer*, **28**, 3–13.
21. Burkitt, D.P., Walker, A.R.P. and Painter, N.S. (1972) Effect of dietary fibre on stools and transit times and its role in the causation of diseases. *Lancet*, **ii**, 1408–1411.
22. Bussey, H.J.R. (1975) Familial Polyposis Coli. Baltimore and London: Johns Hopkins University Press.
23. Bussey, H.J.R., Wallace, M.H. and Morson, B.C. (1967) Metachronous carcinoma of the large intestine and intestinal polyps. *Proceedings of the Royal Society of Medicine*, **60**, 208–213.
24. Cannon-Albright, L.A., Skolnick, M.H., Bishop, D.T., Lee, R.G. and Burt, R.W. (1988) Common inheritance of susceptability to colonic adenomatous polyps and associated colorectal cancers. *New England Journal of Medicine*, **319**, 533–537.
25. Carroll, S.E. (1963) The prognostic significance of gross venous invasion in carcinoma of the rectum. *Canadian Journal of Surgery*, **6**, 281–286.
26. Carter, S.K. and Friedman, M. (1974) Integration of chemotherapy into combined modality treatment of solid tumours. II. Large bowel carcinoma. *Cancer Treatment Reviews*, **1**, 111–115.
27. Castleman, B. and Krickstein, H.I. (1962) Do adenomatous polyps of the colon become malignant? *New England Journal of Medicine*, **267**, 469–474.
28. Cheng, Ming-Chai, Chuang Chi Yuen, Chang Pei-Yu and Hu Jen-Chun (1980) Evolution of

colo-rectal cancer in schistosomiasis. *Cancer*, **46**, 1661–1675.

29. Cheng Ming Chai, Chuang Chi Yuen and Wang Fu Pen *et al*. (1981) Colo-rectal cancer and schistosomiasis. *Lancet*, **ii**, 971–973.

30. Cleave, T.L. (1974) *The Saccharine Disease*. Bristol: Wright.

31. Clemmesen, J. (1977) Statistical studies in the aetiology of malignant neoplasms. Volume V. *Trends and Risks in Denmark* 1943–72. Supplement 261. *Acta Pathologica, Microbiologica, et Immunologica Scandinavica*, Copenhagen: Munksgaard.

32. Cohen, A.M. and Wood, W.C. (1979) Carcino-embryonic antigen levels as an indicator for re-operation in patients with carcinoma of the colon and rectum. *Surgery, Gynecology and Obstetrics*, **149**, 22–27.

33. Cole, W.H., Packard, D. and Southwick, H.W. (1954) Carcinoma of the colon with special reference to prevention of recurrence. *Journal of the American Medical Association*, **155**, 1549–1554.

34. Cooke, R.V. (1956) Advanced carcinoma of the colon with emphasis on the inflammatory factor. *Annals of the Royal College of Surgeons of England*, **18**, 46–51.

35. Cooley, R.N., Agnew, C.H. and Rios, G. (1960) Diagnostic accuracy of the barium enema study in carcinoma of the colon and rectum. *American Journal of Roentgenology*, **84**, 31–35.

36. Cooper, E.H., Turner, R., Steele, L. *et al*. (1975) The contribution of serum enzymes and carcino-embryonic antigen to the early diagnosis of metastatic ano-rectal cancer. *British Journal of Cancer*, **31**, 111–116.

37. Copeland, E.M., Miller, L.D. and Jones, R.S. (1969) Prognostic factors in carcinoma of the colon and rectum. *Diseases of the Colon and Rectum*, **10**, 415–420.

38. Crile, G., Jr and Deodhar, S.D. (1971) Role of pre-operative irradiation in prolonging concomitant immunity and preventing metastases in mice. *Cancer*, **27**, 629–634.

39. Cripps, W.H. (1880) *Cancer of the Rectum*. London: J. & A. Churchill.

40. Cripps, W.H. (1882) *Transactions of the Pathological Society* (*London*), **33**, 165–170.

41. Crowther, J.S., Drasar, B.J., Hill, M.J. *et al*. (1976) Faecal steroids and bacteria and large bowel cancer in Hong Kong by socioeconomic groups. *British Journal of Cancer*, **34**, 191–196.

42. Cummings, J.H. (1983) *Recent Advances in Gastroenterology No. 5* (Ed.) Bouchier, I.A.D. Edinburgh, London, Melbourne & New York: Churchill Livingstone.

43. Cummings, J.H. (1978) Influence of diets high and low in animal fat on bowel habit in gastrointestinal transit time, faecal microflora, bile acid and fat excretion. *Journal of Clinical Investigation*, **61**, 953–958.

44. Cutait, D.E. and Figlioni, F.J. (1961) A new method of colo-rectal anastomosis in abdominoperineal resection. *Diseases of the Colon and Rectum*, **4**, 335–340.

45. Dales, L.G., Friedman, G.D., Ury, H.K. *et al*. (1978) A case control study of relationships of diet and other traits to colorectal cancer in American Blacks. *American Journal of Epidemiology*, **109**(2), 132–144.

46. Devlin, H.B., Plant, J.A. and Griffen, M. (1971) Aftermath of surgery of ano-rectal cancer. *British Medical Journal*, **iii**, 413–418.

47. Devroede, G. (1980) Risk of cancer in inflammatory bowel disease. In *Colo-rectal Cancer: Epidemiology and Screening. Progress in Cancer Research* (Ed.) Winawer, S.J., Sherlock, P. and Shottenfeld, D. New York: Raven Press.

48. Dobbins, W.O., III and Appelman, H.D. (1980) Difficulties in interpretation of dysplasia. In *Colo-rectal Cancer: Epidemiology and Screening. Progress in Cancer Research* (Ed.) Winawer, S.J., Sherlock, P. and Shottenfeld, D. New York: Raven Press.

49. Dockerty, M.B. (1958) Pathologic aspects in the control of spread of colonic carcinoma. *Proceedings of the Staff Meetings of the Mayo Clinic*, **33**, 157–162.

50. Drasar, B.S. and Irving, D. (1973) Environmental factors and cancer of the colon and breast. *British Journal of Cancer*, **27**, 167–172.

51. Dukes, C.E. (1926) Simple tumours of the large intestine and their relation to cancer. *British Journal of Surgery*, **13**, 720–725.

52. Dukes, C.E. (1930) The spread of cancer of the rectum. *British Journal of Surgery*, **17**, 643–648.

53. Dukes, C.E. (1937) Histological grading of rectal cancer. *Proceedings of the Royal Science of Medicine*, **30**, 371–376.

54. Dukes, C.E. (1940) Cancer of the rectum; an analysis of 1000 cases. *Journal of Pathology and Bacteriology*, **50**, 527–532.

55. Dukes, C.E. (1957) Discussion on major surgery in carcinoma of the rectum, with or without colostomy, excluding the anal canal and including the rectosigmoid. *Proceedings of the Royal Society of Medicine*, **50**, 1031–1036.

56. Durdey, P., Weston, P.M.T. and Williams, N.S. (1987) Colonoscopy of barium enema as initial investigation of colonic disease. *The Lancet*, **ii**, 549–551.

57. Dwight, R.W., Humphreys, W.E., Higgins, G.A. and Keehn, R.J. (1973) FUDR as an adjuvant to surgery in cancer of the large bowel. *Journal of Surgical Oncology*, **5**, 243–248.

58. Ekelund, G. and Lindström, C. (1974) Histopathological analysis of benign polyps in patients with carcinoma of the colon and rectum, *Gut*, **15**, 654–659.

59. Ekelund, G., Lindström, C. and Rosengren, J.E. (1974) Appearances and growth of early carcinoma of the colon–rectum. *Acta Radiologica*, **15**, 670–679.

60. Ellis, H. (1971) Curative and palliative surgery in advanced carcinoma of the large bowel. *British Medical Journal*, **iii**, 291–296.

61. Engell, H.C. (1955) Cancer cells in the circulating blood: a clinical study on the occurrence of cancer cells in the peripheral blood and in venous blood draining the tumour area at operation. *Acta Chirurgica Scandinavica* (Supplement), 201.

62. Enström, J.E. (1975) Colo-rectal cancer and consumption of beef and fat. *British Journal of Cancer*, **32**, 432–437.

63. Enterline, H.T., Evans, G.W., Mercado-Lugo, R. *et al.* (1962) Malignant potential of adenomas of colon and rectum. *Journal of the American Medical Association*, **179**, 322–327.

64. Ewing, M.R. (1951) Inflammatory complications of cancer of the caecum and ascending colon. *Postgraduate Medical Journal*, **27**, 515–520.

65. Fearon, E.R., Hamilton, S.R. and Vogelstein, B. (1987) Colonal analysis of human colorectal tumours. *Science*, **238**, 193–197.

66. Feingold, S.M., Sutter, V.L., Sugihara, P.T. *et al.* (1977) Faecal microbial flora in Seventh Day Adventist population and control subjects. *American Journal of Clinical Nutrition*, **30**, 1781–1786.

67. Ferguson, J.A. (1957) Management of villous tumours of the rectum. *Journal of the Kentucky Medical Association*, **55**, 996–1001.

68. Finlay, I.G., Meek, D.R., Gray, H.W. *et al.* (1982) Incidence and detection of occult hapatic metastases in colo-rectal carcinoma. *British Medical Journal*, **284**, 803–805.

69. Fisher, E.R. and Castro, A.F. (1953) Diffuse papillomatous polyps (villous tumours) of the colon and rectum. *American Journal of Surgery*, **85**, 146–151.

70. Fisher, E.R. and Turnbull, R.B., Jr (1952) Malignant polyps of rectum and sigmoid; therapy based on pathological considerations. *Surgery, Gynecology and Obstetrics*, **94**, 619–624.

71. Fisher, E.R. and Turnbull, R.B. (1955) The cytologic demonstration and significance of tumour cells in the mesenteric venous blood in patients with colo-rectal carinoma. *Surgery, Gynecology and Obstetrics*, **100**, 102–107.

72. Fowler, J.W., Bremner, D.N. and Moffat, L.E.F. (1978) The incidence and consequences of damage to the parasympathetic nerve supply to the bladder after abdomino-perineal excision of the rectum for carcinoma. *British Journal of Urology*, **50**, 95–97.

73. Fraser, Sir John (1938) Malignant disease of the large intestine. *British Journal of Surgery*, **25**, 647–648.

74. Friedman, P., Park, W.C. and Afonya, I.I. (1978) Adjuvant radiation therapy in colo-rectal cancer. *American Journal of Surgery*, **135**, 512–517.

75. Frugmorgen, P. (1980) Colonoscopy. In *Endoscopy and Biopsy in Gastroenterology. Technique and Indications*. pp. 87–99. Berlin, Heidelberg and New York: Springer-Verlag.

76. Gabriel, W.B. and Morson, B.C. (1956) Carcinoid of rectum with lymphatic and liver metastases. *Proceedings of the Royal Society of Medicine*, **49**, 472–477.

77. Gabriel, W.B., Dukes, C. and Bussey, H.J.R. (1935) Lymphatic spread in cancer of the rectum. *British Journal of Surgery*, **23**, 395–400.

78. Gardner, E.G. (1951) A genetic and clinical study of intestinal polyposis, a predisposing factor for carcinoma of the colon and rectum. *American Journal of Human Genetics*, **3**, 167–172.

79. Gerber, A., Thompson, R.J., Reiswig, O.K. and Vannix, R.S. (1962) Experiences with primary resection for acute obstruction of the large intestine. *Surgery, Gynecology and Obstetrics*, **123**, 593–598.

80. Gilbertson, V.A. (1959) Adenocarcinoma of the large bowel: 1340 cases with 100 per cent follow up. *Surgery*, **46**, 1027–1032.

81. Gilchrist, R.K. and David, V.C. (1947) A consideration of pathological factors influencing 5-year survival in radical resection of the large bowel and rectum for carcinoma. *American Surgeon*, **126**, 421–426.

82. Ginzburg, L. and Dreiling, P.A. (1956) Successive independent (metachronous) carcinoma of the colon. *Annals of Surgery*, **143**, 117–119.

83. Goldberg, M.J., Smith, J.W. and Nicholls, R.L. (1977) Comparison of the faecal microflora of Seventh Day Adventists with individuals consuming a general diet. *Annals of Surgery*, **186**, 97–102.

84. Goligher, J.C. (1941) The operability of carcinoma of the rectum. *British Medical Journal*, **ii**, 393–398.

85. Goligher, J.C. (1980) *Surgery of the Anus, Rectum and Colon*. 4th Edition, London: Baillière Tindall.

86. Goligher, J.C., Dukes, C.E. and Bussey, H.J.R. (1951) Local recurrences after sphincter saving excisions for carcinoma of the rectum and rectosigmoid. *British Journal of Surgery*, **39**, 199–204.

87. Goulston, K. (1980) The role of diet in screening with faecal occult blood tests. In *Colo-rectal Cancer, Epidemiology and Screening. Progress in Cancer Research* (Ed.) Winawer, S.J. Sherlock, P. and Schottenfeld, D. New York: Raven Press.

88. Gray, R., James, R. and Mossman, J. (1992). AXIS – a suitable case for treatment. UKCCCR Colorectal Cancer Sub Committee. (In press).

89. Greegor, D.H. (1967) Diagnosis of large bowel cancer in the asymptomatic patient. *Journal of the American Medical Association*, **201**, 943–948.

90. Grinnell, R.S. (1939) The grading and prognosis of carcinoma of the colon and rectum. *Annals of Surgery*, **109**, 500–533.

91. Grinnell, R.S. (1953) Results in treatment of carcinoma of the colon and rectum. *Surgery, Gynecology and Obstetrics*, **96**, 31–36.

92. Grinnell, R.S. (1954) Distal intramural spread of carcinoma of the rectum and rectosigmoid. *Surgery, Gynecology and Obstetrics*, **99**, 421–430.

93. Grinnell, R.S. (1966) Lymphatic block with atypical retrograde lymphatic metastases and spread in carcinoma of the colon and rectum. *Annals of Surgery*, **163**, 272–277.

94. Grinnell, R.S. and Lane, N. (1958) Benign and malignant adenomatous polyps and papillary adenomas of the colon and rectum. *International Abstracts of Surgery*, **106**, 519–524.

95. Grossi, C.E., Wolff, W.I., Nealand, T.F. *et al.* (1977) Intraluminal fluorouracil chemotherapy adjuvant to surgical procedure for resectable carcinoma of the colon and rectum. *Surgery, Gynecology and Obstetrics*, **145**, 549–554.

96. Guialdi, G.F., Poppalardo, G., Biase, C.D. and Pitasi, F. (1982) The use of computerised tomography in the study of recurrent pelvic malignancy after surgical treatment of the rectum. *Italian Journal of Surgical Sciences*, **12**, 33–38.

97. Habib, N.A., Peck, M.A., Sawyer, C.N. *et al.* (1983) Does fixity affect prognosis in colo-rectal tumours? *British Journal of Surgery*, **70**, 423–424.

98. Haenszel, W. and Carrea, P. (1971) Cancer of the colon and rectum and adenomatous polyps. *Cancer*, **28**, 14–24.

99. Haenszel, W., Berg, J.W., Segi, M. *et al.* (1973) Large bowel cancer in Hawaiian Japanese. *Journal of the National Cancer Institute*, **51**, 1765–1779.

100. Halkin, H., Meytes, D., Militeanu, J. and Ramot, B. (1973) Multiple lymphomatous polyposis of the gastrointestinal tract. *Israel Journal of Medical Sciences*, **9**, 648–653.

101. Hardcastle, J.D. (1990) Population screening for colorectal cancer. In *UKCCCB Screening for Colorectal Cancer* (Ed.) Hardcastle, J.D. pp. 102–110. Hamburg: Normed Verlag.

102. Hawley, P.R. (1981) quoted by Goligher, J.C. In *Results of Operations in Large Bowel Cancer* (Ed.) De Casse, J.J. Edinburgh: Churchill Livingstone.

103. Heald, R.J. (1980) Towards fewer colostomies – the impact of circular stapling devices in the surgery of rectal cancer in a district hospital. *British Journal of Surgery*, **60**, 198–208.

104. Heald, R.J. and Bussey, H.J.R. (1975) Clinical experience at St Mark's Hospital with multiple synchronous cancers of the colon and rectum. *Diseases of the Colon and Rectum*, **18**, 6–11.

105. Heald, R.J. and Leicester, R.J. (1981) The low stapled anastomosis. *British Journal of Surgery*, **68**, 333–337.

106. Herter, F.P. (1972) Preparation of the bowel for surgery. *Surgical Clinics of North America*, **52**, 859–870.

107. Hewitt, J., Rigby, J., Reeve, J. and Cox, A.G. (1973) Whole gut irrigation in preparation for large bowel surgery, *Lancet*, **iii**, 337–340.

108. Higgins, G.A., Dwight, R.W., Smith, J.V. and Keehn, R. (1971) Fluorouracil as an adjuvant to surgery in carcinoma of the colon. *Archives of Surgery*, **102**, 339–344.

109. Higgins, G.A., Humphrey, E., Juler, G.L. *et al.* (1976) Adjuvant chemotherapy in the treatment of large bowel cancer. *Cancer*, **38**, 1461–1466.

110. Hill, M.J. (1975) The role of colon anaerobes in the metabolism of bile acids and steroids and its relation to colon cancer. *Cancer*, **36**, 2387–2400.

111. Hill, M.J. (1981) Metabolic epidemiology of large bowel cancer. In *Gastrointestinal Cancer* (Ed.) De Cosse, J. and Sherlock, P. pp. 187–226. The Hague: Martinus Nijhoff.

112. Hill, M.J. (1983) Bile bacteria and bowel cancer. *Gut*, **24**, 871–875.

113. Hill, M.J. and Aries, V.C. (1971) Faecal steroid composition and its relationship to cancer of the large bowel. *Journal of Pathology*, **104**, 129–134.

114. Holden, W.D., Dixon, W.J. and Kuzma, J.W. (1967) The use of this topic as an adjuvant to the surgical treatment of colo-rectal carcinoma. *Annals of Surgery*, **65**, 481–486.

115. Hughes, E.S.R. (1966) Carcinoma of the right colon, upper left colon and sigmoid colon. *Australian and New Zealand Journal of Surgery*, **35**, 183–188.

116. Irvin, T.T. and Greaney, M.G. (1977) The treatment of colonic cancer presenting with intestinal obstruction. *British Journal of Surgery*, **64**, 741–746.

117. James, R.D., Johnson, R.J., Eddleston, B. *et al.* (1983) Prognostic factors in locally recurrent rectal carcinoma treated by radiotherapy. *British Journal of Surgery*, **70**, 468–472.

118. Jensen, H.E., Balslev, I. and Nielsen, J. (1970) Extensive surgery in treatment of carcinoma of the colon. *Acta Chirurgica Scandinavica*, **136**, 431–436.

119. Jensen, O.M. (1979) Cancer morbidity and causes of death among Danish brewery workers. *International Journal of Cancer*, **23**, 454–463.

120. Jensen, O.M. and MacLennan, R. (1979) Dietary factors and colo-rectal cancer in Scandinavia. *Israel Journal of Medical Sciences*, **15**, 329–334.

121. Jensen, O.M., Masbech, P., Salaspuro, M. and Ihumaki, T. (1974) A comparative study of the diagnostic basis for cancer of the colon and cancer of the rectum in Denmark and Finland. *International Journal of Epidemiology*, **3**, 183–186.

122. Judd, E.S. (1924) A consideration of lesions of the colon treated surgically. *5th Medical Journal of Nashville*, **17**, 75–80.

123. Keighley, M.R.B. (1977) Prevention of wound sepsis in gastrointestinal surgery. *British Journal of Surgery*, **64**, 315–340.

124. Killen, J.Y., Holyoke, E.D., Moertel, C.G. *et al.* (1981) Adjuvant therapy of adenocarcinoma of the colon following clinically curative resection: an interim report from the Gastrointestinal Tumour Study Group. In *Adjuvant Therapy of Cancer III* (Ed.) Jones, E. and Solman, S.E. New York: Grune and Straton.

125. Kirklin, J.W., Dockerty, M.B. and Waugh, J.M. (1949) The role of peritoneal reflection in the prognosis of carcinoma of the rectum and sigmoid

colon. *Surgery, Gynecology and Obstetrics*, **88**, 326–331.

126. Koprowski, H., Herlyn, M. and Steplewski, Z. (1981) Specific antigen in serum in patients with colon carcinoma. *Science*, **212**, 53–55.

127. Korte, W. (1900) Erfahrungen uber die operative Behandlung der malignen Dickdarm-Geschwulste. *Archiv. für Klinische Chirurgie*, **61**, 403–408.

128. Kussin, S.Z., Lipkin, M. and Winawer, S.J. (1979) Inherited colon cancer: clinical implications. State of the art. *American Journal of Gastroenterology*, **72**, 448–453.

129. Lane, R.H.S. and Parks, A.G. (1977) Function of the anal sphincter following colo-anal anastomosis. *British Journal of Surgery*, **64**, 596–597.

130. Lauer, S.D., Carlson, H.C. and Wollaeger, E.E. (1965) Accuracy of roentogenologic examination in detecting carcinoma of the colon. *Diseases of the Colon and Rectum*, **8**, 190–195.

131. Law, D.J., Olschwang, S. and Monpelat, J.P. (1988) Concerted non syntemic allelic loss in human colorectal carcinoma. *Science*, **241**, 961–964.

132. Lawrence, W., Terz, J.J., Horsley, S. *et al.* (1975) Chemotherapy as an adjuvant to surgery for colo-rectal cancer. *Annals of Surgery*, **181**, 616–621.

133. Lennard-Jones, J.E., Morson, B.C., Ritchie, J.K. *et al.* (1977) Cancer in colitis: assessment of the individual risk by clinical and histological criteria. *Gastroenterology*, **73**, 1280–1289.

134. Leppert, M., Dobbs, M., Scambler, P. *et al.* (1987) The gene for familial polyposis to the long arm of chromosome 5. *Science*, **238**, 1411–1412.

135. Le Quesne, L.P. and Thompson, A.D. (1958) Implantation recurrence of carcinoma of the rectum and colon. *New England Journal of Medicine*, **258**, 578–583.

136. Li, M.C. and Ross, S.T. (1976) Chemoprophylaxis for patients with colo-rectal cancer. *Journal of the American Medical Association*, **235**, 2825–2830.

137. Linos, D.A., O'Fallon, W.M., Beart, R.W. *et al.* (1981) Cholecystectomy and carcinoma of the colon. *Lancet*, **ii**, 379–381.

138. Localio, S.A. and Baron, B. (1973) Abdomino transsacral resection and anastomosis for mid rectal cancer. *Annals of Surgery*, **178**, 540–546.

139. Localio, S.A., Eng, K., Gouge, T.H. and Ransome, J.H.C. (1978) Abdominosacral resection for carcinoma of the mid rectum. Ten years experience. *Annals of Surgery*, **188**, 745–780.

140. Lockhart-Mummery, J.P. (1925) Cancer and hereditary. *Lancet*, **i**, 427–432.

141. Lockhart-Mummery, H.E. and Dukes, C.E. (1952) Surgical treatment of malignant rectal polyps with notes on their pathology. *Lancet*, **ii**, 751–756.

142. Lockhart-Mummery, H.E., Ritchie, J.K. and Hawley, P.R. (1976) The results of surgical treatment for carcinoma of the rectum at St Mark's Hospital from 1948–1971. *British Journal of Surgery*, **63**, 673–678.

143. Levett, E. (1976) Family studies in cancer of the colon and rectum. *British Journal of Surgery*, **63**, 13–18.

144. Lynch, H.T. and Krush, A.J. (1971) Cancer family G revisted 1895–1970. *Cancer*, **17**, 1505.

145. Lynch, H.T. and Krush, A.J. (1971) The cancer family syndrome and cancer control. *Surgery, Gynecology and Obstetrics*, **132**, 247.

146. Lynch, H.T., Lynch, J. and Lynch, P. (1977) Management and control of familial cancer. In *Progress in Cancer Research and Therapy. Genetics of Human Cancer* (Ed.) Mulvihill, J.J., Miller, R.R. and Fraumeni, J.F., Jr. Volume 3. New York: Raven Press.

147. Lynch, H.T., Harris, R.E., Lynch, P.M. *et al.* (1977) Role of heredity in multiple primary cancers. *Cancer*, **40**, 1849–1854.

148. Lynch, H.T., Lanspa, S.J., Boman, B.M., Smyrk, T. *et al.* (1988) Hereditary nonpolyposis colorectal cancer – Lynch Syndromes I and II. *Gastroenterology Clinics of North America*, **17**, 679–713.

149. Macklin, M.T. (1966) Inheritance of cancer of the stomach and large intestine. *American Journal of Human Genetics*, **10**, 42.

150. MacLennan, R. (1977) Dietary fibre transit time, faecal bacteria, steroids and colon cancer in two Scandinavian populations. *Lancet*, **ii**, 207–212.

151. Madden, J.L. and Kandalaft, S. (1971) Clinical evaluation of electrocoagulation in the treatment of cancer of the rectum. *American Journal of Surgery*, **122**, 347–352.

152. Maier, B.R., Flyren, M.A., Burton, G.C. *et al.* (1974) Effects of a high beef diet on bowel flora. *American Journal of Clinical Nutrition*, **27**, 1470–1475.

153. Mair, W.S.J., McAdam, W.A.F., Lee, P.W.R. *et al.* (1977) Carcinoma of the large bowel presenting as a subcutaneous abscess of the thigh: a report of 4 cases. *British Journal of Surgery*, **64**, 205–210.

154. Martin, E.W., Cooperman, M., King, G. *et al.* (1979) A retrospective and prospective study of serial CEA determinations in the early detection of recurrent colon cancer. *American Journal of Surgery*, **137**, 167–169.

155. Mastromarino, A.J., Reddy, B.S. and Wynder, E.L. (1978) Faecal profiles of anaerobic microflora of large bowel cancer patients and patients with non hereditary large bowel polyps. *Cancer Research*, **38**, 4458–4463.

156. Mayo, C.W. and Fly, O.A. (1956) Analysis of 5 years survival in carcinoma of the rectum and recto sigmoid. *Surgery, Gynecology and Obstetrics*, **103**, 94–99.

157. McDermott, F., Hughes, E.S.R., Pihl, E. *et al.* (1982) Long term results of restorative resection and total excision for carcinoma of the middle third of rectum. *Surgery, Gynecology and Obstetrics*, **154**, 833–837.

158. Mendiando, O.A., Wang, C.C., Welch, J.P. and Donaldson, G.A. (1976) Post-operative radiotherapy in carcinomas of the rectum and distal sigmoid colon. *Radiology*, **119**, 673–678.

159. Miles, W.E. (1910) The radical abdomino-perineal operation for cancer of the rectum and of the pelvic colon. *British Medical Journal*, **ii**, 941–946.

160. Miles, W.E. (1926) *Cancer of the Rectum.* London: Harrison.

161. Miln, D.C. and McLoughlin, I.S. (1969) Carcinoma of proximal large bowel associated with acute appendicitis. *British Journal of Surgery*, **56**, 143–148.

162. Minton, J.P., James, K.K., Hartubise, P.E. *et al.* (1978) The use of serial carcinogenic antigen determinations to predict recurrence of a carcinoma of colon and the second look operation. *Surgery, Gynecology and Obstetrics*, **147**, 208–213.

163. Modan, B. (1979) Patterns of gastrointestinal neoplasms in Israel. *Israel Journal of Medical Sciences*, **15**, 301–304.

164. Modan, B., Barell, V., Lubin, F. *et al.* (1975) Low fibre intake as an aetiological factor in cancer of the colon. *Journal of the National Cancer Institute*, **55**, 15 and 18.

165. Moertel, C.G. (1976) Fluorouracil as an adjuvant to colo-rectal cancer surgery. The breakthrough that never was. *Journal of the American Medical Association*, **236**, 1935–1940.

166. Moertel, C.G., Shutt, A.J. and Go, V.L. (1978) Carcinoembryonic antigen test for the detection of recurrent colo-rectal carcinoma – inadequacy for early detection. *Journal of the American Medical Association*, **239**, 1065–1070.

167. Moertel, C.G., Fleming, T.R., Macdonald, J.S. *et al.* (1990). Levamisole and fluorouracil for adjuvant therapy of resected colon cancer. *New England Journal of Medicine*, **322**, 352–358.

168. Moore, G.E., Sanberg, A. and Schuborg, S.R. (1957) Clinical and experimental observations on the occurrence and fate of tumour cells in the blood stream. *Annals of Surgery*, **76**, 755–760.

169. Moore, G.E., Sako, K., Kando, T. *et al.* (1961) Assessment of the exfoliation of tumour cells in the body cavities. *Surgery, Gynecology and Obstetrics*, **112**, 469–474.

170. Morgan, C.N. (1932) Endothelioma of the rectum. *Proceedings of the Royal Society of Medicine*, **25**, 1020–1025.

171. Morson, B.C. (1962) Precancerous lesions of the colon and rectum. *Journal of the American Medical Association*, **179**, 316–321.

172. Morson, B.C. (1966) Factors influencing the prognosis of early cancer of the rectum. *Proceedings of the Royal Society of Medicine*, **59**, 607–612.

173. Morson, B.C. and Dawson, I.M.P. (1979) *Gastrointestinal Pathology*, 2nd Edition, Oxford, London, Edinburgh & Melbourne: Blackwell Scientific Publications.

174. Murday, V. (1990) The family cancer clinic. In *UKCCCR Screening for Colorectal Cancer* (Ed.) Hardcastle, J.D. Hamburg: Normed Verlag.

175. Muto, T., Bussey, H.J.R. and Morson, B.C. (1975) The evolution of cancer of the colon and rectum. *Cancer*, **36**, 2251–2270.

176. Nemer, F.D., Stoeckinger, J.M. and Evans, O.T. (1977) Smooth muscle rectal tumours. A therapeutic dilemma. *Diseases of the Colon and Rectum*, **20**, 405–410.

177. Nicholls, R.J., Ritchie, J.K., Wadsworth, J. *et al.* (1979) Total excision of restorative resection for carcinoma of the middle third of the rectum. *British Journal of Surgery*, **66**, 625–627.

178. Norbury, L.E.C. (1952) Specimen of endothelioma of rectum. *Proceedings of the Royal Society of Medicine*, **25**, 1021–1026.

179. *Office of Population Censuses and Surveys* (1981) Cancer statistics: incidence, survival and mortality in England and Wales. Studies on medical and population subjects. No. 43. London: HMSO.

180. *Offices of Population Censuses and Surveys* (1981) Cancer statistics: registration 1976. London: HMSO.

181. Orda, R., Bawbik, J.B., Wiznitzer, T. and Schujman, E. (1976) Fibroma of the caecum. Report of a case. *Diseases of the Colon and Rectum.* **19**, 626–631.

182. Orloff, M.J. (1971) Carcinoid tumours of the rectum. *Cancer*, **28**, 175–180.

183. Pack, G.T., Miller, T.R. and Trinidad, S.S. (1963) Pararectal rhabdomyosarcoma: report of two cases. *Diseases of the Colon and Rectum*, **6**, 1–6.

184. Papillon, J. (1974) Endocavitary irradiation in the curative treatment of early rectal cancer. *Diseases of the Colon and Rectum*, **17**, 172–177.

185. Parks, A.G. (1972) Transanal technique in low rectal anastomosis. *Proceedings of the Royal Society of Medicine*, **65**, 975–976.

186. Parks, A.G. and Percy, J.P. (1982) Resection and sutured colo-rectal anastomosis for rectal carcinoma. *British Journal of Surgery*, **69**, 301–304.

187. Patterson, H.A. (1956) The management of caecal cancer discovered unexpectedly at operation for acute appendicitis. *Annals of Surgery*, **143**, 670–675.

188. Peskin, G.W. and Orloff, M.J. (1959) A clinical study of 25 patients with carcinoid tumours of the rectum. *Surgery, Gynecology and Obstetrics*, **109**, 673–678.

189. Pollett, W.G. and Nicholls, R.J. (1983) The relationship between the extent of distal clearance and survival and local recurrence rates after curative anterior resection for carcinoma of rectum. *Annals of Surgery*, **198**, 159–163.

190. Pomare, E.W. and Heaton, K.W. (1973) Alteration of bile salt metabolism by dietary fibre. *Gut*, **14**, 826–831.

191. Pomeranz, A.A. and Garlock, J.H. (1955) Postoperative recurrence of cancer of colon due to

desquamated malignant cells. *Journal of the American Medical Association*, **158**, 1434–1439.

192. Quan, S.H.W. (1959) Cul de sac smears for cancer cells. *Surgery*, **45**, 258–263.

193. Quer, E.A., Dahlin, D.C. and Mayo, C.W. (1953) Retrograde intramural spread of carcinoma of the rectum and rectosigmoid. *Surgery, Gynecology and Obstetrics*, **96**, 24–30.

194. Rankin, F.W. and Olsen, P.F. (1953) The hopeful prognosis in cases of carcinoma of the colon. *Surgery, Gynecology and Obstetrics*, **56**, 366–371.

195. Reddy, N.S. and Wynder, E.L. (1977) Metabolic epidemiology of colon cancer: faecal bile acids and neutral steroids in colon cancer and patients with adenomatous polyps. *Cancer*, **39**, 2533–2539.

196. Renton, P. and Blackshaw, A.J. (1976) Colonic lymphoma complicating ulcerative colitis. *British Journal of Surgery*, **63**, 542–547.

197. Roberts, S., Johassan, O., Long, L. *et al.* (1961) Clinical significance of cells in the circulating blood: two to five years survival. *Annals of Surgery*, **154**, 362–367.

198. Rogers, B.H.G. (1981) Complications of hazards of colonoscopy. In *Colonoscopy: Techniques, Clinical Practice and Colour Atlas* (Ed.) Hunt, R.H. and Waye, J.D. pp. 237–264. London: Chapman and Hall.

199. Sanders, G.B., Hazen, W.H. and Kinnaird, P.W. (1958) Adult intussusception and carcinoma of the colon. *Annals of Surgery*, **147**, 796–801.

200. Sanger, B.J., and Leckie, B.D. (1959) Plain muscle tumours of the rectum. *British Journal of Surgery*, **47**, 196–201.

201. Shucksmith, H.S. (1963) Subcutaneous abscesses as the first evidence of carcinoma of the colon. *British Journal of Surgery*, **50**, 514–519.

202. Sizer, J.S., Frederick, P.L. and Olborn, M.P. (1967) Primary linitis plastica of the colon. *Diseases of the Colon and Rectum*, **10**, 339–344.

203. Slanetz, C.A., Herter, F.P. and Grinnell, R.S. (1972) Anterior resection versus abdomino-perineal resection for cancer of the rectum and rectosigmoid. An analysis of 524 cases. *American Journal of Surgery*, **123**, 110–117.

204. Slaney, G. (1971) Results of treatment of carcinoma of the colon and rectum. In *Modern Trends in Surgery 3* (Ed.) Irvine, W.T. London: Butterworth.

205. Smiddy, F.G. and Goligher, J.C. (1957) Results of surgery in treatment of cancer of the large intestine. *British Medical Journal*, **i**, 793–798.

206. Solomon, E., Vossr Hall, V. *et al.* (1987) Chromosome 5 allele loss in human colorectal carcinomas. *Nature*, **328**, 616–619.

207. Spratt, J.S. and Ackerman, L.V. (1962) Small primary adenocarcinomas of the colon and rectum. *Journal of the American Medical Association*, **179**, 337–342.

208. Spratt, J.S., Ackerman, L.V. and Moyer, C.A. (1958) Relationship of polyps of the colon to the development of colonic cancer. *Annals of Surgery*, **148**, 682–687.

209. Staszewski, J., McCall, M.G. and Stenhouse, N.S. (1971) Cancer mortality in 1962–1966 among Polish migrants to Australia. *British Journal of Cancer*, **25**, 599–604.

210. Stearns, M.W., Jr and Binkley, G.E. (1953) The influence of location on prognosis in operable rectal cancer. *Surgery, Gynecology and Obstetrics*, **96**, 368–373.

211. Stemmerman, G.N., Nomura, A.M.Y., Mower, H. and Glober, G. (1981) Clues to the origin of colo-rectal cancer. In *Large Bowel Cancer* (Ed.) DeCosse, J.J. Edinburgh, London, Melbourne & New York: Churchill Livingstone.

212. Stewart, M.J. (1931) Precancerous lesions of the alimentary tract. *Lancet*, **ii**, 565, 617, 669–674.

213. Stout, A.P. (1959) Tumours of colon and rectum (excluding carcinoma and adenoma). In *Diseases of the Colon and Ano-rectum* (Ed.) Turell, R. Volume 1. Philadelphia & London: W.B. Saunders.

214. Strauss, A.A., Strauss, S.F., Crawford, R.A. and Strauss, H.A. (1935) Surgical diathermy of carcinoma of the rectum; its clinical end results. *Journal of the American Medical Association*, **104**, 1480–1485.

215. Swinton, N.W. and Counts, R.L. (1956) Cancer of the colon and rectum: statistical study with end results. *Journal of the American Medical Association*, **161**, 1139–1144.

216. Swinton, N.W., Neissner, W.A. and Soland, W.A. (1955) Papillary adenomas of the colon and rectum: a clinical and pathological study. *Archives of Internal Medicine*, **96**, 544–549.

217. Talbot, I.C., Ritchie, S., Leighton, M. *et al.* (1980) The clinical significance of invasion of veins by rectal cancer. *British Journal of Surgery*, **67**, 439–442.

218. Taylor, I., Bennett, R. and Sheriff, S. (1978) The measurement of blood flow into colo-rectal metastases. *British Journal of Cancer*, **36**, 749–754.

219. Taylor, I., Rowling, J.T. and West, C. (1979) Adjuvant liver perfusion for colo-rectal cancer. *British Journal of Surgery*, **66**, 833–838.

220. Teague, R.H., Salmon, P.R. and Read, A.E. (1973) Fibre optic examination of the colon; a review of 255 cases. *Gut*, **14**, 139–144.

221. Thomas G.D.H., Dixon, M.F., Smeeton, N.C. and Williams, N.S. (1983) Observer variation in the histological grading of rectal carcinoma. *Journal of Clinical Pathology*, **36**, 385–389.

222. Thorlakson, R.H. and Ross, H.M. (1961) Leiomyosarcoma of the rectum. *Annals of Surgery*, **154**, 979–984.

223. Turcot, J., Després, J.P. and St Pierre, F. (1959) Malignant tumours of the central nervous system associated with familial polyposis of the colon. Report of two cases. *Diseases of the Colon and Rectum*, **2**, 465–470.

224. Turnbull, R.B., Jr, Kyle, K., Watson, F.R. and

Spratt, J. (1967) Cancer of the colon: the influence of the no touch isolation technic on survival rates. *Annals of Surgery*, **166**, 420–425.

225. Turunen, M.J. and Kivilaakso, E.O. (1981) Increased risk of colo-rectal cancer after cholecystectomy. *Annals of Surgery*, **194**, 639–641.

226. Umpleby, H.C., Femor, B., Symes, M.O. and Williamson, R.C.N. (1984) Viability of exfoliated colorectal carcinoma cells. *British Journal of Surgery*, **71**, 659–663.

227. Utsunomiya, J. (1977) Present status of adenomatous coli in Japan. In *Pathophysiology of Carcinoma in Digestive Organs* (Ed.) Forber, E. Tokyo: University Tokyo Press, Baltimore: Parks Press.

228. Veale, A.M.O. (1965) *Intestinal Polyposis.* London: Cambridge University Press.

229. Vernick, L.J. and Kuller, L.H. (1982) A case control study of cholecystectomy and right sided colon cancer. *American Journal of Epidemiology*, **116**, 86–101.

230. Villemin, F., Huard, P. and Montagne, M. (1925) Recherches anatomiques sur les lymphatiques du rectum et de l'anus: leurs applications dans le traitement chirurgical du cancer. *Revista Chirurgie (Paris)*, **63**, 69–74.

231. Vogelstein, B., Fearon, E.R. and Hamilton, S.R. (1988) Genetic alterations during colorectal tumour development. *New England Journal of Medicine*, **319**, 525–532.

232. Walker, R.M. (1971) *Annual Report of South Western Regional Cancer Bureau*, UTF House, King Square, Bristol BS2 8HY.

233. Waterhouse, J.A.H., Muir, C.S., Carrea, P. and Powell, J. (Ed.) (1976) *Cancer Incidence in Five Continents*. Volume III. Lyon, *International Agency for Research in Cancer*. IARC Scientific Publications No. 15.

234. Welch, C.E., McKittrick, J.B. and Behringer, G. (1952) Polyps of the rectum and colon and their relation to cancer. *New England Journal of Medicine*, **247**, 959–964.

235. Welin, S. (1958) Modern trends in diagnostic roentgenology of the colon. *British Journal of Radiology*, **31**, 453–458.

236. Werf, S.D.J. van der, Nagengast, F.M., Henegouwan, G.P. van berge *et al.* (1982) Colonic absorption of secondary bile acids in patients with adenomatous polyps and matched controls. *Lancet*, **i**, 759–762.

237. Werf, S.D.J. van der, Nagengast, F.M., Henegouwan, G.P. van berge, *et al.* (1983) Intracolonic environment and the presence of colonic adenomas in man. *Gut*, **24**, 876–880.

238. Whittaker, M. and Goligher, J.C. (1976) The prognosis after surgical treatment for carcinoma of the rectum. *British Journal of Surgery*, **63**, 384–388.

239. Wildrick, D.M. and Bodman, B.M. (1988) Chromosome 5 allele loss at the glucocorticoid receptor locus in human colorectal carcinomas. *Biochemical and Biophysical Research Commission*, **150**, 591.

240. Williams, N.S. and Johnston, D. (1983) The quality of life after rectal excision for low rectal cancer. *British Journal of Surgery*, **70**, 460–462.

241. Williams, N.S. and Johnston, D. (1984) Survival and recurrence after sphincter saving resection and abdominoperineal resection of the rectum for carcinoma of the middle third rectum. *British Journal of Surgery*, **71**.

242. Williams, N.S., Price, R. and Johnston, D. (1980) The long term effect of sphincter preserving operations for rectal carcinoma on the function of the anal sphincters in man. *British Journal of Surgery*, **67**, 203–208.

243. Williams, N.S., Neal, D.E. and Johnston, D. (1980) Bladder function after excision of the rectum for low rectal carcinoma. *Gut*, **21**, A453–454.

244. Williams, N.S., Dixon, M.F. and Johnston, D. (1983) Re-appraisal of the 5 centimetre rule of distal excision for carcinoma of the rectum; a study of distal intramural spread and of patients' survival. *British Journal of Surgery*, **70**, 150–154.

245. Willis, R.A. (1948) *The Pathology of Tumours.* London: Butterworth.

246. Winawer, S.J., Sherlock, P., Schottenfeld, D. and Miller, P.G. (1976) Screening for colon cancer. *Gastroenterology*, **70**, 783–788.

247. Winawer, S.J., Fleisher, M., Green, S. *et al.* (1977a) Carcino embryonic antigen in colonic lavage. *Gastroenterology*, **73**, 719–722.

248. Winawer, S.J., Leidner, S.D., Miller, D.G. *et al.* (1977b) Results of a screening programme for the detection of early colon cancer and polyps using faecal occult blood testing. *Gastroenterology*, **72**, A-127, 1150–1155.

249. Winawer, S.J., Ginther, M., Weston, E. *et al.* (1978) Impact of modification in faecal occult blood test on screening programme for colo-rectal neoplasia. *Gastroenterology*, **74**, 1140–1145.

250. Winawer, S.J., Leidner, S.D., Boyle, C. and Kurtz, R.C. (1979) Comparison of flexible sigmoidoscopy with other diagnostic techniques in the diagnosis of rectocolon neoplasia. *Digestive Diseases & Sciences*, **24**(4), 277–281.

251. Woolfe, C.M. (1958) A genetic study of carcinoma of the large intestine. *American Journal of Human Genetics*, **10**, 42–47.

252. Wood, W.Q. and Wilkie, D.P.D. (1933) Carcinoma of the rectum. An anatomico pathological study. *Edinburgh Medical Journal*, **40**, 321–326.

253. Wood, C.B., Gillis, C.R., Hole, D. *et al.* (1981) Local tumour invasion as a prognostic factor in colo-rectal cancer. *British Journal of Surgery*, **68**, 326–328.

254. Wychulis, A.R., Beahrs, O.H. and Woolner, L.B. (1966) Malignant lymphoma of the colon. A study of 69 cases. *Archives of Surgery*, **191**, 169–174.

255. Wynder, E.L. (1975) The epidemiology of large bowel cancer. *Cancer Research*, **35**, 3388–3394.

256. Wynder, E.L. and Reddy, B.S. (1974) Metabolic epidemiology of colo-rectal cancer. *Cancer*, **34**, 801–806.

257. Yudkin, J. (1972) *Pure White and Deadly*. London: Davis.

258. Youker, J.E., Welin, W. and Main, G. (1968) Computer analysis in the differentiation of benign and malignant polypoid lesions of the colon. *Radiology*, **90**, 794–797.

RADIATION DAMAGE *(R.B. Galland)*

The pathophysiology of radiation damage to the gut, together with predisposing factors and preventive measures have been discussed earlier (Chapter 3, Radiation enteropathy). This chapter deals mainly with the effect of radiation on the large bowel.

CLINICAL FEATURES

Most patients undergoing abdominopelvic radiotherapy experience abdominal symptoms. Nausea and vomiting are common and watery diarrhoea, possibly with abdominal colic, suggest small intestinal involvement. Proctosigmoiditis may produce a mucous discharge and mucosal ulceration can lead to rectal bleeding. Tenesmus suggests rectal involvement. Sigmoidoscopy shows a dusky, hyperaemic, oedematous mucosa which is extremely friable. The radiographic findings using barium enema at this time include muscle spasm and mucosal irregularity. These symptoms generally subside spontaneously within a week or so of completion of the course of radiotherapy and most patients have no further trouble.[28] Whereas these acute affects tend to be transient, the later problems are relentless and progressive. Patients experiencing the worst acute symptoms may be at greater risk of developing late gastrointestinal complications,[9] but even patients who experience no acute problems are still at risk of developing chronic radiation damage.

Subclinical effects

It is now apparent that gut can be damaged while the patient remains apparently asymptomatic. Newman *et al.* found that in 17 consecutive patients attending a radiotherapy follow-up clinic, 12 had a permanent alteration in bowel habit and 16 had evidence of malabsorption.[34]

There are a number of reports in the literature of patients who, having had radiotherapy previously, underwent a laparotomy for a totally unrelated course. Their postoperative course was complicated by a perforation or necrosis of the previously irradiated bowel. Presumably, this emphasizes the precarious nature of the intestinal blood supply in these patients.[14,23]

Late effects

The accepted incidence of late radiation damage following abdominopelvic radiotherapy is between 2% and 5% although higher rates have been reported.[2] There has been a progressive increase in the number of patients presenting with radiation damage over the last few years. At the Hammersmith Hospital, London, over half of the patients presenting with radiation damage did so within the last 10 years of a study extending over 26 years.[15] Other authors have described similar findings.[2,33]

The latent period between the course of radiotherapy and the clinical manifestation of symptoms is usually between 6 months and 2 years. In some patients however, symptoms only become apparent 20 or more years after the radiotherapy. The diagnosis of radiation damage should always be considered when the patient who has had previous radiotherapy presents with abdominal problems. The clinical picture may also vary with time from the initial radiotherapy. Rectal bleeding and tenesmus tend to occur within a few months of treatment finishing, whereas fistula formation, and obstruction due to stricture, occur much later.

The major differential diagnosis lies between radiation damage and recurrence of the original tumour. Misdiagnoses are by no means uncommon. Gilinsky *et al.* described 88 patients with a diagnosis of radiation proctosigmoiditis.[18] Some were overtly Cushingoid as a result of steroids given for presumed ulcerative colitis, two had undergone haemorrhoidectomy and others had been treated with antibiotics, a diagnosis of diverticulitis having been made. It should be remembered, however, that pre-existing inflammatory disease may be exacerbated by radiotherapy.

Proctosigmoiditis appears to be the commonest clinical manifestation of radiation damage, being present in nearly three quarters of the cases in one series.[4] Most patients can be treated conservatively: of 720 cases diagnosed at the Mayo Clinic, only 8.6% required an operation.[26] Most of these had a stricture, fistula or necrosis, and in only six patients (0.8%) was the operation performed for intractible proctitis. Gilinsky *et al.* found that spontaneous remission of proctosigmoiditis was usual in those patients in whom blood transfusions were not required and who had little or no bowel disturbance or abdominal pain. By contrast, those patients in whom transfusion was required, or in whom abdominal pain or bowel disturbance was an important feature, were more likely to need an operation. Furthermore, the radiation-induced mortality was significantly higher in these latter patients.[18]

The overall prognosis of patients with established radiation enteritis is poor.[22] In the author's series, of 51 patients followed up for one year, only 24 (47%) remained symptom free.[15] Of the remainder, 20 had developed new radiation-related gastrointestinal problems. Those patients presenting with fistula or perforation were more likely to go on to develop metachronous lesions than those initially presenting with haemorrhage. It is possible that if only a part of the gut wall is damaged (i.e. the mucosa) to produce bleeding, the radiation effect is less widespread than when the whole thickness of the gut is involved to produce stricture, fistula or perforation. The presence of a fistula does seem to indicate particularly widespread disease. The study revealed that multiple synchronous lesions were more common in patients presenting with a fistula compared with those presenting with stricture.[16] Furthermore, patients with a fistula are more likely to die of recurrent malignancy.[24]

Another study showed that of 34 patients having an operation for radiation enteritis, only 10 were alive 1 year later. Four of these patients had a recurrence of their original tumour. Only two were able to work, four suffered from intermittent abdominal pains, all had diarrhoea and all were below average weight, half having low haemoglobin or serum B12 levels, or both.[32]

Damage to adjacent organs is another main cause of both morbidity and mortality. Urinary tract injuries are common. Radiation myelitis, major pelvic vessel occlusion and liver, pancreatic and bile duct damage have all been described.

Colonic adenocarcinomas can be induced experimentally by exposing rats to abdominal radiation.[12] Patients who have had abdominopelvic radiotherapy appear to have a slightly greater chance of developing colorectal malignancy than the rest of the population.[39] The risk in negligible until 10 years have elapsed from the time of radiotherapy.

Figure 4.72 shows the survival of 70 patients with radiation damage to the large and small bowel treated at the Hammersmith Hospital. The 5-year survival was 42%. The difference between the two curves represents those patients who died of radiation-related causes. Over one third of the patients who died as a result of radiation damage were free of their original tumour.[15]

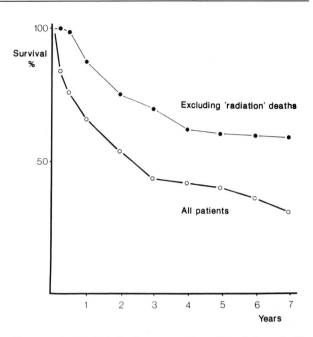

Figure 4.72 Survival of patients presenting with radiation enteritis. (From Galland and Spencer,[15] with permission.)

TREATMENT

Acute symptoms

Acute radiation symptoms usually subside spontaneously within a few weeks of completion of a course of radiotherapy. Should symptoms be severe, a 10% reduction in the daily dose of radiation should relieve symptoms without compromising tumour control.[28] The only other treatment required at this point is likely to be symptomatic control with antispasmodics, anticholinergics or mild opiate analgesics.

Hydrophilic stool softeners may help to control the mucous diarrhoea of proctitis. Sitz baths and perianal compresses have been used in an attempt to ease tenesmus if simple analgesics fail. Steroid retention enemas also appear useful in both acute and chronic radiation proctitis.

Chronic radiation damage

Both medical and surgical management of established radiation enteritis is complex and will vary widely from one patient to the next. It is very easy to underestimate the extent of radiation damage, as much of it is subclinical. Large bowel injury rarely exists in isolation, and it is not uncommon to find patients having symptoms related both to small and large bowel involvement. The differential diagnosis between recurrent malignancy and radiation damage may ultimately only be made on the histology of tissue taken at a laparotomy. Clearly, then, the management of radiation damage to the colorectum cannot be considered without mention of the management of the patient as a whole, and particularly in terms of the management of small bowel problems as discussed by Morganstern in Chapter 3.

Management of colitis and proctitis

General measures include the avoidance of constipation by advising a high residue diet, combined if necessary with osmotic laxatives.

Anti-inflammatory drugs

Topical corticosteroids, either as enemas or foam preparations, have been shown to be effective in the management of acute coloproctitis. However, as yet, there are no controlled trials to confirm their efficacy.

Sulphasalazine (Salazopyrin) and systemic corticosteroids are probably also of value, although again, control studies are currently lacking. Jacobs *et al.* found that the administration of oral or rectal Salazopyrin alleviated the symptoms of acute and chronic radiation proctitis in 37 of 40 patients so treated.[25]

Rectal bleeding

Generally, the bleeding is mild and can be controlled with the measures outlined above. When conventional treatment fails endoscopic laser therapy may be effective. Ahlquist *et al.*, using an Nd:YAG laser, treated four cases of haemorrhagic proctitis.[1] Between one and three sessions per patient were needed with intervals of at least 3 months between each session. Six months after the

end of the course of treatment, all patients were symptomatically and endoscopically improved. Argon lasers seem to produce similar results[8] and may have the theoretical advantage of having a shallower depth of penetration than Nd:YAG lasers.

Colostomy alone, in the treatment of tenesmus or haemorrhage is unlikely to be successful. Irrigation of a defunctioned rectum with a solution of formalin has also been described in a case of intractible haemorrhagic proctitis. The bleeding was controlled and had not recurred 14 months later.[38]

SURGERY

There are two main problems which face a surgeon when operating on a patient with radiation colitis. Firstly, irradiated gut heals poorly and, secondly, bowel that appears normal may be damaged microscopically.

The poor healing potential of irradiated gut has been frequently shown. By the late 1970s many authors had described series of patients in whom resection and anastomosis were followed by a high rate of anastomotic dehiscence (up to 50%) with a corresponding high mortality. This applied equally, to both large and small bowel anastomoses. Ideally, the two ends of bowel used for an anastomosis should have been outside the irradiated field and free of disease. Bowel which appears normal, however, may be microscopically damaged. *Figure 4.73* shows the findings at laparotomy of a patient with both a terminal ileal and sigmoid colon stricture. There appears to be a fairly clear line of demarcation (D) between diseased and normal terminal ileum. In

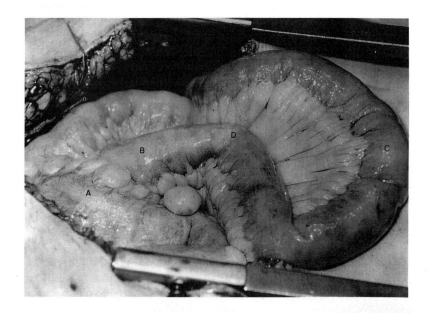

Figure 4.73 Operation photograph showing irradiated sigmoid colon A and terminal ileum B. The distal ileum C, appears normal. (From Galland, R.B. and Spencer, J. (1986) General principles of surgical management. In *Radiation Enteritis* (Eds) Galland, R.B. and Spencer, J., pp. 206–214. London: Edward Arnold Ltd, with permission.)

fact, histological examination of the resected specimen confirmed microscopic evidence of radiation damage 20 cm beyond the line of demarcation. A frozen section is not helpful in these circumstances.

Before considering an elective operation on patients with radiation enteritis, a full assessment of the extent of disease and correction of any underlying biochemical or septic complications should be performed. Some of the general principles that have evolved in operating upon patients with radiation-damaged gut, in order to avoid the pitfalls already mentioned, are described below.

'Wide' resection of irradiated bowel is the ideal and is frequently advocated. There is little attempt, however, to define these wide limits. Schofield *et al.* suggest that in ileal resection, at least 50 cm of gut should be removed.[40] The problem of anastomotic leakage following primary anastomosis can be largely overcome by using gut for one end of the anastomosis which is taken from outside the original radiation field. In patients who presented to the Hammersmith Hospital, most radiation-induced lesions were in the distal ileum, sigmoid colon or rectum. This is not surprising, as the original radiotherapy is mostly undertaken for pelvic pathology. Thus the caecum, ascending colon and descending colon were never involved and only one lesion was encountered in the transverse colon.

Between 1977 and 1984 we followed the above principles and, for recto-sigmoid resection, the splenic flexure was mobilized to bring it down for anastomosis (*Figure 4.74*). Using these techniques, there was a significant improvement in our results, there being only one radiological, anastomotic leak in 14 anastomoses, with no patients dying.[17] Using similar techniques, Marks and Mohiudden described no leaks in intraperitoneal anastomoses and only four in 52 extraperitoneal anastomoses.[31]

Resection followed by an ileostomy and colostomy and mucous fistula may be appropriate in certain circumstances, particularly if there is peritoneal contamination from perforation. If histology confirms the presence of radiation damage at the resection lines, it is clear that further resection is necessary before subsequent anastomosis. Even when the resection margins are apparently healthy, however, a safe anastomosis at a later date cannot be necessarily guaranteed as the disease may progress in the meantime.

In 1976 Palmer and Bush[36] described 31 anterior resections performed on irradiated bowel, with only two anastomotic leaks. The only apparent difference in their technique compared with that of others was that 'a pedicle of omentum was sutured around the anastomosis in all patients'. The importance of having non-irradiated tissue surrounding an anasto-

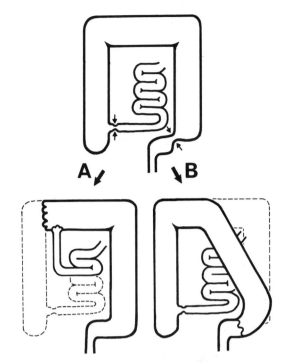

Figure 4.74 Terminal ileal lesions treated by right hemicolectomy and ileotransverse anastomosis. A; and rectosigmoid lesions treated by left hemicolectomy bringing the splenic flexure down for anastomosis. B. (From Galland and Spencer,[17] with permission.)

mosis has been described by Ormiston.[35] In rats, the anastomotic dehiscence rate was higher if both gut and fatty appendages of the epididymis (equivalent to the omentum) were irradiated than if the gut alone were irradiated.[35] This may partially explain why using transverse colon for one end of the anastomosis, as described earlier, is so effective, the anastomosis being surrounded by non-irradiated omentum.

In the face of extensive distal disease, where even the anal canal may be damaged, any attempt at restorative resection could be dangerous. Under such circumstances, an abdominoperineal excision of the rectum may be all that is possible. Of 47 patients with colonic damage, in the series described by Schofield *et al.*, no less than 15 required such an operation.[40] All of these patients made a satisfactory postoperative recovery and about half were well at the time of follow-up.

Bypass or exclusion procedures should be avoided whenever possible. Swan *et al.* described over 200 patients, largely selected from the literature, in whom bypass procedures were apparently better than primary resection and anastomosis.[42] They found that with resection and anastomosis, over one third of the anastomoses leaked, with one fifth of the patients dying. On the other hand, with bypass procedures the leakage rate was less than 10% with a similar reduction in mortality. Bowel which is bypassed or defunctioned, and therefore left in-situ, however, can go on to produce further problems.[17,41] Furthermore, other authors have failed to show a benefit of bypass compared with a resection and anastomosis. Bypass procedures should now only be used when multiple resections would otherwise be necessary, or in the face of a difficult or dangerous dissection.

Should a *stoma* prove necessary it must be carefully sited. In those patients who are unfit for extensive surgery, or in those with a frozen pelvis, a simple colostomy may be all that is feasible. Harling and Balslev found that 63 of their 75 patients with recto-sigmoid injury ultimately required a permanent colostomy.[21]

In these circumstances, it is important to raise the colostomy in bowel which is likely to have been outside the original radiation field. The likelihood of stenosis, gangrene or haemorrhage from colostomies raised in the sigmoid colon is higher than that of those raised in the transverse colon.[11,26] Should there be any chance of reconstructive surgery following the initial colostomy, then the stoma should be sited in the right transverse colon so that the splenic flexure can be mobilized for anastomosis as described earlier.

The importance of avoiding *unnecessary extensive dissection* and division of adhesions, the use of intraluminal tubes, gastrostomies and delayed enteral feeding has all been described and are discussed in chapter 3, Radiation enteropathy.

MANAGEMENT OF RECTOVAGINAL FISTULAS

Conservative treatment of radiation-induced fistulas is unlikely to be successful. Rectovaginal fistulas are the commonest and most challenging of such fistulas to be encountered. The surgical options available can broadly be considered as being perineal procedures, abdominal procedures or some sort of combination of the two. Whatever method is employed, a defunctioning colostomy is advisable.

Perineal procedures

These operations are usually performed in the lithotomy position. There are two main features to the operation. Firstly, the fistula is exposed, the fibrotic margins excised and the vaginal and rectal defects are closed separately. For a high fistula or a large fistula, it may not be possible to close the rectal defect without mobilizing the rectosigmoid junction. This may need to be carried out through the separate abdominal incision. Secondly, healthy tissue is interposed between the rectum and vagina. The use of

mobilized gracilis muscle (the gracilis flap), bulbospongiosus or a labial fat pad (Martius technique) and a flap of skin[27] have all been described. The results of these techniques are difficult to evaluate fully as few people have much experience of them. Of 18 gracilis flap procedures performed by Graham, however, satisfactory results were achieved in 15. Furthermore, in one other patient whose first operation was unsatisfactory, a good result was obtained following a second operation using the gracilis muscle from the opposite side.[20]

Boronov claimed an 84% success rate for rectovaginal and a 50% success rate for vesicovaginal fistulas using the Martius technique,[3] although, only 22 patients were studied.

Abdominal procedures

Pedicle flap

Use of a greater omentum pedicle flap has been described.[19] The fistula is exposed and repaired using an abdominal approach. The greater omentum is then mobilized based on either a left or right gastroepiploic artery and is then tucked down between the rectum and vagina. This type of technique would seem to be suitable for high fistulas with a small fistulous opening.

Rectal excision

Anterior resection or abdominopelvic pull-through operations are often unsatisfactory because of the poor healing potential of the irradiated rectal stump. The 'abdominotransanal sleeve' procedure overcomes this problem.[10,37] The principal features of the operation are firstly, transection of the rectal stump above the fistula. Secondly, the rectal mucosa is removed down to the dentate line, the fistula being left in situ. Thirdly, healthy, mobilized proximal colon is pulled through the tube of rectal muscle, to be anastomosed to the anal verge.

The results of this type of procedure are encouraging. Of approximately 100 patients, taken from six series described in the literature, good bowel function was achieved in approximately two thirds with only 14% being regarded as failures.[29] Frequency and urgency, however, may be troublesome. Although the external sphincter appears to be normal, the internal sphincter may be impaired and there may be marked reduction in the compliance of the neorectum.[43] Anal sphincter function may also be impaired simply as a result of the radiotherapy.[44] A further, theoretical disadvantage of this operation would seem to be that the muscular tube, through which the colon is brought down, may form a stricture at a later date. This technique has also been successfully used in the management of severe haemorrhage from proctitis.[44]

Rectal reconstruction

Bricker from Columbia, Missouri, has developed a technique of rectal reconstruction for both rectovaginal fistulas and rectal strictures.[5,6] This type of reconstruction should only be considered in a fit, well-motivated patient with normal rectal continence. The operation is performed with a minimal degree of rectal mobilization and dissection. The principle of the operation is to dissect between the rectum and vagina in order to expose and open the fistula. The rectal end of the fistula is then closed by suturing the divided end of distal sigmoid colon into it. Colonic continuity is restored by anastomosing proximal, non-irradiated colon, end to side, onto the reconstructed rectum.

MANAGEMENT OF RECTAL STRICTURES

Radiation-induced rectal stenosis will not respond to simple measures such as dilatation. The choice seems to be between simple colostomy or rectal excision on the one hand, and either anterior resection or reconstruction on the other. Should anterior resection be attempted, then as low an anastomosis as possible should be performed; it should be surrounded by omentum and covered with a defunctioning colostomy.

Rectal reconstruction

A linear rectal stricture, with or without a combined fistula, can be repaired using the Bricker fillet and fold-over technique. The stricture is incised longitudinally through its anterior surface. The incision is extended proximally into normal colon. The transected proximal colon is then folded down and the sides of the colon are sutured to the sides of the rectum. Continuity of the bowel is restored as described previously.

Bricker reconstructions lead to good or satisfactory results, in terms of rectal function, in about 70% of cases.[29]

Because surgeons are more likely to be familiar with an abdominotransverse sleeve technique, this would seem to be the best sphincter-saving operation. If the fistula is small, however, with little surrounding radiation damage, then a perineal procedure may be tried first. Should this fail, then the Bricker reconstruction would be adopted although, in some cases, permanent stoma may be a preferred option.

References

1. Ahlquist, D.A., Gostout, C.J., Viggiano, T.R. and Pemberton, J.H. (1986) Laser therapy for severe radiation-induced rectal bleeding. *Mayo Clinic Proceedings*, **61**, 927–931.
2. Allen-Mersh, T.G., Wilson, E.J., Hope-Stone, H.F. and Mann, C.V. (1986) Has the incidence of radiation-induced bowel damage following treatment of uterine carcinoma changed in the last 20 years? *Journal of the Royal Society of Medicine*, **79**, 387–390.
3. Boronow, R.C. (1986) Repair of the radiation induced vaginal fistula using the Martius technique. *World Journal of Surgery*, **10**, 237–248.
4. Bosch, A. and Frias, Z. (1977) Complications after radiation therapy for cervical carcinoma. Acta Radiologica (Therapeutics) (Stockholm) 16, 53–62.
5. Bricker, E.M., Johnston, W.D. and Patwardhan, R.V. (1981) Repair of postirradiation damage to colorectum. A progress report. *Annals of Surgery*, **193**, 555–564.
6. Bricker, E.M., Kraybill, W.G. and Lopez, M.J. (1986) Functional results after postirradiation rectal reconstruction. *World Journal of Surgery*, **10**, 249–258.
7. Browning, G.G.P., Varma, J.S., Smith, A.N., Small, W.P. and Duncan, W. (1987) Late results of mucosal proctectomy and colo-anal sleeve anastomosis for chronic irradiation rectal injury. *British Journal of Surgery*, **74**, 31–34.
8. Buchi, K.N. and Dixon, J. A. (1987) Argon laser treatment of hemorrhagic radiation proctitis. *Gastrointestinal Endoscopy*, **33**, 27–29.
9. Buchler, D.A., Kline, J.C., Peckham, B.C., Boone, M.L.M. and Carr, W.F. (1971) Radiation reactions in cervical cancer therapy. *American Journal of Obstetrics and Gynecology*, **111**, 745–750.
10. Cooke, S.A.R. and Wellsted, M.D. (1986) The radiation damaged rectum: Resection with colo-anal anastomosis using the endoanal technique. *World Journal of Surgery*, **10**, 220–227.
11. DeCosse, J.J., Rhodes, R.S., Wentz, W.B., Reagan, J.W., Dworken, H.J. and Holden, W.D. (1969) The natural history and management of radiation induced injury of the gastrointestinal tract. *Annals of Surgery*, **170**, 369–384.
12. Denman, D.L., Kirschner, R. and Osborne, J.W. (1978) Induction of colonic adenocarcinoma in the rat by X-irradiation. *Cancer Research*, **38**, 1899–1905.
13. Futh, H., Ebeler, F. (1915) Rontgen und radiumtherapie des uteruskarzinoms. *Zentralblatt Gynacologie*, **14**, 217–227.
14. Galland, R.B. and Spencer, J. (1985) Spontaneous postoperative perforation of previously asymptomatic irradiated bowel. *British Journal of Surgery*, **72**, 285.
15. Galland, R.B. and Spencer, J. (1985) The natural history of clinically established radiation enteritis. *The Lancet*, 1257–1258.

16. Galland, R.B. and Spencer, J. (1986) Radiation-induced gastrointestinal fistulae. *Annals of the Royal College of Surgeons of England*, **68**, 5–7.

17. Galland, R.B. and Spencer, J. (1986) The surgical management of radiation enteritis. *Surgery*, **99**, 133–138.

18. Gilinsky, N.H., Burns, D.G., Barbezat, G.U., Levin, W., Myers, H.S. and Marks, I.N. (1983) The natural history of radiation-induced proctosigmoiditis: an analysis of 88 patients. *Quarterly Journal of Medicine*, **205**, 40–53.

19. Goligher, J.C. (1984) Irradiation proctitis and enteritis. In *Surgery of the Anus, Rectum and Colon*, pp. 871–874. London: Baillière Tindall.

20. Graham, J.B. (1965) Vaginal fistulas following radiotherapy. *Surgery, Gynecology and Obstetrics*, **120**, 1019–1030.

21. Harling, H., Balslev, I. (1986) Surgical treatment of radiation injury to the rectosigmoid. *Acta Chirugica Scandinavica*, **152**, 691–693.

22. Harling, H. and Balslev, I. (1988) Long-term prognosis of patients with severe radiation enteritis. *American Journal of Surgery*, **155**, 517–519.

23. Harling, H., Balslev, I. and Larson, J.F. (1986) Necrosis of the rectum complicating abdominal aortic reconstructions in previously irradiated patients. *British Journal of Surgery*, **73**, 711.

24. Hatcher, P.A., Thomson, H.J., Ludgate, S.N., Small, W.P. and Smith, A.N. (1985) Surgical aspects of intestinal injury due to pelvic radiotherapy. *Annals of Surgery*, **201**, 470–475.

25. Jacobs, H., Rindt, W. and Schmid, N. (1971) Beitrag zür behandlung der strahlenproktitis. *Geburtschaft für Frauenheilkunde*, **31**, 1114–1117.

26. Jao, S.-W., Beart, R.W. and Gunderson, L.L. (1986) Surgical treatment of radiation injuries of the colon and rectum. *American Journal of Surgery*, **151**, 272–277.

27. Keleme, Z. and Lehoczky, G. (1987) Closure of severe vesico-vagino-rectal fistulas using Lehoczky's island flap. *British Journal of Urology*, **59**, 153–155.

28. Kinsella, T.J., Bloomer, W.D. (1980) Tolerance of the intestine to radiation therapy. *Surgery, Gynecology and Obstetrics*, **151**, 273–284.

29. Kraybill, W.G. and Lopez, M.J. (1990) Management of radiation damage to the rectum. In *Radiation Enteritis* (Eds) Galland, R.B. and Spencer, J. pp. 242–267. London: Edward Arnold Ltd.

30. Levi, S. and Hodgson, H.J. (1990) The medical management of radiation enteritis. In *Radiation Enteritis* (Eds) Galland, R.B. and Spencer, J. pp. 176–198. London: Edward Arnold Ltd.

31. Marks, G. and Mohiudden, M. (1983) The surgical management of radiation-injured intestine. *Surgical Clinics of North America*, **63**, 81–96.

32. Miholic, J. Schlappack, O. Klepetko, W., Kolbl, H., Szepesi, T. and Moeschl, P. (1987) Surgical therapy of radiation-induced small bowel lesions. *Archives of Surgery*, **122**, 923–926.

33. Morgenstern, L., Thompson, R. and Friedman, N.B. (1977) The modern enigma of radiation enteropathy: sequelae and solutions. *American Journal of Surgery*, **134**, 166–172.

34. Newman, A., Katsaris, J., Blendis, L.M., Charlesworth, M. and Walter, L.H. (1973) Small-intestinal injury in women who have had pelvic radiotherapy. *The Lancet*, **ii**, 1471–1473.

35. Ormiston, M.C.E. (1985) A study of rat intestinal wound healing in the presence of radiation injury. *British Journal of Surgery*, **72**, 56–58.

36. Palmer, J.A. and Bush, R.S. (1976) Radiation injuries to the bowel associated with the treatment of carcinoma of the cervix. *Surgery*, **80**, 458–464.

37. Parks, A.G., Allen, C.L.O., Frank, J.D. and McPartlin, J.F. (1978) A method of treating post-irradiation rectovaginal fistulae. *British Journal of Surgery*, **65**, 417–421.

38. Rubinstein, E., Ibsen, T., Rasmussen, R.B., Reimer, E. and Sorensen, B.L. (1986) Formalin treatment of radiation-induced hemorrhagic proctitis. *American Journal of Gastroenterology*, **81**, 44–45.

39. Sandler, R.S., Sandler, D.P. (1983) Radiation induced cancers of the colon and rectum. Assessing the risk. *Gastroenterology*, **84**, 51–57.

40. Schofield, P.F., Carr, N.D. and Holden, D. (1986) Pathogenesis and treatment of radiation bowel disease: discussion paper. *Journal of the Royal Society of Medicine*, **79**, 30–32.

41. Smith, S.T., Seski, J.C., Copeland, L.J., Gershenson, D.M., Edwards, C.L. and Herson, J. (1985) Surgical management of irradiation-induced small bowel damage. *Obstetrics and Gynecology*, **65**, 563–567.

42. Swan, R.W., Fowler, W.C. and Boronow, R.C. (1976) Surgical management of radiation injury to the small intestine. *Surgery, Gynecology and Obstetrics*, **142**, 325–327.

43. Varma, J.S. and Smith, A.N. (1986) Anorectal function following colo-anal sleeve anastomosis for chronic radiation injury to the rectum. *British Journal of Surgery*, **73**, 285–289.

44. Varma, J.S., Smith, A.N. and Busuttil, A. (1986) Function of the anal sphincters after chronic radiation injury. *Gut*, **27**, 528–533.

45. Walsh, D. (1897) Deep tissue traumatism from Roentgen ray exposure. *British Medical Journal*, **ii**, 272–273.

ENDOMETRIOSIS

R.N. Allan

DEFINITION

Endometriosis is characterized by the presence of extrauterine endometrial tissue. It is a disease of women predominantly in childbearing years with a peak incidence between 30 and 40 years but may occur occasionally in the elderly.[9] The extrauterine endometrial tissue is under hormonal influence so that the normal cycle occurs with maturation, shedding of the surface endometrial epithelium and bleeding.

PATHOLOGY

The lesions involving the gastrointestinal tract are usually small and multiple and may be an incidental finding during laparotomy for endometriosis. Occasionally larger extramural and intramural lesions are found in the intestine. These lesions, if large enough, can produce luminal obstruction usually in the sigmoid colon, particularly at the rectosigmoid junction.[2] They occur less frequently in the appendix,[4] caecum,[8] or ileum.[2]

Occasionally patients present with perianal sepsis, a mass in the rectovaginal septum or the ileocaecal region, or with multiple strictures. Ileocaecal involvement may extend to the right ovary and uterus, and an ovarian chocolate cyst may be adherent to the rectum and ileum.[7]

Reviews of the earlier literature, including historical perspectives, have been reported by Kratzer and Salvati[3] and Gray.[2] Kratzer and Salvati[3] studied 225 patients with endometriosis diagnosed at laparotomy of whom 77 (34%) had involvement of the sigmoid colon and rectum. The involvement was minor in most cases. In 44 the sigmoid and rectum were adherent to the posterior wall of the uterus, and in 15 to the left tube and ovary. Thirteen had endometrial implants on the surface of the large intestine, but only four had endometriosis in two of whom there were signs of intestinal obstruction from lesions involving the sigmoid colon.

CLINICAL FEATURES

Symptoms arising from the underlying endometriosis include dysmenorrhoea, pelvic pain, sterility, dyspareunia and low backache. Pelvic examination usually reveals tender nodules with areas of irregular induration. The presence of both gynaecological and gastrointestinal symptoms in women of childbearing years should raise the possibility of endometriosis. The diagnosis should be considered particularly in patients where radiological examination has shown an obstructing lesion at the rectosigmoid junction. Although exacerbation of the gastrointestinal symptoms at the time of menstruation may occur this is not a consistent feature.[7]

TREATMENT

The largest reported series[2] described 179 cases of endometriosis of the gastrointestinal tract from among 1500 patients undergoing surgical treatment for endometriosis. Most (142) were superficial lesions on the surface of the large bowel, of which 81 were completely excised. There were only 37 patients aged between 25 and 49 years where the involved bowel required resection. In 27 the resection was confined to the anterior wall of the sigmoid or rectosigmoid colon. Ten patients required resections of gut with an end-to-end anastomosis (the lower sigmoid was involved in eight and the terminal ileum in two). The intestinal mucosa was not breached in any patient and none presented with rectal bleeding. Meyers and his colleagues[5] described seven examples of colonic endometriosis all in the sigmoid and rectosigmoid colon. They advocated surgical excision of the involved colon as the appearances could mimic colorectal cancer or even complicated diverticular disease and because the diagnosis can often only be made on histological grounds.

A recent review of 32 patients with a diagnosis of colonic or rectal endometriosis includes an excellent resumé of the therapeutic options.[1]

Women without bowel symptoms or obstruction can be observed without therapeutic intervention. Hormone therapy may be offered to patients with pain, partially obstructing lesions and where the number of endometrial nodules are too extensive for surgical removal. Androgens, progestin agents and the antigonadotrophin agent danazol have all been used. Danazol has fewer side-effects and high efficacy.[1,5]

Surgical intervention may be required for diagnosis where the cause for acute abdominal symptoms is unclear. Surgical removal of constricting lesions is necessary; it is often possible to dissect small impants from the bowel wall without resection of the colon. In women with extensive symptomatic disease who have failed to respond to surgical or hormonal therapy, bilateral oophorectomy may be necessary.[6]

Symptoms arising from endometriosis affecting the small bowel, caecum or appendix are uncommon but the principles of treatment are similar to those for colonic endometriosis.

REFERENCES

1. Graham, B. and Mazier, W.P. (1988) Diagnosis and management endometriosis of the colon and rectum. *Diseases of Colon and Rectum*, **31**, 952–956.
2. Gray, L.A. (1973) Endometriosis of the bowel: role of bowel resection superficial excision and oophorectomy in treatment. *Annals of Surgery*, **177**, 580–587.
3. Kratzer, G.L. and Salvati, E.P. (1955) Collective review of endometriosis of the colon. *American Journal of Surgery*, **90**, 866–869.
4. Lane, R.E. (1960) Endometriosis of the vermiform appendix. *American Journal of Obstetrics and Gynaecology*, **79**, 372.
5. Matta, W.H. and Shaw, A.W. (1987) A comparative study between buserelin and danazol in the treatment of endometriosis. *British Journal of Clinical Practice*, **41**, 69–72.
6. Meyers, W.C., Kelvin, F.M. and Jones, R.S. (1979) Diagnosis and surgical treatment of colonic endometriosis. *Archives of Surgery*, **114**, 169–175.
7. Parr, N.J., Murphy, C., Holt, S., Zakhour, H. and Crosbie, R.B. (1988) Endometriosis and the gut. *Gut*, **29**, 1112–1115.
8. Swann, M. (1962) An endometrioma of the caecum causing an intussusception. *British Journal of Surgery*, **50**, 199.
9. Williams, C. (1963) Endometriosis of the colon in elderly women. *Annals of Surgery*, **157**, 974–979.

PNEUMATOSIS COLI (PNEUMATOSIS CYSTOIDES INTESTINALIS)

A.P. Wyatt

DEFINITION

Pneumatosis coli, also known as pneumatosis cystoides intestinalis, or gas cysts of the colon, is a disorder in which there are multiple collections of encysted gas in the submucous and subserous regions of the colon and rectum, which persist for weeks or many years. A similar condition may be seen in the small bowel but in these cases there is always a recognizable associated pathology, usually a peptic ulcer or other ulcerative lesion, which can explain tracking of gas into the bowel wall or the invasion of the wall by gas-forming organisms. A classification of pneumatosis coli is given in *Table 4.18*. In colonic cases it is most unusual for any other bowel pathology to be demonstrated and thus the condition is often referred to as primary pneumatosis coli.

AETIOLOGY

Gas collections in the tissues are normally rapidly absorbed because the total pressure of gases dissolved in venous capillaries is 7.2 kPa (54 mmHg) below atmospheric pressure owing to the removal of O_2. The explanation of persistent gas collections must be either local gas formation in the cysts by

Table 4.18 Classification of pneumatosis coli

Catastrophic infective type
   Neonatal necrotizing enterocolitis seen in premature and sick newborn infants
   Adult: in association with alcoholism, amoebiasis or ischaemia, necrotizing colitis, etc.

Subacute small bowel (secondary to mucosal ulceration, disease or other abnormality)
   Gastric or duodenal ulcer
   Scleroderma
   Vasculitis
   Systemic lupus erythematosus
   Crohn's disease
   Leukaemia
   Transplantation of kidney, liver, marrow
   Trichlorethylene inhalation
   Jejunoileal bypass
   Pyloric stenosis
   Cystic fibrosis
   Polyarteritis
   Polymyositis
   Tuberculosis
   Myeloma
   Cytomegalovirus infections
   Colonoscopy

Chronic 'primary' pneumatosis coli (associated with obstructive airways disease in 50% of patients)

bacteria or constant replenishment from the bowel lumen. In the absence of a mucosal defect in pneumatosis the replenishment is presumably by diffusion from the bowel lumen. There is no convincing evidence in man of bacterial contamination within the cysts. Cyst gas closely resembles bowel gas on analysis, often containing quite large proportions of H_2,[5] and it is conceivable that the cysts grow and multiply because insoluble bowel gas diffuses into the cysts more quickly that it can diffuse from the cysts into the capillaries. The well-known variations in bowel gas with various dietary components[12] probably explains the spontaneous waxing and waning of the size of the cysts and the symptoms they cause. Keyting et al.[6] proposed that gas originated in the chest as mediastinal emphysema and tracked along the periaortic areolar tissue into the mesentery and then along the mesenteric vessels into the bowel wall. They showed that submucosal colonic cysts could be produced by injection of air into the base of the dogs' mesentery although they failed to persist. The author has observed gas in the juxtacolonic mesentery in a patient dying with mediastinal emphysema in association with fibrosing alveolitis. A further piece of evidence has been provided by Gillon et al.[3] and Read et al.[10] who showed that many patients with pneumatosis coli during a fast have unusually high levels of breath H_2. This indicates abnormal bowel gas formation in the presence of unusual bowel organisms, colonic stasis or some form of malabsorption.

Pneumatosis coli probably occurs in patients who form unusually large amounts of H_2 and other relatively insoluble bowel gases. Following the trauma of coughing, anaesthetic intubation, road accident or some other mechanical insult, they develop surgical emphysema which tracks into the colon wall. The bowel gas then diffuses into gas cysts more quickly than it can be absorbed into the capillaries and so,

instead of resolving, the bubbles grow, split into further bubbles and spread around and along the colon wall.

There is little evidence to suggest that the gas in these chronic cases originates from gas-forming organisms in the bowel wall. It is not the result of colonic ischaemia and is not a neoplastic process, although these suggestions have been seriously proposed.

Haboubi et al.[4] believe, following electron microscopy, that the gas is accumulating in lymphatics but this has not been generally accepted by other pathologists.

PATHOLOGY

Pneumatosis coli usually affects the left side of the colon, especially the splenic flexure and the sigmoid colon. The right side is rarely affected unless there is concomitant small bowel pneumatosis when secondary pneumatosis with an ulcerating intestinal lesion should be suspected. Treatment of the underlying lesion will be followed by resolution of the gas cysts. In most chronic cases the gas cysts extend from the mid-transverse colon to the rectum. Sometimes cysts travel through the wall of the bowel into the omentum and may even occur in the wall of the bladder or vagina.

Macroscopically (*Figure 4.75*) the gas bubbles are spherical with a typically blue tinge and are situated in the submucosa and subserosa. They produce considerable thickening and stiffening of the bowel wall. The condition can be mimicked by injecting air from a syringe into the submucosa of freshly excised colon. Cysts may vary in diameter from a few millimetres to 2 cm but are never larger. Spontaneous pneumoperitoneum is sometimes seen with small

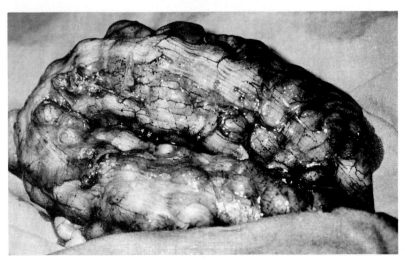

Figure 4.75 Macroscopic appearance of pneumatosis coli. Sigmoid colon exposed at time of surgery. Note the large subserosal blebs of gas.

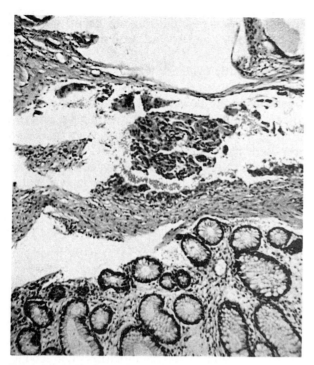

Figure 4.76 Histological section of biopsy specimen. Submucosal gas cyst above, granuloma in centre and mucous membrane inferiorly (H and E).

bowel cysts but not with primary pneumatosis coli. The mucosal surface of the colon sometimes appears haemorrhagic in the region of the cysts but is not otherwise inflamed and with sigmoidoscopy small submucosal vessels can be seen coursing over the gas bubbles.

Microscopically (*Figure 4.76*) the cystic spaces are lined with endothelial cells and are associated with granulomas consisting of collections of endotheloid and foreign body giant cells. There is no acute inflammatory reponse.

Patients are usually middle-aged or elderly and often with multiple pathology. In most large series half the patients suffer from obstructive airways disease.[8] Myocardial infarction and multiple operations are also common and the condition is reported at the distal end of small bowel following bypass operations for obesity.[9]

Untreated the condition may persist for many years. It may recur after apparently successful medical treatment or surgical excision.[11] On the other hand, spontaneous and prolonged remission may occur without any specific treatment, but usually only in recently diagnosed cases.

CLINICAL FEATURES

The presenting features are diarrhoea, excessive flatulence, abdominal pain, bleeding or inconti-

nence. Patients may go to the toilet 20 times a day but only to pass mucus with flatus and perhaps some blood. Despite repeated mucous incontinence the patient will sometimes complain of passing constipated faeces. The symptoms fluctuate considerably and most patients are unable to relate this fluctuation to diet or other factors. The pain is usually in the lower abdomen and colicky but occasionally intestinal obstruction or volvulus will complicate the condition when severe pain is associated with distension and vomiting. In a slim patient it is often possible to see the diseased colon through the abdominal wall and to palpate it as a sausage-shaped mass covered with knobbly bubbles of gas. Rectal examination will reveal the cysts as rubbery blobs protruding into the lumen in about half the cases.

INVESTIGATIONS

In almost all cases the cysts can be seen with sigmoidoscopy as multiple blue-domed swellings (*Figure 4.77*). Biopsy should be carried out for confirmation when a typical 'pop' will be heard as the cyst ruptures. The biopsy will float in the fixative because of its air content.

A plain radiograph of the abdomen is diagnostic because the multiple radiolucent gas-filled cysts are

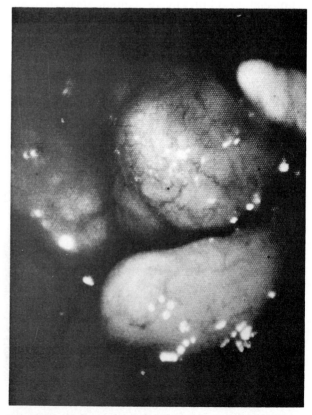

Figure 4.77 Colonoscopic appearance of multiple gas cysts in sigmoid colon. Note small vessels running over the cysts.

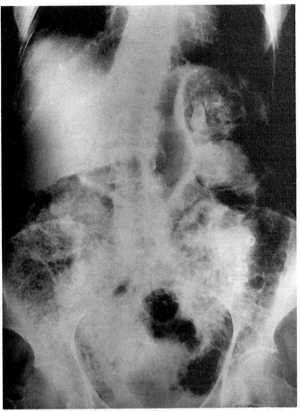

Figure 4.78 Gas cysts of the colon seen on plain radiograph of the abdomen. Note the cystic collections especially on the left side of the colon.

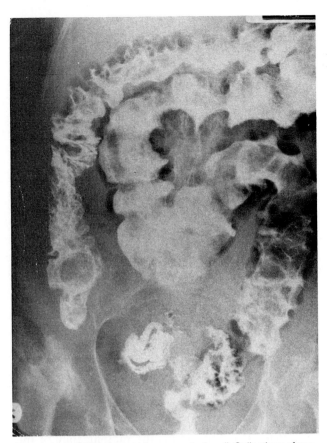

Figure 4.80 Barium enema in pneumatosis coli. Collections of gas lying in the wall of the colon outside the barium-coated mucosa can be easily appreciated.

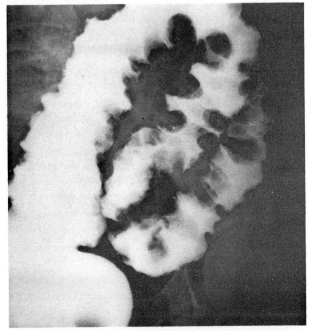

Figure 4.79 Barium enema in pneumatosis coli. This film shows the characteristic scalloped appearance in the sigmoid colon.

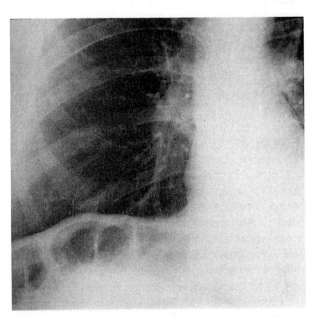

Figure 4.81 Chilaiditi's sign seen on a chest radiograph. The gas-filled colon lies between the liver and the diaphragm .

evident; this proves to be a simple way to document the course of the disease (*Figure 4.78*). A barium enema examination shows the classical scalloped appearance of cysts, protruding into the bowel lumen (*Figures 4.79* and *4.80*). A chest radiograph should be performed in view of the common association with chest disease. The gas-filled colon may also be seen lying between the right lobe of the liver and the diaphragm (the Chilaiditi's sign) (*Figure 4.81*). If cysts are present on the right side of the colon, suggesting the secondary type of pneumatosis, the stomach and small bowel should be investigated by endoscopy and barium studies.

DIFFERENTIAL DIAGNOSIS

The frequent diagnostic difficulty in these cases is related to its rarity. Few specialists will see more than one example in a lifetime. When the gas cysts are palpable per rectum the patient is commonly thought to have a rectal neoplasm.

The barium enema appearances, although characteristic, are commonly interpreted as being those of polyposis, pseudo-polyposis or the thumb-printing of ischaemic colitis, unless the radiolucency of the filling defects is appreciated. Linear gas shadows in the bowel wall are associated with fulminating clostridial infections as in necrotizing colitis or frank gangrene. Solitary giant gas cysts of the sigmoid colon are probably due to the distension of a diverticulum because of valve formation at its neck. Pathologists unfamiliar with pneumatosis coli may interpret biopsies as oleogranulomas because spaces, assumed to have previously contained lipid, in fact contained gas and are associated with granuloma formation.[13]

TREATMENT

MEDICAL

As this is a benign disease with some spontaneous remissions and a low incidence of serious complications, a conservative approach should be adopted initially. Antidiarrhoeal drugs help to some extent as well as antibiotics (such as metronidazole) but these have never been effective in our hands. The advice of a dietician should be sought to advocate food which produces less flatus. Patients placed on water alone or an elemental diet rapidly lose their symptoms but, of course, cannot tolerate this for long. A low residue diet avoiding bran, beans and vegetable fibre, and other foods containing long chain polysaccharides, the fermentation of which is responsible for gas production, seems desirable and often helps. For the same reason lactulose is not the aperient of choice and magnesium salts are to be preferred if the patient is constipated.

OXYGEN

Breathing 70% oxygen at atmospheric pressure for a sufficient period will always result in resolution of colonic gas cysts.[14] First described in 1973,[2] this method of management has now gained wide acceptance and will result in prolonged remission if pursued energetically. There is a high rate of recurrence within 2 years but the treatment may be repeated. Anxiety about the toxic effects of 70% oxygen have proved unfounded in the author's experience. Some authors have used hyperbaric oxygen therapy, but theoretically this is unnecessary and practically it is more expensive. The results of treatment are probably inferior in terms of length of remission as it is difficult to give a sufficient number of treatments to induce complete remission. The essential steps in normobaric oxygen treatment are outlined in *Table 4.19*. It is useless to simply ask the nurse to 'administer oxygen'. Inspired oxygen at 70% is quite difficult to achieve and a close fitting

Table 4.19 Steps in the treatment of pneumatosis coli with oxygen breathing

1 Empty the bowel, e.g. sodium picosulphate (Picolax) two sachets or magnesium sulphate mixture 20 ml two-hourly until diarrhoea

2 Elemental diet or fluid diet only

3 Oxygen by close-fitting mask (humidify or patient will not tolerate) 8–10 litres per minute or more

4 Estimate Pao_2 after 30 minutes and if below 40 kPa (300 mmHg) increase oxygen flow, replace mask or otherwise adjust until desired Pao_2 is obtained

5 Continue oxygen breathing day and night with only 20-minute breaks for food and toilet – the more the patient wears the mask the quicker the treatment will be completed

6 Monitor progress by plain radiograph of abdomen each day

7 When radiological 'cure' is complete, repeat sigmoidoscopy

8 When all cysts have disappeared on the radiograph plate and on sigmoidoscopy, continue oxygen therapy for a further 48 hours

9 Arrange a post-treatment barium enema or colonoscopy to exclude other colonic pathology

Equipment required
- O$_2$ cylinder with flowmeter
- Large nebulizer with O$_2$ concentration dial
- 2 T Pieces
- Rebreathing bag (2L)
- 2 × length of elephant tubing
- 1 cushion-flex anaesthetic mask
- 1 very low pressure one-way valve or flap of Paul's tubing.

Instructions for setting up
1. Connect nebulizer filled with sterile water to O$_2$ cylinder and dial in required O$_2$ concentration.
2. Connect T piece to outlet with rebreathing bag attached to vertical of T piece.
3. Run length of elephant tubing from other side of T piece to second T piece which is connected to face mask.
4. Run second length of tubing (about 45 cm long) off other side of this T piece.
5. Fit valve or Paul's tubing to free end of elephant tubing.

To use
Turn on flow meter on O$_2$ cylinder until a good mist can be seen coming out of face mask. Put mask on patient and tell patient to breathe normally. If patient has difficulty breathing out, the pressure in the one-way valve is too high and should be replaced either with a lower pressure valve or a flap of Paul's tubing.

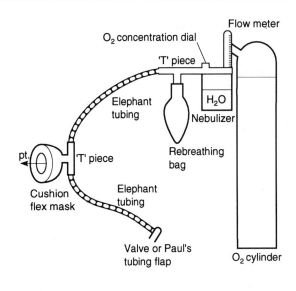

Figure 4.82 Assembly of normobaric oxygen equipment.

mask designed to give high concentrations, together with high flow rates of humidified oxygen (often 10 litres per minute), are essential. An anaesthetist or anaesthetic technician should be asked to assemble the equipment and the author has found the scheme set out in *Figure 4.82* to be most efficient. Adequacy of administration must be monitored by Pao_2 estimations 30 minutes after commencing treatment. In the author's experience, maintained levels of Pao_2 of 40 kPa (300 mmHg) always result in disappearance of the cysts within 5 days. Diarrhoea usually ceases immediately treatment is started. Oxygen therapy may be difficult in patients with obstructive airways disease but Klausen *et al.*[7] have used doxapram hydrochloride successfully in this situation. Oxygen breathing is continued day and night with only 20 minute breaks for refreshment.

Response to therapy is simply monitored by daily abdominal radiography and the resolution of the cysts can be confirmed with sigmoidoscopy. It has been the author's practice to continue oxygen treatment for 48 hours after all evidence of the cysts has disappeared because if any cysts remain, rapid recurrence of the full syndrome occurs. After therapy a barium enema or colonoscopy should be performed to ensure that there is no underlying colonic pathology.

SURGICAL

In secondary pneumatosis coli, surgical management of the primary lesion is frequently necessary and emergency surgery is occasionally required for obstruction or volvulus. Subtotal colectomy may occasionally be required in severely symptomatic patients with recurrent pneumatosis coli despite adequate oxygen therapy.

Case and Hall[1] advocate a rather aggressive surgical approach but one of their four patients suffered recurrent disease and, in the author's experience, patients with subtotal colectomy are symptomatically little better off than those who are managed medically.

REFERENCES

1. Case, W.G. and Hall, R. (1985) Surgical treatment of pneumatosis coli. *Annals of the Royal College of Surgeons*, **67**, 368–369.
2. Forgacs, P., Wright, P.H. and Wyatt, A.P. (1973) Treatment of intestinal gas cysts by oxygen breathing. *The Lancet*, **i**, 579–582.
3. Gillon, J., Tadesse, K., Logan, R.F.A. *et al.* (1979) Breath hydrogen in pneumatosis cystoides intestinalis. *Gut*, **20**, 1008–1011.
4. Haboubi, N.Y., Honan, R.P., Hasleton, P.S., Ali, H.H., Anfield, C., Hobbiss, J. and Schofield, P.F. (1984) Pneumatosis coli: a case report with ultrastructural study. *Histopathology*, **8**, 145–155.
5. Hughes, D.T.D., Gordon, K.C.D., Swan, J.C. and Bolt, G.L. (1966) Pneumatosis cystoides intestinalis. *Gut*, **7**, 553–557.
6. Keyting, W.S., McCarver, R.R., Kovarik, J.L. and Daywitt, A.L. (1961) Pneumatosis intestinalis: a new concept. *Radiology*, **76**, 733–741.

7. Klausen, N.O., Agner, E., Tougaard, L. and Sorensen, B. (1982) Pneumatosis coli in chronic respiratory failure. *British Medical Journal*, **284**, 1834–1835.
8. Koss, L.G. (1952) Abdominal gas cysts. *American Medical Association Archives of Pathology*, **53**, 523–549.
9. Martyak, S.N. and Curtis, L.E. (1976) Pneumatosis intestinals: a compilation of jejunoileal bypass. *Journal of the American Medical Association*, **235**, 1038–1039.
10. Read, N.W., Al-Janabi, M.N. and Cann, P.A. (1984) Is raised breath hydrogen related to the pathogenesis of pneumatosis coli? *Gut*, **25**, 839–845.
11. Sames, C.P. (1964) Pneumatosis cystoides intestinalis (pelvic colon). *Proceedings of the Royal Society of Medicine*, **57**, 400.
12. Sutalf, L.O. and Levitt, M.D. (1979) Follow-up of a flatulent patient. *Digestive Diseases and Sciences (New Series)*, **24**, 652–654.
13. Wyatt, A.P. (1972) Pneumatosis cystoides intestinalis. *Proceedings of the Royal Society of Medicine*, **65**, 780–782.
14. Wyatt, A.P. (1975) Prolonged symptomatic and radiological remission of colonic gas cysts after oxygen therapy. *British Journal of Surgery*, **62**, 837–839.

ANAL AND PERIRECTAL DISORDERS

PHYSIOLOGY OF DEFAECATION AND SPHINCTER CONTROL

R. Farouk, G.S. Duthie and D.C.C. Bartolo

The continence mechanism is a complex one involving local and spinal reflex arcs with a cerebral input acquired by learning. Somatic and visceral muscle formation is integrated with a sensory input to attain continence. Achieving continence involves having the ability to discriminate between flatus, liquids and solids as well as the ability to decide about the appropriateness for the passage of rectal contents.

The internal anal sphincter, the external anal sphincter, the pelvic floor and anorectal mucosa have been identified as factors that are integral for the maintenance of continence. Interaction between these variables result in the complex physiological mechanism that converts the pelvic floor into a functioning sphincter which opposes rises in intra-abdominal pressure thereby maintaining continence without herniation of the rectum.

Previous attempts to investigate the continence mechanism and its disorders tended to consider individual physiological variables allowing only a fragmented picture. Further understanding can only be achieved by an integrated study of these variables in dynamic function rather than in static, unphysiological laboratory environments.

THE INTERNAL ANAL SPHINCTER

The internal anal sphincter is a terminal specialization of the circular colonic muscle. It is thicker than the layer of circular muscle from which it arises, measuring 1.5–5 mm wide and has a length of 2.5–4 cm. Its length is greater in males but there is no relationship with age. It is surrounded by the external anal sphincter throughout its length.

Electromyography (EMG) is an important technique used in the investigation of the anal sphincter muscles. The electrical activity of these muscles can be recorded using surface electrodes, monopolar electrodes, concentric needle electrodes or single fibre EMG electrodes. Individual muscle fibres derived from a motor unit summate to form the motor unit action potential which can be recorded at a greater distance than the close proximity that is required to record individual muscle fibre activities, which have small action potentials of brief duration.

Surface electrode recordings are somewhat unreliable because the electrode is at some distance from the muscular activity which is to be assessed, and the recordings may include the activity of adjacent muscles which may also be contracting.

Monopolar electrodes consist of a solid steel electrode insulated to the tip with resin with a single leading-off surface. The electrode is placed on the skin at a distance from the muscle undergoing assessment. The results are variable, partly depending on the diameter of the tip of the recording electrode. The method is relatively unhelpful for sphincter assessment.

Concentric needle electrodes are commonly used and consist of bare tipped steel wire of 0.1 mm diameter with an insulating resin. The area of uptake of the electrode is small and any electrical

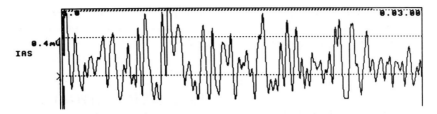

Figure 4.83   Normal internal sphincter EMG appearance.

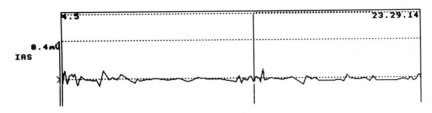

Figure 4.84   Sphincter electrical silence in idiopathic faecal incontinence.

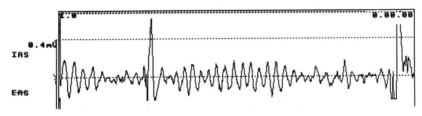

Normal internal sphincter EMG

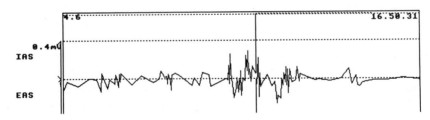

Pre-rectopexy internal sphincter EMG

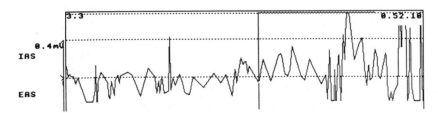

Post-rectopexy internal sphincter EMG

Figure 4.85   Internal sphincter EMG recovery is associated with recovery of continence following rectopexy for rectal prolapse.

activity recorded is that into which the electrode is inserted. Individual muscle fibre action potentials, however, cannot be identified reliably using concentric needle electrodes.

The single fibre EMG electrode, which has an uptake radius of 270 μm can record the activity of individual muscle fibres within a motor unit.

An ambulatory method of assessing individual patients has been developed using fine wire electrodes to assess the EMG activity of the sphincter muscles and puborectalis. Two Teflon coated steel wires, each 0.13 mm in diameter, with tips bared to a diameter of 1 mm, are barbed and introduced through a 21 gauge sterile hypodermic needle into these muscles. The small diameter of these wires and the prior introduction of a local anaesthetic to the area ensures that the procedure is not uncomfortable. Electrical detection is related to a ground electrode placed low on the patient's back.

The morphology of the internal anal sphincter is displayed using intra-anal ultrasonography. A rotating transducer is surrounded within a fluid chamber to provide a visual display of the anal sphincters and puborectalis.

Examination of the internal sphincter reveals electrical slow wave activity which is sinusoidal in nature at a frequency of 15–35 cycles per minute in normal controls.[49] This electrical activity is disrupted, however, in patients with full-thickness rectal prolapse and neurogenic faecal incontinence (*Figures 4.83–85*). Restoration of continence following rectopexy is associated with recovery of the internal sphincter EMG (*Figure 4.85*). Several groups of pacemaker cells are present within the lower sphincteric portion, each group generating a slightly different frequency.[49] This slow-wave activity is not disrupted by general anaesthesia or by pudendal nerve blockage.[21] The frequency of the internal sphincter slow-wave has a linear relationship with resting anal canal pressures and is reduced in patients with neurogenic faecal incontinence,[12] and full thickness rectal prolapse (personal observations). No such correlation was found between the amplitude of slow-waves and resting anal pressures.

The internal sphincter is continuously active.[31] Examination of isolated strips of sphincter muscle in vitro reveal it to be in a continuously tonic state.[8] This indicates that a pure myogenic origin is partially responsible for basal activity during sleep which is accompanied by a fall in resting anal canal pressures. Abolition of internal sphincter electrical activity occurs during rectal distension.[10] Should the rectal distension be sufficient, this abolition in activity becomes prolonged. Passage of flatus, faecal impaction within the rectum and a rectal prolapse[18] conceivably cause sufficient rectal distension with resulting internal sphincter relaxation. In the case of the latter two conditions, faecal incontinence may result.

THE EXTERNAL ANAL SPHINCTER

The external anal sphincter represents the terminal continuation of the longitudinal muscle of the colon. It is a striated muscle which has, in cadaveric dissections, been shown to be arranged in three loops separated from each other by a fascial septum.[54] The external sphincter is continuously active even in subjects who are asleep but the amount of activity is dependent on posture and activity.[20] It is a fatigable muscle, however, and voluntary contraction to maintain maximal squeeze and therefore continence lasts for less than a minute. The muscle is supplied by the pudendal nerve (synonymous with the inferior haemorrhoidal nerve) and external sphincter activity can be abolished by blockade of this nerve.[21]

Rectal distension with 50 ml of air results in the recruitment of external sphincter EMG activity which precedes internal sphincter inhibition.[23] Continued distension of the rectum results in sustained external sphincter EMG activity until 150–200 ml of air has been used to inflate the rectal balloon. This results in complete inhibition of external sphincter activity (constant relaxation is achieved). Such activity of the EAS can be inhibited by a pudendal nerve block.[21] It is, however, present in patients with thoracolumbar spinal transection suggesting a spinal rather than a cortical reflex arc. Other examples of the role of spinal reflex pathways in external sphincter activity include the effect of perianal cutaneous stimulation which can be elicited in paraplegic patients. Furthermore, patients with spinal transection above the third lumbar segment have normal resting external sphincter EMG activity with good recruitment while the patient is coughing.[46,50]

Traction on the anal canal using a digit results in recruitment of the external sphincter and puborectalis EMG activity.[50] In paraplegics this is followed by ensuing complete inhibition for the period of anal canal traction. In normal subjects this EMG activity is sustained and followed by a sharp burst of EMG activity when traction is released. This sharp burst of activity is termed the 'closing reflex'. Such evidence supports a cortical input to this reflex which is abolished by spinal injury.[50] The 'normal' response to defaecation involves pelvic muscle relaxation in most subjects and it is unlikely that there is sustained recruitment of the external sphincter during defaecation. The closing reflex is however commonly seen at the end of defaecation and appears to be a physiological entity.

The puborectalis muscle forms a part of the pelvic floor musculature and exhibits almost identical electrophysiological characteristics with the external anal sphincter during coughing and straining. Indeed, the two muscles appear to function as a single unit during such activity. The puborectalis muscle receives its innervation directly from the anterior rami of the third and fourth sacral nerves. Pudendal nerve blockade does not abolish pelvic floor contraction.[21] Concern is expressed regarding the assumption that puborectalis and the external anal sphincter function is a single unit, based on differing responses of these muscles to rectal distension in the cat.[11] Ambulatory monitoring in humans, however, confirm to a large extent that these muscles often act in concert.

Chronic straining or injury sustained during childbirth can result in pudendal nerve neuropathy.[56] Pudendal nerve stimulation transanally provides for a method of assessing such a neuropathy. An intrarectal, glove-mounted technique is used to stimulate the pudendal nerve on either side of the pelvis and the latent period between pudendal nerve stimulation and electromechanical response of the muscle measured using an oscilloscope.[48] Prolonged pudendal nerve terminal motor latency is seen in most patients with idiopathic faecal incontinence, patients with a rectal prolapse, double anorectal and urinary incontinence and in certain neurological disorders. Damage to the pudendal nerves is thought to occur in 60% of women who have sustained injury to the external sphincter. Furthermore, 20% of women undergoing vaginal delivery with no apparent injury to the external sphincter have prolonged pudendal nerve terminal motor latencies with recovery occurring in 15%.[56]

Determination of pudendal nerve conduction velocity is often complemented by the estimation of single muscle fibre density. Fibre density is calculated using single fibre EMG electrodes to estimate the mean number of single fibre action potentials recorded within an uptake area in 20 different positions within the muscle. This is done by inserting four separate electrodes into the muscle and adjusting the position of the electrode within these individual insertions. Following injury to the motor unit, reinnervation will result in an increase in fibre density, as there will be more fibres innervated by a single axon within the uptake area. In normal subjects the fibre density of most muscles is less than two, although this increases slightly with age.[42]

The degree of correlation between straining in the laboratory setting and normal defaecation remains uncertain. Ihre studied pressure and EMG changes during evacuation of a rectal balloon in 11 patients.[28] External sphincter and puborectalis activity was inhibited in eight subjects while the remainder exhibited continued sphincter activity during straining. The authors have studied 15 patients who displayed inappropriate pelvic muscle contraction exceeding 50% of basal activity of these muscles while straining in the laboratory. Ambulatory monitoring did not exhibit such inappropriate contraction on defaecation in 13 of these patients during defaecation.[13] Such observations should dictate caution in interpreting laboratory based findings, particularly in the diagnosis of anismus.

Eighty per cent of Kerreman's subjects showed temporary sustained increase in external sphincter EMG activity during straining.[31] Other observers have described initial external sphincter recruitment followed by complete inhibition while straining.[46] Paraplegic patients who are able to voluntarily raise their intra-abdominal pressures also exhibit initial recruitment of pelvic floor activity followed by inhibition.[38]

ANAL CANAL PRESSURE

Anal canal pressures may be measured in a number of ways. Each method is subject to its own disadvantages. Methods available include water-filled perfusion catheters, water-filled or air-filled balloons, sleeve catheters and pressure microtransducers.[27] Perfusion systems are dependent on the compliance of the system and the rate of perfusion. Furthermore, the pressure generated may induce contractions. Similar alterations in anorectal contractility may arise when using balloon systems. The sleeve catheters are unable to distinguish between internal and external sphincter activities. Microtransducers avoid many of these problems by minimizing distension of the anus.

Resting anal canal pressures using a pressure microtransducer system in normal subjects vary between 70–110 cm H_2O in this laboratory. The resting pressure undergoes regular fluctuations with an amplitude of 5–25 cm H_2O and a frequency of 10–20 per minute.[31] These fluctuations are termed 'slow-waves' and are thought to be generated by the internal sphincter.[6] The frequency of the slow wave is higher in the lower anal canal providing for a mechanism that propels small amounts of anal canal contents cephalad into the rectum.[31] A gender difference does exist with males generally having higher pressures. No relationship with age has been convincingly demonstrated.[34] Studies to date which do suggest lower pressures in the elderly have been performed in the chronically ill or on those taking multiple medication.[2] Other studies are flawed by a lack of information on their normal subjects.[37,36]

A zone of high pressure does exist approximately 2 cm from the anal verge[21] which is caudal to the puborectalis sling. Zones of low pressure have also been identified within the anal canal.[57] The anterior aspect of the upper one third of the anal canal, which corresponds to the area not closely applied to the puborectalis sling, and the posterior aspect of the lower one third of the anal canal are areas of relatively low pressures.

The relative contributions of the various sphincters has been identified by pudendal nerve block.[21] The authors have shown a direct relationship between internal sphincter EMG frequency and resting anal canal pressures.[12] Division of the internal sphincter results in a fall of anal resting pressures. The internal sphincter contributes to 85% of resting anal tone.[17] The haemorrhoidal plexuses have a minor contribution to resting anal pressures. This increases in patients with haemorrhoids who generally have high resting anal pressures and exhibit ultra-slow anal pressure waves.[25] Anal dilation abolished this ultra-slow wave activity in 39% of one cohort of patients with haemorrhoids and this was associated with a fall in resting anal pressures.[25] Patients with anal fissures[26] and those with idiopathic chronic constipation[1] have also been shown to have such ultra-slow wave activity.

When a subject is asked to voluntarily contract their anal sphincters, the anal canal pressures rise by between 175–270%. There are longitudinal and radial variations as previously described for resting anal pressures.[57] The distribution of the contraction is generally symmetrical except at about 3 cm anteriorly where it is significantly lower compared with the pressures posteriorly at a similar level.

The length of the anal canal can be assessed by manometric measurements.[43] The pressure probe is inserted and allowed to rest for 30 s to allow the pressure to fall to a steady level. The probe is then slowly withdrawn and the pressure will rise sharply, whence the anal canal is entered. This is termed the 'pull-through' technique. The anal canal using this method is 2.5–5 cm long. Males have a longer canal in general. Patients with idiopathic faecal incontinence and full thickness rectal prolapse have a shorter anal canal length which is not reversed by surgery.[4]

RECTAL PRESSURE

Basal pressures within the rectum range between 5–25 cm H_2O. The inflation of an intrarectal balloon is associated with an initial rise in pressure, often followed by a secondary increase in pressure secondary to rectal contraction. A degree of accommodation then occurs and the rectal pressure gradually falls to a baseline value. Increasing the distending volume eventually results in a failure to further accommodate and a large increase in rectal pressure results which may be associated with pain. The contractile response of the rectum to distension is decreased or absent in patients with a spinal cord lesion suggesting a spinal input to this reflex.[10]

ANORECTAL SENSATION

Rectal filling is perceived as a fullness felt in the pelvis. Ability to appreciate this filling is thought to be related to stretch receptors within the rectal wall and pelvic floor. Such sensation therefore persists after rectal excision.[24] Balloon distension up to approximately 15 cm from the anal orifice results in a rectal sensation of fullness whereas distension above this level elicits a colicky discomfort in the left iliac fossa.[22] Rectal sensation is thought to be related to rectal contractile activity.

The anal canal mucosa is richly innervated from the anal canal margin to the dentate line.[16] A sensory input is received from the pudendal nerve.[21] Pudendal nerve block results in loss of sensation of the perianal and genital area with no impairment of rectal sensation. Maximal anal perception is thought to occur at the mid-anal canal encompassing the transitional epithelium.[16] Discrimination of sensation by the anal epithelium is less precise than that of adjacent perianal skin.

Rectal temperature is lower than the anal canal. The anal canal mucosa is highly sensitive to temperature changes between 32–42°C,[39] but the temperature gradient between the rectum and anal canal is only 0.2°C. There is a regional thermal gradient between the rectum and lower, mid and upper anal canal of 0.4, 0.2 and 0.1°C respectively. There is some debate regarding the importance of thermal sensitivity in health although in patients with neurogenic faecal incontinence, the lower rectum has been shown to be significantly less sensitive to temperature changes.[53]

Anal sensation is usually assessed by measuring anal mucosal electrosensitivity.[52] Impaired anal sensitivity has been documented in all patients with anorectal disorders except those with anal fissures. Sensation improves following surgery for sphincter repair and after rectopexy for prolapse.[43] The authors attribute this improvement in anal sensation to the restoration of the prolapsed anal transition zone to anatomical normality.

The role of anal sensation in the maintenance of continence has previously been questioned. Read and Read applied topical lignocaine into the anal canal of normal subjects, who did not show any resulting faecal incontinence.[51] There was, however, a significant reduction in the ability to maintain external sphincter contraction. Sensation may therefore prove crucial to patients with impaired sphincteric mechanisms in providing sufficient warning of impending incontinence.[41]

ANORECTAL SAMPLING

The transitional zone within the anal canal is lined with a specialized sensory epithelium which is able to discriminate with a high index of accuracy variables such as temperature, pain and light touch.[16] This epithelium is exposed in normal subjects on average seven times per hour to rectal contents.[41] Rectal contents cause distension of mechanoreceptors within the rectal wall which, by means of intrinsic nerve pathways, results in inhibition of the internal sphincter. The cephalad anal canal opens and rectal contents are exposed to the anal transition zone. Such events are 'covered' and continence maintained by the external sphincter. Each episode lasts for less than 10 s and therefore recruitment of the fatigable external sphincter is easily achieved. This process is termed 'sampling' and allows for differential appreciation of rectal contents (*Figure 4.86*). The number of sampling episodes are reduced during sleep and prolonged fasting.[32]

Sampling is not seen in patients who have undergone complete rectal excision during restorative proctocolectomy.[30] Such patients frequently are unable to discriminate between flatus and faeces. Preservation of the anal transitional zone does not alter this finding.[30]

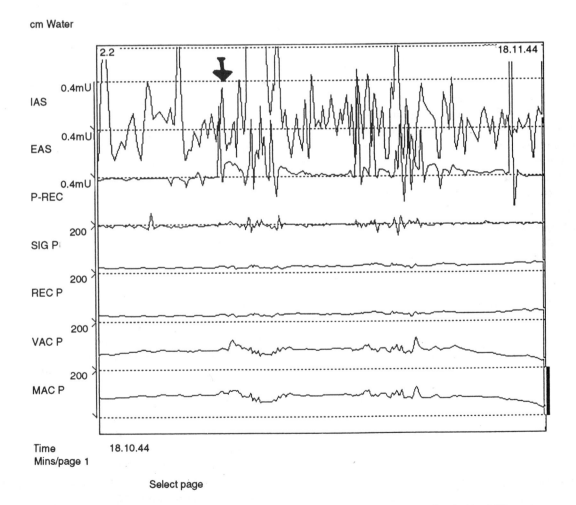

Figure 4.86 Anorectal sampling in a normal subject. (arrowed). Internal sphincter relaxation is associated with a fall in anal pressure and recruitment of the external sphincter and puborectalis. IAS = internal sphincter EMG; EAS = external sphincter EMG; PREC = puborectalis EMG; Sig P = sigmoid pressure; Rec P = rectal pressure; UAC = upper anal canal pressure; MAC P = mid-anal canal pressure.

THE RECTOANAL INHIBITORY REFLEX

Distension of the rectum with a small volume of air causes transient internal sphincter relaxation.[4] This is accompanied by a transient but significant fall in resting anal pressures. Increasing the amount of air/water instilled will result in prolonged inhibition of the internal sphincter accompanied by a similar fall in anal pressures. This reflex is termed the rectoanal inhibitory reflex. It is conceivable that such laboratory investigations simulate defaecation and anorectal sampling.[41]

This reflex is absent after circumferential rectal myotomy and in patients with Hirschsprung's disease[35] suggesting that intrinsic myenteric nerve plexuses play a major role in this reflex. Rectal distension results in descending inhibition of the muscle fibres mediated possibly by vasoactive intestinal peptide.[9] The role of the extrinsic autonomic system in this reflex is less clear.

Distension of the rectum resulting in relaxation of the internal sphincter results in the anal canal becoming funnel shaped to allow rectal contents access to the specialized sensory epithelium. This allows for sampling, a process which is usually covered by external sphincter recruitment. Further rectal distension with increasing volumes results in the anal sphincter not recovering. The external sphincter, if intact, will maintain continence for a short period of time before defaecation ensues. If defaecation is not appropriate and the external sphincters have avoided incontinence, the lower rectal contents are returned cephalad by contraction of the pelvic floor muscles. This allows for internal sphincter recovery from the rectoanal inhibitory reflex. Interestingly, internal sphincter relaxation will also occur following propulsive activity in the lower sigmoid colon in the presence of an empty rectum.[41] Some of the falls in anal pressures recorded during ambulatory recordings may be related to such episodes of sigmoid contractions in the absence of sampling.

RECTAL COMPLIANCE

Rectral capacity determines the frequency and degree of urgency for defaecation. Appreciation of rectal filling occurs with volumes as small as 10 ml but its capacity often approaches 300 ml before there is an urgent desire to defaecate. This can be assessed physiologically by instilling air or water at a steady rate into a rectal balloon and compared with the rate of change of rectal pressure. Initially the proctometrogram shows small increases in rectal pressure per unit volume instilled but the rise in pressure becomes progressively steeper as the maximum tolerated volume is approached. Thus, values can be recorded of volumes causing the initial sensation of distension, a desire to defaecate, urgency and the maximum tolerated volume. This provides for the estimation of rectal compliance which is calculated by plotting volume versus pressure and calculating the gradient. Low compliance is seen in patients with a rectal prolapse,[14] radiation proctitis,[58] colitis[15] and rectal neoplasms.

Restoration of normal compliance can be achieved by excision of the non-compliant rectum and construction of a neorectum. This is possible by forming a pouch from a suitable length of colon following anterior resection or using terminal ileum in restorative proctocolectomy.

Patients with rectal prolapses experience sustained internal sphincter inhibition with only minimal rectal distension. This may either be the result of the rectum being full by virtue of it being occupied by the prolapse or to actual disruption of the sphincter. Attempts to repair the prolapse by use of implantation of foreign material may not improve the situation as such materials make the rectum rigid and therefore non-compliant. The authors' early experience with simple suture rectopexy with resection of redundant colon for full thickness rectal prolapse reveals evidence of internal sphincter recovery based on EMG and anal resting pressure measurements.[19] This method of treatment is further advantageous as it does not leave the patient with an iatrogenic non-compliant rectum.

THE ANORECTAL ANGLE

The sling of puborectalis results in an anorectal angle which alters during defaecation to a more obtuse angle, i.e. the rectum and anal canal lie in a straighter line during defaecation. This change in the anorectal angle is facilitated by the 'squatting' position which is usually adopted during defaecation. This finding has been proposed as a flap valve mechanism to preserve continence.[47] We and others have questioned the importance of the anorectal angle following studies on the liquid-filled rectum using imaging techniques combined with anorectal manometry and EMG. Contact between the anterior rectal wall and the top of the anal canal was never observed during the Valsalva manoeuvre. Continence was associated with recruitment of the external sphincter and puborectalis EMG with rectal pressures consistently being lower than anal pressures.[5] These findings have been subsequently confirmed by other investigators.[3] A further study comparing outcome from sphincter repair for incontinence revealed that resting and squeeze anal pressures rose significantly in patients with a successful outcome whereas the anorectal angle did not significantly alter.[40]

The anorectal angle can be assessed by proctography or scintigraphy. It is often assessed by proponents of the 'flap valve theory' and for the assessment of patients other problems related to defaecation such as the perineal descent syndrome, suspected rectal prolapse, rectoceles and the solitary ulcer syndrome. The interpretation of results is notoriously plagued by a large overlap of results with apparently normal, symptomless subjects.[55] It is therefore a possibility that these findings may represent an epiphenomenon in patients with defaecation problems. There is also a lack of uniformity on defining the anorectal angle. The variation in technique requires normal values to be generated individually. The authors feel that the anorectal angle should be measured between the axis of the anal canal and the central axis of the rectum.

Using the central anorectal angle, the average angle at rest between the axis of the rectum and that of the anal canal is around 80° with hip flexion increasing this angle to over 90°. During defaecation this angle opens to about 115°. Squeezing the anus and the Valsalva manoeuvre decreases the anorectal angle to between 85 and 100°, with the angle being more acute in the former action. Changing position from lateral decubitus to sitting straightens the resting angle, with no change from sitting to standing.

Proctography does have several applications despite the doubt concerning the value of estimating the anorectal angle. Its application used to be with the patient at rest but now a more dynamic examination is usually used termed defaecography.

Dynamic attempts to assess defaecation were devised using the barium-starch bolus and cine-radiography.[7] Fluoroscopic techniques are generally used with cine-radiographic or video recording to reduce radiation dosage in defaecography. The technique is coupled with synchronous anorectal manometry and striated muscle EMG to allow integrated assessment. A dilute solution of barium sulphate is infused into the rectum until the subject reports a desire to defaecate. The anorectum is visualized using a 100 mm camera (Sircam 106, Siemens), 0.6 mm focus from a radiographic source generating 125 kV at 1000 mA. The image, in addition to being displayed on the image intensifier, is stored for further study on a Sony Umatic videotape recorder.

The position of the anorectal junction is another parameter that may be assessed by defaecography or scintigraphy in the measurement of perineal descent. Similar problems as for the anorectal angle exist for the assessment of the perineal plane because of varying interpretations about which anatomical landmarks should be used. The anorectal angle at rest lies closest to a line joining the tip of the coccyx to the most anterior part of the symphysis pubis and this is the line of the perineal plane used in this unit. Radiological assessment of descent is superior to use of a perineometer.[44] Perineal descent of between 1 and 3 cm is seen on straining in most subjects. Descent in excess of this range is defined as a clinical entity, i.e. the 'descending perineal syndrome' which is thought to be a risk factor for the development of neurogenic faecal incontinence.[29]

INTEGRATED ANORECTAL PHYSIOLOGICAL ASSESSMENT

Most current attempts to assess healthy and diseased subjects are not physiological. As a result, increasingly sophisticated attempts are being made to assess these patients in a physiological setting. Baseline measurements such as anal canal sensation and rectal compliance can still be a reliable indicator of anorectal disease. This can be supplemented by neurophysiological investigations such as estimation of pudendal nerve terminal latencies and estimation of single fibre density of individual nerve motor units. A relatively recent and apparently useful technique of assessing sphincter injuries in the laboratory setting is the use of endoanal ultrasound.[33] This investigation allows for identification of gaps within sphincters as well as sites of fistulas and abscesses.

Ambulatory recording systems usually include fine wire EMG recordings of the internal anal sphincter, external anal sphincter and puborectalis muscle. Rectal and anal pressures are recorded by inserting a probe 3 mm in diameter with single pressure microtransducers mounted at 2 cm and 6 cm from the probe tip, and two microtranducers 10 cm from the tip. The single microtransducers record sigmoid and rectal pressures respectively, while the two channels at 10 cm record upper and mid-anal canal pressures. This allows for integrated ambulatory recordings in seven channels (three EMG, four pressure channels) for a period of between 12–24 hours. The recording is digitalized by the recorder and can be viewed in real-time mode or be subsequently transferred for viewing and storage on disc facilities. This recording enables assessment of sphincter and pressure changes during sampling, passage of flatus, defaecation, and micturition as well as various other events which are not reproducible in a laboratory setting. These results are reproducible and have identifiable variables for patient groups. Progress in understanding the physiology and pathology of the continence mechanism may come from such integrated assessment.

ACKNOWLEDGEMENTS

Mr R. Farouk is supported by a grant from the Medical Research Council. Mr G.S. Duthie is supported by a grant from the Wellcome Trust.

REFERENCES

1. Arhan, P., Devroede, G., Jehannin, B. *et al.* (1983) Idiopathic disorders of faecal incontinence in children. *Paediatrics*, **77**, 774–779.
2. Bannister, J.J., Abouzecky, L. and Read, N.W. (1987) Effect on aging on anorectal function. *Gut*, **28**, 353–357.
3. Bannister, J.J., Gibbons, C. and Read, N.W. (1987) Preservation of faecal continence during rises in intra-abdominal pressure: is there a role for the flap-valve? *Gut*, **28**, 1242–1245.
4. Bartolo, D.C.C. and Duthie, G.S. (1990) The physiological evaluation operative repair for incontinence and prolapse. In *Neurobiology of Incontinence*. pp. 223–245. Wiley: Chichester (Ciba Foundation Symposium 151).
5. Bartolo, D.C.C., Roe, A.M., Locke-Edmunds, J.C. *et al.* (1986) Flap valve theory of anorectal incontinence. *British Journal of Surgery*, **73**, 1012–1014.
6. Bouvier, M. and Gonella, J. (1981) Nervous control of the internal anal sphincter of the cat. *Journal of Physiology*, **310**, 457–469.
7. Burhenne, H.J. (1964) Intestinal evacuation study: a new roentgenologic technique. *Radiology Clinics*, **33**, 79–84.
8. Burleigh, D.E., D'Mello, A. and Parks, A.G. (1979) Responses of isolated human internal anal sphincter to drugs and electrical field stimulation. *Gastroenterology*, **77**, 484–490.
9. Burleigh, D.E. (1983) Non-cholinergic, non-adrenergic inhibitory in human internal sphincter muscle. *Journal of Pharmacy and Pharmacology*, **35**, 258–260.
10. Denny-Brown, D. and Robertson, E.G. (1935) An investigation of the nervous control of defecation. *Brain*, **58**, 256–310.
11. Dubrovsky, B. (1988) Effects of anal distension on the sphincter ani muscles in cats. *American Journal of Physiology*, **254**, G100–G106.
12. Duthie, G.S., Miller, R. and Bartolo, D.C.C. (1990) Internal sphincter electromyographic frequency is related to anal canal resting pressure. Both are reduced in idiopathic faecal incontinence. *Gut*, **31**, A619.
13. Duthie, G.S., Bartolo, D.C.C. and Miller, R. (1991) Laboratory tests grossly overestimate the incidence of anismus. *British Journal of Surgery*, **78**, 747.
14. Duthie, G.S. and Bartolo, D.C.C. (1991) Pathophysiology and management of rectal prolapse. In *Recent Advances in Surgery*. Oxford: Butterworth-Heinemann.
15. Duthie, G.S. and Bartolo, D.C.C. Nocturnal leakage is related to high pressure pouch waves following restorative proctocolectomy. *British Journal of Surgery*.
16. Duthie, H.L. and Gairns, F.W. (1960) Sensory nerve endings and sensation in the anal region of man. *British Journal of Surgery*, **47**, 585–595.
17. Duthie, H.L. and Watts, J.M. (1965) Contribution of the external anal sphincter to the pressure zone in the anal canal. *Gut*, **6**, 64–68.
18. Farouk, R., Duthie, G.S., Pryde, A., Bartolo, D.C.C., MacGregor, A.B. and Miller, R. High rectal pressure waves in rectal prolapse are associated with internal sphincter inhibition. *Gut*, (in press).
19. Farouk, R., Duthie, G.S., Bartolo, D.C.C., MacGregor, A.B. and Miller, R. Restoration of continence following rectopexy for prolapse is associated with recovery of the intestinal anal sphincter. *British Journal of Surgery* (in press).
20. Floyd, W. and Walls, E. (1953) Electromyography of the sphincter ani externus in man. *Journal of Physiology*, **16**, 638–644.
21. Freckner, B. and von Euler, C. (1975) Influence of pudendal block on the function of the internal sphincter. *Gut*, **16**, 482–489.
22. Freiling, T., Enck, P. and Weinbeck, M. (1989) Cerebral evoked responses by electrical stimulation of the rectosigmoid in normal subjects. *Digestive Diseases Science*, **34**, 202–205.
23. Gaston, E.A. (1948) The physiology of faecal continence. *Surgery, Gynecology and Obstetrics*, **87**, 280–290.
24. Goligher, J.C. and Hughes, E.R.S. (1951) The sensibility of the colon and rectum. *The Lancet*, **i**, 543–547.
25. Hancock, B.D. and Smith, K. (1975) The internal anal sphincter and Lords procedure for haemorrhoids. *British Journal of Surgery*, **62**, 833–836.
26. Hancock, B.D. and Smith, K. (1977) The internal anal sphincter and anal fissure. *British Medical Journal of Surgery*, **64**, 92–95.
27. Henry, M.M. and Swash, M. (1985) In *Coloproctology and the Pelvic Floor: Pathophysiology and Management*. London: Butterworth.
28. Ihre, T. (1974) Studies in anal function in continent and incontinent patients. *Scandinavian Journal of Gastroenterology*, **9**(suppl.25).

29. Jones, P.N., Lubowski, D.Z., Swash, M. and Henry, M.M. (1984) Relation between perineal descent and pudendal nerve damage in idiopathic faecal incontinence. *International Journal of Colorectal Diseases*, **2**, 93–95.

30. Keighley, M.R.B., Winslet, M.C., Yoshioka, K. and Lightwood, R. (1987) Discrimination is not impaired by excision of the anal transition zone after restorative proctocolectomy. *British Journal of Surgery*, **74**, 1118–1121.

31. Kerremans, R. (1982) *Morphological and Physiological Aspects of Anal Continence and Defecation*. Brussels: Editions Arscia.

32. Kumar, D., Waldron, D., Williams, N.S., Browning, C., Hutton, M.R.E. and Wingate, D.L. (1990) Prolonged anorectal manometry and external sphincter EMG in ambulant humans. *Digestive Diseases Science*, **35**, 641–648.

33. Law, P.J., Kamm, M.A. and Bartram, C.I. (1991) Anal endosonography in the investigation of faecal incontinence. *British Journal of Surgery*, **78**, 312–314.

34. Loening-Buck, V. and Anuras, S. (1984) Anorectal manometry in healthy elderly subjects. *Journal of the American Geriatric Society*, **32**, 636–639.

35. Lubowski, D.Z., Nicholls, R.J., Swash, M. and Jordan, M.J. (1987) Neural control of internal anal sphincter function. *British Journal of Surgery*, **74**, 668–670.

36. Martelli, H., Devroede, G., Arhan, P., Duguay, G., Dornic, C. and Faverdin, C. (1978) Some parameters of large bowel motility in man. *Gastroenterology*, **75**, 612–618.

37. Matheson, D.M. and Keighley, M.R.B. (1981) Manometric evaluation of rectal prolapse and faecal incontinence. *Gut*, **22**, 126–129.

38. Melzack, J. and Porter, N.H. (1964) Studies on the reflex activity of the external anal sphincter ani in spinal masn. *Paraplegia*, **1**, 277–296.

39. Miller, R., Bartolo, D.C.C., Cervero, F. and Mortensen, N.J. McC. (1987) Anorectal temperature sensation: a comparison of normal and incontinent patients. *British Journal of Sciences*, **74**, 511–515.

40. Miller, R., Bartolo, D.C.C., Locke-Edmunds, J.C. and Mortensen, N.J.McC. (1987) A prospective study of conservative and operative treatment for faecal incontinence. *British Journal of Surgery*, **75**, 101–105.

41. Miller, R., Lewis, G.T., Bartolo, D.C.C., Cervero, F. and Mortensen, N.J.McC. (1988) Sensory discrimination and dynamic activity in the anorectum: evidence using a new ambulatory technique. *British Journal of Surgery*, **75**, 1003–1007.

42. Neill, M.E. and Swash, M. (1980) Increased motor unit fiber density in the external anal sphincter muscle in anorectal incontinence; a single fibre EMG study. *Journal of Neurology, Neurosurgery and Psychiatry*, **43**, 343–347.

43. Nivatongs, S., Stern, H.S. and Fryd, D.S. (1981) The length of the anal canal. *Diseases of the Colon and Rectum*, **24**, 600–601.

44. Oettle, G.J., Roe, A.M., Bartolo, D.C.C. and Mortensen, N.J.McC. (1985) What is the best way of measuring perineal descent? A comparison of radiographic and clinical methods. *British Journal of Surgery*, **72**, 999–1001.

45. Ortiz, J., Oya, M., Kumar, D. and Keighley, M.R.B. Neuropathic faecal incontinence, a combination of anal pressures and anal sensitivity. *British Journal of Surgery* (in press).

46. Parks, A.G., Porter, N.H. and Melzack, J. (1962) Experimental study of the reflex mechanism controlling the muscles of the pelvic floor. *Diseases of the Colon and Rectum*, **5**, 407–414.

47. Parks, A.G. (1975) Anorectal incontinence. *Proceedings of the Royal Society of Medicine*, **68**, 681–689.

48. Parks, A.G., Swash, M. and Urich, H. (1977) Sphincter denervation in anorectal incontinence. *Gut*, **18**, 656–667.

49. Pennickx, F. (1981) *Morphological and Physiological Aspects of Anal Function*. Leuven: Acco.

50. Porter, N.H. (1962) Physiological study of the pelvic floor in rectal prolapse. *Annals of the Royal Society of Medicine*, **286**, 379–404.

51. Read, M.G. and Read, N.W. (1982) Role of anorectal sensation in preserving continence. *Gut*, **23**, 345–347.

52. Roe, A.M., Bartolo, D.C.C. and Mortensen, J.J.McC. (1986) New method for assessment of anal sensation in various anorectal disorders. *British Journal of Surgery*, **73**, 310–312.

53. Rogers, J., Hayward, M.P., Henry, M.M. and Misiewicz, V.J. (1988) Temperature gradient between the rectum and anal canal: Evidence against the role of temperature sensation as a sensory modality in the anal canal of normal subjects. *American Journal of Surgery*, **78**, 1083–1085.

54. Shafik, A. (1975) A new concept of the anatomy of the anal sphincter system and the physiology of defecation. The external anal sphincter: a triple-loop system. *Investigative Urology*, **12**, 412–419.

55. Shorvon, P.J., McHugh, S., Diamant, N.E., Somers, S. and Stevenson, G.W. (1989) Defecography in normal volunteers: results and implication. *Gut*, **30**, 1737–1749.

56. Snooks, S.J., Swash, M., Setchell, M. and Henry, M.M. (1984) Injury to innervation of pelvic sphincter musculature in childbirth. *The Lancet*, **ii**, 546–550.

57. Taylor, B.M., Beart, R.W. and Phillips, S.F. (1984) Longitudinal and radial variations of pressure in the human anal canal. *Gastroenterology*, **86**, 693–697.

58. Varma, J.S., Smith, A.N. and Busuttil, A. (1985) Correlation of clinical and manometric abnormalities of rectal function following chronic radiation injury. *British Journal of Surgery*, **72**, 875–878.

PELVIC FLOOR DISORDERS

M.M. Henry

Pelvic floor disorders appear to be forming an increasing element of the workload in centres dealing with colorectal disease. As a consequence, over the last decade new methods of investigating anorectal function in the normal and abnormal states have been introduced in the hope that improved comprehension of the aetiological processes might, in turn, lead to advances in therapy. In the author's opinion, although it is certainly true that we now know more about anal function, sadly, the last 10 years, with a few exceptions, have not seen many significant therapeutic advances.

RECTAL PROLAPSE

Rectal prolapse may be observed within any age group. Prolapse of the mucosa alone commonly occurs in childhood, particularly within the first two years of life; thereafter it becomes increasingly rare.[11] In adults, mucosal prolapse may be due to haemorrhoids or may be associated with perineal descent (see below). The term rectal prolapse is customarily taken to imply extrusion beyond the anus of both rectal wall and its mucosa (full thickness prolapse) (*Figure 4.87*). Full thickness prolapse occurs most commonly in women of advanced age, the maximum incidence being in the fifth, sixth and seventh decades.[16] It is rarely a condition of childhood and, where it is observed, mucoviscidosis must be the first consideration requiring exclusion.

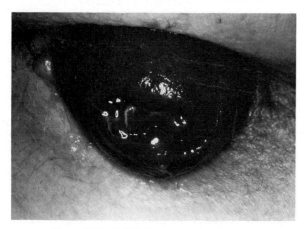

Figure 4.87   Full thickness rectal prolapse.

AETIOLOGY

Mucosal prolapse

In childhood, mucosal prolapse is usually the consequence of an abnormal pattern of defaecation whereby high ultra-abdominal pressures sustained during straining lead to extrusion of mucosa of the lower rectum. In the adult, mucosal prolapse may either be due to extensive hamemorrhoids or may be prolapse principally of the anterior rectal wall (anterior mucosal prolapse) in association with perineal descent.

Full thickness prolapse

A variety of hypotheses have been advanced based on the following observations:

1. An abnormally deep pouch between the rectum and the vagina (or bladder in men) is often observed in these patients. Moschcowitz[29] claimed that this was a true hernia of the pouch of Douglas through a defect in the endopelvic fascia onto the rectal wall and subsequently into the rectal lumen. It seems probable that these are more likely to be secondary events as there is no evidence of primary weakness (or biochemical abnormality) of the supporting connective tissue of the pelvis which might permit such herniation to develop.
2. Cineradiography of the rectum during defaecation in patients with rectal prolapse has demonstrated that prolapse is nearly always initiated by an intussusception of the rectum 6–8 cm from the anal verge.[6] This would appear to be a clear account of the dynamics involved in prolapse but does not explain what pathological processes are established which permit initiation of the intussusception.
3. The internal anal sphincter tone is usually greatly diminished in patients with prolapse as a consequence of being stretched by the four layers of the prolapse as it advances through and beyond the anal canal. Of even greater interest is the observation that the external anal sphincter and puborectalis muscles are deficient. By employing specialized histochemical staining techniques, structural changes consistent with denervation have been identified in these muscles in patients with complete prolapse.[3,37] These histological changes may result from localized damage to the

neuronal supply, as indicated by prolongation of the pudendal nerve terminal motor latency[21] and by changes observed using single fibre electromyography.[32] Further clinical evidence in support of a neurological factor in the development of rectal prolapse is the observation that prolapse is extremely common in patients with cauda equina lesions.[52]

Hence, in some patients, denervation of the pelvic floor results in increased obliquity of the anorectal angle, which, in turn, permits prolapse of the anterior rectal wall. The latter sets up a circumferential intussusception of the rectal wall which may eventually extend beyond the anal canal. There is a small subgroup of patients who develop prolapse but who display no features of denervation of the pelvic floor; the aetiology of the prolapse in these patients remains unexplained.[32]

CLINICAL FEATURES

Mucosal prolapse

The symptoms of mucosal prolapse may be indistinguishable from those observed in patients with haemorrhoids. The specific problem of anterior mucosal prolapse and perineal descent is discussed below. In children, the symptoms are usually of a minor nature and are accompanied by a history of constipation (in the absence of mucoviscidosis).

Full thickness prolapse

Symptoms
The prolapse may appear only during defaecation with spontaneous reduction; alternatively the prolapse may be permanent and require manual replacement. Although the physical presence of prolapsing bowel can be the origin of some distress, particularly if associated with anal incontinence, it is rarely a source of discomfort, although mucous discharge is common. In some patients, the prolapse itself is asymptomatic.

The most serious and disabling sequel is anal incontinence. Penfold and Hawley[38] reported that 62% of patients were incontinent of liquid stool and 42% were incontinent of formed stool. Apart from weakness of the sphincters and pelvic floor some patients cannot distinguish impending prolapse from a faecal bolus.

Irregular bowel function, particularly constipation, often precedes the onset of prolapse[25] and may play a role in the causation of the denervation which subsequently gives rise to the prolapse. It has now become well established that prolonged straining[24]

and long periods of constipation[48] both lead to stretch-induced injury to the pudendal nerves.

Physical findings
The diagnosis is not always readily realised, either because patients are not examined during straining, or because some patients are reluctant to reproduce a defaecatory effort on the examination couch. Examination with the patient in the squatting position may help to establish the diagnosis where the left lateral position fails.

Inspection of the perineum may reveal signs of soiling, absence of the anal reflex (evidence of pudendal neuropathy), abnormal perineal descent and a patulous anus. Digital examination of the anal canal may reveal poor resting tone, a deficient anorectal angle and a poor squeeze. Sigmoidoscopic examination of the rectum and lower sigmoid colon may be normal but the macroscopic appearances of a mild proctitis due to trauma is commonly observed. Such patients may be easily misdiagnosed as having inflammatory bowel disease.

TREATMENT

Mucosal prolapse

Treatment is rarely indicated in children as spontaneous resolution is usually seen once bowel function has improved. Local measures can be applied to the prolapsing mucosa but these are rarely necessary. In the adult, mucosal prolapse may be treated by surgical excision, rubber band ligation or injection sclerotherapy. Where there is a history of defaecatory disorder, this may require treatment in addition, to prevent an early recurrence.

Full thickness prolapse

Once a complete prolapse has developed, resolution of the problem cannot usually be achieved by medical treatment alone. The only effective means of controlling the prolapse and improving anal continence is by surgery which can, in most cases, be offered irrespective of the patient's age.

The Thiersch operation
This is the most minor procedure available for treating prolapse and consists of the insertion of silver wire or Teflon subcutaneously around the lax anus; this may be performed under local anaesthesia. The procedure is associated with a 68% recurrence rate, however, and complications such as secondary infection, faecal impaction and wire fractures are common. The procedure has now generally

been abandoned because it does not cure the prolapse but merely contain it just inside the anus.

Rectosigmoidectomy

Excision of the upper rectum and sigmoid colon was initially advocated by Miles[26] and more recently by Muir.[30] This is a major procedure, however, with all the attendant risks of anastomotic leakage. The chief criticism is the high recurrence rate which Porter[40] found to be of the order of 58% within the first 3 years.

Rectopexy (use of implants)

Ripstein[41] devised a technique whereby a rectangular implant is sutured onto the anterior aspect of the rectum leaving two lateral flaps which are sutured onto the anterior surface of the sacrum. A sling is thus created which is in contact with the anterior two thirds of the circumference of the rectum and which fixes it to the sacrum. The implanted material was initially fascia lata and later changed to Teflon mesh.

A similar technique was later divised by Wells[54] who tethered the rectum to the hollow of the sacrum by means of a strip of polyvinyl alcohol (Ivalon) sponge. The technique differs from the Ripstein approach, in that the mid-point of a rectangle of sponge is first sutured to the anterior surface of the sacrum, thereby creating two flaps which are sutured to the anterior surface of the rectum in such a way as to leave the anterior third uncovered by the material. Similar techniques have also been described using the more inert polypropylene (Marlex) mesh with excellent functional results[19] (*Figure 4.88*).

Both procedures appear to be safe and relatively free of complications. Recurrence seems to be more common with the Ripstein operation (2–6%) than with the Wells operation and the former may be associated with stricturing at the site of the rectopexy.[12] Ripstein and Lanter[42] recorded one recurrence in a series of 45 operations although the recurrence rate recorded at the Lahey Clinic was of the order of 7.5%.[18] In a series of 150 patients treated by Wells' operation, Morgan and his colleagues noted a recurrence rate of 3.2%.[28] There were no recurrences in the Marlex mesh posterior rectopexy procedures performed in Birmingham.[19]

Not all authorities accept that it is essential to insert foreign material to achieve a good result from rectopexy. Similar results have been claimed by simple suture of the rectum to the presacral fascia. Goldberg combines this approach with excision of the redundant sigmoid colon.[53] Of 102 patients treated by this method, the incidence of recurrence was only 1.9% although 4% developed complications directly related to the anastomosis.

It is important to recognize that rectopexy is successful in controlling prolapse but other problems may persist postoperatively and require further medical/surgical management. In particular, anal incontinence may persist in up to 18.6% of patients postoperatively and constipation is often made worse by surgery.[25] The latter may be the consequence of damage inflicted by the pelvic dissection on the pelvic parasympathetic supply to the rectum.

Delorme's operation

There has been renewed interest in the procedure first described by Delorme[9] in which the rectal

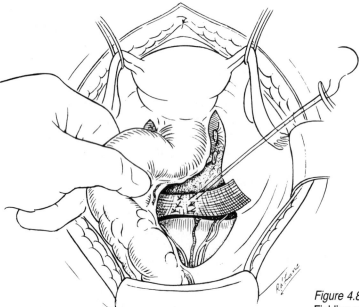

Figure 4.88 Abdominal rectopexy. (From Keighley, Fielding and Alexander-Williams,[19] with permission.)

mucosa is peeled off the muscle wall which is then plicated. The operation has been advocated in patients at high risk because the approach is trans-anal, thereby reducing the risks associated with an abdominal procedure. Christianssen and Kirke-gaard reported satisfactory results in a small series of 12 patients[8] and Monson and colleagues reported a series of 27 patients with only two recurrences at a mean follow-up of 35 months.[27] Recurrence rates of up to 31% have been reported however, following this procedure.[51]

FAECAL INCONTINENCE

Those afflicted by faecal incontinence rapidly de-velop a sense of social alienation and imprisonment and is a symptom frequently concealed by the patient because of embarrassment. The prevalence has never been accurately assessed in the younger age groups although it is widely recognized to be a common disorder in the elderly, in whom the inci-dence may approach 60%.[5] Although both sexes may be affected, of those patients treated by sur-gery, the condition appears to be more prevalent in women by a ratio of 4:1. The age groups most commonly affected are the fifth and sixth decades.[15]

MECHANISMS OF CONTINENCE

The preservation of anal continence is dependent on several factors, the most important of which are listed below.

1. The angle between the lower rectum and upper anus (anorectal angle) created by contraction of the puborectalis muscle. Continuous electrical activity maintains tone in this muscle even during sleep[10] and is facilitated by means of a spinal reflex arc.[34] It is not known why the creation of an angle is so important in the creation of conti-nence but it would appear that the puborectalis is essential for gross continence; reasonable con-trol, for example, can be maintained even if both sphincters are divided provided the puborectalis is intact.
2. The internal sphincter is probably implicated in providing fine 'tuning', i.e. continence to flatus and to liquid stool.[4]
3. The external sphincter assists in maintaining con-tinence over short periods. When the sphincters become threatened by copious liquid stool, vigorous contraction, which can be maintained for approximately one minute, may provide suf-ficient time to prevent soiling.
4. The sensation of rectal filling and appreciation of the nature of rectal contents are important for faecal continence. The former probably depends on sensory receptors in the levator muscles and the latter depends on a locally mediated visceral reflex (the rectosphincteric inhibitory reflex). When the rectum is distended by a bolus of air or faeces, the internal sphincter reflexly relaxes. This permits a sample of rectal contents to enter the anal canal and provide an afferent stimulus to the sensory receptors in the midanal canal.

AETIOLOGY OF FAECAL INCONTINENCE

Diarrhoea

Copius liquid stool from whatever cause may over-whelm the normal anal sphincter mechanisms and lead to incontinence. Diarrhoea may commonly be secondary to infestation or infection of the gut, to inflammatory bowel disease or to extensive intesti-nal resection.

Faecal impaction

In the elderly, and in some patients with upper motor neurone lesions, incontinence may be the consequence of faecal impaction. The latter causes chronic rectal distension and overstimulation of the rectosphincteric inhibitory reflex so that internal sphincter tone is permanently reduced.

Internal anal sphincter deficiency

Rectal prolapse, and certain surgical procedures such as anal sphincterotomy and manual dilatation of the anus, may render the internal sphincter de-ficient. The degree of disability is usually slight and is confined to loss of control to liquid stool and to flatus. Recent pharmacological studies have re-vealed that some patients have intrinsic damage to the internal sphincter (and possibly to its nerve supply) and these patients may describe significant degrees of incontinence.[50] Examination of the patient may reveal scarring from previous surgery or the presence of a rectal prolapse.

External sphincter deficiency

The striated muscle component of the anal sphincter musculature can be affected alone or in combination with deficiency of the internal sphincter. Such damage may occur in full thickness rectal prolapse as well as following operations for anal fistulas, perineal trauma and obstetric injuries (third degree tear). Rarely, some infections such as lymphogranuloma or Crohn's disease and, occasionally, malignant tumours can cause severe destruction of the sphincter.

Traumatic disruption of the external sphincter ring may lead to incontinence, particularly if the puborectalis muscle is damaged. Such may arise following an impalement injury or road traffic accident, or be iatrogenic following inexpert fistula surgery.

Neurological

Spinal cord lesions such as tumours involving the anterior horn cells supplying the pelvic floor muscles may lead to a lower motor neurone lesion. The history is often brief and may be attended by a history of perineal pain. There are usually other neurological features with disturbance of bladder function. Incontinence may also be a significant feature of generalized neurological disorders such as multiple sclerosis and diabetes mellitus.

Congenital

Congenital anorectal atresias are associated with incontinence particularly if the levator plate fails to develop normally (*Figure 4.89*).

Idiopathic

In most patients with faecal incontinence, none of these aetiological factors apply. Histochemical

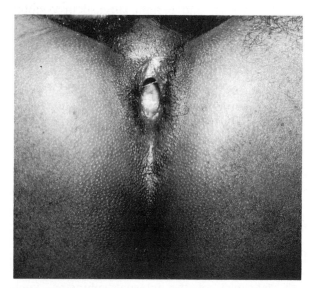

Figure 4.89 Imperforate anus, treated at birth but the anal canal was open outside the sphincter. Continence was restored after re-routing the anal canal.

staining of biopsies from pelvic floor muscles in patients with idiopathic anal incontinence show the same denervation changes as observed in patients with rectal prolapse.[37] Supportive evidence for a neuropathy has also been provided by detailed electrophysiological investigation of these patients.[31,21] The cause of the nerve damage remains speculative. Many women provide a history of preceding difficult or prolonged labour, or both. Neuronal damage in these patients may be the consequence of undue compression by the fetal head of the nerves supplying the pelvic floor. Research has shown that vaginal delivery (rather than the pregnancy itself) is indeed associated with pudendal nerve damage and that this is most marked in women (a) with large babies; (b) who have a forceps assisted delivery; and (c) who undergo a second stage of labour in excess of one hour.[46,49] Perineal descent may be another factor (see below).

CLINICAL FEATURES

Because of embarrassment experienced by the patient, there is often a considerable delay between the onset of symptoms and presentation. Pads may be required and have to be changed frequently throughout the day. The degree of incontinence and the amount of dislocation of normal life is of importance because this will determine treatment. Where the history is of short duration and accompanied by pain, myelography to exclude spinal tumour should be considered.

A full proctological examination, including sigmoidoscopy, should always be performed. Local examination will reveal perianal soiling, a gaping anus and possibly failure to elicit the anal reflex. Local scarring may indicate previous anal surgery or obstetric injury. Digital examination of the anal canal may reveal reduced resting tone if the internal sphincter is deficient and a reduced squeeze tone if the external sphincter/pelvic floor are deficient. The posterior 'bar' created by the puborectalis may be less obvious or absent.

TREATMENT

Conservative measures

Partial incontinence
Where the problem is one of soiling due to faecal impaction, treatment with aperients supported, where necessary, by an irritant suppository is usually successful in restoring full continence. Those patients with internal sphincter deficiency alone (following manual dilatation of the anus, for

example) can be adequately managed by constipating agents.

Severe incontinence

Simple measures can rarely be applied with success to this group of patients, particularly if there is a rectal prolapse or gross sphincter deficiency.

Operative measures

In the surgical treatment of congenital anorectal disorders, it is most important that the neo-anus and rectum should be sited accurately in relationship to the pelvic floor muscles and the external sphincter if continence is to be restored.[33] Where incontinence is secondary to disruption of the external sphincter ring, sphincter reconstruction (*Figure 4.90*) will restore continence in approximately 70% of patients.[36] A poor clinical result may be expected, however, if there is preoperative evidence of denervation within the external sphincter.[23]

A variety of procedures have been devised to treat idiopathic (neurogenic) incontinence. The gracilis sling procedure has been advocated, particularly in North America.[39] Both gracilis tendons are transplanted so as to encircle the anus and thereby act as a sphincter substitute. The results are variable, probably because the gracilis is electrically silent at rest and hence there is no muscle tone at rest and during sleep. Williams *et al.*[55] have approached this problem by inserting an electrical implant into the muscle capable of providing tetanic stimuli. The long-term results of this technique are awaited.

As the anorectal angle is of considerable importance to normal control, procedures which attempt to restore this angle should prove helpful. Hakelius and colleagues[13] described an operation to transplant the palmaris longus or sartorius muscle around the rectum as a U-shaped sling. The transplanted muscle could be shown to be capable of function, possibly due to re-innervation from collateral sprouting of nearby axons supplying healthy muscle.

Parks[7] and others[20] have achieved the same ideal using a simpler technique. The anorectal angle is restored by the insertion of a lattice of sutures into the pubococcygeus and puborectalis muscles behind the rectum via the intersphincteric plane (*Figure 4.91*).

When all other measures fail, most patients find an incontinent abdominal wall stoma preferable to an incontinent perineal stoma. The clinical value of a colostomy in this condition should not be undervalued.

PERINEAL DESCENT

A syndrome associated with abnormal descent of the pelvic floor was described by Parks and colleagues.[35] They described a condition in which pelvic floor descent caused disruption of the anorectal angle which, in turn, favoured prolapse of the anterior rectal wall mucosa into the anal canal. These patients then experienced pronounced difficulty with defaecation since the anterior mucosal prolapse obstructed the passage of stool during straining and some patients describe the need to insert a finger into the anal canal to push the mucosa aside before defaecation may proceed. At the completion of defaecation, the mucosa may remain in contact with the sensory rich zone at the dentate line and so gave rise to the false impression that stool remains within the rectum (incomplete evacuation). Patients then

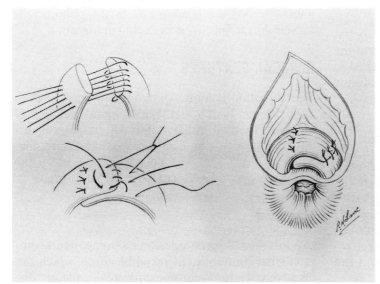

Figure 4.90 Sphincter reconstruction. (From Keighley and Fielding,[20] with permission.)

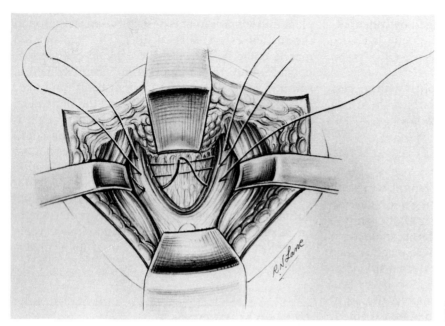

Figure 4.91 Postanal repair. (From Keighley and Fielding,[20] with permission.)

embark on further excessive straining in fruitless attempts to empty a perceived full rectum.

Since the description of this syndrome, it has become apparent that perineal descent is merely a physical sign associated with a wide range of pelvic floor disorders (commonly observed in urinary/faecal incontinence, constipation and solitary rectal ulcer syndrome, for example) and is not a specific syndrome. Anterior mucosal prolapse is only associated with perineal descent in 20% of patients on initial presentation; the commonest symptoms being bleeding, pain and a sense of localized prolapse or 'block' within the anus.[1]

DEFINITION

Using the perineometer, perineal descent is defined as being present if the plane of the perineum descends below that of the bony outlet of the pelvis during a straining effort.[14] By the application of the more accurate radiological methods, it is defined as descent of greater than 3 cm during a straining effort.[2]

DENERVATION

It is apparent that the common factor in the manifestation of this physical sign is denervation of the pelvic floor. Perineal descent hence correlates with the denervation associated with vaginal delivery[46] and with long-term constipation.[22] It has also been demonstrated that there is a linear and direct relationship between the degree of descent and the degree of nerve damage as determined by increases in the pudendal nerve terminal motor latency.[17]

SOLITARY RECTAL ULCER SYNDROME

The solitary rectal ulcer syndrome is a complex of symptoms related to the presence of a shallow ulcer usually sited anteriorly on the midrectal wall.

AETIOLOGY

In company with patients with anterior mucosal prolapse, many patients with rectal ulcer syndrome strain excessively with defaecation and can be shown to have denervation of the pelvic floor musculature.[47] The histological features are non-specific with smooth muscle hypertrophy.[44] Ulceration may arise either from ischaemia when the tip of the prolapse becomes impacted within the anal canal or alternatively from trauma due to the puborectalis muscle which fails to relax during defaecation.[43]

CLINICAL FEATURES

The condition is most common in women in their third decade. Rutter and Riddell found that 68% of ulcers were sited either anteriorly or anterolaterally,[44] Fourteen per cent were situated laterally, whereas only 18% were posterior. Almost all the ulcers were found 4–10 cm from the anal verge.

Symptoms

In addition to disordered defaecation, patients commonly have intermittent rectal bleeding, which can be severe causing chronic anaemia. Mucous discharge and soiling are common and a high proportion of patients complain of perineal pain, probably due to inflammation and stimulation of the sensory receptors in the pelvic floor.

Examination

There may be perineal descent, and occasionally a complete prolapse is observed during straining. On digital examination, both sphincters may be deficient and the ulcers with a surrounding area of induration may be palpable on the anterior rectal wall. With sigmoidoscopy, the ulcer is seen usually as a shallow well-demarcated lesion with a grey coloured slough over its base. The outline may be irregular and the edge may be polypoidal.

TREATMENT

In the first instance, attempts should be made to improve defaecation by a combination of bulking agents and an irritant suppository. In the belief that internal intussusception is a major aetiological factor, Schweiger and Alexander-Williams[45] treated patients by rectopexy and have reported success in 10 of 12 patients. It is known that the results of rectopexy are poor in the absence of intussusception and the long-term results in those who can be shown to have internal prolapse have not been reported.

Clinicians must be aware of this condition. Sometimes the macroscopic appearances closely resemble a carcinoma and patients have in the past been incorrectly treated by rectal excision. It is therefore mandatory that all ulcers in the rectum should be biopsied before excisional surgery is considered.

REFERENCES

1. Allen-Mersh, T.G., Henry, M.M. and Nicholls, R.J. (1987) Natural history of anterior mucosal prolapse. *British Journal of Surgery*, **74**, 679–682.
2. Bartram, C.I., Turnbull, G.K. and Lennard-Jones, J.E. (1988) Evacuation proctography: an investigation of rectal expulsion in 20 subjects without defecatory disturbance. *Gastrointestinal Radiology*, **13**, 72–80.
3. Beersiek, F., Parks, A.G. and Swash, M. (1979) Pathogenesis of ano-rectal incontinence: a histometric study of the anal sphincter musculature. *Journal of the Neurological Sciences*, **42**, 111–127.
4. Bennett, R.C. and Duthie, H.L. (1964) The functional importance of the internal anal sphincter. *British Journal of Surgery*, **51**, 111–127.
5. Brocklehurst, J.C. (1975) Management of anal incontinence. *Clinics in Gastroenterology*, **4**, 479–487.
6. Broden, B. and Snellman, B. (1968) Procidentia of the rectum studied with cineradiography: a contribution to the discussion of causative mechanism. *Diseases of the Colon and Rectum*, **11**, 330–347.
7. Browning, G.G.P. and Parks, A.G. (1983) Post anal repair for neuropathic faecal incontinence: correlation of clinical results and anal canal pressures. *British Journal of Surgery*, **70**, 101–104.
8. Christianssen, J. and Kirkegaard, P. (1981) Delorme's operation for complete rectal prolapse. *British Journal of Surgery*, **68**, 537–538.
9. Delorme, R. (1900) Sur le traitement des prolapsus du rectum totaux pour l'excision de la muquese rectable au rectocolique. *Bulletin Membres Societé Chirurgical Paris*, **26**, 498–499.
10. Floyd, W.F. and Walls, E.W. (1953) Electromyography of the sphincter ani externus in man. *Journal of Physiology*, **122**, 599–609.
11. Goligher, J.C. (1980) *Surgery of the Anus, Rectum and Colon,* 4th Edn, London: Baillière Tindall.
12. Gordon, P.H. and Hoexter, B. (1978) Complications of the Ripstein procedure. *Diseases of Colon and Rectum*, **21**, 277–280.
13. Hakelius, L., Gierup, J. Grotte, G. and Jorulf, H. (1978) A new treatment of anal incontinence in children: free autogenous muscle transplantation. *Journal of Paediatric Surgery*, **13**, 77–82.
14. Henry, M.M., Parks, A.G. and Swash, M. (1982) The pelvic floor musculature in the descending perineum syndrome. *British Journal of Surgery*, **69**, 470–472.
15. Henry, M.M. and Simson, J.N.L. (1985) The results of postanal repair: a retrospective study. *British Journal of Surgery*, **72** (Suppl.), 17–19.
16. Hughes, E.S.R. and Gleadell, L.W. (1966) Complete prolapse of the rectum. *British Journal of Surgery*, **53**, 760–765.
17. Jones, P.N., Lubowski, D.Z., Swash, M. and Henry, M.M. (1987) Relation between perineal descent and pudendal nerve damage in idiopathic faecal incontinence. *International Journal of Colorectal Disease*, **2**, 93–95.
18. Jurgeleit, H.C., Corman, M.L., Coller, J.A. and Veidenheimer, M.C. (1975) Procidentia of the rectum: Teflon sling repair of rectal prolapse, Lahey Clinic experience. *Diseases of Colon and Rectum*, **18**, 464–467.
19. Keighley, M.R.B., Fielding, J.L. and Alexander-Williams, J. (1983) Results of abdominal rectopexy using polypropylene (Marlex) mesh in 100 consecutive patients. *British Journal of Surgery*, **70**, 229–232.
20. Keighley, M.R.B. and Fielding, J.L. (1983) Surgical management of faecal incontinence. *British Journal of Surgery*, **70**, 463–468.
21. Kiff, E.S. and Swash, M. (1984) Slowed conduction in the pudendal nerves in idiopathic (neurogenic) faecal incontinence. *British Journal of Surgery*, **71**, 614–616.
22. Kiff, E.S., Barnes, P.R.H. and Swash, M. (1984) Evidence of pudendal neuropathy in patients with perineal descent and chronic straining at stool. *Gut*, **25**, 1279–1282.
23. Laurberg, S., Swash, M. and Henry, M.M. (1988)

Delayed external sphincter repair for obstetric tear. *British Journal of Surgery*, **75**, 786–788.

24. Lubowski, D.Z., Swash, M., Nicholls, R.J. and Henry, M.M. (1988) Increase in pudendal nerve terminal motor latency with defaecation straining. *British Journal of Surgery*, **75**, 1095–1097.

25. Mann, C.V. and Hoffman, C. (1988) Complete rectal prolapse: the anatomical and functional results of treatment by an extended abdominal rectopexy. *British Journal of Surgery*, **75**, 34–37.

26. Miles, W.E. (1933) Recto-sigmoidectomy as a method of treatment for procidentia recti. *Proceedings of the Royal Society of Medicine*, **26**, 1445–1452.

27. Monson, J.R.T., Jones, N.A.G., Vowden, P. and Brennan, T.G. (1986) Delorme's operation: the first choice in complete rectal prolapse? *Annals of the Royal College of Surgeons of England*, **68**, 143–145.

28. Morgan, C.N., Porter, N.H. and Klugman, D.J. (1972) Ivalon (polyvinyl alcohol) sponge in the repair of complete rectal prolapse. *British Journal of Surgery*, **59**, 841–846.

29. Moschcowitz, A.V. (1912) The pathogenesis, anatomy and cure of prolapse of the rectum. *Surgery, Gynecology and Obstetrics*, **15**, 7–21.

30. Muir, E.G. (1954) Rectal prolapse. *Proceedings of the Royal Society of Medicine*, **48**, 33–44.

31. Neill, M.E. and Swash, M. (1980) Increased motor unit fibre density in the external anal sphincter muscle in ano-rectal incontinence: a single fibre EMG study. *Journal of Neurology, Neurosurgery and Psychiatry*, **43**, 343–347.

32. Neill, M.E., Parks, A.G. and Swash, M. (1981) Physiological studies of the pelvic floor in idiopathic faecal incontinence and rectal prolapse. *British Journal of Surgery*, **68**, 531–536.

33. Nixon, H.H. (1980) Congenital deformities of the anorectal region. In *Surgery of the Anus, Rectum and Colon* 4th Edn (Ed.) Goligher, J.C. pp. 259–278. London: Baillière Tindall.

34. Parks, A.G., Porter, N.H. and Melzak, J. (1962) Experimental study of the reflex mechanism controlling the muscles of the pelvic floor. *Diseases of the Colon and Rectum*, **5**, 407–414.

35. Parks, A.G., Porter, N.H. and Hardcastle, J.D. (1966) The syndrome of the descending perineum. *Proceedings of the Royal Society of Medicine*, **59**, 477–482.

36. Parks, A.G. and McPartlin, J.F. (1971) Late repair of injuries of the anal sphincter. *Proceedings of the Royal Society of Medicine*, **54**, 1187–1189.

37. Parks, A.G., Swash, M. and Urich, H. (1977) Sphincter denervation in anorectal incontinence and rectal prolapse. *Gut*, **18**, 656–665.

38. Penfold, J.C.B. and Hawley, P.R. (1972) Experiences of Ivalon-sponge implant for complete rectal prolapse at St Mark's Hospital, 1960–1970. *British Journal of Surgery*, **59**, 846–848.

39. Pickrell, K.L., Broadbent, T.R., Masters, F.W. and Metzger, J.T. (1952) Construction of a rectal sphincter and restoration of anal continence by transplanting the gracilis muscle. *Annals of Surgery*, **135**, 853–862.

40. Porter, N.H. (1962) Collective results of operations for rectal prolapse. *Proceedings of the Royal Society of Medicine*, **55**, 1087–1091.

41. Ripstein, C.B. (1952) Treatment of massive rectal prolapse. *American Journal of Surgery*, **83**, 68–71.

42. Ripstein, C.B. and Lanter, B. (1963) Etiology and surgical therapy of massive prolapse of the rectum. *Annals of Surgery*, **157**, 259–264.

43. Rutter, K.R.P. (1974) Electromyographic changes in certain pelvic floor abnormalities. *Proceedings of the Royal Society of Medicine*, **67**, 53–56.

44. Rutter, K.R.P. and Riddell, R.H. (1975) The solitary ulcer syndrome of the rectum. *Clinics in Gastroenterology*, **4**, 505–530.

45. Schweiger, M. and Alexander-Williams, J. (1977) Solitary ulcer syndrome of the rectum: its association with occult rectal prolapse. *Lancet*, **i**, 170.

46. Snooks, S.J., Swash, M., Henry, M.M. and Setchell, M. (1984) Injury to innervation of pelvic floor sphincter musculature in childbirth. *Lancet*, **ii**, 546–550.

47. Snooks, S.J., Nicholls, R.J., Henry, M.M. and Swash, M. (1985) Electrophysiological and manometric assessment of the pelvic floor in the solitary rectal ulcer syndrome. *British Journal of Surgery*, **72**, 131–133.

48. Snooks, S.J., Barnes, P.R.H., Swash, M. and Henry, M.M. (1985) Damage to the innervation of the pelvic floor musculature in chronic constipation. *Gastroenterology*, **89**, 977–981.

49. Snooks, S.J., Swash, M., Henry, M.M. and Setchell, M. (1986) Risk factors in childbirth causing damage to the pelvic floor innervation. *International Journal of Colorectal Disease*, **1**, 20–24.

50. Speakman, C.T.M., Hoyle, C.H.V., Kamm, M.A., Henry, M.M., Nicholls, R.J. and Burnstock, G. (1990) Adrenergic control of the internal anal sphincter is abnormal in patients with idiopathic faecal incontinence. *British Journal of Surgery*, **77**, 1342–1344.

51. Swinton, N.W. and Palmer, T.E. (1960) The management of rectal prolapse and procidentia. *American Journal of Surgery*, **99**, 144–151.

52. Todd, I.P. (1959) Etiological factors in the production of complete rectal prolapse. *Postgraduate Medical Journal,* **35**, 97–100.

53. Watts, J.D., Rothenberger, D.A. and Goldberg, S.M. (1985) *Coloproctology and the Pelvic Floor*, (Eds) Henry, M.M. and Swash, M. London: Butterworth.

54. Wells, C.H. (1959) New operation for rectal prolapse. *Proceedings of the Royal Society of Medicine*, **52**, 602–603.

55. Williams, N.S., Hallan, R.I., Koeze, T.H. and Watkins, E.S. (1989) Construction of a neorectum and neoanal sphincter following previous proctocolectomy. *British Journal of Surgery*, **76**, 1191–1194.

HAEMORRHOIDS

J.P.S. Thomson and M.R.B. Keighley

Over 50% of patients attending a rectal clinic have haemorrhoids. Although the condition is thus common, it is only recently that surgeons have begun to research the subject.

AETIOLOGY

In his essay 'De Haemorrhois', Parks[15] outlined the surgical history of haemorrhoids over four millenia. More recently W.H.F. Thomson[18] conducted an elegant anatomical study of the nature of haemorrhoids and reviewed some of the theories concerning their origin. He undertook injection studies to demonstrate the arterial and the venous system as well as any arteriovenous communications. He also studied the smooth muscle in the anal submucosa, first described by Treitz in 1853, and gave an account of the anal cushions.

The injection studies showed that the anal canal receives a rich blood supply from the superior, middle and inferior rectal arteries, whose branches reach the anal submucosa in a variety of ways. The previous finding of dilated veins forming the haemorrhoidal plexus was confirmed. This observation was also present in 8 out of 10 neonates that were studied. Using serial section and radiological techniques, the presence of arteriovenous communications was also substantiated.

Treitz described the venous plexus being surrounded by smooth muscle in the submucosa and Thomson[18] verified this finding believing that this muscle acts as a support to the anal lining during defaecation. These anal cushions were also demonstrated even in the neonate. The anal lumen was shown to be a triradiate slit with the stem of the 'Y' directed posteriorly. These anatomical studies demonstrated that the cushions consisted of an area of venous dilatation covered by smooth muscle with intervening elastic and fibrous tissue. These cushions are found in infants and in asymptomatic people and must be regarded as normal structures.

There are a number of theories concerning the aetiology of haemorrhoids; one theory is that they are merely varicose veins, another is that they represent an area of vascular hyperplasia. A small proportion may also represent a true portosystemic communication in the anal submucosa. Thomson considered the nature of haemorrhoids to be due primarily to a lax anal mucosa which slides downward causing distal displacement of the anal cushions. This is especially liable to occur where there is a history of constipation or prolonged straining at stool leading to stretching or disruption of Treitz's muscle and venous engorgement. Once displaced, a tight internal sphincter is liable to perpetuate the venous engorgement.

Haemorrhoids occur at the site of the primary venous cushions and so are found at three sites around the circumference of the anal canal – left lateral, right posterior and right anterior. When the primary haemorrhoids are large, secondary haemorrhoids often develop in between.

Large haemorrhoids usually consist of an internal and external component, the external component having an epithelial lining and lying below the line of the anal valves (dentate line). The portion of the haemorrhoid above the dentate line is covered with columnar epithelium but there are sometimes areas of squamous change in patients with a long history of prolapse. Below the dentate line the haemorrhoid is covered with stratified squamous epithelium and skin (*Figure 4.92*). The external component is frequently overlooked by the clinician but is often responsible for the symptoms. Skin tags also occur which may be troublesome and can impair cleaning of the perineum after defaecation.

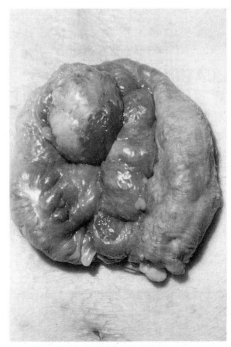

Figure 4.92 Prolapsed haemorrhoids. Note the squamous epithelial change on the right anterior haemorrhoid.

PREDISPOSING FACTORS

Reference has already been made to the role of constipation and straining at defaecation in the pathogenesis of haemorrhoids. A study of consecutive new patients attending a rectal clinic, however, found a history of straining in only 1 out of 8 patients (unpublished data). A family predisposition to haemorrhoids (50%) seemed to be more important.

Pregnancy is often accompanied by the onset of haemorrhoidal symptoms (see below) which are aggravated during labour. This often contributes to marked discomfort in the early puerperium. A few patients with pelvic disease, such as large ovarian or uterine masses, present with haemorrhoids but the symptoms usually disappear after removal of the pelvic mass. Certain hormones, such as follicle-stimulating hormone, prolactin and glucocorticoids, may be responsible for initiating some of the symptoms in female patients.[17]

The relationship between carcinoma of the rectum and haemorrhoids is probably coincidental rather than causal. Haemorrhoids do not occur any more commonly in patients with portal hypertension than in those without. When anal varices do occur they are quite different in appearance from true haemorrhoids.

Haemorrhoids are very unusual below the age of 20 and, if they do occur, the diagnosis of an haemangioma of the rectum should be considered. It must be recognized that, in most patients, no explanation for the onset of symptoms due to haemorrhoids can be found.

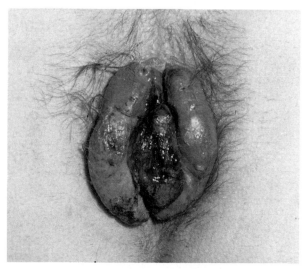

Figure 4.93 Circumferential,   thrombosed,   prolapsed haemorrhoids. Note the groove between the internal and external components.

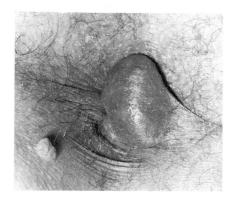

Figure 4.94 Clotted venous saccule (perianal haematoma).

COMPLICATIONS

A fissure may complicate prolapsing haemorrhoids. Other complications include a prolapsing polyp or a hypertrophied anal papilla.

Thrombosis is a frequent, painful occurrence in patients with haemorrhoids and may occur in the external venous plexus or in the internal and external venous plexus of a prolapsed haemorrhoid (*Figure 4.93*). This condition is somewhat confusingly referred to as a strangulated haemorrhoid. This process may involve one or more of the primary sites of haemorrhoids, and in its most severe form the whole circumference of the anal canal. A very localized form of thrombosis is now called a clotted venous saccule[19] or thrombosed perianal varix having previously been incorrectly called perianal haematoma (*Figure 4.94*) see page 918.

CLINICAL FEATURES

Haemorrhoids occur in either sex and usually present in patients over 20 years of age. Often there is a long history of symptoms before the patient seeks advice. The symptoms of haemorrhoids may be similar to those with neoplastic and inflammatory bowel disease. The widespread custom by some physicians to prescribe treatment for symptoms with one of the many proprietary brands of suppository without a full proctological assessment will achieve very little and is to be condemned as other more sinister diseases may be missed. The patient must be fully assessed to establish the exact diagnosis and, if the haemorrhoids warrant it, appropriate treatment instituted. In many instances the patient merely wishes for some reassurance that the symptoms do not indicate that there is underlying colitis or cancer.

Table 4.20 Traditional classification of haemorrhoids

First degree	Bleeding
Second degree	Prolapse (with or without bleeding)
Third degree	Prolapse (with or without bleeding) requiring replacement

The traditional classification of haemorrhoids (*Table 4.20*) is based on two symptoms only: bleeding and prolapse. Although it is clear that these are important, there are others which, if present, may trouble the patient more. These symptoms, together with the frequency of their occurrence as the first symptoms, are shown in *Table 4.21*.

Anorectal bleeding is a most important feature, particularly as it may be the only presenting symptom of adenomas, adenocarcinomas and inflammatory bowel disease. It always requires full assessment. Bleeding from haemorrhoids is at the time of defaecation, often after passage of the stool, when there is a spurt of bright red blood. The bleeding usually drips into the pan especially during straining at stool. The bleeding may be episodic or continuous, but iron deficiency anaemia only occurs in about 1% of patients. Sometimes haemorrhoidal bleeding occurs into the rectum, rather than externally after defaecation. This may result in dark blood being passed at the next time of defaecation or dark blood being noted on the rectal mucosa at sigmoidoscopy at levels up to 15 cm from the anus. Although bleeding from haemorrhoids may present in this way, it is rare and a tumour in the colon must always be excluded by barium enema, flexible sigmoidoscopy or colonoscopy.

Discomfort and pain are different degrees of the same symptom and, contrary to what is often taught, are relatively common in patients with haemorrhoids.[14] In most patients this is due to engorgement of the external haemorrhoidal component with stretching of the sensitive overlying epithelium or due to excessive internal sphincter overactivity. Pain

may also be due to an associated fissure, thrombosis of the external plexus or a clotted venous saccule.

Pruritis ani commonly occurs in association with haemorrhoids and is mainly due to the swelling of the external component or to skin tags leading to inability to achieve perfect cleansing after defaecation. The patient will often give a history that there is faecal staining of his underwear. Faeces contain bacteria which produce endopeptidases and these chemicals are some of the most powerful itch-producing substances known. Mucous discharge may also be responsible. Other possible causes of pruritus must be excluded.[1]

Prolapse of haemorrhoids occurs usually at the time of defaecation, although patients with large haemorrhoids may experience prolapse at other times of exertion such as when lifting heavy objects or playing certain sports. As prolapse is often associated with external haemorrhoidal venous engorgement, discomfort or pain may also be present.

A swelling at the anal margin may be the way a patient describes prolapse, but more usually it is due to the external component of a haemorrhoid. Such a swelling can reach a considerable size, particularly if there has been straining at stool and there is a tight sphincter. Thrombosis of the external plexus will result in a painful swelling.

Discharge is from excessive mucus production as a consequence of a reddened mucosa (traumatic proctitis) or from the prolapsed internal pile. Discharge is often a cause of pruritus in these patients.

In all patients a full rectal examination, consisting of inspection, palpation, sigmoidoscopy and proctoscopy, is essential.

With inspection, skin tags, a thrombosed external haemorrhoidal plexus or permanent prolapse will be detected. Gentle parting of the anal margin should indicate whether or not a fissure is present. An essential step in this part of the examination is to ask the patient to strain as on defaecation (Valsalva manoeuvre). A good indication of the degree of prolapse and engorgement of the external plexus can be obtained in this way. Any descent of the perineum also will be detected. This finding may suggest a long history of straining at defaecation with consequent weakening of the pelvic floor.

Palpation will detect areas of thrombosis, or an hypertrophied anal papilla or fibrous anal polyp (*Figure 4.95*). Uncomplicated haemorrhoids are impalpable.

Sigmoidoscopy is always the next part of the examination which is aimed not at assessing the haemorrhoids, but excluding other more serious diseases. It must be remembered that more of the rectum can be felt with the finger than seen with the proctoscope, so it is logical to pass the sigmoido-

Table 4.21 The symptoms of haemorrhoids

Symptoms	Occurrence (%)	Incidence as first symptom (%)
Bleeding	81	39
Discomfort	64	13
Pruritus ani	62	8
Prolapse	50	20
Swelling	49	11
Pain	35	9
Discharge	29	Nil

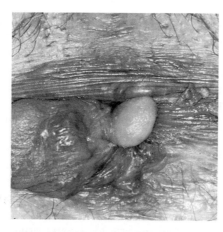

Figure 4.95 Prolapsed fibrous anal polyp.

scope after the digital examination. The presence of inflammatory bowel disease will modify the approach to any haemorrhoids that may require treatment and tumours must be excluded. Haemangioma of the rectum may be detected.

Proctoscopy is only of value to examine the lowermost rectum and the anal canal but is essential for outpatient treatment. Proctoscopy will allow examination of the anal cushions for enlargement and prolapse and squamous epithelial change may be detected, as may reddening of the mucosa. Hypertrophied anal papillae and anal polyps occur in approximately 20% of patients and bleeding may be produced by the examination in about 5%.

INVESTIGATIONS

Barium enema, flexible sigmoidoscopy and colonoscopy may be required to complete the assessment, particularly in patients with bleeding, or in whom blood is found on sigmoidoscopy. Anal canal manometry has been recommended to define treatment groups, but more work is required to determine if this has any useful routine clinical application.

TREATMENT

Some patients with haemorrhoidal symptoms do not require any specific treatment – it is an explanation for their symptoms that is required and reassurance that they do not have a serious problem. If the patients have constipation and difficulty with defaecation, they require advice about fluid intake and diet or the use of laxatives and suppositories to ensure a regular, easy bowel movement without excessive straining.

Table 4.22 The methods for treating haemorrhoids

Fixation of the mucosa	Injection sclerotherapy; infrared coagulation
Fixation of the mucosa and removal of redundant internal component	Elastic band ligation; cryotherapy
Relaxation of internal sphincter	Maximal anal dilatation; partial internal sphincterotomy
Radical excision of internal and external component	Haemorrhoidectomy

Many patients, will require treatment of the actual haemorrhoids. Proprietary suppositories are widely used but of dubious value, although critical assessment is lacking.[3] There is, a wide range of different techniques (*Table 4.22*) available and these will be discussed but there is some difficulty in evaluating the effectiveness of the various treatment methods because there is no acceptable method of classifying patients. The traditional classification of first, second and third degree haemorrhoids only takes into account two of the symptoms, and does not indicate the state of the external component. There is no way at present to assess treatment other than taking each symptom in turn. Furthermore, most available studies only report short-term results. It should also be stressed that treatment should be directed towards control of symptoms and not anatomical perfection. A patient whose symptoms have disappeared requires no more treatment even if there are still abnormal signs on proctoscopy. It must be remembered that anal cushions are normal.

INJECTION SCLEROTHERAPY

A submucosal injection of 5% phenol in arachis oil is given at the anorectal junction, usually at the three primary sites. This induces submucosal inflammation and fixation of the mucosa and perhaps occlusion of some of the haemorrhoidal vessels. This technique may cause some discomfort and can be complicated by mucosal ulceration if the injection is too superficial. Other complications include oleogranuloma formation and prostatitis if the injection is too deep. Injection is a simple outpatient procedure and can be repeated. The only administrative burden is in preparing the syringes with the sclerosant. Injection sclerotherapy has been used for over 100 years and is effective in controlling bleeding, but of little value in patients with prolapse[4] (and unpublished data). Injection is comparable to elastic band ligation but is more invasive, nevertheless, complications are less common after injection than band ligation.[5]

INFRARED COAGULATION

Infrared coagulation is a recent innovation. A small controlled area of coagulation to tissue is created at the anorectal junction by a light beam. The area becomes fibrosed and leads to mucosal fixation. This treatment is as effective as injection sclerotherapy and elastic band ligation and has the advantage of being less invasive and causing fewer side-effects. The risk of secondary haemorrhage is small and postoperative pain is rare, but the equipment required is more expensive. Long-term results suggest that infrared coagulation is inferior to injection and band ligation.[4]

ELASTIC BAND LIGATION

The principle of elastic band ligation is to apply a tight elastic band above the internal (insensitive) haemorrhoid and the mucosa above it (*Figure 4.96*). Not only does this remove some of the redundant mucosa, but also fixes the mucosa at the site of banding to the underlying muscle by scar tissue, thereby preventing the haemorrhoid from sliding down the anal canal.

This procedure can be done in the office or on an outpatient basis, but it is usual to band above only two haemorrhoids at any one time. Further bands may be applied after four weeks. Elastic band ligation reduces many of the symptoms of haemorrhoids, including prolapse, for several years. A complication of treatment is pain, which occurs about one week after therapy and may be severe even when the band is correctly placed. If the band is placed too low in the anal canal, onto the sensitive epithelium, it causes immediate pain and a general anaesthetic may be necessary to remove it. Secondary haemorrhage may also be a problem and is reported in 10% of patients, occurring any time up to 3 weeks after application.

CRYOTHERAPY

Cryotherapy freezes living tissue. The application of a closed probe in which liquid nitrogen ($-180°C$) is allowed to boil off, or in which pressurized nitrous oxide is allowed to expand rapidly ($-75°C$), may be employed to achieve this. As the tissues freeze they become solid and white. When rewarming occurs, the tissues look normal. Six hours later swelling occurs, followed in 24 hours by thrombosis and infarction. The area then becomes black and over a

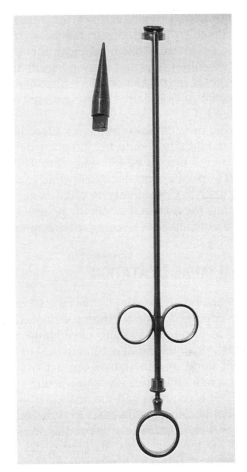

(a)

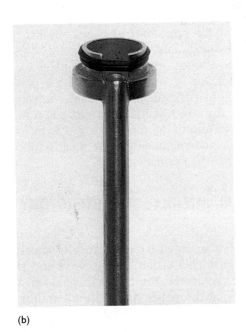

(b)

Figure 4.96 The banding of haemorrhoids. (a) One design of band applicator. The loading cone is to the left. (b) Enlargement showing the band stretched around the ring of the applicator.

10–14-day period separates from the surrounding healthy tissue. Although this technique is probably suitable for internal haemorrhoids, the external component often does not respond well. Internal haemorrhoids can be treated on an outpatient basis, but external piles usually require general or local anaesthesia.[20]

Freezing of haemorrhoids has its advocates who are pleased with the results, but it is not widely used. Cryotherapy is associated with considerable discomfort and a troublesome discharge while the frozen area sloughs.[10] Cryosurgery is often incapable of eradicating the external component and has the further disadvantage of needing special apparatus.

MAXIMAL ANAL DILATATION

It has been argued that the displaced anal cushions become engorged not only during defaecation but also as a result of a tight unyielding internal sphincter. Maximal and dilatation is used to disrupt this tight band and to reduce the activity of the internal anal sphincter. A short-acting general anaesthetic is required and the anal canal is gently dilated until it accommodates six to eight fingers. A sponge is then inserted to exert gentle pressure on the wall of the anal canal to reduce the risk of haematoma. A postoperative regimen of a regular bulk laxative and the passage of an anal dilator is recommended by some for six months[12] but others have found no benefit from postoperative dilatation[8]

There is no doubt that this procedure reduces many of the symptoms of haemorrhoids, particularly in young male patients. It should be used with extreme caution in the elderly and in women; it should never be used in those with a pelvic floor neuropathy (descending perineum syndrome). It is specifically contraindicated if there is a history of obstetric trauma as there is a 2–4% incidence of incontinence (of not only flatus but also solid faeces) which may be permanent.

PARTIAL INTERNAL SPHINCTEROTOMY

Surgical division of the tight unyielding distal internal sphincter only is an alternative to maximal anal dilatation. This avoids dilatation of the proximal internal sphincter, the external sphincter and also muscles of the pelvic floor. The operation is best performed in the lateral rather than the midline position, under general anaesthesia. This simple and safe procedure has been widely adopted in the treatment of fissure, but its use in the management of haemorrhoids is inferior to anal dilatation.[10]

HAEMORRHOIDECTOMY

There is no doubt that a correctly performed haemorrhoidectomy is sometimes the best treatment for curing a patient of haemorrhoids. Often, though, it is not done well and symptoms persist or return early. In most series only 5–10% of all patients with haemorrhoids need this operation. The following criteria are used in the selection of patients for haemorrhoidectomy: those who have large prolapsing haemorrhoids with areas of squamous epithelial change and a large external component (see *Figure 4.92*); those whose symptoms have not responded to other treatments; and those who have recurrent episodes of thrombosis in the external component.

The principle of the operation is the removal of the three primary haemorrhoids, taking care not to damage either of the underlying sphincters and to preserve a bridge of mucosa and skin between each wound to ensure healing without stenosis. However, the mucocutaneous bridges often cover secondary haemorrhoidal tissue and are often redundant themselves. This secondary haemorrhoidal tissue can be dissected from under the bridges, which are then sewn into the anal canal so that there is no external redundancy. The operation is based on that described by Milligan and Morgan in 1934[13] and is widely used.

The first bowel movement and dressings on the first few postoperative days are painful and although this can be dealt with quite simply with analgesics, surgeons have developed other operations aimed at reducing this problem, such as the Parks' submucous haemorrhoidectomy[16] and Ferguson's closed haemorrhoidectomy.[6] Because they are more complicated, however, they have not been widely adopted in the UK but closed haemorrhoidectomy is now regarded to be the optimum form of excision for piles in the USA.

Apart from pain, other complications of haemorrhoidectomy include retention of urine, which may occur in 2% of patients, faecal impaction, secondary haemorrhage, occurring also in 2%, and impaired healing of the anal wounds which is often due to excessive granulation tissue that can be cauterized readily with silver nitrate. Once the anal canal has healed, most patients are delighted with the result.

CRITIQUE OF AVAILABLE THERAPY

Which of these various treatments are generally used? Injection sclerotherapy is still the most popular first treatment for internal haemorrhoids and elastic band ligation is becoming widely used for other patients, often avoiding the need for operation. The place of infrared coagulation, cryotherapy, maximal and dilation and internal sphincterotomy still requires evaluation. Although less radical methods of treatment for haemorrhoids should be tried first, haemorrhoidectomy has a definite place in the treatment of persistent or complicated piles, provided the patient requests it.

TREATMENT OF COMPLICATIONS

A fissure sometimes accompanies large prolapsing haemorrhoids. It is usual to treat these patients with a haemorrhoidectomy and a partial internal sphincterotomy.

Thrombosed external and thrombosed prolapsed haemorrhoids may be treated by bedrest, the application of an evaporating and therefore cooling lotion (lead and spirit lotion) or ice packs, and the administration of non-constipating analgesics and a lubricant laxative (liquid paraffin). It may take as long as 10 days for the acute symptoms to resolve. Definitive treatment for the haemorrhoids will subsequently be required in most patients. Some surgeons therefore advocate an emergency haemorrhoidectomy, when dealing with thrombosis which involves the whole circumference of the anal canal. Maximal dilatation of the anus or partial internal sphincterotomy may reduce the patient's pain, but the cosmetic results are bad and most patients require a haemorrhoidectomy later.

Clotted venous saccule may be treated in the first 24 hours by evacuation of the clot under local anaesthesia. Most cases are allowed to resolve spontaneously.

HAEMORRHOIDS IN PATIENTS WITH INFLAMMATORY BOWEL DISEASE

All patients with haemorrhoids should be assessed to determine whether or not there is evidence of underlying inflammatory bowel disease. Patients with Crohn's disease often have oedematous skin tags (*Figure 4.97*) which are not seen in any other condition and must be distinguished from ordinary skin tags or thrombosed external haemorrhoids. In fact haemorrhoids are relatively uncommon in Crohn's disease.

There is a low incidence of complications in patients with idiopathic proctocolitis (ulcerative colitis) who require outpatient or operative treatment of haemorrhoids.[9] This is not the case with Crohn's

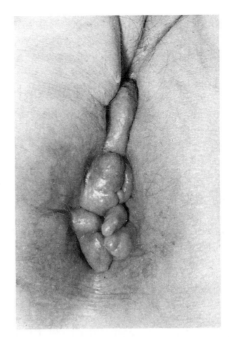

Figure 4.97 Crohn's disease. Oedematous skin tags should not be operated on.

disease where such treatments may lead to severe ulceration and sepsis. Local treatment of haemorrhoids is rarely necessary and is rarely advised in Crohn's disease.

REFERENCES

1. Allan, A. and Keighley, M.R.B. (1988) Treatment for pruritis ani. *Surgical Rounds*, **July**, 69–76.
2. Alexander-Williams, J. (1981) Haemorrhoids. In *Colorectal Disease* (Ed.) Thomson, J.P.S., Nicholls, R.J. and Williams, C.B. pp. 331–344. London: Heinemann.
3. Alexander-Williams, J. (1982) The management of piles. *British Medical Journal*, **285**, 1137–1139.
4. Ambrose, N.S., Hares, M.M., Alexander-Williams, J. and Keighley, M.R.B. (1983) Prospective randomised comparison of photocoagulation and rubber band ligation in treatment of haemorrhoids. *British Medical Journal*, **286**, 1389–1391.
5. Ambrose, N.S., Morris, D., Alexander-Williams, J. and Keighley, M.R.B. (1985) A randomised trial of photocoagulation or injection sclerotherapy for the treatment of first and second degree haemorrhoids. *Diseases of the Colon and Rectum*, **28**, 238–240.
6. Goldberg, S.M. (1983) Closed haemorrhoidectomy. In *Rob and Smith's Operative Surgery* (Ed.) Todd, I.P. and Fielding, L.P. 4th Edn. Alimentary Tract and Abdominal Wall. 3. Colon, Rectum and Anus pp. 489–494. London: Butterworth.
7. Goligher, J.C. (1980) *Surgery of the Anus, Rectum and Colon*. pp. 93–135. 4th Edn. London: Baillière Tindall.
8. Greca, F., Nevah, F., Hares, M. and Keighley, M.R.B. (1981) Value of an anal dilator after anal

stretch for haemorrhoids. *Journal of the Royal Society of Medicine*, **74**, 368–370.

9. Jeffrey, P.J., Ritchie, J.K. and Parks, A.G. (1977) Treatment of haemorrhoids in patients with inflammatory bowel disease. *Lancet*, **i**, 1084–1085.

10. Keighley, M.R.B., Alexander-Williams, J., Buchmann, P. *et al.* (1979) Prospective trials of minor surgical procedures and high fibre diet for haemorrhoids. *British Medical Journal*, **ii**, 967–969.

11. Leicester, R.J., Nicholls, R.J. and Mann, C.V. (1981) Infrared coagulation – a new treatment for haemorrhoids. *Diseases of the Colon and Rectum*, **23**, 602–605.

12. Lord, P.H. (1983) Maximal anal dilatation. In *Rob and Smith's Operative Surgery* (Ed.) Todd, I.P. and Fielding, L.P. 4th Edn. Alimentary Tract and Abdominal Wall. 3. Colon, Rectum and Anus. pp. 474–479. London: Butterworth.

13. Mann, C.V. (1983) Open haemorrhoidectomy (St. Mark's ligation/excision method). In *Rob and Smith's Operative Surgery* (Ed.) Todd, I.P. and Fielding, L.P. 4th Edn. Alimentary Tract and Abdominal Wall. 3. Colon, Rectum and Anus. pp. 495–502. London: Butterworth.

14. Murie, J.A., Sim, A.J.W. and Mackenzie, I. (1981) The importance of pain, pruritus and soiling as symptoms of haemorrhoids and their response to haemorrhoidectomy or rubber band ligation. *British Journal of Surgery*, **68**, 247–249.

15. Parks, A.G. (1956) De Haemorrhois – a study in surgical history. *Guy's Hospital Reports*, **104**, 135–156.

16. Parks, A.G. (1983) Haemorrhoidectomy. In *Rob and Smith's Operative Surgery* (Ed.) Todd, I.P. and Fielding, L.P. 4th Edn. Alimentary Tract and Abdominal Wall. 3. Colon, Rectum and Anus. pp. 480–488. London: Butterworth.

17. Saint-Pierre, A., Treffot, M.J. and Martin, P.M. (1982) Hormone receptors and haemorrhoidal disease. *Colonproctology*, **4**, 116–120.

18. Thomson, W.H.F. (1975) The nature of haemorrhoids. *British Journal of Surgery*, **62**, 542–552.

19. Thomson, W.H.F. (1982) The real nature of 'perianal haematoma'. *Lancet*, **ii**, 467–468.

20. Williams, K.L. (1983) Cryosurgery of haemorrhoids. In *Rob and Smith's Operative Surgery* (Ed.) Todd, I.P. and Fielding, L.P. 4th Edn. Alimentary Tract and Abdominal Wall. 3. Colon, Rectum and Anus. pp. 503–508. London: Butterworth.

ANAL FISSURE

J.P.S. Thomson and M.R.B. Keighley

An anal fissure (fissure-in-ano) is a disruption in the lining of the anal canal usually beginning at or distal to the pectinate line and extending to or beyond the anal verge.

CLASSIFICATION

Fissures may be classified as either acute or chronic and further subdivided as either primary or secondary.[8] A primary fissure is 'idiopathic' as there is no satisfactory explanation for its occurrence. A secondary fissure is either linked to a known disorder, such as Crohn's disease or leukaemia, or to a cause and effect relationship, such as following damage from a foreign body, childbirth or previous anal surgery.

An acute fissure is superficial and amounts to a crack in the anoderm without any surrounding fibrosis. The floor of the acute fissure is formed by the longitudinal fibres of the muscularis mucosa. It resolves spontaneously or after conservative treatment. On the other hand the chronic fissure rep-resents true ulceration of the anoderm with surrounding fibrosis, exposure of the underlying transverse fibres of the internal sphincter muscle and/or the triad of ulcer, hypertrophied papilla, and a sentinel pile. Chronic fissures do not usually heal with conservative treatment.

AETIOLOGY

Despite the common occurrence and 'apparent simplicity' of anal fissure, its aetiology remains an enigma. The concept that all fissures result from the passage of a constipated stool is an oversimplification. In one report only 20% of patients gave a history of constipation.[18] Other possible causes include cryptitis, venous stasis and diarrhoea.

PRIMARY FISSURE

There has been much discussion about spasm or hypertonicity of the internal sphincter and its relationship to anal fissures. Many studies show an

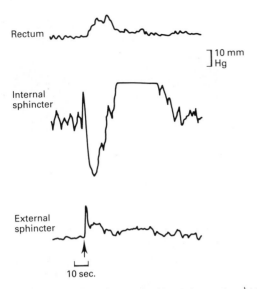

Figure 4.98 Contraction of internal sphincter in a patient with anal fissure. (From Nothmann and Schuster,[22] with permission.)

increase in the resting internal sphincter pressures in patients with anal fissure.[2,11]

Nothman and Schuster[22] have recognized 'overshoot' contraction occurring in the internal sphincter after receptive relaxation of the rectum in patients with anal fissure (*Figure 4.98*). This phenomenon is almost certainly related to spasm of the internal sphincter in patients with anal fissure. These changes disappear after successful treatment. It is impossible at present to know whether these findings represent cause or effect. The concept of internal sphincter spasm, however, provides a rationale for the present day medical and surgical treatments.

Eisenhammer[7] postulated a number of reasons for the common posterior occurrence of anal fissure. He put forward the idea that the posterior midline was the most unsupported point of the anal skin because of the V-shaped divergence of the subcutaneous external sphincter and undermining of the anoderm in the posterior quadrant by deep crypts. He felt, however, that the most important factor was the bilateral pull by the corrugator cutis ani in the posterior midline superimposed on a loss of elasticity and mobility of the anoderm by acute or chronic irritation. Oh[23] believes that acute primary fissures occur in the posterior or anterior midline because of greater expansibility in this direction and the elliptical shape of the anus.

SECONDARY FISSURE

Crohn's fissures are probably much more common than is generally recognized because they are often painless. Fielding reported a 51% incidence of fissures in Crohn's disease[5] and found them to be asymptomatic in over 90%. Other causes of secondary fissures include syphilis, tuberculosis, leukaemia, anorectal surgery, anal carcinoma, childbirth and prolonged diarrhoea secondary to laxative abuse.

CLINICAL FEATURES

Although the peak incidence is in the second and third decades, all age groups are affected. Both sexes are equally affected. Approximately 10% of fissures in females are anterior compared with only 1% in males.[10]

The principal symptom is painful defaecation. The pain is described as sharp or burning and may persist for hours after defaecation. Pain can lead to constipation and symptoms are aggravated by the eventual passage of a constipated stool thus creating a vicious circle.

Bleeding is also a common symptom. It is usually scanty and is always bright red in colour. Frequently bleeding is noticed only on the toilet paper. A chronic discharge may lead to soiling of the underclothes and pruritus ani. Urinary tract symptoms, such as frequency, dysuria and even urinary retention, may occur. Dyspareunia has also been reported.

Anal fissures can almost always be detected by inspection alone. A few words of reassurance followed by slow, gentle separation of the buttocks will usually reveal the fissure and the associated 'sentinel pile'. If an acute fissure is seen, no further examination is necessary, conservative treatment should be instituted if appropriate and the patient brought back a few weeks later for completion of the examination. Occasionally there is such severe spasm that the fissure cannot be visualized and in such cases intersphincteric abscess must be considered in the differential diagnosis. If in doubt, a gentle digital examination aided by a topical, local or even a general anaesthetic may be necessary.

For chronic fissures, a complete anorectal examination can usually be performed at the initial visit. Occasionally, a topical or local anaesthetic may be necessary. Any chronic fissure in which Crohn's disease or carcinoma is suspected should be biopsied. Beware of the laterally placed fissure as this usually is a secondary fissure. Broad-based or multiple fissures, regardless of location, should arouse suspicion. Tuberculosis fissures are rare and may be difficult to distinguish from Crohn's. Leukaemic fissures are usually a sign of advanced disease and can be extremely painful. No treatment is indicated except occasionally to drain an abscess.[9]

TREATMENT

Conservative therapy is the treatment of choice for acute primary fissure, whereas operative intervention is indicated for chronic primary fissure. The treatment of a secondary fissure is directed to the underlying problem.

ACUTE FISSURE

Conservative treatment consists of avoiding constipation by the use of bulk laxatives (psyllium seed or bran) and symptomatic measures such as a warm bath.[3] An additional advantage of increased dietary fibre is the resulting dilatation of the anal sphincter as a consequence of increased stool weight. Anaesthetic ointments, suppositories, anal dilators and injection of long-acting local anaesthetics are of unproven effectiveness but nevertheless play a role in conservative therapy.

CHRONIC FISSURE

Although there are no satisfactory explanations for why some acute fissures become chronic, once chronicity occurs, further conservative treatment is usually unsuccessful. The basis for present-day surgical treatment of chronic anal fissure is 'pectenotomy'.[19] Eisenhammer[6] later recognized that 'pectenotomy' is actually an internal sphincterotomy.

Excision of anal fissure was popularized by Gabriel.[10] He excised a triangle of skin with the ulcer, removed a small triangle of internal sphincter muscle and stretched the anal sphincter. However, a 'keyhole' deformity sometimes develops, resulting in soiling, and the popularity of the procedure has waned.

In many centres, sphincterotomy gave way to anal stretching.[17] Following reports of high failure rates and occasional incontinence, however, the value of sphincter stretching was questioned. As is so often the case, it is not so much the form of treatment which is questioned but its method. Hence gentle dilatation is often effective and uncomplicated, whereas forceful dilatation may cause incontinence in postpartum patients.

Lateral internal sphincterotomy subsequently became the most popular form of therapy. This sphincterotomy ignored the fissure site and thus the 'keyhole' deformity was avoided. Variations in the basic technique have been described by Parks (*Figure 4.99*)[24] and Notaras (*Figure 4.100*).[21] These techniques avoid an anal incision, thus theoretically reducing postoperative discomfort. Many reports have shown that lateral internal sphincterotomy

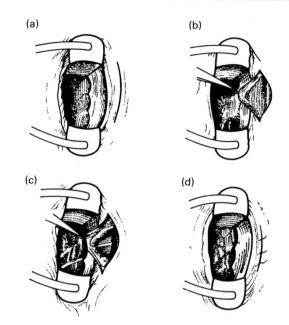

Figure 4.99 Lateral internal sphincterotomy, perianal incision (after Parks[24]): (a) lateral skin incision; (b) division of the lower border of the internal sphincter; (c) division of the internal sphincter to dentate line; (d) closure of wound.

achieves the best results with the least morbidity (*Table 4.23*).[1,4,10,12] A major advantage is that it can be performed under local anaesthesia. Minor degrees of incontinence, such as mucous drainage and staining of the underclothes, appear to be rare and recurrence rates are low (see *Table 4.23*).

Theuerkauf[26] introduced bilateral superficial distal internal sphincterotomy. In this procedure, the internal sphincter muscle is superficially incised in two quadrants through half of its thickness rather than a full thickness one-quadrant division as in the conventional lateral internal sphincterotomy. Results in his first 100 patients have been excellent with a recurrence rate of 1% and a 1% incidence of incontinence.

At the present time, the authors favour one-quadrant lateral internal sphincterotomy. Keighley, Greca and Nevah[15] achieved better results when lateral internal sphincterotomy was performed under general anaesthesia compared with local anaesthesia. We believe, however, that with proper patient selection the use of local anaesthesia is satisfactory. The technique described by Nivatvongs[20] allows the local anaesthesia to be performed with minimal or no discomfort (*Figure 4.101*).

ANAL FISSURE IN CHILDREN

Anal fissure is the most common cause of rectal bleeding in infants[13] but the bleeding is rarely profuse. Anal fissure is extremely rare in breast fed

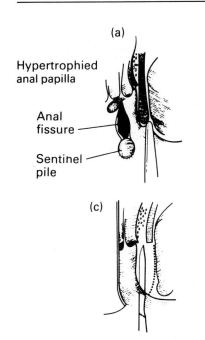

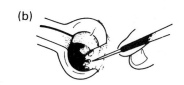

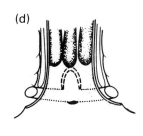

Hypertrophied
anal papilla

Anal
fissure

Sentinel
pile

(a)

(b)

(c)

(d)

Figure 4.100 Lateral internal sphincterotomy, stab wound technique (after Notaras[21]): (a) anal fissure; (b,c) insertion of blade between the epithelium of the anal canal and the internal sphincter as far as the dentate line; (d) after the subcutaneous sphincterotomy, the divided sphincter separates under a bridge of skin.

infants.[25] The fissures in children are almost always acute and therefore superficial. Unlike adults, acute primary fissures in children are often multiple and commonly located laterally.[16] In older children, the presence of a fissure-in-ano should signal the possibility of leukaemia.[25]

As a rule, the diagnosis can easily be confirmed by inspection. Sometimes the fissure will have healed by the time the parents seek medical attention for the child. The characteristic history and lack of symptoms at the time of examination usually make the diagnosis obvious.

Medical therapy consists mainly of bulk laxatives, stool softeners, mineral oil, or simple dietary regulation. Only approximately 1% of acute fissures in children become chronic.[25] These are treated quite

Table 4.23 Comparisons of procedures for anal fissure

	No. of patients	Impaired control for:		Faecal soiling (%)	Unhealed or recurrence (%)
		Flatus (%)	Faeces (%)		
Lateral internal sphincterotomy					
Hoffman and Goligher[14]	99	6	1	7	3
Hawley[12]	24	?	0	0	0
Abcarian[1]	150	30[a] 0[b]	0	0	1.3
Collopy and Ryan[4]	86	17	12	19	15
Sphincter stretch					
Watts, Bennett and Goligher[27]	95	12	2	20	16
Hawley[12]	18	?	0	0	28
Abcarian[1]	ND	ND	ND	ND	ND
Collopy and Ryan[4]	74	30	16	34	30
Posterior internal sphincterotomy					
Bennett and Goligher[8]	127	24	11	28	7
Hawley[12]	32	?	0	8	8
Abcarian[1]	150	40[a] 5[b]	5	5	1.3
Collopy and Ryan[4]	ND	ND	ND	ND	ND

[a]Temporary; [b]permanent.
ND = no data.

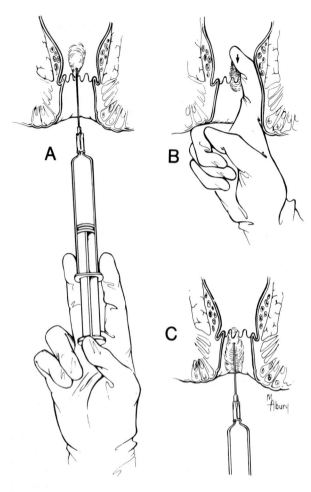

Figure 4.101 Technique of local anaesthesia. A: injection of the anaesthetic solution 2 mm proximal to the pectinate line. B: the anaesthetic solution is squeezed into the anoderm. C: injection of the anaesthetic solution 2 mm distal to the pectinate line. (From Nivatvongs,[20] with permission.)

successfully under general anaesthesia by dilatation of the anus with excision of any chronic scar tissue or papilla if necessary.[16,25] Dilatation alone is usually the only form of treatment required in children who develop a chronic fissure.

REFERENCES

1. Abcarian, H. (1980) Surgical correction of chronic anal fissure: results of lateral internal sphincterotomy vs. fissurectomy-midline sphincterotomy. *Diseases of Colon and Rectum*, **23**, 31–36.
2. Arabi, Y., Alexander-Williams, J. and Keighley, M.R.B. (1977) Anal pressures in hemorrhoids and anal fissure. *American Journal of Surgery*, **134**, 608–610.
3. Bennett, R.C. and Goligher, J.C. (1962) Results of internal sphincterotomy for anal fissure. *British Medical Journal*, **2**, 1500–1503.
4. Collopy, B. and Ryan, P. (1979) Comparison of lateral subcutaneous sphincterotomy with anal dilatation in the treatment of fissure-in-ano. *Medical Journal of Australia*, **2**, 461–462 and 495.
5. Crapp, A.R. and Alexander-Williams, J. (1975) Fissure-in-ano and anal stenosis. Part I: Conservative management. *Clinics in Gastroenterology*, **4**, 619–628.
6. Eisenhammer, S. (1953) The internal anal sphincter: its surgical importance. *South African Medical Journal*, **27**, 266–270.
7. Eisenhammer, S. (1959) The evaluation of the internal anal sphincterotomy operation with special reference to anal fissure. *Surgery, Gynecology and Obstetrics*, **109**, 583–590.
8. Eisenhammer, S. (1974) Internal anal sphincterotomy plus free dilatation versus anal stretch with special criticism of the anal stretch procedure for hemorrhoids: the recommended modern approach to hemorrhoid treatment. *Diseases of the Colon and Rectum*, **17**, 493–522.
9. Goldberg, S.M., Gordon, P.H. and Nivatvongs, S. (1980) Fissure-in-ano. In *Essentials of Anorectal Surgery*. 1st edn, pp. 86–99. Philadelphia: J.B. Lippincott.
10. Goligher, J.C. (1980) Anal fissure. In *Surgery of the Anus, Rectum and Colon*, 4th edn, pp. 136–153. London: Baillière Tindall.
11. Hancock, B.D. (1977) The internal sphincter and anal fissure. *British Journal of Surgery*, **64**, 92–95.
12. Hawley, P.R. (1969) The treatment of chronic fissure-in-ano: a trial of methods. *British Journal of Surgery*, **56**, 915–918.
13. Holder, T.M. and Ashcraft, K.W. (1980) Acquired anorectal lesions-fissure-in-ano. In *Pediatric Surgery*. 1st edn, p. 429. Philadelphia: W.B. Saunders.
14. Hoffman, D.C. and Goligher, J.C. (1970) Lateral subcutaneous internal sphincterotomy in treatment of anal fissure. *British Medical Journal*, **3**, 673–675.
15. Keighley, M.R.B., Greca, F., Nevah, E. *et al.* (1981) Treatment of anal fissure by lateral subcutaneous sphincterotomy should be under general anaesthesia. *British Journal of Surgery*, **68**, 400–401.
16. Kleinhaus, S. (1979) Miscellaneous anal disorders. In *Pediatric Surgery* (Ed.) Ravitch, M.M. 3rd edn, p. 1078. Chicago: Year Book Medical Publishers.
17. Lord, P.H. (1969) A day-case procedure for the cure of third-degree haemorrhoids. *British Journal of Surgery*, **56**, 747–749.
18. Mazier, W.P., De Moraes, R.T. and Dignan, R.D. (1978) Anal fissure and anal ulcers. *Surgical Clinics of North America*, **58**, 479–485.
19. Miles, E.W. (1939) Anal fissure. In *Rectal Surgery: A Practical Guide to the Modern Surgical Treatment of Rectal Diseases*. 1st edn, pp. 147–157. London: Cassell.
20. Nivatvongs, S. (1982) An improved technique of local anesthesia for anorectal surgery. *Diseases of the Colon and Rectum*, **25**, 259–260.
21. Notaras, M.J. (1971) The treatment of anal fissure

by lateral subcutaneous internal sphincterotomy – a technique and results. *British Journal of Surgery*, **58**, 96–100.

22. Nothmann, B.J. and Schuster, M.M. (1974) Internal anal sphincter derangement with anal fissures. *Gastroenterology*, **67**, 216–220.

23. Oh, C. (1975) Lateral subcutaneous internal sphincterotomy for anal fissure. *Mount Sinai Journal of Medicine*, **42**, 596–601.

24. Parks, A.G. (1967) The management of fissure-in-ano. *Hospital Medicine*, **1**, 737.

25. Raffensperger, J.G. (1980) Gastrointestinal hemorrhage. In *Swenson's Pediatric Surgery*. 4th edn, pp. 425–458. New York: Appleton-Century-Crofts.

26. Theuerkauf, F.J. (1981) Bilateral superficial distal internal sphincterotomy. *Presentation at American Society of Colon and Rectal Surgeons Meeting*, Colorado Springs, Colorado, 1981.

27. Watts, J.M., Bennett, R.C. and Goligher, J.C. (1964) Stretching of anal sphincters in treatment of fissure-in-ano. *British Medical Journal*, **2**, 342–343.

ANORECTAL SEPSIS

J.P.S. Thomson and M.R.B. Keighley

Anorectal sepsis is a common surgical emergency. The latest available figures show that 6970 patients were admitted to hospital in 1978 in England and Wales with anorectal sepsis.[12] There is also a population which is treated outside hospital practice and which is not referred until the patient presents with a fistula or further episodes of sepsis. Sepsis is commoner in men than women and, although occurring in the young and the old, it is commonest in the third and fourth decades.[12] Two to three per cent of all admissions with anorectal sepsis are associated with underlying inflammatory bowel disease: the primary diagnosis is more likely to be Crohn's disease than ulcerative colitis. Perianal abscess is about three times more common than ischiorectal abscess. Supralevator abscess is rare despite Prasad's claim that supralevator sepsis accounted for 9.1% of their series.[19]

Anorectal sepsis usually begins with an infection of the anal glands to form an intermuscular abscess,[4,5,6,18] this abscess then tracks through or around the sphincter to present at one of the standard sites. (*Figure 4.102*). Although there is strong evidence for this aetiology, Goligher[9] was able to identify only eight intermuscular abscesses in 28 patients carefully explored. In addition, recent microbiological studies have suggested that an intermuscular abscess or fistula is only likely to be present when culture of the pus has demonstrated a bowel-derived organism.[11] Staphylococcal abscesses originate from skin and not from anal glands. It is not known why these abscesses should be commoner in men than in women and why the anal glands should be more susceptible to sepsis in the third and fourth decades.

Although this is a common problem, management may be poor and the recurrence rate is high. Correct management depends upon:

1. An understanding of the anatomy of the anal canal with particular reference to the anatomy of abscesses and fistulas.
2. The correct diagnosis.
3. Microbiology.
4. An understanding of the objectives of surgical management.

PATHOLOGY

ABSCESS

An understanding of the anatomy of the anal canal is essential when considering the management of all abscesses, but especially those which originate in the

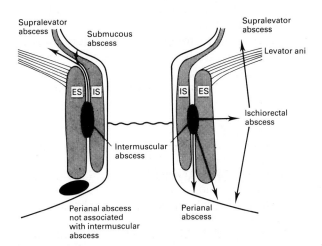

Figure 4.102 Anatomy of anorectal abscess. IS = internal sphincter; ES = external sphincter.

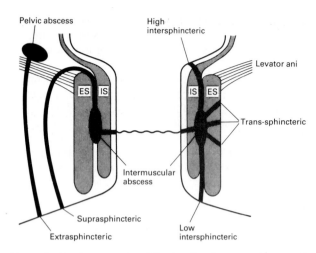

Figure 4.103   Anatomy of anal fistulas. IS = internal sphincter; ES = external sphincter.

intermuscular plane. The potential space between the internal and external sphincters contains the anal glands whose ducts open into the anal canal at the dentate line. The type of abscess depends upon the direction that the pus takes from the intermuscular space. The pus may track along three planes (*Figure 4.103*):

1. Between the internal and external components of the sphincter, or sometimes through the lowermost fibres of the external sphincter, to present as a perianal abscess.
2. Laterally through the external sphincter to present as an ischiorectal abscess. Occasionally an ischiorectal abscess may also track through the levator ani to present with a supralevator component.
3. Proximally between the sphincters to present as a submucous abscess or very rarely in the supralevator space as a supralevator abscess.

Any abscess which does not originate in the intermuscular space will lie subcutaneously and will be perianal rather than ischiorectal.

CLINICAL FEATURES

ABSCESS

The diagnosis of sepsis is usually easy with the patient complaining of a painful lump in the region of the anal canal. On examination there is erythema overlying an obviously tender swelling. A large area of erythema, however, does not necessarily mean that the abscess is ischiorectal; those abscesses which are close to the anal canal are likely to be

perianal. Occasionally a patient may complain of acute anal pain but, despite tenderness, there is nothing abnormal to see. An examination under anaesthetic is required to make the diagnosis, and usually pus may be identified either under the submucosa of the anal canal or in the intermuscular plane, which is more difficult to detect. An intersphincteric abscess may defy diagnosis and must always be considered in a patient with anal pain and no evidence of an anal fissure.

MICROBIOLOGY

Until recently very little interest has been taken in the microbiology of anorectal sepsis. Coliforms have been the most commonly isolated organism but recent surgical interest in the obligate anaerobes has demonstrated *Bacteroides fragilis* in a high proportion of anorectal abscess. The incidence of isolating *B. fragilis* varies, Abcarian[1] found occasional colonies, but Meislin[16] suggested that the incidence was as high as 47%; however, his study was small with only 21 patients. Whitehead[22] reported that 32/74 patients had 'gut-specific' *Bacteroides*. Other authors have emphasized the frequency with which skin organisms such as *Staphylococcus aureus* are identified; they are responsible for 15–25% of the organisms cultured.[2,8,17,23] A recent study confirmed this incidence and then suggested that associated fistulas are only found when a bowel-derived organism is grown in culture.[11] This view was supported by Wilson[23] who related recurrent sepsis to the original organism cultured; there were seven recurrent fistulas and, in each case, the original was bowel-derived. In contrast, however, Whitehead[22] claimed that fistulas were found when skin organisms were cultured but his study does not say whether or not the *Staphylococci* were found in pure culture and the operations in his study were performed by surgeons of varying experience.

TREATMENT

PRINCIPLES OF MANAGEMENT

The aims of surgical management are threefold:

To relieve symptoms;
To achieve rapid healing, thereby ensuring early return of the patient to work;
To avoid recurrent sepsis.

There are two distinct schools of thought concerning immediate surgical management. One argues that the relief of symptoms with an early return to work is of prime importance, while suggesting that even if the recurrence rate is high, the remaining patients have no further trouble. It is further claimed that definitive surgery in the acute phase to an associated fistula may cause damage to the sphincter and thereby incontinence. It is suggested that this approach is associated with an unacceptable risk of incontinence particularly as the surgery for ano-rectal sepsis is often performed by surgeons in training. This concept of management prevails in the USA and may reflect the very large number of surgeons operating on small numbers of patients. This view, however, also has support in the UK.

The second and more positive school argues that, whatever the surgical diagnosis, a high recurrence rate is unacceptable as a principle of correct surgical management. Surgery should therefore aim to prevent recurrence as well as alleviate symptoms and ensure an early return to work.

The relief of symptoms

The pain of anorectal sepsis is caused by the pressure of pus within the abscess cavity; any surgical manoeuvre that removes the pus will relieve the symptoms.

Rapid healing

The smaller the wound, the more rapid will be the healing providing that the pus does not re-collect; healing may be aided by antibiotics.

The prevention of recurrent sepsis

An anorectal abscess will recur or the patient will be left with an anal fistula if the presenting abscess is secondary to an intermuscular abscess and if a fistula is not laid open during the acute episode. Most of these recurrences will present within two years but the time interval may be much longer.

There are few good studies of recurrence since the length of follow-up is either inadequate or the number of patients successfully followed is too small.[7,14,15] The incidence of recurrent sepsis reported in Cardiff was 25%[2] which was comparable to that of Wilson.[23] In 1982 the authors showed that 68/165 (41.2%) of the patients presenting with ano-rectal sepsis had had a previous abscess;[11] 30 of these patients had a fistula demonstrated at operation. Chrabot, Prasad and Abcarian[3] demonstrated fistulas in 53 out of 68 patients presenting with recurrent anorectal sepsis.

SURGICAL TECHNIQUES

Aspiration of the pus

This will relieve the acute symptoms but the pus will almost certainly recollect unless aspiration is followed by a more definitive surgical procedure. Successful aspiration may be associated with an immediate return to work but does nothing to prevent recurrent sepsis.

Drainage of the abscess

Simple drainage will relieve the acute symptoms, and is associated with rapid healing and an early return to work, but does not prevent recurrence.

Incision and primary suture (under antibiotic cover)

This will relieve the symptoms and is associated with rapid healing and an early return to work but it does nothing to prevent recurrence. Originally described by Ellis,[8] Wilson[23] demonstrated a recurrence rate of 22% within the relatively short mean follow-up period of just over 2 years while a later study from the same unit[14] showed a recurrence rate of 8/66 patients successfully followed over one year; 44 patients, however, were lost to follow-up. These studies emphasize the problems associated with inadequate follow-up. It has been suggested that suture of the wound after drainage of soft tissue abscesses holds no advantage over simple drainage provided that each procedure is covered by systemic antibiotic therapy.[20] This study and that of Leaper[14] used clindamycin as the antibiotic of choice.

Saucerization

This previously popular management was based on the misconception that the large wound would 'heal from the bottom' and would be associated with a low incidence of recurrence. This concept, however, ignored the presence of the intermuscular cavity and the internal opening. The technique is associated with a large wound, slow healing and a long period of time off work. That it does nothing to prevent recurrence was demonstrated by Leaper[14] with 23 (21.1%) recurrences in 109 patients within one year.

Incision and drainage/laying open the fistula

Drainage relieves the symptoms; laying open of the fistula prevents recurrent sepsis, but the patient has to accept slower healing of the wound and a longer period lost from work.

It is suggested that the correct management of anorectal abscess is as follows:

1. Examination under anaesthesia, drainage of abscess (laying open of fistula). The patient is examined under anaesthetic and the abscess is drained. A search is made for a fistula remembering that this should be done with great care as the tissues are friable and false tracks can easily be produced. Pressure on the abscess from outside before drainage may define the internal opening by demonstrating pus at the dentate line.
2. Microbiology of the pus. The pus should be sent for both aerobic and anaerobic culture. No further surgical procedure will be required if culture grows a skin-derived organism.[11]
3. Second examination under anaesthesia (laying open of fistula). A second procedure is performed particularly if any organisms are isolated after 7–10 days and any fistula track demonstrated is laid open.

These techniques have been described in *Rob and Smith's Operative Surgery*.[10]

It is emphasized that the laying open of any fistula in a patient with acute anorectal sepsis should be approached with caution and is the province of experienced surgeons rather than surgeons in training.

INFLAMMATORY BOWEL DISEASE

Anorectal sepsis is commoner in Crohn's disease than ulcerative colitis and commoner in Crohn's colitis than small bowel disease.

CROHN'S DISEASE

Management of anorectal sepsis in Crohn's disease is never easy. The basic principle is that surgical intervention should be the minimal required to relieve symptoms while remembering that anal Crohn's disease is merely a manifestation of total gut disease which may require systemic therapy as well as local treatment. Abscesses should be drained and very low fistulas may be laid open; however, the wounds do not heal well and laying open of high fistulas should be avoided if possible. Partial internal anal fistulotomy with curettage of the track has recently been advocated with some success.[21] The presence of multiple fistulas and recurrent sepsis may be an indication for excision of the rectum. There may be a place for azathioprine and it has been suggested that a combination of metronidazole and trimethoprim/sulphamethoxazole (Septrin) will

help to control the problem but no data are yet available.

ULCERATIVE COLITIS

Abscesses should be drained and low fistulas may be laid open with reasonable confidence that the wound will heal. High fistulas are uncommon in ulcerative colitis and should be approached with caution.

TUBERCULOSIS

Tuberculosis perianal disease is usually associated with systemic disease and in the UK this is usually only seen in the immigrant population. Surgical drainage, combined with antituberculosis therapy, will control the problem.

HIDRADENITIS SUPPURATIVA

Hidradenitis is a curious problem which may cause debilitating disease; the pus can be very offensive. Sepsis arises in abnormal apocrine sweat glands and anal manifestations are often associated with axillary, cervical, groin and scrotal disease. The infecting organism is usually *Staphylococcus aureus* but *Bacteroides* has recently been implicated.[13] Surgical management varies from wide excision of the affected areas to simple laying open of the tracks with careful postoperative nursing care.

FULMINATING GANGRENE

This is not a common condition but the extent of the sepsis is generally so severe that diagnosis is easy; management, however, is more difficult. There is a high incidence of associated disease, particularly diabetes mellitus. This problem is variously described as acute dermal gangrene, invasive necrotizing infection, or loosely associated with scrotal gangrene (Fournier's disease). Surgical excision should be vigorous, with excision of the involved tissue leaving healthy, bleeding wound edges. The infecting organism is not necessarily clostridial but there may be a place for hyperbaric oxygen.

REFERENCES

1. Abcarian, H. (1976) Acute suppurations of the anorectum. *Surgery Annual*, **8**, 305–333.
2. Buchan, R. and Grace, R.H. (1973) Anorectal suppuration: the results of treatment and the factors influencing the recurrence rate. *British Journal of Surgery*, **60**, 537–540.
3. Chrabot, C.M., Prasad, M.L. and Abcarian, H.

(1983) Recurrent anorectal abscesses. *Diseases of the Colon and Rectum*, **26**, 105–108.

4. Eisenhammer, S. (1956) The internal anal sphincter and the anorectal abscess. *Surgery, Gynecology and Obstetrics*, **103**, 501–506.
5. Eisenhammer, S. (1958) A new approach to the anorectal fistulous abscess based on the high inter-muscular lesion. *Surgery, Gynecology and Obstetrics*, **106**, 595–599.
6. Eisenhammer, S. (1961) The anorectal and anovulval fistulous abscess. *Surgery, Gynecology and Obstetrics*, **113**, 519–520.
7. Eisenhammer, S. (1978) The final evaluation and classification of the surgical treatment of the primary anorectal cryptoglandular intermuscular (intersphincteric) fistulous abscess and fistula. *Diseases of the Colon and Rectum*, **21**(3), 237–254.
8. Ellis, M. (1960) Incision and primary suture of abscesses of the anal region. *Proceedings of the Royal Society of Medicine*, **53**, 652–653.
9. Goligher, J.C., Ellis, M. and Pissidis, A.G. (1967) A critique of anal glandular infection in the aetiology and treatment of idiopathic anorectal abscesses and fistulas. *Diseases of the Colon and Rectum*, **17**, 357–359.
10. Grace, R.H. (1983) Ano-rectal sepsis. In *Rob and Smith's Operative Surgery* (Ed.) Todd, I.P. and Fielding, L.P. 4th Edn, Section 3 – Colon, Rectum and Anus. pp. 516–523. London: Butterworth.
11. Grace, R.H., Harper, I.A. and Thompson, R.G. (1982) Ano-rectal sepsis: microbiology in relation to fistula-in-ano. *British Journal of Surgery*, **69**, 401–403.
12. HIPE (1978) Hospital in-patient enquiry.
13. Leach, R.D., Eykyn, S.J., Phillips, A. *et al.* (1979) Anaerobic axillary abscess. *British Medical Journal*, **ii**, 5–7.

14. Leaper, D.J., Page, R.E., Rosenberg, I.L. *et al.* (1976) A controlled study comparing the conventional treatment of idiopathic anorectal abscess with that of incision, curettage and primary suture under antibiotic cover. *Diseases of the Colon and Rectum*, **19**, 46–50.
15. McElwain, J.W., Alexander, R.M. and MacLean, M.D. (1966) Primary fistulectomy for anorectal abscess: a clinical study of 500 cases. *Diseases of the Colon and Rectum*, **9**, 181–185.
16. Meislin, H.W., Lerner, S.A., Graves, M.H. *et al.* (1977) Anaerobic and aerobic bacteriology and outpatient management. *Annals of Internal Medicine*, **87**, 145–149.
17. Page, R.E. and Freeman, R. (1977) Superficial sepsis: the antibiotic of choice for blind treatment. *British Journal of Surgery*, **64**, 281–284.
18. Parks, A.G. (1961) Pathogenesis and treatment of fistula-in-ano. *British Medical Journal*, **i**, 463–469.
19. Prasad, A.L., Read, D.R. and Abcarian, H. (1981) Supralevator abscesses: diagnosis and treatment. *Diseases of the Colon and Rectum*, **24**, 456–461.
20. Simms, M.H., Curran, F., Johnson, R.A. *et al.* (1982) Treatment of acute abscesses in the casualty department. *British Medical Journal*, **284**, 1827–1829.
21. Sohn, N., Korelitz, B.I. and Weinstein, M.A. (1980) Anorectal Crohn's disease: definitive surgery for fistulas and recurrent abscesses. *American Journal of Surgery*, **139**, 394–397.
22. Whitehead, S.M., Leach, R.D., Eykyn, S.J. and Phillips, I. (1982) The aetiology of perirectal sepsis. *British Journal of Surgery*, **69**, 166–168.
23. Wilson, D.H. (1964) The late results of anorectal abscess treated by incision, curettage, and primary suture under antibiotic cover. *British Journal of Surgery*, **51**, 828–831.

FISTULA-IN-ANO

P.J. Lunniss and J.P.S. Thomson

EPIDEMIOLOGY

Fistula-in-ano may be found in association with a variety of specific conditions, but most are non-specific, and are thought to be due to infection in one of the anal glands in the intersphincteric space (the cryptoglandular hypothesis).[13] Fistulas, however, complicate Crohn's disease, tuberculosis, carcinoma, actinomycosis, lymphogranuloma venereum, presacral dermoids, rectal duplication, trauma and foreign bodies. The incidence of tuberculous fistulas has fallen during the 20th century, Lockhart-Mummery[40] in 1929 suggesting that up to 20% of fistulas seen at St Mark's Hospital, London, at that time were tuberculous in nature; now the incidence is less than 2%. By contrast, particularly with an increasing awareness of the disease, fistulas complicating Crohn's disease have increased in frequency.

Epidemiological studies in Scandinavia have shown that the incidence of non-specific fistulas is about 10:000 000, with a significant male preponderance.[17,62] The reported male to female ratio varies from 1.8:1[62] to 8:1.[15] This difference is even more striking in the neonatal period, where there is an overwhelming (over 90%) male preponderance, raising the possibility of a different aetiology from that seen in adults.[2,12,19,70]

The condition most commonly affects patients in the third, fourth and fifth decades of life. There is no particular occupational predisposition. No relation between complexity of the fistula and racial origin has been found.[42]

It is evident that a variable proportion of fistulas are preceded, in some instances, many years earlier, by a history of acute perineal suppuration.[7] Marks and Ritchie[42] in their review of 793 patients with fistulas treated at St Mark's, found that 27% had had an abscess drained surgically on at least one occasion, and 12% gave a history of a discharging abscess. In the study by Shouler et al.,[72] 69% of patients with a fistula gave a history of a previous anorectal abscess, while Misra and Kapur[46] reported that all their patients with fistulas had a history of a previous perianal abscess needing drainage.

The incidence of the different types of fistula-in-ano depends on the classification used. The most widely adopted classification is one in which the course of the primary track and any secondary extensions are classified according to their position relative to the anorectal sphincter complex. Most fistulas are simple and, as such, are relatively easy to treat with little or no functional disturbance incurred. The high proportion of more complex fistulas seen at St Mark's, as shown by Parks, Gordon and Hardcastle[54] and Marks and Ritchie[42] indicates that the more simple types are managed locally whereas complex fistulas are referred to the specialist centres.

AETIOLOGY AND PATHOGENESIS

CHILDHOOD FISTULAS

Childhood fistula-in-ano is usually simple, with a single track running directly between an anal crypt and the external opening. These are generally superficial and practically always intersphincteric.[12] The onset in the first months of life, the almost exclusive male preponderance, and the simple nature of the tracks appear to indicate a developmental abnormality of the anal crypts and ducts.

Shafer et al.[70] considered the developmental abnormality to consist of an irregular and thickened dentate line which contained abnormally deep crypts. The work of van de Putte[78] suggests that these abnormal crypts may result from some defect in the dorsal portion of the cloaca membrane. Parks[53] demonstrated cystic dilatation of ducts which he thought could either be acquired duct obstruction or a congenital abnormality.

Pople and Ralphs,[59] surprised by the finding of transitional and columnar epithelium within infant fistulas, suggested that they might form from the urogenital sinus which had become misplaced during development of the perineum. The fact that childhood fistulas occur almost universally in boys may be explained by the much more extensive fusion of the genital folds in boys compared with girls.

Takatsuki[75] believed the primary cause of childhood fistulas to be abnormal hyperfunction of perianal sebaceous glands stimulated by neonatal and maternal androgenic hormones.

ADULT FISTULAS

The aetiology of adult fistula-in-ano has been the subject of debate for over a hundred years. It was widely held that fistulas were caused by infection penetrating the wall of the anal canal through a fissure or other wound and that the track, once established, is maintained by faecal contents entering the internal opening. This may be disputed on the grounds that internal openings are sometimes not clinically detectable (13% in the study by Choen et al.),[8] and any break in the mucosa which cannot be palpated, seen, or probed is unlikely to allow sufficient contamination to perpetuate infection.

Most authors subscribe to the view that fistula-in-ano are caused by an infection in the anal glands.[53] Anal glands may be found in the submucous and intermuscular space. Shropshear[73] considered that only those anal glands located in the submucosa participated in the transmission of infection. Thus sepsis spread across into the internal sphincter, into the intermuscular space along the medial extensions of the conjoined longitudinal muscle. Approximately 50% of anal sinuses do not have glands discharging into them, although occasionally more than one gland may discharge into the same sinus.[35,53] Rarely glands may communicate with the anal lumen above the level of the anal sinuses.[80] There are rarely more than 10 anal glands in an individual anal canal,[29] of which between one to two thirds are found to penetrate the internal sphincter to lie in the intersphincteric space.[32,43] The anal ducts are 30–40 μm in diameter, and 2–8 mm in length;[55] the larger ducts are lined by stratified columnar epithelium,[29,53,77] and the terminal branches by one or two layered cuboidal epithelium.[39,43] Mucin secretion has been demonstrated in a variable proportion of the glands,[39,53] although their actual function is disputed.

How then, may these intermuscular anal glands be involved in the pathogenesis of fistula-in-ano? Nesselrod[49] advanced a theory that infection which had penetrated the anal sinus, duct and gland led to oedema and obstruction of the duct, resulting in an infected retention cavity: rupture of this cavity caused spread of infection into the surrounding tissue and thence into the perianal or perirectal spaces. It is mainly to Eisenhammer[13] and Parks[53] that the cryptoglandular hypothesis has been attributed. Eisenhammer[14] considers all non-specific fistulas to be the result of an abscess originating in a deep anal or intramuscular gland. Parks proposed that once an acute abscess involving the anal gland had developed, the diseased gland became the seat of chronic infection with subsequent fistula formation. The fistula is thus a track of granulation tissue which is perpetuated by a chronic infective source.

Parks[53] thought that it was unlikely that a normal anal gland became infected; noting cystic dilatation in 8 out of 30 specimens, he attributed this change to either acquired duct obstruction or a congenital abnormality.

Histological evidence that the anal gland was implicated in fistula pathology was provided by Gordon-Watson and Dodd.[24] Later Parks[53] demonstrated anal gland epithelium in 23 or 30 fistulas. By contrast, Goligher et al.[23] found evidence of an intersphincteric abscess in only 8 of 28 patients with anorectal sepsis, and an intersphincteric abscess in only 14 of the 28 fistula cases examined. Though Goligher did not reject the possibility of anal gland involvement in the causation of some fistulas, he suggested that this did not apply in all cases.

The internal opening of fistulous abscesses is most commonly at the posterior and anterior commissures; Eisenhammer[13] thought that infective diarrhoea and heavy purgation might be causative factors in intermuscular gland infection. Parks[53] considered that anal fissures were sometimes a cause of intersphincteric abscess; also that the inflammation and fibrosis resulting from this condition may lead to stenosis of the anal duct, causing stasis and infection in the posterior gland.[26] Specific centres of anal gland infection are occasionally identified, such as Enterobius vermicularis.[48]

In the series reported by Henrichsen and Christiansen,[28] 50% of fistulas investigated microbiologically were sterile; this was attributed to previous antibiotic therapy. Seow-Choen et al.[69] however, in a study of the bacteriology of chronic anal fistulae, found a relative paucity of organisms, most of which were cultured only on incubation in enriched media. This is rather surprising, and casts doubt on our assumptions about how or why a fistula track is maintained.

CLASSIFICATION OF FISTULA-IN-ANO

The surgical management of fistula-in-ano is dependent upon an accurate knowledge both of the anatomy of the anorectal sphincter complex and the course of the fistula through the sphincter. Failure to accurately identify the course of the fistula leads to either fistula recurrence or disturbances to anorectal function if the track is laid open with devastating consequences. At the beginning of this century, fistulas were divided into two main groups, those in which the track did not pass through the external sphincter, and those in which the sphincter was penetrated by the track. Milligan and Morgan[45] having emphasized the importance of the anorectal ring in the maintenance of continence, classified fistulas according to their relation with the anorectal ring.

The classification in widespread use at present in this country is that devised at St Mark's, based on a study of 400 fistulas treated at that hospital,[54] and on the premise that the primary site of infection is in the intersphincteric space (Table 4.24). Thus a fistula is classified by its course in both the vertical and horizontal planes, with circumferential spread in any of the three spaces also being acknowledged (Figure 4.104). It is evident that sepsis above the levator muscles can arise from three sources:

1. Pelvic disease
2. Cephalad extension of an intersphincteric fistula
3. Cephalad extension of a trans-sphincteric fistula.

Parks et al.[54] stressed the importance of accurately determining the origin of supralevator sepsis because:

1. Drainage of a pelvic abscess through the ischiorectal fossa results in an extrasphincteric fistula which, if laid open, would lead to total incontinence.
2. Drainage of a supralevator extension of an intersphincteric abscess into the rectum is safe and appropriate, whereas drainage through the ischiorectal fossa would create a suprasphincteric fistula.
3. Drainage of a supralevator extension of a transsphincteric fistula must be through the perineum, as drainage into the rectum would result in an extrasphincteric fistula.

Eisenhammer,[13] as long ago as 1956, introduced the term cryptoglandular abscess–fistula, the acute

Table 4.24 The St Mark's classification applied to 793 consecutive patients presenting to St Mark's (1968–1973) with idopathic fistula-in-ano[54]

Type of fistula		No. of patients	%
Superficial		126	
Subcutaneous	54		
With fissure	56	520	65.6
Surgical wound	16		
Intersphincteric			
Simple	394		
With extension below puborectalis	22		
With extension above puborectalis	11	36	4.5
With entry into rectum	3		
Transsphincteric			
Simple	56		
With ischiorectal fossa extension	87	164	20.7
With supralevator extension	21		
Suprasphincteric			
Simple	5		
With ischiorectal fossa extension	1	26	3.3
With supralevator extension	20		
Extrasphincteric		23	2.9
Multiple		17	2.1
Unclassified		7	0.9

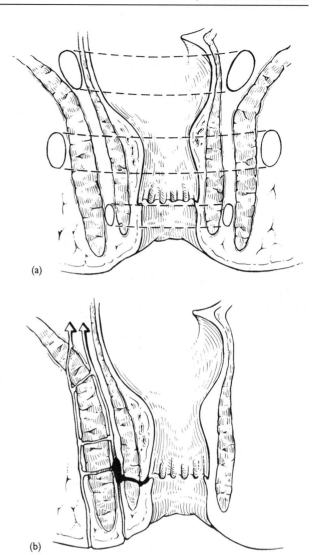

(a)

(b)

Figure 4.104 The upper diagram shows the routes along which fistulas may track from the seat of infection in the intersphincteric space in the vertical and horizontal planes. Spread may also occur circumferentially in the intersphincteric, ischiorectal and supralevator spaces (lower diagram).

abscess resolving into the chronic fistula and the two meriting the same classification. He divided abscess–fistulae into those confined to the area within the intermuscular space and those which had spread laterally out into the ischiorectal space. These groups were further subdivided according to vertical and circumferential spread (*Figures 4.105– 107*). Eisenhammer[20] was struck by the relatively high incidence of complex anal fistulas described by the surgeons at St Mark's, his own work suggesting that fistulas ran along relatively simple, predetermined paths.

chronic abscess and an area of induration along the fistula track. There may also be scarring from previous surgical treatment.

CLINICAL FEATURES

Most anorectal fistulas initially present as an anorectal abscess which continues to intermittently discharge after initial drainage. Sometimes there is no history of an abscess and the main symptom is of anal discharge and pruritis ani. Inspection reveals an external opening. Rectal examination may identify a

INVESTIGATIONS

To achieve the goals of surgery, namely cure of the fistula without recurrence and preservation of function, the exact anatomical location of the fistula must be carefully established. Although it is rightly claimed[8] that careful examination of a fistula under anaesthetic by a surgeon experienced in this field is the most important part of the assessment, other

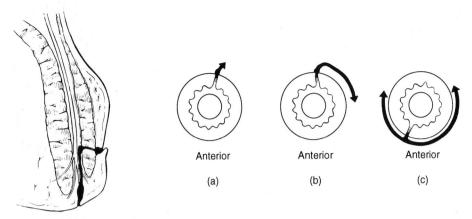

Figure 4.105 The low intermuscular fistulous abscess and fistula, representing 85% of Eisenhammer's cryptoglandular anorectal suppurative conditions.[15] Ninety per cent occur posteriorly (a), and may rarely spread anteriorly in the superficial ischiorectal space as a unilateral horseshoe (b). Ten per cent occur anteriorly (c) and these very rarely may spread bilaterally.

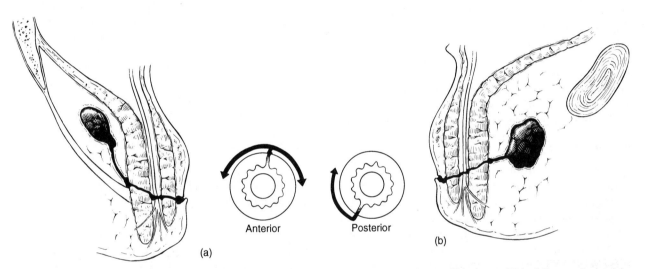

Figure 4.106 The intermuscular transsphincteric ischiorectal fistulous abscess and fistula. This forms 13% of the cryptoglandular pathologies according to Eisenhammer.[15] Ninety per cent occur posteriorly, the abscess developing in the deep postanal space and spreading initially unilaterally but later bilaterally (a). The corresponding anterior lesion is more superficial and only spreads in one direction (b).

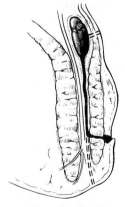

Figure 4.107 The high intermuscular fistulous abscess, representing 2% of cryptoglandular infections.[15] This posterior lesion arises from an anal gland situated above the level of the dentate line, and spreads upwards in the intermuscular space above the anorectal ring. Spontaneous rupture (dotted lines) will result in the corresponding fistula.

methods have been proposed in order to provide accurate anatomical delineation before surgery.

The distance from the external opening to the anal verge will give an idea as to whether a fistula crosses the external sphincter, and the application of Goodsall's rule will help in determining where the internal opening is likely to be. Several methods have been employed to identify a 'concealed' internal opening, the simplest of which is to digitally massage the track and look for a bead of pus emanating at the anorectal mucosa. Glen[21] described the use of hydrogen peroxide which, injected into the external opening, may mark the internal opening but complications have been reported using this technique.[18] Saline, instilled into the track through a vascular catheter inserted into the external opening has also been reported as demonstrating most of internal openings.[20] Dyes such as methylene blue and indigo carmine have also been used, both to identify internal openings and the course of fistula tracks.[14] These have the disadvantages of staining the anorectal mucosa which may blur the location of the internal opening, if the initial appearance of the dye is missed, and also of staining the tissues once a track is cut into.[68]

The primary track can usually be inferred by identifying the internal and external openings and feeling between these two points with a well-lubricated finger. Careful probing can help delineate primary and secondary tracks; if internal and external openings are easily detected but the probe cannot easily traverse the path of the track, it is possible that a high extension exists, and a probe passed via each opening may then delineate the primary track.[18] High induration should also alert the surgeon to the possibility of a supralevator extension.[68]

The usefulness of preoperative fistulography was critically assessed by Kuijpers and Schulpen[33] in 1985. Not only were fistulograms incorrect in 90% of cases, but misleading information suggesting high internal openings and high extensions occurred in 12%. The authors concluded that the investigation was therefore inaccurate, unreliable and even potentially harmful to the patient, should false-positive information be acted upon. Pommeri[58] on the other hand, found fistulography in conjunction with radioopaque markers to aid anatomical definition of the anorectum, very helpful in demonstrating the relations of fistulous tracks to puborectalis, and the presence of secondary tracks and abscesses.

A more recent investigation has been anal endosonography.[36] Revised criteria have improved on the accuracy of this examination in the determination of the internal openings.[8] At present, however, the technique has several drawbacks:[37] sepsis lateral to the external sphincter is not always identified, as it is beyond the focal range of the probe; and disease above the levators cannot be assessed because of lack of acoustic contact at this level. The technique therefore fails to image those aspects of fistulas that are most likely to cause difficulties in management. Cotte et al.[10] were impressed, however, with anal endosonography in the delineation of complex fistulous tracks and abscesses, with good correlation with fistulographic and operative findings.

Descalzo et al.[11] described the use of scintigraphy with radiolabelled leukocytes as an aid to transrectal echography in locating otherwise undetected accumulations in difficult anal fistulas.

Patients with fistula-in-ano at St Mark's Hospital are currently being assessed by magnetic resonance imaging: fistula pathology was revealed brightly in the infra- and supralevator compartments on STIR

(short tau inversion recovery) sequences. The results of initial studies are promising and it is hoped that, with wider availability of scanning machines, a useful assessment of the more complex fistulas may be made before surgical intervention.

SURGICAL TREATMENT

Operations for fistula-in-ano are associated with the very earliest records of surgical literature. Instruments unearthed at Pompeii, buried in AD 79, indicate that the treatment of the condition by operation was well known by that time. One of the earliest descriptions of the treatment of fistula-in-ano is the 15th century manuscript by John of Arderne, who described complete division of the main track in one clean cut of a knife and leaving the wound to granulate without applying caustic agents, the practice hitherto.[3] Peter Lowe, in 1612, described three methods of curing the condition: burning the fistula away with a cautery, cutting it open into the bowel, and ligature. He considered treatment with ligature the safest in terms of avoiding incontinence, but suggested that in very complicated fistulae it was wiser not to operate.

TIMING OF OPERATION IN ACUTE ANORECTAL SEPSIS

Eisenhammer, a strong advocate of the cryptoglandular hypothesis, considered the optimal time of surgery to be during the acute septic stage, and therefore proposed primary fistulectomy in which the abscess–fistula is drained via both openings, internal drainage through a distal internal sphincterotomy. In his series of 400 patients thus treated[15] there was a 99% cure rate. McElwain et al.[44] reported his series of 1000 patients with anorectal sepsis treated in a similar manner, and claimed a recurrence rate of only 3.6%.

Schouten et al.,[65] in accordance with Eisenhammer, believed division of the internal sphincter overlying the intermuscular abscess essential in the treatment of acute anorectal sepsis if recurrent abscess and fistula formation were to be avoided; he reported a 100% cure rate by this method, although a third of patients underwent a second drainage procedure. A later study, however, this time prospective in nature,[66] showed that a recurrent or persistant fistula occurred in 41% of patients treated by simple incision and drainage, and this fact, together with the increased incidence of functional disturbances associated with primary partial internal sphincterotomy led the authors to conclude that definitive surgery should be reserved as a second stage procedure if necessary. Vasilevsky and Gordon[79] reported a 48% rate of recurrent or persistent fistula following simple incision and drainage, reinforcing similar evidence[67] to support a policy of secondary fistulotomy in order to avoid sphincter division in most patients, who would not need it.

MANAGEMENT OF ESTABLISHED FISTULA-IN-ANO

Irrespective of any opinion as to whether primary fistulotomy obviates the need for surgery for fistulas, established, chronic fistulas will continue to present. Treatment of a low, simple fistula-in-ano remains traditional fistulotomy, incurring minimal sphincter damage and little risk of recurrence. Parks[53] in 1961 described his operative treatment, the crux of which was removal of the infecting source, the diseased anal gland in the intersphincteric space; this is most easily approached by internal sphincterectomy. Any part of the track lying outside the intersphincteric space is curetted, thus preserving the external anal sphincter, although some division of the external sphincter may be necessary if high infralevator or supralevator extensions are to be adequately drained.[56] Parks stressed the importance of leaving at least the upper one third of the internal sphincter intact to avoid incontinence of flatus and fluid faeces.

Manometric studies

What then, are the manometric consequences of sphincter division? The internal anal sphincter normally contributes up to 85% of the resting anal pressure; the external anal sphincter increases the pressure when faeces enters the upper part of the canal or upon voluntary contraction. Bennett and Duthie[5] demonstrated a significant reduction in anal pressure after internal anal sphincterotomy, and later published evidence that pressure was reduced in the distal 2 cm of the anal canal in patients who had undergone surgery for fistula.[6] Belliveau, Thomson and Parks[4] in 1983 similarly found reduced resting pressures in the distal anal canal, although the mean maximal resting pressure in patients who had undergone surgery for intersphincteric fistulas did not differ significantly from controls. Voluntary contraction pressures were similar in patients whose internal sphincters had been laid open, compared with controls, but patients with trans-sphincteric fistulas in whom the external sphincter was divided had significantly lower resting and contractile anal pressures than those in whom the muscle had been left intact. Preservation of muscle with a loose seton in those patients in whom the track crossed the external sphincter or levators led to no fall in resting or squeeze pressures. There is an association between the incidence of impaired continence, division of the external anal sphincter and reduced anal pressures.

Sainio and Husa[64] showed that patients with postoperative functional defects, mainly women, already had lower resting, squeeze and contractile pressures before surgery than patients who subsequently had no problems with continence. Furthermore, the reduction in pressures incurred by identical surgery was greater in women than in men. In a larger study,[63] it was demonstrated that internal anal sphincter division, especially the more extensive division performed in the treatment of transsphincteric fistulas, resulted in the lowest resting anal pressures and the highest incidence of defective anal control. Pescatori et al.[57] showed that a more conservative approach, as indicated by low pressures recorded at preoperative manometry, led to a significantly lower rate of soiling, and also a lower recurrence rate.

Other factors

Although sphincter preservation appears to be the predominant factor in the maintenance of continence, the exquisitely precise function of the anal canal must be the result of many factors. The rectoanal inhibitory reflex has been found by some[6] to be disturbed after fistula surgery, but not by others.[63] Similarly, scar shape and consistency have on occasions been found to be associated with changes in degrees of continence. Disturbance of the function of the conjoint longitudinal muscle, consequent upon its division during fistula surgery, may augment functional problems but which, at present, have not been quantified. This little understood muscle binds and braces the components of the anal canal together,[47] and some believe that the consequences of sphincter muscle division would be very different if the mesh formed by the longitudinal muscle and perianal connective tissue were not present.[25] Thomson and Ross[76] raised the suggestion that disordered anal control in patients with fistulas may also be contributed to by nerve damage to the sphincters by sepsis or by surgical dissection. The wide variety of factors which may impair anal function therefore make it impossible to predict exactly the functional changes after fistula surgery. The consequences of puborectalis or extensive external sphincter division are known and accordingly more 'conservative' approaches have been sought which are aimed to preserve anorectal function.

SPHINCTER PRESERVING TECHNIQUES

Excision and primary closure

Primary closure was attempted by Chaissagnac in 1856 and by Stephen and Smith in 1879, but was later discontinued because of the fear of persistant infection.[22] Rygich, however, claimed a 96% success rate in the 1700 cases treated by him since 1953, his closure consisting of repair of all divided tissues except the skin.[61] Parkash et al.[52] reviewed a series of 120 cases treated in a similar manner; after identification of the tracks, these were excised, with stay sutures inserted into the muscles to hold and identify the divided structures. The internal opening was cored out and the mucosal defect closed. All divided muscle layers were then meticulously repaired (except in some cases the skin). Eighty per cent healed within 2 weeks, and three recurrences were successfully treated using the same manner.

Lewis[38] advocated 'coring out' the fistula track and its branches from the external opening inwards, stopping well short of the anal margin. The anorectal wall was then closed in two layers followed by closure of the tunnel in the sphincter or pelvic floor. The external wound was lightly packed. Using this method, Lewis reported one recurrence in 18 transsphincteric and suprasphincteric fistulas.

Setons

Wollfers[82] reported the highly successful ayurvedic treatment of fistula-in-ano as practised in Columbo; a thread, impregnated 21 times for 15 minutes in a caustic solution prepared from the ashes of herbs, is inserted into the fistula track and changed weekly until healing is complete (up to 12 weeks for 'large' fistulas). In the cases of multiple fistulas, no more than two threads are inserted at any one session. There were no recurrences in the series of 80 patients who, quite apart from avoiding hospital admission were able to continue their employment during the treatment. Misra and Kapur[46] working in a similar environment, in a less developed country, advocate outpatient treatment involving the passage of a braided stainless steel wire seton through the track which is tied securely and tightened weekly until it cut through. A 4% recurrence rate was reported, with no complaints of temporary or permanent incontinence to flatus or faeces.

Thomson and Ross[76] assessed the results in patients with trans-sphincteric fistulas in whom the external sphincter is preserved as much as possible by using a loose seton, which acts as both a marker and drain for the track and to stimulate fibrosis around it. The intersphincteric space was drained by internal sphincterotomy, any secondary tracks curetted, and a loose seton then passed to encircle the primary track. The seton was removed at a later date after examination under anaesthesia had revealed that the rest of the wound had fully healed. Complete healing after seton removal and without recourse to external sphincter division occurred in 44% of patients, with a better functional outcome in those patients in whom the external sphincter had been preserved. Kennedy and Zegarra[31] using a similar technique reported recurrence or a persistent fistula in 34% of posterior fistulas but in only 12% of anterior fistulas.

Other workers have found good functional results with low rates of recurrence when a tight seton is used.[27] A tight elastic seton converts an acute abscess into a chronic draining fistula, and tightening of the seton at intervals leads to severance with fibrosis and little separation of the sphincter musculature. Christensen et al.,[9] using this method and tightening the seton every second day so that it had cut through by a maximum of 12 days, were disturbed to find a 63% incidence of some impaired continence.

Other methods

Excisional advancement flap

A different approach is that of fistulectomy and mucosal advancement flap, initially applied to the treatment of rectovaginal fistulas and with the theoretical advantages of involving just a single surgical procedure and a shorter healing time.[16,50] The track is excised together with the crypt-bearing tissue in the intersphincteric space and the overlying anoderm. A proximally based flap of variable thickness is then mobilized and anastomosed to a site distal to the (excised) internal opening. The success of this technique has been reported by several workers[1,30,51,60,71,81] but the numbers studied have been relatively small, and there seems little uniformity over details such as management of the external wound and thickness of the advancement flap. Although it is generally agreed that drainage of an acute abscess and its conversion into a chronic draining track should be achieved before performing this method, interestingly, outcome does not appear to be influenced by the presence or absence of a covering stoma. Work at St Mark's suggests that the technique carries a high risk of external wound breakdown and flap necrosis, but the theoretical advantages and success reported by others make it an attractive alternative.

Re-routing

Mann and Clifton[41] avoided sphincter division by a staged re-routing of a well established chronic track inwards to a site where it may be laid open without any sacrifice of external sphincter.

Gentamicin beads

Kupferberg et al.[34] in a small group of patients described the successful use of gentamicin impregnated beads; these were inserted into the wound after the track had been excised to the level of the sphincter and the track closed as close to the rectal wall as possible.

Laser excision

Slutki et al.[74] tried to minimize sphincter damage by coring out the fistula with a carbon dioxide laser beam.

REFERENCES

1. Aquilar, P.S., Plasencia, G., Hardy, T.G. et al. (1985) Mucosal advancement in the treatment of fistula-in-ano. *Diseases of the Colon and Rectum*, **28**, 496–498.
2. Arakawa, K., Arakawa, J. and Ooi, M. (1973) Symposium on infantile anal fistula. *Journal of the Japanese Society of Colo-Proctology*, **26**, 69.
3. Arderne, J. (1910) *Treatment of Fistula-in-ano, Haemorrhoids and Clysters*. From an early 15th Century manuscript translation, Power, D. (Ed.) London: Kegan Paul, Trench, Trubner.
4. Belliveau, P., Thomson, J.P.S. and Parks, A.G. (1983) Fistula-in-ano: a manometric study. *Diseases of the Colon and Rectum*, **26**, 152–154.
5. Bennett, R.C. and Duthie, H.L. (1964) The functional importance of the internal anal sphincter. *British Journal of Surgery*, **51**, 355.
6. Bennett, R.C. and Duthie, H.L. (1965) Pressure and sensation in the anal canal after minor anorectal procedures. *Diseases of the Colon and Rectum*, **8**, 131–136.
7. Buchan, R. and Grace, R.H. (1973) Anorectal suppuration: the results of treatment and the factors which influence the recurrence rate. *British Journal of Surgery*, **60**, 537–540.
8. Choen, S., Burnett, S., Bartram, C.I. and Nicholls, R.J. (1991) Comparison between anal endosonography and digital examination in the evaluation of anal fistulae. *British Journal of Surgery*, **78**, 445–447.
9. Christensen, A., Nilas, L. and Christiansen, J. (1986) Treatment of transphincteric anal fistulas by the seton technique. *Diseases of the Colon and Rectum*, **29**, 454–455.
10. Cotte, L., Bujol, B., Valette, P.J., Grandjean, J.P. and Souquet, J.C. (1990) Fistule anale complexe: apport de l'endosonographie. *Gastroenterology and Clinical Biology*, **14**, 510–511.
11. Discalzo, L., Dal BoR. and Cacace, G. (1990) Scintigraphy using Indium-111-oxine as an aid to transrectal echography in the diagnosis of perianal abscess. *Minerva Clinics*, **45**, 1371–1373.
12. Duhamel, J. (1975) Anal fistulae in childhood. *American Journal of Proctology*, **26**, 40–43.
13. Eisenhammer, S. (1956) The internal anal sphincter and the anorectal abscess. *Surgery, Gynecology and Obstetrics*, **103**, 501–506.
14. Eisenhammer, S. (1978) The final evaluation and classification of the surgical treatment of the primary anorectal, cryptoglandular intermuscular (intersphincteric) fistulous abscess and fistula. *Diseases of the Colon and Rectum*, **21**, 237–254.
15. Eisenhammer, S. (1985) Emergency fistulectomy of the acute primary anorectal cryptoglandular intermuscular abscess–fistula in ano. *South African Journal of Surgery*, **23**, 1–7.
16. Elting, A.W. (1912) The treatment of fistula in ano with especial reference to the Whitehead operation. *Annals of Surgery*, **56**, 744–752.
17. Ewerth, S. Ahlberg, J., Collste, G. and Holmstrom, B. (1978) Fistula-in-ano. A six year follow up study of 143 operated patients. *Acta Chirurgica Scandinavica*, Suppl. 482, 53.
18. Fazio VW. (1987) Complex anal fistulae. *Gastroenterology Clinics of North America*, **16**, 93–114.
19. Fitzgerald, R.J., Harding, B. and Ryan, W. (1985) Fistula-in-ano in childhood: A congenital aetiology. *Journal of Paediatric Surgery*, **20**, 80–81.
20. Gingold, B.S. (1983) Reducing the recurrence risk of fistula-in-ano. *Surgery, Gynecology and Obstetrics*, **156**, 661–662.
21. Glen, D.L. (1986) Use of hydrogen peroxide to identify internal openings of anal fistula and perianal abscess. *Australian and New Zealand Journal of Surgery*, **56**, 433–435.
22. Goligher, J.C. (1961) *Surgery of the Anus, Rectum and Colon*. (1st Edn) 166–196. London: Cassel.
23. Goligher, J.C., Ellis, M. and Pissidis, A.G. (1967) A critique of anal glandular infection in the aetiology and treatment of idiopathic anorectal abscesses and fistulas. *British Journal of Surgery*, **54**, 977–983.
24. Gordon-Watson, C. and Dodd, H. (1935) Observations on fistula in ano in relation to perianal intermuscular glands. *British Journal of Surgery*, **22**, 703–709.
25. Haas, P.A. and Fox, T.A. (1977) The importance of the perianal connective tissue in the surgical anatomy and function of the anus. *Diseases of the Colon and Rectum*, **20**, 303–313.
26. Hawley, P.R. (1975) Anorectal fistula. *Clinics in Gastroenterology*, **4**, 635–649.
27. Held, D., Khubchandani, I., Sheets, J. et al. (1986) Management of anorectal horseshoe abscess and fistula. *Diseases of the Colon and Rectum*, **29**, 793–797.
28. Henrichsen, S. and Christiansen, J. (1986) Incidence of fistula-in-ano complicating anorectal sepsis: a prospective study. *British Journal of Surgery*, **73**, 371–372.
29. Johnson, F.P. (1914) The development of the rectum in the human embryo. *American Journal of Anatomy*, **16**, 1–57.

30. Jones, I.T., Fazio, V.W. and Jagelman, D.G. (1987) The use of transanal rectal advancement flaps in the management of fistulas involving the anorectum. *Diseases of the Colon and Rectum*, **30**, 919–923.

31. Kennedy, H.L. and Zegarra, J.P. (1990) Fistulotomy without external sphincter division for high anal fistula. *British Journal of Surgery*, **77**, 898–901.

32. Kratzer, G.L. and Dockerty, M.B. (1947) Histopathology of the anal ducts. *Surgery, Gynecology and Obstetrics*, **84**, 333–338.

33. Kuijpers, H.C. and Schulpen, T. (1985) Fistulography for Fistula-in-Ano. *Diseases of the Colon and Rectum*, **28**, 103–104.

34. Kupferberg, A., Zer, M. and Rabinson, S. (1984) The use of PMMA beads in recurrent high anal fistula: a preliminary report. *World Journal of Surgery*, **8**, 970–974.

35. Kuster, G.G. (1965) Relationship of anal glands to lymphatics. *Diseases of the Colon and Rectum*, **8**, 329.

36. Law, P.J. and Bartram, C.I. (1989) Anal endosonography: technique and normal anatomy. *Gastrointestinal Radiology*, **14**, 349–353.

37. Law, P.J., Talbot, R.W., Bartram, C.I. and Northover, J.M.A. (1989) Anal endosonography in the evaluation of perianal sepsis and fistula-in-ano. *British Journal of Surgery*, **76**, 752–755.

38. Lewis, A. (1986) Excision of fistula-in-ano. *International Journal of Colorectal Disease*, **1**, 265–267.

39. Lilius, H.G. (1968) Fistula-in-ano: a clinical study of 150 patients. *Acta Chirurgica Scandinavica*, **383**, 3–88.

40. Lockhart-Mummery, J.P. (1929) Discussion on fistula-in-ano. *Proceedings of the Royal Society of Medicine*, **22**, 1331–1341.

41. Mann, C.V. and Clifton, M.A. (1985) Re-routing of the track for the treatment of high anal and anorectal fistulae. *British Journal of Surgery*, **72**, 134–137.

42. Marks, C.G. and Ritchie, J.K. (1977) Anal fistulas at St Mark's Hospital. *British Journal of Surgery*, **64**, 84–91.

43. McColl, I. (1965) The comparative anatomy and pathology of anal glands. *Annals of the Royal College of Surgeons*, **40**, 36–67.

44. McElwain, J.W., Maclean, M.D., Alexander, R.M. *et al.* (1975) Anorectal problems: experience with primary fistulectomy for anorectal abscesses. A report of 1,000 cases. *Diseases of the Colon and Rectum*, **18**, 646–649.

45. Milligan, E.T.C. and Morgan, M.C. (1934) Surgical anatomy of the anal canal with special reference to anorectal fistulae. *The Lancet*, **ii**, 1150–1156, 1213–1217.

46. Misra, M.C. and Kapur, B.M.L. (1988) A new non-operative approach to fistula-in-ano. *British Journal of Surgery*, **75**, 1093–1094.

47. Morgan, C.N. and Thomson, H.R. (1956) Surgical anatomy of the anal canal with special reference to the surgical importance of the internal sphincter and conjoint longitudinal muscle. *Annals of the Royal College of Surgeons of England*, **19**, 88–114.

48. Mortensen, N.J. and Thomson, J.P.S. (1984) Perianal abscess due to *Enterobius vermicularis*. *Diseases of the Colon and Rectum*, **27**, 677–678.

49. Nesselrod, J.P. (1957) *Clinical Proctology* (2nd Edn). Philadelphia: W.B. Saunders.

50. Noble, G.H. (1902) New operation for complete laceration of the perineum designed for the purpose of eliminating danger of infection from the rectum. *Transactions of the American Gynecological Society*, **27**, 357–363.

51. Oh, C. (1983) Management of high recurrent anal fistula. *Surgery*, **93**, 330–332.

52. Parkash, S., Lakshmiratan, V. and Gajendran, V. (1985) Fistula-in-ano: treatment by fistulectomy, primary closure and reconstitution. *Australian and New Zealand Journal of Surgery*, **55**, 23–27.

53. Parks, A.G. (1961) Pathogenesis and treatment of fistula-in-ano. *British Medical Journal*, **1**, 463–469.

54. Parks, A.G., Gordon, P.H. and Hardcastle, J.D. (1976) A classification of fistula-in-ano. *British Journal of Surgery*, **63**, 1–12.

55. Parks, A.G. and Morson, B.C. (1962) The pathogenesis of fistula-in-ano. *Proceedings of the Royal Society of Medicine*, **55**, 751–754.

56. Parks, A.G. and Stitz, R.W. (1976) The treatment of high fistula-in-ano. *Diseases of the Colon and Rectum*, **19**, 487–499.

57. Pescatori, M., Maria, G., Anastasio, G. and Rinallo, L. (1989) Anal manometry improves the outcome of surgery for fistula-in-ano. *Diseases of the Colon and Rectum*, **32**, 588–592.

58. Pommeri, F., Pittarello, F., Dodi, G., Pianon, P. and Muzzio, P.C. (1988) Diagnosi radiologica delle fistole anali con reperi radiopachi. *Radilogikal Medicine*, **75**, 632–637.

59. Pople, I.K. and Ralphs, D.L.N. (1988) An aetiology for fistula-in-ano. *British Journal of Surgery*, **75**, 904–905.

60. Reznick, R.K. and Bailey, H.R. (1988) Closure of the internal opening for treatment of complex fistula-in-ano. *Diseases of the Colon and Rectum*, **31**, 116–118.

61. Rygich, A.N. (1965) *Atlas of the Operations on the Rectum and Colon*. p. 80, Moscow.

62. Sainio, P. (1984) Fistula-in-ano in a defined population. Incidence and epidemiological aspects. *Acta Chirurgica Gynaecologica*, **73**, 219–224.

63. Sainio, P. (1985) A manometric study of anorectal function after surgery for anal fistula, with special reference to incontinence. *Acta Chirurgica Scandinavica*, **151**, 695–700.

64. Sainio, P. and Husa, A. (1985) A prospective manometric study of the effect of anal fistula surgery on anorectal function. *Acta Chirurgica Scandinavica*, **151**, 279–288.

65. Schouten, W.R., van Vroonhoven, T.J.M.V. and van Berlo, C.L.J. (1987) Primary partial internal

sphincterotomy in the treatment of anorectal abscess. *Netherlands Journal of Surgery*, **39**, 43–45.

66. Schouten, W.R. and van Vroonhoven, T.J.M.V. (1991) Treatment of anorectal abscess with or without primary fistulectomy: results of a prospective randomized trial. *Diseases of the Colon and Rectum*, **34**, 60–63.

67. Scoma, J.A., Salvati, E.P. and Rubin, R.J. (1984) Incidence of fistulas subsequent to anal abscesses. *Diseases of the Colon and Rectum*, **17**, 357–359.

68. Seow-Choen and Phillips, R.K.S. (1991) Insights gained from the management of problematical anal fistulae at St Mark's Hospital, 1984–88. *British Journal of Surgery*, **78**, 539–541.

69. Seow-Choen, F., Hay, A.J., Heard, S. and Phillips, R.K.S. (1992) Bacteriology of anal fistulae. *British Journal of Surgery*, **79**, 27–28.

70. Shafer, A.D., McGlone, T.P. and Flanagan, R.A. (1987) Abnormal crypts of Morgagni: The cause of perianal abscess and fistula-in-ano. *Journal of Paediatric Surgery*, **22**, 203–204.

71. Shemesh, E.I., Kodner, I.J., Fry, R.D. and Neufeld, D.M. (1988) Endorectal sliding flap repair of complicated anterior anoperineal fistulas. *Diseases of the Colon and Rectum*, **31**, 22–24.

72. Shouler, P.J., Grimley, R.P., Keighley, M.R.B. and Alexander-Williams, J. (1986) Fistula-in-ano is usually simple to manage surgically. *International Journal of Colorectal Disease*, **1**, 113–115.

73. Shropshear, G. (1960) Surgical anatomic aspects of the anorectal sphincter mechanism and its clinical significance. *Journal of the International College of Surgeons*, **33**, 267–287.

74. Slutzki, S., Abramsohn, R. and Bogokowsky, H. (1981) Carbon dioxide laser in the treatment of high anal fistula. *American Journal of Surgery*, **141**, 395–396.

75. Takatsuki, S. (1976) An etiology of anal fistula in infants. *Keio Journal of Medicine*, **25**, 1–4.

76. Thomson, J.P.S. and Ross, A.H.McL. (1989) Can the external sphincter be preserved in the treatment of trans-sphincteric fistula-in-ano? *International Journal of Colorectal Diseases*, **4**, 247–250.

77. Tucker, C.C. and Hellwig, C.A. (1935) Anal ducts: comparative and developmental anatomy. *Archives of Surgery*, **31**, 521–530.

78. Van de Putte, S.C.J. (1986) Normal and abnormal development of the anorectum. *Journal of Paediatric Surgery*, **21**, 434–440.

79. Vasilevsky, C-A. and Gordon, P.H. (1984) The incidence of recurrent abscess or fistula-in-ano following anorectal suppuration. *Diseases of the Colon and Rectum*, **27**, 126–130.

80. Walls, E.W. (1958) Observations on the microscopic anatomy of the human anal canal. *British Journal of Surgery*, **45**, 504–512.

81. Wedell, J., Meier, Z.U., Eissen, P., Banzhaf, G. and Kleine, L. (1987) Sliding flap advancement for the treatment of high level fistulae. *British Journal of Surgery*, **74**, 390–391.

82. Wollfers, I. (1986) Ayurvedic treatment for fistula-in-ano. *Tropical Doctor*, **16**, 44.

PRURITUS ANI

T.R. Russell

Pruritus ani is a symptom of itching and irritation in the perianal region but does not designate a specific aetiology. The symptom complex is exceedingly common as the skin is covered, often moist, and soiled by faeces. Often the patient enters a cycle of irritation which leads to scratching of the area and continued irritation. The mainstay of treatment must be directed at breaking this cycle.

AETIOLOGY

Most cases are idiopathic and a specific cause cannot be determined.[2] The known causes are:

1. *Proctologic disorders*: Skin tags, mucin-producing prolapsing internal hemorrhoids or polyps, draining fistulas or sinuses, fissures, condylomata acuminatum, hidradenitis suppurativa.

2. *Dermatological conditions*: psoriasis, seborrheic dermatitis, atopic eczema.

3. *Contact dermatitis*: soaps with irritating chemicals and alkaline pH, local analgesic compounds with 'caine', other topical ointments.

4. *Fungal*: Candidiasis, dermatophytosis.

5. *Bacterial*: Secondary to scratching and infection.

6. *Parasitic*: pinworms (*Enterobius vermicularis*), pediculosis, scabies.

7. *After oral antibiotic therapy*: frequently related to diarrhoea and irritating bowel movements.

8. *Systemic diseases*: diabetes.

9. *Neoplasms*: intraepithelial carcinoma (Bowen's disease), extramammary Paget's disease.

10. *Hygiene*: poor hygiene as well as over-meticulous hygiene using excessive soap.

11. *Warmth and hyperhidrosis*: related to under-clothing, obesity, moisture and climate.
12. *Dietary*: excessive consumption of coffee, alcohol, milk, fruit juices.
13. *Psychogenic*: perpetuation of the cycle of anxiety–itch–anxiety may be significant in certain patients.
14. *Idiopathic*: represent around 50%.

CLINICAL FEATURES

The symptoms of pruritus ani may range from mild to severe, for periods of days to years. Careful history must be obtained regarding the onset of the problem and associated factors, such as diet, drugs, stool consistency and skin eruptions.[5] A careful dietary history should be taken, paying particular attention to excessive coffee consumption. Other dermatological problems should be sought as well as the use of drugs or chemicals applied to the perianal area. It is important to note a prior history of anorectal surgery.

Examination of the perianal area may reveal, on the one hand, normal-appearing skin and, at the other extreme, severe inflammation with thickening and lichenification. Specific dermatological conditions may be recognized (such as psoriasis) by its gross appearance or biopsy.

Specific anorectal diseases should be identified and corrected, that is, causes that allow moisture to escape from the rectum, keeping the area moist. These include chronic abscesses and fistulas which drain pus, as well as prolapse of mucosa from the rectum which allows mucus to continually seep onto the perianal skin. Evaluation of the sphincter is important because the prime physiological disorder explaining pruritus ani appears to be decreased continence.[1] This allows seepage of proteolytic enzymes onto the perianal skin.

Following anorectal surgery (fistulotomy) where a portion of the sphincteric ring is cut, incontinence may also play a significant role. A sulcus may result which allows continuous seepage from the rectum with concomitant moisture. Studies have not confirmed changes in the faecal microflora in patients with pruritus ani.[3]

INVESTIGATIONS

Laboratory tests are rarely helpful but should be performed in refractory cases. Specifically, scrapings may reveal yeast and a tape test may disclose pinworm infestation. Biopsy of the involved skin may be useful to exclude a malignancy or other specific dermatological conditions.

TREATMENT

Because, in most cases, no cause is identified, patients should understand that a specific cause does not exist. Frequently, there is concern about cancer or other serious conditions.

SECONDARY PRURITUS ANI

In cases where a specific aetiology is determined, treatment is so directed. This includes medical treatment of fungal, yeast and parasitic involvement as well as surgical treatment of anorectal disease which permits moisture accumulation. Band ligation or sclerotherapy of prolapsing internal hemorrhoids may control mucin production by decreasing redundant tissue without resorting to hemorrhoidectomy. Drainage of abscesses, fistulectomy, removal of condylomata and fissurectomy with lateral internal sphincterotomy are directed towards other surgical problems which account for 5–10% of all patients.

PRIMARY PRURITUS ANI

In cases where a specific aetiology has not been determined, a more general approach must be used. Dietary restrictions may be indicated and specifically directed towards coffee and alcohol. Hygiene is also a precipitating cause of pruritus ani as many patients, when they begin to have irritation, shower and bathe the area more vigorously, which may perpetuate the cycle. Refraining from the use of soap in the perianal region is important as soap is slightly alkaline in pH and often remains in contact with the skin after bathing. Soap should not be used in the perianal region during the active treatment phase. All other topical medications in use should be stopped, to avoid contact dermatitis. Following bathing, the area must be thoroughly blotted and dried to prevent masceration. Frequently, dry cotton is useful during the day to prevent accumulation of moisture. Bathing should be performed after bowel movements, if possible, or the area cleansed thoroughly with moistened tissue paper.

Suppositories and analgesic agents should be avoided. A water-soluble 0.25% or 1% steroidal cream with an acid pH may be helpful if used sparingly, twice a day, in the involved area.[4]

In certain individuals, tension and stress may promote this condition, as may an irritable bowel with irritating, loose, frequent bowel movements. These patients will benefit from counselling, dietary restrictions to firm the loose bowel movements and the use of hydrophilic bulk agents.

In difficult and refractory cases, dermatological consultation may be of value. There is no role for wide surgical excision of the involved skin, or radiation which was used in the past.

REFERENCES

1. Allan, A., Ambrose, N.S., Silverman, S. and Keighley, M.R. (1987) Physiological study of pruritus ani. *British Journal of Surgery*, **74**, 576–579.
2. Friend, W.G. (1977) The cause and treatment of idiopathic pruritus ani. *Disease of the Colon and Rectum*, **20**, 40–42.
3. Silverman, S., Youngs, D., Allan, A. *et al.* (1989) The fecal microflora in pruritus ani. *Diseases of the Colon and Rectum*, **32**, 466–468.
4. Smith, L.E., Henrichs, D. and McCullah, R.D. (1982) Prospective studies on etiology and treatment of pruritus ani. *Diseases of the Colon and Rectum*, **25**, 358–363.
5. Sullivan, E.S. and Garnjobst, H. (1978) Pruritus ani: A practical approach. *Surgical Clinics of North America*, **58**, 505–512.

PROCTALGIA FUGAX

T.R. Russell

AETIOLOGY

CLINICAL FEATURES

The cause of this painful syndrome is unknown with no anatomical or physiological defects recognized. It may be related to stress, fatigue or functional gastrointestinal disorders, or both. A number of reports support the association of functional disorders with loose frequent bowel movements, passage of mucous and abdominal bloating and pain with proctalgia fugax.[2] Other causes of pain in the rectum should be excluded such as coccydynia, infections of the rectum and perianal area, thrombosed hemorrhoids, fissure-in-ano and tumour. Consideration should also be given to radicular pain originating in the back.

Proctalgia fugax (fleeting rectal pain) or levator muscle spasm is a common symptom, but often not recognized.[3] The pain is described as sudden, sharp, and electrical in nature and lasts from seconds to hours. The pain may awaken patients at night and may be incapacitating.

On performing digital rectal examination, tenderness may be elicited in the pubococcygeous muscle which may mimic the pain of proctalgia fugax. Proctoscopic evaluation reveals normal mucosa with no evidence of proctitis.

TREATMENT

Treatment is non-specific and is begun only after excluding other possible causes. Patients must be reassured and instructed as to the harmless nature of the attacks. Because the aetiology is unknown, treatment is non-specific and may include warm baths, muscle relaxants or periodic massage of painful spastic muscle of the levator mechanism. Individual patients may express relief by bowel passage.

Recent experience using electrogalvanic muscle stimulation has proved effective in refractory cases.[1] The rationale of this treatment is based on applying a low frequency oscillating current to muscle. This causes fatigue of the muscle, thereby breaking the spastic cycle.

REFERENCES

1. Oliver, G.C., Rubin, R.J., Salvati, E.P. and Eisenstat, J.E. (1985) Electrogalvanic stimulation in the treatment of levator syndrome. *Diseases of the Colon and Rectum*, **28**, 662–663.
2. Pilling, L.F., Swenson, W.M. and Hill, J.R. (1972) The psychologic aspects of proctalgia fugax. *Diseases of the Colon and Rectum*, **32**, 466–468.
3. Thompson, W.G. (1981) Proctalgia fugax. *Digestive Diseases and Sciences*, **26**, 1121–1124.

MALIGNANT TUMOURS OF THE ANUS

R.W. Beart, Jr

GENERAL CONSIDERATIONS

TYPES OF ANAL MALIGNANCY

Carcinoma of the anus represent about 1–4% of cancers of the large bowel. The distribution of malignant types in this region was noted by Beahrs:[4] squamous cell carcinoma (55%), basaloid carcinoma (31%), Paget's disease (4%), melanoma (3.5%), basal cell carcinoma (3.5%), and adenocarcinoma (3.5%). Additional tumours include lymphosarcoma, leiomyosarcoma, rhabdomyosarcoma, hemangiopericytoma, plasmocytoma and endothelioma. The complexity and multiplicity of cellular elements involved in formation of the anal canal is responsible for this diversity of tumour types. Although first described in detail by the French anatomists Hermann and Desfosses,[31] Grinvalsky and Helwig[29] are generally credited for the clear anatomical and histological descriptions used today.

SEX INCIDENCE

Anal cancer has been perceived as being more prevalent in women. The Mayo Clinic experience noted a 3:1 ratio of females to males (*Table 4.25*). More recently, however, the disease is reported to be equally divided between males and females and occurs predominantly in the fifth and sixth decades.[11] Cancers of the anal margin are more common in males, whereas cancer of the anal canal is slightly more common in females.

PREDISPOSING FACTORS

Anal cancer can be associated with chronic irritation of the anal canal such as fistulas, fissures or abscesses.[8,9,37,62] Recent changes in the epidemiology of anal cancer have been associated with the prevalence of HIV infection.[13] The association of viral infection with malignant transformation has been well documented and immunosuppressed patients need to be watched for anal cancers.[18,33,54]

ORIGIN OF MALIGNANCY: CLASSIFICATION

The basaloid squamous type of cloacogenic carcinoma and its glandular variants (adenocystic or mucoepidermoid) take their origin from the 'transit-ional zone' between the non-keratinized squamous portion of the anal canal and the keratinized epithelium (anoderm) of the anus. The anal canal is 1–6 cm in length and is limited by the puborectalis cephalad and the anal verge distally. The 'transitional zone' results from remnants of the embryonal cloacal membrane and closely resembles the lining of the urinary tract. Stratified squamous epithelium commonly extends into this region and can give rise to squamous cell carcinomas. The rare adenocarcinoma of the anal canal arises from the anal glands located in the crypts of Morgagni. The keratinized, stratified, squamous epithelium below the anal verge is the perianal skin. Cancers of this area need to be recognized as arising from outside the anal canal as they are treated differently.

Morson initially grouped all tumours arising in the anal canal as non-keratinizing or keratinizing tumours. Tumours arising within the anal canal

Table 4.25 Characteristics of squamous cell and non-keratinizing basaloid cell carcinoma

	Number
Sex	
Male	46
Female	125
Total	171
Age	
Median	59
Range	34–84
Treatment	
Local	19
AP Resection	118
Palliative	23
Radiation	12
Stage	
A	17
B1	33
B2	14
B3	32
C	41
D	23
Unknown	12
Histology	
Squamous 1–2	30
Squamous 3–4	76
Basaloid 3–4	66

Table 4.26 Small-cell carcinoma versus squamous cell carcinoma

	Small cell	Squamous
Presentation with unresectable disease	5/13 (38%)	23/173 (13%)
Median survival	2.2 months	7.5 months
5-year survival	1/7 (14%)	81/114 (71%)

show keratin production in 45% of tumours.[38] Keratin production is generally related to the differentiation of the tumours. Small-cell variants of anal cancer were recently documented and have a dramatically poorer prognosis than other anal cancers (Table 4.26). Although cell type may have prognostic significance, it has little effect upon treatment.[25,50,53]

SPREAD

The unique anatomy of the anal canal can give rise to several patterns of metastatic spread. Patterns of spread depend largely upon the location of the tumour within the anal canal. This can be by direct extension through the anal wall, regionally to pelvic or inguinal lymph nodes, or via venous routes of the canal or portal systems. The rarity of these tumours, the diverse nature of histological types, tumour nomenclature, and the anatomical variance from other areas have made standard regimens of treatment of these carcinomas difficult to develop and assess.

In assessing the location of tumours within the canal, Kuehn[7] noted that 2% of epidermoid cancers were in the rectum and likely resulted from malignant change in stratified squamous epithelium extending along the columns of Morgagni. Fifty-eight per cent of tumours were adjacent to the pectinate line; 14% were within the anal canal; 11% abutted the anal verge, and 15% were on the perianal skin. In reviewing pathologic specimens, Wolfe[62] noted that the route of invasion correlated with the location of the tumour. Prognosis is related to the size and depth of invasion of the tumour.[6] Various staging systems exist and the one by Boman et al.[6] has been documented in a large series to be helpful. TNM classification should be used in all reports.

CLINICAL FEATURES

Most patients with anal cancer present with symptoms similar to other anal disorders. Common symptoms include bleeding, pain, mass, constipation, diarrhoea, and pruritis.[6,10,16,30] Because these are common symptoms, diagnosis is often delayed. In addition, the disease may be difficult to diagnose if it occurs in a chronic fistula. Examination under anesthesia may be necessary to make a definitive diagnosis.

TREATMENT

Traditionally, surgery alone, either by local excision for low grade squamous lesions or abdominal perineal resection for other types, has been the primary mode of treatment and radiation reserved for salvage therapy.[28,45,60] Beginning with the report of Nigro,[40] therapeutic planning has now reversed and radiation therapy is the most common mode of therapy for most anal tumous.

Anal cancer is a rare neoplasm. The management of this cancer has changed dramatically in the past decade. Management depends upon site, histology, size and biological characteristics. It is important for the physician to recognize the variable histology possible in this tumour and be prepared to offer appropriate therapy.

SQUAMOUS CELL CARCINOMA, BASALOID CARCINOMA

Typically squamous carcinoma of the anal margin and perianal region is well differentiated and of low metastatic potential leading to wide local excision as the treatment of choice. Squamous carcinoma of the anal canal, however, is generally poorly differentiated and more malignant, necessitating more aggressive therapy. Most studies today consider 'transitional cell carcinoma', basaloid carcinoma and cloacogenic carcinoma to be the same non-keratinizing squamous carcinoma.

The aetiology remains unclear but recently, high proportions of these tumours have been associated with papilloma virus.[33,49,54] This finding has potential diagnostic, epidemiological and therapeutic implications.

Early lesions may present as a localized ulcer or warty growth with raised, irregular and ulcerated borders. Later the lesion is more often hard and protuberant, with or without ulceration. The smaller tumours may be confused with condylomata, papilloma, a primary chancre, an anal fissure or prolapsed and thrombosed internal hamorrhoids. Any indurated lesion should be sampled for biopsy.

TREATMENT

Squamous carcinomas of the anus and perianal region, if superficial, well differentiated and small (1–2 cm) are frequently well treated by local excision alone.[2,4,24,34,35,45] The use of new staging modalities such as ultrasound[26] and flow cytometry[25,52] may help to identify candidates for local management more accurately. In a Mayo Clinic series of 194 patients, 19 patients were candidates for local excision.[6] Twelve patients with tumour not invasive into anal muscle were cured by local excision. Al-Jurf, Cuthbertson and Eby also noted good survival in selected patients treated with local excision.[2,16,20]

Traditional management is well reflected in the Mayo Clinic series of 194 patients treated between 1950 and 1976.[6] Until 1974, the standard therapy for epidermoid carcinoma of the anus was surgical (*Table 4.27*). Radiation treatment was considered ineffective in eradicating disease and associated with long-term effects on anal function. Damage to the perianal skin and anal sphincters necessitating colostomy was not unusual.[17] In the Mayo Clinic series, treatment was retrospectively stratified by depth of penetration into the anal musculature. Radiation therapy in this series was selected as primary treatment in 11 patients, who presented with clinically resectable disease (surgical refusal, poor condition). Survival was poor although 4 of the 11 lived longer than 5 years free of disease. Survival was also poor (1 of 13) in a group of patients in whom very extensive disease was present, and were treated with a variety of radiation techniques. No judgement should be made as to efficacy of radiation therapy in these small, select populations.

One hundred and thirty patients underwent abdominoperineal resections, for potential cure. Fifty-one of 130 patients developed recurrent disease (*Table 4.28*). Survival was related to the stage of disease. In addition to stage, tumour size was a

Table 4.27   Recurrence after abdominoperineal resection

Stage	No. of patients	Recurrences	%
A	4	0	
B1	26	6	23
B2	13	3	23
B3	31	16	52
C	40	21	53
Cell type			
Squamous Grade 1–2	19	7	37
Squamous Grade 3–4	51	22	43
Non-keratinizing basaloid	44	17	39

Table 4.28   Initial sites of recurrence

Local		27 (84%)
Pelvic	12	
Inguinal	8	
Pelvic + Ing	7	
Distant only		6 (29%)

significant factor in survival. Four centimetres was found to represent the size between good and poor survival. Tumour histology was a third significant factor in survival, with low-grade squamous cell carcinoma having the best (approximately 90%) followed by high-grade squamous and basaloid (approximately 63%), with small-cell carcinoma having poor survival (approximately 13%) (see *Table 4.27*). It is important to note that most recurrences were local rather than distant which has significant implications towards the use of adjuvant therapy (*Table 4.28*). Patients with small cell tumours tend to develop local and distant metastases.

Surgery has traditionally been the most common therapy for squamous cell cancer of the anus as reflected in the Mayo series. Beginning with the report of Nigro[39] surgery has increasingly been relegated to salvage therapy and primary therapy consists of radiation and chemotherapy.[11,14,15,23,30,32,41,42,44] Epidermoid anal cancers are generally radiosensitive, much like other epidermoid tumours. Therapy has generally not been controlled for histology, size or stage. Not all patients are successfully treated with radiation therapy. Current efforts of research are directed towards defining the histological, morphological, cellular and biological features which will help predict those patients most amenable to radiation or surgical therapy. External irradiation is limited by the sensitivity of the perineal tissues and requires protracted treatment.

Current treatment consists of 3500–5000 cGy and additional chemotherapy. Nigro described using 5-fluorouracil plus mitomycin but this can be a toxic regimen and current investigation is focused on the necessity of using mitomycin and the use of alternative chemotherapeutic regimens. It is clear that larger tumours tend to do less well than smaller ones (less than 5 cm) with this therapy. In reviewing the combined results of most reports where information is available, it appears that the tumour will fail to resolve in about 25% of patients and about 30% of the successfully treated patients (about 25% of the entire group) will have complications of therapy which require proctectomy or diversion. Thus,

Table 4.29 Five-year cancer related deaths after radiation therapy

Series	Ref.	Year	Survival (%)
Sischy et al.	56	1985	30
Salmon et al.	50	1986	59
Frost et al.	22	1984	38
Papillon et al.	43	1983	18

about 50% of the treated patients will be spared a colostomy if radiation therapy is used routinely on all patients with anal canal squamous cancers (*Table 4.29*).

MELANOMA

Melanoma of the anorectum was first described in 1812 and first diagnosed in 1857. There are only about 250 cases described in the literature.[55] Next to the skin and eyes, the anal canal is the most common site, although less than 1% of all melanomas arise here. In a recent review from the Mayo Clinic, a total of 37 cases were found which were carefully documented, analysed and followed for at least 5 years.[12] Twenty-four were females and 13 were males. Age ranged from 22 to 79 years with an average of 62 years. Symptoms include bleeding (25), pain (15), mass (14), constipation (10), diarrhoea (4), tenesmus (1) and averaged 40 days before presentation. Melanoma of the anal canal may present as a polypoid, bluish-black lesion which may be mistaken for a thrombosed hemorrhoid, or there may be ulceration and marked induration. Most tumours (19/37) were larger than 2 cm. Twelve were ulcerating, 11 were verrucous and 4 were flat. Twenty-four of 37 were amelanotic.

TREATMENT

Of the 31 patients treated surgically (wide local excision, 12; abdominoperineal resection, 19), only four are alive, three of these four for more than 5 years. Six patients had distant disease at presentation and there was no attempt made for cure. It has been the author's general policy that radical surgery has a very limited role in the management of anorectal melanoma. If dissemination has already occurred at the time of presentation, then lymphadenectomy will not save the patient. If the tumour is localized, lymphadenectomy will add nothing to local excision.

Ross et al.[48] and Ward (1337) noted a 6% 5-year survival in most series. He also favours local excision as the primary therapy but noted local recurrence less frequently in patients undergoing abdominoperineal resection. The author does not favour an elective groin dissection because of the increased morbidity associated with inguinal dissections.

BASAL CELL CARCINOMA

Basal cell carcinomas occur typically as a firm lesion with irregular raised edges with a central ulceration. They comprise less than 1% of anorectal neoplasms.[6,47,61] They occur three times more commonly in men than women. They must not be confused with basaloid carcinoma, and are similar to basal cell carcinoma located elsewhere. They are slow growing and of very low malignant potential. Metastasis is very rare. Wide local excision is the treatment of choice.

BOWEN'S DISEASE

Bowen's disease, described by the pathologist of that name in 1912, is a low grade intraepidermal squamous carcinoma in situ. These most often appear as discrete, scaly, erythematous plaques. Itching or burning may accompany this lesion. Histologically there are multinucleated giant cells with vacuolation. This lesion may be a harbinger of other cutaneous, respiratory, gastrointestinal, genitourinary or other malignancies which occur within 10 years of the diagnosis of Bowen's disease in up to 40% of cases.[58] A more recent survey of members of the American Society of Colon and Rectal Surgery suggests that the incidence of associated cutaneous or internal malignancy may be substantially lower.[36] Only 4.7% of patients in this review developed associated malignancy, whereas 9.4% developed recurrent Bowen's disease and 5.7% developed invasive disease. It was concluded that an extensive and invasive work-up of patients with perianal Bowen's disease was not warranted. Ten per cent of patients with Bowen's disease will develop invasive squamous cell carcinoma in that lesion, and 35% of those tumours will go on to metastasize unless treated. Local excision with careful follow-up is the treatment of choice.[36,46,59] Split-thickness skin grafting may be necessary after excising larger lesions.

PERIANAL PAGET'S DISEASE

Paget's disease presents as a pruritic, scaling, plaque-like area similar to Bowen's disease in appearance. The distinction must be made on the basis of content of acid mucosubstance,[5,19] among other histological grounds. The lesion may chronicle a carcinoma of a local apocrine gland[51,57,3] or may be associated with a *de facto* or future visceral carcinoma.[51] These associations are less frequent than previously thought but should be eliminated in the evaluation of Paget's disease. For localized lesions, a wide local excision controlled by frozen section margin evaluation is recommended.[54,57] For more extensive lesions or for patients with underlying carcinoma, abdominoperineal resection is the treatment of choice.

BUSCHKE-LOWENSTEIN TUMOUR

The Buschke-Lowenstein tumour is a variant of squamous cell carcinoma. This low-grade squamous carcinoma is frequently mistaken for exuberant condyloma acuminata. Radiation and chemotherapy have been conspicuously ineffective, and radical excision is the treatment of choice.[21,1]

REFERENCES

1. Alexander, R.M. and Kaminsky, D.B. (1979) Giant condyloma acuminatum (Buschke-Lowenstein tumor) of the anus: case report and review of the literature. *Diseases of the Colon and Rectum*, **21**, 561–565.
2. Al-Jurf, A.S., Turnbull, R.B. and Fazio, V.W. (1979) Local treatment of squamous cell carcinoma of the Anus. *Surgery, Gynecology and Obstetrics*, **148**, 576–578.
3. Armitage, N.C., Jass, J.R., Richman, P.I., Thomson, J.P. and Phillips, R.K. (1989) Paget's disease of the anus: a clinicopathological study [see comments]. *British Journal of Surgery*, **76**, 60–63.
4. Beahrs, O.H. and Wilson, S.M. (1976) Carcinoma of the anus. *Annals of Surgery*, **184**, 422–428.
5. Bielefeldt, K., Enck, P. and Wienbeck, M. (1990) Diagnosis and treatment of fecal incontinence. *Digestive Diseases*, **8**, 179–188.
6. Boman, B.M., Moertel, C.G., O'Connell, M.J. *et al.* (1984) Carcinoma of the anal canal. A clinical and pathologic study of 188 cases. *Cancer*, **54**, 114–125.
7. Boulos, P.B. and Araujo, J.G.C. (1984) Adequate internal sphincterotomy for chronic anal fissure: subcutaneous or open technique? *British Journal of Surgery*, **71**, 360–362.
8. Brennan, J.T. and Stewart, C.F. (1972) Epidermoid carcinoma of the anus. *Annals of Surgery*, **176**, 787–790.
9. Bretlau, P. (1967) Carcinoma arising in anal fistula. *Acta Chirurgica Scandinavica*, **133**, 496–500.
10. Brown, D.K., Oglesby, A.B. and Scott, D.H. (1988) Squamous cell carcinoma of the anus: A twenty-five year retrospective. *American Surgeon*, **54**, 337–342.
11. Cantril, S.T., Green, J.P., Schall, G.L. and Schaupp, W.C. (1983) Primary radiation therapy in the treatment of anal carcinoma. *International Journal of Radiation, Oncology, Biology and Physics*, **9**, 1271–1278.
12. Chiu, Y.S., Unni, K.K. and Beart, R.W. Jr. (1980) Malignant melanoma of the anorectum. *Diseases of the Colon and Rectum*, **23**, 122–124.
13. Croxson, R., Chabon, A.B., Rorat, E. and Barash, I.M. (1984) Intraepithelial carcinoma of the anus in homosexual men. *Diseases of the Colon and Rectum*, **27**, 325–330.
14. Cummings, B.J., Keane, T.J. and Thomas, G.M. (1984) Results and toxicity of the treatment of anal canal carcinoma by radiation therapy and chemotherapy. *Cancer*, **541**, 2062–2066.
15. Cummings, B.J. (1987) Treatment of primary epidermoid carcinoma of the anus. *Colorectal Disease*, **2**, 107–112.
16. Cuthbertson, A.M. and Kaye, A.H. (1978) Local excision of carcinomas of the rectum, anus, and anal canal. *Australian and New Zealand Journal of Surgery*, **48**, 412–414.
17. Dalby, J.E. and Pointon, R.S. (1961) The treatment of anal carcinoma by interstitial irradiation. *American Journal of Roenterology*, **858**, 515.
18. Daling, J.R., Weiss, N.S. and Hislop, T.G. (1987 Sexual practices, sexually transmitted diseases, and the incidence of anal cancer. *New England Journal of Medicine*, **317**, 973–977.
19. Dwight, R.W., Higgins, G.A., Roswit, B., LeVeen, H.H. and Keehn, R.J. (1987) Preoperative radiation and surgery for cancer of the sigmoid colon and rectum. *Gastroenterology Clinic of North America*, **16**, 35–45.
20. Eby, L.S. and Sullivan, E.S. (1969) Current concepts of local excision of epidermoid carcinoma of the anus. *Diseases of the Colon and Rectum*, **12**, 332–337.
21. Elliot, M.S., Werner, I.D., Immelman, E.J. and Harrison, A.C. (1979) Giant condyloma (Buschke-Lowenstein tumor) of the anorectum. *Diseases of the Colon and Rectum*, **22**, 497–500.
22. Frost, D.B., Richards, P.C., Montague, E.D., Giacco, G.G. and Martin, R.G. (1984) Epidermoid Cancer of the Anorectum. *Cancer*, **533**, 1285–1293.
23. Glimelius, B., Graffman, S.H., Pahlman, L. and Wilander, E. (1983) Radiation therapy of anal carcinoma. *Acta Radiologica Oncology*, **22**, 273–279.
24. Golder, G.T. and Horsler, J.S. (1976) Surgical

management of epidermoid carcinoma of the anus. *American Journal of Surgery*, **131**(3), 275–280.

25. Goldman, S., Gerz, S., Erhardt, K. and Seligson, U. (1987) Prognostic significance of clinical stage, histologic grade, and nuclear DNA content in squamous-cell carcinoma of the anus. *Diseases of the Colon and Rectum*, **306**, 444–448.

26. Goldman, S., Glimelius, B. and Norming, U. (1988) Transanorectal ultrasonography in anal carcinoma. *Acta Radiologica*, **29**, 337–341.

27. Goldman, S., Glimelius, B. and Glas, U. (1989) Management of anal epidermoid carcinoma – an evaluation of treatment results in two population-based series. *International Journal of Colorectal Diseases*, **4**, 234–243.

28. Grenall, M.J., Quan, S.H.Q., Urmacher, C. and DeCosse, J.J. (1985) Treatment of epidermoid carcinoma of the anal canal. *Surgery, Gynecology and Obstetrics*, **161**, 509–517.

29. Grinvalsky, H.T. and Helwig, E.B. (1956) Carcinoma of the anorectal junction: histological considerations. *Cancer*, **9**, 480–488.

30. Habr-Gama, A., DaSilva, E., Sousa, A.H., Nadalin, W., Gansi, R., Hyppolito da Silva, J. and Pinotti, H.W. (1989) Epidermoid carcinoma of the anal canal: results of treatment by combined chemotherapy and radiation therapy. *Diseases of the Colon and Rectum*, **32**, 773–777.

31. Hermann, G. and Desfosses, L. Sur la muquese de la Region Cloacale de Rectum. *C R Acadamy Science*, **90**, 1201–1203.

32. Hughes, L.L., Rich, T.A. and Delclos, L. (1989) Radiotherapy for anal cancer: experience from 1979–1987. *International Journal of Radiology, Oncology, Biology and Physics*, **12**, 1153–1160.

33. Kato, T., Saijyo, S., Hatchome, N., Tagami, H. and Kawashima, M. (1988) Detection of human papillomavirus type 16 in bowenoid papulosis and invasive carcinoma occurring in the same patient with a history of cervical carcinoma. *Archives of Dermatology*, **124**, 851–852.

34. Kuehn, P.G. Jr, Beckett, R.T.E., Eisenberg, H. and Reed, J.F. (1964) Epidermoid carcinoma of the perianal skin and anal canal. *New England Journal of Medicine*, **270**, 614–617.

35. Madden, M.V., Elliot, M.S., Botha, J.B.C. and Louw, J.H. (1981) The management of anal carcinoma. *British Journal of Surgery*, **68**, 287–289.

36. Marfing, T.E., Abel, M.E. and Gallagher, D.M. (1987) Perianal Bowen's disease and associated malignancies. Results of a survey. *Diseases of the Colon and Rectum*, **30**, 782–785.

37. McAnnally, A.K. and Dockerty, M.B. (1949) Carcinoma developing in chronic draining cutaneous sinuses and fistulas. *Surgery, Gynecology and Obstetrics*, **88**, 87–96.

38. Morson, B.C. (1960) The pathology and results of treatment of squamous cell carcinoma and adenoacanthoma of the colon. *Cancer*, **53**, 414–420.

39. Nigro, N.D., Vaitkevigius, V.K. and Considine, B. (1974) Combined therapy for cancer of the anal

canal: a preliminary report. *Diseases of the Colon and Rectum*, **17**, 354–356.

40. Nigro, N.D., Seydel, H.G., Considine, B., Vaitkevicius, V.K., Leichman, L. and Kinzie, J.J. (1983) Combined preoperative radiation and chemotherapy for squamous cell carcinoma of the anal canal. *Cancer*, **51**, 1826–1983.

41. Nigro, N.D. (1984) An evaluation of combined therapy for squamous cell cancer of the anal canal. *Diseases of the Colon and Rectum*, **27**, 763–766.

42. Nigro, N.D. (1987) Multidisciplinary management of cancer of the anus. *World Journal of Surgery*, **111**, 446–451.

43. Papillon, J., Mayer, M., Montbarbon, J.F., Gerard, J.P., Chassard, J.L. and Bailly, C. (1983) A new approach to the management of epidermoid carcinoma of the anal canal. *Cancer*, **51**, 1830–1837.

44. Papillon, J. and Montababon, J.F. (1987) Epidermoid carcinoma of the anal canal. *Diseases of the Colon and Rectum*, **305**, 324–333.

45. Pyper, P.C. and Parks, T.G. (1985) The results of surgery for epidermoid carcinoma of the anus. *British Journal of Surgery*, **72**, 712–714.

46. Ramos, R., Salinas, H. and Tucker, L. (1983) Conservative approach to the treatment of Bowen's disease of the anus. *Diseases of the Colon and Rectum*, **26**, 712–715.

47. Rosenthal, D. (1967) Basal cell carcinoma of the anus: report of two cases. *Diseases of the Colon and Rectum*, **10**, 397–400.

48. Ross, M., Pezzi, C., Pezzi, T., Meurer, D., Hickey, R. and Balch, C. (1990) Patterns of failure in anorectal melanoma. A guide to surgical therapy. *Archives of Surgery*, **125**, 313–316.

49. Rudlinger, R. and Buchmann, P. (1989) HPV 16-positive bowenoid papulosis and squamous-cell carcinoma of the anus in an HIV-positive man. *Diseases of the Colon and Rectum*, **32**, 1042–1045.

50. Salmon, R.J., Safrani, B., Labib, A. Asselain, B. and Girodet, J. (1986) Prognosis of cloacogenic and squamous cancers of the anal canal. *Diseases of the Colon and Rectum*, **294**, 336–340.

51. Sasaki, M., Terada, T., Nakanuma, Y., Kono, N., Kasahara, Y. and Watanabe, K. (1990) Anorectal mucinous adenocarcinoma associated with latent perianal Paget's disease. *American Journal of Gastroenterology*, **85**, 199–202.

52. Scott, N.A., Beart, R.W. Jr, Weiland, L.H., Cha, S.S. and Lieber, M.M. (1989) Carcinoma of the anal canal and flow cytometric DNA analysis. *British Journal of Cancer*, **60**, 56–58.

53. Shepard, N.A., Scholefield, J.H. and Love, S.B. (1990) Prognostic factors in anal squamous carcinoma: a multivariate analysis of clinical, pathological and flow cytometric parameters in 235 cases. *Histopathology*, **16**, 545–555.

54. Shutze, W.P. and Cleysteen, J.J. (1990) Perianal Paget's disease. Classification and review of management: report of two cases. *Diseases of the Colon and Rectum*, **33**, 502–507.

55. Siegal, B., Cohen, D. and Jacob, E.T. (1983)

Surgical treatment of anorectal melanomas. *American Journal of Surgery*, **146**, 336–338.

56. Sischy, B., Remington, J.H., Hinson, J. *et al.* (1982) Definitive treatment of anal canal carcinoma by means of radiation therapy and chemotherapy. *Diseases of the Colon and Rectum*, **25**, 685–688.

57. Stacy, D., Burrell, M.O. and Franklin, E.W. III. (1986) Extramammary Paget's disease of the vulva and anus: use of intraoperative frozen-section margins. *American Journal of Obstetrics and Gynecology*, **155**, 519–523.

58. Strauss, R.J. and Fazio, V.W. (1979) Bowen's disease of the anal and perianal area. *American Journal of Surgery*, **137**, 231–234.

59. Strauss, R.J. and Fazio, V.W. (1979) Bowen's

disease of the anal and perianal area. A report and analysis of twelve cases. *American Journal of Surgery*, **137**, 231–234.

60. Syed A.M.N., Puthawala, A., Niblett, D. *et al.* (1978) Primary treatment of carcinoma of the lower rectum and anal canal by a combination of external irradiation and interstitial implant. *Radiology*, **128**, 199–203.

61. White, W.B., Schneiderman, H. and Sayre, J.T. (1984) Basal cell carcinoma of the anus: clinical and pathological distinction from cloacogenic carcinoma. *Journal of Clinical Gastroenterology*, **6**, 441–446.

62. Wolfe, H.R.I. and Bussey, J.H.R. (1968) Squamous cell carcinoma of the anus. *British Journal of Surgery*, **553**, 295–301.

ANAL AND PERIRECTAL PROBLEMS

A. Allan

PILONIDAL SINUS

Pilonidal sinus is a common condition. It affects young adults and is more common in men than in women. Such sinuses are usually situated in the sacrococcygeal area and although true pilonidal sinus is most common in the sacral area, a similar condition caused by implantation of hair may occur at other sites. These sites include the web of the fingers or toes, the perineal scar after abdominoperineal excision or the anal canal.[29,30] Unlike true pilonidal sinus, these foreign body granulomas involve direct penetration of skin by hair and represent a separate pathology.

AETIOLOGY

Whether pilonidal sinus is a congenital or acquired disease is controversial but, currently, an acquired aetiology seems most probable.[12] The sequence of events leading to the formation of a sacrococcygeal pilonidal sinus is initiated by the keratin plugging of a pilosebaceous follicle. Keratin plugging is followed by stasis in the follicle with sepsis and subsequent rupture of the infected follicle into the surrounding subcutaneous fat. From this septic area the primary sinus usually extends in a cephalad direction and hair and skin debris accumulate within it. In any event, the direction of the sinus track always correlates with the orientation of the normal hair follicles in the vicinity of the inflamed follicle.[17] Some subcutaneous side tracks may ramify laterally

into the buttocks where abscess formation may occur. Rarely a pilonidal sinus can form tracks towards the anus and this may be confused with an anal fistula.[28]

Most of the sinus track is lined with granulation tissue. Hair fragments surrounded by foreign body giant cells are frequently seen within this tissue. Hair is found inside the track in approximately two thirds of cases of pilonidal sinus in men and one third of cases in women.[20]

CLINICAL FEATURES

A pilonidal sinus may be discovered on routine inspection of the natal cleft. The patient is unaware of its presence, but on inspection of the natal cleft there are one or more midline pits. When the lesion becomes inflamed the patient may present with either a chronic discharging sinus or an acute abscess. Approximately equal numbers of cases present in each of these two ways. The discharging sinus is easily identified by its characteristic midline position and there may be hair tufts protruding from its orifice. When an abscess forms it may not be possible to identify the infected hair follicle because of oedema and inflammation. The position of the abscess to one side of the natal cleft is the clue to the correct diagnosis.

TREATMENT

A wide variety of methods are used to treat pilonidal sinus. The optimal treatment for a particular sinus depends upon the complexity of its tracks and the degree of associated sepsis. Although the ideal treatment has probably not yet evolved, the older methods of treating pilonidal sinus by wide excision of tissue down to the presacral fascia have largely been discarded.

Currently the most conservative approach is injection of the pilonidal sinus with 80% phenol.[23] Phenol remains in the sinus track for one minute before the sinus is curetted. This procedure can be repeated. Such phenolization of pilonidal sinus is associated with a 35% relapse rate within 6 months, but a second injection with phenol lowers this rate to 25%. A similarly conservative technique in which the primary sinus is excised with cleaning of the side tracks is accompanied by a similar relapse rate of 23%.[8] These conservative techniques probably represent a useful approach to uncomplicated pilonidal sinus with minimal sepsis.

Pilonidal sinus with more significant sepsis requires more extensive operative treatment and the choice lies between excision of the primary sinus together with unroofing of the side tracks, the wound being left open to granulate, or else excision with primary closure. Primary closure is most suitable for small non-suppurating lesions. Even when cases for primary closure are carefully selected, however, the recurrence rate following closure is higher than after simply laying open the sinus.[4,20] Furthermore, when the costs of outpatient attendances and of treating recurrences after failed primary closure are considered, then laying open is a cheaper treatment.[2,4] If the sinus is excised and the wound left to granulate, then during the healing phase the wound edges should be kept shaved to prevent hair growing into the wound and impeding healing by forming a hair granuloma.

Although the procedures described above are the most commonly used in the treatment of pilonidal sinus, attempts have been made to decrease the recurrence rate. Generally this has been by a primary closure with alteration of the contours of the natal cleft.[3,14] Most probably these techniques are successful because they flatten the skin of the natal cleft thus decreasing the physical forces predisposing to a recurrence of the sinus. Karydakis[14] reports a series of 754 pilonidal sinuses treated by his method with only nine recurrences. An alternative approach is to avoid a natal cleft wound altogether and to create a transverse incision cranial to the natal cleft. The natal cleft skin being undermined and the pilonidal sinus being cored out from a cephalad to a caudal direction.[22] There are interesting approaches but generally are more invasive with greater morbidity than the more widely used and simpler procedures.

Many patients with pilonidal sinus present with an established pilonidal abscess. Simple drainage of these is associated with a cure rate of 58% of cases.[13] Those sinuses with fewer pits and lateral side tracks have a greater chance of healing with this treatment than more complex sinuses. There is some evidence that the recurrence rate of a pilonidal abscess following incision, curettage and primary closure with instillation of 2% fucidic acid gel may be associated with as low a recurrence rate as 13%.[6]

HIDRADENITIS SUPPURATIVA

Hidradenitis suppurativa is a chronic suppurative disorder of the skin. The pathogenesis involves occlusion and ectasia of apocrine ducts and glands. Ectasia is followed by secondary bacterial infection of the glands with subsequent inflammation, sinsus formation and eventually healing with scarring. The disease is associated with other poral occlusion disease such as acne vulgaris and comedones as well as pilonidal sinus.[9] Factors suggesting that hidradenitis is an androgen dependent disease include the rarity of the disease before pubity as well as its improvement during pregnancy. Recent studies show that women with hidradenitis suppurativa have a higher serum testosterone level than normal individuals,[19] and there may be an increased ability of apocrine glands to convert testosterone to its metabolic products in women with hidradenitis.[11]

DISTRIBUTION

Only skin bearing apocrine glands is affected by the disease and, therefore, hidradenitis most commonly affects the axillas and inguinogenital region. The perianal skin, submammary skin and ear lobes also may be affected. When all anatomical sites are considered, hidradenitis is more common in women with a preponderance of 5:2. Perianal disease is more common in men with a preponderance of 5:1. This may represent a difference between sexes in the density of the perianal apocrine glands.

CLINICAL FEATURES

Hidradenitis suppurativa is an important clinical problem because it causes very severe morbidity and for which no entirely satisfactory treatment exists. It is often at an advanced stage before it is diagnosed, by which time undermining abscesses and sinus tracks are established. Although the disease may become quiescent at an early stage, it more commonly continues relentlessly for years until waning in female patients at the climacteric.

Once established, the disease has a characteristic appearance including cylindrical areas of skin undermined with ulcers and fistulas. It may be mistaken for perianal Crohn's disease but in hidradenitis there is no track connecting the abscesses with the anal canal, though there is often a track connecting one abscess with another.

TREATMENT

Based on the possible relationship of hidradenitis suppurativa to excess circulating androgens, Mortimer and colleagues,[19] have suggested treatment of the early lesions with the anti-androgen cyproster-one acetate. Unfortunately early presentation is rare and excision of diseases and suppurating areas of skin is required, Traditionally, this consists of excision of the affected area followed by either skin grafting or else healing by granulation. Treatment of the established lesion should never be allowed to become a greater burden to the patient than the disease itself. A localized abscess should be incised and the granulations within curetted, the resulting wounds being left open to heal by secondary intention. Where there is extensive involvement of skin, a wider excision is necessary. Incision and laying open of tracks can be repeated and it is often best to do this by stages. Attempts to lessen the magnitude of the surgical treatment of hidradenitis include limited excision of the lesions using a carbon dioxide laser which probably causes less damage to surrounding tissues than other techniques.[7]

CONDYLOMATA ACUMINATA

Infection of perianal or endoanal skin with human papilloma virus (types, 6, 11, or 16) can result in condylomata acuminata (viral warts). Ninety percent of cases are found in males.[1] More than two thousand years ago the Romans recognized these lesions which they called 'figs', and regarded them as a sign that the patient practiced anoreceptive intercourse. More recent observers record that 50% of male sufferers admit to anal coitus. The presence of condyloma acuminata, however, is not solely the preserve of the male homosexual (unpublished data).

CLINICAL FEATURES

Condylomata acuminata generally have a dome-shaped appearance and this distinguishes them from condylomata lata, lesions of secondary syphilis which are flat or saucer shaped. The density of condylomata acuminata on the perianal skin and the size of each individual lesion is very variable. Usually these lesions gradually increase in size and number with time but, occasionally, spontaneous regression may occur over several months. Such regression follows the appearance of a purple or dark lesion among the usual pink ones. Besides regression, malignant change in condylomata acuminata may occur but is exceptionally rare.

Some 80% of patients presenting with condylomata acuminata present complaining of anorectal bleeding. Forty-five per cent also complain of pruritus ani and anal discomfort.[26] The presence of warts on the perianal skin is not difficult to detect and usually the diagnosis can be made on naked eye appearances. The lesions may extend over wide areas of skin, as well as the genitalia, including the urethral meatus in the male and the cervix in the female. Proctoscopy may reveal lesions in the anus and, in 2% of cases, condylomata may be present on squamous cell rests in the rectum (unpublished data).

Before surgical treatment, patients with condylomata acuminata should be referred to a genitourinary clinic so that other forms of sexually transmitted disease can be detected if present. It is important to know the hepatitis and HIV status of the patient before operation so that the necessary precautions can be taken if these tests are positive. A recent report suggests that in patients presenting with condylomata acuminata, there may be an increased incidence of seropositivity to HIV in excess of 70%.[5] This is likely to vary widely according to the population under study. There is also evidence that the incidence of rectal condylomata acuminata is higher in patients with seropositivity to HIV.[5]

TREATMENT

Although perianal condylomata scattered widely on the perianal skin can be treated by the application of podophyllin, most cases require excision.

When podophyllin is used, it is applied once or twice weekly. The skin around the lesion is smeared with vaseline to protect it from the action of podophyllin. Then podophyllin is applied to each wart on the tip of an orange stick. A recent study in which patients with perianal condylomata acuminata were randomly treated by podophyllin or scissor excision shows that at follow-up 18 months later, 21% of the patients treated by scissor excision suffered a recurrence of their condylomata compared with 60% of those patients treated with podophyllin. Furthermore 87% of patients treated by scissor excision were satisfied with their treatment compared with only 37% of those treated with podophyllin, which required regular outpatient attendance.[15]

When there are extensive condylomata acuminata on the perianal skin or in the anal canal, then scissor excision under general anaesthesia is probably the optimal method of treatment. Certainly this method of treatment causes less skin damage than diathermy excision which is associated with prolonged healing time when compared with scissor excision. An elegant technique for scissor excision is described by Thomson and Grace (1978).[26] The perianal skin is infiltrated with adrenaline in saline (1:300 000) in the subcutaneous plane. This is advantageous not only to decrease bleeding from the skin but also to separate the bases of adjacent condylomata. It is then easier to dissect with pointed scissors between adjacent condylomata and leave a skin bridge which might otherwise not be possible. When dissecting perianal skin warts and endoanal warts with the patient in lithotomy, it is best to begin with the perianal condylomata before continuing with the endoanal warts. If the dissection is done in this order, it prevents the excision sites of the endoanal warts bleeding down around the perianal skin where it can obscure the operator's view. Occasionally confluent endoanal and lower rectal condylomata may need to be excised using a rectal mucosal advancement technique with suturing of the rectal mucosa to the level of the dentate line.[27]

The reported occurrence of further warts following scissor excision ranges from 8.8%[10] to 28% (unpublished data). Small isolated recurrences may be dealt with using podophyllin or by excision under local anaesthetic although more extensive recurrent growths may require further operative treatment.

ANAL STENOSIS

Anal stenosis is associated with a variety of underlying causes which are either congenital or acquired.

CONGENITAL

Anorectal stenosis may occur in the newborn either as a solitary defect or in association with an ectopic or covered anus as well as an imperforate anorectal membrane.[24] When a stenosis presents as an isolated defect, the external appearance of the anus is normal and the stenosis may not be noticed for some months. When weaning occurs and the stool thick-ens, constipation may become overt. Treatment of such an isolated defect is by repeated digital dilatation. Where stenosis occurs in association with a covered anus then a cutback operation may be required in addition to digital dilatation.

ACQUIRED

The most common cause of anal stenosis is involvement of the anus with rectal adenocarcinoma spreading distally towards the perianal skin. Less commonly, squamous cell carcinoma of the anal canal may cause anal stenosis but accounts for only 3.5% of cases of carcinoma in the anorectal region.[18] Because of the high incidence of malignant strictures in the anorectal region, a careful examination with biopsy of all anal strictures is necessary. This may be done with the patient anaesthetised.

When considering the non-malignant causes of anal stenosis, the most frequent is stenosis secondary to anal Crohn's disease. In such cases the stenosis is often associated with anal ulcers and fissures. Patients with Crohn's disease may be asymptomatic but can present when anal sepsis forms an abscess or perianal fistulation occurs. Perianal pain, incontinence, constipation or bloody diarrhoea can all be symptoms of anal strictures in these patients.

Treatment of anorectal strictures in patients with Crohn's disease can be managed by repeated gentle dilatation.[16] Approximately 30% of patients treated in this way will require more than two dilatations[16] and on rare occasions this treatment can predispose to the development of a perianal abscess or the exacerbation of symptoms from a perianal fistula. Approximately 16% of patients treated by dilatation for anorectal stricturing will come to proctocolectomy because of severe anorectal disease within 10 years. It should be borne in mind that, on rare occasions, anal Crohn's disease may be complicated by either adenocarcinoma[16] or squamous cell carcinoma of the anorectum.[21]

Other causes of benign anal stenosis include postoperative strictures, which may occur after excision of anorectal mucosa, as occurs in the removal of a large villous adenoma or following coring out of the anal mucosa before construction of a colo- or ileoanal anastomosis. Benign stenosis is also seen following ischaemic or ulcerative proctitis, radiotherapy to the pelvis, rectal injury or as part of the infective process of lymphogranuloma venereum.

In general, benign strictures respond to repeated gentle anal dilatation with a finger or metal sounds. The use of laser photoablation may also have a place in their management. Very occasionally some form of 'Y–V' plasty may be necessary.

SKIN TAGS

Perianal skin tags are seen commonly in patients attending proctological clinics and patients may mistake them for haemorrhoids. Skin tags develop from oedematous squamous epithelium and this oedema may be associated with other anal conditions such as haemorrhoids, perianal haematoma or anal fissure. When the subcutaneous oedema resolves, this leaves redundant skin which forms a tag.

Generally perianal skin tags remain asymptomatic but one indication for their removal is severe pruritus ani. Removal of tags under local anaesthetic may allow better cleansing of the perianal skin after defaecation.

In patients with prolapsing haemorrhoids which include a large cutaneous element, haemorrhoidectomy may become necessary, principally to treat the cutaneous part of the haemorrhoid. In treatment of such cases, care should be taken to ensure preservation of adequate skin bridges between adjacent excision sites. A skin tag (sentinel pile) associated with a chronic anal fissure similarly should be excised. This allows better drainage of the fissure bed and promotes healing. Removal of the tag can be conveniently carried out together with a subcutaneous sphincterotomy.

Oedematous skin tags can be associated with perianal Crohn's disease and removal of one of these tags may reveal epithelioid granulomas on histological examination hence, a diagnosis where this is in doubt. Once a histological diagnosis is established, the remaining tags are best left undisturbed.

PERIANAL HAEMATOMA

Patients suffering from perianal haematoma present with acute anal pain and this may follow an episode of excessive straining at stool. These haematomas are caused by acute thrombosis in the perianal subcutaneous venous plexus.[25] On examination the buttocks are gently parted to reveal a spherical blue mass the size of a garden pea at the anal verge. This mass is often very tender to palpation and is covered by perianal skin.

The method of treatment depends on the degree of pain experienced by the patient at the time of presentation. If the patient presents several days following the onset of the problem, then the pain may be resolving rapidly. It is then reasonable to explain to the patient that spontaneous resolution can be expected and to treat discomfort by simple oral analgesics. Conversely, if the lesion is exquis-

itely tender and the pain shows no sign of rapid resolution, then it is a simple matter to infiltrate it with local anaesthetic and to incise the perianal skin over the haematoma. The haematoma is expressed with digital pressure. One absorbable suture may be necessary to arrest haemorrhage from the incision. The patient is sent home with a supply of oral analgesics, and rectal examination to exclude coexisting haemorrhoids or tumour is done on review in the outpatient clinic.

HYPERTROPHIED ANAL PAPILLA

Hypertrophied anal papilla are the enlarged tips of the dentate line. Normally these are just visible to the naked eye through a proctoscope. These papillas commonly enlarge to 4 or 5 mm in length and occasionally around 2 cm, when they become known as fibroepithelial polyps. The characteristic position of the base of the papilla in the anal canal is the key to their recognition.

The stimulus for hypertrophy of anal papillas is uncertain, but it seems probable that infection of an adjacent perianal crypt may cause a localized acute inflammatory response with hyperplasia of the papilla and subsequent fibrosis.

Hypertrophied anal papillas are of clinical importance because they may be associated with anal fistula. A hypertrophied papilla is often found in association with the internal orifice of an anal fistula and may form a valuable landmark in the search for this orifice. Hypertrophied anal papillas may also be associated with anal fissure. The hypertrophied papilla can prolapse down the anal canal on defaecation and shear the anal mucosa. This prevents healing of the anal fissure. A hypertrophied anal papilla accompanying an anal fissure should be removed for this reason. This can be done conveniently with the diathermy forceps.

Hypertrophied anal papillas, if very large, can present as a prolapsing mass through the anal sphincter. Usually this is interpreted as a prolapsing pile by the patient but proctoscopic examination reveals its true nature. Excision should be carried out with a transfixion stitch to secure haemostasis.

REFERENCES

1. Abcarian, H. and Sharon, N. (1982) The long term effectiveness immunotherapy of anal condylomata acuminata. *Diseases of the Colon and Rectum*, **25**, 648–651.
2. Allen-Mersh, T.G. (1990) Pilonidal sinus: finding the right track for treatment. *British Journal of Surgery*, **77**, 123–132.

3. Bascom, J.V. (1977) Repeat pilonidal operations. *American Journal of Surgery*, **64**, 867–868.

4. Bissett, I.P. and Isbister, W.H. (1987) The management of patients with pilonidal sinus. *Australian and New Zealand Journal of Surgery*, **57**, 939–942.

5. Christen, D., Buchmann, P. and Gernnalos, S. (1988) Condylomata acuminata in HIV positive patients. *Coloproctology*, **2**, 102–103.

6. Courtney, S.P. and Merlin, M.J. (1986) The use of fucidic acid gel in pilonidal abscess treatment: cure, recurrence and failure rates. *Annals of the Royal College of Surgeons of England*, **68**, 170–171.

7. Dalrymple, J.C. and Monaghan, J.M. (1987) Treatment of hidradenitis suppurativa with the carbon dioxide laser. *British Journal of Surgery*, **74**, 420.

8. Edwards, M.H. (1977) Pilonidal sinus: a five year appraisal of the Millar-Lord technique. *British Journal of Surgery*, **64**, 867–868.

9. Frankowiak, J.J. and Jackman, R. (1962) The aetiology of pilonidal sinus disease. *Diseases of the Colon and Rectum*, **5**, 28–36.

10. Gollock, J.M., Slatford, K. and Hunter, J.M. (1982) Scissor excision of anogenital warts. *British Journal of Veneral Diseases*, **58**, 400–401.

11. Harrison, B.J., Read, G.F. and Hughes, L.E. (1988) Endocrine basis for the clinical presentation of hidradenitis suppurativa. *British Journal of Surgery*, **75**, 972–975.

12. Hueston, J.T. (1953) The aetiology of pilonidal sinus. *British Journal of Surgery*, **41**, 307–311.

13. Jensen, S.L. and Harling, H. (1988) Prognosis after simple incision and drainage for a first episode of pilonidal abscess. *British Journal of Surgery*, **75**, 60–61.

14. Karydakis, G.E. (1973) New approach to the problem of pilonidal sinus. *The Lancet*, **ii**, 1414–1415.

15. Khawaja, H.T. (1989) Podophyllin versus scissor excision in the treatment of perianal condylomata acuminata – a prospective study. *British Journal of Surgery*, **76**, 1067–1069.

16. Linares, L., Moreira, L.F., Andrews, H., Allan, R.N., Alexander-Williams, J. and Keighley, M.R.B. (1988) Natural history and treatment of anorectal strictures complicating Crohn's disease. *British Journal of Surgery*, **75**, 653–655.

17. Millar, D.M. (1970) Aetiology of postanal pilonidal disease. *Proceedings of the Royal Society of Medicine*, **63**, 19–20.

18. Morson, B.C. (1959) The pathology and results of treatment of cancer of the anal region. *Proceedings of the Royal Society of Medicine*, suppl. 52, 117.

19. Mortimer, P.S., Dawber, R.P. (1986) Double blind trial of cyprosterone acetate in females with hidradenitis suppurativa. *British Journal of Dermatology*, **115**, 263–268.

20. Notaras, M.J. (1970) A review of three popular methods of treatment of postanal pilonidal sinus. *British Journal of Surgery*, **57**, 886–889.

21. Preston, D.M., Fowler, F., Lennard-Jones, J.E. and Hawley, P.R. (1983) Carcinoma of the anus in Crohn's disease. *British Journal of Surgery*, **70**, 346–347.

22. Roe, F. (1971) A new operative technique for pilonidal sinus. *Surgery, Gynaecology and Obstetrics*, **132**, 291–296.

23. Stansby, G. and Greatorex, R. (1989) Phenol treatment of pilonidal sinus of the natal cleft. *British Journal of Surgery*, **76**, 729–730.

24. Stephens, F.D. and Smith, E.D. (1971) Ano-rectal malformations in children. Chicago: Year Book Medical Publishers.

25. Thomson, H. (1982) The real nature of perianal haematoma. *The Lancet*, **ii**, 467–468.

26. Thomson, J.P.S. and Grace, R.H. (1978) Perianal and anal condylomata acuminata: a new operative technique. *Journal of the Royal Society of Medicine*, **71**, 180–185.

27. Thomson, J.P.S. and Hawley, P.R. (1987) Anorectal surgery. In *General Surgical Operations*, 2nd edn (Eds) Kirk, R.M. and Williamson, R.C.N. pp. 151–170. Edinburgh: Churchill Livingstone.

28. Vallence, S. (1982) Pilonidal fistulas mimicking fistulas-in-ano. *British Journal of Surgery*, **69**, 161–162.

29. Walsh, T.H. and Mann, C.V. (1983) Pilonidal sinuses of the anal canal. *British Journal of Surgery*, **70**, 23–24.

30. Weston, S.D. and Schlachter, I.S. (1963) Pilonidal cyst of the anal canal. *Diseases of the Colon and Rectum*, **6**, 139–141.

INDEX

Note: Page references in *italics* refer to figures; those in **bold** refer to tables